Klaus J. Zülch

Brain Tumors

Their Biology and Pathology

Third, Completely Revised Edition

Foreword by
Percival Bailey

With 165 Figures in 252 Separate Illustrations

Springer-Verlag
Berlin Heidelberg NewYork Tokyo

KLAUS J. ZÜLCH, M.D., Dr. h.c.
Professor emeritus of Neurology University of Cologne,
and former Director, Department of General Neurology of
the Max-Planck-Institute for Brain Research
and the Neurological Department
Municipal Hospital Köln-Merheim
Ostmerheimer Straße 200
D-5000 Köln 91

First and Second American Edition published by Springer Publishing Company, Inc., New York

Library of Congress Cataloging-in-Publication Data. Zülch, K.J. (Klaus Joachim), 1910–
Brain tumors. Translation of: Die Hirngeschwülste in biologischer und morphologischer Darstellung. Includes bibliographies and index. 1. Brain – Tumors. I. Title. [DNLM: 1. Brain Neoplasms. WL 358 Z94h] RC280.B7Z773 1986 616.99′281 85-23285
ISBN-13: 978-3-642-68180-6 e-ISBN-13: 978-3-642-68178-3
DOI: 10.1007/ 978-3-642-68178-3

Softcover reprint of the hardcover 3rd edition 1986

Reproduction of the figures: Gustav Dreher GmbH, Stuttgart

Typesetting : Universitätsdruckerei H. Stürtz AG, Würzburg
2125/3130-543210

This volume is dedicated to my sister G.R. *whose contributions made the work on which it is based possible, and to the memory of Professor* SIR JAMES LEARMONTH, *Aberdeen/Edinburgh and Professor* OTFRID FOERSTER, *Breslau*

Foreword to the First American Edition*

When I began, in 1922, the study of Cushing's collection of tumors of the nervous system, it was my hope and intention to publish with him a comprehensive treatise correlating their biological behavior with their pathology. This ambitious project I was unable to complete because, in 1928, I left his clinic to create one of my own at the University of Chicago. Although I found time there to publish an account of the astroblastomas and, with Bucy, another of the oligodendrogliomas, I was soon forced by the pressure of clinical responsibilities to abandon the project.

Yet such a treatise was greatly needed, and I am happy that the need has been so brilliantly satisfied by the exhaustive study of Dr. ZÜLCH that has appeared in Vol. III of the *Handbuch der Neurochirurgie*. This study, profusely illustrated, is an inexhaustible mine of information concerning tumors of the brain. It is, however, too long and involved to be of everyday use to the busy neurosurgeon and neurologist. For this reason Dr. ZÜLCH has put the essence of his vast experience into the present smaller volume which is equally authoritative but more manageable. Its translation into English makes it more readily utilizable to the American clinician.

One of the things that is learned with advancing age is that one is not going to be able to fulfill all of the dreams of one's youth. I am happy that one of mine has been so admirably realized by Dr. ZÜLCH.

PERCIVAL BAILEY †

* Slightly abbridged from the first edition

Preface to the First American Edition *

Ever since the appearance of BAILEY and CUSHING's monograph in 1930, their new classification of brain tumors has gradually gained acceptance everywhere, including Germany and other German-speaking countries. When the first German edition of this book appeared in 1951, it was intended as an aid in the classification of brain tumors and as a means of dispelling some of the obscurity which seems to surround the subject. Through accurate macroscopic and microscopic examination and especially through a precise differential diagnosis, the classification of these tumors may become a real science, and one readily accessible to anyone prepared to make the necessary effort. The first edition, I may hope, made some progress in this direction. Beyond the mere classification, however, the data thus acquired needed to be compiled and analyzed. Figures on preferential site, age incidence, sex predilection, and general incidence are therefore included. Moreover, the form of the tumor, its manner of growth, and type of spread, as well as such reactions of the surrounding brain as alterations in its shape or shifts in its position have been considered. All of the foregoing data – and their relation to the clinical picture – should be of very real help to the neurologist, radiologist and surgeon in making a preoperative diagnosis. Lastly, some thoughts on the origin of brain tumors have been included.

The special attention given to the clinical aspects of the subject is the result of our close association with the neurosurgical clinics of the late Dr. W. TÖNNIS in Würzburg, Berlin, Bochum-Langendreer, and Cologne. This monograph has benefited greatly from our collaboration, and I am much indebted to him.

The American edition is based on the second German edition, which has been revised and enlarged both to keep abreast of current progress in the field and to record our own increasing experience. In particular, a number of tables concerning biological data on brain tumors have been added.

KLAUS J. ZÜLCH

* Abbridged; for the full text see the first and second editions.

Preface to the Third Edition

The third American edition has been completely revised and expanded, although parts of the text of the second edition have been included. I wish to acknowledge once again the excellent translation of the former two editions by Dr. ALAN B. ROTHBALLER and the late Dr. JERZY OLSZEWSKI.

With this edition I have followed the general theme of the original German edition published in 1951. However, I have tried to consider modern techniques and the many new publications on the subject of brain tumors. Meanwhile, an early desire of mine has been fulfilled by the completion and publication of a classification which can be understood worldwide and hopefully be used widely, namely, the classification of the World Health Organization: *Histological Typing of Tumours of the Central Nervous System* (1979).

The classification which I used in the 1951 edition is very close to the final pattern of that accepted by the World Health Organization (WHO), since both follow the line of the BAILEY and CUSHING classification of 1926/1930.

To consolidate our old concepts and experiences we have reclassified our collection of 9000 cases with the assistance of my co-workers Dr. M. FUKUI, Dr. A. SATO. Dr. E. SCHARRER, Dr. E. SIMON, and Dr. J. SZYMAS. In the last decade two large atlases have been published, one called an *Atlas of the Histology of Brain Tumors*[1] (in six languages) and a second one called an *Atlas of the Gross Neurosurgical Pathology*[2]. In both publications the text is abbreviated. Therefore this book is intended to overcome this fault. On the other hand, we have tried to keep the number of figures in this book to a minimum for economic reasons, hoping that readers will have access to the two atlases, which may be readily available in most medical libraries and are still in stock in the bookshops. Our volume, which appeared as part of the *Handbuch der Neurochirurgie* of 1956 was the most extensive publication of our knowledge up to that time and contained a vast amount of macroscopic and microscopic illustrations, regrettably is not accessible to most people as it is in German. I hope, however, that it may remain in some of the libraries for reference purposes, and that *for the daily use the*

---

[1] ZÜLCH KJ: Atlas of the histology of brain tumors. Springer, Berlin Heidelberg New York 1971

[2] ZÜLCH KJ: Atlas of gross neurosurgical pathology. Springer, Berlin Heidelberg New York 1975

two atlases of 1971 and 1975 and this text may deliver the main data of the aforementioned handbook volume.

For this third edition, I am particularly grateful to Dr. SZYMAS for his undefatigable assistance in preparing the literature and helping me to "digest" it. My wife, Dr. MARIE-LUISE ZÜLCH, also has helped to collect and collate the data of the vast literature on brain tumors. To Mr. HANS and Mrs. MARGOT GÖLDNER, who have supported my literary work for 30 years, I must express my full indebtedness. Finally, my friend Dr. W. S. FIELDS-HOUSTON has undertaken the tiresome work of correcting the English text.

I am particularly appreciative that my friend Dr. HEINZ GÖTZE took this third edition into the program of Springer-Verlag, Heidelberg, and arranged for the excellent form and layout.

KLAUS J. ZÜLCH

Contents

Important Note Regarding "HBT" and "GP"

In the text reference is made to figures in two of my own atlases at Springer Publishers

1. Atlas of the Histology of Brain Tumors.
   Springer-Verlag, Berlin Heidelberg New York, 1971

   abbreviated "HBT"

2. Atlas of Gross Neurosurgical Pathology.
   Springer-Verlag, Berlin Heidelberg New York, 1975

   abbreviated "GP"

1 Classification of Brain Tumors

1.1 Introduction

In the majority of laboratories throughout the world the classification of BAILEY and CUSHING (1926, 1930) has been formerly used with some modifications. In English-speaking countries Kernohan's classification, based on a system of "grading" (KERNOHAN et al. 1949), was most often employed and in the Portuguese- and Spanish-speaking world DEL RIO HORTEGA'S (1945, 1962) system of classification was preferred.

What this means in terms of common usage is illustrated by a table reproducing various names for the "unipolar spongioblastoma" of BAILEY (1927) and by PENFIELD'S (1931) description, which is now termed *pilocytic astrocytoma* (ZÜLCH 1979, p. 44). Here, as in other fields of medicine, we felt obliged to support all attempts to achieve a uniform system. We therefore decided to accept the recommendation of the International Union Against Cancer (UICC) for a new general classification of tumors. This was completed after extensive committee work (in which Kernohan had been a member for some time) and published in 1965 by Springer-Verlag (Berlin-Heidelberg-New York) in five languages (UICC 1965; see also UICC 1966–1969). This work, however, did not find general acceptance. Therefore, the World Health Organization (WHO) set up a project directed toward the histological classification of tumors which included 300 pathologists in over 50 countries. Since 1967 already 25 volumes in the first series of the *International Histological Classification of Tumors* (IHCT) have been published. They are based on the morphologically identifiable cell types and histological patterns as seen by means of light microscopy and conventional staining techniques. The goal of a unified terminology is emphasized in IHCT because "communication in oncology remains complicated by the large number of tumor types. Different terms are often used for the same tumor and sometimes the same term is applied to different lesions. Furthermore the tabulation of tumors can follow a variety of former terms. All of these variables hamper the comparison of data originating in different pathology laboratories and clinical departments and their radiological services" (see SOBIN 1981).

Other classifications with coding schemes exist which raise further confusion as to how they relate to each other (ICD, IHCT, ICD-O, SNOP, and SNOMED); details have been discussed by SOBIN (1981).

Despite the evolution of various new techniques such as electronmicroscopy, histochemistry, and immunology, the diagnosis of cancer remains firmly based on light microscopy and conventional histology. From the global point of view, refinements in sophisticated techniques are less important than reaching an acceptable level of proficiency in routine diagnostic microscopy.

In summary, therefore, we must emphasize the wide discrepancies in terminology and definition of brain tumors in the various schools, countries, subcontinents, and continents. These differences seriously hinder statistical comparison of various forms of treatment, i.e., surgery, radiotherapy and/or chemotherapy, as well as the comparison in experimental tumor production.

Was there any hope that uniformity in classification could ever be achieved? The Symposium on Classification of Brain Tumors in Santander (see OBRADOR ALCALDE and SANZ IBANEZ 1955) led to acceptance of the more common classification of Bailey, by the Spanish pathologists in the same form used by our own group. The only exception was the group of "polar spongioblastoma," for which no universally acceptable name seemed to be available. The compromise term of "isomorphous glioma," suggested at the Symposium, was definitely not adequate for either the morphologist or the clinician (see OBRADOR ALCALDE and SANZ IBANEZ 1955).

The International Symposium on Classification held in Cologne in 1961 (see ZÜLCH and WOOLF 1964) only served to emphasize the differences between the various schemes, and no success in unification was reached although the aforementioned compromise scheme proposed by the *Unio Internationalis Contra Cancrum* (UICC) was discussed. Therefore, we have to elaborate on the details of the suggestions made by the nomenclature commission of the World Health Organization, whose classification has now been published and recommended.

1.2 Historical Development and Present State of Classification

The essential criteria for a classification of tumors according to their intrinsic properties can be found only in the study of their chemical nature, their microscopical structure, and the manner and sequence of their development .... It has always seemed to me that the tumor types most correctly formulated are those that are arranged parallel to normal structures, like the tendinous, fibrous-tissue tumors ... and the enchondroma, whose structure is parallel to that of cartilage [Johannes MÜLLER (1838) *Über den feineren Bau und die Formen der krankhaften Geschwülste*. Reimer, Berlin].

Certainly the neurosurgeon of the present day must take the wide view, if he ever is to attain the goal he should strive for, of foretelling, before the operation, not only the precise situation of a given lesion but its probably character as well ... (Harvey CUSHING: *Intracranial Tumors and the Surgeon.* The Cameron Prize Lectures 1925).

These two quotations seemed to characterize so clearly the development of tumor research over the past 150 years, that I used them to introduce a review article (1939a) appearing in commemoration of Harvey Cushing's 70th birthday. Johannes Müller indicated the direction the development was to take in the following century. Investigations of the chemical nature of a tumor, with the demonstration of protein-like or gelatine-yielding substances, have developed into microchemical demonstrations of the individual components of the tissue, their degeneration products including special proteins and by the use of various dyes, chemical and immunological tests as well as the tissue responses to impregnation with metallic salts. Investigations of the bio- and histochemistry as well as the immunological properties and the metabolism of tumors and their genuine respiration soon followed. The morphological development of tumor tissue has been elucidated to some extent by the application of tissue culture and cloning methods. Müller's idea of comparing tumors with normal tissues was further pursued and enlarged upon by taking into consideration the developmental stages of cells. In the hands of PICK and BIELSCHOWSKY (1911), RIBBERT (1918), and BAILEY and CUSHING (1926, 1930), this approach yielded outstanding results in the classification of brain tumors. Thus it happened that Cushing was not only able to formulate his goal set forth in the above mentioned quotation, but also to witness its realization 10 years later.

To understand the present state of brain tumor classification, we had best begin with a historical review covering the past century. Such a review – as in most fields of pathological anatomy – must commence with VIRCHOW (1847, 1863/65, 1871). Prior to his time there was a lack of basic or systematic knowledge, although, to be sure, there were clear and informative individual descriptions of brain tumors, particularly in the excellent work of CRUVEILHIER (1829/35). Indeed, preliminary attempts at classifications were made before this, but precise histological differentiation was still not possible. Classification according to certain external characteristics, such as cyst formation and fatty degeneration, constantly led to erroneous conclusions. (For details see the second edition, ZÜLCH 1965a).

A new period began with the discovery of the cell by SCHLEIDEN (1838) and SCHWANN (1839). The possibility of microscopical study caught the imagination of Johannes MÜLLER (1838), who was convinced that the development of the normal cell would repeat itself in pathologic processes. Thus he succeeded in taking an essential step forward in the approach to tumor study: he was able to compare tumor tissue with normal tissue and even with the development of cells in "embryonic formations." We find in Müller's work descriptions of the morphology and composition of individual tumor cells and "tailed elements."

We have devoted so much attention to the description of that early period because we see anticipated there the developments during the coming century. This century has brought about a deeper understanding and improved methods of investigation, but it is surprising how few really new ideas about pathogenesis have emerged since such pioneers as Johannes Müller blazed the trail. In LEBERT'S exhaustive study (1851) the most important contribution was the distinction between the two large groups of "cancer" and "fibroblastic" tumors. The real value of this extensive work is that for the first time the differences in biological significance of these groups were appreciated (see p. 31), i.e., that life expectancy was longer for one than for the other.

The period of systematic classification of tumors did not begin until VIRCHOW described in 1846 the neuroglia and related it to brain tumors. He separated the gliomas from the other "sarcomas" of the nervous system (see VIRCHOW 1847, 1863/65, 1900). Furthermore, he recognized hard and soft forms, and cellular medullary, fibrous, and telangiectatic types which occasionally, through mucoid degeneration, assumed the character of myxogliomas. In general, he found that soft forms were more closely related to myxomas and hard forms to fibromas (fibrogliomas). He called soft forms with numerous cells and blood vessels gliosarcomas. They were likely to contain spindle cells with long processes, large round cells with single or multiple nuclei (resembling giant cells, with four to five nuclei), and frequently fatty degeneration and hemorrhages as well. It was often difficult to distinguish them macroscopically from true apoplexy. In addition to fresh hemorrhages, these hemorrhagic gliomas also contained older ones, and in some instances even caseous or fibrinous foci (necrosis?). Moreover, VIRCHOW (1856) recognized gliomas of the ependyma in the form of warty structures, sometimes as large as peas (ependymitis granularis?), and larger when located in the fourth ventricle (our ependymomas). He considered tumors of the acoustic nerve and some of the spinal cord as derivatives of the brain substance originating from perineurium, and therefore also classifiable as neuroglia. Finally, VIRCHOW (1900) offered a new interpretation for the neoplasms of the dura: the presence of psammoma bodies caused him to exclude some of them from the dural sarcomas and to put them into a new group of "psammomas." But in classifying them according to an external characteristic he made an error, inasmuch as he included other "psammomatous" neoplasms as well, e.g., the calcified pinealomas, and "hyperplasias" of the choroid plexus.

This classification by VIRCHOW remained almost unchanged for half a century and found its last major application in BORST's tumor atlas (1902a, 1924). In this form it influenced the teaching of German pathology for a long time (see also RIBBERT 1904).

There were subsequent attempts at further definition of the "glioma" entity. The beginning of such endeavors goes back as far as 1874, when SIMON described the "spider cell glioma." Shortly before, von KÖLLIKER (1859) had discovered the cells with long and short processes, DEITERS (1865) the fiber-forming astrocytes ("connective tissue cells"), BOLL (1874) the "brush cells," and JASTROWITZ (1870, 1872) the "spider cells." Von LENHOSSEK's (1895) investigations of the origin of the ganglion and glial cells of the spinal cord further clarified the subject. We credit him with the concept of "astroma." GOLGI (1884), furthermore, described as "gliomas" only those growths that were composed of fiber-producing spider cells and generally quite benign. Together with Virchow, he defined as "sarcomas" tumors that were composed of round undifferentiated (malignant) elements. Here historical comparison shows very clearly how each new discovery in the field of normal anatomy was soon followed by a corresponding one in oncology (ZÜLCH 1962a, p. 159). A contrast to these views is seen in the isolated opinion of KLEBS (1889) who suspected that the gliomas were "organoid tumors," i.e., a hyperplasia of all parts of the brain (neurogliomas) which explained the different manifestations of gliomas as so many different stages of their development. He nevertheless described certain cases of glioma extremely well, and illustrated them with excellent pictures (for example a temporal oligodendroglioma).

MALLORY (1902) was able to show Weigert's "blepharoplasts" in certain "sacral" tumors which BORST (1902b) also had described. MUTHMANN and SAUERBECK (1903) with the help of serial sections proved the origin of a glioma of the fourth ventricle from the ependyma.

STROEBE (1895) published an observation that attracted considerable attention and influenced the literature for nearly 30 years. He reported on a glioma with cystic spaces formed of cylindrical epithelium, which had supposedly been pinched off from the ventricular wall and thus given rise to the tumor. The search for scattered "germinal rests" became the principal focus of many studies.

Meanwhile, experimental cancerology has taught us that "mixed tumors" from two germ layers actually exist (B. SCHIEFER 1958; KLEIHUES 1965; ZÜLCH and WECHSLER 1968). Yet, during the "classical" period an important contribution was made by STORCH (1899), who was working on the origin and growth of fibroblastic and brain tumors. He investigated them for signs of an "infectious" stimulus (cf. the concept of viral origin, p. 58). Noteworthy, also, is the work of STUMPF (1911), who described the penetration of tumor cells into the glial syncytium and HELD's (1909) views of the reticular (syncytial) arrangement of the glial cell groups also played an important part in this. RANKE (1911), too, expressed similar thoughts. It finally became necessary to separate the gliomas from the sarcomas and to decide whether there was really such a bipotential tumor as the "gliosarcoma" (von LENHOSSEK 1895; STROEBE 1895; LANDAU 1910). This controversy has persisted up to the present day (p. 123ff.), and a compromise has been made in the classification of the World Health Organization (ZÜLCH 1979; see p. 322).

The "field theory" of WILLIS (1960) was supported by KERSTING (1961), but it cannot be based on actual observations of "growth" of intracranial tumors. Since neuroradiology and, particularly, computed tomography (CT) have convincingly shown in recent years that the real growth of tumors from the quantitative point of view is not consistent with the field theory, we have sufficient arguments against its validity. On the contrary, we see the continuing growth of tumors from a central point outward rather than the global increase of volume in a large "field", e.g., the simultaneous onset of neoplastic growth in a larger zone.

Similar important proof comes from experience with transplantations and growth in tissue culture, particularly, by "cloning." For these reasons the field theory can be excluded from our discussions about tumor growth, except perhaps in the case of gliomatosis (p. 341).

Concurrently, the development of modern neurosurgery had begun. This was in the time of the pioneers V. von BRUNS (1854), von BERGMANN (1866–73, 1890), MACEWEN (1885), Sir Victor HORSLEY (1886), WAGNER (1989) and KRAUSE (1892, 1909–12) (see also C.M. BEHREND 1957), when some excellent monographs on the clinical aspects of brain tumors and/or their pathology were written (L. BRUNS 1897, 1904, 1908; BORST 1902a; OPPENHEIM and KRAUSE

1913a). After such original pioneers as MACEWEN[1] (1881, 1888), HAHN (see WERNICKE and HAHN 1882), BENNET and GODLEE (1885), DURANTE (1887), von BRAMANN (1893), and Ernst von BERGMANN (1895) came two European surgeons, who can be considered more specifically as neurosurgeons according to our present definition: Sir Victor HORSLEY (1887, 1906) and Fedor KRAUSE (1908, 1911). Indeed, neurosurgery is indebted to the latter for the first descriptions of innovative operative approaches to the brain (chiasm, cerebellopontine angle, and collicular region). Both, however, lagged far behind in their knowledge of pathological anatomy, which was limited to the information available in the clinical monographs of NOTHNAGEL (1879), BERNHARDT (1881), BRUNS (1904, 1908), and DURET (1905). The excellent chapter by BRUNS on pathologic anatomy accurately reflects the state of knowledge of his time. Compared with this, Fedor KRAUSE (1908, Fig. 132) had a surprisingly good knowledge of the histology of tumors (see OPPENHEIM 1907).

The beginning of the final phase of development in the field of classification is marked by the work of PICK and BIELSCHOWSKY (1911), who considered that the indifferent neurogliocyte previously described by HELD (1909) was the focal point of cell development. Divergent development led from there to the ganglion cell, glia, and Schwann cell. The authors maintained that a separation of such multipotential elements from the normal tissue groups could lead to nerve cells and fibers during the subsequent neoplastic transformation as well as to glial cells and fibers, or even sheath and capsule cells. The differentiation of tumor cells, however, could stop at any given stage. Theoretically, the development of the gliomas would be possible either from embryonic rests of solely glial potential spongioblasts or from an indifferent precursor of these cells. COHNHEIM'S (1882) doctrine of the development of tumors from scattered embryonic rests was obviously still very prevalent and here received even histological support.

Circumscribed developmental malformations of the brain and spinal cord, as reported in the literature of the last 100 years, contain numerous attempts to prove that tumors originate from embryonic rests isolated by developmental disturbance.

In a glioma from a 64-year-old woman, STROEBE (1895) described cystic spaces which were partly lined with "ciliated columnar epithelium," and which he considered to be detached fragments of the neural tube or ventricular epithelium. He presumed that the glioma had developed from these fragments and this concept of tumor origin dominated the literature for a long time. However, Stroebe's findings were not in the least convincing. Neither his illustrations nor his descriptions eliminated the possibility of *secondary* development of these

[1] In addition to the "classic" case of MACEWEN (operated on in 1879, published in 1881), which is usually cited as the first report of a successful brain operation, Oppenheim points especially to the case of WERNICKE and HAHN (1882). While Macewen was led to the tumor by external changes in the skull (exostosis), Wernicke was the first to recommend surgical intervention on a space-occupying lesion (tuberculous) that was localized solely through cerebral symptoms (for details see ZÜLCH 1975b). However, meanwhile I have found a paper on the "successful radical removal of an intracranial meningioma" in 1835 by Professor PECCHIOLI of Siena (see GIUFFRE 1984).

histological structures by regressive changes. Stroebe himself referred to numerous "softenings" in the vicinity. Between those holes, the walls of which were partly softened, were single cystic spaces which stood out because they were lined with regular, simple "high cuboidal of columnar epithelium."

In one of our cases – an oligodendroglioma of the thalamus in a boy of 3.5 years (GP, Fig. 109) – we almost made the same error as Stroebe, since the plexus was incorporated into the blastoma. This had given rise to the formation of "epithelium-lined small cavities, probably representing a developmental error." However, silver impregnations showed the true nature of this tissue, thereby preventing, at the last moment, an erroneous presentation at a neurosurgical meeting in 1939.

Such "cell rests" have been described by COOPER and KERNOHAN (1952; see KERNOHAN and SAYRE 1952, p. 21). These authors considered that the heterotopic localization of such cell rests was the cause for tumor growth.

RIBBERT'S (1918) formulation of the different stages of maturation of the gliomas (spongioneuroblastoma → spongioblastoma → glioblastoma → glioma/neuroblastoma) contained the foundation for present-day classification. With this, the stage was set for a basically new classification – which required, however, the development of completely new methods of research, both clinical and histological.

Neurosurgery, in the meantime, had made rapid strides. CUSHING (1908, 1912, 1917) had developed it into a teachable discipline and it had branched off as a surgical specialty. The concentration of many brain tumor patients in one clinic afforded unusual opportunities for research, especially when the clinician himself was interested in pathology, as Percival Bailey was. This kind of research was urgently needed, since the available pathological information had been insufficient to answer the clinician's principal question regarding the tumor's biological significance: "We were at a loss to know how it could be that a patient, from whose cerebellum a large tumor diagnosed "glioma" was removed as long ago as 1906, might prove to be living and well, whereas another patient from whom a "glioma" happened to be removed in like fashion, supposedly in its totality, might survive for a scant six months before a rapid recurrence took place" (BAILEY and CUSHING 1926, p. 104).

This, then, supplied the impetus for subsequent investigations, which used the work of PICK and BIELSCHOWSKY (1911), RIBBERT (1918), and STRAUSS and GLOBUS (1918) as a starting point. The latter two authors reported a case of "spongioblastoma" with an unusually rapid course and had mentioned some ideas about the cytogenetic origin of this tumor.

A new approach to research now became necessary: a tumor had to be investigated simultaneously from a clinical, surgical, and pathological point of view. This approach had already been anticipated in the works of CUSHING on *The Pituitary Body and its Diseases* (1912), and *Tumors of the Nervus Acusticus* (1917), and by F. HENSCHEN (1910) in his work *On the Tumors of the Posterior Fossa, Especially the Cerebello-Pontine Angle*.

The next advance concerned the "gliomas." BAILEY and CUSHING (1926, 1930) divided this task between them and ultimately achieved a common goal. Bailey, drawing on the descriptions of the German embryologists and the help

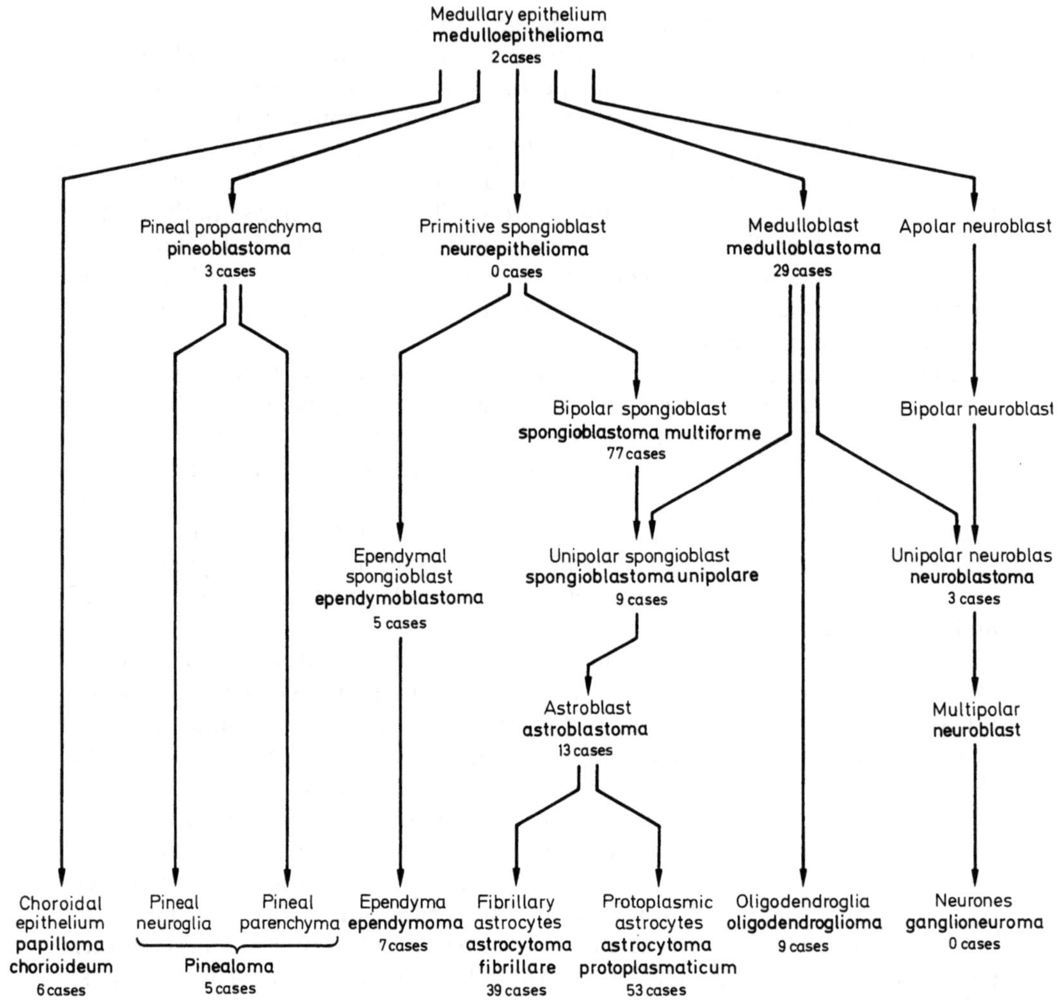

Fig. 1. Maturation of cells from medullary epithelium. (Scheme from Bailey and Cushing 1926, p. 103)

of metallic impregnation techniques developed by the Spanish shool of Ramon y Cajal and Del Rio Hortega, undertook the demonstration of the cell types present in brain tumors. These were compared with the cells of normal tissue and their developmental stages (Fig. 1), according to the cytogenetic principles established by the German (His 1904) and Spanish (Ramon y Cajal 1908, 1952; Del Rio Hortega 1932) schools. It became possible to correlate the different cell types within various gliomas and their stages of development. The result was that 15 (14) groups (spongioblastoma multiforme and unipolare must be considered as two groups) of brain tumors were derived from medullary epithelium, with only a few tumors remaining unclassified.

1. Medulloepitheliomas
2. Medulloblastomas
3. Pineoblastomas
4. Pinealomas
5. Ependymoblastomas
6. Ependymomas
7. Neuroepitheliomas
8. Spongioblastomas
   a) multiforme
   b) unipolare
9. Astroblastomas
10. Astrocytomas
    a) protoplasmic
    b) fibrillary
11. Oligodendrogliomas
12. Neuroblastomas
13. Ganglioneuromas
14. Papillomas of the choroid plexus

This new classification was at first rather detailed probably for theoretical reasons. With increasing experience, however, the desire arose to simplify it, with the result that it was condensed to ten types of neuroepithelial tumors – as in the German edition of 1930 – and finally to the eight types that form the basis of Bailey's contribution to PENFIELD'S *Cytology and Cellular Pathology of the Nervous System* (1932a).

At the same time CUSHING (see below) was reviewing the clinical histories of patients on whom he had operated at least 1 year previously; he noted the earliest localizing symptoms, the general signs of increased intracranial pressure, the postoperative course, and the survival period. A review of 254 cases classified by Bailey (see BAILEY and CUSHING 1926, p. 105) allowed an approximate estimate of the average survival period for each tumor type and, for the first time, of the biological behavior of these brain tumors. It was shown that tumors with little cell differentiation grew quickly while those with more highly developed forms grew slowly (see BAILEY and CUSHING 1926, schemes I and IV).

This was the first time that a satisfactory answer had been found to the above-mentioned question of BAILEY and CUSHING (1926, 1930). Equal clinical importance was attached to the recognition of *sites of preference* of many tumor types and the determination of the *age* at onset of the disease process. The greatest significance of these results was that the Bailey and Cushing classification brought *order* out of the "chaos" previously surrounding the various forms and types of brain tumors. The classification had *biological significance,* since the different forms and types could now be correlated with a presumed postoperative survival period. Moreover, the tumors showed a *preference* for certain *age* groups and *sexes* and for certain *sites* within the brain (CUSHING 1932, 1935; BAILEY 1933, 1936a, 1951).

The comparison with stages of cytogenesis was probably considered more as a working hypothesis than an oncologic dogma for the origin of the tumor cells. It provoked a number of attacks, most of which, however, appeared to have originated in the quiet isolation of the laboratory, and thus were scarcely comparable to the work of the two authors who, in ceaseless efforts at their patients' bedside, had created a new era in neurosurgery and neuropathology. True, in the long run their original theoretical and scientific concepts might not have been entirely adequate, but their new classification was extremely practical as far as clinical work was concerned. It promptly became the basis for the undisputed progress of neurosurgery since 1926. In spite of various attacks – especially from pathologists – this new classification was accepted with only minor changes in all fields where therapy was of primary concern. It may even be considered as the basis for the new *Histological Typing of Tumors of the Central nervous System* of the World Health Organization (ZÜLCH 1979).

Almost simultaneously with these American authors, the French investigators ROUSSY et al. (1924) produced another classification of brain tumors. Since they failed, however, to take impregnation methods into consideration, their scheme proved to be somewhat deficient. As a basis for subdivision, they too utilized the similarity between tumors and mature and embryonic cells. They recognized astrocytomas, cellular and afibrillary gliomas, glioblastomas, and spongioblastomas. More important than the classification itself was the manner of investigation, which resulted in an excellent pathological description of the individual groups, including a thorough appreciation of regressive processes or changes.

In 1928 ROUSSY (see ROUSSY and CORNIL 1928) criticized Bailey's classification, mainly on the grounds that the cytogenesis was still insufficiently substantiated, and that a classification from a cytogenetic point of view was simply hypothetical and could not be proved. Moreover, they took exception to the idea that tumors arose from cells that had been arrested at certain stages of their development rather than from cells that underwent anaplastic transformation. Nevertheless, ROUSSY and OBERLING (1931) in their atlas came very close to BAILEY and CUSHING'S (1926, 1930) classification, the differences being essentially only in nomenclature.

Classification of Gliomas According to ROUSSY and OBERLING (1931)

1. Gliomas: astrocytomas, oligodendrogliomas, glioblastomas
2. "Ependymochoroidal" tumors: ependymocytomas, ependymoblastomas, plexus papillomas
3. Ganglioneuromas
4. Neurospongiomas
5. Neuroepitheliomas

The difference in the principle of classification which the authors wished to emphasize was that they spoke only of a *similarity* to embryonic tissue, and unlike Bailey and Cushing, did not necessarily presuppose a *dysembryogenetic* development (aberrant development of fetal cells). In their atlas, which was carefully composed but slightly confusing because of the welter of terms, they distinguished three main groups of tumors derived from nervous tissue: those from the glia, those from the ependyma and choroid plexus, and finally those from the neuronal elements. In addition, there were tumors which recalled the primitive neurospongium, i.e., neurospongiomas (medulloblastomas). Others, i.e., neuroepitheliomas, duplicated tissues of the earliest development stages.

PENFIELD (1931, 1932b) largely adopted the proposals of Bailey and Cushing. His work contained the same eight main brain tumor groups as Bailey's. In an only slightly altered form, this classification was accepted by the American Neurological Association and the Commission on Nomenclature. Similar was the atlas of tumors by ZIMMERMAN et al. (1956).

Classification of Gliomas According to Penfield (1932)

Astrocytoma
Glioblastoma multiforme
Medulloblastoma
Ependymoma
Astroblastoma
Spongioblastoma polare
Oligodendroglioma and oligodendroblastoma
Neuroepithelioma
Pinealoma

It no longer seems necessary to discuss Schaffer's (1927) classification (for details see Zülch 1965, 2nd edn). Bergstrand's (1932a) suggestions for improvement were understandable from a clinical viewpoint. Olivecrona (1927), whose tumor material Bergstrand had studied, first used a predominantly biological classification of the cerebral gliomas, distinguishing only "malignant" and "benign" forms according to their clinical syndromes. Bergstrand provided a detailed *morphological* basis for this classification.

Classification of Gliomas According to Bergstrand (1932a)

1. *Benign* group
   Astrocytoma fibrillare
   Astrocytoma protoplasmaticum
   Astrocytoma gigantocellulare
2. *Malignant* group
   Glioblastoma multiforme
   Glioblastoma fusiforme
   Glioblastoma protoplasmaticum
3. Ependymoma
4. Oligodendroglioma

He considered a division into two main groups sufficient for the classification of the most common cerebral gliomas, i.e., (a) the *benign* types of astrocytoma (fibrillare, protoplasmaticum, and gigantocellulare) and (b) the *malignant* types of glioblastomas (multiforme, fusiforme, and protoplasmaticum). The third and fourth groups were relatively rare.

Bergstrand aligned the astroblastoma with the gigantocellular astrocytomas and abandoned the term spongioblastoma polare altogether. In one paper Bergstrand (1932b) correctly pointed out the biological and morphological difference between the cerebellar form of astrocytoma and the cerebral tumor of the same name. Later (1937), however, he blurred the picture by extending the description further but including some misleading interpretations. The new names – gliocytoma embryonale and glioneuroblastoma – that he proposed for this tumor (namely pilocytic astrocytoma) were never generally accepted. Moreover, they contradicted his otherwise praiseworthy attempts to simplify the nomenclature.

Cox (1933) and Carmichael (1928) made important additions to the discussion of cytogenetic classification (for details see the 2nd edition, Zülch 1965a).

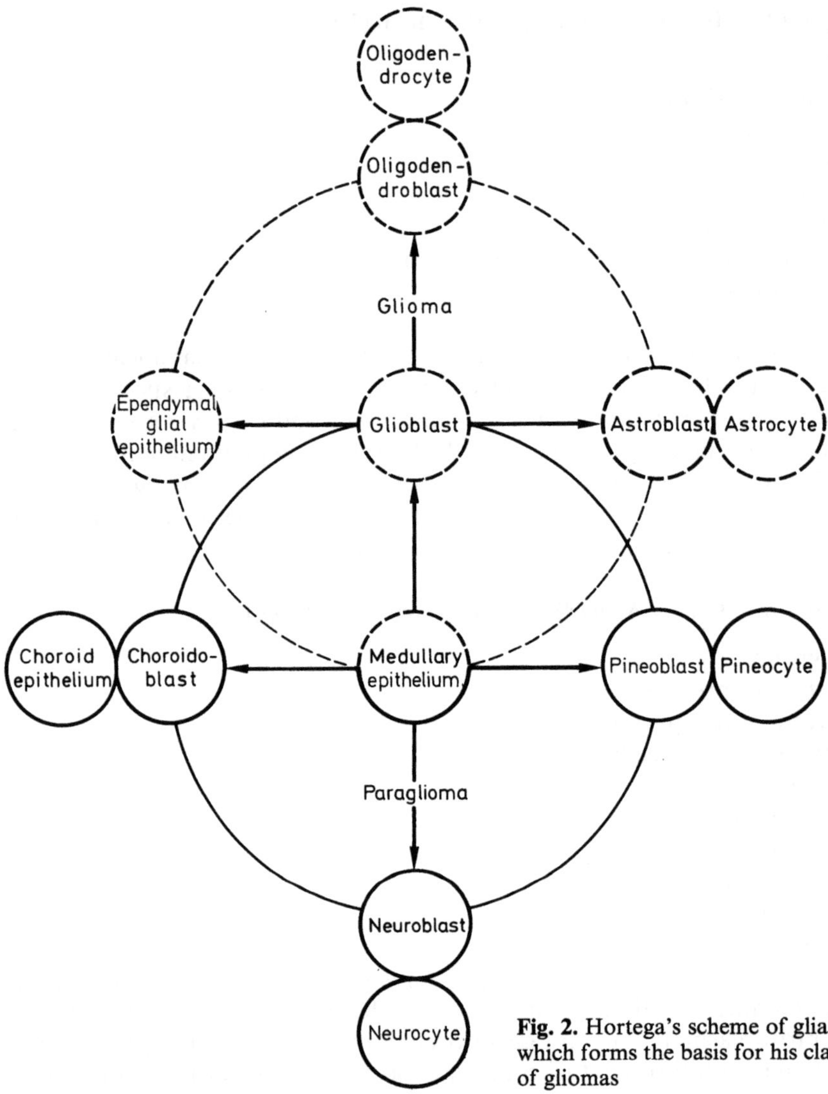

Fig. 2. Hortega's scheme of glial origin, which forms the basis for his classification of gliomas

Finally, we have the work of DEL RIO HORTEGA (1932, 1944, 1945, 1962) who presented his experience with the scientific investigation of intracranial tumors in two monographs and numerous articles published while working in Argentina. From his histogenetic studies he arrived at a developmental system for glia and specific parenchyma which differed from the above system devised by Bailey only superficially and not in principle. An important feature was the division of the developmental lines of medullary epithelium into one cell series related to "gliomas", and another, related to "paragliomas" (Fig. 2).

Del Rio Hortega distinguished two main types of immature glioma (glioblastoma): the isomorphic and the heteromorphic, depending on the uniformity of the tumor cells. In the isomorphic group we find some examples of glioblastoma multiforme, ependymoma, and the medulloblastoma; in the heteromorphic group we find most of the examples of glioblastoma multiforme.

One criticism of Del Rio Hortega's classification must be made, although it in no way detracts from the great service he rendered by his work on cytogenesis of brain tumors. His system fails to include the most essential feature of Bailey and Cushing's classification, in which the main advantage was the parallelism between the *biological* and the *morphological* properties of the different groups based on clinical experience.

Del Rio Hortega (Fig. 2) abandoned this way of classification in favor of a purely histological grouping, and for this reason his work unquestionably represents a step backward. He was often misled by an analysis of cell types based on metallic impregnation, where it is the form of the individual cells that is most striking. He succumbed to the great danger of constructing his classification purely according to histogenesis and cytology, without having it checked constantly against the biological aspects which only clinical examination can provide. Type of growth, general architecture, and especially biological behavior too often remained in the background. (For details see the second edition, ZÜLCH 1965a). The Del Rio Hortega concept has been further discussed and developed by POLAK (1966) and by SCHARRENBERG and LISS (1969). In his review of gliomas, HENSCHEN (1934) aligned himself – with only minor exceptions – with Hortega's classification; but in 1955, Henschen adhered to the scheme of Bailey and Cushing.

H.J. SCHERER (1933, 1935, 1941), who was initially fundamentally opposed to all current classifications, also later (1941) found it to be the most acceptable. At the beginning of his comprehensive study of intracranial tumors, Scherer took up the problem of existing classifications and thought, by the extension from the example of a small special group of tumors (glioblastoma multiforme ganglioides of Foerster and Gagel), that they would all lead to absurdity. He was unwilling to admit that any valid classification was conceivable. He deplored the fact that any valid classification as arrived at by "enthusiasts of histogenesis" had made of the glioma question a pure "problem of cell diagnosis," which had "degenerated more and more into a mere cytological game."

The first objection to H.J. SCHERER's work (1933, 1934, 1935) is that in his early papers he did not employ the terms proposed in the "American" classification. Consequently, it is frequently difficult to understand to which tumor type a given observation refers. The second objection concerns Scherer's approach, which depends *exclusively* upon *morphological* characteristics without any reference to clinical experience. The following "conclusions" (H.J. SCHERER 1940a, b; DE BUSSCHER and H.J. SCHERER 1942) would otherwise have been impossible:

There are no circumscribed astrocytomas; these tumors, because of their diffuse spread, can scarcely be differentiated from brain swelling and brain edema; most of them undergo dedifferentiation spontaneously (without operation); 20% of glioblastomas are sufficiently demarcated to assure a successful operation, so that pessimism on the part of neurosurgeons is not warranted; and finally, ependymomas are the only operable gliomas which do not recur.

This is not true, however, of the glioblastomas or of the ependymomas of the cerebral hemispheres; on the other hand, in every neurosurgical clinic the cerebellar – pilocytic – astrocytomas (spongioblastomas) consistently produce the longest postoperative survivals and even some permanent cures.

It was also possible to apply Bailey and Cushing's system of classification of tumors to the spinal cord without essential change. KERNOHAN et al. (1931) reported a study of 51 primary spinal tumors, among which they found all the intracranial types, after FOERSTER and BAILEY (1936, jubilee volume for Davidenkov) had already described seven primary spinal cord tumors. We are indebted to FOERSTER and GAGEL (1935) also for a condensed description of spinal tumors. A partial attempt to apply the same principles of classification to the tumors of the eye not only seems to be ontogenetically justified, but has actually shown itself to be possible in practice (GRINKER 1932; VERHOEFF 1932) (for details see p. 552).

Meanwhile, tissue culture methods gave new support to the BAILEY and CUSHING classification of gliomas (1926, 1930). Investigations by KREDEL (1928, 1929), BUCKLEY and EISENHARDT (1929), CANTI et al. (1935), COX and CRANAGE (1937), BENEDEK and JUBA (1941a), COSTERO and POMERAT (1955c), LUMSDEN (1971), and KERSTING (1964) were in fact able to show that individual morphological and biological properties (for instance, movement and form) persist in tissue culture of tumor cells. This was shown particularly well by demonstration of growth in time-lapse motion pictures. While very real differences existed, for example, between astrocytomas and oligodendrogliomas, such differences between astrocytomas and glioblastomas were not as striking as might have been expected on the basis of the fixed material.

COX and CRANAGE (1937), LUMSDEN (1971), and KERSTING (1964) succeeded in culturing tumor cells from meningiomas, neurinomas, and angioblastomas, as well as from gliomas in a manner that had been successful previously. The forms of the cultured cells were generally similar to the appearance observed in the usual histological preparations.

Among other articles on classification those by CHIOVENDA (1933), MAFFEI (1937), and JEQUIER-DOGE (1941), together with several by GLOBUS and KUHLENBECK (1944) and GLUSZCZ (1972) are worth mentioning. GLUSZCZ (1972) based his very detailed system correctly on growth dynamics and biomorphological trends; but he produced such a complex nomenclature that it was not applicable for daily routine use.

Strict adherence to the cytogenetic interpretation of tumors just does not seem reasonable and to discuss it in further detail would only be repetitious. This interpretation was intended only as a basis for organization, but the authors never intended to imply – as Bailey later strongly emphasized – that the tumor cells *really consisted* of embryonic spongioblasts, astroblasts, etc. This cytogenetic interpretation has proven to be so defective as a doctrine (most recently through the new classification of astroblastomas and spongioblastomas) *that there is no justification for its further expansion or the introduction of new terms.* Similarly, to deduce a cytogenetic system for normal development by basing it on the findings in tumors seems to be "putting the cart before the horse."

A major step forward was the work of KERNOHAN et al. (1949), who proposed a new simplified classification based upon a revised cytogenetic interpretation. This proposal grew out of the commendable desire to make the classification of brain tumors comprehensible and yet acceptable to pathologists as well (BRODERS 1926). KERNOHAN looked upon the different tumor types as having arisen not from particular tissues and their developmental stages, but from anaplasia of cellular development. The latter had already been assumed by ROUSSY et al. (1924) and COX (1933). KERNOHAN and SAYRE (1952) also believed that there is a continual series of gradations extending from fibrillary and protoplasmic astrocytomas through astroblastomas to glioblastomas, and that a comparable series of stages might be demonstrated for oligodendrogliomas, ependymomas, and other tumor types, although they never worked the latter out in sufficient detail for every group.

Their system reads as follows:

New Names	Old Names (with new names in parentheses)
Astrocytoma grades 1–4	Astrocytoma (astrocytoma grade I) Astroblastoma (astrocytoma grade II) Spongioblastoma polare (left out) Glioblastoma multiforme (astrocytoma grades III and IV)
Ependymoma grades 1–4	Ependymoma (ependymoma grade I) Ependymoblastoma (ependymoma grades II–IV) Neuroepithelioma (left out) Medulloepithelioma (ependymoma grade IV)
Oligodendroglioma grades 1–4	Oligodendroglioma (oligodendroglioma grades I–IV) Oligodendroblastoma (oligodendroglioma grades II–IV)
Neuroastrocytoma	Neurocytoma Ganglioneuroma (neuroastrocytoma grade I) Gangliocytoma Ganglioglioma Neuroblastoma Spongioneuroblastoma (neuroastrocytoma grades II–IV) Glioneuroblastoma
Medulloblastoma	Medulloblastoma

A detailed discussion of Kernohan's proposed classification appears in the section on grading of individual tumor types (p. 31). Suffice it here to make a few general remarks. By and large Kernohan's classification follows cytological criteria, and an overall evaluation of the tumor (as an "organoid" unit) is hinted at only by an occasional reference to the blood vessels. Regressive cell changes were not considered as possible causes for a particular cell or tissue pattern although it has been well demonstrated repeatedly that changes occur in the "normal" tissue of various tumors through *regressive processes* (p. 135ff.). We need only mention that the pilocytic astrocytoma, so decidedly benign, may acquire a very polymorphic structure through purely regressive changes (ZÜLCH 1940a, 1956).

Histological investigation and interpretation of a small area of tissue and a prognosis as to the probable grade of malignancy are very difficult to obtain if the matter of *regressive processes* is not taken into account. In addition, the same tumor can show a different histological appearance in different regions, without this variability necessarily influencing its overall biological significance. This was shown in the oligodendroglioma (ZÜLCH 1941a, 1955a, 1956), where the normal small cell structure and the spindle cell or large cell variant can be found adjacent to one another in the same tumor. It is merely a matter of chance which of these three tissues comes from the operating room to be studied, diagnosed, and graded. The same applies to monster cell sarcomas (ZÜLCH 1953, 1956) and other tumors.

In contrast to the four grade classification of Kernohan a similar classification with three grades has been published by RINGERTZ (1950); it is based on Olivecrona's material and was taken up by W. Müller (see SCHRÖDER et al. 1968a, b, 1970) and his group. In general, Ringertz' concept agrees with that of Kernohan. However, the concept of the origin of glioblastomas from malignant degeneration of ependymomas and oligodendrogliomas will certainly apply only very rare examples of glioblastoma multiforme (see p. 315).

One of the dangers of Kernohan's classification may be conceptual, namely, that grade IV astrocytomas usually develop from astrocytomas grades II and III. This is definitely not the normal case but may occur as an exception to the rule.

1.3 The Basis of Our Present Classification: The Classification of the World Health Organization

Correct classification of intracranial tumors is still fundamental to the creation of a common "language" between neurosurgeons and neurologists on one side and neuroradiologists and neuropathologists on the other. Neither epidemiological nor prognostic studies are relevant without an underlying classification which is equally applied and understood by all groups. We have only to point to the "Babelian confusion" in the terminology which has existed up to now (see Chap. 1).

All of our attempts to promulgate an international classification like that of the UICC (see our two atlases of 1971a and 1975a) or to define a new classification within the various schools at an international symposium in Cologne in 1961 (ZÜLCH and WOOLF 1964) or during the classification meeting of the Spanish school in Santander (OBRADOR ALCALDE and SANZ IBANEZ 1955) failed. Since then we have been intensively occupied in the preparation of the WHO classification (ZÜLCH 1979; see also ZÜLCH 1978, 1980a).

After the general experience with the other WHO "Blue Books" in the world of pathologists, we felt that this classification had a reasonable chance of being universally accepted. We have used it in our daily work, though in some specific aspects our personal opinion differed. This is not surprising since this classification was a compromise between the various schools in the world. Therefore, when we describe fully in the following chapters this "histological typing", we will sometimes add our own concepts, if they differ.

Before discussing the various groups in detail some further remarks seem to be appropriate. Some of them are contained also in the introductory section of the WHO classification.

1. The classification could not solve all the open problems of interpretation, as for example that of the correct position of some tumor types. In this particular situation either one of two classifications will be permissible in the future according to one's own scientific experience or prejudice.
2. It must be taken into account that many tumors are a mixture of cells and yet – if possible – have to be classified according to the prevailing type of cell (e potiori fit denominatio). Classification is sometimes possible only with difficulty because of the admixture of several elements and therefore some "mixed" groups are inevitable.
3. The process of malignant dedifferentiation is accounted for in all groups where such changes occur by the designation of a higher grade of malignancy, which is called "anaplastic." The term "anaplasia" includes all the morphological features associated with malignant biological behavior, such as cellular pleomorphism, increased cellularity, greater amount of mitotic activity, dedifferentiation, abnormal stromal reactions, especially vascular proliferation, and finally necrosis formation with or without pseudopalisading of nuclei or presence of metastases.
4. The terms provided in the book are not always those that are in widest use in the world. However, they seem to be the most acceptable from a scientific point of view. Synonyms are always placed in parentheses in order to make for easier understanding.
5. Finally, the group working on the classification felt it necessary to give a prognosis of the tumor type by grading. However, the difficulties of grading will be emphasized later.

The simplification of using "grades" for "prognosis" might, however, encounter a number of objections since (a) the tissue sample may not be representative of the whole tumor, (b) the cytological grading makes it difficult to interpret correctly tumors with a mixed cell population, and last but not least (c) the fact that the clinical circumstances may influence the prognosis even more than the biological behavior of the new growth. The importance of localization with respect to the influence on cerebro-spinal fluid circulation and on the "vital" centers leads to the final prognosis of "clinical malignancy" (see p. 32).

We have enlarged the text of the "histological typing" of the WHO in some groups, particularly with respect to the description of histologically different space-occupying or neurosurgically important groups, with the expectation that it would be helpful since it had been used in the earlier editions of this book.

Let me illustrate this by citing a particular problem, namely, that of the *pineal tumors* (pp. 283, 414). This is of especial importance because there are such gross differences in epidemiology that the riddle of origin and classification must be further investigated.

My concept ist that there is not only *one* form of "two-cell pattern" pineal tumor, namely, the germinoma; on the contrary, I still hold that there is a second type consisting of cells of the pineal parenchyma, which is the original *pinealoma* of Krabbe (1923). One should be able to distinguish between the two:

1. The *germinoma* not infrequently may have giant – or multinucleated – cells intermingled.

2. It may stain heavily with PAS, and not become impregnated with the De Girolami method.
3. On the other hand, the *pinealoma* has no giant cells, does not stain with PAS and yet it becomes impregnated with De Girolami's method for pineal parenchymal cells (see also pp. 207, 289, 418).
4. Moreover, pinealoma cells in the CNS resemble exactly the cell type described by Del Rio Hortega (see RIVERSON and ZÜLCH 1979, Figs. 3, 4).
5. The pinealoma has a strong tendency to calcify completely, a characteristic feature unknown for the germinoma elsewhere in the body.
6. Finally, there are immunohistochemical indications, that the large cell is a pineal parenchyma cell (MATSUTANI 1976).

Tumors of Neuroepithelial Tissue (for detailed description see Chap. 15)

Astrocytic Tumors

1. The astrocytic tumors will be subdivided into the three well-known groups of fibrillary, protoplasmic, and gemistocytic tumors, all of the same grade II.
2. A special subtype of *pilocytic astrocytoma* is added. This tumor corresponds to the older term "polar spongioblastoma" of BAILEY and CUSHING (1926), which was also used in our own former classification. However, it is separated in the WHO classification from the aforementioned three types of astrocytoma by its better biological prognosis (grade I).

There have always been difficulties with the interpretation of this tumor. It is characterized by mostly fusiform cells which, however, may also be astrocyte-like. Rosenthal fibers and "granular" bodies (ZÜLCH 1937b) are essential characteristics. Del Rio Hortega even came to the conclusion that many of these cases particularly in the optic fascicle and chiasma were oligodendrogliomas; hence his expression "fusiform" oligodendrocytoma. Since Rosenthal fibers appear in the subependymal glia after inflammation, degenerative states, and even syringomyelia, I felt it justified in relating pilocytic astrocytomas to a proliferation of the mature subependymal glia. Morphologically this glia occupies a position between the ependymal cell and the astrocyte, as described by OPALSKI (1934), and it corresponds to the tumor cells of the pilocytic astrocytoma, whose main representative has always been the "cerebellar astrocytoma."

3. Included in the astrocytic group is the ventricular tumor of tuberous sclerosis; it is termed *subependymal giant cell astrocytoma*. In tuberous sclerosis the ventricular tumors near the foramen of Monro may have neurosurgical importance, whereas in other sites, although always in local relation to the ventricles, they are of less significance clinically. The gross nodules of the cortex (tubera) and other malformations are rarely genuine space-occupying lesions and virtually never develop into autonomous neoplasms.
4. The term *"astroblastoma"* is still subject to discussion. This diagnosis will be restricted to growths of astrocytic cells arranged in a perivascular pattern with thick processes radiating toward a central blood vessel. These cells resemble astrocytes, and they are demonstrated with gold sublimate and other impregnations. Yet, since similar patterns of radiating processes may occur in glioblastomas (without this positive impregnation) and other groups this term of astroblastoma should be used only in the above "narrow" sense and with strong reservations.
5. The malignant form of astrocytoma has long been well recognized and is referred to as the *anaplastic astrocytoma* (grade III). This anaplastic transformation can occur in parts of an astrocytoma or may undergo transition into an adjacent tumor of the glioblastoma type (as described by TELTSCHAROW and ZÜLCH 1948) (Fig. 41; see also GP, Fig. 95; HBT, Fig. 27). We have found this regional transformation into anaplasia in about 10% of our series (TELTSCHAROW and ZÜLCH 1948).

If, as in our case, a large anaplastic tumor mass has developed and an astrocytic origin has been demonstrated, this can be referred to as a *secondary* glioblastoma as against a *primary* glioblastoma. If the anaplasia is only regional we prefer the term of *anaplastic astrocytoma*.

There is no experience which supports the proposition that *most* glioblastomas arise from preexistent astrocytomas as might be suggested by the Kernohan way of "grading glioblastomas as astrocytoma III and IV."

Oligodendroglial Tumors

1. The typical pattern of the oligodendroglioma is accepted widely (grade II). We must emphasize, however, that apart from the cases with classical honeycomb architecture and characteristic round cells other types are observed such as a spindle cell type reminiscent of pilocytic astrocytomas, and large cell types with a certain resemblance to the giant cell astrocytoma.
2. Not infrequently a conspicuous mixture of genuine oligodendroglial cells and astrocytes may occur and then the term of *mixed oligoastrocytoma* is applicable in this case.
3. For the "anaplastic" variant of the oligodendroglioma (grade III) pleomorphism is characteristic. There may be *two different forms* of *pleomorphism,* namely, the occurrence of multinucleated giant cells of the Langhans type ("cellular anaplasia") and/or abundant necrotic zones with pseudopalisading, proliferation of vessels, and other features of "tissular" anaplasia, as seen in most glioblastomas.

The question whether genuine oligodendrogliomas occur in the cerebellum has not yet been solved. There are cases reported in the literature, though it may be a very rare occurrence. The majority of tumors described as oligodendrogliomas of the cerebellum are probably in fact pilocytic astrocytomas undergoing mucoid degeneration with architectural patterns which because of regressive changes are deceptively similar to those of oligodendrogliomas (HBT, Fig. 55d).

Ependymal and Choroid Plexus Tumors

1. The ependymal tumors comprise the typical mass within the ventricles with true ependymal rosettes, perivascular rosettes, blepharoplasts, and ependymal canals (grade I).

Large extraventricular ependymomas constitute one of the most frequent tumors of childhood and can be more malignant (grade II–III).

The subdivision into ependymoblastomas and ependymomas has been discarded already by Bailey since it does not reflect a difference in biological behavior. Furthermore, we have to point out that in some ependymomas the architecture and cell form may be different, particularly in the ependymomas near the foramen of Monro and the third ventricle, where the usual architecture of a "nucleus free space around the blood vessel" is seen to a lesser extent than in other variants. On the other hand, ependymal tubules can be observed in *large numbers* only in the ependymomas near the aqueduct, 4th ventricle and spinal cord. However, among these there do not appear to be any biological difference between the subtypes.

a) The *myxopapillary ependymoma* (grade I) occurs almost exclusively in the cauda equina, however, where the stroma is highly vascular and mucin is often demonstrable. The stroma may be changed to such an extent that the original architecture is blurred.
b) *Papillary ependymoma* is a rare papillary variant, which may mimic the features of choroid plexus papilloma in some areas (papillotrabecular type).
c) *Subependymomas* are intraventricular tumors of varying size composed of nests of uniform ependymal cells, situated in a stroma of dense acellular glial fibers. These tumors have also been termed "subependymal glomerate astrocytomas." Typical ependymomas, particularly in the fourth ventricle, may also contain areas of "subependymoma" architecture, possibly as an atrophy subsequent to local pressure (grade I).

2. Rare forms of *anaplastic ependymomas* may resemble glioblastoma or medulloblastoma, although features of ependymal differentiation can still be recognized (grade III).
3. *Choroid plexus papillomas* are composed of a papillary pattern of low columnar or cuboidal cells covering a delicate core of vascular connective tissue (grade I). Some of these tumors are heavily calcified (usually in the temporal horn).
4. There may be – although rarely – anaplastic forms of this tumor (grade III) with a blurred achitecture, pleomorphism, and mitoses.

Care must be taken not to misinterpret metastases from cancer elsewhere as choroid plexus papillomas.

Pineal Cell Tumors

The WHO classification distinguishes between the *pineocytoma*, which is a rare isomorphous tumor with uniform cytology and processes radiating toward the vascular stroma (grades I–III), and the *pineoblastoma*, which is also a rare and highly cellular, malignant pineal neoplasm, very closely resembling the medulloblastoma (grade IV).

In Europe the traditional way of classifying, since KRABBE (1923), is to distinguish the pinealoma (the "two-cell-type" tumor) and the malignant counterpart. In the United States the concept, that the large majority of tumors of the pineal gland are actually germinomas, is prevalent. The same is true for the "ectopic" two-cell-pattern tumor near the chiasm. My personal belief, which is supported by my own investigations of some 30 pineal parenchymal tumors, is that there are two entities: (a) a real tumor of the great cells of the pineal parenchyma, which shows the typical cell processes with club-like expansions at their tips as described by Del Rio Hortega (e.g., CLARA 1959, Fig. 320, intermingled with "lymphoid" cells and formerly called "anisomorphous pinealoma" in our institution) and (b) the *germinoma*, a common tumor at this site, which does not originate in the pineal epithelium (this will be discussed later on p. 414).

Neuronal Tumors

1. *Gangliocytomas* consist of mature ganglion cells and are well defined. They are situated in various parts, preferably in the brainstem apart from one group that occurs in the medial basal temporal lobe, which has been described by TÖNNIS and ZÜLCH (1939), and is readily amenable to surgical treatment.

A dysplastic variant of this tumor (Lhermitte-Duclos) occurs in the cerebellum (all grade I).

2. Gangliocytomas containing both mature ganglion cells and neoplastic glial cells have to be classified as *gangliogliomas* (grade I and II).
3. If the spectrum of neuronal cells is larger and immature neuroblasts occur as well as mature ganglion cells, the term of *ganglioneuroblastoma* (grade III) seems appropriate.
4. There are rare *anaplastic gangliocytomas* and *gangliogliomas* (grade II–IV) in which the cells or the tissue can show forms of anaplasia.
5. *Neuroblastoma* is a cerebral tumor composed of small dark staining poorly-differentiated cells with slender processes and a tendency to form pseudorosettes (grade IV). It is closely related to retinoblastoma and sympathoblastoma.

This grouping may overcome the considerable confusion prevailing about the definition, grouping, and biological evaluation of ganglion cell tumors.

We must emphasize even at this early stage how difficult it may be to prove the neuronal nature of a cell or of a tumor. The "ganglioid" nucleus does not suffice (p. 122). Even impregnation frequently does not show the specific form of neuroblasts. In mature ganglion cell tumors axons are sometimes not as common as expected. The classification of the neuronal tumors will still remain a battlefield for young investigators.

Poorly Differentiated and Embryonal Tumors

1. The most prominent tumor in this class is the *glioblastoma multiforme* with its variegated architecture of necrosis, pseudopalisading, fistulous vessels, vascular endothelial proliferation and both old and fresh hemorrhages (grade IV). There are two further subgroups:

a) If the stroma appears to consist of many malignant transformed hyperplastic mesodermal elements, the tumor may be classed as *glioblastoma with sarcomatous component* or *mixed glioblastoma* and *sarcoma* (grade IV).
b) On the other hand, if a glioblastoma shows a predominance of bizarre multinucleated (even "monstrous") giant cells, the term of *giant cell glioblastoma* may be appropriate (grade IV).

My interpretation of this last group is different. Since 1940 I have described these tumors as a special form of the sarcomas (monstrocellular sarcoma), because they differ not only in structural elements but also in their biology. They have no sex or age preference nor preferential site (as the glioblastomas; see p. 307).

2. The second, also very frequent, tumor in this group of the undifferentiated blastomas is *medulloblastoma* (grade IV), characterized by poorly differentiated cells and a tendency to form pseudorosettes (Homer-Wright). There are two variants:
a) *Desmoplastic medulloblastoma*, in which the architecture has abundant reticulin fibers in its stroma. It occurs preferentially in the cerebellar hemispheres and corresponds to what has been referred to by FOERSTER and GAGEL (1939) as a "circumscribed arachnoidal sarcoma of the cerebellum." This is an undifferentiated tumor with a particular architecture containing lightly stained reticulin-free islands between strands of a specifically desmoplastic character (grade IV).
b) *Medullomyoblastoma* can be applied if a medulloblastoma contains either striated or non-striated muscle fibers. These are very rare tumors (grade IV).
3. *Medulloepithelioma* is also a very rare tumor of undifferentiated columnar cells with a characteristic tubular or papillary pattern resembling a primitive medullary epithelium (grade IV). This entity has been accepted by the WHO classification but the *neuroepithelioma* has been omitted.

Neuroepitheliomas were included in the classification of BAILEY and CUSHING (1926, 1930) for theoretical reasons. Certain structures in rare tumors of the retina, for instance, were interpreted as medullary epithelium and the "true rosettes" of the retinoblastomas considered neuroepithelial rests. However, only part of the retinoblastomas form true rosettes (and those only in the eye and never in metastases) and most of the cases in the literature have actually been ependymomas with ependymal canals or true rosettes. Therefore there seems to be no justification for this group.

4. *Primitive polar spongioblastoma* is a very rare tumor of unipolar or bipolar cells with delicate processes, forming an unusual palisading pattern (grade IV).
5. *Gliomatosis cerebri* is a rare entity with diffusely spread glial cells resembling either spongioblasts, astrocytes or oligodendroglia. These diffuse cell populations infiltrate large parts of the cerebrum but may contain circumscribed foci resembling glioblastoma.
These diffuse neoplastic proliferations have been referred to as glioblastosis, gliomatosis, lemmoblastosis and central diffuse schwannosis. They ought to be distinguished from *diffuse* gliomas, *multicentric* gliomas, and *multiple* brain tumors (see pp. 112, 341).

Tumors of the Nerve Sheaths (for detailed description see Chap. 16)

1. *Neurilemmomas* are the well-known tumors composed of Schwann cells (grade I).
2. *Anaplastic neurilemmomas* rarely occur (grade III).
3. *Neurofibromas* are either localized or diffuse tumors consisting of a mixture of Schwann cells and fibroblasts with abundant collagen fibers and usually occur as a component of von Recklinghausen's disease (grade I).
4. *Anaplastic malignant neurofibroma* (grade III and IV) is the malignant counterpart of the neurofibroma. This malignant transformation is also described as a neurosarcoma.

The term "neuroma" should be dropped, because this is a non-neoplastic overgrowth of nerve fibers, Schwann cells and other components of *scar tissue*.

The term of *neurilemmoma* was accepted only after some hesitation since in European neurosurgery the term of "neurinoma" was prevalent. However, the other term, "schwannoma," contravened the rule that an author's name should not be used in connection with cells and tumors.

Tumors of Meningeal and Related Tissues (for detailed description see Chap. 17)

In the *meningioma* group some of the traditional entities are given as subgroups, as are some of the later forms. For tumors of the meninges the term *meningioma* seems to be appropriate as a general heading, based on the broad view that the meninges, including the dura, the capsular elements of the arachnoid, the arachnoid granulations, the subarachnoid blood vessels, and fibroblasts in the pia, is the point of origin. Some meningiomas arise from the connective tissue of the choroid plexus while some others begin within the bone and/or invade the bone and occasionally invade muscle as well. Most meningiomas are encapsulated but finger-like projections may occur. Occasionally they grow diffusely and flat like a carpet.

1–4. Microscopically the following additional subtypes are recognized, namely, the *meningotheliomatous*, *fibrous*, *transitional*, and *psammomatous*.
5–7. If a meningioma shows predominantly vascular channels the term *angiomatous meningioma* is used, while if it is indistinguishable histologically from a hemangioblastoma, although encapsulated and non-invasive, it may be termed a *hemangioblastic* variant of meningioma. The *hemangiopericytic* subgroup is indistinguishable from hemangiopericytoma elsewhere in the body, except that it is encapsulated and non-invasive. All meningiomas are grade I tumors apart from the last-mentioned, which may have a worse prognosis.
8. *Papillary meningioma* is a rare form, also with a poorer prognosis.
9. The typical *anaplastic meningioma* can occur in many of the subgroups and displays anaplastic features; however, its anaplastic changes are not yet as far developed (grade II–III) as in the primary fibrosarcoma of the dura mater.

Meningeal Sarcomas

1. The *primary fibrosarcoma* of the dura mater is histologically well-defined, invasive, yet fairly well-circumscribed (grade III–IV).
2. *Polymorphic cell sarcoma* is rarely seen and there is wider variation in size and shape of the cells (grade III–IV).
3. *Primary meningeal sarcomatosis* is a diffuse sarcomatous neoplasm in the subarachnoid space (grade IV), which has to be distinguished from seeding from a medulloblastoma.

At this point in the text a few other rare types of sarcoma will be mentioned, although some of them will be discussed in greater detail in other groups (e.g., the *periadventitial sarcoma* and the *reticular sarcoma*, with the *lymphomas*, the *monstrocellular sarcoma*, with the *tumors of the blood vessels*, etc.).

Xanthomatous Tumors

1–2. The *fibroxanthomas* and their malignant counterpart are rare forms in which the xanthomatous component is prominent. Recent investigations suggest a glial origin.

Primary Melanotic Tumors

1–2. *Primary melanomas* and *meningeal melanomatosis* are rare in the central nervous system. For proper classification the nature of the pigment has to be investigated. They are highly malignant.

Others

A large variety of fibromas, chondromas, chondrosarcomas, etc. are included in this group.

Primary Malignant Lymphomas (for detailed description see Chap. 18)

This category includes reticulum cell sarcoma, reticulosarcoma, microglioma, microgliomatosis, periadventitial diffuse sarcoma, and all other types of lymphoma which occur primarily in the central nervous system. They will be described broadly only when they are of neurosurgical importance, since there is a WHO *Blue Book* dealing specifically with the classification of the lymphomas.

Of these special entities the spinal *epidural reticulosarcoma* (or *lymphosarcoma*) is well known to the neurosurgeon and neuroradiologist and therefore will be more broadly discussed in detail (grade III–IV).

Tumors of Blood Vessel Origin (for detailed description see Chap. 19)

1. The *hemangioblastoma* of Lindau is a well defined tumor of blood vessel origin and its existance has long been known. Semantically, the *Lindau syndrome* is a combination of retinal and cerebellar tumors, while *von Hippel-Lindau disease*, in contrast, is an inherited form of this syndrome (grade I).
2. *Monstrocellular sarcoma*. This group has been mentioned with reference to the differential diagnosis of giant cell glioblastomas. In our experience these tumors seem to be relatively well-demarcated; they occur at any age and site and equally in both sexes, contain an abundant reticulin stroma and are characterized by monster cells of enormous size, which have many nuclei and inclusions (grade IV). These "monstrous" cells cannot be compared with any other cells in the body. Therefore, these tumors may be easily distinguished from glioblastoma.

Germ Cell Tumors (for detailed description see Chap. 20)

The tumors in this group occur most often in the pineal region.

1. *Germinomas* are tumors composed of large primitive spheroidal cells indistinguishable from the testicular seminoma and the ovarian dysgerminoma. The *two-cell-pattern* tumor of the pineal gland, with large epithelial and many *lymphoid* cells in its stroma, is the representative of this group. Multinucleated giant cells are sometimes found.

Our own concept has been mentioned already in the discussion of pineal cell tumors (see pp. 20, 286ff.).

According to prominent authors *germinomas* are not only the most frequent tumors of the pineal region but also the type of mass encountered in the hypothalamic region and referred to as *ectopic pinealomas*. Histologically they are grade II and III tumors.

2–3. *Embryonal carcinomas* and *choriocarcinomas* are rare tumors so sufficiently defined in general pathology (grade IV) as to make further discussion here unnecessary.

4. *Teratomas* occur in many regions of the central nervous system (grade I). They are typically composed of several types of tissue, representing more than one germinal layer.

Other Malformative Tumors and Tumor-Like Lesions
(for detailed description see Chap. 21)

1. *Craniopharyngiomas* are the most common tumors of childhood in the sellar region. They can be cystic and calcified. The group is biologically benign (grade I). The cell pleomorphism, which arises as a regressive process – resulting from cholesterin irritation – does not justify the interpretation as *anaplastic*.
2. *Rathke's cleft cysts* are intrasellar epithelial cysts.
3. *Epidermoid cysts* are lined with a keratin producing squamous epithelium. Their contents are typically brittle, white and pearly. Malignant transformation is very rarely seen.
4. *Dermoid cysts* are lined with keratin-producing squamous epithelium. Their contents are more smeary and cheesy than brittle; they contain skin appendages, and hair and rarely teeth may be included.
5. *Colloid cysts of the third ventricle* occur in the foramen of Monro and their origin has not yet been clarified. They are ciliated and lined with columnar or cuboidal epithelium.
6. *Enterogenous cysts* are lined with epithelium which secretes mucin and are located intraspinally.
7. *Other cysts* may occur in the arachnoid system or be ependymal, lined, and sited in various regions.
8. *Lipomas* also benign, have a dangerous trend to grow into the stroma septa, for instance in the region of the spinal cord, cauda equina, or the corpus callosum.
9. *Choristomas*, *pituicytomas*, or *granular cell myoblastomas* are found in the pars nervosa of the pituitary gland.
10. The hypothalamic *neuronal hamartomas* are rare and of a malformative origin. However, they may also grow and take on the feature of a space-occupying lesion. They are usually associated with a typical clinical syndrome of precocious puberty, etc.
11. *Nasal glial heterotopia* or *nasal gliomas* are rare.

Vascular Malformations (for detailed description see Chap. 22)

1–5. Vascular malformations contain the very well-known entities of *capillary teleangiectasia*, *cavernous angiomas*, *arteriovenous malformations*, *venous malformations*, and *Sturge-Weber disease*.

The Tumors of the Anterior Pituitary (for detailed description see Chap. 23)

1–2. The tumors of the anterior pituitary can be classified according to the traditional systems with the subgroups of *acidophil* (*eosinophil*), *basophil* (*mucoid*), *mixed acidophil/basophil* and *chromophobe* entities. The malignant form of these would be the *pituitary adenocarcinoma*.

The *oncocytic* adenoma is a new subgroup of the chromophobe adenoma.

Today, however, the classification is more sophisticated and based upon the endocrinological behavior of the various subtypes (e.g., prolactin-secreting adenomas, which may be *microadenomas*, etc.).

Local Extensions from Regional Tumors (for detailed description see Chap. 24)

1–7. Among the local extensions from regional tumors into the cranial cavity the *glomus jugulare tumor* (*chemodectoma*) is well known because of its high vascularization and "clinical" malignancy, whereas the *chordoma* and *chondroma* are less well known and very slow growing neoplasms. More malignant are the *chondrosarcoma*, the rare *olfactory neuroblastoma* (*neuroesthesio-epithelioma*), and the not infrequent *adenoid cystic carcinoma* (*cylindroma*). These entities have to be well known because of their projection about the brain and/or spinal cord.

Metastatic Tumors (for detailed description see Chap. 25)

Metastatic tumors do not need any definition here since there will be a relevant report provided later.

Unclassified Tumors (for detailed description see Chap. 26)

The term *unclassified tumors* will be used for the entities that cannot placed in any of the above categories with sufficient certainty. We still maintain this miscellaneous group because it seems to us practical to call a tumor unclassified when its nature is not clear despite of quite sophisticated staining techniques and other investigations. It seems to us better to call a tumor *unclassified* and perhaps point to some resemblance to a well-known tumor group than to "force" it into such a group. Since the grading and the biological behavior is so well known for all the entities described here, a *false prognosis* may be given when one forces the tumor into an inappropriate group.

No other entities are contained in the WHO classification.

Since this book is meant to meet the needs of pathologists, clinicians, and radiologists worldwide, some other entities are added that are still of clinical importance particularly in Third World countries. These include the parasitic cysts, the granulomas, the scarring processes of arachnoiditis and ependymitis, and finally the syndrome of *pseudotumor cerebri*. In this respect we have followed the lines of the former editions of this book. A survey on certain regional tumors such as tumors of the spinal cord and the orbita, is also added (pp. 532, 552).

1.4 Critical Evaluation of the Present State of Classification of Tumors of the Nervous System

With the completion of the classification of the World Health Organization we have achieved our desired goal. We must bear in mind that this is a compromise reached through the discussion by members of most of the pertinent schools working on classification of CNS tumors. We, the members of the WHO Study Group, are aware that there are still weaknesses and perhaps even minor failures in the present pattern. But after working on this project, we have all finally agreed to accept the pattern we have given to it. It is important not only that a classification using simple technical methods has been developed, but a gross estimation is presented also of the biological behavior of the tumor groups by grading. Moreover, the World Health Organization is prepared to re-establish another study group after 10 or 20 years to evaluate (a) whether this classification has been accepted by relevant members of the neurological sciences and their clinical departments, and (b) what amendments are desirable on the basis of experience acquired with it in daily teamwork.

Up to now, none of the "other" classifications of the UICC (1958, 1965), of the ICD-O (1975) or the Anderson Hospital Nomenclature (1974), have been promoted in such a way as to make its acceptance throughout the world likely.

In an attempt to promote the UICC nomenclature (1958, 1965), I unfortunately based two of our atlases (1971 a, 1975 a) on this classification. This definitely limited their use (GP, HBT).

The anticipated acceptance of the WHO classification, for instance in the field of neuroradiology (WENDE et al. 1977; KAZNER et al. 1981), leads us to hope that there will be improved understanding among the various specialists working in the field of oncology from now on.

2 Biological Behavior and Grading (Prognosis)

2.1 Malignancy – Anaplasia – Dedifferentiation

The following chapter will deal with the prognosis of the patients with an intracranial tumor. It had to be based on both the morphology and the corresponding biological behavior of the particular tumor. The classification of tumors has already been discussed, and it is clear that their biological behavior has to be defined by morphological characteristics of the tumor tissue and its clinical consequences. This kind of discussion started in general pathology long ago with the problem of the "malignancy of cancer" (von HANSEMANN 1898, 1920). Malignancy was ascertained in a tumor if *anaplasia* (von HANSEMANN) was observed. Anaplasia was defined for this author by the low grade of differentiation of a cell in comparison with the mother cell, and this dedifferentiation together with a higher capacity to metastasize caused a reduced survival capacity to live. The morphological phenomenon of anaplasia has now to be more broadly described with reference to discussions over the last century.

Earlier CRUVEILHIER (1829/35) had defined a neoplasm as "malignant" when it "recurred and killed the patient" even if the tumor were "cut and burnt out"; this was also the concept of Johannes von MÜLLER (1838). On the other hand, TOOTH (1912) had referred to histological malignancy when he observed undifferentiated nuclei in a tumor which was rich in cells. These neoplasms were possibly polynucleated, the vessels were either proliferated or multiform. Tooth probably conceived these characteristics from his study of tumors of the glioblastoma multiforme type.

2.1.1 Definition of Benignity and Malignancy

In an earlier edition of this book we have tried to summarize the characteristics of benignity and malignancy by the histological evaluation of a neoplasm.

Benignity was thought to be recognizable in the gross morphology by expanding growth respecting organ boundaries, formation of capsules, absence of metastases, and recurrence only after incomplete removal. The *histology* of benign tumors was thought to be characterized by regular cell structures, slow growth without mitoses, low cell density with differentiation of structures (parenchyma, stroma, etc.), and an orderly arrangement of the vascular stroma without new formations.

Signs assumed to be indicative of *relative malignancy* (anaplasia) in the *gross morphology* were infiltrating and destructive expansion without regard for organ boundaries, rapid growth, tendency toward formation of metastases and recurrence despite supposedly total removal. The *histology* in such cases was thought to be characterized by increased cellularity; pleomorphism with disorderly arrangement of cells and tissues – deficient differentiation of cells – disturbance in the ratio of nucleus to cytoplasm; multinucleation and formation of giant cells with disproportionate nuclei; rapid growth and/or high rate of mitoses; short life span of cells with either diffuse disintegration or rapidly proceeding broadly extended regressive processes in the form of necroses; abnormally prominent, incomplete and disorganized arrangement of stroma, particularly of vascular origin; pathologic overgrowth and neoformation, particularly in the form of fistulas and sinusoidal vessels (arteriovenous shunts). The latter are angiographically demonstrable as early filling veins or observed during surgery as "red" veins.

A few features will be discussed in more detail. In the formation of *metastases* we differentiate seeding by way of the CSF (meningeal and ventricular) and through the blood system (hematogenous). The latter is a sign of high malignancy and is observed particularly in medulloblastomas and occasionally even in glioblastomas, as well as in rarer entities such as monstrocellular sarcomas. It will be described below that spontaneous seeding along the CSF pathway – so common in medulloblastomas, pineoblastomas, meningeal sarcomas – occasionally also occurs in relatively benign tumors such as oligodendrogliomas, ependymomas, and choroid plexus papillomas, etc.

Local *invasion* of neighboring tissues by infiltration occurs even in the most benign glioma types as will be demonstrated later. SCHALTENBRAND and BAILEY (1928) emphasized the "breaching" of the blood-brain or CSF barrier as a sign of relative malignancy. Earlier (1940a) we reported the invasion of the leptomeninges by pilocytic astrocytomas of the cerebellum and the optic nerve, that is to say by gliomas of the most benign biological nature. This also will be reported for the oligodendrogliomas, where a particular feature is formed, viz. warts.

A last question to be briefly discussed here is the occurrence and/or number of *mitoses* (see p. 132). More than 50 years ago investigations showed that the number of mitoses in neoplastic tissue did not change in different temperatures such as that in the refrigerator, at room temperature or body temperature (EVANS 1926).

The Cologne team led by W. MÜLLER (see R. SCHRÖDER 1964, 1967; SCHRÖDER and KAESS 1972; MÜHLICHEN 1974) has made a very thorough study of the occurrence and form of mitoses in various tumors. However, they apparently did not devote any attention to the problem of variation by the kind and time of fixation ("the tissue came from surgical specimens and was immediately placed in fixative, in order to avoid postmortem changes"). The data on atypical features and differences in astrocytomas, oligodendrogliomas, medulloblastomas, glioblastomas, and mesodermal tumors are interesting (see the special sections).

The number and disordered form (atypicality) of mitoses cannot be estimated quantitatively, nor can the fact of formation of the *typical* structures of mitoses be assumed to indicate a lesser malignancy. Mitoses of normal structure occur in oligodendrogliomas which are relatively benign and quite in a higher percentage also in the medulloblastomas, which are one of the most malignant tumors. Despite its high malignancy atypical mitotic figures never occur in this latter tumor.

Finally, the feature of *pleomorphism* must be discussed briefly. Pleomorphism occurs sometimes in the same tumor entity in various forms, e.g., in the *cells* or in the *tissue*. This may or may not indicate anaplasia. In oligodendrogliomas we may have the phenomenon of multinucleation and formation of giant cells. These most often take the form of the so-called Langhans type. Where the *iso*morphism of *cells* is maintained but acute regressive phenomena such as necroses in the tissue are observed coincidentally with a disorderly formation of vascular stroma with neoformations, hyperplasia, etc., this is the "tissular" form of pleomorphism. However, we have not been able to distinguish a difference in the degree of anaplasia (or biological behavior) between these two types of pleomorphism, despite the variable "cellular" or "tissular" differentiation and/or a possible atypicality of the stroma.

After our characterization of malignancy by the phenomenon of morphological anaplasia some reports from the literature will be cited where this problem has been discussed on the basis of the malignancy of neoplasms (see GLOBUS 1931; MÜLLER 1933; H.J. SCHERER 1940a; EARNEST et al. 1950; REYMOND and RINGERTZ 1950).

We lay particular emphasis here on the two discussions of ARENDT (1964a, 1965), where he raised the problem of whether small anaplastic foci in a tumor entitle us to assume malignant dedifferentiation of the whole neoplasm and hence accept a higher degree of malignancy. We will take up this problem again when discussing the "intermediate" forms of malignancy (grade III; see p. 37ff.).

At this point we have to state that anaplasia may actually be noted on examination of a tumor: (a) in the *total* tissue, or (b) as a *focus*, as discussed by ARENDT (1964a, 1965).

These different forms of global or focal development of anaplasia are typical in the course of some tumors and will be illustrated by reference to some case histories:

1. In the famous case of Dorothy May Russell (see CUSHING and EISENHARDT 1938) in the collection of Cushing's patients with meningiomas, where finally *total* anaplasia with formation of the papillary type of meningioma (see p. 373) and metastases in the lung occurred after the 17th operation.
2. We may add here the case of ZÜLCH et al. (1954) of a patient with meningioma in which, 23 years (!) after the first biopsy, malignant transformation took place with finally a 1 kg tumor metastasis into the lung (!). *Total* anaplasia was also evident in the pulmonary lesion.
3. Our case with an astrocytoma (described by TELTSCHAROW and ZÜLCH 1948) (Fig. 41; see also GP, Fig. 95; HBT, Fig. 27) showed the growth of a circumscribed, hard, highly fibrillary astrocytoma with a thinning of the overlying bone (a very rare occurrence) and its final transformation into a tumor resembling a glioblastoma multiforme. It took its origin from the astrocytoma which continued to have its original benign histologic appearance. From there it grew

into the white substance of the entire hemisphere and across the corpus callosum to the contralateral side; however, this was a focal anaplasia.

4. A similar transformation was observed in one of our cases of oligodendroglioma (SCHUIER 1976) in which focal seizures developed in a 21-year-old woman patient without any detectable radiologic focus. The seizures were medically controlled for 8 years after which a temporal oligodendroglioma was diagnosed and surgically removed. The histologic appearance was that of an isomorphous oligodendroglioma. At autopsy $2\frac{1}{2}$ years later the appearance in some areas still persisted with the same pattern but in other areas was transformed into a neoplasm which almost entirely consisted of nuclear material where the highest degree of pleomorphism and anaplasia was visible; yet, it was a *focal* anaplasia.

After very long postoperative survivals anaplastic changes were also reported by RUSSELL and RUBINSTEIN (1962), for example, 23 years after biopsy of a ganglioglioma.

Such – though less dramatic – *foci* of malignant transformation were reported by ourselves in oligodendrogliomas (ZÜLCH 1941a, 1955a, 1956), in gangliocytomas (TÖNNIS and ZÜLCH 1939), in ependymomas (ZÜLCH 1940b), in pilocytic astrocytomas (ZÜLCH 1940a). COURVILLE and ABBOTT (1955) considered such anaplastic foci a "regular occurrence" and noted it also in gangliogliomas. TELTSCHAROW and ZÜLCH (1948), in their paper on astrocytomas, reported the existence of such foci in 10% when the examination of large block sections included the "total" tumor. Similarly ESCALONA-ZAPATA (1966) showed in 15% of his cases anaplasia, however, this author referred to the statement of H.J. SCHERER (1940a) that all astrocytomas showed signs of anaplasia, and pointed out that RUBINSTEIN (cited in RUSSELL and RUBINSTEIN 1959, 1977) found anaplasia in 53% of cases.

2.1.2 Other Characteristics of Anaplasia and Malignancy

We have summarized above the gross characteristics of anaplasia and malignancy. We shall now emphasize that for instance the degree of functional tightness of the *blood-brain barrier* in a new growth was accepted as a characteristic of malignancy by R. SCHRÖDER et al. (1970; see p. 124) and also by O'CONNOR and LAWS (1969), who investigated the breakdown of the blood-brain barrier in brain tumor. This has also been examined by K.-A. HOSSMANN et al. (1965).

Further pieces of evidence came from *histochemistry* as demonstrated, for example, by BINGAS (1966, 1970), who showed a decrease of alkaline and an increase of acid phosphatase in progressive anaplasia, although the dihydrogenase increased. Histochemically, he found the separation of glioblastoma on one hand and astrocytoma and oligodendroglioma on the other possible when based on these criteria. Later efforts were reported, for instance, by ODA (1974), who tried to find tumor specific antigens. HEIENBROCK et al. (1978) tried to define malignancy by objective parameters such as the cytometric measurements of DNA. Abnormal inhibition of pyruvate kinase by alanine also was observed, namely the M2 type. This did not occur in normal brain tissue (VAN VEELEN et al. 1979) and could be used for evaluating malignancy.

Most of these attempts are still in the test situation but may later be helpful in determining the degree of malignancy in particularly difficult problems of anaplasia, that cannot be solved by conventional morphology.

In summary we can state at the moment that since BERNHARD'S (1961) attempt to define malignancy by ultrastructural characteristics has been frustrated our efforts to achieve a definition have to be continued in every direction. However, since most of these histochemical methods are still under investigation, they have not replaced as yet the gross characterization of anaplasia by light microscopy, which we have to explore systematically.

2.2 Prognosis – Biological Evaluation – Postoperative Survival Time – The Problem of Grading

Prognosis of tumor growth is intended to define the probable course of the disease (VIRCHOW 1888), or more specifically the possible survival time of a patient with or without various forms of therapy. Prognosis is based (a) on the diagnosis of the tumor and its *morphological* pattern, and (b) on the probable *biological* behavior according to clinical experience.

Attempts to define prognosis in intracranial tumors go back to 1851, when LEBERT distinguished intracranially "fibroblastic" neoplasms and "cancer," the former having a better life expectation in his experience. Later attempts were more theoretically based. PICK and BIELSCHOWSKY (1911) were the first to try to define the position of the tumor cells in their hierarchy of growth. They suggested that the more undifferentiated and immature the cells were in their development, the more rapid and disorderly would be their growth. This concept was followed and further developed for the gliomas by the pathologist RIBBERT (1918; see p. 7). The same assumption later formed the basis of the meticulous work of BAILEY and CUSHING (1926, 1930) at the time when neurosurgery was developing into a modern specialty. Bailey's efforts led to a most refined system of classification and prognosis. This was necessary since VIRCHOW'S (1847, 1863/65) gross subdivision of tumors in the more "benign" (psammomas and gliomas) and the "malignant" (sarcomas and gliosarcomas) still existed, and was no longer adequate for clinical purposes. A finer classification was possible because the glia had already been subdivided following the research of the German and Spanish anatomical schools and particular types of gliomas had been correspondingly described (see ZÜLCH 1962a, Fig. 1 and p. 159).

Bailey's attempts (BAILEY and CUSHING 1926, 1930) to subdivide the various tumors of Cushing's patients and to classify them "histogenetically" after metallic impregnation helped him to bring order into the chaos which existed in classification and nomenclature. Cushing's contribution was to evaluate the average survival time for every group of patients with the same tumor type as classified by Bailey. Although in this biological classification scheme "histogenesis" played an important role, the prognosis actually was derived from the *clinical survival data*. It quickly became obvious that some of the biological and prognostic deductions in the histogenetic classification scheme were no longer tenable.

This can be explained by applying it to the group of tumors classified as polar spongioblastoma. In the maturation scale the spongioblast was still pretty unadvanced and accordingly the prognosis for such tumors was thought to be bad. On the other hand, the polar spongioblastoma of Bailey (which is now classed as pilocytic astrocytoma) was actually one of the most benign gliomas. So CUSHING's (1931) data corrected the merely hypothetical assumptions of prognosis and gave this classification the proper value.

In summary: BAILEY and CUSHING (1926, 1930) provided the first exact and rational cytohistogenetic classification and definition of biological prognosis of intracranial tumors, particularly of the gliomas.

2.2.1 Clinical Malignancy

But there were pitfalls not connected with the conception of histogenesis as a basis of classification but stemming from the old *clinical* experience that in the long run *every intracranial* tumor would be malignant, that is to say it will lead to the patient's death due to increased intracranial pressure and herniation caused by the particular characteristics of the neoplasm within the intracranial and intraspinal cavities.

The final prognosis can therefore only be defined if we add a new dimension, namely the evaluation and consideration of the *clinical* data. We must consider the various factors in intracranial tumor growth that cause the actual problems of "clinical malignancy" (see Table 1).

Table 1. "Clinical" malignancy of intracranial tumors

Histological malignancy *plus* biological behavior, as induced by
1. Volumen auctum (effective volume, e.g., tumor and edema)
2. Mass movements with herniation
3. Action on CSF pathway: hydrocephalus
4. Action on arteries (infarcts)
5. Action on vital centers: hypothalamus, brain stem, etc.

To make it clear one must distinguish:
1. Histological malignancy, based on morphological data
2. Biological malignancy, based on average survival time of the particular tumor group
3. Clinical malignancy, e.g., histological plus biological malignancy plus particular clinical features of the tumor in question.

The *final prognosis* is then based on the following steps:

First step: Histological diagnosis based on the WHO classification

Second step: Ascertaining grade and postoperative statistical survival time for the group

Third step: Application of the concept of clinical malignancy to the particular case

Fourth step: Definition of the final prognosis by summation of all available data

2.2.2 Tumor Groups With Identical Histology and Similar Location, Age and Sex

We found this defining of particular "tumor groups" (classification, age, site, and even sex) convincing and clinically very useful and tried ourselves to describe typical tumor groups which were characterized by age, localization of the tumor and histology.

In 1937 Tönnis and I described the extraventricular ependymomas of childhood and adolescence (GP, Fig. 64) which grew within the frontal, parietal, and temporal lobes. We also described the temporobasal very benign gangliocytomas (GP, Fig. 51) occurring in the same age group (Tönnis and Zülch 1939). In addition I was able to add here the ependymomas of the foramen of Monro in middle age (GP, Fig. 55), described with Schmid (Zülch and Schmid 1955); the typical oligodendrogliomas (Zülch 1941a) of middle age (Figs. 57, 59), located in the second and third frontal convolution; and finally the thalamic oligodendroglioma of adolescence (GP, Fig. 109), and various other types of typical gliomas. In addition, with the help of various students working for their doctorates (Esslen 1950; Krause 1950; Engel 1951), the various tumors in the frontal lobes (Zülch 1951a) were described. Finkemeyer (1961) in Hamburg has continued this line of research – tumors in particular age groups and at particular sites – describing the glioblastomas in various localizations and thus defining their clinical malignancy. Although pathological and neuroradiological data were available, this line of study has apparently not been followed further.

There is no need to discuss the excellent work of Cushing and Eisenhardt (1938) concerned with the various groups of *meningiomas*. The terms, which they used, have a recognized part of daily clinical jargon as, for example, *olfactory meningiomas*, *meningiomas of the sphenoidal ridge*, *meningiomas of the third frontal convolution* (Ectors 1945), and *parasagittal meningiomas* (Olivecrona 1947). In summary, Bailey and Cushing were able to bring order into the various morphological classifications and succeeded in characterizing biologically (clinically) the morphological intracranial tumor groups by adding the average postoperative survival times of the patients.

In other words, the biological evaluation of brain tumor prognosis has to be based on a statistical determination of the postoperative *average survival period of patients within the same tumor group, and not merely on particularities of morphology*.

In *individual* cases, however, even these figures were insufficient and inadequate as long as the *localization* of the tumor was not considered. For example, the prognosis of a small *inoperable* pilocytic astrocytoma in the aqueductal region could not be evaluated in accordance with the average survival time of this tumor type because its "clinical malignancy" is so high. On the other hand, the average survival period of a group as benign as the pilocytic astrocytomas in the cerebellum would be falsely defined when the survival data obtained from pilocytic astrocytomas in other regions such as the chiasm or brainstem were used as a basis.

A final point had to be considered as well. Even histologically identical tumors could have different biological (not clinical) behaviors in different locations. ZÜLCH and KLEINSASSER (1957) have emphasized that there is a decisive difference in the growth of ependymomas of the fourth ventricle, the spinal cord, the foramen of Monro, the cerebellopontine angle and the cauda equina on one hand and those of the extraventricular region of the cerebrum on the other.

2.2.3 Statistical Data on the Postoperative Survival of Patients

The recently reported data of postoperative survival occasionally include also the percentage of patients returning to work. The early data came from Cushing's co-workers, e.g., VAN WAGENEN (1934), who reported on 149 patients among whom the 80 with gliomas had an average 38.8 months of survival and 24.4 months of working capacity. The papers of EISENHARDT (1935), CAIRNS (1936), CAIRNS and ADELAIDE (1936), HENDERSON (1939), and DAVIDOFF (1940) were partly devoted to the survival of patients operated on during one year at Cushing's clinic or they reported the postoperative survival within an entire specific tumor group. Louise EISENHARDT (1935), however, collected from Cushing's series 476 patients who survived 5 years and grouped them according to the various types of tumors; she showed that pilocytic astrocytomas, other forms of astrocytomas and even oligodendrogliomas were those most frequently represented in this group of 5-year survivors (Tables 2 and 3).

The fate of the patients with astrocytomas in Cushing's series was evaluated by ELVIDGE and MARTINEZ-COLL (1956). They reported on 112 astrocytomas observed during an 11-year period, of which 90% could be followed-up. They formed three subgroups, viz.:

1. Diffuse astrocytomas (25.8% of the series); of these patients 42.1% lived longer than 8 years, with an average survival time of 5 years and 4 months.
2. Gemistocytic astrocytomas (21.4% of the series) with an average survival of 1.5 to 7 years.
3. Pilocytic astrocytomas (47.3% of the series), of which 48.7% survived more than 5 years, and even up to 23.5 years with an average of 8.5 years.

Table 2. Average survival period of different histological tumor types. (BAILEY and CUSHING 1926, 1930)

1. Medulloepithelioma	8 months
2. Pineoblastoma	12 months
3. Glioblastoma	12 months
4. Medulloblastoma	17 months
5. Pinealoma	18 months
6. Ependymoblastoma	19 months
7. Neuroblastoma	25 months
8. Astroblastoma	28+ months
9. Ependymoma	32+ months
10. Spongioblastoma	46+ months
11. Oligodendroglioma	66+ months
12. Astrocytoma protoplasmaticum	67+ months
13. Astrocytoma fibrillare	86+ months

Table 3. Postoperative survival of 5 years or more. (EISENHARDT 1935)

Type of tumor	No. of patients	Approx. percent of 476 survivors
Astrocytomas, cerebellar	39	8.0
Astrocytomas, cerebral and pontine	24	5.0
Spongioblastoma polare	11	2.0
Oligodendrogliomas	6	1.2
Ependymomas	7	1.4
Medulloblastomas	6	1.2
Plexus papillomas	4	0.8
Pituitary adenomas	152	30.0
Meningiomas	119	24.0
Acoustic neurinomas	77	15.0
Craniopharyngiomas	24	5.0
Epidermoids and dermoids	7	1.4
Total	476	

GERMAN (1961a) reported survivals of 3–4 years for the astrocytomas, up to 14 years for their pilocytic subgroup in the cerebellum, and 6 months for the glioblastomas. Among the medulloblastomas the survival was only 1 year. BUCY (1942, 1946) has repeatedly emphasized the benignity of pilocytic astrocytomas of the cerebellum, which have a curability rate of at least 50%. An excellent, though only general, review article on postoperative survival was published by NAFFZIGER and BOLDREY (1948). In this further details can be found.

Particularly long survivals have been reported by MCCORMICK et al. (1967): astrocytoma 30 years; DAVIS et al. (1950): 20 years and 3 months; BOUCHARD and PEIRCE (1960): 15–18 years; WEIL and ROSENBLUM (1952): 15 years; GRANT (1956): 20 patients with 15–20 years' survival; ROBERTS and GERMAN (1969): 40-year survival of a patient with a temporal oligodendroglioma 39 years after craniotomy; HARA and TAKEUCHI (1975, 1977): pontine gliomas: after diagnosis of 10, 20, and 22 years.

Similar articles reporting very long survivals in patients with cerebellar pilocytic astrocytoma appear in the literature. For instance, GJERRIS and KLINKEN (1978) noted a 25-year cumulative survival rate of 94% among their patients with this type of astrocytoma, in contrast to 38% of their patients with the diffuse type of astrocytoma.

VAN GEHUCHTEN and BRUCHER (1965; VAN GEHUCHTEN et al. 1967) made a survey of hemispheric tumors (245 personal cases), with survival times of 6 months to 10 years with ependymomas; 6 months to 12 years with oligodendrogliomas; and 6–10 months with glioblastomas. They also reported on the ability of their patients to return to part- or full-time work in a similar way to FINKEMEYER et al. (1965), who examined a personal series of 748 cases for postoperative survival (see *their* Figs. 1–13).

BETTY (1964) reported his 260 cases of which 12.6% returned to work, 53.4% "remained at home", and 18.4% were chronically incapacitated. They recommended extensive lobectomies; radical procedures which were also advised in the review of Hitchcock and Sato (1964). Pia (1977) stated that of the patients operated on by Tönnis, 60%–70% of those with benign gliomas and meningiomas were capable of working.

The fate of the patients with medulloblastomas is very different, although the conclusions are made from series accumulated in recent years. Bloom et al. (1969) reported on 68 unselected cases of medulloblastomas among which 32% had survived for 5 years, and of the remaining cases 26% were still alive after 10 years. These results should be compared with the results in the series reported by Cushing (1930), who had operated on 61 cases of medulloblastoma with a case mortality of 32% and only 1 patient living after 3 years.

The earlier poor results are consistent with the experience of Pool (1968), who stated that patients with glioblastomas had an average survival of only 9 months.

We found also a report on glioblastomas by Di Lorenzo et al. (1977). 50% of their patients died within the first 6 months after surgery, 26% survived for over 1 year, and only 4% survival for more than 4 years. A brief report of Grumme and Bingas (1969) stated that 2 of their cases with cerebral sarcomas were surviving 5.6 and 10 years.

One wonders about the validity of some of the statistical data. Differences in histological classification still seem to play a major role. In the series of glioblastoma patients reported on by Di Lorenzo et al. (1977), eight patients survived for between 4.5 and 10 years. Although they all received radiotherapy one wonders about the actual classification, particularly since there were gross disparities in age from the average age of occurrence of the well-known tumor groups; for instance, there was one patient aged 13 with a glioblastoma multiforme.

According to the "All Japan Brain Tumor Registry" (Takeuchi 1983, p. 42) the following survival data are apparently characteristic for that country:

	1	3	5 years
Gliomas	60%	35%	29%
Glioblastomas	45%	12%	8%
Takeuchi's series	46%	18%	7%

Takeuchi is of the opinion that neither surgery, radiotherapy nor drugs can improve these survival rates at the present time.

Operative Mortality

Operative mortality has definitely decreased for various reasons:

1. Better localization by angiography, later by technetium scan and more recently by computed tomography.
2. Better pre- and postoperative care by the anesthesist.
3. Use of the operating microscope.

Yet, Cushing's figures were astounding; CAIRNS in 1936 found the mortality as low as 11% for the gliomas and 8.5% for the entire series of intracranial tumors in Cushing's series of the year.

After these very satisfactory figures, it is surprising to find two papers reporting operative mortality of 23.5% for temporal lobe tumors (PIA 1953) and 20.7% in 188 cases of WEICKMANN (1969). Similarly, a paper published by BONNAL et al. (1966) gave a mortality of 20.3% in patients under 55 years, and 42.3% of those over 55 years. In contrast GULLOTTA and BETTAG (1967), GULLOTTA and WÜLLENWEBER (1968), GRANT (1956), and JELLINGER and SLOWIK (1975) published data corresponding to the more conventional figures.

Further References: KINO (1935), SCHEINKER (1938a), NETSKY et al. (1950), LØKEN (1952), LEVY and ELVIDGE (1956), PIA (1957), FRANKEL and GERMAN (1958), LAPHAM (1959), PAILLAS and COMBALBERT (1964), ZÜLCH (1966/67), ELVIDGE (1968), WEIR (1973), KLEINMAN et al. (1978), FLOSSDORF et al. (1981), SANO (1983b).

2.2.4 The Problem of Grading

We return to the classification of BAILEY and CUSHING (1926, 1930) and their definition of *postoperative survival time* particularly in the neuroepithelial tumors with their 14 subtypes. This seemed to be too sophisticated to many neurosurgeons particularly with the extremely precise definition of postoperative survival time given in months and years. Up to then general pathologists had used such terms as "benign," "semibenign," "relatively malignant," or "highly malignant" (see RÖSSLE 1950; HAMPERL 1952). Therefore, KERNOHAN et al. (1949) found a rapid and enthusiastic reception when they introduced a simplified biological classification. For the well-known glioma forms they adopted the four-grade system of BRODERS (1920, 1926).

Some scientists, for example, RINGERTZ (1950) and the team of Walter MÜLLER (particularly SCHRÖDER et al. 1970 in Cologne), as also KHOMINSKY (1969 in Russia on the basis of 3720 personal cases) have preferred a *three grade* system.

RINGERTZ (1950) was of the opinion that typical "intermediate grades" existed between benign and malignant; furthermore, that astrocytic, oligodendroglial and ependymal tumors – when becoming anaplastic – would converge into one type, namely the glioblastoma multiforme. Undoubtedly such "secondary glioblastomas" do occasionally occur (see pp. 312, 321), but the common glioblastoma is a "primary" tumor "sui generis". It is the "primary cancer of the brain" and, as I have called it, a "disease rather than a neoplasm" (ZÜLCH 1959, 1969).

Unfortunately R. SCHRÖDER et al. (1968) and W. MÜLLER and R. SCHRÖDER (1968a, b) did not only use a three-grade system of prognosis but also "grade" the common astrocytomas and oligodendrogliomas "grade I". This presents some difficulties if other scientists use the four grade scheme provided by KERNOHAN. Consequently, the equation of R. SCHRÖDER et al. (1970, p. 4) astrocytoma III = glioblastoma = Oligodendroglioma III is not only highly confusing but misleading.

Certainly, the pilocytic astrocytoma (the former polar spongioblastoma) is a more benign glioma than most of the other astrocytomas and should be graded I. Most astrocytomas therefore correspondingly should be graded II, anaplastic astrocytomas should be graded III and glioblastomas are now well-accepted worldwide as grade IV tumors.

For only a short time there has existed a discrepancy with the "grading" by the neuroradiologists based on computed tomography. This has been corrected (WENDE et al. 1980) mainly by an article discussing the real concepts of KERNOHAN and the WHO grading (ZÜLCH 1980).

However, when choosing a system for uniform use by the various schools (see p. 1) around the world, we had to bear in mind that among neurosurgeons and neuropathologists in the English speaking countries the four grade system of KERNOHAN et al. (1949) had already been widely accepted.

We personally had difficulty in applying the methods and recommendations of KERNOHAN and SAYRE (1952) and SAYRE (1964) with respect to grading. The new method of grading malignancy merely on the basis of the histology involved counting the dedifferentiated tumor cells in a given neoplasm. If 25% of all the tumor cells were dedifferentiated then the tumor's grade of malignancy was I, if 50% it was grade II, if 75% it was grade III; and the presence of 100% undifferentiated cells meant grade IV.

We needed to know exactly how to define a "dedifferentiated astrocyte." Was it one in which the nuclear-cytoplasmic relationship was disorderly? Did it have to be richer in cytoplasm, have fewer processes and not form fibrillae? Had it lost its normal form? Was the gemistocytic type already dedifferentiated and were plasmatic astroglia without processes ("protoplasmic" type) more malignant than the fibrillary type? What about the oligodendroglia and their possible polymorphism and dedifferentiation (p. 240ff.)? Were the large, cytoplasmic, eosinophilic oligodendroglial cells, seen in some of these tumors and also in brain edema (ZÜLCH 1943, Fig. 13) dedifferentiated? What was the significance of the number of mitoses in the process of dedifferentiation and anaplasia or of other proliferative phenomena within the stroma (see p. 123ff.)?

In our laboratory we could not answer these questions and thereby could not provide a basis for grading in the manner of Kernohan. Therefore we returned to the old procedure of Bailey and Cushing in (a) *classifying* tumors histologically in groups and for this purpose readily accepted the classification of the World Health Organization (see ZÜLCH 1979); and (b) we then evaluated the *probable degree of malignancy* (Table 4) by employing the average postoperative survival time (see Table 5) as determined by the clinicians.

For our daily routine work – as stated above – we used the WHO classification.

Differences in Terminology

Scientists have criticised our use of the term grading for this process of determining a prognosis. They are correct insofar as we do not grade strictly in the manner of Kernohan by evaluating the percentage of dedifferentiated cells, as described above.

Table 4. Modified grading for the most frequent tumors of the brain and related structures (After ZÜLCH, GP p. 34)

Tumors	Grade I benign	Grade II semibenign	Grade III relatively malignant	Grade IV highly malignant
Astrocytoma		+		
Astrocytoma, anaplastic			+	
Pilocytic astrocytoma	+			
Pilocytic astrocytoma, anaplastic			+	
Oligodendroglioma		+		
Oligodendroglioma, anaplastic			+	
Ependymoma	+	+		
Ependymoma, anaplastic			+	+
Choroid plexus papilloma	+			
Choroid plexus papilloma, anaplastic			+	+
Pinealocytoma	+	+	+	
Pinealoblastoma				+
Germinoma		+	+	
Gangliocytoma	+	+		
Gangliocytoma, anaplastic			+	+
Glioblastoma				+
Medulloblastoma				+
Neurilemmoma	+			
Neurilemmoma, anaplastic			+	
Meningioma	+			
Meningioma, anaplastic			+	+
Hemangioblastoma (Lindau)	+			
Sarcoma				+
Craniopharyngioma	+			
Pituitary adenoma	+			
Pituitary adenoma, anaplastic (Adenocarcinoma)			+	

However, since in the WHO classification grades of malignancy are given for every tumor group but the grades are not more closely defined in terms of survival time; we attempted such a definition early (Tables 4 and 5).

We based our concepts on Bailey and Cushing's experience and the results obtained in the great neurosurgical clinics of the world, particularly those of the Mayo Clinic, Olivecrona's Serafimer Hospital and Tönnis' clinic. Moreover, we considered the data reported in the various publications from the Americas, Europe, and the Far East (see below).

First, I will emphasize here the data I produced in 1951 b (see ZÜLCH 1958, p. 99), since I believe that they are still valid as long as radiotherapy and chemo-

Table 5. Correlation of the various brain tumors with their corresponding malignancy grading[a] (After ZÜLCH, GP p. 35)

Degree of malignancy	Prognosis after "total" removal	Tumors	
		Extracerebral	Intracerebral
Grade I benign *	Cure or at least survival time of 5 and more years	Neurilemmoma Meningioma Craniopharyngioma Pituitary adenoma Others	Astrocytoma, pilocytic Ependymoma of the ventricles Choroid plexus papilloma Gangliocytoma (temporobasal) Hemangioblastoma
Grade II semibenign **	Postoperative survival time: 3–5 years	Neurilemmoma, anaplastic Meningioma, anaplastic	Astrocytoma Oligodendroglioma Ependymoma (cerebral, extraventricular) Choroid plexus papilloma Ganglioglioma
Grade III relatively malignant ***	Postoperative survival time: 2–3 years	Pituitary adenocarcinoma Meningioma, anaplastic "Neurosarcoma"	Astrocytoma, anaplastic Oligodendroglioma, anaplastic Ependymoma, anaplastic Gangliocytoma, anaplastic Germinoma
Grade IV highly malignant ****	Postoperative survival time: 6–15 months	Sarcomas and other highly malignant local extensions	Glioblastoma Medulloblastoma Sarcoma, primary

[a] The data reflect biological behavior without radiation and chemotherapy

therapy are not applied in order to define their efficiency (see pp. 142ff., 150ff.). Furthermore, we have abbreviated the results in Table 5, where we have defined the grades in terms of survival times.

3 The Origin of Brain Tumors

3.1 Current Concepts

In the preceding historical review (p. 2ff.) I have presented the most important classic conceptions concerning the origin of brain tumors. I shall repeat here only the key features of what knowledge of brain tumors can contribute to general oncology. Cohnheim's theory regarding the origin of tumors is still applied to some subgroups of tumors, in particular the *dysontogenetic* tumors. Cohnheim stated "that the real cause of the subsequent development of tumors should be sought in a fault, an anomaly of the embryonic anlage ... and that tumors often develop at sites where certain complications have occurred at some stage of embryonic development ...." Yet this theory has not been proved generally but is only applied to some dysontogenetic types. The demonstration of "split-off embryonic rests" was repeatedly attempted during the "classical period" (STROEBE 1895), but the general thinking has gradually moved away from any further consideration of this theory of Cohnheim, although it was later elaborated by RIBBERT (1910, 1918) and has survived to some extent in FISCHER-WASELS' (1927) "misregeneration theory" (see also BRZUSTOWICZ and KERNOHAN 1952).

On the other hand, the hypothesis, advanced especially by VIRCHOW (1847, 1863/65), that tumor growth is induced by chronic internal and external irritation has been largely confirmed for some particular types of neoplasm and confirmed also in modern experimental neuro-oncology. Apart from the classic "carcinogens," i.e., parasites, poisons, viruses, chemical and physical irritants, especially radiation of various kinds, and other environmental factors may be listed here. Experimental neuro-oncology, in particular, has revealed that in addition to external factors which are involved in tumor origin there are also internal, predisposing factors that are necessary for the induction of a tumor. We have learned about these particularly from experimental neuro-oncology (fundamental differences in the various animal models, differences in transplantability, and other factors, see p. 79). For a long time it seemed as though genetic factors, at least for animal tumors, were playing a decisive role and even now they cannot be entirely excluded. In man, genetic influences have been demonstrated in particular in the familial hamartoblastomatoses (phakomatoses) (p. 63ff.) and in retinal neuroblastomas (see STRONG 1978).

According to some authors' concepts concerning tumor growth, numerous internal and external carcinogenic factors are *simultaneously* involved in the induction of the tumor, e.g., a multifactorial genesis is likely (*syncarcinogenesis*; see p. 49).

Before we begin to discuss modern sophisticated concepts of various kinds about the origin of cancer, we have to list some particulars of brain tumor growth.

Site of predilection. There is no doubt that the majority of intracranial and most spinal tumors have a predilection *site* (see p. 531 ff.). This was worked out in detail by CUSHING and EISENHARDT (1938) for the meningiomas and has been roughly sketched by OSTERTAG (1936b, 1941, 1952) and P. SCHWARTZ (1932, 1936) for gliomas. Their basic statements were detailed and depicted in our first edition (1951) with all the various types of tumors with a preferential site and also particularly by KAUTZKY-ZÜLCH et al. (1982) (see Fig. 14).

This predilection of the various tumor types for a particular localization, so that they appear with "photographic identity," is one of the factors that must be explained in any theory of cancer involving the brain tumors.

Age predilection. It has been well known since BAILEY and CUSHING's publications (1926, 1930, and various other papers) that there is an age range usually with a marked peak, which characterizes the clinical manifestation of each tumor group. During the years from age 15–20 there is a border zone beyond which the tumors of infancy and adolescence no longer occur, whereas the tumors of middle age gradually increase in frequency (pp. 85 ff., 91, 92, Figs. 11, 12). This characteristic phenomenon of brain tumors has also to be considered in a modern cancer theory including tumors of brain and spinal cord.

Sex. There are striking sex predilections in specific malignant tumor groups. For example, the medulloblastomas have a male preponderance of 7:3 and glioblastomas a male preponderance of 6:4 (see p. 93).

On the other hand, there are also sex predilections for the tumors of the pineal gland, the craniopharyngiomas, and for the meningiomas and among the latter, particularly, for some spinal forms; I emphasized that a *male predominance* is found among highly malignant tumors, such as medulloblastoma and glioblastoma, whereas a *female preponderance* is more common among benign tumors, such as neurilemmomas and some meningiomas, particularly those of the spinal cord.

There is one exception from the predilection rule: the sarcomas, which may occur in or near the CNS in either sex, at any age, or in any location. This also has to be considered if a general statement is to be considered about the growth of tumors of the brain and spinal cord. In our earlier editions we favored a concept that was fully explained therein, that there was a local factor within the brain (perhaps of a chemoarchitectural nature?) and a general factor (puberty? sexual involvement?), which would interact to induce tumors with the aforementioned predilections. The only exception was the sarcomas where I held a viral genesis to be must likely.

We do not yet have at our disposal sufficient knowledge of the chemoarchitecture of the brain to explain predilection sites among the various tumor groups (FRIEDE 1966).

Finally, in man there are tumors with a familial predilection, the so-called hamartoblastomatoses (phakomatoses), neoplastic disease entities in which the genetic factor can be followed either in one or through various generations (see Sect. 3.3.2).

Particular Features of Experimental Neuro-oncology

In the last several decades experimental induction of tumors in the nervous system has been realized in many laboratories around the world and we, in collaboration with the group of Druckrey (Druckrey et al. 1972), have become familiar with various models and have worked also to some extent on the biochemical concepts of chemical induction of tumors (Kleihues 1972; Kleihues and Magee 1973; Kleihues et al. 1976).

Taking into consideration the results of this experimental work and the various concepts proposed for the origin of brain tumors, I shall emphasize the most important points to be considered in developing a theory of cancer of the nervous system.

The Possible Causal Factors. We have investigated very thoroughly every possibility of existing causal factors that could elucidate the problem. An extensive collection of the pertinent data is found in *Biology of Brain Tumors* (Workshop Report No. 5, Vol. 30, UICC, Geneva 1978; see Laerum et al. 1978). Mulcahy and Harlan (1976) have also reviewed the data. The latter authors emphasize that each type of brain tumor has a distinct age- and sex-specific pattern of incidence, which suggests specific etiological features.
Factors eliciting tumor growth:
1. Misregeneration
2. Trauma
3. Inheritance (genetically)
4. Hormonal factors
5. Immunological disorders
6. Environmental influences
7. Physical and chemical agents
8. Viral induction or
9. Mutation

1. Misregeneration (see pp. 6, 7). We have stated previously that only a few dysontogenetic tumors like the epidermoids, dermoids, craniopharyngiomas, teratomas, and sympathoblastomas (Beckwith and Perrin 1963) could start from developmental defects. Other examples owe not discussion at any length in Cohnheim's theory of the splitting off of germinal tissue.

2. Trauma. In a separate chapter we will discuss (p. 70ff.) the possibilities in the literature that apparently support the notion of a traumatic origin for brain tumors. Though we accept this possibility for a few cases, trauma certainly does not play any practical role in the majority of brain tumors.

3. Heredity. We will analyze later in more detail the possibility that an inherited factor may induce tumor growth in the nervous system and its coverings as in the case of neurofibromatosis, tuberous sclerosis, hemangiomatosis, and other hamartoblastomatoses. Furthermore a number of familial or inherited brain tumors have been described for which a similar genetic factor must be responsible (pp. 61, 63). Intensive studies have been also conducted in identical twins (see p. 60). However, Kurland concluded that neither familiar occurrence nor the evidence obtained from identical twins provided a decisive clue regarding the origin of brain tumors in man (KURLAND et al. 1962; KURLAND 1972; KURLAND and KURTZKE 1972; KURLAND et al. 1973; see also KURTZKE 1969).

4. Hormonal Factors. There may be some link between the inheritance of tumor growth and hormonal disorder which may also have some relationship to potential disturbances of the immune system. Earlier we have discussed a possible "internal" factor inducing tumor growth and this could be of a hormonal nature. We have emphasized a sex predilection of malignant medulloblastomas, glioblastomas, and many other tumors (see p. 93) and stressed the peak of the age curve, which for medulloblastomas is around puberty and for glioblastomas at the beginning of sexual changes with senescence. We have stressed also the preponderance of neurilemmomas and some types of meningiomas among females. One of the most convincing pieces of evidence of the action of a hormonal factor is the example of stilbestrol. In a large series of pregnant women treatment with stilbestrol induced an unusually high incidence of vaginal cancer in their daughters, which is a very rare form of cancer in female offspring (see p. 57).

5. Immunological Disorders. It has been evident in all investigations concerning metastases and particularly in the discrepancies in tumor growth after transplantation that immunology can play a very important role. Moreover, it has been observed in the recent decades that the recipients of renal transplants with complete immunosuppression occasionally growth of cerebral neoplasms occurs. In most cases these have been lymphomas and sarcomas (SCHNECK and PEN 1970, 1971; HOOVER and FRAUMENI 1973; VARADACHARI et al. 1978). Tumor growth under such circumstances is explained by the "loss of a surveillance mechanism" for foreign cells. However, MULLAN (1975) stated firmly that immunology is not far enough along to permit proper evaluation.

6. Environmental Influences. One of the main fields of investigation in the past several decades has been the possibility of environmental influences. We will discuss some of the data available below (see also BEHREND's chapter on "Epidemiology," 1974).

One of the potential examples was the situation in Guam, where cycasin food is eaten by the natives and forms part of the daily meals. Cycasin has been found to be carcinogenic in rats when incorporated into a basic diet (LAQUEUR et al. 1963; LAQUEUR 1964; SPATZ and LAQUEUR 1967). The experimentally induced tumors were almost identical with those in rats after transplacental application of ethylnitrosourea. However, an elevated incidence of cancer or brain tumors has not been encountered in the human population of Guam.

Another example has been published by WAXWEILER et al. (1976), who among workers exposed to vinylchloride for 20–30 years, found brain and other CNS cancer in three cases, whereas the expected rate was 0.9.

Has there been an increase in the incidence at all of cancer generally, or of particular tumors, or in the nervous system? POCHE and HOFFMANN (1968) counted cancer frequency and age distribution of cancer in various organs at the Pathological Institute in Düsseldorf between 1908 and 1964. There appeared to have been an increase in the incidence of brain tumors from 1% to 2.5% in the male and 0.9% and 2.8% in the female sex.

I have cited these data in order to provide a basis for discussion of the above-posed question. Since they point to a causative action of environmental factors, particularly, external chemical or physical agents. However, I should cite also PERCY et al. (1972) who found after examining comparable data that the overall incidence of CNS tumors in Rochester/Minnesota in the same period had remained stable.

In the first edition of this book it was emphasized that the influence of the "modern industrial age," with its enormous increase in chemical pollution of every kind, has left at least the spectrum of tumors of the CNS unchanged. When we compare the tumors depicted and mentioned in the atlases of CRUVEILHIER (1829/35), Johannes von MÜLLER (1838), VIRCHOW (1847, 1863/65) with our own material we find no significant difference.

There are also reports of an increased frequency of CNS tumors in the region of the rubber industry in Ohio. SWENBERG (1976), in his review article about "chemical induction of brain tumors," also states that epidemiological studies demonstrated an eightfold increase in brain tumor incidence for residents of Summit County, Ohio (MANCUSO 1963). SWENBERG also introduces his paper by stating that "it has been estimated that 80% to 90% of all human cancer is caused by chemicals." In contrast to this, VICK (1975) emphasizes in his paper that "at present with experimental work progressing in many directions, we still lack proof that human brain tumors are caused by any of the known carcinogenic agents."

OESER (1982), a prominent radiologist in the Federal Republic of Germany, has conducted careful statistical investigations of the period from 1873 to 1978 and proved that in West Berlin the cancer mortality in both sexes and in the various age groups had been constant since the beginning of this century. The sole well-known exception is in the older age groups of the male sex where there is a higher lung cancer mortality due to an increase in cigarette smoking (see also KOEPPE and OESER 1982).

However, the most dramatic single observation was that of MAGEE and BARNES (1956), who were informed of the increased incidence of liver cancer in workmen in a chemicals factory in Britain and discovered the action of some chemical products of the nitrosourea group.

This discovery initiated modern experimental neuro-oncology using transplacental and resorptive carcinogens. The original chemical product rarely induced experimental tumors of the CNS. However, after modifications in its structure by DRUCKREY et al. (1967) and particularly after the discovery of its transplacental action (DRUCKREY et al. 1966; IVANKOVIC and DRUCKREY 1968), the number of chemically induced brain tumors was so much increased that this is now the standard model for chemically induced CNS neoplasms. (For more details see Sect. 3.2.)

7. Physical and Chemical Agents. In this field of investigation, the classical examples of *physical* induction of skin cancer by ultraviolet and other rays (sunshine, high altitude, etc.) provided practical examples which created great interest and also induced the obligation to prevent such detrimental effects. In the last 20 years a number of neoplastic processes have been induced artificially by x-rays [usually fibrosarcomas and often meningiomas (see p. 148) and even astrocytomas (COHEN et al. 1981)]. One of the early experiments was that of HAYMAKER et al. (1972), who induced glioblastomas in monkeys by heavy irradiation. Apparently, most of these kinds of induction can now be prevented by modification of the technique of administration.

The *chemical* induction of tumors (see Environmental Effects, p. 44ff.) has been produced by chronic tar irritation experimentally during the early years of the 20th century and continued later by SELIGMAN and SHEAR (1939) and ZIMMERMAN and ARNOLD (1941), using more sophisticated chemical compounds. In spite of progress made following notification of the tragic incident in Britain as mentioned above, a large number of problems is still entirely unsolved and urgently deserves clarification. We will mention only a few of the problems here:

a) Why are there changes in the spectrum of tumor induction depending on the time administration of the carcinogen, i.e., between the 15th and 21st day of gestation and after birth? Why at this latter time is there such a high incidence of neurilemmomas, immediately after birth? Does that reflect the inherent capacity for proliferation?

b) Why do certain subgroups of tumors fail to occur by experimental induction in animals? For instance, medulloblastomas have been seen only after adenovirus 12 application. Gangliocytomas, of which only one or two examples are known, and all the benign tumors such as meningiomas and malignant sarcomas, which arise in man after radiation, do not occur in animals. This is also true of glioblastomas, craniopharyngiomas, pinealomas, choroid plexuspapillomas, and pilocytic astrocytomas. With the latter there is the exception in a particular model of induction by Rous sarcoma in the Schmidt-Ruppin strain of rats.

c) Why are only rodents so specifically susceptible to chemical tumor induction (e.g., rat, mouse, Syrian hamster, and rabbit) whereas all higher mammals up to the present have rarely shown any experimental tumors when this model is employed? As shown by IVANKOVIC and DRUCKREY (1968), the sensitivity of embryos is practically zero *before* the 12th day of pregnancy for nitrosamine carcinogens administered by resorption and in the intraplacental manner. However, from the 15th day of pregnancy onward the young are almost 50 times more sensitive then the normal adult rat and the same holds true for the newborn up to the 19th day after birth.

d) Why is there this difference in the spectrum of tumors after a single dose on the one hand and after chronic or transplacental administration of the carcinogen?

e) Why is there a fundamental difference between experimental tumors and the corresponding tumors in man: e.g., the preponderance in localization, age, and sex? All our endeavors to at least *localize* tumor growth by "co-carcinogenesis" (see MENNEL et al. 1971) failed when we administered a stab wound after initiating the process of resorptive general chemical tumor induction.
f) Why is there such a difference in response between the various strains of rats, e.g., Sprague-Dawley, Fischer rats, BN Druckrey strain?
We could add to this series other questions and problems ad infinitum and have done so in various papers (see ZÜLCH 1969e; MENNEL and ZÜLCH 1972a; ZÜLCH and MENNEL 1974; ZÜLCH and MENNEL 1977; ZÜLCH and MENNEL 1978). Some of the problems have found at least a probable or reasonable explanation in the differences in "susceptibility" of liver and brain. Apparently it is dependent on different "repair" mechanisms in action. It was possible to examine the enzymatic repair of alkylated DNA in brain, while the "capacity" to extract O^6 alkylguanine enzymatically from DNA was found to be higher in liver than in any other rat organ particularly the brain (see KLEIHUES 1978). This may assist in understanding at least part of the molecular mechanism underlying malignant transformation of a particular cell.

There have certainly been great advances in basic neurobiology on both the molecular and the cellular level, yet the familial, genetic predisposition for neural neoplasia, which occurs in man, has not been found in animals. Certainly, it has been proved that the most actively proliferating cells, namely the ependymal and subependymal cells, are the ones that are susceptible to chemical induction of neoplasms. Yet, these cells do not preferentially give rise to *brain tumors* in later life in man (except probably to the pilocytic astrocytomas). The developing nervous system may have a pronounced susceptibility to tumor growth as long as it is still in a proliferative and differentiating state. Why has this matrix have such a different susceptibility to various slightly differently structured chemical agents of the same general nitrosourea group? Neuro-oncology in this area must cultivate close links with general oncology, although the peculiarities of *neural* neoplasia must nonetheless be kept in mind and explained when a *general* model of cancer induction is conceived and formulated.

8. Viral Induction. Virus-like particles in human brain tumors have been found in the cerebellar arachnoidal sarcoma (RAMSEY and KERNOHAN 1964), in neurofibromas, and in neurilemmomas (HOSIBUCHI 1970). Yet, in intensive studies in our own laboratory by HOSSMANN and WECHSLER (1971b), who examined very thoroughly by electron microscopy more than 120 tumors from Dr. Tönnis' neurosurgical department, found virus-like particles only in an intracerebral fibroma (see also BRUCHER et al. 1971). (For further literature see the papers of YOHN 1972; STOCKER 1975; BIGNER and PEGRAM 1976; BIGNER and SWENBERG 1977; BIGNER 1978.)

Up to now, the evidence that brain tumors in man are virus induced, has very little support. On the other hand, the potential for inducing brain tumors by viruses in experimental animals is evident. GROVE et al. (1967) were able to induce brain tumors by Rous sarcoma virus in dogs. We already mentioned adenovirus 12 as a possible agent for inducing medulloblastomas (personal demonstration by OGAWA; see also OGAWA et al. 1969). Moreover, avian adenovirus, papova viruses, polyoma virus, simian virus (SV40), BK viruses, oncorna viruses (pavian, murine and simian sarcoma viruses) and other viruses have been successful in animals. BIGNER (1978, p. 95) has a table listing the predominant brain tumor types induced in vivo by oncogenic viruses.

9. Mutation. The somatic mutation theory of cancer postulates that it is a reversible cellular change that follows either spontaneous or induced mutation and permanently alters the stable nuclear pattern of a somatic cell. This concept was early formulated by K.H. BAUER (1928, 1949). RUBINSTEIN (1976) discussed the various cancer theories based on mutation. However, neither the mechanism of gene interaction nor the change in the genetic code, nor the disturbance of the epigenetic regulatory mechanisms have been clarified as yet (see KLEIHUES 1978). There have been mainly general ideas, which suggest that (a) it is a multistage process, (b) the number of stages may be reduced in inherited cancer, and (c) neoplasia is a stepwise progression. However, these concepts by no means explain the permanent change of code information.

KLEIHUES (1978) has discussed in detail the "somatic mutation theory," the changes in nucleotide sequences resulting from alteration, deletion or arrangement in the primary structure of cellular DNA. He emphasizes that this concept originated with BOVERI (1914) and later K.H. BAUER (1928) (see also KLEIHUES and MARGISON 1974, 1976; BÜCHELER and KLEIHUES 1977; KLEIHUES 1978, p. 113 ff.). Whereas KLEIHUES and his group focused their interest particularly on the chemical carcinogens, RUBINSTEIN (1976) in his discussion pointed to the possibility of mutagenic induction by x-rays, viruses, and immunological factors. Epigenetic regulatory mechanisms would fail and excessive growth could ensue.

Conclusions

It is difficult, after this listing of possible mechanisms and models of origin of brain tumors, to summarize and formulate a concept which is completely acceptable.

It is a general law in neuropathology that even if the results in two cases are identical or even comparable, one must be careful in assuming that this infers that the etiology and formal pathogenesis are also identical. There are scientists who believe that all neoplastic growth is virally induced. There is no proof as yet that this is the case, at least for the tumors of the nervous system. The spectrum of human brain tumors has not changed in the last century even with the advent of the industrial era. There is no significant difference between the spectrum of brain tumors found in highly industrialized countries and that observed in regions not yet much influenced by technological progress. There are, however, apparent differences in the spectrum of brain tumors among different races (see p. 99ff.), but other regional, climatic, or nutritional factors are not yet evident. With a few rare exceptions (see p. 97ff.), apparently spontaneous brain tumors in the human have the same distribution throughout the world. On the other hand, animal experiments have proven that tumors of the nervous system can be due to exogenous factors. Our concepts about the origin of human brain tumors are purely speculative, and therefore, we have to take all possible preventive measures to protect man from exogenous carcinogens as long as the pathogenesis of spontaneous tumors remains an unsolved problem. One of the pitfalls is that premalignant hyperplasia, so often observed in other body organs, is rarely encountered in the brain, where hundreds of thousands of slices and blocks have been investigated carefully for other reasons in the neuropathological laboratories of the world.

Even the possibility is not yet proven that, if rather than a single factor is not clearly responsible, co-carcinogenesis or multiple factors may be involved and must be investigated (see our own attempt: MENNEL et al. 1971). There is no doubt that experience in neuro-oncology has made remarkable progress in the last three decades, particularly since refinements in experimental design and resources provide the possibility of following various stages of differentiation of tumor growth. The initial importance for therapy is obvious already in the application of radio-, chemo-, and immunotherapy.

Further References: ALBRECHT (1907a, b), HIGGINSON (1968), BELLER et al. (1972).

3.2 Experimental Brain Tumors (Carcinogenic Substances – Viral Induction – Others)

Experiments With Carcinogenic Substances (Chemical)

It has been noted in Sect. 3.1 that both the etiology and pathogenesis of brain tumors have not yet been clarified. Therefore, the experimental production of neoplasms by using carcinogenic substances could provide tools for the elucidation of such open questions. Two major objectives for experimental neuro-oncology can be proposed: (a) development of experimental models with a reproducible high rate of tumor incidence and (b) examination of the etiology and pathogenesis of these models with the objective of developing new therapeutic regimens.

A number of authors have succeeded in producing a variety of tumors in mice (in which species spontaneous gliomas are almost unknown) and other animals, predominantly rodents (see ZIMMERMAN 1961, 1969; DRUCKREY et al. 1972; JÄNISCH and SCHREIBER 1969, 1974; IVANKOVIC and PREUSSMANN 1970; KLEIHUES et al. 1970, 1976; KLEIHUES 1972; MENNEL and ZÜLCH 1972; RABOTTI 1972; IKUTA and KUMANISHI 1973; BIGNER and PEGRAM 1976; BIGNER and SWENBERG 1977; MENNEL 1977).

A variety of tumors have been induced in the mouse and other animals by the local implantation of pellets containing the classic hydrocarbons, e.g., benzpyrene and methylcholanthrene (SELIGMAN and SHEAR 1939: methylcholanthrene; and PEERS 1940). ZIMMERMAN and ARNOLD (1941) instituted this work and were helpful in the histological classification of brain tumors, which developed after 227–511 days. Moreover, FREEMAN and ZIMMERMAN (1944), ZIM-

MERMAN (1962), and NETSKY (1964) continued to pursue this kind of experimental research. According to ALEXANDER (1939) predominantly gliomas such as glioblastoma, oligodendroglioma, ependymoma, pinealoma, and pilocytic astrocytoma developed, but fibrosarcomas also were found. PEERS (1940) too was able to produce 32 tumors in 87 mice (specifically 15 gliomas and 17 mesodermal tumors). Some of these could be transplanted and were still growing after 5 to 11 passages. ZIMMERMAN (1943, 1955) has reported similar results in tumor transplantation (ependymoblastoma).

There existed an interesting relationship between the type of tumor which arose and the site at which the carcinogenic agent had been applied. When the agent was put on the ventricular wall, ependymomas developed whereas, when applied to the white matter, glioblastomas or more rarely astrocytomas arose. Oligodendrogliomas usually grew in the occipital lobe, pilocytic astrocytomas in the corpus callosum and medulloblastomas in the cerebellum. In this respect, the distribution of experimental tumors resembled that of spontaneous tumors in man (ZIMMERMAN and ARNOLD 1941, 1943; ARNOLD and ZIMMERMAN 1943). This method of production was followed up by Bruno SCHIEFER (1962) in our institute who came to the same successful result apart from one additional feature: he was able to induce an oligodendroglioma-like tumor with some intermixed features of a monstrocellular sarcoma, e.g., monster cells developing from the capillaries of the otherwise mainly glial tumor. This then was a "composition tumor" (see p. 77).

Unfortunately, for more sophisticated research on the origin of brain tumors this model of local "traumatic" implantation was not suitable. One could not define the beginning of autonomous growth of a blastoma and then follow it and could not exclude, morphologically, the local action of trauma and scar formation. Little new information relating to actual pathogenesis had been gained.

The real progress came from the investigations conducted by MAGEE and BARNES (1956) (see p. 45). Thereafter, a wide range of different *N*-nitroso-compounds with a carcinogenic effect were developed by Druckrey (DRUCKREY et al. 1965, 1972). Also different species of animals were found to be susceptible (DRUCKREY 1975). The carcinogens acted after "resorption", e.g., after "systemic" application in vivo (feeding, breathing, i.v. injection, etc.). Apparently the carcinogens were rapidly decomposed – mainly in the liver – where they were locally enzymatically activated (BRODIE et al. 1958), until they formed the "ultimate carcinogen." The process of carcinogenic transformation of the cell was apparently induced by the decomposition of the neuro-oncogenic agent with liberation of alkylating intermediates.

The first results, however, were still somewhat disappointing, since depending on the chemical structure, tumors arose mainly, even almost exclusively, in extraneural body organs such as esophagus, kidney, bladder, lung, or the nasal cavity, depending upon the specific carcinogen. This "organ specifity" depended upon the distribution and metabolism of the compound. CNS tumors, however, had so far been few with this model.

The first positive results of "multiple" (chronic) administration after resorption of the carcinogen in adult BD rats were achieved with *N*-nitrosopiperidine and *N*-piperazine applied in the olfactory region after s.c. injections (medulloepitheliomas, carcinomas, MENNEL 1966). True brain tumors were found, when alkylated nitrosamides were used. The results depended somewhat on the kind of carcinogen used, ethylnitrosourea (ENU) and methylnitrosourea (MNU) being the ones used most frequently. When chronic i.v. administration of MNU was carried out by the Freiburg group (DRUCKREY et al. 1966, 1967) tumors of the brain, spinal cord, cranial and peripheral nerves were achieved also in adult rats. Similarly chronic tumors were produced by oral doses of MNU by JÄNISCH and SCHREIBER (1967) in rabbits, and STROOBANDT and BRUCHER (1968) in rats. The latter investigations gave very high doses four or five times a week and thus produced not only oligodendrogliomas, but surprisingly medulloblastomas and a gangliocytoma also. These tumors otherwise are only exceptionally seen in experimental model systems.

KLEIHUES et al. (1970), in our institute, also succeeded in experimental induction of malignant tumors of a particular kind, namely, pleomorphic oligodendrogliomas or mixed gliomas with varying degrees of cellular dedifferentiation, and occasionally ependymomas as well. These tumors appeared when he injected i.v. MNU to rabbits in chronic experiments which led to tumor growth after 252 to 293 days. Meanwhile the single injection method (for example of MNU) in adult rats also had given good results and was therefore preferred. In addition to using MNU, di-MNU, tri-MNU, and ENU as carcinogens, different species of animals were used, namely, rats, Syrian hamsters (MENNEL and ZÜLCH 1972), rabbits etc. Dogs and monkeys failed for a long time to give a positive result.

It seemed possible at least in principle to induce tumors of the nervous system in different species of animals by systemic administration of chemical carcinogens of the nitrosourea type. However, the percentage of CNS tumors produced was limited.

Further progress came from a particularly interesting observation made by chance, viz. that when a carcinogenic substance was administered to a pregnant mother rat, it also induced tumors in young. Nearly all the animals in the litter died of brain tumors or tumors of the peripheral nervous system over the course of a year or more (IVANKOVIC et al. 1966). Moreover, the "transplacental transmission" showed that the immature nervous system was approximately 50 times more sensitive to the action of carcinogenic substances than mature tissue. Furthermore, the transplacental induction of tumors in growing embryos was only possible at a certain stage of gestation, i.e., after the 12th day with a maximum around the 22nd day. After birth the sensitivity to carcinogens decreased appreciably, though it was still possible to induce neurogenic tumors regularly by single injection (IVANKOVIC and DRUCKREY 1968). Great progress was noted in the high frequency of CNS tumors presumed to be due to the "organ specifity" of this transplacental model. In fact, 92% of the offspring showed nervous system tumors while only 2% of the tumors occurred in other organs. They were also very commonly multiple.

The sensitivity of embryonic tissue is substantiated by comparison of the single doses needed for tumor production; in adult rats 140 to 200 mg/kg body weight is required while for the fetuses as little as 5–80 mg/kg body weight of the mother rat is enough.

In summary, this new *transplacental* model showed several advantages:

1. It showed a very high organ specifity of the carcinogenesis, namely for CNS tumors.
2. Commonly these tumors were multiple and of different ages, allowing closer studies of tumor growth.
3. Any tendency towards correlation between age or sex and specific tumor growth could be defined.
4. The number of perineural tumors was very high and the variation in their location very great. The neurilemmomas induced by this method turned out later to be excellent tools for tissue culture and transplantation.

Nature of the Experimental Tumors Induced

Multiplicity

In contrast to man, experimental animals frequently displayed multiple tumors; this was particularly a prominent feature of the transplacental model. The multiplicity depended somewhat upon the doses given.

The occurrence of several tumors per animal – the multiplicity – had already been observed in the postnatal experiments of DRUCKREY et al. (1970). The values ranged from 2.4 to 4.7 and depended on the model and the kind of search, which was made (naked eye, microscopy). In man, however, multiplicity is seen only in the hamartoblastomatoses such as von Recklinghausen's disease (see p. 63) except for rare multiple tumors like meningiomas or other rare combinations (p. 112).

Isomorphism and Pleomorphism

When the various kinds of tumor induced were tabulated, it was observed that "pure growths" were found mostly in the early stages. As the tumor grew a mixing of the tumor elements, in particular parenchyma and stroma, was found. Nonetheless, the architecture and pattern usually remained comparable to those in the corresponding species in human pathology.

Signs of dedifferentiation or pleomorphism were frequently found in the larger growths. Sometimes real foci of anaplasia were encountered such as small medulloblastoma-like islands in the middle of the tissue of an ependymoma or other gliomas. Moreover, a higher vascularization, stromal proliferation and formation of necroses were observed. These growths were classified as anaplastic (or pleomorphic) examples of that particular tumor entity.

In the larger neoplasms, particularly, a mixture of oligodendrocytes and astrocytes was found, so that after a short time these neoplasms were genuine "mixed" oligoastrocytomas. Mixed ependymomatous and gliomatous architectures also occurred.

Location

We have reported a rough analysis of the location of 1731 neoplasms (ZÜLCH 1969a, b; ZÜLCH and MENNEL 1970, 1971a). Without going into detail we

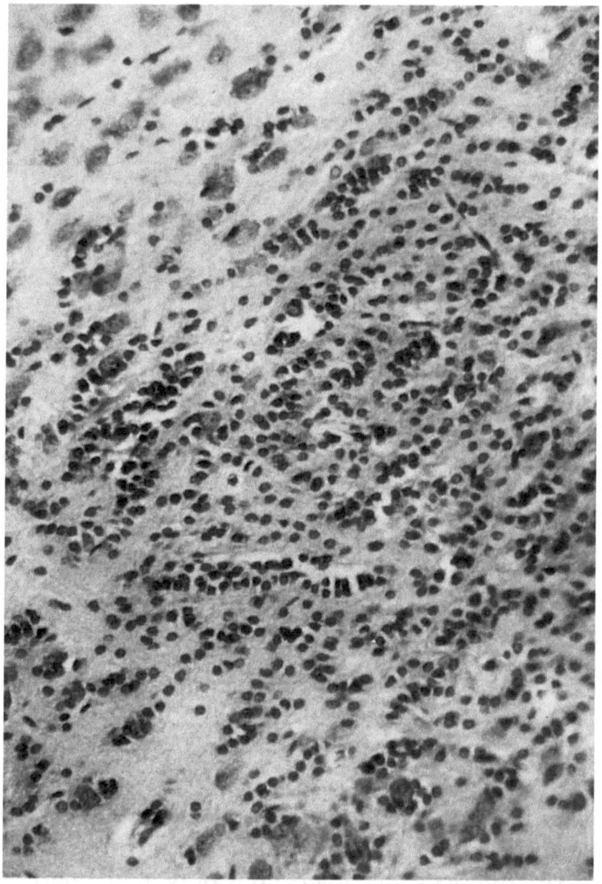

Fig. 3. First stage of neoplastic transformation of oligodendroglia cells near hippocampus

can state that 42.2% of the tumors were located in the brain, 13.2% in the spinal cord, and 35.2% in the peripheral nervous system. Less frequent locations were 2.7% pituitary gland, 1.8% meninges, 2.8% olfactory bulb, and 2.3% in other locations. Within the cerebral hemispheres, tumors demonstrated a preferential occurrence for the periventricular white matter. This is understandable, since the subependymal zones maintain a prolonged and persisting proliferation of glial cells and therefore, probably a susceptibility for the carcinogen. Fifty percent of the brain tumors grew in the white matter, less than one in five (16% overall) were localized to the subependymal glial layer, tumors of the brainstem accounted for 6.5% and were situated near the third or fourth ventricle. No tumors occurred in the hemispheres of the cerebellum. Among all experimental tumors of the brain 20% grew within the ventricular system (ependymomas). These, however, could infiltrate the white matter through the ventricular wall. In contrast only about 10% of tumors occurred solely in the cerebral cortex, and more than half (6.5%) of these were in the hippocampal cortex (Fig. 3). In the spinal cord preferential sites were found, first near the

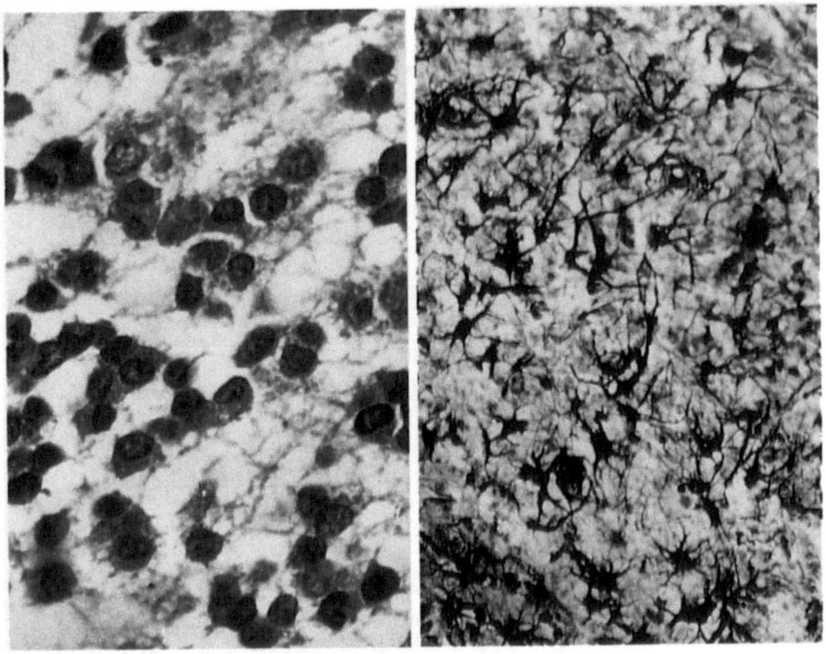

Fig. 4a, b. Microscopical pictures of small astrocytoma. **a** H & E, ×420; **b** gold sublimate, ×125

central canal (predominantly ependymomas) and second in the region of the dorsal septum. Some growths extended over the whole spinal cord as "pencil-like" tumors while others grew only in one part of the spinal cord. Neurilemmomas occurred on the cranial nerves in 38%, with a surprising preference for the trigeminal nerve (other nerves only 4%). The large nerve plexuses [cervicobrachial (12%) and lumbar (18%)] were the next most frequent sites of tumor growth.

Classification

From the Druckrey collection and from the experiments of our own institution, we had classified approximately 3000 of these experimental tumors (see ZÜLCH and MENNEL in *Biology of Brain Tumors:* LAERUM et al. 1978, p. 7) in accordance with the new classification of the World Health Organization. There were typical *astrocytomas* (Fig. 4), sometimes undistinguishable from their human counterparts, but they were not common. They tended to occur in the white matter and the cellular elements were much larger than in oligodendrogliomas. There were tumors with a mixed population of cells comparable to mixed oligoastrocytomas in man, as previously mentioned.

The *oligodendrogliomas* were sometimes typical, particularly when they were microtumors, in which case they were frequently in the hippocampus. The elements of the oligodendrogliomas produced by MNU in rabbits (chronic experi-

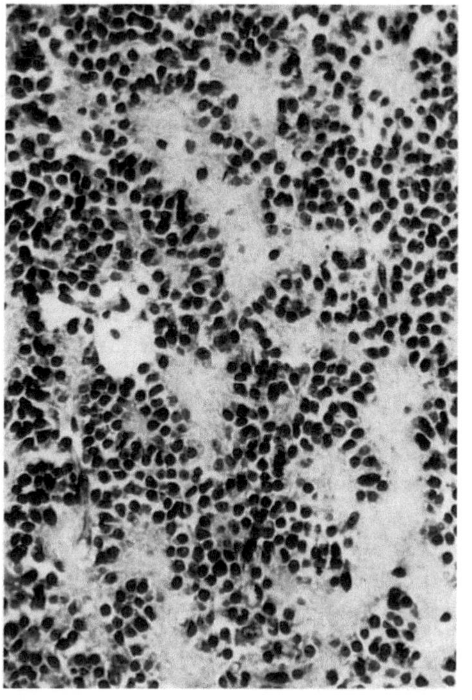

Fig. 5. Perivascular cuffs in an ependymoma of the rat

ment, KLEIHUES et al. 1970) were identified as oligodendroglia, using the impregnation method (Grinyo). Typical anaplastic, polymorphous oligodendrogliomas with the characteristic Langhans type of multinuclear cell were also induced.

Tumors classed as *ependymomas* (Fig. 5) had the same typical architecture and arrangement as in the human counterpart when located in the spinal cord. In the ventricles the ependymomas were of a more malignant variant than the spinal forms which were well differentiated. The distribution is shown in Fig. 1 of MENNEL and ZÜLCH (1971a). In a classification of 1442 experimental tumors produced by ENU only 22 cases were nonneural, so that neurotropism was paramount in this model. It was of considerable interest that the relative frequency of neurilemmomas (mostly anaplastic) in *transplacental* carcinogenesis depended significantly on the day of injection of the pregnant mother, the frequency of occurrence being 23.2% on the 15th day, 57.5% on the 20th day, and 87.5% on the 22nd day, and finally 57.6% on the 23rd day. *Single-dose* experiments produced only 68% of neurilemmomas when injected at birth, around 50% at 10 days after birth, and 35.2% at 30 days after birth.

Some classes of tumors were *never encountered*, in particular, most of the very *benign* tumors on one hand and of the more *malignant* ones at the other. There were no medulloblastomas, only two gangliocytomas (both in the autonomic nervous system) and no benign meningiomas, craniopharyngiomas, or pinealomas, for example. All experimental tumors had to be classified as semibenign or relatively malignant, e.g., grade II or III.

Predilection of Age and Sex

In man tumors have particular tends of preference for an age group such as childhood or adolescence, middle age, elderly, or senescence (see p. 85ff.). It is interesting to see that such trends are not visible in experimental tumors. Even such tumors as grow in a particular age group in man, such as the malignant medulloblastomas and the benign pilocytic astrocytomas, are almost completely absent. Furthermore, glioblastomas, the typical "cancer" of the nervous system in the older human patient, were also never induced.

With regard to a sex preference, we tried to determine whether there was any predilection among the different tumor entities. We classified the tumors in various litters and did not find any correlations (ZÜLCH and MENNEL 1973).

The Time of Transplacental Induction

There is a clear defined period for the action of carcinogens in experimental animals when one uses the transplacental model, namely, after the 12th day and up to the 22nd day of gestation. The susceptibility of the embryo to the carcinogen increases considerably toward the end of pregnancy. After birth a much higher dose of the same carcinogen will never produce tumors in a similar high percentage.

Type of Action of the Carcinogen

WECHSLER et al. (1969) have shown that the action of a carcinogen develops in three different stages, the first, when it is toxic and kills the animal, the second, in which toxic and carcinogenic effects are seen together equally, and the third after the 12th day of gestation, when the carcinogenic action prevails.

In the second stage there may be a trend toward malformations. We saw three cases of obstructive hydrocephalus after some proliferation of tissue near the aqueduct. WECHSLER et al. (1969) observed a series with microcephaly.

Latency

In the chronic experiment there is also a time-dose relationship. There is usually a latency of 300–500 days for tumor formation. By rule of the thumb, the time lag appears to be fairly dependent on the quantity of carcinogen although not in a linear relation. The problem of the latency has not yet been clarified but remains obscure and cannot be compared with any known human tumor biology phenomena.

Transplantation

The large number of neurilemmomas resulting from the transplacental experiment turned out to be an excellent tool for transplantation and tissue culture. The neurilemmomas had two different types, one type consisting almost totally of cellular and fibrous elements, the other developing into large cysts at an early stage. Both types of neurilemmoma, and the well-differentiated gliomas, such as oligodendrogliomas as well, could be preserved in tissue culture for a long time. In the first three passages the induction time of tumors was about

60 days. After that the induction times varied widely in the next ten passages, which finally became stabilized at about 20–30 days.

During this time a progressive morphological *anaplasia* took place. The tumors of the peripheral nervous system became less cystic and began to resemble sarcomas in morphology. Among the entities of the central nervous system, highly differentiated formations such as honeycomb architecture, piling of cells in columns, and perivascular cuffing, were replaced by a uniformly poor differentiation of structures. Such tumors which preserve their highly differentiated architecture over 20 passages, also still maintained considerably longer induction times of 40–50 days (MENNEL et al. 1975).

Further investigations with these transplanted tumors in rats show that the length of induction times was not only dependent on the morphology of the tumor, but also, curiously enough, on the age of the animal and the size of the inoculated tissue. The tumors grew more rapidly in younger animals than in adults. The number of cells inoculated influenced the latent period before the appearance of the tumor but did not accelerate the subsequent growth of the tumor itself, measured after that date. Such measurements and calculations of the inoculated tumors were possible only with s.c.-grafted peripheral nerve tumors.

Does Transplacental Carcinogenesis Also Occur in the Human?

We have mentioned the observation in man that after therapeutic administration of stilbestrol, a synthetic estrogen, to pregnant women vaginal carcinomas were later found in a series of female children (HERBST et al. 1971). We tested this problem experimentally and administered stilbestrol to pregnant rats, without any such effect, apart from benign proliferations of the mammary gland. The administration of a female sex hormone, in *addition* to systemically acting carcinogens, somehow blocks brain tumor production in the animal, and the incidence in these cases is somewhat lower than in control experiments (KALVELAGE 1976).

Tissue Culture

Further studies were conducted with experimental tumors to investigate the mode of growth. For instance, tumors of the brain, spinal cord, and peripheral nervous system were successfully transplanted over several passages (MENNEL and BÜCHELER 1974a, b), following which a sort of sarcomatous growth has been observed after transformation, particularly in anaplastic gliomas and neurilemmomas.

In the large series of transplantations (430 cases) with primary tumors, performed by H.D. MENNEL (1980) in BD-IX rats in our laboratories, certain stereotyped results were achieved: (a) apolar, round cells were rare and occurred in tumors of the nasal cavity; (b) bipolar types were observed in two forms, bipolar fibroblasts and slender bipolar cells such as are seen in malignant neurilemmomas; (c) semipolar cells as determined as fibroblasts in locomotion; and (d) multipolar cells were observed in transplanted gliomas exclusively. Long processes were seen in the early passages only; in later generations, short branching processes prevailed.

Carcinogenesis

The process of carcinogenesis has not yet been clarified. KLEIHUES (1972) performed a series of experiments with interesting results indicating to the mechanism.

We have cited above (p. 47) the fact that there are apparently different repair capacities in the various organs which have a different potential for excision of alkylating (carcinogenic) substances (for example O^6-alkylguanine) from DNA. This repair capacity seems to be different for the brain and for the liver for example, thus explaining the different "organ specifity" of the particular carcinogen. How far this concept of the "excision repair of alkylated bases" can be extrapolated into the mechanism of cancerization of the cell in man still remains open.

At the end of this discussion of work on experimental brain tumors in animals, we now cite the summary of our UICC workshop on *Biology of Brain Tumors* (LAERUM et al. 1978):

The induction of tumors in the animal's brain is possible despite the protection of the cranium. That this does not prove that "systemic" administration of chemical substances also induces nervous system tumors in man. However, because of the severity of the problem a common mechanism has to be considered, and has to be intensively investigated. Useful tools in neurobiology and neurooncology have been developed by the induction of experimental tumors particularly in the transplacental way and the models of transplantations are now stable after some passages and deliver the tools for therapeutic attempts as also do the tissue cultures after clinical isolation.

Further References: POMERAT and GOLDBLATT (1961), ZIMMERMAN (1969), KIRSCH et al. (1972), WECHSLER (1972a, b), KLEIHUES and MAGEE (1973), TOMATIS and MOHR (1973), WECHSLER et al. (1973), BARBOSA-COUTINHO et al. (1974), JÄNISCH and SCHREIBER (1974), MENNEL et al. (1974), WECHSLER and ZÜLCH (1974), MAGEE et al. (1975), KLEIHUES and COOPER (1976), KLEIHUES and MARGISON (1976), MENNEL and ZÜLCH (1976), KLEIHUES and BÜCHELER (1977), MENNEL and GRONECK (1977), MENNEL (1978), JELLINGER et al. (1981).

Virus-Induced Tumors

Since the first observations of virus-induced lymphomas by BURKITT and WRIGHT (1970), the research for a virus active in the production of tumors of the CNS has been intensified and is the subject of specific studies. All sorts of viruses have been tested, including the human adenovirus 12, the simian adenovirus and simian virus 20, the avian adenovirus, the bovine papilloma virus, the polyoma virus, the human papova virus (for details see LAERUM et al. 1978, p. 85).

I have only had experiences of tumors induced by Ogawa in mice using adenovirus 12. These were medulloblastoma-like tumors, with a very typical character in some parts, but having the tendency to a surprising degree of anaplasia with formation of giant cells consisting more or less only of nuclear material, culminating in accumulations of pure nuclear substance with no cytoplasm. The same virus induced neurofibromas in the peripheral nerve (OGAWA et al. 1969).

The interesting tumors induced by VANDEPUTTE and BRUCHER (1962) with polyoma virus formed a sort of meningeal sarcomatosis (as I can confirm from a personal study of the slides). Medulloblastoma-like tumors were induced by the JC virus in Syrian hamsters of ZU RHEIN and VARAKIS (1975). In other models all sorts of tumors have been induced (see loc. cit., Table 1, p. 95), such as anaplastic astrocytomas or even glioblastoma multiforme, medulloblastomas, neuroblastomas/retinoblastomas, ependymomas, choroid plexuspapillomas, pineocytomas, sarcomas, and other meningeal highly undifferentiated tumors. According to certain authorities the ASV-induced anaplastic astrocytoma in the rat is the most profitably and widely employed virus-induced brain tumor for all types of experimental work. These tumors can be transferred into cell cultures in vitro and through many passages the histologic appearance will remain the same.

The intensive search for viruses in human brain tumors has been entirely negative. Virus-like particles have been detected naturally in large number.

Our own electron microscope studies (WECHSLER and HOSSMANN, personal communication) in more than 120 brain tumors of Tönnis' patients did not reveal under the electron microscope either virus or virus-like particles or other similar particles, which have been searched for since the first description of intranuclear inclusions in glioblastoma multiforme by Dorothy RUSSELL (1932).

IBELGAUFTS (1982) condensed his concepts based on investigations performed partly in our laboratories (IBELGAUFTS et al. 1980) and partly in Edinburgh (IBELGAUFTS et al. 1982) to the following statements: "Although final proof of a causal relationship between DNA viruses and the pathogenesis of certain types of human neurogenic tumors is still lacking, there are numerous reasons for assuming this (see IBELGAUFTS 1982). Moreover, the viruses in question are ubiquitous in the human population, lead to persistent infection, can cross anatomical barriers (BBB, placenta) and are either sporadically or frequently involved in human CNS infections". IBELGAUFTS then discussed the possible proof by using antigens, antibodies, etc. and pointed to the results of isolation and visualization of tumor viruses from human brain neoplasms.

It is certainly important to be informed about these concepts, although I personally am still reluctant to accept them.

We can probably summarize the present state of knowledge by the statement made by BIGNER at the UICC workshop in 1978 that "despite a massive effort in viral oncology over the last 30 years, there has been no etiological association of any human viruses with any human tumors." We stated further that "none of the above studies have presented any conclusive evidence for tumor virus particles, genomes or antigens in human brain tumors."

Traumatic Brain Tumors (Experimental)

We have also tried to attack the problem of traumatic brain tumors (see also Sect. 3.4). We "directed" the carcinogen to a point of increased cell proliferation caused by an acute stab wound on the brain of a rat, which was thought to be suitable for this purpose. We combined trauma of the brain with the effect of ENU in the same organ in two models (MENNEL et al. 1971): (a) by giving an ENU transplacentally and shortly after birth making a stab wound in the right hemisphere; (b) by causing trauma in rats immediately after birth and then administering ENU some days later. Both models had negative results, with no tumors growing locally.

3.3 Hereditary Factors

3.3.1 Tumors in Twins

Twin studies have been widely used in the investigations of the pathogenesis of brain tumors. Statistics in the older literature on brain tumors are unfortunately often of only limited value, because the pathologic and genetic diagnoses are sometimes obsolete. However, already the report of LEAVITT (1928) of one pair of twins is one of the best known. This report also mentioned another set of twin girls, originally reported by JOUGHIN (1928), each of whom developed a glioma of the base of the brain. THUMS (1939) reported to the World Congress of Neurology in Copenhagen 45 verified cases of intracranial tumors in twins, among one pair of identical twins, both of whom were operated on for brain tumor at about the same time, and an instance of triplets of the same sex, two of whom developed pituitary tumors.

Among the early accurate observations one must mention the report of GEYER and PEDERSEN (1939), who reviewed six pairs of identical twins with concordant disease. They added a new pair of nonidentical twins, a brother and sister, who at almost the same age (43 and 44 years) developed cerebral gliomas, probably glioblastomas. In addition, the authors collected three identical but discordant pairs from the Berlin clinic of Tönnis. One member of the first pair of twins developed a sphenoid wing meningioma at the age of 40; one of the second pair had a ganglion cell tumor at the age of 12 (erroneously classified by us at first as an astrocytoma); and one of the third pair developed a pituitary tumor (diagnosed only by x-ray) at the age of 24, while their twins apparently had no tumor at that time. However, the brother of the patient with the sphenoid wing meningioma subsequently became concordant and died of a glioblastoma in 1951 (see HOPPE 1952).

Furthermore GEYER and PEDERSEN (1939) reported the first case of identical twins with von Recklinghausen's disease (28 years old at that time, but affected since puberty). They also referred to discordant occurrence of brain tumors in identical twins (PETERSEN and GEYER 1938).

Our colleague LÜDERS/Berlin (see GRIEPENTROG and PAULY 1957) was kind enough to send us the histologic sections from a pair of identical female twins both of whom had died of medulloblastoma in the midline of the cerebellum at slightly less than three months of age. One of the partners also had a pigeon egg-sized metastasis in a supraclavicular lymph node with spread to the pulmonary apex, as well as other small lymph node metastases. The other partner had remained free of metastases.

There is a review of 54 publications by SCHOENBERG et al. (1975) including 8 cases of glioma in twins. CLARENBACH et al. (1979) reported on subependymomas and FAIRBURN and ULRICH (1971) on malignant gliomas. However, only G. KOCH (1954) followed this problem extensively from the beginning and summarized in a table all cases known until 1951. He was able to find in the literature 12 pairs of twins affected with brain tumors, among them 9 identical pairs of which the concordant occurrence of brain tumors was observed in 5. He reported his results at the Cologne Symposium on Brain Tumors (KOCH 1957, 1964, 1981), and later on in several papers (for instance, 1972a). Furthermore he followed the so-called series of twins of Berlin (450 monozygotic and bizygotic twin pairs) and reported in 1957 and again in 1981 on the end results (at that time there were 3 brain tumors in *monozygotic* twins).

In summary, concordant and disconcordant identical twins and even concordant nonidentical twins with intracranial tumors have been reported in the literature.

3.3.2 Familial and Hereditary Brain Tumors

The well-known "hereditary" brain tumor reports from BENDER and PANSE (1932), and from HALLERVORDEN (1936, on the G siblings) are the best introductions into the subject.

Of the three brothers, Hermann G appears to have suffered from pilocytic astrocytoma or a tumor very similar to diffuse astrocytosis. Reinhold G obviously had a diffuse oligodendroglioma. The other brother had some sort of changes related to tuberous sclerosis. A similar case had already been reported by BÖHMIG (1918).

Already in the former edition of this book, I mentioned the B brothers in our own series, both of whom died of glioblastomas in the parieto-occipital region, Willi B at the age of 54 and Georg B at the age of 61.

The family reported by GARDNER and FRAZIER (1930; see also GARDNER and TURNER 1940) is also considered a particularly impressive example of familial brain tumor disease. This was a study of five generations with 217 members, in whom bilateral deafness was inherited as a Mendelian dominant. In the entire family 38 individuals were affected; of these 15 became blind and 4, on close investigation, proved to have optic atrophy secondary to papilledema. Two members were autopsied and both had bilateral acoustic neurilemmomas. The authors were able to study 7 of the deaf members, among whom 5 were unresponsive to the Barany test. It is interesting that the average age of death of the members affected in each succeeding generation declined rapidly. The second generation died at an average age of 72 years, the third at 63 years, the fourth at 42 years, and the fifth at 28 years. Surprisingly, there were never any signs of von Recklinghausen's disease.

G. KOCH (1954, pp. 176 ff.) has tabulated familial brain tumors observed up to that date. He was able to find six instances of familial brain tumor.

Among the numerous reports on familial brain tumors that reported by DELLEMAN et al. (1978) must be mentioned, in which family meningiomas were found in 5 members over two generations. NOETZEL (1959), KJELLIN et al. (1960), GAINER et al. (1975) also reported on familial neoplastic disease in the CNS. Frontal oligodendrogliomas in two siblings were seen by PARKINSON and HALL (1962), astrocytomas in three sisters by PELGROM von MOTZ et al. (1977), medulloblastomas in two brothers by YAMASHITA et al. (1975), in cavernous angiomas by CLARK (1970); familial gliomas were recorded by ARMSTRONG and HANSON (1969), GROSZ and PLASCHKES (1960), and BICKERSTAFF et al. (1967); tumors of the pineal region in brothers by KIDO et al. (1984).

Among the cases collected between 1950 and 1960 there were 26 families reported and the tumors most frequently encountered were astrocytomas.

AITA (1968a, b) proposed that of all the "hereditary" cases 50% were in siblings, leaving 17% in mother and child, 4% in father and child; in 20% more than two immediate family members had brain tumors.

It can be seen then, that the least frequent combination was father and child. SCHARRER and BRUNNGRABER (1973) published a very interesting report from our own institute of gliomas in a father and son.

Familial frontonasal (epidermoid) cysts have been described by PLEWES and JACOBSON (1971). HAUGE and HARVALD (1957) screened the families of 179 patients with glioblastoma and found 5 cases of intracranial tumors among 1813 siblings.

VAN DER WIEL (1960), in an interesting monograph, based on an investigation of the population of the Netherlands, made a detailed study of the significance of hereditary factors in the origin of gliomas. In comparison with the general population the death rate from gliomas in his group was 4 times higher than would be expected, and the frequency of dysraphias was apparently also uncommonly high. This statistical study supports the concept that an inborn "hereditary or inherited factor" plays a role in the origin of gliomas. In another study of 643 patients with CNS tumors in childhood parents, siblings and offspring were compared with 360 controls. 11 nervous system tumors occurred in relatives of cases, whereas none occurred in relatives of controls. Nine relatives of cases but no relatives of controls had cancer of the hematopoietic system (FARWELL and FLANNERY 1984).

On the other hand, HARVALD and HAUGE (1956) screened the siblings of 169 patients with glioblastoma and concluded that heredity did not play any role.

KOCH (1954), after studying and tabulating a vast number of reported cases, suggested that a local (hereditary) and a general factor (perhaps of a hormonal nature) could play a role in inducing intracranial blastomatous growths. My own almost identical concept (see ZÜLCH 1951b) differs inasmuch as I would prefer "congenital" rather than "hereditary."

The question of hereditary carcinomas has been studied in general cancerology and the term "cancer family" has been coined (cancer family syndrome; see LYNCH et al. 1976, pp. 355 ff., and KOCH 1980, pp. 577 ff.). This is defined as tumor growth in nonrelated families, widely dispersed geographically and presenting an increased occurrence of various types of cancer.

Further References: HOFFMANN (1919), MCKCRAIG (1937), MUNSLOW and HILL (1955), METZEL (1963, 1964), CHOI et al. (1970a), BICKNELL et al. (1978), SCHIANCHI and KRAUS-RUPPERT (1980), TIJSSEN et al. (1982).

3.3.3 Familial Systematic[1] Hamartoblastomatoses (Phakomatoses)

We recognize three systematic tumor groups that are either definitely or at least in part familial and/or hereditary: (a) neurofibromatosis (von Recklinghausen's disease), (b) tuberous sclerosis (Bourneville's disease), and (c) angiomatosis of the CNS (von Hippel-Lindau disease).

In the WHO classification these appear (a) as neurofibroma, the most common tumor entities of von Recklinghausen's disease, (b) as subependymal giant cell astrocytoma in Bourneville's disease (see p. 68), and (c) as hemangioblastoma in von Hippel-Lindau disease (see p. 69).

For the sake of completeness, the calcifying capillary and venous angiomas of the face and brain should be added as a fourth entity, although the hereditary nature of this latter condition is not prominent: in the WHO classification it is designated as Sturge-Weber disease (see p. 70).

VAN DER HOEVE (1933) called these entities phakomatoses, but we prefer the well-known pathologico-anatomic terms of hamartoma and hamartoblastoma (for the latter cases with autonomous growths), and apply the term hamartoblastomatosis to the widespread systematic occurrence of developmental abnormalities combined with partly autonomous neoplastic growth, in order to keep in conformity with general pathology.

3.3.3.1 Neurofibromatosis

Historical Note and Definition

Von Recklinghausen in 1882 recorded his experience with this entity in his basic monograph, from which the association of his name with this disease was then derived. First examples of bilateral tumors in central neurofibromatosis were published by WISHART (1822) and KNOBLAUCH (1843).

Since the epochal work of von Recklinghausen hundreds of papers have been published, so that the entity is now well characterized. It is a systematic hamartoblastomatosis of various connective and supporting tissues of the body. In the full-blown syndrome we find neurofibromas of myelinated and unmyelinated nerves, plexiform neurofibromas of the skin, racemous angiomas, pigmented nevi, and a variety of intracranial tumors, particularly multiple meningiomas, neurilemmomas of the cranial nerves, pilocytic astrocytomas of the midline, ependymomas, and numerous heterotopic rests of the parenchyma.

---

[1] Translators' note (first American edition): The term "systematic" used here pertains to the tendency of these disorders to manifest themselves regularly in certain characteristic organs or tissues rather than to appear throughout the body at random. It is used in preference to the term "systemic," which suggests involvement of the entire organism.

Many families with single or multiple tumors and other signs of von Recklinghausen's disease are well-known from the literature (see below).

Epidemiology (Age – Sex – Frequency – Site)

The first manifestations of neurofibromatosis are sometimes seen in early adolescence, although RODRIGUEZ and BERTHRONG (1966) reported an average age of 27 years. Some authorities think that neurofibromatosis is supposed to show a female preponderance. However, in Rodriguez' 48 cases females and males were equally affected.

In the Krakow series of 2250 tumors, reported by GLOWACKI (1963), 25 cases of von Recklinghausen's disease (1.1%) were observed, out of which 9 cases were of the central type (0.4%). It is impossible to describe preferential sites of the tumors in this disease, however, RODRIGUEZ and BERTHRONG (1966) recorded 82 bilateral acoustic neurilemmomas (Fig. 6) and 18 unilateral cases, as well as 54% intracranial multiple meningiomas (42% intraspinal and intracranial combined and only 4% merely intraspinal neoplasms). Associated gliomas occurred in 45%.

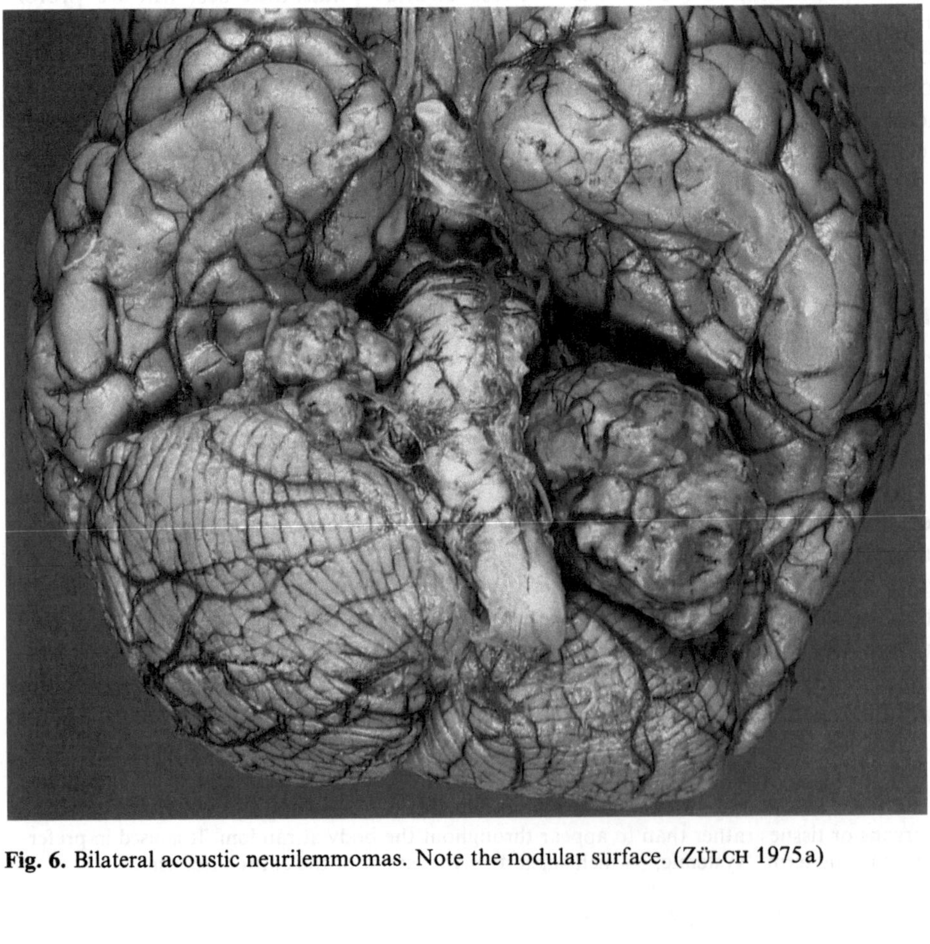

Fig. 6. Bilateral acoustic neurilemmomas. Note the nodular surface. (ZÜLCH 1975a)

Gross Pathology

The gross pathology is well-known for the single entities of which the syndrome consists, i.e., meningiomas, neurilemmomas, pilocytic astrocytomas. The peripheral forms, namely, the neurofibromas, are well-known from textbooks of neurology and general pathology. One can observe hundreds of nodular enlargements along the course of the peripheral nerves, intermingled with pigment nevi and plexiform angiomas where the skin hangs down in large folds and pockets. Moreover, café au lait patches are characteristic and common.

Histologic Appearance

The histologic picture corresponds to that of the neurilemmomas, meningiomas, ependymomas and pilocytic astrocytomas elsewhere in the body. The neurofibromas, on the other hand, are tumors that can be localized, either ball-like or fusiform, more diffuse and consist of a mixture of Schwann cells and fibroblasts. The mesodermal portion consists of collagen fibers, which may undergo mucoid degeneration and form an interesting architecture of wavy fascicles in which the neurites of the former nerves may appear as local remnants. The typical appearance of the neurilemmoma with its A and B pattern does not appear in the neurofibroma.

The pilocytic astrocytoma, in particular, can frequently grow in the chiasm or optic fascicle, similar to the *forme fruste* of this entity (see p. 232), which involves pigmented nevi as the only sign of kinship to neurofibromatosis (see RETTELBACH and SCHUTZBACH 1942; DAVID et al. 1956).

Biologic Behavior (Grading), Metastasis, and Recurrence

The peripheral neurofibromas can be categorized as grade I, the problem in treating them is their multiplicity and deep location and moreover, the trauma to the peripheral nerve when they are excised. The other tumors behave biologically as described for their entities elsewhere in this volume. Neurofibromas can undergo malignant degeneration, and they then will correspond to anaplastic neurofibromas or neurofibrosarcomas which are categorized as grades III and IV. Finally, one of the greatest problems with neurofibromatosis is the combination of multiple intracranial and peripheral tumors (see FOERSTER and GAGEL 1932c: five tumor entities; KATZENSTEIN 1932; GAGEL 1936; BRACKEN 1957; OBRADOR ALCALDE and ESCALONA 1963).

General Radiological Changes

Cases of full-blown von Recklinghausen's disease have been described by HOLT and WRIGHT (1948); the syndrome consists in adjacent erosions of bone, bending of bones, pseudoarthroses, interosseal cystic lesions and congenital anomalies, etc. There may be several groups of cranial changes: orbital defects, suture defects, dysplastic temporal bone, enlargement of optic foramen, sellar changes, enlargement of the internal acoustic meatus and of the orbits, and finally, nonspecific changes that have been similarly described by GALANSKI and BENZ

(1978) and KLAUS et al. (1978). KLAUS et al. drew attention to the changes in the bony carotid and ophthalmic vascular channels.

Origin of von Recklinghausen's Disease

The heredity and genetics of this disease have not been adequately clarified. In the early basic work, particularly of the German neuropathologists, the relation of central neurofibromatosis to tuberous sclerosis on the one hand (BIELSCHOWSKY and HENNEBERG 1922; BIELSCHOWSKY and ROSE 1927; GAMPER 1929; PENFIELD and YOUNG 1930; KERNOHAN and PARKER 1932; MONRO and SMITH 1968) and the relation of peripheral neurofibromatosis to hypertrophic neuritis and neural muscular atrophy on the other, are worthy of mention (KRÜCKE 1942).

The scientific discussion started with the variant disease of so-called central changes, i.e., rachischisis, syringomyelia, heterotopias of nerve cells, displacement of the cortical layers, plaques fibromyeliniques, excessive atypical glia, and small angiomatous malformations, as well as connective tissue inclusions (see FOERSTER and GAGEL 1932c). These changes sometimes showed a loose kinship with tuberous sclerosis and familial hypertrophic neuritis, as already mentioned. There is also some relation to the diffuse gliomas (see p. 112) whose origin can be better understood on the basis of BIELSCHOWSKY's (see above) description of the migration of cells from the neural crest and the disturbances that occur during this process. It may be stated that in neurofibromatosis disturbances of *cytogenesis* and *cytokinesis* occur, which lead in part to static and in part to neoplastic malformations. It is of interest to note that the diffuse infiltration of misdirected and malformed cells was indicated by the finding of Rosenthal fibers scattered diffusely through the white matter (HALLERVORDEN 1952; HALLERVORDEN and KRÜCKE 1956). These fibers ordinarily occur only as degenerative forms of the subependymal glia (see p. 229).

The question of why, in this combination of neoplasia and disturbed cytogenesis, only some should have received the stimulus for autonomous growth, and why this stimulus does not lead to tumor growth immediately, but only years later (GAMPER 1929), remains open. We have not been able to shed any new light on this problem by thorough study of a number of cases from our own collection.

3.3.3.2 Tuberous Sclerosis

Synonym: Bourneville's disease

Introduction

Tuberous sclerosis shows a series of central and peripheral changes characterized mainly by the triad of adenoma sebaceum, tumors of heart and kidneys, and central changes in the brain. The brain changes consist of the well-known gross nodules of the cortex (tubers), macro- or microgyria, maldevelopment of the histologic structure including heterotopias, glial nests and monster cells developing into either glial or ganglion cells or cells of ambivalent character, and ependymal nodules. In some instances the ependymal tumors reach the size of large mass lesions. These tumors are listed in the WHO classification as *subependymal giant cell astrocytoma* or *ventricular tumor of tuberous sclerosis* (see p. 232).

Historical Note and Definition

Apparently the first case of tuberous sclerosis was described by von Recklinghausen at a meeting of the Obstetric Society in Berlin in 1862 (see GAGEL 1942). However, von Recklinghausen had apparently not understood the correlation between the cerebral and the cardiac changes. Therefore BOURNEVILLE (1880), who described a series of such observations between 1880 and 1898, was the first to recognize these correlations and coined the new term of "tuberous sclerosis." In GAGEL'S (1942) paper we find a more detailed history of the development of these concepts by various authors who described similar observations at about the same time. Indeed, in the absence of the otherwise characteristic clinical syndrome (as shown by STENDER and ZÜLCH 1943) such a large mass lesion as mentioned above can appear merely as a ventricular tumor in the foramen of Monro and produce a general increase in intracranial pressure associated with hydrocephalus of the lateral ventricles. The cortical changes, however, particularly the "tubers," are indicative of the disease process.

Epidemiology (Age – Sex – Frequency – Site)

Age. The typical skin lesions (adenoma sebaceum) and accompanying epileptic seizures mark the beginning of the condition's clinical syndrome in early youth.

Sex. Apparently males are more commonly involved than females (BIELSCHOWSKY and GALLUS 1913:46:26).

Frequency. The frequency has not been determined.

Site. The central changes within the brain have no local predilection, although the large ependymal tumors have their predilection site at the foramen of Monro (GP, Figs., 78, 79; see also Fig. 53).

Other sites for these ventricular tumors are less common, yet we may cite an example our own collection in a 9 year old boy. In addition to multiple tubers and numerous small or minute ventricular nodules of no neurosurgical significance, he had a cylindrical tumor the size of a hen's egg along the wall of the lateral ventricle in the parieto-occipital region, where it did not produce a significant obstructive hydrocephalus.

Gross Pathology

The tubers are easily recognized by their whitish, hard, circumscribed appearance, whereas the ventricular tumors may be either small and multiple and/or larger, usually starting from the floor of the lateral ventricle near the foramen of Monro and increasing to the size of a hen's egg. These are nodular, bluish-red, sharply delineated tumors, which separate easily from the brain tissue (GP, Figs. 78, 79).

Histologic Appearance

The histology of ventricular tumors (HBT, Fig. 15a–d) will be described p. 233. The heterotopias are histologically interesting, consisting of nests of astrocytic cells that form abundant glia fibrils, and of monster cells which may develop either toward the glia, toward the neurons or may have an ambivalent character. There may be small angioma-like formations (NOETZEL 1952). Retinal tumors may have a different histology.

Does tuberous sclerosis have a hereditary nature? Familial occurrence of tuberous sclerosis is not been mentioned in the older literature; however, later relevant cases have since been proved. Tuberous sclerosis in identical twins has been described by FABING (1934). GAGEL (1942) cites three families in which heredity was easily proven and supports the doctrine that tuberous sclerosis is a hereditary disease. This would mean that tuberous sclerosis should be considered an autosomal dominant disorder, in which lesions of the CNS and skin are combined with tumors of body organs, such as rhabdomyoma of the heart, renal tumors, and additional lesions of the eye and other organs. Nevertheless, the frequent brain tumors are only one partial expression of the disease (KAPP et al. 1967).

Radiological Changes

Calcification within the tubers, particularly the ventricular tumors, strongly suggests the presence of tuberous sclerosis, if the corresponding clinical symptoms are present. The pneumoencephalographic appearance of these tumors has been reported by KAUTZKY and ZÜLCH (1955, Figs. 57, 58; KAUTZKY-ZÜLCH et al. 1982).

Biologic Behavior (Grading), Metastasis, and Recurrence

The ventricular tumor can be categorized as grade I. Malignant/anaplastic changes are unknown. If only partly excised they are likely to recur. In general, the prognosis of these patients is poor. Most rarely they reach the fourth decade, although isolated cases survive even to their 70ieth year; HOLANDA and HOLANDA (1980) gave a better prognosis.

Operability

Surgical treatment of the ventricular tumor is specifically indicated in cases of the "forme fruste" (see STENDER and ZÜLCH 1943; HOLANDA and HOLANDA 1980), whereas excision does not seem indicated for single tubers. In cases of the "forme fruste" the changes in the cortex are usually minor, although, as seen in our own cases, sufficient to make the diagnosis. However, the appearance of the ventricular tumor is so characteristic that the diagnosis of tuberous sclerosis can be made from this pattern alone.

Further References: BIELSCHOWSKY (1914), GUNTHER and PENROSE (1935), VAN BOGAERT (1933, 1949), DENNY-BROWN (1938), ROSS and DICKERSON (1943), GAGEL and KREISSEL (1948), PARR (1948), VAGOS and GOMEZ (1967), KOCH (1972b), SEITELBERGER (1972), WARKANY (1977).

3.3.3.3 Systematic Angiomatosis of the CNS and Eye (von Hippel-Lindau Disease)

Synonyms: Hemangioblastoma, retinal angioma, angioreticuloma

Introduction

One subgroup of this entity is described as hemangioblastoma (p. 400) in accord with the classification of the WHO. For clarification of terminology, however, it must be emphasized that small angiomas of the retina are called *retinal angiomatosis of von Hippel*, whereas the hemangiomatous tumors in the cerebellum are named *hemangioma or hemangioblastoma of Lindau*. The term *von Hippel-Lindau syndrome* referring to a combination of both, has been accepted generally. When this occurs as an autosomal dominant disorder, with an intracranial neoplasm as an integral part of the syndrome, it is called "von Hippel-Lindau disease."

Historical Note and Definition

When studying cerebellar cysts, Arvid LINDAU (1926) noticed that some of them had hemangiomatous tumors (angioplastic tumors or capillary angiomas) in their walls and furthermore that these frequently were combined with small angiomas of the retina, the well-known angiomatosis retinae or von Hippel's disease. He called the combination of these two lesions "angiomatosis of the CNS."

There is no total coincidence of these two lesions, since the retinal angioma occurs only in one-fifth of the cases. BERBLINGER (1928) had previously noted the relationship between spinal angioblastomas and cysts of the pancreas.

In this often systematic disease the genetic component is of importance, since most cases with a solitary neoplasm are beyond the scope of a hereditary factor. For example, there is a study by SILVER and HENNIGAR (1952), who reported that 9 of 40 patients in their series had the combined von Hippel-Lindau syndrome.

Among the *hereditary* cases of von Hippel-Lindau disease, the MÖLLER family (1929, 1944) is particularly well-known. Out of 27 patients with hemangioblastosis there were only 3 with retinal involvement. This family can be traced through four generations; in the last three generations six male and four female members have been affected. Of these, five had cerebellar angioblastomas and four had combined retinal and cerebellar disease, while in one the retina alone was involved. The site of the angioma in the affected member of the first generation could not be accurately established. Among the reports of familial involvement those of BONEBRAKE and SIQUEIRA (1964, three siblings with solitary hemangioblastomas), of HOFF and BRONSON (1968), and also of TONNING et al. (1952) deserve particular attention.

A rare combination was seen in the case of MCKCRAIG and HORRAX (1949) of a *cerebral* hemangioblastoma and the von Hippel-Lindau syndrome and similarly in the three cases of THOMAS et al. (1978) with neurofibromas and retinal angiomatosis.

KOCH (1960a, b, 1964) who was particularly familiar with the genetic aspects of blastomatous growth in the CNS, restudied the heredity of the Sturge-Weber syndrome and the von Hippel-Lindau disease. He came to the conclusion that the latter has a dominant, or irregularly dominant mode of inheritance. It seems evident that the heredity of the various patterns of the von Hippel-Lindau syndrome must be further studied on members of such families.

3.3.3.4 Sturge-Weber Disease

BROUWER, VAN DER HOEVE, and MAHONEY (1937) have added Sturge-Weber disease to the three mentioned above as a fourth type of familial systematic hamartoblastomatosis (phacomatosis). (For a detailed description of this condition see p. 457). The manifestation of a "port-wine nevus" in the distribution of one or more branches of the trigeminal nerve and calcified angiomatosis of the meninges (see p. 458) probably occur either as a sporadic lesion, or as a familial one, as some cases in the literature have indicated.

Sturge-Weber syndrome is now often categorized as a systematic blastomatosis or "neuroectodermal dysplasia" (VAN BOGAERT 1935; KOCH 1940). Some authorities have formed the opinion that Sturge-Weber disease originates as a mesodermal malformation, as described in the third phase of G.L. STREETER'S schematic division of development (see TÖNNIS, p. 89 in BERGSTRAND et al. 1936). It can therefore be accepted as a multiple congenital angiomatosis of skin, chorioidea, leptomeninges, and brain (PETERS 1939).

We have observed a similar angiomatosis of the leptomeninges in a malformed newborn (see ZÜLCH 1956, Fig. 403d; HBT, Fig. 81 a–d); the condition had some pathogenetic relationship to Sturge-Weber angiomatosis. The pia was densely covered throughout with a network of small and medium-sized blood vessels, predominantly of venous structure, whose morphology was similar to that of the blood vessels in Sturge-Weber syndrome.

3.4 Traumatic Brain Tumors

We are currently faced with the problem as to whether or not head injury can stimulate or enhance the development or growth of brain tumors, a problem, long discussed, in classical neurology and neuropathology (GERHARDT 1882; GOWERS 1888; STARR 1889, 1894; BRAMWELL 1894; ADLER 1898; E. MÜLLER 1903; BUCK 1909; VON MONAKOW 1924; COURVILLE 1956; MANUELIDIS 1971).

As the result of head injuries in two World Wars and those stemming from highly developed industrialization and dense traffic conditions this question has long been a matter of conjecture (ZÜLCH 1951b, 1953b, 1984; PETERS 1952; ZÜLCH and MENNEL 1971b, c). It is not only a legal problem but is even more clearly a medical and biological problem. Therefore, its clarification seems necessary. The causal relationship between trauma and the development of tumors has been emphasized in the title of many publications and particularly in MARBURG's book *Unfall und Hirngeschwulst* (Trauma and Brain Tumors), Springer, Vienna 1934.

The scientific evidence for a correlation between trauma and tumor growth may be provided on the base of three separate lines of argument:

1. Examination of individual human cases in the light of modern cancer theory
2. Experimental investigation.
3. Statistical data concerning the occurrence of brain tumors in series of brain-injured persons who are examined adequately.

Causation

This term has to be defined according to a modern concept of cancerogenesis. The results of modern experimental neuro-oncology facilitate the discussion, and particularly with respect to the "resorptive" and even "transplacental" carcinogens. Nonetheless the question is not yet solved since it is not yet known whether a traumatic alteration of neuroepithelial tissue can trigger blastomatous autonomous growth during the regenerative process. This was called the "misregeneration" theory by the classical pathologists (BENEKE 1926, 1932; FISCHER-WASELS 1927, 1932). However, the effects of scar formation in infected brain wounds and also the normal scarring around foreign bodies such as metal fragments, bone splinters, gauze sponges etc. were in many cases apparently the precursors of such traumatic brain tumors. This "misregeneration" theory (see p. 41) has been discussed in detail in our earlier papers (ZÜLCH 1953b; see also ZÜLCH 1984).

Co-Carcinogens

A second way by which to assess the possibility of a traumatic origin of brain tumors is the introduction of trauma as a co-carcinogen as applied in the experiment. This has been applied by MENNEL et al. (1971) and by MORANTZ and SHAIN (1978).

In experiments in our laboratory the typical model of the transplacental carcinogenesis was employed and a trauma was made with a needle 2 mm into the right hemisphere. "Trauma evidently did not influence the location of the tumors which were induced by an urea compound" (MENNEL et al. 1971) (see p. 59ff.).

In MORANTZ and SHAIN's (1978) experiment a left cerebral stab wound was made in Fisher rats. The experiment seems at first sight to be positive: in the trauma cases 73% gliomas were induced and in the controls only 47%. On the other hand, the distribution of gliomas between the left and right sides of the brain was *equal* in the control group.

Statistical Analysis

From an early date the study of "traumatic" brain tumors was approached very early through statistical analysis. P. SCHEID (1938) and A. DIETRICH (1941, 1950) reviewed very critically the cases reported during the first World War and at that time a connection was considered likely in only 12 cases. OSTERTAG and BUSCHMANN (1941) repeated this type of analysis and found 8 gliomas in 14400 brain-injured subjects.

A reverse deduction, namely, the analysis of the number of traumas suffered in a series of patients with brain tumors was undertaken by CUSHING and EISENHARDT (1938), who reported 101 positive cases in 313 meningiomas. However, this correlation was not considered convincing, and DUNSMORE and ROBERTS (1974) called the argument "nebulous." Moreover, GUIDETTI and MOSCATELLI (1958) could not definitely accept any such correlation. In 500 cases of brain tumor, 6.6% had suffered a trauma, but the authors recorded the "impossibility of a sufficiently definite explanation of this question," and they called it only a "theoretical hypothesis."

The most important contribution toward this problem was provided quite early by PARKER and KERNOHAN (1931). They reviewed critically the possible significance of head injury in the development of brain tumors, adopting an exceptionally critical attitude; in a large series of tumor cases they found that 13.4% had sustained a head injury. In the evaluation of these cases, however, they found that there could be serious consideration of trauma in only 4.8%. For comparison, however, they produced a group of 431 patients of corresponding age with other diseases, 10.4% of whom had a history of antecedent head trauma. Finally, in a corresponding group of healthy individuals of the same age and occupation, 71 (being 35.5% of the total group) had a similar history of cranial trauma.

Retrospective Analysis of Reports in the Literature

One might add a fourth way, namely analysis of cases in the literature where according to the authors traumatic alteration of brain tissue and its covering had led to a regenerative process, which eventually turned into an autonomous blastomatous growth. The most convincing cases are those of REINHARDT (1928), and of SCHMIDT and JAQUET (1963), in each of which a metallic foreign body was discovered within the blastoma, e.g., a meningioma.

Meningiomas. REINHARDT'S case was a 57 year old man who had a four-year clinical history of brain tumor. At autopsy the brain was adherent to the cribriform plate, where an extracerebral tangerine-sized tumor extended from the frontal pole to the chiasma (olfactory groove meningioma?). A 1 cm long and $\frac{1}{3}$ cm wide metal wire lay within the center of the tumor. As it turned out later this wire had been driven in during a boiler explosion 20 years before. Histologically, the lesion was classed as a "sarcomatous meningeal tumor" (meningioma?).

In a case of SCHMIDT and JAQUET (1963) a foreign body shaped like a needle was observed by x-ray in the middle fossa 1 cm above the cranial base. In examining this tangerine-sized tumor (meningioma) actually revealed an old needle, which, according to analysis by the Federal Institute of Criminologic Investigation in Wiesbaden, had probably been driven into the skull of the child soon after birth in an attempt at murder.

The following cases from the *meningioma* group are also convincing: LIEBALDT (1957): depressed fracture with tumor growth after a 14 year interval; LOEW and PLOGSTIES (1964): skull trephine with operative cyst followed by tumor formation 6 years later; HOWARTH and BUNTS (1950): $\frac{3}{8}$ in. deep depressed fracture with tumor formation 21 years later; HUNG et al. (1972): postoperative brain lesion followed 3 years later by encapsulated elastic tumor even though the edge of the bone flap had previously been inspected for 1.5–2 cm; TURNER and LAIRD (1966): comminuted fracture of the skull with tumor formation beneath 13 years afterwards; SCHAEFER (1965): superficial cranial defect with small metallic splinter and a meningioma beneath 21 years later; WALSH et al. (1969): scalp bruised in the midline with meningioma confined to bone discovered 26 years later; WALSHE (1961): metal penetrating the skull and trepanation followed by meningioma beneath defect 16 years later.

The two cases published by BUSHE (1958) are among the most convincing observations with regard to the growth of meningiomas in an old skull fracture line. SCHULZE and BINGAS (1968) noted the growth of a beansized meningioma around a silver clip at a second operation two years after the original one.

In the earlier edition of this book, I mentioned the case reported by H.R. MÜLLER (1939) of a healed, depressed fracture of the left temporal bone and a meningioma the size of a small apple. The critical analysis may be found in the earlier edition. I emphasized the radiologic feature of a so-called depressed fracture, an exostosis, which can be, and often has been, misinterpreted as a fracture of the inner table (see the case of LESZINSKY 1907; CUSHING and EISENHARDT 1938; CALVO 1952; NIZZOLI and BRIZZI 1964; DUNSMORE and ROBERTS 1974), whereas such an osteoblastic reaction is not uncommon with meningiomas.

In summary, in my experience traumatic tumors are very rare, if and when they occur, are most likely to arise after lesions of the dura and the arachnoid. Neuropathologic evidence to support this concept and the report on an own case will be presented on p. 75.

Neuroepithelial Tumors. FINKEMEYER and BEHREND (1956) published a case of a "protoplasmic astrocytoma", which after viewing the pictures, I would prefer to classify as an oligoastrocytoma (which grew during 9.8 years after a small splinter missile lesion to the brain beneath a hole in the skull). I would accept this more readily than the famous case of HALLERVORDEN (1948), which I have cited in the earlier edition (1951 b). I said at that time that the diagnosis did not seem well substantiated and not beyond criticism. This tumor was an oligodendroglioma containing bony splinters and plant fiber. Information about an "open brain wound" was unavailable, the case history was not known, and the brain was forwarded without the general autopsy findings, and was wrapped in straw.

HALLERVORDEN later, in a letter to me, agreed that "the idea that this plant fiber got into the brain at autopsy is most likely. I am sorry that I did not have this interpretation before..." However, he maintained the opinion "that an oligodendroglioma had developed from a focal contusion."

STAEMMLER'S (1938) case was well described and it still seems possible. More acceptable are the cases of N. WOLF (1951), NOETZEL (1953: glioblastoma of the posterior corpus callosum in contact with the margin of an old bullet track) and finally HEYCK (1954: anterior butterfly glioblastoma multiforme within the scar of a bilateral frontal leucotomy after 5 years). After the experience we have had so often with meningiomas, I am now inclined not to regard this tumor growth as coincidental.

The last case that should be mentioned is that of H.R. MÜLLER (1939) of a 57 year old man who had several trepanations following a brain injury in the right parietal region. He died 22 years later during status epilepticus. Autopsy showed a meningocerebral cicatrix together with a missile track from the temporal region to the falx, along which lay grenade splinters. The tumor was situated occipitally with "two cherry-sized nodules directly in the missile track." Histologically it was a typical monstrocellular sarcoma. Since missile tracks have a considerable admixture of connective tissue in the scar this particular kind of mesodermal tumor *might* have developed from a scar.

I would still hesitate to accept evidence from the reports of von MONAKOW (1924), P. SCHEID (1938), DIEZEL (1949), and FLENKER (1972), as I have hesitated in my critical reviews (1951b, 1953a) with regard to the cases of RÖSSLE (1911), NEUBUERGER (1925), BECKMANN (1930), DAMMER (1930), von HASSELBACH (1931), and FISCHER-WASELS (1932).

One case will be portrayed in more detail because it is, so to speak, the introduction to MARBURG'S book (1934): *Unfall und Hirngeschwulst* (Accident and Brain Tumor). A 10 year-old boy who fell striking back of his head while skating, but did not lose consciousness or vomit. Neurological symptoms appeared 14 days later. His condition deteriorated rapidly during the next two weeks and he died slightly more than 4 weeks after the fall. Autopsy revealed a medulloblastoma of the cerebellum (4.5 × 5 cm), which was quite hemorrhagic. There was subpial spread, which was considered by Marburg to be a "persistent external granular layer." He also had the opinion that this "embryonic germ" was "proliferated" by the trauma. The time elapsed between fall and the growth of the medulloblastoma is inadequate, and the concept of a persisting external granular layer indefensible. Moreover, subpial spread is very characteristic of medulloblastoma.

Before ending this discussion I would like to emphasize two personal observations, the first of which has been included briefly and with figures in the paper of TÖNNIS and GRIPPONISSIOTIS (1939, Figs. 1 and 6). Two different stages of granuloma formation within old brain scars are described and illustrated in this paper. The first, 2 years after the trauma, showed a cellular granulomatous tissue consisting of large arachnoidal flecks and islands, which are often seen coincidentally in the normal leptomeninges. In the second, seen 13 years after the trauma, similar but more fibrous tissue, found on the edge of the scar, contained abundant psammoma bodies, which probably had been formed as remnants of the former granulomatous arachnoidal tissue.

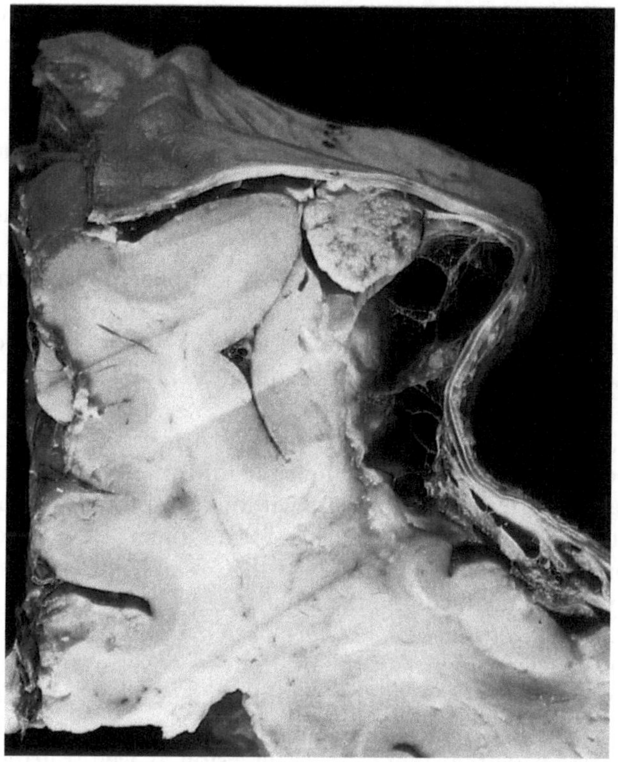

Fig. 7. Small meningioma at edge of traumatic scar

My interpretation would be that in this case the arachnoidal tissue within the scar had been displaced inward and had begun to proliferate years before. Although the stimulation ended, the scar remained with the psammoma bodies as vestiges of the former arachnoidal granulation tissue. In very rare cases this regenerative process, stimulated by an unknown factor, continues and results in the formation of a meningioma.

For further support of this concept I had a specific case, which I presented in a Washington symposium in 1969c (Fig. 46-11), where I described the growth of a cherry-like meningioma at the edge of an old brain contusion with scarring and adhesion between dura and leptomeninges (Fig. 7). A glial scar is probably far less suitable for such "misregeneration," which ends in autonomous tumor growth.

Juridical Causation. As stated earlier, the assessment of a possible relationship between trauma and its effect is dependent on the definition of "causation". At Washington in 1969c we discussed the field of "medical causation" (see Spielmeyer 1969). Medical causation (Zülch 1969c, p. 453) is based on the actual state of medical and biological knowledge and therefore is understood internationally. "Juridical causation" must be considered independently since it depends upon "artificial" correlations established through regulations and laws which are differently defined in each country and therefore not internationally applicable.

Further References: JORDAN (1901), THIEM (1912, 1916), VON MONAKOW (1924), REINHARDT (1928), MASSON (1934), EWING (1935), P. SCHEID (1938), R. FROWEIN (1949).

Legal Evaluation of Cases With "Posttraumatic" Tumors

In order to facilitate the medico-legal evaluation of questionable cases of "traumatic brain tumors", we have proposed the following checklist.

We have listed above the classical papers in which the possibility of "posttraumatic" tumors has been discussed. Taking into consideration both these discussions and our own experience as well as the knowledge of the aforementioned theses the following requisites should be met before the "posttraumatic origin" of a tumor is accepted:

1. *The patient should have been well before the trauma.* This requirement should be insisted upon even though the information may be difficult to obtain. Brain tumors often grow for years without symptoms and can elude diagnosis (ventriculographic demonstrations in former times: PENNYBACKER and MEADOWS 1938) but modern neurodiagnosis with CT and nuclear magnetic resonance (NMR) imaging may facilitate the situation.
2. *The head trauma must have been adequate,* i.e., sufficiently severe to produce destruction of parts of the brain or its coverings leading to chronic regenerative processes. Even a minor trauma can lead to considerable pathologic change but on the other hand contusions or lacerations of the scalp do not suffice to conclude that there is a *brain* lesion as well. Furthermore, loss of consciousness and other signs of concussion are not mandatory, since severe brain damage can occur without them. Consequently, thorough investigation of each individual case is necessary (ZÜLCH 1951b, 1953b, 1965a; ZÜLCH and MENNEL 1971b, c).
3. *The site of tumor formation must correspond to that receiving the trauma.* It is not enough merely to state that the tumor lies at the site of external skull injury or in the region of supposed contrecoup injury (see PACK and ARIEL 1958, who emphasized that "cancer can be in the line of force of the injury as in the contrecoup lesions of the brain"). The proof of injury to the bone, meninges, or brain substance, must be based upon morphological findings, which are now more easily determined by CT.
4. *The time interval between the trauma and the development of the tumor should be adequate.* At present we know enough about the rate of brain tumor growth to provide accurate information. Criticism based on this point led for example to the rejection of Marburg's case referred to above. In individual cases where a meningioma, pilocytic astrocytoma, or even a large medulloblastoma has been encountered only a few weeks after the incident, trauma can be dismissed as a cause. On the other hand, glioblastomas or medulloblastomas might *theoretically* develop from a scar as a result of trauma even many years after the accident.
5. *The tumor has to be proved histologically at autopsy or by biopsy.* We must caution, particularly, against misinterpretation of the simple glial or connective tissue portions of the scar. The meningocerebral cicatrix is a good example

of this problem since very frequently small regions of the glial scar cannot be definitely distinguished from low grade astrocytoma.

6." *The external force should be defined as sufficient to be considered true trauma.* The definition might be as follows: An accident is a single externally inflicted mechanical bodily injury, which produces alterations in the structure and function of the body and was not intended by the victim. The trauma must be proved without question. Interval (bridging) symptoms are of little significance, since we would not anticipate the onset of the tumor immediately after the trauma. However, they can be of some value in linking the trauma to the tumor growth. Trauma need not be the result of an "accident."

If one adheres to these strict criteria a traumatic etiology can be accepted for only a few brain tumors (AUSTER 1961).

Trauma may call attention to or provoke symptoms in an already existing tumor, so this possibility has to be excluded. Finally, one might observe *aggravation* of the clinical picture or actual *participation* of the trauma in causing premature clinical manifestations. This possibility is illustrated by the following professional opinion on one of Tönnis' patients (SPROCKHOFF 1940).

A previously healthy 41-year-old truck driver received a blow to the back of his head while working. This trauma produced headaches but no loss of consciousness. On the following day the man was admitted to hospital because of a series of epileptic seizures. The attacks recurred regularly and he became an invalid. After eight years his condition became worse, and one year later he was referred for operation by the neurological department.

The operation revealed "peculiar changes in the form of many large cysts lying anterior to a parasagittal meningioma the size of a small apple." No such changes were seen posterior to the tumor where the brain was noted to be atrophic. The cysts were opened, the tumor extirpated along with "cicatricial strands of the surrounding tissue and the damaged portions of the brain" and the patient got well. It was assumed that the blow to the back of the head had caused compression of the brain when it was pressed against the tumor. The proof lay in the immediate appearance of the clinical symptoms and in the operative findings. The accident was thought to have had a definite influence upon the "clinical course" of the disease.

We hope that the delineation of these six points for the medico-legal evaluation of cases with posttraumatic tumors (first published in the German edition of this textbook in 1951) will serve as a guide for the handling of cases in litigation.

3.5 "Composition" and "Mixed" Tumors

Synonyms: Concurrent, composition, collision, juxtaposition, combination, and mixed tumors originating from different germ blades

Introduction

Apart from the not infrequent glioblastoma with a sarcomatous component there are tumors in which tissue originating from two different germ layers appear to be intermixed in the mantle zone.

The definition can be clarified with reference to two published cases from our institute. PROBST (1971) has reported the very close mixing of two tumor types in the sellar region, namely a pituitary adenoma (leading to Cushing's syndrome) and a meningioma. This is a genuine "collision" ("combination") tumor according to the definition. I have also described personally a pituitary adenoma and a meningioma occurring simultaneously at different sites in the same patient (ZÜLCH 1956, p. 489). This, naturally, is not a case of combination tumor.

Composition tumors are not mentioned as an entity in the WHO classification.

Historical Note and Definition

In 1919/20 R. MEYER discussed nomenclature and coined the name of "composition tumor" for those blastomas, in which tissue elements from different germ layers showed blastomatous growth.

Epidemiology (Age – Sex – Frequency – Site)

Since the various reported cases of combined neoplastic growths originate from such different "mother" tissues one cannot assume a typical epidemiology.

Gross Pathology

Similarly, the appearance to the naked eye is quite different in the various forms.

Histologic Appearance

The histologic evaluation and the diagnosis must be made on the grounds that the two tissues are really intermixed or interwoven and not that one was only growing side by side. In this regard KLEIHUES (1965), for example, described the intermixed growth of an ependymoma and a monstrocellular sarcoma, where the ependymoma was perivascularly infiltrated by the sarcoma. It is interesting in this case that the vascular stroma was apparently transformed and introduced into the sarcomatous growth. Similarly, as we have seen in our institute (B. SCHIEFER 1958, 1964) in an experimental oligodendroglioma the vessels followed a sarcomatous pattern with formation of monster cells.

KLEIHUES in his survey found 28 cases in the literature, and later SACKETT et al. (1974) collected 52 tumors, 24 of which showed a real mixture whereas in 28 the tissue types were separate. In the majority of these cases the histologic diagnosis was meningioma and astrocytoma, but there were also a chordoma and hemangioblastoma (FUKAYA et al. 1976), blastocytoma and meningioma (BANERJEE and BLACKWOOD 1971), craniopharyngioma and eosinophilic pituitary adenoma (TZONOS and PFINGST 1964) as well as many others.

Further References: STROEBE (1895), FEIGIN and GROSS (1955).

3.6 Transplantability of Human Brain Tumors – Immunological Aspects

The brain has proved to be a good host not only for homologous but also for heterologous tissues, especially tumors. Only the anterior chamber of the eyes provides an equally suitable site (GREENE 1951 a, b). Following homologous transplantation, mature and embryonic tissue and malignant tumors grow, whereas benign tumors and precancerous tissue do not "take". After heterologous transplantation, however, only embryonic tissue and malignant tumors survive. These experiments were carried out on rabbits, guinea-pigs, rats and mice. Since this early work of GREENE (1951 a, b; KREMENTZ and GREENE 1953) and his later investigations of transplantation of neural tumors subcutaneously and into the vitreous chamber the question regarding immunization of the host against neoplastic tissue has arisen.

GREENE had first used transplantability tests for the definition of malignancy. Later, it was also demonstrated that one could culture neuroepithelial tumors on chick embryos and transplant them for eight generations. However, it was noted that the tumor lost its characteristic architecture in the process and regained it only upon being transplanted back into mice (COHN and ZIMMERMAN 1955).

A transplant of anaplastic astrocytoma into the subcutaneous tissue in *man* has been successfully performed by BATTISTA et al. (1961). The histologic characteristics remained similar to those of the original brain tumor. The response of these transplants to x-ray therapy and chemotherapy was studied and this provided some hints as to the most effective form of treatment.

Of considerable interest were the experiments performed by MITTS and WALKER (1964), in which glioblastoma tumor cells were injected into the subcutaneous tissues of five patients, and into normal brain tissue in two others. In the latter cases, no survival or growth was observed. On the other hand, in two of the five tumor transplants, microscopic study showed evidence of growth and adhesion to surrounding tissue. Growth of reticulin fibers was a prominent feature. Malignant glial cells grew but were not as active as the reticulin producing cells.

I had been reported previously that a certain degree of immunity against such transplantations of experimental ependymomas had been achieved when the tumor was used as an antigen together with Freund's adjuvant. The incidence of tumor "take" was lowered to 50% as compared with 100% in the controls. Investigations have also been made into the possibility of stimulation of an antibody response to tumors implanted in animals or even in man. Such immunological studies have been performed by MAHALEY et al. (1977a, b) and HASS (1966). MAHALEY, from his studies since 1963, reported results pointing to the antigenic potential of human gliomas and tried to determine the feasibility of producing heterologous antiglioma "carrier" antibodies, capable of preferentially hitting a glioma *in vivo*. The possible consequences of such investigations for treatment of human neoplastic disease soon became evident. However, he was forced to conclude at the time that there has been no proof of specific glioma antigens or specific antiglioma antibody production, autogenous or heterologous, despite continuing interest in utilization of antibodies for the treatment of tumors either by direct antigen – antibody action – or as carriers of therapeutic agents. The report of ODA (1974) on neuroepithelial tumor groups bearing a tumor specific antigen in a protein layer of the cell membrane and the deduction also that patients have serum-blocking factors has not found any practicality in therapy. In fact autotransplantation is possible in man and has been known since the observation of Cairns after an operation during which parts of an oligodendroglioma were accidentally transplanted into the scalp and began to grow as an implant (CAIRNS 1929).

Another report of such tumor autografts was published by GRACE et al. (1961), in which serological studies revealed no evidence of humoral antibody against brain antigens in any of the patients. It was interesting that in two patients with successful takes there was no positive reaction to a skin test using the same antigen, whereas in two patients who rejected the tumor there were strongly positive delayed-type skin responses. This fact may have played a role in determining the success or failure of the autografts.

What then was the deciding factor in the immunological behavior of animals or man towards tumors and the possibility of their antigenic action? In searching for glia specific antigens in intracranial tumors (CGSA), i.e., in attempting to assess the antigenic properties of neoplastic tissue, LACH and WEINRAUDER (1978) found that there probably existed a deficiency of normal antigenic material in neoplastic glia and that this was particularly noticeable in the case of oligodendrogliomas and anaplastic gliomas.

The entire problem of immune suppression of neoplastic tissue growing in the brain is by no means clarified yet. MORANTZ et al. (1978) stated that "immune surveillance," which is one function of the immune system which eliminates small numbers of malignant cells that arise spontaneously within the organism, apparently does not operate in the rat with respect to the ENU tumors. They concluded that the brain possibly has an "immunologic privilege."

With progress in immunology and particularly the identification of different lymphocytic cells in the immunologic and antigenic process, investigations have been made into the occurrence and behavior of lymphocytes in various kinds of brain tumor. RIDLEY and CAVANAGH (1971), in a study of 93 cases of glioma, found significant lymphocytic infiltration in 30% and a slight infiltration in 28%, which they interpreted as an attempt toward "host resistance" against the growing neoplasm.

DI LORENZO et al. (1977) noted in 200 patients with glioblastoma multiforme that 8 survived more than four years. In 6 of these cases a heavy perivascular lymphocytic infiltration was present, which they interpreted as an immune defense reaction. A re-examination of the histology in these cases with longer survival and "lymphocytic infiltration" appears to be necessary. The mean age of these long survivors was only 29 years. This also may have some particular significance. It is important to note that this phenomenon of "lymphoid perivascular accumulation" (see p. 248) is more often seen with oligodendrogliomas. PALMA et al. (1978) found definite lymphocytic infiltration in 11.5% of 200 patients operated for glioblastoma. They also had a significantly longer preoperative history and postoperative survival than two other groups, which presented with only slight or no infiltration.

To make certain that the "lymphocytes" in such cases actually were T lymphocytes, an indirect immunofluorescence method was applied in human and rat gliomas by STAVROU et al. (1977). They interpreted their results as evidence for the occurrence of tumor-specific and/or tumor-associated antigens in parenchymal cells of spontaneous and chemically induced gliomas.

For in depth studies of immunologic mechanisms it seemed necessary to investigate the protein structure of various neuroepithelial cells, including both normal and neoplastic ones. Indeed, a "nervous tissue" specific antigen (MOORE and MCGREGOR 1965) was isolated; this substance was given the name protein S-100 and was found localized in cells of normal brain and of neoplasms as well, including astrocytomas, glioblastomas, some oligodendrogliomas, and neurilemmomas (BENDA 1968; PFEIFFER and WECHSLER 1972; HAGLID et al. 1973) (see p. 30). Its existence even seemed useful for the definition of a tumor's degree of malignancy, since the levels of S-100 were apparently inversely proportional to the degree of malignancy (HAGLID and STAVROU 1973).

Furthermore, another protein, i.e., 14-3-2, was identified by MOORE and PEREZ (1966). It was later further isolated as NSP – neuron specific protein – (PICKEL et al. 1975). This has been considered as indicator of neuronal differentiation (ZOMZELY-NEURATH and WALKER 1980). An acidic protein was found in the glial fibrillae (GFAP) by ENG et al. (1970). The glial nature of tumors such as astrocytomas could be established by histochemical staining for GFAP. It was even possible to differentiate such glial fibrillae in medulloblastoms (RUBINSTEIN and BRUCHER 1981). Moreover, it was concluded that a low level of GFAP was found more often in malignant forms while a higher level was noted, understandably, in astrocytic elements within the tumor.

WARECKA (1975) found "α_2 glycoprotein" in all lower grade astrocytomas, while no glioblastoma contained it. In the tumor astrocytes, however, this protein was contained in a form containing less neuraminic acid. In those glioblastomas investigated one could accept that, if devoid of "α_2 glycoprotein," the tumor did not contain any astrocytes or only relatively few slowly proliferating cells. Furthermore, "surface antigens", "common glioma antigens", and "glioembryonic antigens" (PFREUNDSCHUH et al. 1978) were detected independently from "α_2 glycoprotein" and "neurofilament protein." For detailed references on immunologic cell surface markers see GORIDIS and SCHACHNER (1978).

There is continuing interest in production and application of antibodies for the treatment of tumors either by direct antigen – antibody action or as carriers of therapeutic agents. However, a general conclusion can probably be formulated, that there has been no proof to date of specific glioma antigens or specific antiglioma antibody production, autogenous or heterologous.

Further References: SCHEINBERG and TAYLOR (1968), TROUILLAS and LAPRAS (1970), WHO (1973a, b), TAKAKURA et al. (1973), MAUNOURY et al. (1975), SOBUE et al. (1976), VELASCO et al. (1980).

Interesting results have been also obtained from tissue cultures and from transplantations. In conventional homologous transplantation MENNEL (1972) and MENNEL and BÜCHELER (1974b) found a preservation of pattern and cells until the 10th serial subtransplantation (mean induction time, 3rd to 9th generations: 47 days, later only 24 days). From the 11th generation on the cells were closely packed and more chromatin dense, and there were abundant mitoses.

Further Reference: STAVROU et al. (1980).

3.7 Spontaneous Brain Tumors in Animals

Brain tumors in animals are fairly rare; however, we should use every opportunity to make a comparison between human brain tumors and those found in animals. Mice are considered to be *almost free* of spontaneous gliomas (see MORGAN et al. 1984), and intracranial tumors are *very rare* in monkeys; nonetheless, in the last 30 years large collections of animal tumors have been classified, so that their spectrum of occurrence is now fairly well-known (see Fig. 8).

This section is based very closely on the work of Hans-Ruedi LUGINBÜHL (LUGINBÜHL 1962a, b, 1963, 1964a, b; FANKHAUSER and LUGINBÜHL 1968;

	Spontaneous tumors																Experiment tumors
	Dog	Cow	Cat	Pig	Mouse	Goat	Kangaroo	Rat	Horse	Zebra	Fox	Sheep	Hen	Elephant	Budgerigar	Parrot	Rat
Astrocytoma	●	●	●														●
Pilocytic astrocytoma	●	○				○											
Oligodendroglioma	●	○	○		○		○										●
Ependymoma	○	○	○		○			○									●
Plexus papilloma	●		○						●								
Pinealoma		○				○		○	○	○	○						○
Gangliocytoma	○																○
Glioblastoma	●	●		○	○												○
Medulloblastoma	●	●	○	○	○												
Neurilemmoma	●	●							○					○			●
Meningioma	●	○	●		○				○			○					
Hemangioblastoma	○			○					○				○				
Pituitary adenoma	●	●			●			●	●						●	●	●

● regular
○ sporadic

Fig. 8. Occurrence of tumors in animals. ●, regular; ○, sporadic. (After FRAUCHIGER and FANKHAUSER (1957) and LUGINBÜHL et al. (1968)

LUGINBÜHL et al. 1968), who started his particular work on spontaneous brain tumors in animals in Frauchiger's laboratory. He began this work in close collaboration with our laboratory and kept in touch with us for a long time. Therefore we are familiar with most of his work and can estimate its value when making comparison with any observations in man. Furthermore, the work of B. SCHIEFER (1964; B. SCHIEFER and DAHME 1962) is very close to us in the concepts regarding spontaneous brain tumors in animals since he started with an experimental doctoral thesis in our laboratory (see B. SCHIEFER 1958). Also KOESTNER (see KOESTNER and ZEMAN 1962) was a frequent guest in our laboratory when we had basic discussions about the genesis of tumors. Therefore his work is well-known to us and his concepts closely parallel our own.

Before these aforementioned authors dedicated most of their work to the study of brain tumors, a large amount of data had been collected by classical neuropathologists such as GRÜN (1936), JUNGHERR and WOLF (1939), BARBONI (1940), H.J. SCHERER (1944), and last but not least FRAUCHIGER and FANKHAUSER (1949, 1957) in whose laboratory LUGINBÜHL had started his work.

Epidemiology (Age – Sex – Frequency – Site)

To date statistics on the absolute and relative frequency of tumors of the nervous system in domestic and wild animals are lacking. It is generally assumed that they are rare. However, some of them seem to occur at least as frequently as in man; e.g., oligodendrogliomas in brachycephalic dogs. MCGRATH (1962) found 173 intracranial tumors (2.83%) in 6175 dogs. Of these, 119 were primary (82 gliomas, 10 meningiomas, 3 cranial nerve tumors, 24 miscellaneous tumors) and 57 were metastatic (see also LUGINBÜHL 1964a; SCHIEFER 1964).

A collection of approximately 500 intracranial neoplasms was classified at the University of Bern (FANKHAUSER and LUGINBÜHL 1968), and another 400 neoplasms investigated at the Pennsylvania School of Pathology (MCGRATH 1962). These tumor entities have been described in detail with excellent pictures in the paper of LUGINBÜHL et al. (1968).

LUGINBÜHL (1963) in Frauchiger's institute had undertaken earlier an extensive comparative study of CNS neoplasms in animals, the details of which are reported here. He was able to collect 80 cases of his own and 250 cases from other sources, which he analyzed according to our classification. Unfortunately, the accompanying biological data were rather incomplete, so the series is being continued.

The majority of the animal brain tumors occurred in dogs (183 out of 330), and among those in whom the gender was known (160), 85 were males, and 75 were females. Fifty-seven of these 160 dogs were brachycephalic.

In this series of 330 cases. LUGINBÜHL (1964a, presented at the International Symposium in Cologne 1961) found 8 medulloblastomas, 4 tumors resembling (polar) spongioblastomas, 35 oligodendrogliomas, 5 astrocytomas, 10 glioblastomas, 4 ependymomas, 18 neurinomas, 1 pinealoma, 1 gangliocytoma, 8 plexus papillomas, and 2 neoplasms, which resembled those seen in human tuberous sclerosis.

There were in this series 50 meningiomas, the majority of which (32 cases) occurred in cats, arising predominantly from the tela chorioidea of the third ventricle. Eight animals had malformations and neoplasms of the blood vessels, and 54 had either sarcomas (one-third) or reticuloendothelioses (two-thirds). There were 46 pituitary tumors in this series, 10 of which were eosinophilic adenomas.

In his summary, LUGINBÜHL pointed out that of his 330 cases 30% were neuroectodermal, 41% mesodermal, 14% ectodermal in origin, and 15% were metastases. The incidence of oligodendroglioma in dogs was particularly high (48%) in comparison with approximately 14% among the *neuroectodermal* tumors in man. This was also true of sarcomas, which were found in 17%, as compared with 2.7% in man. Of all neuroectodermal tumors 15% remained unclassified. This number is significantly higher than that seen in man.

This extremely interesting study by Luginbühl, based on the largest collection of such cases available in the world and later tested after considerable enlargement of the collection, will continue to provide valuable information on the biology of intracranial tumors. The reason for making this assumption is the fact that he has been analyzing his material according to the same criteria that have been used in collecting and analyzing tumors in man, i.e., with reference to each tumor type's incidence and prevalence according to species, location, age, and sex.

Figure 8 presents a survey of the occurrence of intracranial tumors in various species. A column with corresponding experimental tumors has been added.

We personally observed the famous elephant "Jumbo" in the Cologne Zoo, who, during the last years of his life was blind, due to corneal scarring, and showed more and more disagreeable behavior. At autopsy, a tumor of the size of a man's fist was found in the corresponding trigeminal ganglion. It was identified histologically as a neurosarcoma (HBT, Fig. 83d). Since this tumor ultimately had become malignant although the history went back many years, a secondary anaplastic change must be assumed.

Further References: NEUBUERGER and DAVIS (1943), KLÜVER and WEIL (1948), DOBERSTEIN (1955), GILBERT and GILLMAN (1958), KENT and PICKERING (1958), SPAAR and WILLE (1959), DAHME and SCHIEFER (1960), WIGHT and DUFF (1964), BOTS et al. (1968b), FRAUCHIGER (1968), FANKHAUSER et al. (1974), HAYES et al. (1975), KOESTNER (1975), WHO (1976).

4 Epidemiology of Brain Tumors – General Statistical and Biological Data

Epidemiology ("geographic pathology") is a medical science that deals with the incidence, distribution and control of a disease in a population or a region. Furthermore, the correlation between social and biological environment and pathogenesis is also examined.

As early as 1886, HIRSCH in the first handbook of geographic pathology, regretted the paucity of scientific material and the fact that very few observers had extended their inquiry into the prevalence and incidence of disease of the nervous system. R.C. BEHREND (1974) in his chapter on the "epidemiology of brain tumors" in the *Handbook of Clinical Neurology* gives an excellent review of our knowledge on this very important topic up until 1972. When we discuss the international data on incidence and prevalence of CNS tumors below, we may assume that in the populations of technologically developed countries probably 1 out of 25000 inhabitants each year manifests an intracranial tumor (ZÜLCH 1951b; KURLAND 1958). Furthermore, we must remember as a rule of thumb that approximately one third of the patients with CNS tumors may be "cured" by surgery, radiation, and chemotherapy, one third may have a survival time of 3–5 years, while the remaining one third will die within the 12 months following onset. Furthermore, according to reliable data tumors of the CNS account for about 2% (NAFFZIGER and BOLDREY 1948) of all cancer deaths.

Terminology

In the following discussion the term "incidence" means the number of *newly* observed cases *during* a specific period of time, usually 1 year, in a *specified* population, commonly 100000 individuals.

The "prevalence", on the other hand, is the number of patients per unit population presenting with a particular tumor at a specific time.

4.1 Age Incidence

Determination of the age incidence of individual tumor types was one of the most important achievements in the study of biology of brain tumors. The fact that in the last 50 years specific chapters or books have been published dealing exclusively with this specific subject could have two causes:

1. The diagnosis and therapy in these particular age groups needed special discussion.

2. Although some intracranial tumors occur at *all* ages, others develop preferentially or sometimes even exclusively in *childhood* and *adolescence* or in *senescence* and their pathology will differ.

O.T. SCHULZ (1926) appears to have been one of the first to strongly emphasize that the nature and distribution of neoplasms that occur during childhood and adolescence varies widely from that of tumors of adult life (see CUSHING 1930, 1931). Since "the pecularities of intracranial tumors during infancy and childhood lacked precision," BALLEY et al. (1948) decided to collect their data and condense them in a monograph. Other large contributions to this subject were made by CUNEO and RAND (1952) and INGRAHAM and MATSON (1954). The highly instructive monographs of RAND and RAND (1960), BUSHE and GLEES (1968), KOOS and MILLER (1971), and finally, an important volume on the pathology of CNS tumors in fetuses and infants by JÄNISCH et al. (1980) must also be mentioned. A symposium in 1981 (Mainz/FRG) on CNS tumors in childhood provided an excellent review of the subject (see VOTH et al. 1982).

Our interest was aroused particularly by an observation of Tönnis, who had operated on a large series of mostly cystic, frequently calcified, extraventricular tumors in children, most of which to our surprise turned out to be ependymomas (TÖNNIS and ZÜLCH 1937). The comparison of the 262 tumors in childhood and adolescence observed in the series of Tönnis (ZÜLCH 1940b, Table 2) on the one hand and the cases in the mid-life and older age groups on the other gave support to the above cited concept that the spectrum of pathology in this age group was distinctive.

Distribution of Age Groups

The first problem was to define the age limits of "childhood and adolescence." It was necessary to decide whether to accept the conventional upper limit for the admission to children's hospitals, namely, the 14th or 15th year, or the end of the 20th year. The latter seems more adequate to us for the specific reason that, when the age of incidence is plotted against the frequency of all tumor groups, the resulting curves show characteristic age peaks (Figs. 9, 11, 12).

Since the actual time of tumor onset cannot be determined we use the age at the time of admission to the hospital, or where there has been no hospital treatment, the time of death.

With all the age groups plotted together on a single ordinate we find that many of the curves cross around the age of 20, i.e., the ascending and descending limbs of a number of the curves cross one another at that point. This indicates a special biological significance for this age period which represents the end of childhood and adolescence.

The age curves of individual tumor types, however, may not be "pure" inasmuch as they include groups with mixed age incidences. For example, oligodendroglioma, which occurs mostly in the third and fourth decades, also includes a type that definitely occurs mostly in "adolescent" type, oligodendroglioma of the thalamus, which blurs the age peak to some extent.

We found some earlier scientific support for our use of the age limit "year 20" in the report by STARR (1894) as well as those of CUSHING and EISENHARDT in their age limit for some meningiomas (1938), and also in the work of SORGO (1940 b) and many others.

We note that certain tumor types show a predilection for the third and fourth decades, and others the fifth and sixth decades (p. 88 ff., Fig. 9). Thus, we defined "childhood and adolescence" as the time between 1 and 20 years of age; "middle age" as 21–45 years; the "age of involution" as 46–65 years, and "old age" from 66 on (ZÜLCH 1949 b; BORCK and ZÜLCH 1951; ZÜLCH and BORCK 1952).

Many neurosurgeons in their reports (LEY and WALKER 1936; STERN 1937) have limited "youth" to below the age of 16, when the incidence of neoplasms typical of childhood *falls off* rapidly as was evident from CUSHING'S graphs (1927). However, at this age those tumor types characteristic of adult life have scarcely begun to make themselves apparent.

I am aware of the fact that our limit stands in contrast to the ordinary limitation of childhood and adolescence and to that used in most of the tumor series published in the literature for this age group. However, O. FOERSTER gave a report about "101 tumors under the age of 20" (1937, unpublished) to the "British Society of Neurological Surgeons" (cited by BAILEY et al. 1948). DOHRMAN and FARWELL (1976) also reported on 49 ependymomas up to 20 years.

The incidence of CNS tumors in childhood and adolescence relative to the incidence of childhood tumors in general bears some discussion at this point. DARGEON (1947) found 370 neoplasms of the CNS (20.9%) in 1770 cases. FUKUYAMA et al. (1957) noted among 19529 autopsies that there were 0.6% tumors of the CNS in childhood. ARENDT and MÖLLER (1973) in their surgical series found 19.8% tumors in children up to 14 years.

It is also important to ask whether there is a significant difference in tumor incidence in various parts of childhood and adolescence. There is a large number of reports on what have been considered to be congenital tumors. JÄNISCH et al. (1980) reported on a series of 722 such cases. Tumors in the first year of life, according to SCHREIBER et al. (1982), are not any rarer than those occurring later on. JELLINGER and MACHACEK (1982) observed in their series 35 cases presenting in the first year (4.3%). JOOMA and KENDALL (1982) in a series of 1296 patients found 8% with first symptoms during the first year of life. SATO et al. (1975) in their series of 2832 patients, encountered between 1933 and 1973, observed 10 cases in which symptoms occurred during the first year. There are also other individual case reports such as those of MENDIRATTA et al. (1967) about a congenital meningioma, of LUYENDIJK and STAAL (1964) on an ependymoma in a child of 2 months, of SUNDER-PLASSMANN and JELLINGER (1972) about two cases in the first year, of KOOS and LAUBICHLER (1967) and many others.

The last problem is that of the *location* where we find different figures mentioned about infra- und supratentorial sites. For example there is the series of SUNDER-PLASSMANN and GRUNERT (1971), in which 67% of the tumors in infants were supratentorial and 25% infratentorial, while 8% were in both

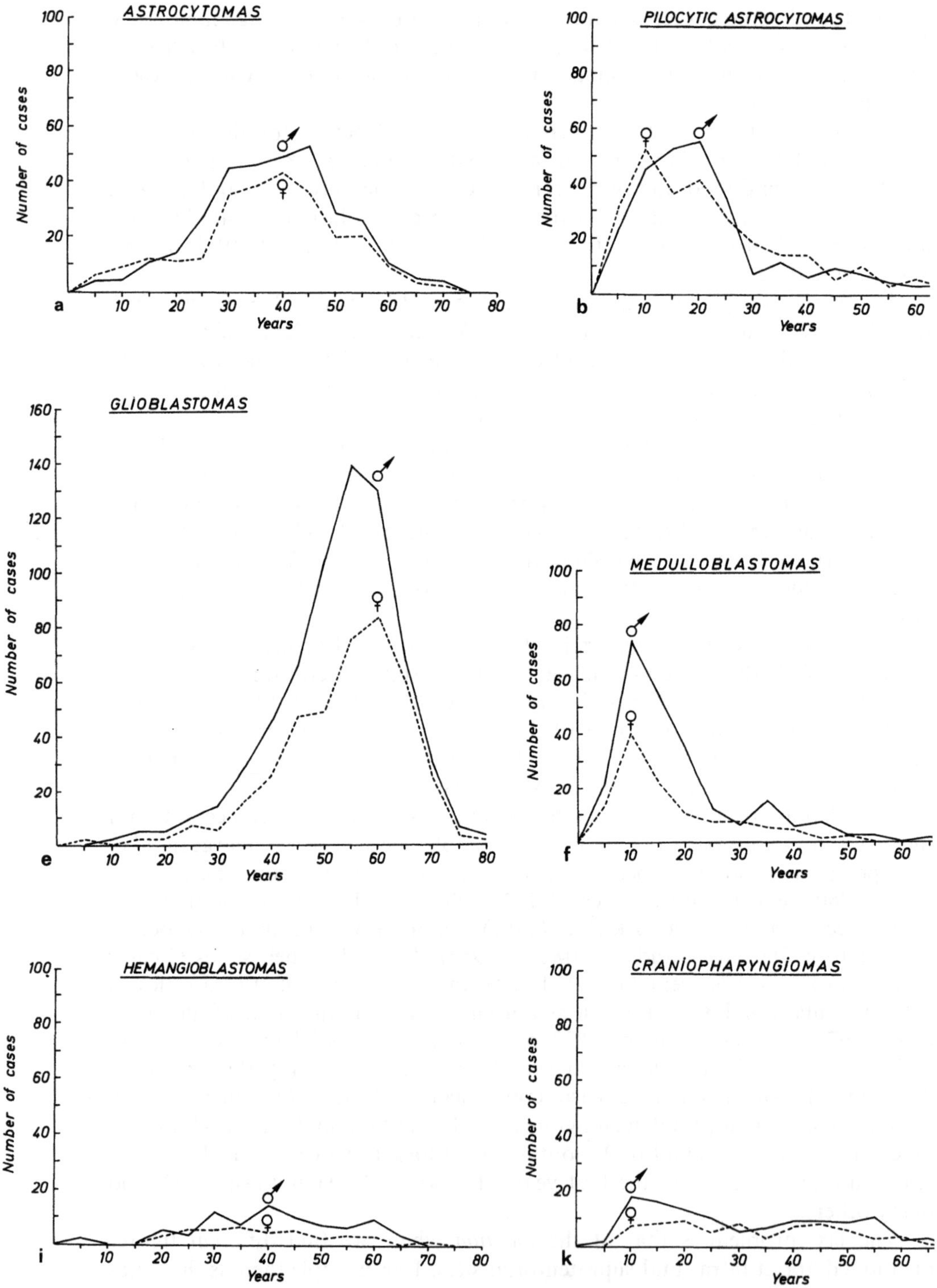

Fig. 9a–m. Frequency of different tumor types for the various age groups for each sex

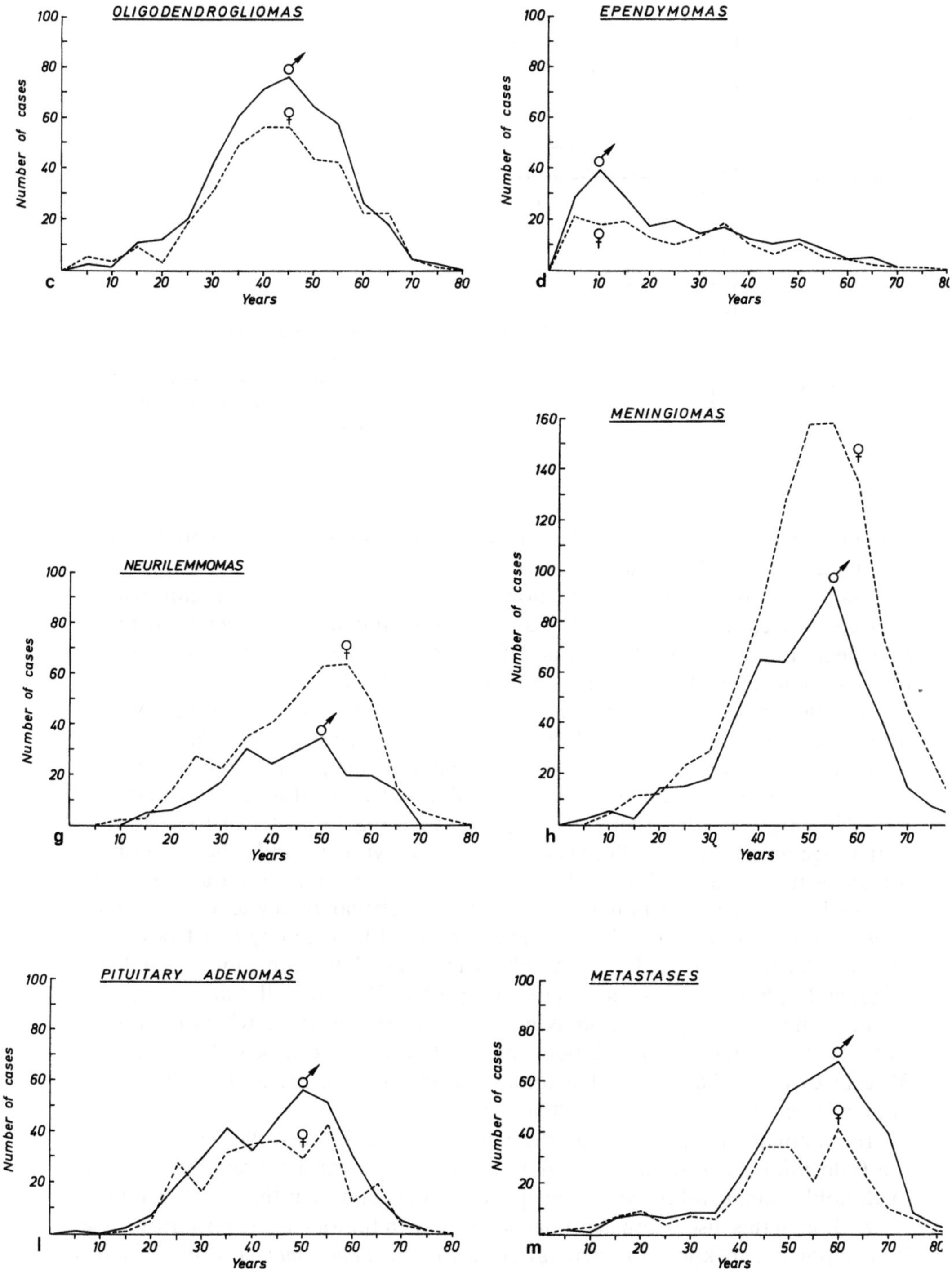
OLIGODENDROGLIOMAS
EPENDYMOMAS
NEURILEMMOMAS
MENINGIOMAS
PITUITARY ADENOMAS
METASTASES
Number of cases
Years
c
d
g
h
l
m

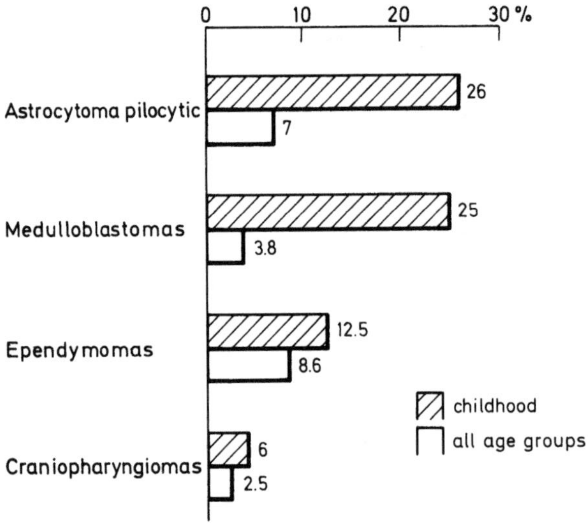

Fig. 10. Frequency of occurrence (as percentages) of different types of brain tumors in childhood and all age groups. (After BEHREND 1974)

locations at the same time. In the series of SATO and SANO (1975) 50.7% were infratentorial and 44.3% supratentorial.

The question of whether, and how many, tumors were spinal can also be answered. According to JÄNISCH et al. (1980) no spinal tumors occurred in the first year. In the series of ROSS and O.T. BAILEY (1953) 13 out of 63 spinal tumors occurred in childhood up until 16 years (21%).

In order to demonstrate *the spectrum* of the most common tumors in childhood I refer here to my series of 263 tumors (published in 1940b, Table 2).

A further interesting problem remains, namely, the *participation* of the various tumor groups *in the spectrum* of childhood and adolescence tumors of the CNS (Fig. 10). MECHTIJEVA (1954) found among 46 posterior fossa tumors in that age group, 26 medulloblastomas, 12 astrocytomas, and 3 hemangioblastomas. ARENDT and MÖLLER (1973) gave a very precise subgrouping of the tumors in their series: Among others 22.6% cerebellar pilocytic astrocytomas, 20.9% medulloblastomas, 11.1% ependymomas, 10.4% pilocytic astrocytomas of other localizations, 5.8% craniopharyngiomas, 3.4% pinealomas, and 2% oligodendrogliomas. MORI et al. (1977) reported 51% medulloblastomas, 31% astrocytomas, 18% ependymomas near the fourth ventricle, which comprised 29% of their tumors in childhood and adolescence. HOOPER (1976) observed 36 astrocytomas, 28 medulloblastomas, 18 ependymomas, and 16 brainstem gliomas (see also COHEN and DUFFNER 1983).

In summary, it appears that the average ratio for medulloblastomas and the (pilocytic) astrocytomas is almost equal, with a certain preference for the medulloblastomas, followed by the ependymomas and then the lesser groups.

Although this discussion dealt particularly with tumors of the posterior fossa, it is important to know the general rules for the *tumor incidence in childhood and adolescence* for the entire intracranial cavity. If we evaluate a large series of patients from this point of view we come to the conclusion that in childhood

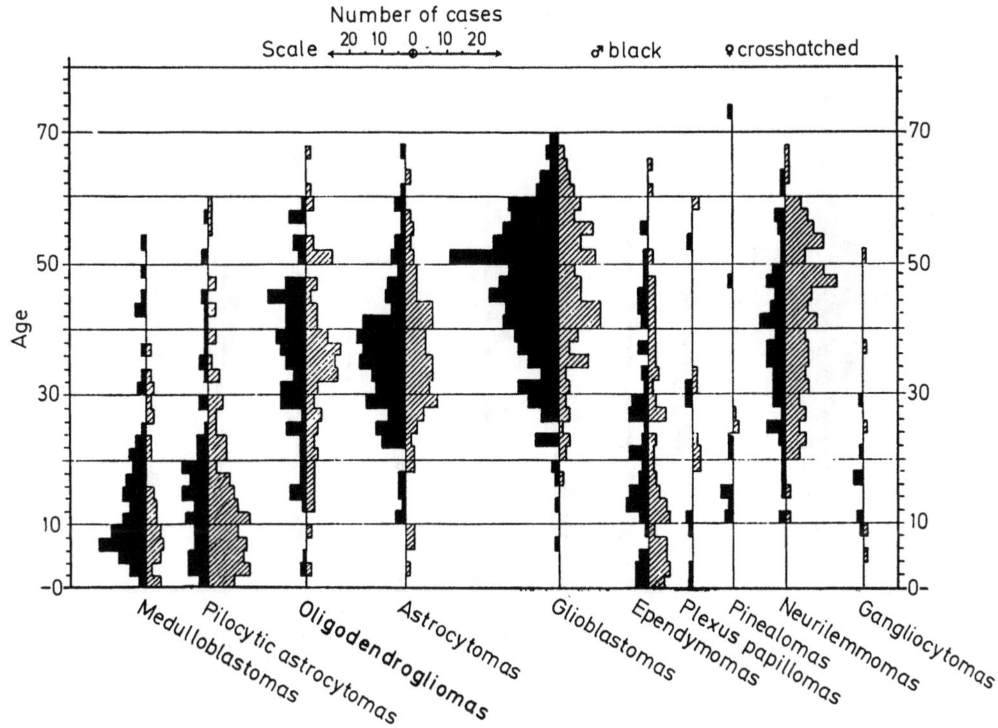

Fig. 11. Distribution of different tumor types by sex and age (in 1-year groups) (cf. Figs. 12, 13)

and adolescence the most common tumors in the cerebral hemispheres are ependymomas, whereas the other gliomas and ganglion cell tumors appear less frequently. Monstrocellular sarcomas are also encountered. On the other hand, we see only a few of meningiomas which form the single largest tumor group in the older age groups. In the chiasmal region craniopharyngiomas and pilocytic astrocytomas are frequent, while pituitary adenomas are rare. The complete absence of neurilemmomas is striking while in the cerebellum itself the bulk of all tumors occurring in the younger age group consists of medulloblastomas and pilocytic astrocytomas. Angioblastomas of the fourth ventricle are not very evident as yet. Teratomas and germinomas/pinealomas occur in this age group in the region of the quadrigeminal plate. Nearly all pilocytic astrocytomas around the aqueduct occur in patients under the age of 20. Other tumors of childhood and adolescence are the oligodendrogliomas of the thalamus and astrocytomas, particularly their pilocytic forms, in the pons.

The *middle decades* of life (third and fourth) are characterized by the frequent occurrence of gliomas of the cerebral hemispheres (astrocytomas and oligodendrogliomas), the meningiomas of various sites, pituitary adenomas, the neurilemmomas of the cerebellopontine angle, and the angioblastomas of the cerebellum. The two cerebellar tumor types seen in the younger age groups are encountered only rarely.

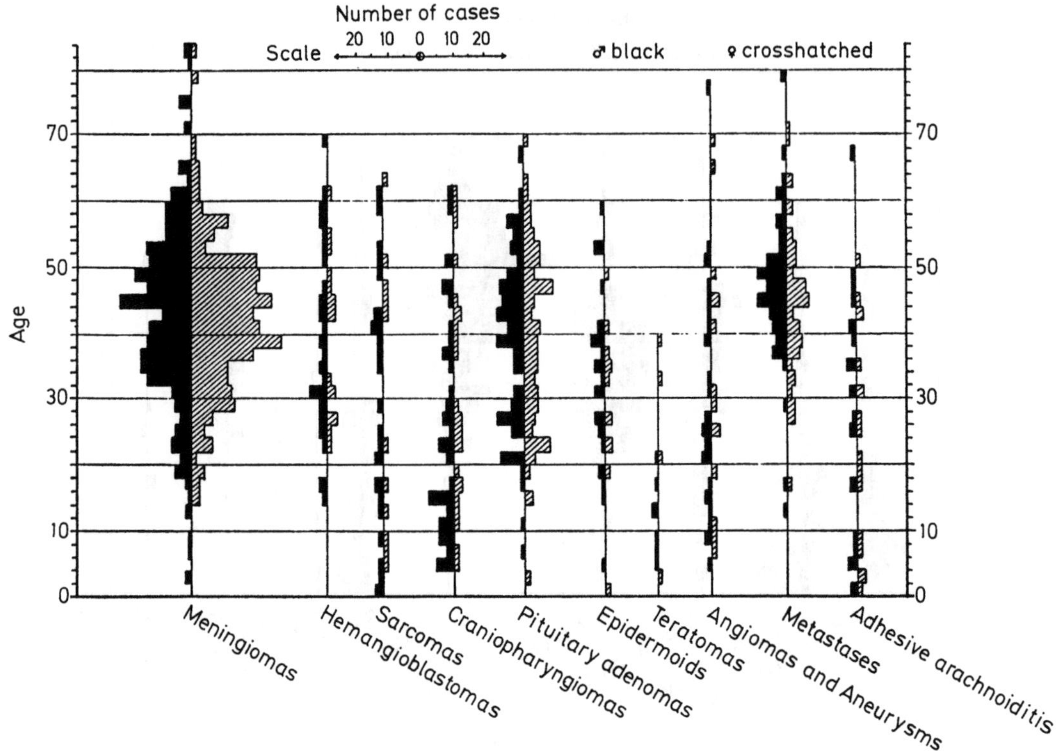

Fig. 12. Distribution of different tumor types by sex and age (in 1-year groups). (cf. Figs. 11, 13)

The *fifth and sixth decades* of life show a more frequent occurrence of malignant glioblastomas and of metastatic tumors, while oligodendrogliomas and astrocytomas, as well as meningiomas, angioblastomas, and neurilemmomas are still encountered. In the *seventh and eight decades* glioblastomas, meningiomas, and neurilemmomas comprise 82% of all CNS tumors found, and together with the metastatic tumors they clearly predominate. According to MOERSCH et al. (1941) 20% of all brain tumors occur in the sixth decade and 8% beyond the age of 60 (see also KLOSS 1952). VAN DER DRIFT and MAGNUS (1961) have plotted the distribution of the various tumors seen between the decades 51–60 and 61–70.

The relative frequency of the various tumor types within each age group and their sex distribution can be read from the three graphs in Figs. 11 and 12 (see also ZÜLCH and BORCK 1952). The above-mentioned predilection of tumors for childhood, middle age, involution and old age is very evident in these graphs.

Further References: ZÜLCH (1937c, 1938a, 1951d, 1965b, 1982b), BUCY (1947), BERKHEISER (1956), DEL REGATO (1958), RASKIND and BEIGEL (1964), WALTZ and BROWNELL (1966), LASSMAN and ARJONA (1967), CROUSE and BERG (1972), WECHSLER and ZÜLCH (1974), YOUNG et al. (1975), LIU et al. (1976), THOMPSON and GREEN (1976), COULON and TILL (1977), RICHMOND and WILSON (1978), DOHRMANN et al. (1978), FARWELL et al. (1978).

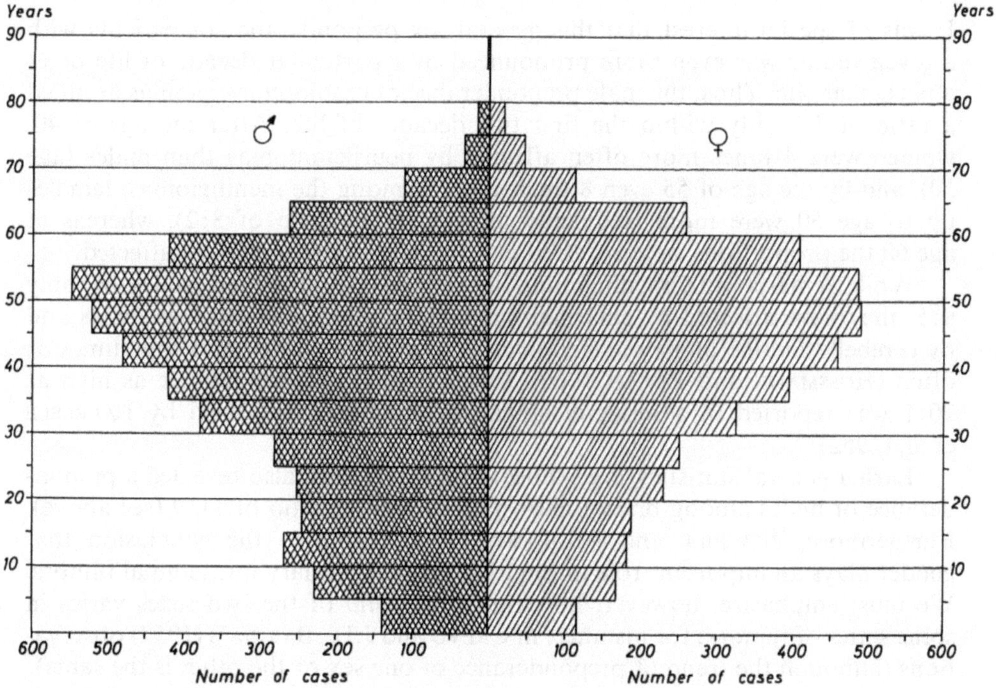

Fig. 13. Block diagram depicting the correlation between brain tumors of all types and patient age for each sex. (KAUTZKY, ZÜLCH et al. 1982)

4.2 Sex Distribution of Patients With Brain Tumors

Sex distribution and the discovery of a clear sex predilection of certain tumor types have proved to be particularly significant (ZÜLCH 1949; BORCK and ZÜLCH 1951; ZÜLCH and BORCK 1952).

An analysis of our total series has resulted in the general conclusion (Fig. 13) that there is a slight preponderance of males over females (52.8% to 47.2% or approximately 11:9), which corresponds to results previously mentioned in the literature. Moreover, certain brain tumors showed a particularly pronounced sex predilection.

Male predominance was found in a selected group of tumor cases as follows (ZÜLCH 1975a, p. 44):

Astrocytomas	7:5	Glioblastomas	6:4	Epidermoids	5:2
Oligodendrogliomas	5:4	Medulloblastomas	7:3	Angiomas and aneurysms	4:3
Ependymomas	6:4	Angioblastomas	2:1	Metastases	7:4
Pinealomas/ germinomas	2:1	Teratomas	4:3		
		Craniopharyngiomas	2:1		

Female preponderance was noted for:

Neurilemmomas	2:1	Pilocytic astrocytomas	11:9
Meningiomas	9:5		

It was of special interest that this general sex preponderance of patients with a given tumor was even more pronounced in a particular decade of life or at a particular site. Thus, the male preponderance of craniopharyngiomas attained a ratio of 4:1 only within the first two decades of life. After the age of 40, women were 4 times more often affected by neurilemmomas than males (age 50), and by the age of 55 even 8 times more. Among the meningiomas, females up to age 50 were more frequently affected (at a ratio of 3:2), whereas at age 60 the proportions were reversed and twice as many men were affected.

While females with meningiomas in general outnumbered males by only 9:5, they were affected by chiasmal meningiomas twice as often as males and by cerebellopontine angle meningiomas and spinal meningiomas four times as often (HOSSMANN and ZÜLCH 1966). Even a female preponderance as high as 20:1 was reported in a series of spinal meningiomas examined by LAPRESLE et al. (1952).

Earlier general statistics, e.g., those of STARR (1894), also revealed a preponderance of males among brain tumor patients with a ratio of 11:9 (see above). Furthermore, NEWBILL and ANDERSON (1944) came to the conclusion that gender plays an important role in the frequency of primary intracranial tumors. We must emphasize, however, how much the *ratio* of the two sexes varies in some series of tumors; for instance, in CALVO and J.L. BARCIA'S (1952) observations (although the trend of preponderance of one sex or the other is the same).

It seems important to us *that generally speaking the more malignant tumors of neuroepithelial origin have a preponderance in the male sex* (Figs. 12, 13), *whereas the benign tumors of the coverings of the brain and spinal cord occur more frequently in female hosts* (Figs. 11, 12). This will be discussed further below (p. 541).

BORCK in his doctorate (1950), BORCK and ZÜLCH (1951), and ZÜLCH (1956) have made a series of statements about particular features of the ratio between the two sexes in various smaller age periods. These were criticized by GÄRTNER (1955a) in a presentation of the biology of 654 intracranial tumors (versus more than 1000 in our collection).There were discrepancies between his statistics and ours. However, it seems to me that the size of his series is too small to show-up these interesting relations with sufficient exactness. We have therefore taken our last 1000 cases and undertaken another statistical analysis with the same results. We will defend these results until other statistics disprove them (Figs. 11, 12).

4.3 Frequency

The figure of 4–5 cases of brain tumor/annum/100000 population, reported by SCHOENBERG and CHRISTINE (1970), probably represents the most commonly cited data, although more recent and more refined studies have revealed higher frequencies. KURLAND et al. (1962) have recorded an incidence initially to be 4.2–5.4 for the United States and Canada. This value coincides with the number of deaths I had counted in 1951 (see above) on the basis of indirect calculations. Later these values were found to vary substantially with race, region, and sex.

Because of these discrepancies, the data collected in a small, but controlled, population such as those obtained in Rochester, Minnesota, are very valuable. Two studies were made there, one over a period of 10 years (1945–1954: KURLAND 1958) and another over 34 years (1935–1968: PERCY et al. 1972). The particular value of these precise and compact epidemiologic studies lies in the fact that half of the residents of the Rochester area were seen annually by a medical examiner. Moreover, the data were very carefully collected in the files of the Mayo Clinic and were available for re-examination. 36% of the primary CNS neoplasms were first diagnosed at autopsy. Annual incidence rates per 100000 population were 12.5 for primary brain neoplasms, 1.9 for pituitary neoplasms, 1.3 for primary spinal cord neoplasms, and 11.1 for metastases to the CNS.

From all these studies one can estimate an age-adjusted prevalence rate of 46/100000 inhabitants in the United States. Also an incidence rate of 10/100000 was estimated for all cases of primary cerebral tumors and the "probable" incidence in the United States was believed to be 15/100000 new cases per year.

However, KURLAND et al. in 1962, on the basis of data collected in Connecticut, Iowa and 10 open districts estimated the prevalence rate to be much lower than for the Rochester area, probably because of the more complete identification of cases in Rochester (autopsies). Equally important is the fact that 36% of the primary CNS neoplasms among the Rochester cases were not diagnosed until autopsy. The clinical diagnoses in these cases had been of something other than neoplasm. The number of asymptomatic tumors in the elderly was apparently large and they were only diagnosed post mortem. This fact is particular significant because the number of autopsies differs remarkably, namely 40% in Rochester versus 16% in Connecticut. Certainly SCHOENBERG and CHRISTINE (1970) were correct in stating that the incidence of brain tumor may increase with merely statistical diagnostic corrections, particularly since so many asymptomatic tumors were only discovered at autopsy (SCHOENBERG et al. 1978).

Other discrepancies concern the ratios of specific intracranial tumor types as observed in the very accurate study at the Mayo Clinic group. The ratio of meningiomas to gliomas, for instance, was 1:3. Amongst the tumors diagnosed during life the ratio was quite different, namely, 1:0.7. Finally, the ratio of all meningiomas to all gliomas in this study was 1.2:1. *This illustrates the appalling differences in the already published data brought about through methods of collecting statistical material which differ substantially from one country and one author to another.* Still more extreme is the reported percentage of 29% meningiomas amongst 1500 intracranial tumors in Iran (AMELI et al. 1979). This major difference may be due to socioeconomic factors such as the long and difficult journey to the capital and its neurosurgical clinics and by stimulation of the growth of meningiomas below areas of x-radiation for ringworm infection in childhood and youth (see p. 148).

Other Possibilities for Collecting Statistical Data. KURLAND (1958; KURLAND et al. 1962), KURTZKE (1969), and R.C. BEHREND (1974) recommended that one should only undertake *prospective* studies. Unfortunately this procedure takes an almost endless amount of time and does not satisfy the demands of today. There are two ways of collecting data which have been used in the past apart from such prospective studies. These must, of course, be properly designed and critically analyzed if they are to be useful.

Autopsy Statistics

In an earlier edition of this book, I cited data available from the past, starting with KLEBS (1877) in Prague, who found 74 brain tumors in 3622 autopsies (1.76%). STARR (1894) reported that in childhood and adolescence (which he, like us, defined as under 20 years of age) tuberculomas were 4 times as frequent as in the older age groups. GRUBER (1935) in Göttingen reported 79 intracranial tumors (1.3%) in 6000 autopsies. SCHMINCKE found 2.07% brain tumors out of 7642 autopsies in Tübingen (see RAPP 1924) and 1.4% primary brain tumors out of 31698 autopsies (1854–1931) in Heidelberg (SCHMINCKE 1933). RUDERSHAUSEN (1932) examined Schmincke's material in detail and found 444 primary tumors of the brain and 102 metastases. Among his 232 cases of gliomas there were 139 males and 93 females; granulomas were not included. GÄRTNER (1955a) continued with the series at the Heidelberg Institute for another 21 years, during which 710 intracranial mass lesions were recorded, in 654 of these proper evaluation was possible. The results have been compared with those obtained in our collection of 4000 cases and differ only in unimportant details. Our figures – stemming from various sources – can therefore be considered as fairly typical, varying in only minor items from those presented by LINK and SCHLEUSSING (1950).

At this point we must emphasize that the nature of the clinical departments, serviced by a pathological institute, is of considerable importance in determining the results of autopsies. It is the "genius loci", as I have called it, which directs many statistics. For instance, CUSHING's skill in operating on tumors of the chiasmatic region led to a high number of pituitary adenomas in his series. Autopsy statistics of an institute servicing a great neurological and neurosurgical department will be different from those of others.

Germany, when it still had a population of 70 million, had at that time about 800000 deaths per year, 140000 of which were due to malignant tumors. Early figures gave a cancer mortality rate of 26/10000, compared to a general mortality rate of 106/10000 (see also FREUDENBERG 1955, for the FRG). Since the central nervous system share of tumors is about 2% (NAFFZIGER and BOLDREY 1948), we can indirectly calculate the mortality rate from brain and spinal cord tumors to be about 1:20000 or 1:25000 population per year, corresponding to the existing age distribution. That was the figure, which I cited above as having it reported in my first edition as early as 1951.

Other data regarding the frequency of brain tumors in autopsy statistics have been uninformative when based on hospital admissions (MCLEAN 1936a: 0.2–2.6%). In 20000 admissions to the Wenzel Hanke Krankenhaus, Breslau (Otfrid FOERSTER 1934) 4.6% of patients had brain tumors (see owing to the "genius loci" above). BAILEY (1933) calculated the corresponding figures for three London hospitals as 1.8% of 15000 admissions. The statistics of the Royal

Infirmary at Leeds revealed 167 brain tumors (1.3%) out of 13000 patients admitted, but the brain was examined only in 27% of the autopsies. From the autopsy figures of PEERS (1936) at Boston City Hospital more information was gained. Autopsies performed on 10592 patients in 38 years showed 16.8% tumors as the cause of death. Among these were 188 CNS tumors with 43.1% gliomas. Apparently PEERS observed no variation over 39 years on his autopsy service. However, he pointed also to the discrepancies between neurosurgical series and those recorded at necropsy.

The question arises as to whether data collected 100 years ago are of any importance, because the classification of the tumor type may have changed. Nevertheless we have stressed since 1951, that the spectrum of tumors since CRUVEILHIER (1829/1835) and Johannes von MÜLLER (1838) through that of VIRCHOW and his monograph (1863/65), and finally up to modern times has not shown a significant variation in the *type* of tumors.

In concluding this review, I would like to draw attention to the statistics of the General Pathological Institute in Düsseldorf and its data from 1908 to 1964 (POCHE and HOFFMANN 1968), which has definitely changed with the establishment of such new specialties as neurology, neurological surgery, and thoracic surgery. There has been a significant shift in the number and ratio of the various tumor types (operable tumors, glioblastomas, metastases). Therefore, such statistics must be adjusted and interpreted according to the structure of the hospital.

Mortality Statistics, National or International

Official mortality statistics are usually based on some international classification, e.g., the International Statistical Classification of Diseases (ISCD) or the classification of the World Health Organization (so-called *Blue Books*), which is now used in many countries (available since 1979 for the classification of CNS tumors; see ZÜLCH 1979). However, in the ISCD the rubrics are so ill-defined that the system preclude making an exact neurologic and neuropathologic classification. This is possible only with the WHO system, which is especially adapted for that purpose.

Kurtzke (1969) noted that the number of spinal and other tumors of the nervous system was so low that it could be safely ignored in many of the general statistical analyses. GOLDBERG and KURLAND (1962) tried to compare age-adjusted mortality rates for all cerebral tumors from 27 countries and found that they were all close to 5/100000. However, some years later KURTZKE (1969) expressed the opinion that the methodologic differences revealed by an analysis of this kind made it difficult to accept any comparative studies, particularly the mortality data for "nonwhites" in the United States. These were open to grave suspicion. Therefore mortality rates had to be adjusted according to the "number of physicians per head of population" which, according to R.C. BEHREND (1974), would give a good index for the re-evaluation of the data.

Perhaps it is possible to use data already collected for a general survey, which showed, for example, that the brain tumor death rate is equal in Denmark and United States (KURTZKE 1969). Furthermore, the, incidence that tumor deaths are fairly uniformly distributed would not favor a unifactorial pathogenesis but rather an endogenous or multifactorial one.

In Israel, COHEN and MODAN (1968) found a brain tumor incidence of 4.4/100000 of which 2.4/100000 were benign. Apparently there was a difference between the European and Israeli born population on the one hand, and the Asiatic and African born population on the other. This was further emphasized by the figures of LEIBOWITZ et al. (1971) who gave a brain tumor incidence of 12.8/100000 with differences between the populations born in Africa, Asia, or Europe.

Another different type of analysis of tumor incidence for the United States can be found in a 1975 editorial (no author cited) in the Archives of Neurology. The following data reported there were remarkable: (a) the incidence was 5.3/100000, (b) of all the patients suffering from cancer, 0.61% had CNS tumors, (c) 665000 new cases in one year of intracranial tumors occurred in a population of 200 million, (d) 18% of the cancer patients had cerebral metastases when they died of cancer; two thirds were mass lesions, one-fifth meningeal seedings, and the rest mixed.

There are excellent data for the incidence and prevalence of brain tumors in the autopsy material available in the German Democratic Republic, where there is an official cancer register with obligatory notification. The towns of Erfurt and Suhl (GDR) with around 1.8 million inhabitants recorded 631 new tumors of the nervous system in one year, of which 381 (60%) were neuroectodermal. There was a 5.1 incidence for all intracranial tumors (see the figures given above). Some general trends were also visible (e.g., a male preference for the neuroectodermal tumors, and a female preference for the mesodermal tumors, which concurs with the data already given p. 93). Some data are also available for the Federal Republic of Germany (WAGNER 1978). The overall mortality figures for West Germany included 20.8% deaths from cancer and related malignant tumors. A new tabulation of data was given for Sweden in 1971 (RINGERTZ et al. 1971). In the years 1959–1965 only 3.2% of all cancer cases were intracranial tumors among males, and 3.1% among females with a mean age of 50.9 and 50.38 years respectively. Data on the histology of the tumors were also given. Roughly 71% of all male cases of histologically verified intracranial tumors were gliomas, but only 51% among the females. The crude type and sex ratio were somewhat different from those in most world statistics. This is in conformity with RINGERTZ et al. (1962). In their data for 1959, tumors of the CNS represented 3.3% of the neoplasms which were designated as "cancer". Of the 3.3%, 349 patients were men, and 326 women. The distribution of these tumors by sex and tumor type is shown in Table 6.

Other lesser information about special population groups came, for instance, from BARKER et al. (1976), who reported on the Southampton area where among 1.5 million people over 15 years of age 894 patients had gliomas (this was the commonest tumor group) with an incidence of 394/100000. CHOI et al. (1970a) reported from the Minnesota area about 760 patients among whom there was an excess proportion of brain tumor deaths in the *immigrants* from Norway,

Table 6. Distribution by age and sex of neoplasms designated cancer in data for 1959

	Total		Intracranial		Intraspinal	
	M	F	M	F	M	F
Medulloblastoma	6	4	6	4	–	–
Malignant glioma	120	86	120	84	–	2
Sarcoma	1	3	1	3	–	–
Astrocytoma, oligodendroglioma	58	45	56	45	2	–
Ependymoma	11	11	11	11	–	–
Choroidal papilloma	–	1	–	1	–	–
Pinealoma	1	1	1	1	–	–
Meningioma	68	94	68	81	–	13
Neurinoma	24	30	17	23	7	7
Angioma	9	9	7	9	2	–
Craniopharyngioma	6	9	6	9	–	–
Other with PAD	4	3	2	3	2	–
No histological examination	41	30	38	28	3	2
	349[a]	326[a]	333	302	16	24

The particular value of this statistical series lies in the accuracy of the classification, which follows closely the one used in this book (Table BB in RINGERTZ et al. 1962, p. 45).

[a] Two pinealoma cases, one in a patient of each sex, were taken from Table 7, p. 72, of the book by RINGERTZ et al. (1962)

Germany, Canada, and Finland. FAN et al. (1977) reported on a higher mortality rate of brain tumors in a Jewish residence in New York compared to that among Protestants and Catholics. FAN et al. (1977), however, provided another important piece of information based on thorough evaluation of the *American Forces Institute of Pathology* data. They noted a higher relative frequency of primary CNS tumors in American Caucasians than in American Negroes. The latter have a population index of 8.4%, however, a tumor index in this tabulation of 13.7%. Furthermore, gliomas were seen significantly more frequently in the Caucasians, and pituitary adenomas and meningiomas in the Negroes. Interesting information has also come from *Japan*, where medical conditions and statistics are very "westernized." KATSURA et al. (1959) screened 3312 cases from 23 surgical clinics and found the incidence of gliomas to be smaller than in the United States and Europe. Meningiomas seem to have been equal while neurilemmomas and pituitary adenomas were more common in Japan. There was also a higher figure for pineal tumors and craniopharyngiomas in Japan (UEKI 1963).

Pinealomas (tumors of the pineal region) were 3.9% in UEKI'S (1963) series of tumors, 8% in ARAKI and MATSUMOTO'S series (1969), 7.5% in ARAI et al. series (1976), 5.6% in ITO'S (1958), and 9.3% in the report of KATSURA et al. (1959). The proportion of pinealomas/germinomas in our series of 9000 cases was 0.5% and in CUSHING'S (1932, 1935) collection 0.6%.

Similar discrepancies were found in the percentage of neurilemmomas, as pointed out by R.C. BEHREND (1974, Table 3, p. 65). GRANT (USA, 1956) found

4.6% in 3326 cases and KATSURA et al. (1959) 12.1% in 3312 cases, whereas in our 6000 case series they comprised 7.6%. According to DASTUR and LALITHA (India, 1968) very different figures came out about the occurrence of ependymomas, which constituted 23.8% of all gliomas in children, in contrast to the lower proportion of medulloblastomas in the same series with 21.8%. This must be a consequence of a considerable divergence in classification (see also DASTUR et al. 1968).

There are also very gross and partly contradictory figures about the occurrence of certain tumor groups in North America, Europe, Africa, and Asia. In an earlier report JANSSEN and PIRAUX (1955) showed that most of the common tumors occur in Blacks. In more specific data about the Bantus FROMAN and LIPSCHITZ (1970) reported 30.3% meningiomas and 16% gliomas, and in 20 years only 1 acoustic neurilemmoma. They also reported a female predilection for spinal meningiomas (sex ratio 12:3), which corresponds to the reports from the United States and Germany (see p. 541 and p. 358 ff.).

PROCTOR (South Africa, 1955) reported that astrocytomas and meningiomas occur 5 to 6 times more commonly in Europeans than in Bantus (7597 autopsy protocols from the Johannesburg area). A report of LEIBOWITZ et al. (1971) inform us about *Israel* where the incidence of CNS tumors was very high (1354 cases or 12.8/100000). Africa-born Jews had the lowest incidence, European-born the highest (15.6/100000) and Asian-born had an intermediate value. COHEN and MODAN (1968) had pointed out earlier that the malignant tumors occurred at a significantly higher ratio in European and Israeli-born individuals.

SHUANGSHOTI et al. (1969) presented a general review from *Thailand* were the spectrum of tumors was quite similar. Astrocytomas were the most common glioma being almost as frequent as meningiomas and twice as common as glioblastomas. SHUANGSHOTI and PANYATHANYA (1974) completed the collection of these data from a series of 2897 cases. YENERMEN (1955) in *Turkey* collected 11318 autopsies with 1669 intracranial tumors, out of which 58.51% were gliomas. ADELOYE and ODEKU (1969) reported that gliomas were less frequent in Africans than in Europeans. In Rhodesia (now Zimbabwe) the relative frequency of astrocytomas in the European and African populations was 30% and 15% respectively. Meningiomas were the commonest histologic variety of brain neoplasms in Africa. They constituted 30% of all brain tumors in Bantus. In Rhodesia meningiomas accounted for 21% and 12% of intracranial tumors respectively among Africans and Europeans. There was a deviation from this general trend in Egypt and even more so in Senegal (Dakar), where the pattern was closer to that of Europe. The probable causes of this high number of meningiomas were discussed by AMELI et al. (1979) (see p. 95).

This compendium of data could be extended endlessly, but I will terminate it with the report of ANNEGERS et al. (1981:1935–1977). These epidemiologists found a tumor incidence in male subjects of 8.3/100000, of which 4 were gliomas, 1.2 meningiomas, and 1.5 pituitary adenomas. In female subjects the incidence was 10.1/100000, with 4.1 gliomas, 2.6 meningiomas, and 1.7 pituitary adenomas. They concluded that these figures, all of which were obtained from cohort studies, could not be compared between places or over time. They stated that conclusions should be only very carefully drawn and pointed out the marked increase in the incidence of pituitary adenomas in girls and women 15–44 years of age among less than 1–7 cases per 100000 population in the various regions.

Finally, I must mention the discussion of GOLDBERG and KURLAND who suggested as long ago as 1962 *that many of the differences were due "to artefacts of reporting and diagnosis."*

Nevertheless, questions of pathogenesis are sometimes of interest when examining such data. The possible inferences for host and environmental influences as well as ethnic peculiarities will be discussed in Chap. 3.

Relative Frequency of Intracranial Tumors in Large Series

The relative frequency for the 9000 case neurosurgical series collected in our institute was published in 1975 (GP, p. 48) (Table 7).

ZIMMERMAN (1969) tabulated the relative frequency for the large collections in New Haven, New York, and Boston as well as those of West Germany (ZÜLCH), India (DASTUR), and the ITO series in Japan. The relative frequencies in these combined series were as follows (ZIMMERMAN 1969, Table 2):

Gliomas	36.5%
Meningiomas	12.5%
Neurilemmomas	4.9%
Medulloblastomas	4.1%

On the other hand, the tabulation in ZIMMERMAN'S personal series (neuroepithelial; ZIMMERMAN 1969, Table 3) was:

Glioblastomas	51.3%
Astrocytomas	24.5%
Ependymomas	6.4%
Oligodendrogliomas	5.5%
Astrocytomas, pilocytic	3.4%

Further References: EARLE et al. (1957), RINGERTZ (1971).

4.4 Preferential Sites of Brain Tumors

Brain tumors can occur singly or in multiple sites, can be diffuse, and are usually restricted to the CNS. Most, however, are single growths (KRAUSE and ZÜLCH 1951).

Long experience has shown (and it is easily understandable from what we know of embryology) that pituitary adenomas, germinomas/pinealomas, and craniopharyngiomas occur only at particular sites, and that the neurilemmomas (of the cerebellopontine angle) prefer the *acoustic* nerve (although experimentally *trigeminal* neurilemmomas are preponderant). Meningiomas and cerebellar tumors also show a similar regularity in preferential occurrence (CUSHING 1930/31; CUSHING and EISENHARDT 1938).

Table 7. Review of the classification of 4000, 6000 and 9000 brain tumors compared with Cushing's (1932) and Jänisch's et al. (1976) series. (After Zülch 1975a)

	Personal series of 4000		Personal series of 6000		Personal series of 9000[a]		Cushing's series	Jänisch's et al. series	
	Cases	% of total	Cases	% of total	Cases	% of total	% of total	Cases	% of total
Astrocytomas	283	7.1	381	6.4	591	6.6	9.8	408	24.1
Pilocytic astrocytomas	292	7.1	419	7.0	538	6.0	6.1	–	–
Oligodendrogliomas	312	7.8	490	8.2	859	9.6	1.3	24	1.4
Ependymomas	184	4.6	259	4.3	384	4.3	1.3	55	3.3
Plexus papillomas	20	0.5	30	0.5	52	0.6	0.6	11	0.7
Pinealomas	16	0.4	25	0.4	48	0.5	0.7	10	0.6
Gangliocytomas	15	0.4	27	0.4	38	0.4	0.2	1	0.06
Glioblastomas	530	13.3	738	12.3	1093	12.2	10.3	473	28.0
Medulloblastomas	161	4.0	230	3.8	373	4.2	4.3	58	3.4
Neurilemmomas	297	7.5	451	7.6	614	6.8	8.7	85	5.0
Meningiomas	723	18.1	1079	18.0	1492	16.6	13.4	326	19.3
Hemangioblastomas	60	1.5	78	1.3	119	1.3	1.2	14	0.8
Sarcomas	74	1.9	162	2.7	372	4.3	0.7	44	2.6
Epidermoids, Dermoids[a], Teratomas	78	1.8	128	2.1	166	1.8	0.9	24	1.4
Craniopharyngiomas	107	2.7	150	2.5	185	2.1	4.6	24	1.4
Chondromas, Osteomas[a], Lipomas	20	0.7	53	0.9	–	–	0.8	6	0.4
Fibromas	5	0.1	7	0.1	–	–	–	–	–
Angiomas and aneurysms[a]	83	2.1	151	2.5	337	3.8	1.0	–	–
Pituitary adenomas	282	7.1	478	8.0	596	6.6	17.8	76	4.5
Chordomas	9	0.2	14	0.2	75	0.8	0.1	–	–
Cylindromatous epitheliomas	8	0.2	12	0.2	–	–	–	–	–
Metastases	163	4.1	242	4.0	636	7.1	3.2	–	–
Unclassified tumors	151	3.8	221	3.7	286	3.2	9.6	48	2.9
Parasites[a]	6	0.2	9	0.1	–	–	0.1	–	–
Granulomas	32	0.8	45	0.7	–	–	2.2	–	–
Arachnoiditis and ependymitis[a]	53	1.3	92	1.5	–	–	1.1	–	–
Miscellaneous (myelomas, Schüller-Christian disease etc.)	28	0.8	39	0.6	146	1.6	–	–	–

OSTERTAG (1936b, 1952) and P. SCHWARZ (1932, 1936) are credited with having demonstrated similar relationships for some other types of glioma. Unfortunately, however, in their regional classification both authors paid little attention to the characteristic that is most decisive for the neurosurgeon, namely, the tissue type of the tumor. Moreover, occasionally tumors in the same location but of a different type were grouped together which was an understandable oversight since the idea of dysontogenetic origin was uppermost in Ostertag's mind.

I have reversed the former procedure by starting with the histologic tumor type and then establishing its site of predilection. On this basis and after considerable experience, I can confirm the concept of a preferential site for each type of brain tumor in the overwhelming majority of instances and have found it to be especially pronounced with respect to glioblastomas.

Whereas the figures (Fig. 14) only illustrate the types commonly in particular sites occurring the subsequent *text lists them according to the relative frequency at which they occur in each of the various intracerebral locations*. The intracranial extensions from the base and vault of the skull will be demonstrated in a special schematic drawing (Fig. 15).

Special characteristics or little frequencies are added in parentheses/brackets.

Frontal lobes

Frontodorsal: Astrocytomas, glioblastomas, meningiomas (parasagittal, uni- or bilateral)
Frontolateral: Oligodendrogliomas, glioblastomas, meningiomas (of the convexity), astrocytomas (with spread to the insula)
Frontomedial: Oligodendrogliomas (parasagittal with extension into the corpus callosum), astrocytomas (with spread to the septum), meningiomas (of the falx, uni- or bilateral)
Frontobasal: Glioblastomas, meningiomas (of the olfactory groove)
Diffuse: Astrocytomas

Temporal lobes

Temporolateral: Oligodendrogliomas, glioblastomas, meningiomas (Sylvian fissure), astrocytomas
Temporobasal: Gangliocytomas, meningiomas, chordomas
Temporomedial: Glioblastomas, oligodendrogliomas

Parietal lobes

Parietolateral: Astrocytomas, oligodendrogliomas, glioblastomas, ependymomas and pilocytic astrocytomas (in adolescence), meningiomas (of the convexity)
Parietodorsal: Glioblastomas, astrocytomas, meningiomas (parasagittal)
Parietomedial: Astrocytomas

Occipital lobes. Glioblastomas spreading from the corpus callosum or its radiation, meningiomas (posterior third of the sagittal sinus, tentorium/torcular) [astrocytomas and oligodendrogliomas spreading from the temporal or parietal region]

---

[a] This last classification comprises the earlier series of 4000 and 6000; the recent series of 9000 however, was compiled according the scheme proposed by the UICC. Therefore some alterations between the earlier and the last series were necessary: dermoids and epidermoids were put into one rubric. Some entities which were not contained in the UICC classification, were deleted and the tumors summarized under the heading "miscellaneous". Some of the percentages are grossly rounded off

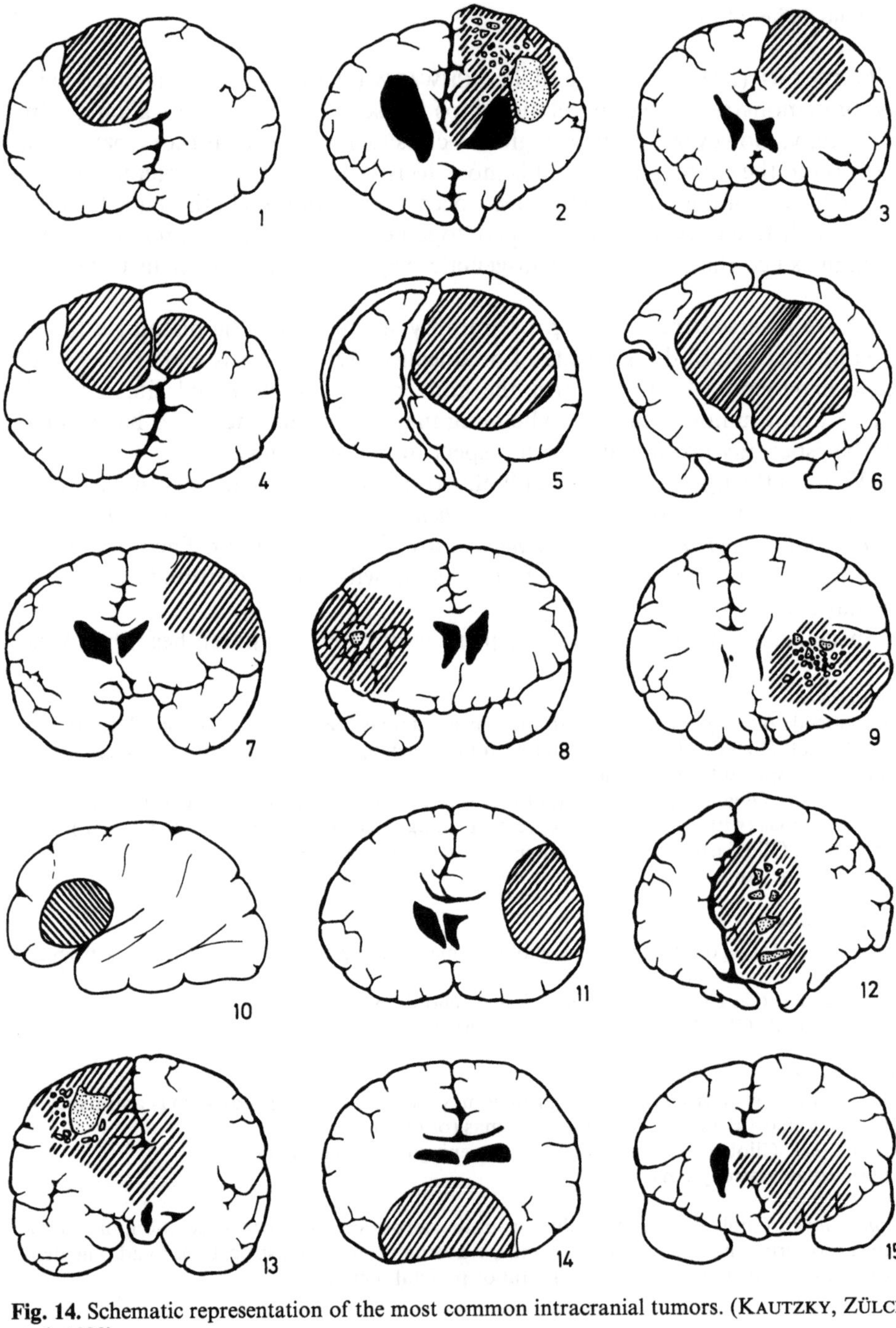

Fig. 14. Schematic representation of the most common intracranial tumors. (KAUTZKY, ZÜLCH et al. 1982)

Frontal tumors: *1,* Meningioma of the anterior third of the sagittal sinus – frontodorsal meningioma; *2,* frontodorsal astrocytoma; *3,* frontodorsal glioblastoma; *4,* meningioma of the anterior third of the sagittal sinus (bilateral); *5,* falx meningioma (frontomedial meningioma); *6,* bilateral falx meningioma; *7,* frontolateral glioblastoma; *8,* frontolateral oligodendroglioma; *9,* frontolateral astrocytoma; *10,* frontolateral (F3) meningioma; *11,* frontolateral meningioma (also known as the convexity meningioma); *12,* frontomedial astrocytoma; *13,* frontomedial oligodendroglioma (parasagittal oligodendroglioma); *14,* olfactory groove meningioma (frontobasal meningioma); *15,* frontobasal glioblastoma.

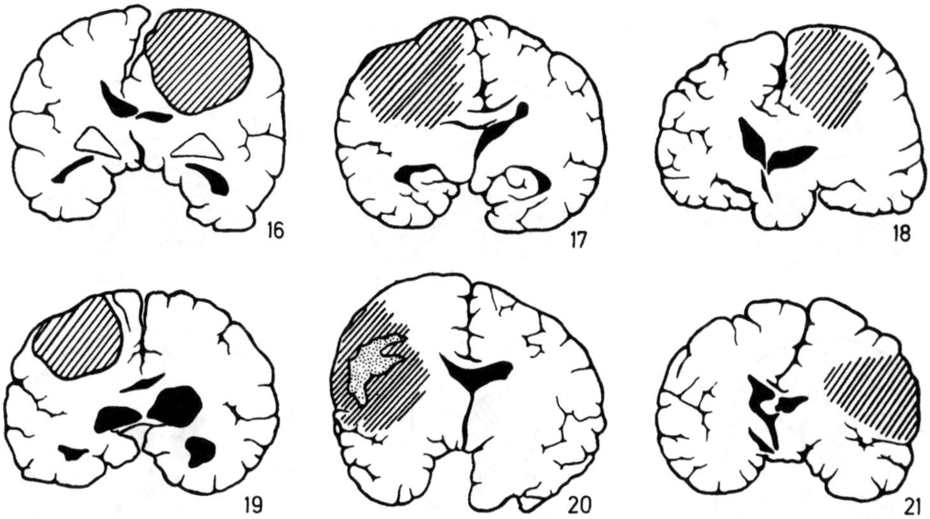

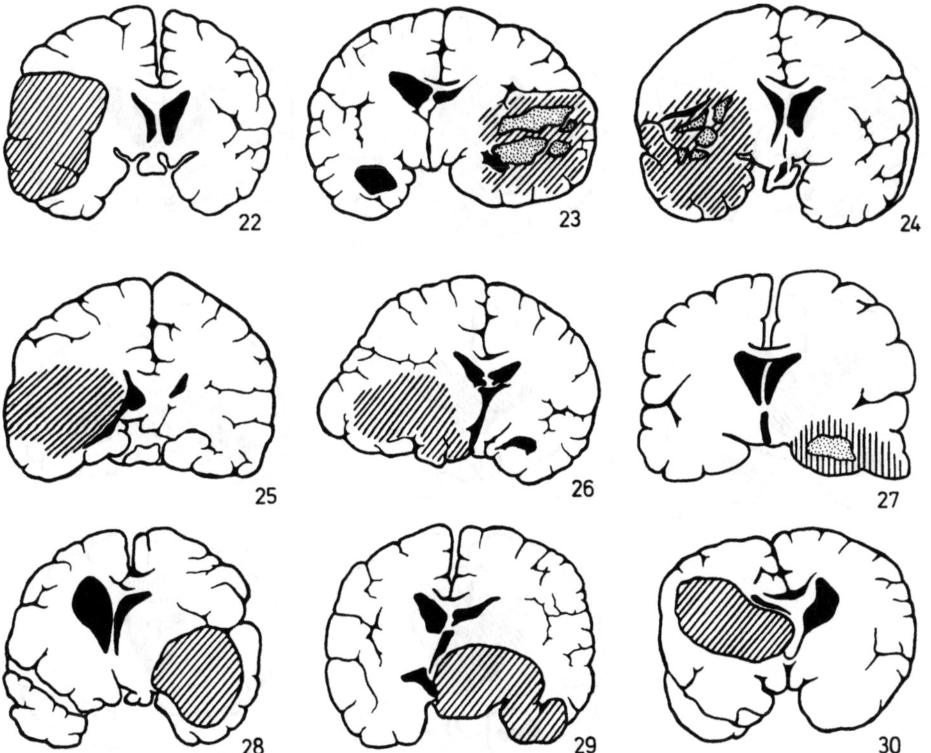

Parietal tumors: 16, Parietodorsal meningioma (meningioma of the middle third of the sagittal sinus); *17,* parietodorsal oligodendroglioma; *18,* parietodorsal glioblastoma; *19,* meningioma of the convexity; *20,* parietolateral astrocytoma; *21,* parietolateral glioblastoma.

Temporal tumors: 22, Meningioma of the sylvian fissure; *23,* temporal astrocytoma; *24,* temporal oligodendroglioma; *25,* temporolateral glioblastoma; *26,* temporomedial glioblastoma; *27,* temporobasal gangliocytoma; *28,* sphenoid wing meningioma; *29,* meningioma-en-plaque of the sphenoid wing; *30,* ependymoma of the cerebral hemisphere (cerebral ependymoma).

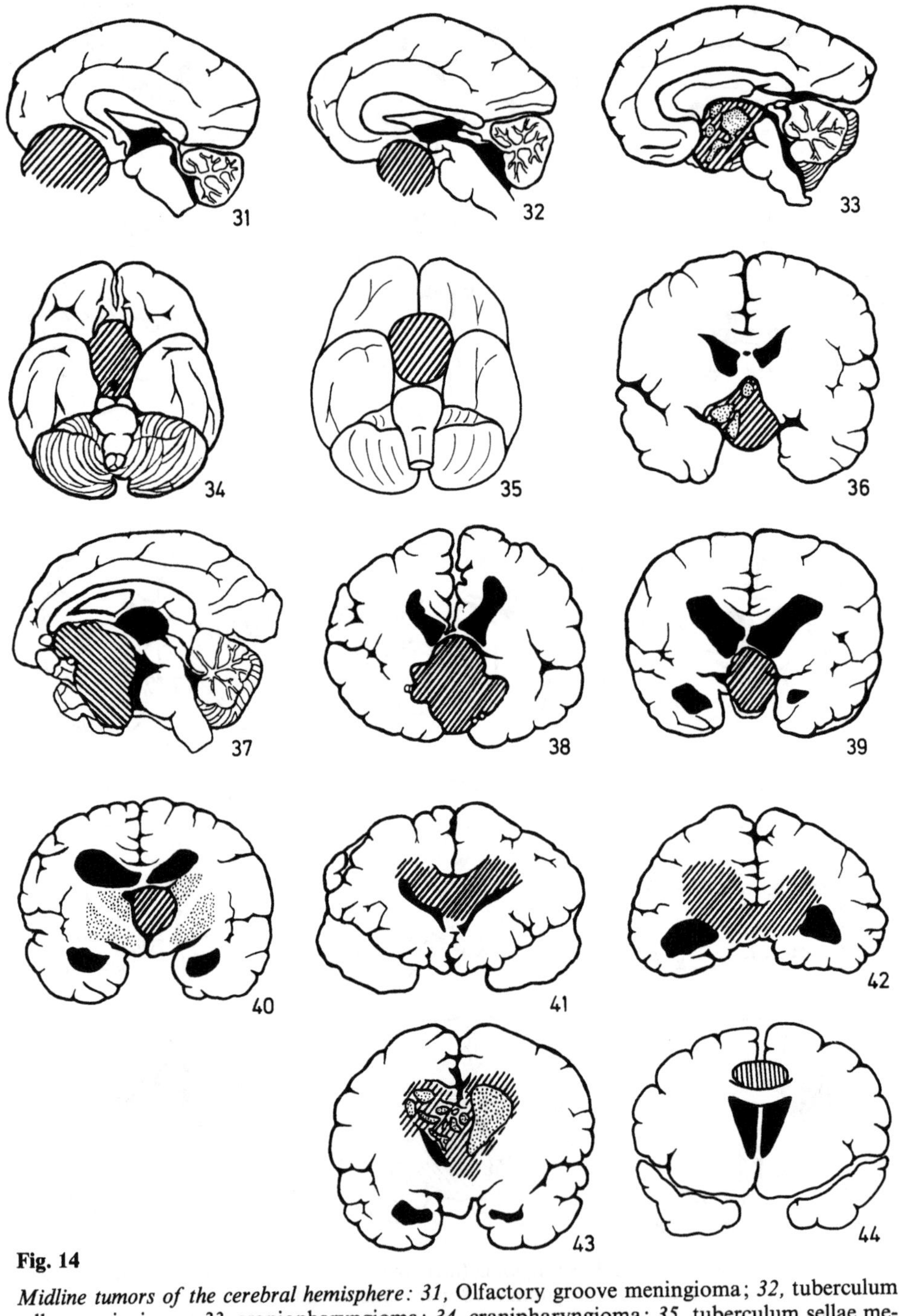

Fig. 14

Midline tumors of the cerebral hemisphere: 31, Olfactory groove meningioma; *32,* tuberculum sellae meningioma; *33,* craniopharyngioma; *34,* cranipharyngioma; *35,* tuberculum sellae meningioma; *36,* craniopharyngioma; *37,* pituitary adenoma; *38,* pituitary adenoma; *39,* pilocytic astrocytoma of the chiasm; *40,* ependymal (colloid) cyst of the foramen of Monro; *41,* glioblastoma of the rostral corpus callosum; *42,* glioblastoma of the caudal corpus callosum; *43,* oligodendroglioma of the corpus callosum; *44,* lipoma of the corpus callosum.

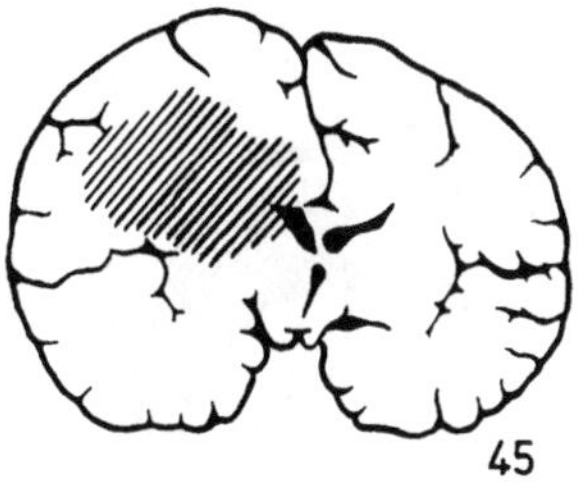
45

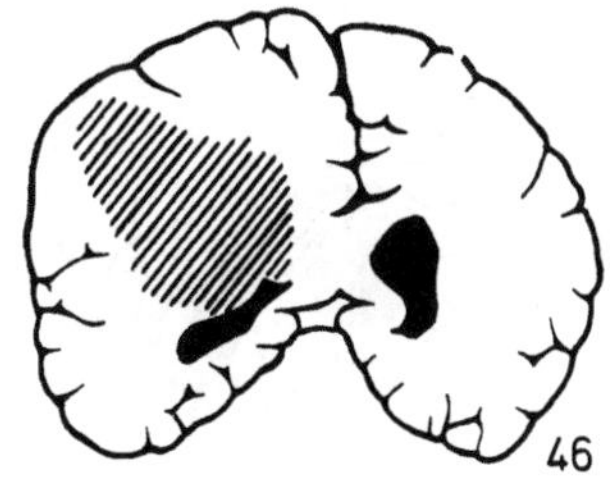
46

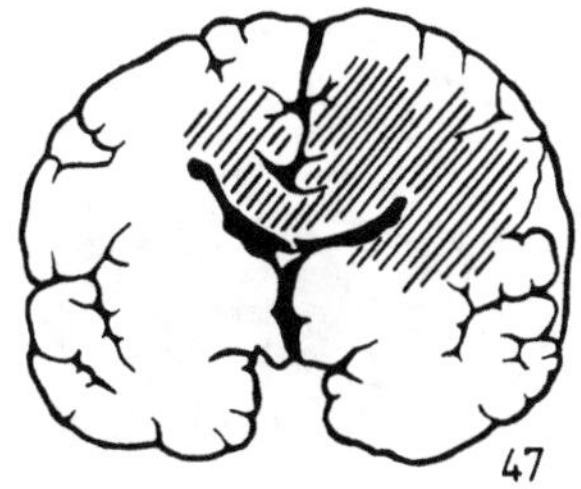
47

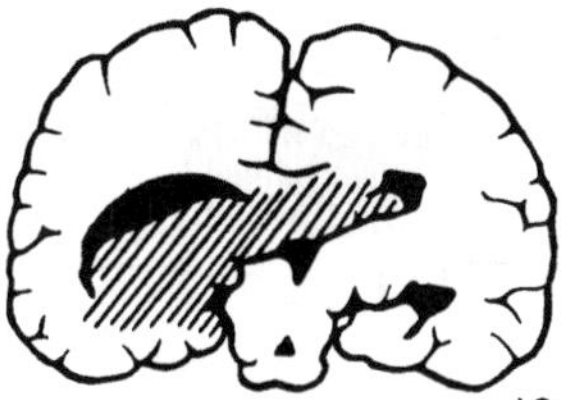
48

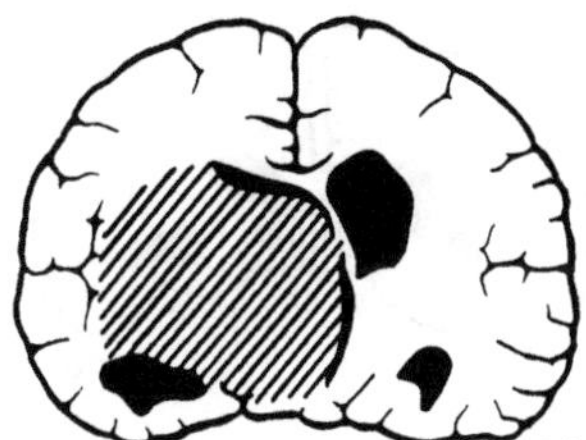
49

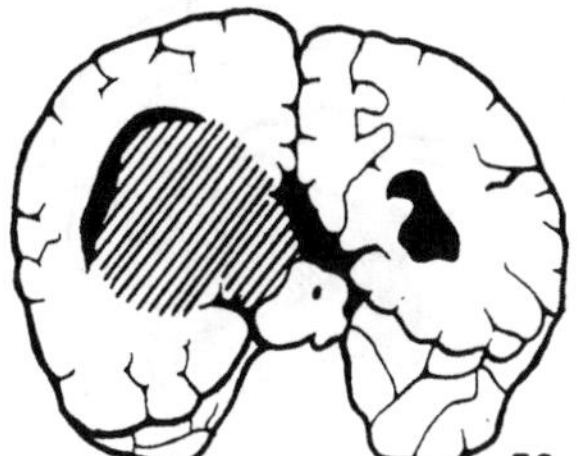
50

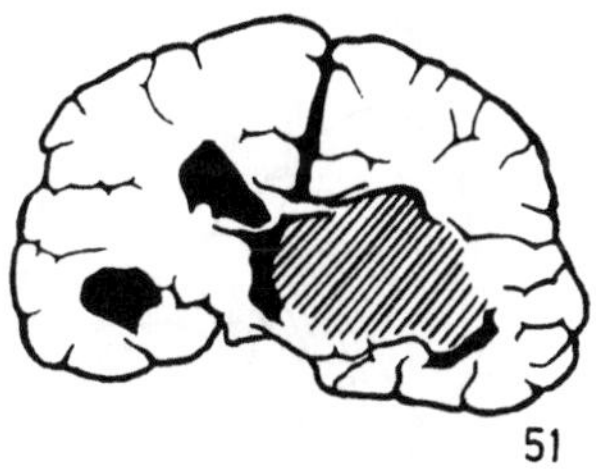
51

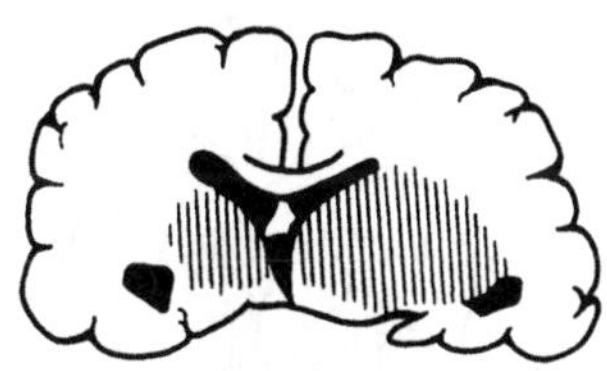
52

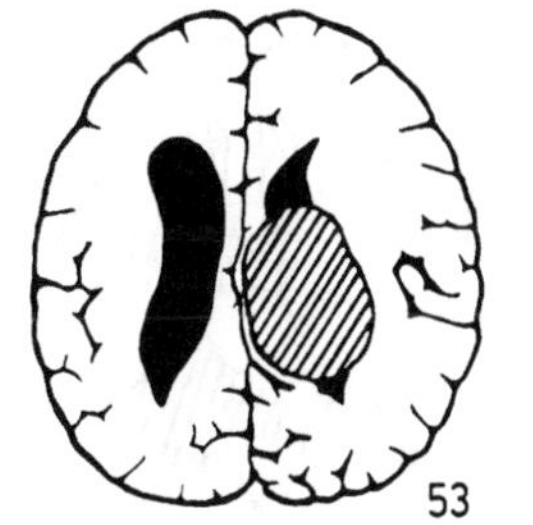
53

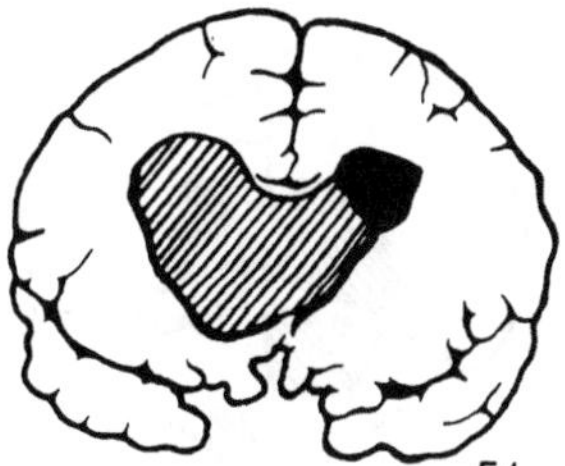
54

Paramedian tumors of the cerebral hemisphere: 45, Glioblastoma of the rostral radiation of the corpus callosum; *46,* glioblastoma of the caudal radiation of corpus callosum; *47,* diffuse astrocytoma; *48,* glioblastoma of the fornix; *49,* oligodendroglioma of the thalamus; *50,* glioblastoma of the thalamus; *51,* astrocytoma of the thalamus; *52,* glioblastoma of the thalamus (bilateral); *53,* meningioma of the lateral ventricle; *54,* ependymoma of the lateral ventricle (at the foramen of Monro).

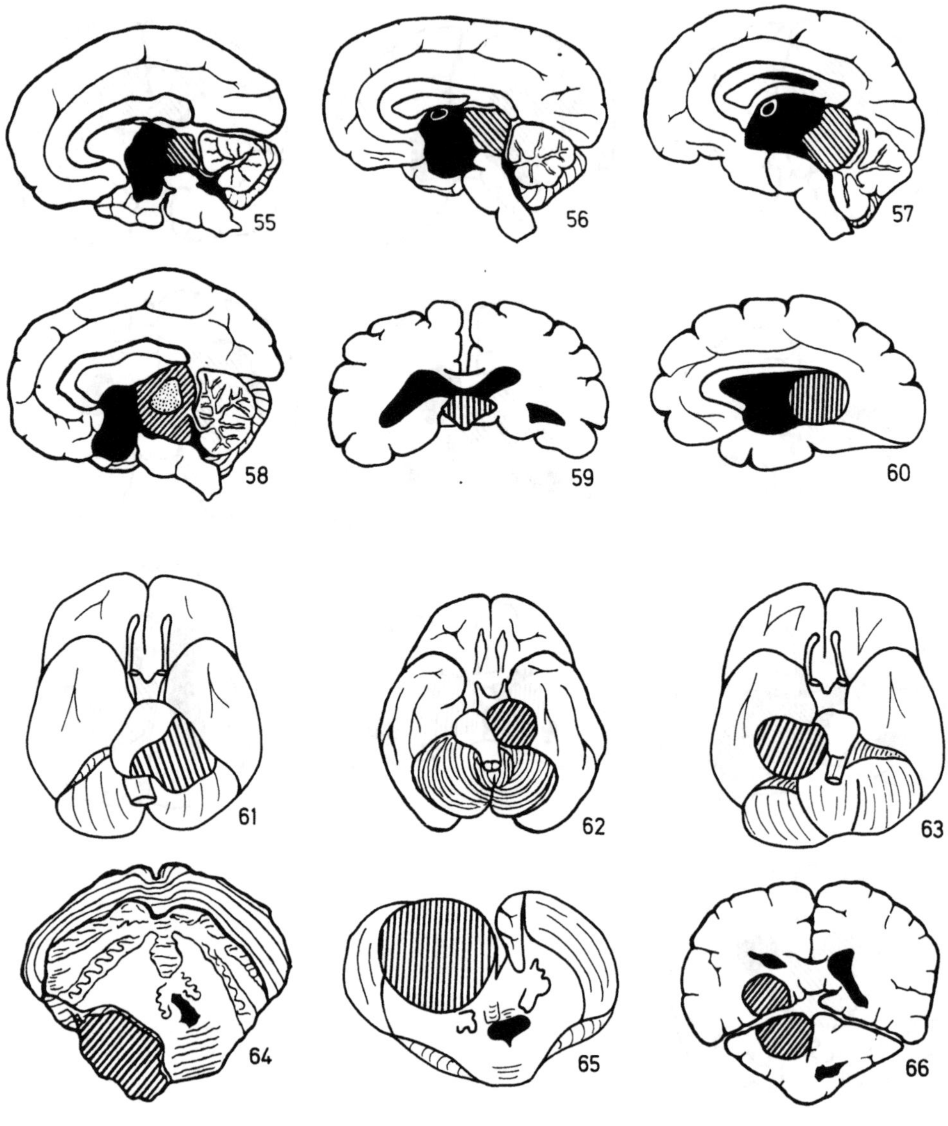

Fig. 14

Midline tumors (mesencephalic): 55, Pinealoma – germinoma; *56,* ependymoma of the posterior third ventricle (quadrigeminal plate region); *57,* glioblastoma of the midbrain; *58,* pilocytic astrocytoma of the midbrain; *59,* pinealoma – germinoma; *60,* meningioma of the quadrigeminal plate (of the tentorial hiatus).

Paramedian tumors of the posterior fossa: 61, Epidermoid of the cerebellopontine angle; *62,* meningioma of the tip of the petrous pyramid (cerebellopontine angle); *63,* neurilemmoma of the cerebellopontine angle; *64,* neurilemmoma of the cerebellopontine angle; *65,* peritorcular meningioma; *66,* meningioma of the tentorium.

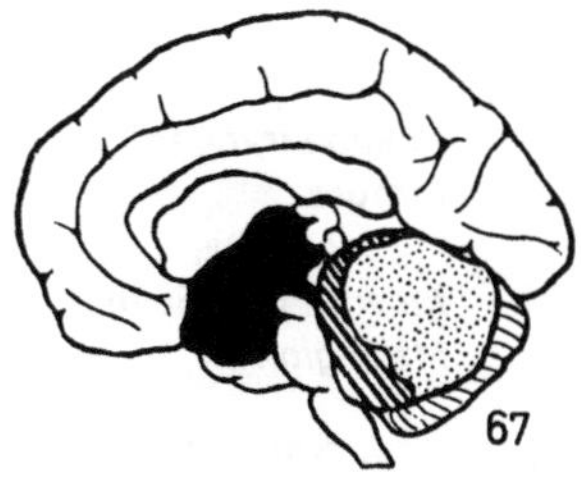
67

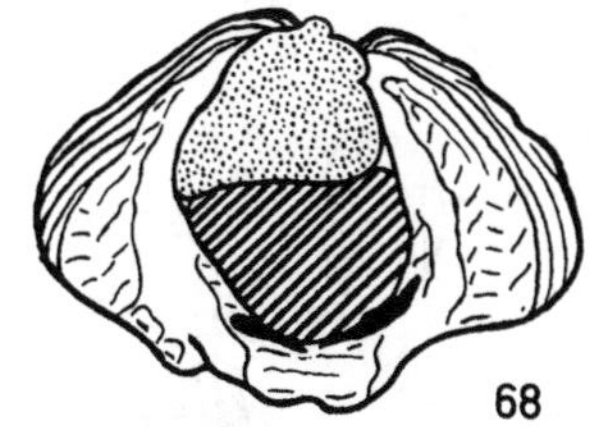
68

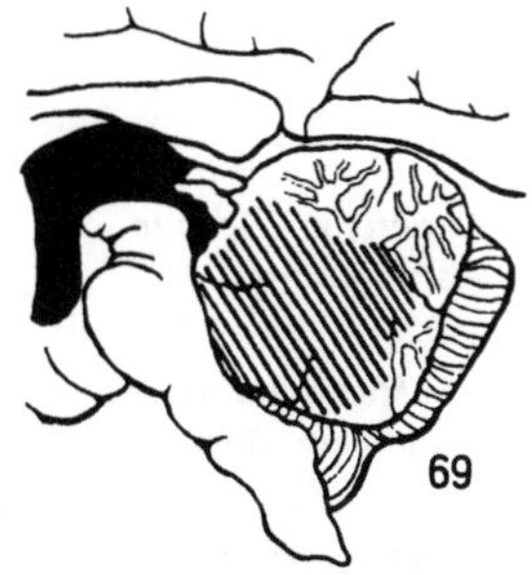
69

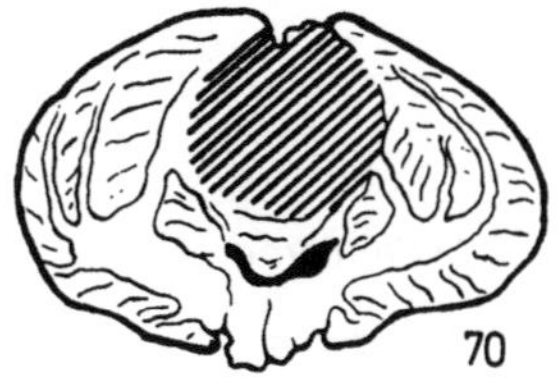
70

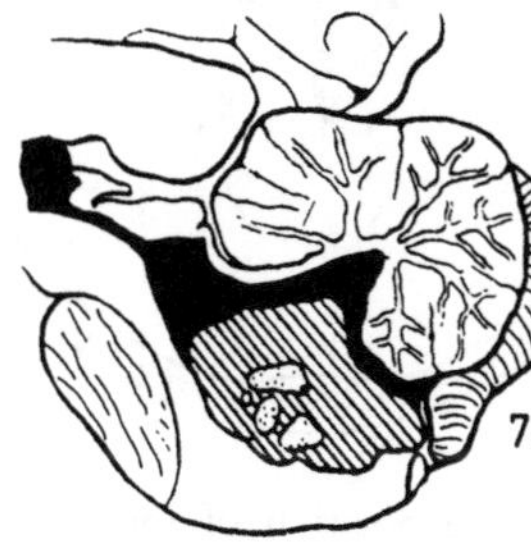
71

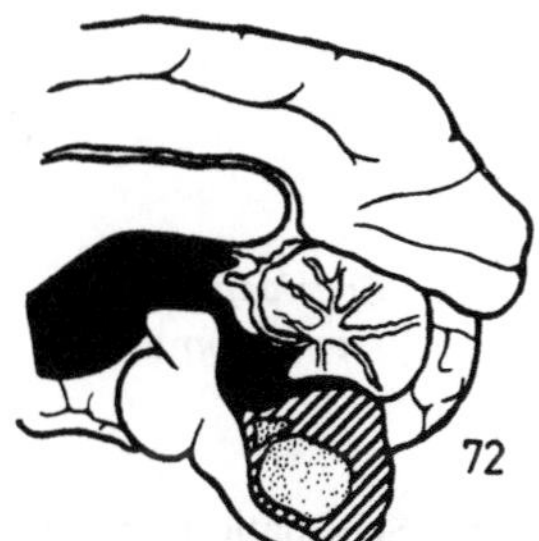
72

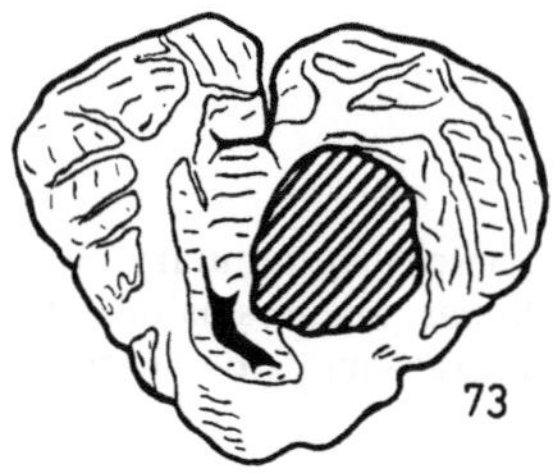
73

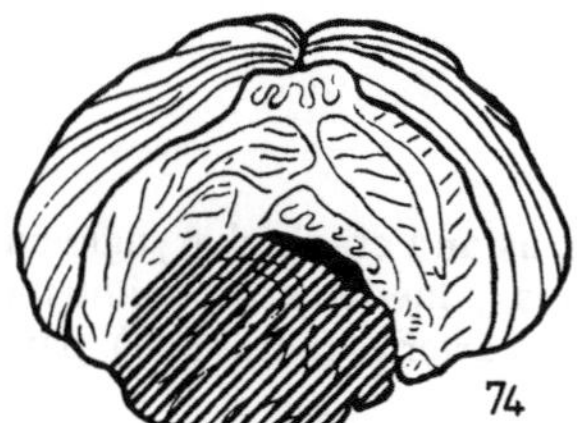
74

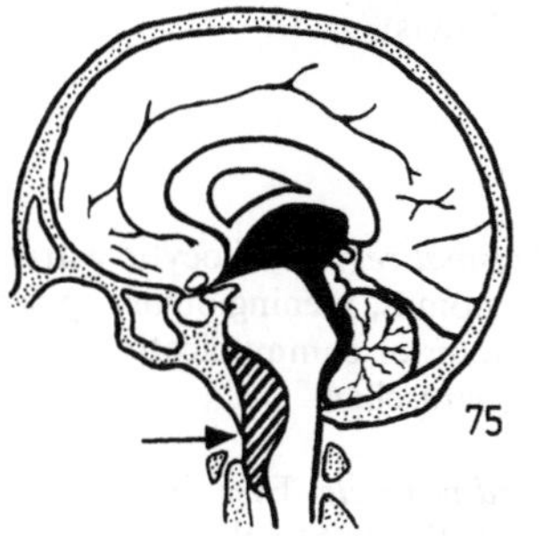
75

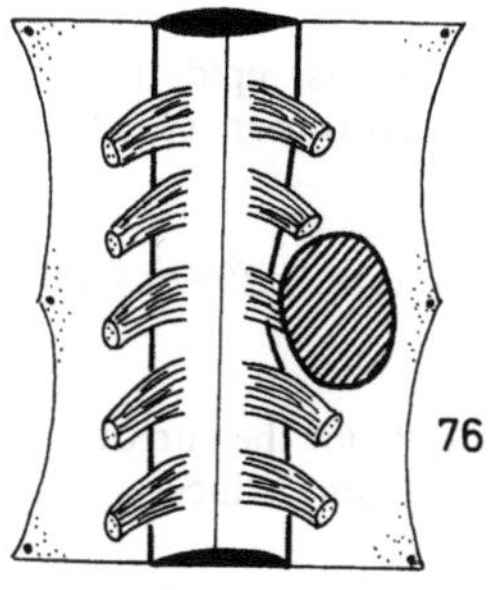
76

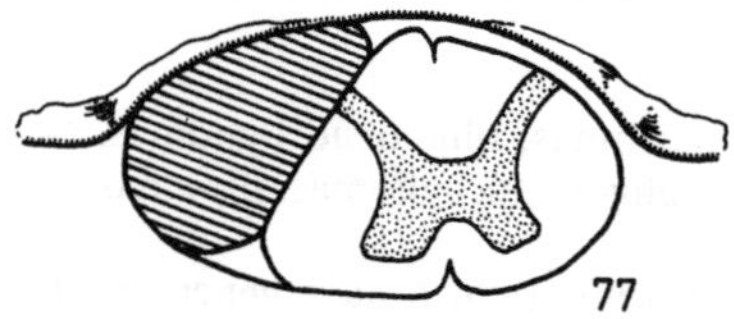
77

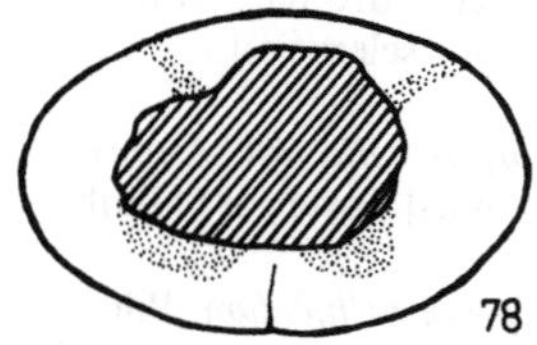
78

Midline tumors of the posterior cranial fossa: 67, Pilocytic astrocytoma of the cerebellum; *68,* pilocytic astrocytoma of the cerebellum; *69,* medulloblastoma of the cerebellum; *70,* medulloblastoma of the cerebellum; *71,* ependymoma of the fourth ventricle; *72,* hemangioblastoma of the fourth ventricle; *73,* hemangioblastoma of the cerebellar hemisphere; *74,* astrocytoma of the pons; *75,* meningioma of the clivus (craniospinal meningioma).

Spinal tumors: 76, Spinal neurilemmoma; *77,* spinal meningioma; *78,* spinal ependymoma/pilocytic astrocytoma

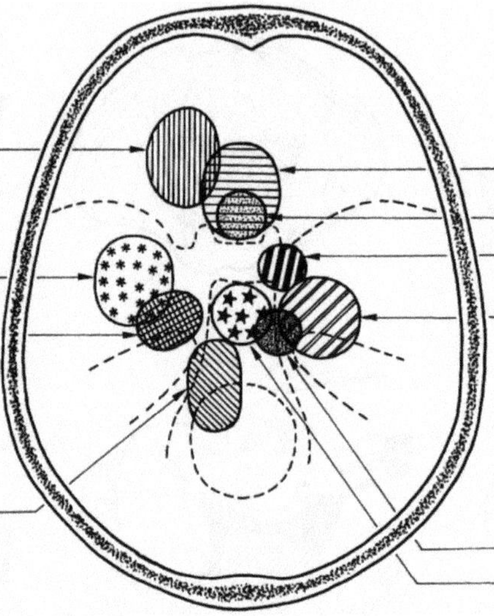

Fig. 15. Schematic representation of the position of the less common tumors involving the base of the skull (excluding pituitary adenomas, craniopharyngiomas, and sphenoid wing meningiomas)

Chiasmal region. Pilocytic astrocytomas and craniopharyngiomas (adolescence), pituitary adenomas, meningiomas, epidermoids, adhesive arachnoiditis, chordomas, aneurysms of the anterior communicating and carotid arteries (parasellar), parasellar teratomas, cavernomas (parasellar)

Third ventricle. Ependymal cysts (foramen of Monro), ependymomas, pilocytic astrocytomas (of the hypothalamus), choroid plexus papillomas [epidermoids], meningiomas of the velum interpositum

Lateral ventricles[1]. Ependymomas, meningiomas, choroid plexus papillomas, epidermoids [chondromas, teratomas, lipomas, glomerate astrocytomas (the ventricular tumors of tuberous sclerosis)]

Corpus callosum. Anterior: Glioblastomas, oligodendrogliomas, astrocytomas (diffuse) [lipomas] Posterior: Glioblastomas, oligodendrogliomas, [lipomas]

Septum pellucidum. Pilocytic astrocytoma (which have generally grown in from the surroundings), astrocytomas, oligodendrogliomas, glioblastomas, cysts of the septum pellucidum

Rostral brain stem and basal ganglia. Glioblastomas, oligodendrogliomas (adolescence), astrocytomas (often bilateral, growing across the massa intermedia)

---

[1] We subdivide these tumors as follows: *Primary*, true tumors of the lateral ventricle are those that develop from the ventricular lining (the ependyma and subependymal glia), from the epithelium of the choroid plexus and its arachnoidal supporting tissue, or from misplaced tissue – epithelium, adipose tissue, or embryonic rests. They leave the ventricular wall intact except for their place of attachment.
Secondary tumors are infiltrating tumors of the brain substance that bulge into the ventricular lumen.

Region of the quadrigeminal plate. Pinealomas/germinomas/pineoblastomas, pilocytic astrocytomas [glioblastomas, ependymomas (aqueduct and posterior third ventricle), ependymal cysts, arachnoidal cysts, teratomas, meningiomas, capillary angiomas]

Aqueduct. Pilocytic astrocytomas (adolescence), ependymitis, malformations, [ependymomas]

Cerebellar vermis. Medulloblastomas, pilocytic astrocytomas [epidermoids, dermoids, teratomas], meningiomas (torcular)

Cerebellar hemispheres. Medulloblastomas, pilocytic astrocytomas, angioblastomas, meningiomas (tentorial)

Fourth ventricle. Ependymomas, choroid plexus papillomas, pilocytic astrocytomas, angioblastomas (calamus scriptorius), adhesive arachnoiditis/arachnoidal cysts

Cerebellopontine angle. Neurilemmomas, meningiomas, epidermoids, choroid plexus papillomas, ependymomas, ependymal cysts, adhesive arachnoiditis

Caudal brain stem (pons and medulla). Astrocytomas, pilocytic astrocytomas [glioblastomas, gangliocytomas, chordomas] meningiomas (clivus/craniospinal)

Spinal tumors. See p. 532

Orbit. See p. 552

Optic foramen. Pilocytic astrocytomas, meningiomas

Retina. Retinoblastomas, melanoblastomas, pilocytic astrocytomas

Peripheral nerves. Neurilemmomas and neurofibromatosis (von Recklinghausen's disease), plexiform neurilemmomas, sarcomas, [neuroepitheliomas?]

Sympathetic trunks. Sympathoblastomas, gangliocytomas, paragangliomas

Leptomeninges. Primary sarcomas, diffuse and circumscribed, melanomatosis, carcinomatosis (secondary)

Diffusely growing tumors. Astrocytosis, oligodendroblastosis, sarcomatosis of the vessels

Tumors without preferential location. Metastases, primary circumscribed sarcomas of the brain, granulomas, parasites

Pathology of the Cranial Base

Figure 15 shows the most prominent types of tumors of the base of the skull. However, since not all of them have predilection sites which can be illustrated, they will be listed in the following lines: Osteomas and osteoid osteomas, fibromas, giant cell tumors, glomus jugulare tumors, "[cylindromatous] adenoid carcinomas," carcinomas and sarcomas of the nasopharynx all occur, as do more superficially hemangiomas (cavernomas), lipomas, teratomas, epidermoids and dermoids.

Different osteomatous tumors may be encountered in the orbits as may dermoids, cavernomas, meningiomas, epitheliomas, sarcomas, lymphomas (reticulosarcomas). One may also find pilocytic astrocytomas at the optic disc, retinoblastomas and melanosarcomas of the retina (see above).

Pathology of the Cranial Vault

Neoplasms occurring in the vault of the skull will also only be summarized and figures not given since there are no recognizable predilections apart from a tendency for eosinophilic granulomas (see p. 511 ff.) to appear more commonly in the frontal bone.

Among the tumors, meningiomas, osteomas, epidermoids and particularly metastases, myelomas and cavernous hemangiomas must be mentioned. Among the rare lesions are the cystic "brown" tumors of von Recklinghausen's *ostitis fibrosa cystica* and granulomas (Schüller-Christian) or the diffuse increase in thickness seen in Paget's disease.

"Chronic" inflammatory lesions are now rare in western countries. These include syphilomas (gummas) encountered more commonly in the aged, and also tuberculomas of the vault, which are more frequent in the young. Finally, malformations occur at the suture lines in the forehead and occiput and may be pea- to plum-sized. The volume may differ in relation to the intracranial pressure (encephalocele, meningocele).

A detailed description can be found in the sections dealing with each specific tumor.

4.5 Diffuse and Multiple Brain Tumors

The name "diffuse glioma" has been applied to a variety of pathologic processes. In a broad sense, this term includes gliomas, growing diffusely throughout one or both hemispheres, such as oligodendrogliomas (Landau 1910) and astrocytomas (Scherer 1940a). In a narrower sense, it is presently also understood to include diffuse neoplastic proliferation (not circumscribed lesions), such as has been described under the terms gliosis, glioblastosis, lemmoblastosis, and central diffuse schwannosis (see p. 341 ff.). This subject, however, needs further study and clarification.

Historically Borst (1902a, Vol. I, p. 55–57) provided the first logical subdivision and distinguished:
1. Multiple organ tumors located symmetrically in bilateral organs
2. Tumors of one organ system
3. Tumors of functionally related organs
4. Tumors of unrelated organs

On the basis of this schema Courville (1936) differentiated:
1. Multiple gliomas in one lobe or hemisphere
2. Multiple gliomas in both hemispheres
3. Multiple gliomas within the CNS
4. Multiple tumors in CNS and meninges or nerves
5. Multiple tumors in the brain and distant organs

As logical this classification is, it may still be too complicated. However, it was thoroughly discussed by Courville (1936) in a report based on the presentation of 21 of his own cases and cases from the world literature, which were demonstrated in schematic drawings.

The subdivision used by BUDKA et al. (1980) seems to be even more complex and the change for it to be commonly accepted seems to be remote.

To improve both the understanding and the classification of these conditions I would like to propose the following less complicated grouping:

1. Diffuse glioblastosis (spongioblastosis etc.) as an independent entity (see p. 341 ff.)
2. Diffuse gliomas, i.e., diffusely growing astrocytomas, oligodendrogliomas, etc.
3. Multicentric gliomas, i.e., tumors of a single type with multiple independent growth centers where careful histological examination reveals no continuous cellular connection
4. Multiple brain tumors
   a) Multiple tumors of similar type, e.g., multiple meningiomas
   b) Multiple tumors of different type, e.g., meningiomas, combined with gliomas, etc.
   c) Multiple tumors in the brain and in one of the body organs

Multicentric Gliomas

Certain gliomas can grow in the form of multiple nodules, connected by thin cellular bridges (ZÜLCH 1941 a) or with no cellular bridges being found during thorough histologic examination (KÖHLMEIER 1943).

The distinction between multicentric and multiple tumors is not too sharp. Ordinarily, the term of "multicentric" gliomas is used even if there is a demonstrable cellular interconnection, but several meningiomas in a single case are called "multiple".

In our own material we have seen four cases of glioblastoma multiforme occurring simultaneously in the second and third frontal convolutions and in the occipital lobe (see also BERTHA 1942, who placed his case of a 40 years old man at our disposal (GP, Fig. 134a and b).

We have no explanation for the form of growth in these cases nor in another peculiar, unclassified pilocytic astrocytoma-like tumor in a 37 year-old woman, which was found growing in one temporal pole and in the superior cerebellar vermis without any cellular interconnection.

Some authors appear to have observed these cases frequently. COURVILLE (1936) states that 10% of glioblastomas and 6% of astrocytomas are multiple. Whether they are ever "multicentric" without any cellular connections, remains open. The apparent "multiplicity" of many of these tumors can be explained by the growth of the tumor along winding fiber bundles. For instance, the glioblastoma multiforme, reported by HASENJÄGER (1938), which lay close to the lateral ventricle and seemed to be multicentric, was proved to be growing along the fornix. The possibility of metastasis along some pathway as yet unknown, perhaps via the subarachnoid cerebrospinal fluid, also must be considered (see our cases in the frontal and occipital lobe mentioned above).

COURVILLE (1936) found among his own series of 269 tumors 21 with multiple growth and he also collected 120 observations from the literature. MANZINI and SERRA (1952) presented 16 multiple gliomas from the literature and 6 of their personal cases. I have collected further reports from the literature in 1956 (p. 114).

Multiple Brain Tumors

Multiple tumors of different types occur most frequently in the systematic hamartoblastomatoses (phacomatoses), such as von Hippel-Lindau disease and von Recklinghausen's disease. In the latter condition, meningiomas, neurilemmomas and pilocytic astrocytomas form a well-known triad and are sometimes associated in addition with ependymomas and angiomatous malformations (FOERSTER and GAGEL 1932c).

Many other combinations have been described and are many reported in the literature. These include (a) meningiomas with astrocytomas, (b) glioblastomas, oligodendrogliomas and other undefined gliomas, and (c) monstrocellular sarcomas with pituitary adenomas (personal observations). Other combinations reported are melanoma and neurilemmoma; chordoma and craniopharyngioma; pilocytic astrocytoma and gangliocytoma; epidermoid, dermoid or teratoma in one case; fibrosarcoma and pituitary adenoma in another. In CUSHING'S series (1932, 1935), according to L. EISENHARDT, pituitary adenoma and cerebellar angioblastoma, and finally, astrocytoma and granular cell myoblastoma were seen in combination. The case of CASTAIGNE et al. (1974) of gliomatous foci in a focal leucoencephalopathy has to be mentioned as a special observation. For the sake of completeness some cases have to mentioned in which a brain tumor was combined with a tumor elsewhere in the body, as in our case of a 64 year-old woman, in whom there was the combination of a malignant tumor of the brain (monstrocellular sarcoma) and an ovary carcinoma.

In oncology the frequent occurrence of multiple malignant tumors in the same patient in different organs has been pointed to (for instance GULEKE 1946; EBHARDT and HEISS 1984). However, the meaning of this observation has to be more thoroughly studied and clarified.

Meningeal Gliomatosis

The entity "meningeal gliomatosis" (KERNOHAN and SAYRE 1952) was believed to be identical with "gliosarcoma of the meninges" or "meningeal sarcomatosis", yet later on it was considered as always of glial origin, being the result of the spread of gliomas. In a series reported by POLMETEER and KERNOHAN (1947) tumor cells growing in the arachnoid were seen in 42 cases of which 20 were medulloblastomas while others were malignant astrocytomas or glioblastomas. These were nothing else besides particularly heavy seedings and do not require assignment to a special entity.

Further References: CONNOR and CUSHING (1927), MYERSON (1942), FEIRING and DAVIDOFF (1947), ALEXANDER (1948), GASS and VAN WAGENEN (1950), WISE et al. (1953), FENYES and KEPES (1956), GREENWOOD and MCGUIRE (1957), KRÜGER (1961), SOLITARE (1962), BATZDORF and MALAMUD (1963), NAGASHIMA et al. (1963), BINGAS and BRUNNGRABER (1964), KUNFT and PIOTROWSKI (1964), PINEDA (1964a), FINKEMEYER and TZONOS (1965), BELZA (1966), WELCKER and SEIDEL (1966), LEWIS (1968), WAHL and DILLARD (1972), BHRANY et al. (1974), ARSENI et al. (1975), BOROVICH et al. (1976), STRONG et al. (1976), BHANGUI et al. (1977), RUSSO (1979), BUDKA et al. (1980).

5 Gross Pathology of Brain Tumors

5.1 The Process of Tumor Diagnosis

In the following presentation of the gross and histologic structure of brain tumors, pure description takes precedence over interpretation. The need for a certain amount of caution in setting up *hypotheses* becomes apparent upon reading the older literature, since some of the earlier notions, e.g., that of concerning the problem of "infiltrating" versus "induced" growth (p. 128ff.), are now useless. This is largely because the findings themselves were relegated to the background and the interpretations were overburdened with hypotheses. On the other hand, good descriptions of classical pathology still allow diagnoses of tumor types according to present classifications (e.g., KLEBS 1877, 1889).

We must make every attempt not to confine ourselves too much to a study of the individual cell, an exercise that was, and still is, the guiding principle in many schools and is certainly the background for ultrastructural studies. In his later work on tumors BAILEY (1932a) adopted the detailed study of the whole tissue, though it was he who had previously stressed so much the single cell approach.

In Germany, the tradition of the Nissl school prevented any such one-sided approach. We have early examples from Olga LOTMAR (1918) in whose publications tumors were presented as case reports and then, one by one, nuclei, cells, architecture (syncytium), vessels, growth and fibers were dealt with. The method that was customarily used in that school for the elucidation of a pathologic process, emphasized particularly by SPIELMEYER (1922, 1927), was a study of serial sections with a variety of stains. Applied to the study of tumors, this technique resulted quite naturally in consideration of the tumor growth as an "organoid" entirety ("ensemble"). This explains why H.J. SCHERER (1940a), a disciple of SPIELMEYER, demanded a "complete" investigation.

A systematic tumor study alone can form the foundation for an accurate diagnosis. The site of the tumor, and the appearance of the tumor cells, the rate of growth and viability of the cells, the intercellular substances, the stroma, and finally, regressive processes such as necrosis and necrobiosis (hyalinization, fatty degeneration, mucoid degeneration and cyst formation, calcification and hemorrhages) are all precisely established.

By correlating this information with the age and sex of the patient yields a concept that must be consistent with the knowledge already accumulated. By this means, we arrive at a diagnosis of the tumor type. Moreover, the most important points of differential diagnosis are already available since they are based on the evaluation of the morphologic characteristics mentioned above. The prognosis is obtained from clinical knowledge of the behavior of the specific tumor type after radical operation, radiotherapy and/or chemotherapy (see pp. 142, 150).

I have emphasized here the study of the "whole" tumor to which I have referred as the "ensemble". This must be stressed because modern techniques, particularly electron microscopy, point to the particular image of the cell or parts of it, as was done in the beginning of Bailey's earlier studies. It is agreed that this investigation of the cell in all its details has provided much basic information about its origin, composition and nature and has solved many scientific problems. Its importance for routine diagnosis is limited, however, because many, if not most, tumors have an admixture of other cells ("e *potiori* fit denominatio") and therefore we have to study *tissue* for diagnosis and not *cells* alone.

5.2 Form, Color, Consistency, and Appearance to the Naked Eye

The form or shape of a brain tumor depends very much on the manner of growth, described below. The shape of those tumors that grow by expansion is determined not only by their intrinsic growth properties, but also by the restrictions imposed on them by the surrounding tissue. Tumors within the ventricles, for instance, readily assume the ventricular shape (GP, Figs. 54, 56), those in the fourth ventricle taking on the shape of a flattened pyramid (Fig. 67), those in the third ventricle becoming round (Fig. 78) or pear-shaped and those in the lateral ventricles are elongated.

In the cerebellopontine angle the extra-axial tumors are usually shaped like a chestnut (GP, Fig. 194) or a plum (Fig. 109; GP, Fig. 200); in the spinal canal they assume the form of a kidney bean (GP, Fig. 209) or grow in long, finger-like shapes (Fig. 122).

The meningiomas assume a hemispherical shape (Fig. 119, GP, Fig. 192) over the convexity and are round when attached to the falx (GP, Fig. 189). If they grow into two intracranial fossae (tentorium) they are dumbbell shaped (GP, Fig. 196) or saddle shaped along the sphenoid bone (GP, Fig. 179) and occasionally spread out like a carpet (en plaque). In addition to the main types of meningiomas with round, peaked, or flat growth, there are mixed forms in which a peaked projection of tumor emerges from a broad, flat base (GP, Fig. 211).

Little is known about the form and infiltrating tendencies of intracerebral tumors, such as the glioblastomas (see Figs. 16–19). In cross sections oligodendrogliomas have a garland-like form (Fig. 59, 60; GP, Fig. 106) since they spread along the gyri and expand them. The white matter at the center often undergoes cystic degeneration. By and large the circumscribed astrocytomas assume a spherical form (Fig. 40; GP, Fig. 95) and grow concentrically from the inside out. This tendency is particularly pronounced in the pilocytic forms which, although they infiltrate at the periphery, grow essentially by expansion. The intramedullary growths in the spinal cord usually assume the shape of a pencil (GP, Fig. 159) and extend over many segments.

Color

The color of a brain tumor depends on the main type of tissue present and on the amount of blood it contains. The fibrous astrocytomas are whiteyellow and glassy both before and after fixation, during which they lose little but the slight coloration from their blood they contained. The oligodendrogliomas, on the other hand, are pinkish, since they are relatively vascular and contain no fibers. Blood-vessel tumor, such as angioblastomas, resemble dark red cherries. Fatty degeneration of a tumor results in a yellow to ochre color (a patchy or striped pattern in neurilemmomas and glioblastomas). Hyalinization produces a grayish-translucency (neurilemmomas and meningiomas), mucoid degeneration a clear glassy appearance (chordomas). Old and fresh hemorrhages produce brown to dark or bright red coloration in glioblastomas. The cyst walls of piloid astrocytomas take on the dark brown color of hemosiderin as the result of hemorrhages, which are common. Chondromas may look as white ivory.

Consistency

The consistency of brain tumors depends upon the relative amount of cells, fibers, intercellular substances and blood vessels, as well as on the firmness of the invaded tissues. Cellular tumors poor in fibers, such as medulloblastomas, are soft and almost granular. On the other hand, relatively acellular tumors containing abundant fibers, such as astrocytomas, particularly the pilocytic ones, are often as hard as cartilage.

These characteristics are readily apparent even on the cut surface. Astrocytomas, because of the sparse cells and abundant fibers, have a smooth cut surface while oligodendrogliomas, which are cellular but have few fibers, have a "velvety" raw surface. Mucoid tumors, such as some pilocytic astrocytomas, are sometimes correspondingly soft whereas tumors bearing many fibers, such as fibrous meningiomas, are elastic and firm and depending upon the amount of blood vessels they contain, they feel springy or flabby. In certain meningiomas and craniopharyngiomas, and also in some regions of oligodendrogliomas, calcification can lead to hardening, even to the consistency of chalk. The cut surface of monstrocellular sarcomas looks like asbestos.

Size and Weight

The weight of tumors depends on their size. The largest tumor removed in our clinic was a true meningioma in an 11-year-old girl which weighed 618 g. In the literature a meningioma is reported which measured 18 × 14 × 9 cm, and weighed 1300 g, including the involved bone (Kerschner 1928).

6 Histology of Brain Tumors

6.1 Architecture and Cell Formation

The historical development of the study of gliomas explains the serious confusion over problems of nomenclature. The neurosurgical/clinical group of investigators split off rather early from the anatomical/pathological group. The different works on tumors therefore contain varying terms and all-too-individual descriptions and classifications. Reviews of large series of tumors, that were collected in some American and European institutes finally led to considerable degree of agreement in the oncological nomenclature. This has come to finality in the WHO monograph entitled *Histological Typing of Tumors of the Central Nervous System* (ZÜLCH 1979).

The confusion of terms was worst in the description and naming of the tissue architecture. The evolution of a cell pattern must be clearly understood

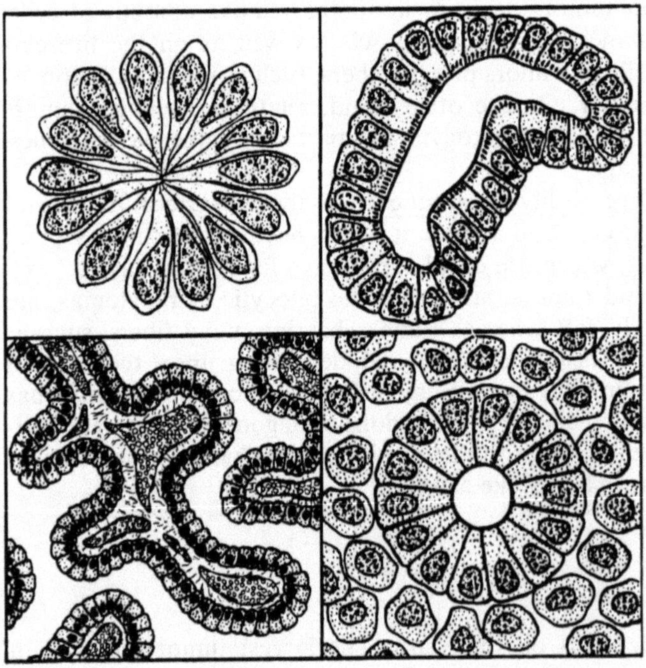

a b c d

Fig. 16a–d. Arrangement of cells in: **a** pseudorosettes, i.e., radial arrangement around an imaginary center; **b** ependymal tubules, i.e., large lumen similar to the central canal, lined with ependyma: **c** papillae, i.e., fingerlike processes of stroma covered by epithelium; **d** true rosettes, i.e., radial arrangement around the minute true lumen

before assigning it a name. Investigation of form and pattern of these architectural arrangements makes it possible to use the following classification (similar to that of H.J. SCHERER 1933, 1935).

Genuine ("Primary") Architectures

These are genuine tendencies toward pattern formation, which are so to speak atavistic, being so deeply rooted that they "break through" whenever growth is unhindered.

We can distinguish a tendency to a particular arrangement: pseudorosettes, i.e., radiating around an imaginary center (Fig. 16a); true rosettes, i.e., radiating around a minute true lumen (Fig. 16d); ependymal tubules, i.e., the formation of epithelial tubules similar to the central canal (Figs. 16b, 20b) with a large true lumen (Figs. 16d, 20b); the form of palisades (Fig. 18d; HBT, Fig. 70a), phalanges, files, and rows, i.e., parallel cell arrangement in columns; onion-skin arrangement, i.e., concentric cell layers around a center (Fig. 17c); radial or crown-like patterns, i.e., radial arrangement around a blood vessel (Fig. 17a); a satellite arrangement of the tumor cells around neurons, etc. (HBT, Fig. 35a,

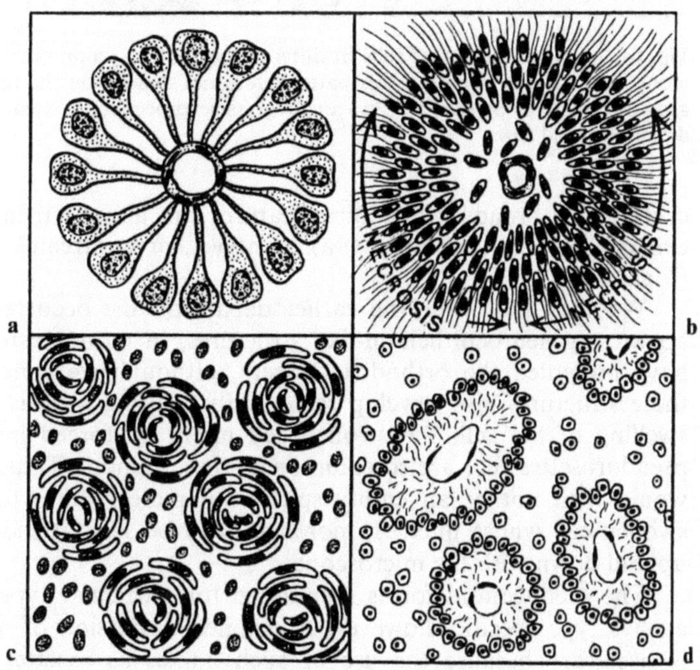

Fig. 17a–d. Arrangement of cells in: **a** crownlike pattern, i.e., radially around a blood vessel to whose wall the cells are attached by vascular feet; **b** perivascular cell cuffs, i.e., in a multicellular layer around the vessel, while the tissue further away from the vessel is destroyed by necrosis; **c** onionskin arrangements, i.e., concentric layers around an imaginary center; **d** pseudopapillae, i.e., structures similar to papillae containing a vessel in the center and covered with one layer of cells. These structures develop "secondarily," i.e., through mucoid degeneration of the tissue between the vessels

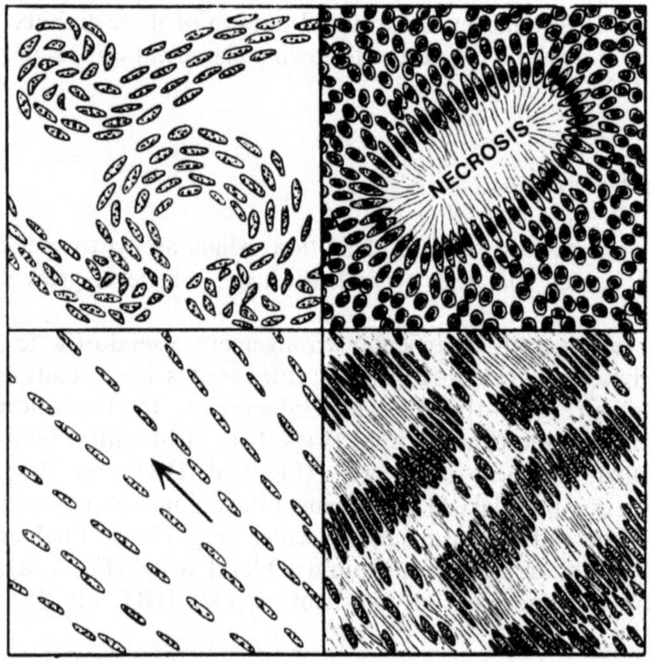

Fig. 18a–d. Arrangement of cells in different patterns: **a** whorls or loops; **b** pseudopalisades along the bands of necrosis; this pattern does not depend on the intrinsic properties of cell growth but develops secondarily from regressive processes; **c** streams like a school of fish; **d** palisades and rows

c, d). Some broad architectural features can also be mentioned here, such as orientation in whorls (Fig. 18a) or hooks, or in streams like a school of fish (Fig. 18c).

We shall pass over the earlier debate on the occurrence of true rosettes, apparently neuroepithelium-like structures, in retinoblastomas (Fig. 16d). We have presented the orthodox concept, although we consider it possible that these structures also develop secondarily. During mitosis or during regressive swelling of the cell, the swollen cell might be forced into the center of the pseudorosettes that are so common in these tumors. Thus, the so-called lumen would then not be an empty space, but merely the cytoplasm of a severely swollen cell whose nucleus, moreover, can be seen at the edge when focusing up and down with the microscope.

The architectural forms mentioned for particular types of tumors are not always type specific, however. A detailed discussion of architectural features is necessary because the use of such names as rosettes and pseudorosettes (Homer Wright rosettes) has resulted in great confusion. These terms have been employed interchangeably for the pseudorosettes of medulloblastomas, the ependymal tubules in ependymomas, the true rosettes in retinoblastomas, the perivascular arrangement of cells in glioblastomas, the pseudopapillae in pilocytic astrocytomas, and the radial pattern in ependymomas. Furthermore, it is necessary that true palisading in neurilemmomas (Fig. 18d) be distinguished

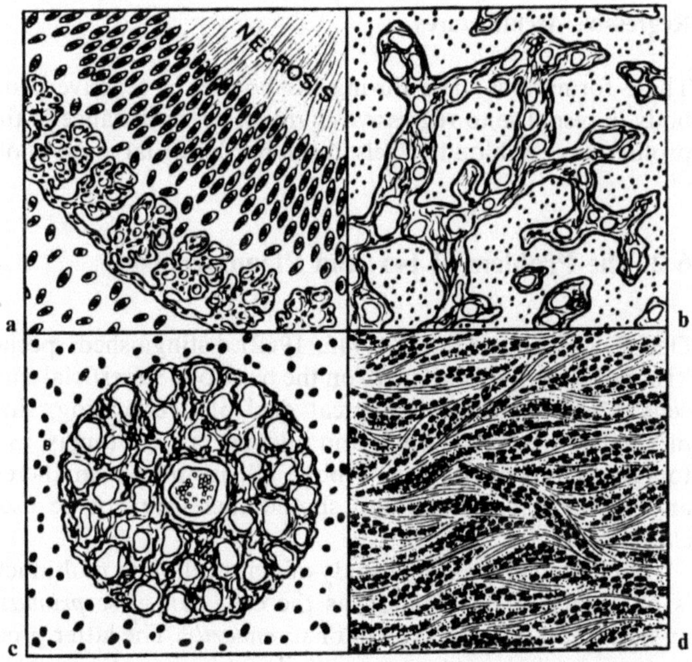

Fig. 19a–d. Architecture of the stroma: **a** a barrier of blood vessels in the marginal zone of a necrotic area; **b** network of proliferating blood vessels in a glioblastoma; **c** perivascular proliferation around a large blood vessel in a glioblastoma; **d** feltwork of arachnoid infiltrated by the cells of a medulloblastoma. This stroma imposes a typical architectural pattern upon the tumor

from other cell alignments, such as those along the border of a band of necrosis of glioblastomas (Fig. 18b) (pseudopalisading). A clear grasp of this concept is essential for adequate understanding of tumor cell histology.

"Induced" (Secondary) Architectures

These are secondary features that arise from the action upon the tumor of external influences, e.g., through the orienting effect of the local tissue on the tumor cells [fibers of the corpus callosum or other commissures, U fibers, meshwork of the arachnoid, dendrites of the Purkinje cells (Fig. 102b)]. These features may also arise secondarily from regressive processes (Figs. 18b, 19a). Examples may be found in the honey comb picture resembling the oligodendroglioma seen in the pilocytic astrocytoma (HBT, Fig. 55d) after mucoid degeneration (Fig. 51) and in the neurilemmoma after fatty degeneration (HBT, Fig. 68d). Further examples include the pseudopalisading along the bands of necrosis (Fig. 18b) in glioblastomas (HBT, Fig. 50b); the perivascular cell arrangement after the same process (HBT, Fig. 50a), when the cells surrounding the nutrient vessels are preserved the longest (Fig. 94a); and the pseudoependymal tubules in some choroid plexus papillomas and hypophyseal adenomas, where after mucoid degeneration of the supporting stroma only the covering epithelium persists.

Regressive Architectures

These formations arise during the course of reactive processes set up by the body in response to regressive changes, as for instance in the case of endothelial proliferation of blood vessels at the border or large areas of necrosis (Fig. 19a).

6.2 The Problem of Iso- and Pleomorphism

DEL RIO HORTEGA (1932, 1945, 1962) distinguished special tumor groups like "isomorphic glioblastomas" on the basis of a superficial similarity of constituent cells. However, there is a great deal of overlapping, since these criteria are met by many glioblastomas and pilocytic astrocytomas, as well as medulloblastomas and ependymomas. Above all, isomorphism therefore cannot provide any basis for prognosis and should therefore not be used as a criterion for classification.

On the other hand, the study of giant cells and multinucleated cells in tumors is of particular importance, as the cells can arise *primarily,* and then can be an indication of rapid growth or *secondarily*. The latter process occurs especially in tumors of the astrocytoma (pilocytic variant) series that have undergone mucoid degeneration. The cell nuclei stick together and become hyperchromatic (HBT, Figs. 20d, 54d); and sometimes assume a "carpet-like" appearance. We also find considerable cellular dysplasia in rather benign meningiomas (type IV, 2 of CUSHING and EISENHARDT 1938 – a transitional form between the meningothelimatous and the angiomatous subtypes). In all likelihood these features arise through regressive changes and should not be interpreted as signs of malignancy (see KERNOHAN and SAYRE 1952; MARCOS 1954).

6.3 Nuclei of the Cells

Despite claims to the contrary (SCHMINCKE, personal communication), the nucleus in the light microscope cannot be considered proof of the origin of the cell; it may change depending on the cell's state of vitality. Neuron-like vesicular nuclei with a distinct membrane and large nucleolus-like chromatin clumps appear during the rapid growth of astrocytes and fibroblasts, as well as in certain large cells of oligodendrogliomas and in many cancers. They can even be produced artificially if the tumor tissue fixed in formol-ammonium-bromide is later stained with Nissl's method. They stand out exceptionally well with Bouin or Susa fixation and after staining with cresyl violet. Recent studies of the nucleus have shown that the nucleolus and the nuclear membrane are closely interdependent in their metabolism. It is erroneous to conclude, simply from the appearance of the nucleus, that a cell originates from the ganglion cell series, since the form of the nucleus is subject to many external influences. In the case of a tumor growing in white matter, for instance, not only can the cell assume an elongated form (i.e., the astrocyte becomes "piloid"/"pilocytic") but the nucleus, too, may be drawn out to a cigar-like shape. This point is particularly well illustrated in general pathology by the growth of certain forms of sarcoma (HEINE 1931) and by the appearance of leucocytes when they infiltrate the cornea. The nuclei of the tumor cells usually adapt to the structure of the infiltrated tissue.

The monstrocellular sarcoma elements, and to a lesser extent those of glioblastomas, consist sometimes of very little besides nuclear chromatine, show particularly numerous atypical nuclear forms, which are described in the special Sect. 19.2 (see also ACHUCARRO 1912). The presence of inclusion bodies has been described in the literature (D. RUSSELL 1932; WOLF and ORTON 1933), and was found in malignant glioblastomas with impressive frequency. We have seen them especially in monstrocellular sarcomas. Other inclusions have been considered to be plasma intrusions into the nucleus (ROBERTSON and MACLEAN 1965, in meningiomas; see also p. 369). Whether the assumption of Dorothy RUSSELL (1932) that this feature is a sign of the tumor's origin from virus infection is correct remains undecided for the present (see also KRYNAUW and JACKSON 1948). Why and how large giant-sized cells or nuclei are formed is not generally clarified. In meningiomas it seems that they occur when the nutritional conditions are most likely to be poor. There are older (KIMURA 1921; ALPERS 1931) as well as more recent (ALTMANN 1961) investigations reported, but the result of which, however, cannot be generalized.

The cell body and nucleus can be altered, as already mentioned, by external influences. I should like to call attention to the action of electrical currents applied during the cutting and coagulation of brain and tumor tissue, which can change the architecture artificially into one of loops, whorls, and streams; cells can be coagulated and can assume a hyperchromatic appearance (ZÜLCH 1940 d). Even the drying-out process between operating table and laboratory leads to similar severe changes near the surface of the tumor, where the tissues may become condensed and hyperchromatic. The appearance of tumor cells can also be considerably changed by x-ray therapy (for further details see p. 142).

Meanwile chromosome studies have been performed, for instance, in glioblastoma multiforme (deviations in groups 6–12, near diploid karyotype: WILSON et al. 1970; extra chromosomes in medulloblastoma cells: LUBS and SALMON 1965; double minutes (dms) in all or most of the cells in human gliomas: MARK and GRANBERG 1970).

6.4 Stroma

The mutual influence of parenchyma and stroma in tumors has been frequently studied. If infiltration occurs, vessels and other forms of stroma are assumed to be part of the host tissue and primarily nonneoplastic, so that there no voluminous growth of tumor is possible without sufficient vascularization. In recent decades this issue has again received considerable attention, while during the era of purely cytological analysis of tumors (as in Hortega's time) interest in it had diminished. Our modern conceptions started with the work of SCHALTENBRAND and BAILEY (1928).

The vascular pattern depends to some extent on the biological behavior of a tumor. It can be orderly patterned and mostly resembling capillaries in astrocytomas and oligodendrogliomas and disorderly, as in glioblastoma multiforme. The original working hypothesis on the interpretation of blood vessels was that the degree of maturity of the blood vessels of the stroma rather paralleled that of the tumor cells (BERTHA 1940). The more embryonic the cell type and the more malignant the tumor, the greater the amount of connective tissue, and the more diffuse its distribution throughout the tumor. SCHALTENBRAND and BAILEY (1928) thought that, in brain tumor particularly, the tendency to respect glial barriers and the restriction of the connective tissue to the blood vessels walls could be regarded as evidence of comparative benignity. In the same way, the crossing of the glial membrane by tumor cells, i.e., the mixing of ectodermal and mesodermal elements or the invasion of the leptomeninges, could be considered characteristic of malignancy. This rule of thumb, however, has frequently been broken (see p. 226). For example, in oligodendrogliomas and in gangliocytomas of the temporal lobe, which are extremely benign, circumscribed tumor nodules and islands occur in the meninges. Indeed in the pilocytic astrocytoma of the cerebellum this invasion leads to the formation of a surgically important "capsule" (GP, Fig. 146). The same process in medulloblastomas, however, leads to widespread metastases via the CSF (Fig. 103). A hasty conclusion based on morphology alone would therefore contradict biological behavior.

The same applies to statements on the mixing of the stroma with the tumor tissue in the form of diffuse interpenetration. In medulloblastomas, the diffuse permeation by reticulin fibers has been taken rightly as evidence of disruption of the glia-connective tissue barrier and therefore a sign of malignancy. The connective tissue, however, is as much confined to the blood vessels in medulloblastomas as it is in most other neuroepithelial tumors. In those portions (with the exception of the desmoplastic type), where there is diffuse mixing of tumor cells and reticulin fibers, we are dealing with remnants of the leptomeninges of the cerebellar folia which have been included in the tumor and diffusely spread. This, on the one hand, can easily be recognized in the architecture (ZÜLCH 1940 a; see also Figs. 19d, 101b). On the other hand, in the desmoplastic type the mixing of the two germ layers has not been explained, as is also true in glioblastomas with a sarcomatous component. Up to now the assertions about the connective tissue in glioblastomas are not biologically unequivocal. If the presence of "glomerulus-like" vascular formations (PENFIELD 1932 a; HBT, Fig. 45a, b) is to be accepted as a generally valid sign of malignancy (BREM 1976), examination of other gliomas and paragliomas would quickly show up some contradictions, since these loops and glomerulus-like formations (HBT, Fig. 57a, b) occur in nearly all neuroepithelial tumors as a reaction to cystic degeneration or necrosis (ZÜLCH 1940 a). I have seen them develop even around a cyst in neurilemmomas, and since *necrosis* occurs mainly in malignant brain tumors, and *cysts* in benign ones, these formations lose their *absolute* biological value. We must therefore assume that the number and the growth rate (fresh mitoses, HBT, Fig. 45c) of such formations, which are otherwise so similar, offer a basis for biological evaluation (HBT, Fig. 45). In glioblastomas we must take into consideration the overall behavior of the blood vessels, which then reveals findings that are quite type specific for malignant tumors. These formations are again not restricted to glioblastomas, but can be observed in certain other malignant tumors. We shall discuss these structures more fully in our systematic description of the stroma. They must somehow be dependent on the metabolism of the malignant tumors – something that can easily be observed in the vicinity of small metastases of glioblastomas (GP, Fig. 133) and other tumors, and also as a general phenomenon in gastric cancer (GOLDMANN 1911) or osteosarcomas (DOS-SANTOS 1950).

Structure of the Stroma in Various Tumors

New methods of demonstrating blood vessels [staining of the red blood cells in the vessels in thick sections according to the methods of Lepehne-Pickworth (BERTHA 1939, 1940, 1955; SAHS and ALEXANDER 1939; HARDMAN 1940; LUZZATO 1942; WILKE 1943; ESSBACH 1943; ZÜLCH 1956; SCHÖCHE et al. 1980)] have given us a better overall picture of the distribution of blood vessels in tumors than was possible with conventional stains in thin sections (DEERY 1932, 1934; ELSBERG and HARE 1932; H.J. SCHERER 1933, 1935; MONIZ 1940; CERVOS-NAVARRO and MENOZZI 1959; KHOMINSKY and SCHAMAEV 1971). These methods have complemented our own investigations on specimens cleared according to the method of SPALTEHOLZ (see ROMEIS 1968), which have supplied good general survey material (HBT, Fig. 49). Errors are likely to arise only in the case of thrombosed vessels, as seen in glioblastomas (ZÜLCH 1939b, 1956, 1959a, 1969a) where the erythrocytes can no longer be stained.

In astrocytomas of the cerebral hemispheres we usually find only a few inconspicuous vessels, predominantly capillaries, which can scarcely be distinguished from the normal capillaries of the brain. An increased density of vessels can be seen further into the center of the tumor. The gigantocellular subtype inclined, in our experience, toward the formation of repeatedly coiled, reduplicated vessels within the adventitial covering (ZÜLCH 1956, Fig. 156b). The astroblastoma-like type of astrocytoma is distinguished by a dense, uniform vascular bed within its "pseudopapillary" architecture (Fig. 17d). Its vessel walls are widened by the marked production of reticulin fibers, whereas the mesodermal cells proliferate only slightly. Astroblastoma-like astrocytomas occasionally advance along their growth zone by peculiar, fingerlike buds (HBT, Fig. 23) which consist of coils of vessels surrounded by tumor cells ("gliovascular system").

The ependymoma also has a dense regular vasculature like that of the astroblastoma-like astrocytoma. The blood vessels tend to show intimal proliferation progressing to complete occlusion (resulting in cyst formation). In pilocytic astrocytomas there are regions with numerous, frequently coiled blood vessels. Some astrocytomas (pilocytic?) have such a high degree of vascularization that they have been considered as angiomatous mixed tumors (BERGSTRAND 1937). This applies especially to the subfornical region (WEISS 1932) and to the outlet of the fourth ventricle, where one of our cases showed the presence of a tangle of vessels resembling a cavernoma. Both regions have their own special vascular architecture (WISLOCKI and PUTNAM 1924).

In oligodendrogliomas the vascular architecture is not characteristic; there are densely packed capillary networks in the zone of growth and also larger vessels with proliferation of their walls, all of which tend to show hyalinization and calcification (HBT, Fig. 36a). In neurilemmomas we often see small accumulations of vessels resembling cavernomas, particularly in the marginal zone. In medulloblastomas, the capillaries are not very numerous and only exceptionally show proliferation of their walls. The structure of the vessels in glioblastomas is exceptionally interesting, when growth has been precipitous and the vessels are abnormally formed (Fig. 19c).

Systematic classification and description of vascular patterns are best achieved by introduction of the following eight types (see also UDVARHELYI et al. 1955; SCHIEFER et al. 1955b):

1. Large lacunar vessels of venous or arterial structure (according to the part of the vascular limb being studied). These are partly pre-existing and partly new-formed vessels ("vascular fistulae, lacunae"), which ultimately grow to the thickness of a knitting needle and surround the tumor (GP, Figs. 132–136) like a mantle (HBT, Fig. 47b).
2. Dense, somewhat disordered capillary networks, which differ from normal capillaries by a definite increase in reticulin fibers and dilatation of their lumina (Fig. 19b).
3. Long vascular barriers of proliferating capillaries, which frequently take the forms of loops and tangles (Fig. 94b). They also occur in single small groups, usually close to the necrotic areas (Fig. 19a).
4. Organized vascular systems reminiscent of cavernomas (Fig. 19c).
5. Glomeruli, either single or in systems, with definite, recognizable efferent and afferent limbs, especially close to areas of reactive and neoplastic proliferation (Fig. 19a).
6. Proliferation of the adventitia of pre-existing blood vessels, resulting in the growth of sprays and clusters of newly formed vascular loops around the central vessel (Fig. 19c).
7. Large recently thrombosed vessels (HBT, Fig. 47a, d).
8. Vessels disintegrating after endothelial proliferation or possibly as late stage of thrombosis. Frequently large swarms of fibroblasts spread out from these foci (HBT, Figs. 47c, 48a; see also DEERY 1932, 1934).

The changes under type 1 are of great interest for the understanding of glioblastomas (HBT, Fig. 49) and account for the arteriographic findings. We have followed the development of these patterns in small metastatic glioblastomas (GP, Fig. 133; see also ZÜLCH 1948). The stimulus of the tumor tissue brings about proliferation of the neighboring capillaries, widens their lumina, subjects them and the veins to arterial pressure, and opens up arteriovenous shunts. In short, a jacket of dilated, aneurysmal "fistuli" (TÖNNIS 1938; GP, Fig. 135) consisting of lacunar or sinusoidal ectatic vessels develops around the tumor. They are most probably type specific for glioblastomas and are responsible for most of the arteriographic findings described by TÖNNIS (1938), LORENZ (1940) and SCHIEFER et al. (1955b). The flow in glioblastomas is usually decreased, may be normal or increased, in contrast to arteriovenous malformations, where it may go up to 4 times the normal flow (GÄNSHIRT and SCHIEFER 1954).

The connective tissue of glioblastomas remains confined to the blood vessels, with the exception of the diffuse swarms of fibroblasts mentioned above and in patches of scarring around necrosis. Accurate studies have been published by ESSBACH (1943) and W. MÜLLER (1962b) on the vascular pattern of meningiomas and by HÄGERSTRAND (1961) on that of metastases.

In the neoplastic regions of the growth zone a stimulus develops that acts upon the vascular bed of the host tissue (ZÜLCH 1951b; GP, Fig. 133; BREM 1976). These vessels subsequently become the stroma of the tumor. In this way the capillaries proliferate and undergo vasodilatation, leading to the capillary pattern described under type 2. The formation of necrosis in the tumor induces reparative reaction of the connective tissue in the marginal zone. Thus, a wall of connective tissue is erected from the neighboring capillary systems (HBT, Figs. 46a, b, 48b), whose action is to limit and surround the tumor. Larger blood vessels are induced to form capillary buds. Under the influence of necrosis the lumen becomes enlarged, and the patterns described under type 3 develop (GP, Fig. 133).

Once a vessel is included in the tumor the stimulus of the tumor tissue induces a proliferation of the wall, which can lead to complete obliteration (HBT, Fig. 47c) of the lumen (pattern in type 6) with consequent necrosis of the dependent tissue. In the center of the larger vessels a peculiar proliferation of capillaries arises, which is either primary or can be interpreted as due to recanalization of thrombi. Such thrombi can also be seen in their fresh state (pattern of type 8; HBT, Fig. 47a).

During consideration of the stroma of glioblastomas, it must be remembered that certain patterns, such as those described under type 5, are also present in brain metastases, in carcinomas of stomach (GOLDMANN 1911), and other malignant tumors, e.g., sarcomas of bone (DOS SANTOS 1950). Consequently glioblastomas and metastases can be differentiated arteriographically only on the basis of the external shape of the tumor, as revealed by the surrounding vascular jacket. Differentiation is an easy task if the metastases are multiple.

It must be stressed once again that the vascular proliferation adjacent to necrosis is not exclusively type-specific for glioblastomas, but can also occur around the cysts and small areas of necrosis of other neuroepithelial tumors. We have even observed it in the subependymal zone in cases of ependymitis (ZÜLCH 1939b).

Our views on tumor blood vessels can be summarized as follows: architecture, quantity and form of the connective tissues of the blood vessels can be largely explained by their function as stroma; otherwise they arise as a consequence of regressive changes. The typical blood vessel pattern for each individual tumor type is known and will be discussed later together with other histologic findings. Type-specific patterns of blood vessels occur most frequently in glioblastomas and can be used as an important sign in angiography for the differential diagnosis from astrocytomas.

Blood vessels, however, are only one component of the organoid total picture of the tumor. It is not yet known why and when the stroma is transformed and begins to grow as an autonomous tissue in the sense of a "composition tumor" (Feigin et al. 1958; see also the section: "Glioblastoma with Sarcomatous Component,", p. 322).

The pathologic phenomena of the vascular stroma in neoplastic processes include several entities that are well-known to the radiologist and should be explained here. *"Blush"* is a hyperemia due either to vasodilatation (arterioles, capillaries, venules) or to a general diffuse hyperplasia of the vascular stroma of small vessels.

This is not the place to discuss the formation all the way from the reticulin fiber (Doljanski and Roulet 1933) to the concepts by Brem (1976) about the inductive influence on the stroma. There are still many questions to be answered. For instance, how in postoperative CSF metastases of an ependymoma the vessel-free leptomeninges could be vascularized to nourish the neoplastic tissue (GP, Fig. 71), as seen in one of our cases.

Similar observations, though not as exceptional, have been made by Hasenjäger (1939b) of the vascularization of small metastases of glioblastomas at the ventricular wall.

In summarizing one can state: Vessels and stroma are thought to be part of the host tissue and are primarily nonneoplastic. Voluminous growth cannot take place without sufficient vascularization. Form and pattern are apparently widely dependent upon tumor type. However, we have no explanation for the marked difference between highly malignant tumors such as medulloblastoma, with a diffuse capillarization and similarly malignant glioblastomas with their markedly variegated patterns (see points 1–8, above).

"Early filling veins" represent an especially rapid filling of the veins on the angiogram. These corresponds to the "red" veins seen during surgery. They are the result of dilated capillary segments of the vasculature, so that they appear "too early" on the angiogram, and also "too red" on the surgically exposed surface ("... found in arteriovenous fistulas, in arteriovenous malformations, and in malignant tumors like glioblastomas and metastases etc."; Zülch, cited in Kautzky, Zülch et al. 1982, p. 166).

Early filling veins in neoplastic disease have been taken as indicators of malignancy. However, Zülch et al. (1973) emphasized that this is only a rule of thumb with certain exceptions. They reported the case of a 41 year old man with a meningioma of the choroid plexus in the lateral ventricle. Angiography revealed a mantle of "pathologic" angiomatous vessels drained by early veins. Histologically the tumor was benign. A preoperative problem arose particularly from the fact that a mandibular "cyst" had been removed several months previously and had been diagnosed as a carcinoma.

Further References: Kung et al. (1969), Khominsky and Schamaev (1971), Kawamura and Kamijyo (1975), Pakula et al. (1978), Schöche et al. (1980).

6.5 Growth

The growth of brain tumors can be described as expanding, infiltrating, or destructive, according to the custom of pathologists. All nonneuroectodermal tumors except for angioblastomas, sarcomas, and metastases, grow in brain tissue by expansion. Neuroepithelial tumors behave in different ways. Neurilemmomas, plexus papillomas, and ependymomas grow by expansion, although occasional ependymomas force themselves into the host tissue by forming papillae (ZÜLCH 1940b) and thus occasionally enclosing islands of parenchyma. Pilocytic astrocytomas and pineocytomas/germinomas grow by infiltration in their marginal zone, but the bulk of the growth takes place from the inside outward, i.e., by expansion. This internal increase in volume is not very pronounced in circumscribed fibrillary astrocytomas. The oligodendrogliomas and medulloblastomas grow predominantly by infiltration, but have considerable cell proliferation at their center so that they also possess an expanding component. Growth is purely diffuse only in diffuse astrocytomas and "diffuse gliomas" or glioblastosis respectively.

Examples of tumors with destructive growth are glioblastomas, sarcomas, and metastases. Neuroepithelial tumors rarely invade the mesodermal tissue in a destructive or infiltrating manner. One exception is the *subarachnoid* space, into which nearly all "central" neuroepithelial tumors (HBT, Fig. 3c, d) (excluding the "peripheral" neurilemmomas) penetrate and where oligodendrogliomas can even form real warts (see p. 244 and HBT, Fig. 34). The penetration and growth of pilocytic astrocytomas (see p. 226) or particular forms of "astrocytosis" (KERNOHAN 1930; WALKER 1941) is most frequently observed. The other exception is the *perivascular* space of the larger vessels (which is probably also permeated by CSF) into which the cells of glioblastomas and medulloblastomas infiltrate and the cells of oligodendrogliomas and gangliocytomas frequently spread in "lymphoid" form. The very nature of these cells has to be clarified and may be part of an immune reaction.

Certain neuroepithelial tumors, such as oligodendrogliomas, adhere to the dura but never infiltrate it (see p. 244). Only meningiomas invade it, and monstrocellular sarcomas permeate it occasionally with nodules (GP, Fig. 239). Meningiomas can grow into muscle after penetration of the bone, e.g., temporal muscle (CUSHING and EISENHARDT 1938; also our own observation).

The statements above are based on findings dealing with growth in the marginal zone. The question of whether "intracerebral tumors" grow by *infiltration* or by *induction* has not been clarified since STORCH (1899) originally raised this question. Illustrative of infiltrating growth are the peculiar "gliovascular" formations (HBT, Fig. 23), which are seen in the marginal zone of some astrocytomas (astroblastoma-like) and which seem to extend finger-like into the tissue, as well as the infiltration of the subarachnoid spaces by oligo-, medullo-, ganglio-, and glioblastomas and even by the seemingly benign pilocytic astrocytomas. Induced growth is illustrated by the findings in monstrocellular sarcomas where, at some distance from the tumor edge, single, obviously neoplastic, cells begin to split off from the blood vessels (ZÜLCH 1953a; HBT, Figs. 86, 87). Our observation of smooth muscle cells in a medulloblastoma, with the cells swarming out from the blood vessels, should also be mentioned here (ZÜLCH 1940b).

Unfortunately, tissue culture has not yet yielded any information about the particular forms of growth of neuroepithelial tumors in the brain. These forms of growth are type-specific only to relatively small degree.

We often see subpial accumulation of tumor cells and further extension under the leptomeninges in medulloblastomas and glioblastomas. Only in oligodendrogliomas, however, is this subpial accumulation pronounced enough – with the formation of tiny nodules and a marked increase of glial fibers – that it can be used by the surgeon as a macroscopic characteristic (little wart-like structures: identified by palpating finger) (HBT, Fig. 34). The oligodendrogliomas are frequently very sharply delineated from the neighboring brain tissue. However, they can infiltrate the leptomeninges, expand them with mushroom-like (Fig. 58) or nodular growths (see the classical case of MERZBACHER and UYEDA 1910), and adhere to the dura (Fig. 57), so that they may easily be mistaken for a meningioma at the first stage of surgery. They can also grow in a patchy manner, which again brings up the question of multicentric origin. They share with many gangliocytomas the tendency to form round cell lymphoid (immunoreactive? neoplastic?) infiltrations around blood vessels of the marginal zone. Whether these are neoplastic and really undifferentiated cells or a "lymphocytic" immunologic reaction will be discussed later (see pp. 80, 247). However, these changes are all that can be listed as somewhat specific for this neuronal tumor. Oligodendrogliomas share certain growth characteristics with all densely cellular tumors, particularly glioblastomas, inasmuch as they follow all the fiber tracts, U fibers and the commissures and yet all these structures can also be spared to a striking degree. The oligodendrogliomas are tumors of white matter which, growing from the deeper structures, can often spare the cortex for a long time. Nonetheless, one of their characteristics may be diffuse distention of the cortex with disintegration of the subjacent white matter (Fig. 59; GP, Fig. 106; garland-like patterns of oligodendrogliomas). The role of the fiber tracts in determining the pattern of tumors has been described above (see p. 121). This applies to some degree to such structures as the latticework of the arachnoid, or Bergmann's glia in the cerebellum, whose formative action brings about rhythmic patterns such as the cell columns of medulloblastomas (Fig. 102b). Not only the myelin sheaths but the blood vessels, as well, can exercise a formative influence. Blood vessels furnish the means of spread for the so-called periadventitial sarcomas (HBT, Fig. 82), diffuse sarcomatosis of the blood vessels, and to a lesser degree, of medulloblastomas (HBT, Fig. 65d). Without doubt perivascular accumulations of cells are also seen around the border of oligodendrogliomas.

The external "infarct-like" appearance of certain glioblastomas (GP, Fig. 120) and metastases, and the similarity of their spread to that of purulent encephalitis following brain wounds (GP, Fig. 138) indicates that a similar *vascular* factor may play a role in the spread of all of these processes.

Special attention should be given to a description of tumor growth when it reaches the leptomeninges. Astrocytomas, particularly their pilocytic variants, oligodendrogliomas, glioblastomas, and pinealomas/germinomas can grow into the leptomeninges. Certain of these tumors, e.g., medulloblastomas and, to a lesser degree pinealomas/germinomas and oligodendrogliomas, can even metastasize (by seeding) diffusely via the CSF (GP, Figs. 111, 112), as can ependymomas after operation (GP, Figs. 70–72). The biologic significance of these facts will be discussed later (see p. 183ff.). Whenever medulloblastomas invade the leptomeninges they expand them slightly but continue with their rapid, unrestricted propagation. Pilocytic astrocytomas expand the leptomeninges considerably and stimulate a marked formation of glial fibers in the arachnoid with the blood vessels in this area becoming hyalinized. An oligodendroglioma greatly expands the subarachnoid space, like a mushroom or a balloon. In this region it frequently attaches itself to the dura (see above). The architecture of these three tumor types, once they have broken into the subarachnoid space, is clearly type-specific.

Whether induction of a cell to neoplastic growth is possible is still unknown, however, especially since even the question as to whether the cells spread by *infiltration* or whether they are *induced* or *transformed* by some agent (see pp. 121, 129) *locally* has not yet been answered for every form. The presence of Rosenthal's fibers in pilocytic astrocytomas distant from the subpendymal glia, even in the meninges, is more suggestive of infiltration. Also unanswered is the question of whether infiltration takes place at an undifferentiated stage, with differentiation occurring subsequently. Such an undifferentiated form could be the lymphoid cells (in gangliocytomas, oligodendrogliomas, and pineocytomas/germinomas; see also KALM and MAGUN 1950). Infiltrations of the walls of the third ventricle as a "pre-stage" of the large cells are nowadays more commonly considered to be a sign of an immunological defense reaction. We actually find around the blood vessels of gangliocytomas, in addition to "lymphoid cells," small elements that resemble nerve cells (HBT, Fig. 1) that appear capable of further maturation (TÖNNIS and ZÜLCH 1939, Fig. 18). The spindle-shaped cell seen in monstrocellular sarcomas is probably a precursor of the monster cell. As far as medulloblastomas are concerned, I am inclined to reject Bailey's concept of the differentiation of cells in two different directions, into ganglion and glial cells (BAILEY and CUSHING 1926; BAILEY 1930), and prefer to consider them as included local parenchyma, although modern literature appears to refute this concept.

The rapidity of growth is a particular problem. It can be determined, for instance, by time of volume doubling of a neoplasm. This time lapse can be measured and the rapidity of growth thus evaluated. However, this really cannot be done, for instance, in meningiomas since they are usually treated surgically soon after the diagnosis is confirmed. A second possibility is the explanation of tumor tissue as has been done in malignant glioma (MENNEL in a personal communication) and measurement of rapidity of cell growth and "doubling". Whether, for instance, growth differs in the same tumor type in children and adults has not yet been clarified particularly since the number of childhood tumors is small (JÄNISCH et al. 1980). More detailed information of growth kinetics (volume doubling time) has been published by STEEL (1978).

The problem of rapidity of growth has become particularly challenging since TAKEUCHI (1983) described the type of "inactive" or "silent" glioma following his CT investigation. He found it present in 10% of 150 histologically proven gliomas. He sometimes found a silent period of an average of 8.5 years, mostly in fibrillary astrocytomas. In such cases the treatment policy had to be carefully considered.

Several attempts have been made to define rapidity of growth, particularly by the form and relative number of mitotic figures. According to early investigations by EVANS (1926) this number did not change in the first 24 hours after removal of the tumor. R. SCHRÖDER (1964) studied the relative frequency of atypical mitoses in astrocytomas and glioblastomas (mitoses are rarer in astrocytomas) and in medulloblastomas and glioblastomas (R. SCHRÖDER and KAESS 1972; see also SWAEN et al. 1964; ARCHANGELSKY et al. 1972). Finer abnormalities have even been looked for in nuclear structures, e.g., chromosomes, by modern techniques (BICKNELL 1967). No abnormal excess nor abnormal extra chromosomes were found and the exposure to radiation had to be excluded in any abnormal cases. A specific study was conducted by HOSHINO et al. (1972, 1975) in which they gave ^{14}C and ^{3}H-thymidine to the patients before operation and then the marked cells were counted and a labeled index determined. In necroses of glioblastomas it was 0, in viable parts of the same tumor up to 20%. An index was found in glioblastomas which went up to 17.8%; that in anaplastic astrocytomas to 11.3%; in astrocytomas to 2.1%; and in metastases to 21.5%. The tumor cell cycle time was 57 h $\pm$ 6 h. This figure has to be considered in the planning of chemotherapy. The DNA distribution has also been examined in benign and malignant tumors.

A different method for determining the rapidity of growth was developed through investigations of the angioarchitecture (SCHÖCHE et al. 1980). PAKULA et al. (1978) repeated early studies of ZÜLCH (1939b) of the instructive growth patterns of experimental malignant neurilemmomas. They discussed their significance for deciding the degree of malignancy and also the possible value in the administration of chemotherapy.

In general pathology the cell death in normal and malignant tissues has been studied also in order to determine the rapidity of growth (COOPER et al. 1975).

Further Reference: FOLKMAN (1976).

6.6 Form and Staining Properties of Tumor Cells

There are no known universal staining, impregnation, or morphological characteristics peculiar to all *tumor* cells. For a long time an imbalance in the nucleus-cytoplasm ratio was considered to be such a characteristic. The cell is thought to lose in differentiation what it gains in intensity of growth. However, this applies only to some malignant tumor cells which are completely dysplastic, e.g., the elements of anaplastic glioblastomas of the multiforme type, or the grotesque giant cells of monstrocellular sarcomas. Other tumor cells – like those in astrocytomas – are often remarkably similar to the tissue of origin. Consequently, the distinction between the tumor cells of the infiltrating neoplasm and those of the host tissue is sometimes difficult [see also LUSE's (1958) attempt to distinguish reactive and neoplastic astrocytes]. It can become nearly impossible when considering cells in the marginal zone of an astrocytoma, unless some local reactive astrocytes are clearly distinguishable due to their impregnation by the gold sublimate method. Certain tumor cells of astrocytomas and oligodendrogliomas cannot be distinguished from host tissue cells – a fact that is of great importance in the evaluation of operative or post mortem tissue as well as needle biopsies. On the other hand, local astrocytes may be included in glioblastomas and transformed, according to Cox (1933). Tumor cells may be identical with the corresponding or analogous cells of the host tissue or with their developmental precursors (astrocytoma: astrocytes; craniopharyngioma: immature corium, etc.). Moreover, they can resemble regressive forms; for instance, the cells of gigantocellular (gemistocytic) astrocytomas may be similar to normal astrocytes that have first actively proliferated and then undergone regressive ("amoeboid") changes. Further difficulties are encountered in differentiation of the perivascular accumulations of small lymphoid hyperchromatic cells, often tumor cells, in the marginal zones of pinealomas/germinomas, oligodendrogliomas, and gangliocytomas, originating from infiltrations of normal lymphocytes or those formed during an immunological defense reaction.

When a tumor engulfs the local host tissue as, for instance, the granule cell layer of the cerebellum, the host cells may be mistaken for small, especially hyperchromatic tumor cells.

Furthermore, the numerous nuclear fragments of disintegrating medulloblastoma cells have often been mistaken for mitoses. That error was particularly striking in a case of glioblastoma where, in additon to describing medium-sized spindle-shaped tumor cells, an author mentioned streams of "hyperchromatic small round cells," which were obviously fresh nuclear fragments along the border of necrosis.

The external cell form can be type specific, like the star shape of astrocytes when stained by the gold sublimate method. This method can be considered upon as specific for astrocytes and other fiber-forming glial cells (e.g., the subependymal glia). Other methods, especially metallic impregnation, are fairly specific for neoplastic cells (GRINYO 1968). Embryonic cells such as neuroblasts, however, can rarely be identified solely on the basis of supposedly selective metallic impregnation methods. Only the tumor cells of ependymomas seem to give a clue about their origin from ependymal cells, in that blepharoplasts can be demonstrated with the Heidenhain or aniline-orange G stain, or with Hortega's fourth variant or other impregnations. However, they can be recognized only with oil immersion and must be distinguished from coarse formalin precipitates or dust. Rosenthal fibers are a type-specific characteristic of the cells of the subependymal glia, though only after the onset of regressive changes. Rosenthal fibers are also frequently found in pilocytic astrocytomas. Therefore, we associate this tumor with the subependymal glia as its tissue of origin. The same accounts for the "granular bodies" (ZÜLCH 1940a, 1956).

Certain tumor cells give evidence of internal secretion, such as those in adenomas. This forms the basis of identification and classification (see p. 463). The same has been assumed for the ganglion cells of the infundibular region (DRIGGS and SPATZ 1939). An excellent contribution to the identification of fibril forming glia is offered by the demonstration of "glial fiber acidic protein" (GFAP).

These glial fibrillae can be marked by immunohistochemical methods, which show up the acidic protein of the fibers (GFA and PAP methods). In the astrocytes one of two staining patterns may be visible, (a) abundant immunoreactive material may be demonstrated in the perikarya and processes of neoplastic

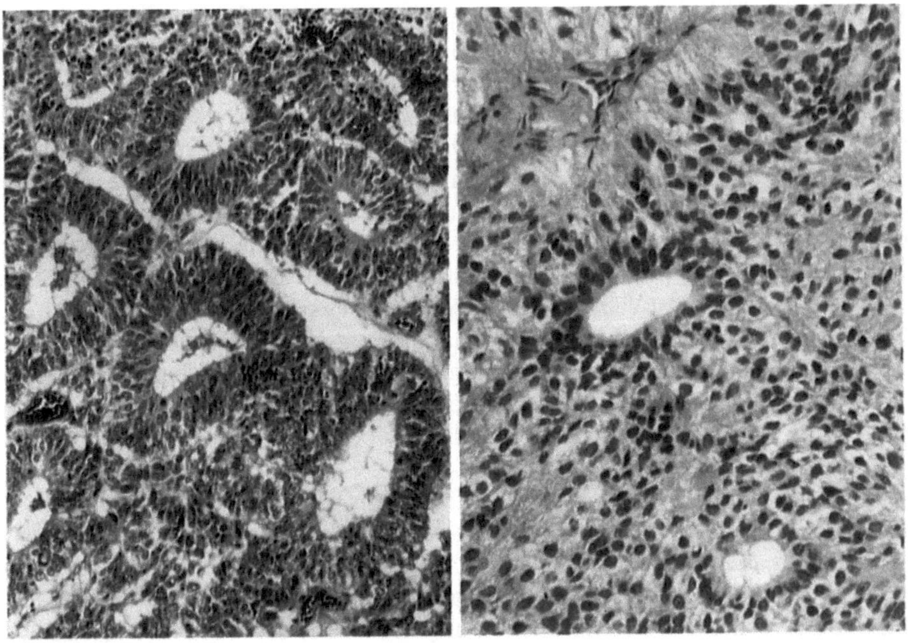

a b

Fig. 20. a Formation of tubules similar to medullary epithelium. Nissl, ×220. **b** Neuroepithelial tubules similar to the central canal. H & E, ×160

astrocytes; or (b) a meshwork of stained fibers with no perikaryal staining may be found.

In astrocytic tumors the cytoplasm of large cells in the gemistocytic form stains intensely, while staining fails in small cellular elements. In pilocytic astrocytomas a dense and loose cellular pattern may be strongly accentuated by immunostaining. Rosenthal fibers stain either as solid masses or only peripherally. In the subependymal giant cell astrocytoma of tuberous sclerosis intense perikaryal immunostaining is visible. Yet, some of the cells may remain totally unstained. Glioblastoma multiforme may have a strong reaction in the gemistocytic cells as is also the case in most of the elongated bipolar cells. Small round cells show little or no staining. Areas of necroses and macrophages remain unstained.

Ependymomas show very distinct staining in the cell processes traversing the perivascular space. Perikaryal immunostaining can be observed in only a few. A subependymoma shows a distinct immunostained material in multipolar cells, particularly in the perikarya and extending into a few thick cell processes. Oligodendrocytes in oligodendrogliomas do not stain at all, apart from some reactive astrocytes admixed with the neoplastic cells. Primitive neuroepithelial tumors (Fig. 20a, b) show no GFAP reactivity. In some medulloblastomas areas of distinct astrocytic cell differentiation can be found, but they are readily distinguished from reactive astrocytes whithin the tumor mass. Ganglion cells show no immunoreactive appearance (Eng and Rubinstein 1978; Friede and Pollak 1978; Van der Meulen et al. 1978; Velasco et al. 1980).

7 Regressive Processes

Regressive changes are by no means rare in brain tumors and can make tumor tissue unrecognizable or at least almost unclassificable. Yet, in both type and extent they are quite characteristic for each of the various subtypes of neuroepithelial tumors. Knowledge of these processes is therefore both necessary and helpful in evaluating biopsies from altered tissues. Regressive changes, such as calcification, necrosis, and cyst formation, may permit localization of a tumor by x-ray or CT. They can also be used in differential diagnosis, since as stated above, the degenerative processes are to a certain extent type specific.

7.1 Necrosis

Necrosis arises most commonly through sudden vascular occlusion. It occurs mainly in glioblastomas where endothelial proliferation and thrombosis are particularly common (HBT, Figs. 47, 48). It may be widespread or confined to small areas which appear in the form of streaks on histologic section (Fig. 18b). The marginal cells may undergo pseudopalisading (see p. 120). If the vascular lumina are not completely blocked, wreaths of cells persist around the blood vessels, where they receive nourishment for quite a long time. In addition to glioblastomas, necrosis occurs very frequently in metastases from small cell carcinomas of the bronchus and from malignant retinoblastomas (Fig. 17b). Smaller areas of necrosis also occur in oligodendrogliomas, and less commonly in ependymomas and pilocytic astrocytomas, where cyst formation predominates as is the case in all comparatively benign gliomas. This observation is useful in formulating the rule of thumb that tissue destruction progresses slowly (necrobiosis) in the more benign neuroepithelial tumors, while it occurs suddenly with necrosis in malignant tumors. Only in medulloblastomas is such necrosis rare. There the cells are more apt to disintegrate individually (by karyorrhexis) and to be scattered diffusely throughout the tumor. Reactive formation of glomerulus-like formations around necroses is common. Also inflammatory infiltrates, particularly leukocytes, may appear around the border of necrosis in glioblastomas, and in the stroma of metastases. Round cell infiltrates occur in many tumors (see p. 133), but their origin and significance is uncertain; they are now commonly regarded as a sign of an immunological defense reaction. Single plasma cells can be found in all mesodermal tumors. Superimposed infection from without may cause the whole tumor to putrefy and be densely infiltrated with leukocytes, as in one of our cases, where we saw that the multinuclear monster cells of a sarcoma acted as macrophages by enclosing the inflammatory cells.

A general basic investigation of cell death in normal and malignant tissues has been performed by COOPER et al. (1975). This study was not specifically concerned with malignancies of the CNS.

7.2 Necrobiosis, Mucoid Degeneration, Cyst Formation, Calcification, Hyalinization, and Fatty Degeneration

Mucoid degeneration and liquefaction (HBT, Fig. 25), leading to cystic degeneration, are particularly characteristic for certain brain tumors, generally of a benign nature. Of the neuroepithelial tumors, astrocytomas disintegrate through focal mucoid degeneration leading to the formation of large cysts (GP, Figs. 84, 85), whereas the subtype astroblastoma forms a system of small cysts (HBT, Fig. 24c) around the numerous preserved blood vessels. Oligodendrogliomas can also form small cysts filled with mucoid material (GP, Fig. 106). The most pronounced disintegration is encountered in pilocytic astrocytomas of the cerebellar vermis (Figs. 46, 48; GP, Figs. 143, 145), where often, as also in the case of angioblastomas (GP, Figs. 221–223), only small mural nodules remain (Fig. 137). Ependymomas of the cerebral hemisphere also usually possess a single giant cyst (Fig. 69). Cystic degeneration is infrequent in malignant glioblastomas and neurilemmomas, but when seen in the latter it is most pronounced in the spinal form. Spinal cord tumors often contain large pencil-shaped cavitations.

Cysts are almost never encountered within pineocytomas/germinomas and plexus papillomas; in these papillomas, however, a large cyst may sometimes lie next to the tumor, having developed possibly by transudation (secretion?). Smaller cysts can occur in meningiomas while larger ones are occasionally encountered in monstrocellular sarcomas (Figs. 141, 142; GP, Figs. 235, 236) and in metastases (Fig. 163). The cysts usually arise through mucoid degeneration and liquefaction, which often changes the basic tumor structure in a particular way: it makes a pilocytic astrocytoma at the beginning of cystic disintegration look similar microscopically to an oligodendroglioma (Fig. 51a). In addition to this mucoid disintegration of the tumor tissue, transudation plays a large role in the maintenance of the cyst contents and in the refilling after therapeutic puncture of certain tumors, such as angioblastomas. It is surprising, however, how long large tumor cysts, which have been emptied, can continue to remain empty as observed sometimes in pilocytic astrocytomas. BUCY and GUSTAFSON (1939) reported symptom-free periods of 12 years following puncture (CUSHING's case no. 5), 7 years (case no. 7), and 7.5 years (case no. 17); all these patients had cystic astrocytomas of the cerebellum. The most remarkable case is that of BUCY (1946, case no. 30), in which therapeutic puncture of the cyst resulted in a symptom-free period of 15 years. In craniopharyngiomas, mucoid degeneration leads to cyst formation producing either small networks of cysts or giant solitary cysts with only a small mural nodule of tumor (GP, Fig. 267). Solitary cysts following liquefaction of the tissue frequently develop in chromophobe adenomas of the pituitary (GP, Fig. 251). Mucoid degeneration can be recognized particularly by its metachromatic properties seen with cresyl violet staining. The presence of so-called mast cells in connective tissue tumors has the same significance. We found this commonly in the vascular connective tissue of angioblastomas and less frequently in meningiomas.

According to the literature a cyst can be *defined* as a closed sac filled with fluid and surrounded by a tissue wall of varying nature. Some cysts arise within the tumors themselves (neoplastic cysts) while others arise in the neighboring tissue. In the brain, however, the macroscopic concept „cyst" also includes the following processes, arranged according to pathogenesis:

1. Intracerebral („brain cysts") (Drew and Grant 1948; Lemke 1950):
   a) Parasitic cysts
   b) Brain cysts following vascular occlusion (birth trauma, porencephaly, embolism and thrombosis, earlier radiation)
   c) Posttraumatic cysts
   d) Intraneoplastic cysts
   e) Malformative cysts (septum pellucidum, etc.)
   f) Glandular cysts (pineal, pituitary gland)
2. Extracerebral (arachnoid) cysts:
   g) Cysts resulting from neighboring inflammation (old meningitis)
   h) Cysts resulting from a congenital malformation

(See also Drew and Grant 1948; El Banhawy and Ahmed 1962).

The content of cysts is quite variable. The cyst fluid of craniopharyngiomas resembles brownish black motor oil in which small crystals of cholesterol are dispersed. The contents of arachnoidal cysts which develop from congenital malformations are milky (p. 525), while those resulting from inflammatory processes contain CSF.

In the literature tumor growth and cyst growth have often been regarded as essentially parallel processes. In my opinion, however, cyst formation is usually a regressive process within the tumor. Cysts in spinal ependymomas, pilocytic astrocytomas, and angioblastomas therefore correspond to the large cysts within the same type of tumors in the cerebral hemispheres and cerebellum (not to a concomitant „syringomyelia").

Calcification

Calcification is largely a sign of slow benign growth, seen in CT even when mild. However, it is often sufficiently advanced to be demonstrable on plain x-ray films (in oligodendrogliomas, less often in ependymomas of the hemispheres, plexus papillomas and gangliocytomas, and less frequently so in pilocytic astrocytomas of the cerebellum). Among extracerebral tumors, most of the craniopharyngiomas are calcified, as are a portion of the teratomas and dermoids, many pineocytomas/germinomas, and some meningiomas.

Only rarely does this process lead to ossification (Bebin and Tytus 1955). In the series of Martin and Lemmen (1952) 207 of 1577 tumors (13.1%) were calcified microscopically (see also Schiffer et al. 1961; Schiffer 1971; Tanaka et al. 1975: 12%).

Histologically, calcification occurs in different parts of the tissue in different tumor types (MARTIN and LEMMEN 1952: four patterns). In oligodendrogliomas, the tumor vessels themselves, or the capillary system of the neighboring (overlying) cortex calcify (as in Sturge-Weber's disease; W. MÜLLER 1961), or calcifications appear free in the tissue. A similar pattern of calcification can also occur in pilocytic astrocytomas (not in „brain stem gliomas" (?); DUFFNER et al. 1978), gangliocytomas, and ependymomas. In meningiomas, the best known form of calcification is the „psammoma body", which is the final stage of calcium incrustation of hyalinized balls with a concentric pattern like the skin of an onion (Figs. 17c, 128). Pencil-shaped calcifications are also encountered or, more rarely, calcification of individual capillaries. Calcium deposits are very frequent in craniopharyngiomas where the „keratoid" degenerated parts are involved, and they occur in teratomas and dermoids. Calcification almost never occurs in angioblastomas or astrocytomas but if it is seen in the latter, the possibility that an oligodendroglioma has been misdiagnosed must be considered. The circumstances under which calcification occurs and the role of pseudocalcium and calcium (BOCHNIK 1953) have not yet been well clarified. For instance, a diffuse dusting of the tissue with tiny calcium particles, for instance, in the wall of capillaries is often the precursor of massive calcification (see also SCHIFFER et al. 1961).

Calcification is an interesting phenomenon in the parenchymatous tumors of the pineal gland (pineocytomas/germinomas). The „two-cell" tumors are frequently so heavily calcified that they are as demonstrable on plain x-ray films as the pineal gland itself, which after the age of 8–10 years has a tendency to calcification.

On the other hand, germinomas found elsewhere in the body never manifest that trend. This is one more sign, which indicates to me that the „two-cell" tumors of the pineal region belong only partly to the germinomas.

Hyalinization

Connective tissue tumors, such as meningiomas, undergo hyalin degeneration in large areas. In neuroepithelial tumors such as pilocytic astrocytomas and oligodendrogliomas, blood vessels often show hyalin changes and the larger vessels in glioblastomas can also become hyalinized. A similar degeneration occurs in neurinomas where large sections appear hyalin-like (even though neuroepithelial cells do not form hyalin in the strict sense of the word). x-Ray irradiation also leads to hyalin-like („para-amyloid") changes in vessel walls (see p. 142).

Fatty Degeneration

Slow necrobiotic deterioration of tumor tissue usually leads to diffuse fatty degeneration, which in neurilemmomas can be considered the best example of this. The characteristic yellow color of glioblastomas, and particularly the ochre yellow streaks along the borders of necroses, are signs of locally advancing fatty degeneration. A zone of macrophages is formed close to the necrosis (HBT, Fig. 51c), which not infrequently is made up of rod cells (HBT, Fig. 51d), which rapidly accumulate fat and are often transformed into round, compound granular corpuscles. Inasmuch as they can proliferate and form compound granular corpuscles, for example, some tumor cells still show the normal potentialities of some types of glia or mesodermal tissue. However, gradual fatty degeneration of larger portions of the tumor, with partial vascular occlusion, also occurs in glioblastomas. It is interesting that fatty degeneration almost never occurs in medulloblastomas, which have a meager vascular supply. Moreover, astrocytomas and oligodendrogliomas only show scattered individual compound granular corpuscles. The latter are uncommon in meningiomas, where if they do occur, they lie in the center of islands in the meningotheliomatous type and are diffusely scattered in the fibromatous type. They are seldom seen in craniopharyngiomas and are completely absent from pituitary adenomas. On the other hand, the interstitial cells of angioblastomas often show abundant fatty degeneration with the presence of birefrigent lipids (fatty infiltration?). In the case of neurilemmomas, with their fatty degeneration together with hyalin changes and liquefaction of the tumor cells into round, fat-filled elements with centrally-placed pyknotic nuclei, a histologic picture startlingly similar to the honeycomb pattern of the oligodendrogliomas develops in paraffin-embedded tissue (Fig. 114a, b). [See, however, W. MÜLLER's concept that the lipids are not of a regressive nature, but result from defective myelin formation of the blastomatous Schwann cells (W. MÜLLER 1965)].

7.3 Hemorrhages

Massive hemorrhages (the „glioma apoplecticum" of the classic literature) are rare (0.8%–10.2%, ZUCCARELLO et al. 1981; ALBERT 1982) but they do occur in oligodendrogliomas, glioblastomas and metastases of melanomas and even less often in pituitary adenomas. In the latter, hemorrhages of different ages are often found adjacent to one another. They can result in the death of the patient or in the destruction of the gland with dire consequences. Massive hemorrhages can be explained by pathologic changes in the vessels. In oligodendrogliomas, this takes place through hyalinization and complete calcification (HBT, Fig. 36), and in glioblastomas due to their precipitous growth and hyalinization (HBT, Figs. 46–49). In the past pressure differences following pneumoencephalography or ventriculography or the consequences of arteriography sometimes induced a fatal hemorrhage. Therefore, in markedly calcified oligodendrogliomas caution was necessary when applying any diagnostic method which changed the intracranial pressure. Small hemorrhages are also encountered in other tumors (see also EBHARDT et al. 1983). The blackish brown color of eosinophilic pituitary adenomas, for example, and the red-brown discoloration of the cyst wall in pilocytic astrocytomas indicate frequent hemorrhages. Occasionally, a hemorrhage can occur in a cystic spinal neurilemmoma and induce functional transsection of the spinal cord.

7.4 Other Regressive Processes

The cells of gigantocellular astrocytomas are similar to astrocytes, which have passed first through a progressive and then through a regressive phase (the nuclei are pyknotic and lie peripherally within the tumor). They resemble some forms of amoeboid change (ALZHEIMER 1910). Since the gemistocytic astrocytes of this subtype lie in the central portion of the tumor, and normal cells grow in the marginal zone, it does not seem impossible that the large cells arise from the smaller cell type through a particular kind of regressive process perhaps of a nutritional nature. In pilocytic astrocytomas, we find the well-recognized degenerated forms of Rosenthal fibers (ZÜLCH 1937b, 1940a, 1963a; HBT, Fig. 58). These have been described repeatedly in the literature and have been used as support for certain theories about syringomyelia (BIELSCHOWSKY and UNGER 1920; HALLERVORDEN 1952), derivatives of axis cylinders (TANNENBERG 1924; JUNG 1935), derivatives of blood pigment, and „heme bodies“ (LIBER 1937). The changes described by MCLEAN (1934) and VERHOEFF (1922, 1932) as „cytoid bodies,“ particularly in pathology of the eye, are only in parts identical with Rosenthal fibers. We agree with the view expressed by DEL RIO HORTEGA (1944) that the Rosenthal fibers are the result of regressive alterations in glial cells themselves (OPALSKI 1934; ZÜLCH 1937b; GRCEVIC and YATES 1957; DIEZEL and ROTTMANN 1958; KALM 1959; FOTAKIS 1961b; RAIMONDI et al. 1962; GULLOTTA and KREUTZBERG 1963; ZÜLCH 1963a, Fig. 1, chronic ependymitis; SCHLOTE 1967) (see Fig. 52a).

Our personal extensive but as yet unpublished studies with various staining methods showed that Rosenthal fibers occur almost exclusively among the cells of the subependymal glia. We are apparently dealing with a special form of degeneration of the fibrous part of these cells arising through swelling (ZÜLCH 1940a; ZÜLCH and WECHSLER 1968, Fig. 12b). In our material, the formation of Rosenthal fibers was confined to pilocytic astrocytomas and to the reaction of the subependymal glia in other types of tumors which lie near the ventricle; e.g., ependymomas, angioblastomas, etc. Moreover, they occur diffusely (HALLERVORDEN 1952) in von Recklinghausen's disease. I have described „granular bodies“ (or corpuscles; see ZÜLCH 1940a; HBT, Fig. 59c, d; and ZÜLCH and WECHSLER 1968, Figs. 12a, 13) as another regressive phenomenon in the same kind of tissue or tumors (see Fig. 52b).

SZYMAS/Poznan has actually shown in ultrastructural investigations that glial fibrillae lie in the marginal zone whereas the nucleus of the Rosenthal fiber is formed by some unstructured protein elements (personal demonstration).

In cystic adenocarcinomas or cylindromas, the center of the cell columns and streams undergoes liquefaction, with formation of well-recognized „cylinders“ (see p. 485ff.). Since it would be impractical to mention all the minor alterations of tumor cells, only such artificial changes, which occur through autolysis in the saline solution during surgery will be mentioned. In epithelial tumors such as the pituitary adenomas these alterations can lead to cell swelling, with a high degree of dissociation of the tissue making it difficult to recognize its nature. Immersion of the tissue to remain in normal saline for any length of time should be avoided. Cell alterations due to electrical current and drying have been mentioned on p. 123.

At the cellular level regressive changes in the tumor cells can occur in single elements or in large tissue regions (see also Sect. 7.1). One of the remarkable changes at the cellular level is the atrophy which occurs in ependymomas from chronic pressure. This has been described by GIAMPALMO (1937) in the tongue-like process of an ependymoma of the fourth ventricle reaching down into the cisterna magna and the upper cervical cord. I also showed this process in 1956 (Fig. 226). Whereas this process probably starts with atrophy and post-atrophic disappearance of the cells, a similar process can occur in the so-called mucopapillary ependymomas of the cauda equina. In that location local pressure could also be the acting force in this case. On the other hand, the mucohyaline degeneration of the stroma around the vessels could also be regarded as a causative factor. (This process is shown in Fig. 231c, d in ZÜLCH 1956.)

Although a large part of the tumor tissue undergoes cellular atrophy in gigantocellular astrocytomas, a regressive process may provoke this characteristic feature. In this event the cells in the center of the tumor resemble some forms of so-called „amoeboid“ change. Gemistocytic astrocytes of this subtype of astrocytoma are mainly encountered in the central portion of the tumor while smaller and „more normal-looking“ astrocytes grow in the marginal zone, therefore, it is not unreasonable to assume that the large cells arise from the smaller cell type due to some kind of regressive process.

In gangliocytomas one frequently finds cell „shadows“, i.e., opaque cell bodies free of nuclear material are not infrequently found; these are probably neurons undergoing an atrophic process.

8 Changes Produced by External Factors Such as Radiation

In order to determine the risks of radiotherapy and its effects on various tumors we must investigate the changes within the tumor tissue itself, the possibility of damage to the surrounding brain tissue (so-called "delayed radionecrosis"), and the reaction of the individual patient to the use of ionizing radiation (ZÜLCH 1956, 1960b, c; ZÜLCH and OESER 1974; OESER and ZÜLCH 1974). These investigations have to be considered against the background of results available at the time when only surgery was applied or when combined surgery and radiation were used (POOL and KAMRIN 1966). It is very difficult to determine the incidence, prevalence and course of tumors of the nervous system both untreated and provided with the best possible care of neurosurgery, radiotherapy, and chemotherapy.

POSNER and SHAPIRO (1975) have given an excellent survey on the current status of treatment of brain tumor, its complications and its results (see p. 34ff.) and also a gross epidemiologic study.

Furthermore, the actual effect of radiation on neoplastic tissues has to be thoroughly studied, keeping in mind particularly the question as to whether an effect is brought about through prevention of growth by destruction of *individual cells,* or whether necrosis of the whole tissue is achieved, perhaps as result of interference with the blood supply. The mechanism could be the permeation of certain substances through the vessel wall and their destruction of the tissue either directly or indirectly through an allergic/immunologic process or even by producing complete anoxia and ischemia, as suggested by SCHOLZ (1934; SCHOLZ et al. 1959).

We feel that there is some justification for assuming that the most complete and ideal effect of radiation, i.e., the destruction of growing tumor cells, occurs predominantly in two types of tumor, medulloblastomas and the pineocytomas/germinomas. The possibility of a cure of such tumors by radiation seems to be near in spite of the usual diffuse spread of metastases to the subarachnoid spaces.

The following very brief survey will consider the radiation effect upon the most important types of intracranial neoplasms with a greater emphasis on the more malignant forms (see also TICE and IRVING 1950).

Let us consider here first the general results of the series of BOUCHARD and PEIRCE (1960) of 826 cases. Of the 534 patients, which survived for 5 years or more after radiation, 399 were adequately treated five to twenty years ago.

Astrocytomas. Some authors recommend radiation of astrocytomas very enthusiastically, e.g., WEIR (1973), who called radiation therapy the most important determinant of prolonged postoperative survival. STENBERG and MOBERG (1971), however, felt that the matter should be reviewed first very rationally, both the pros and cons, before forming a final opinion. HERBST (1982) recommended radiation of astrocytomas in children when only subtotally removed. I personally lack the experience necessary to discuss this matter authoritatively.

Oligodendrogliomas. Since the time of recurrence is unpredictable with these tumors, our personal strategy in the radiation of oligodendrogliomas has been to wait until a postoperative recurrence appears. A similar policy was followed by SHENKIN (1965). However, we reported three cases in 1969, treated at times with very high radiation doses (see also the case of EICKE 1952) where after survival for 5–8 years signs of gross delayed radionecrosis with subsequent death was noted. In PEIRCE's (1964) series 77.7% of the patients survived 3 years and 33.3% the 10 years border after radiation.

Our own strategy was to start with radio-/chemotherapy immediately after surgery only in subtotally operated cases.

Pilocytic Astrocytoma. We had no successful results with radiation of pilocytic astrocytomas, and therefore discontinued it because of the benign character of the tumors. This was in accordance with the experience of BOUCHARD (1966). PEIRCE (1964) classed all forms of astrocytomas together and found a survival of 61.7% for more than 3 years after surgery and radiation.

Ependymomas. In patients with ependymomas operation was considered to be indicated in all ventricular (operable) cases, as well as in the extraventricular large cystic cerebral tumors, which were usually calcified. We could see at autopsy the "para-amyloid substance and a certain sclerosing effect" (ZÜLCH 1963c, Fig. 5). PEIRCE (1964) noted that 75% of his patients with ependymomas survived for 3 years, and 50% for more than 10 years, again after surgery and radiation.

Glioblastoma Multiforme. Prolongation of life was reported by SACHS (1954) when he described the results of radium treatment of glioblastoma. KLAR et al. (1954) tried ^{60}Co treatment, however, the longest survival time was only 6 months. In PEIRCE's (1964) series only 20% survived for more than 2 years, and in the series of astrocytoma III and IV patients reported by SEILER et al. (1978) a gain of only 5 weeks resulted from combined radio- and chemotherapy. Histological changes with "scarring" were shown by SHAW et al. (1978) following fast neutron therapy (see p. 149). RAMSEY and BRAND (1973) limited the field of radiation which permitted giving a higher dosage and reported an increase in overall survival time and tumor-free period. Finally YAMASHITA and GILLINGHAM (1975) investigated 560 cases of glioblastoma treated with radiotherapy (45 Gy over 4 weeks). The average survival time was 13.8 months. For comparison they took a second nonradiated group with a survival of 5.2 months.

Probably prolongation over 6–8 months by radiotherapy will be the expected result with, however, deviations from these figures in individual cases according to the "clinical malignancy" (see p. 32) of the tumor.

Our experience with radiation of glioblastoma multiforme was not possible to judge because chemotherapy was given at the same time (see p. 150), but we had interesting morphological results by radiotherapy alone, which we reported in 1969.

Medulloblastomas. One of the most impressive improvements with radiation has taken place in the field of medulloblastomas, when compared with older experiences (CRUE et al. 1967; FAUST et al. 1970).

PEIRCE (1964) had already emphasized that 75% of his patients had a useful life period postoperatively and a prolongation of survival. He found 29% survivors of 3 years, and 14.6% over 10 years. WILSON (1970) believed that almost one-third would survive beyond 10 years after radiation. On the other hand, PROBERT et al. (1973) noted that 27% of their patients had a 5-year survival following megavoltage radiation that included the entire cerebrospinal axis. The results of HOPE-STONE (1970) showed that 75% of patients were still alive after 5 years, and 50% after 10 years when having undergone a whole CNS radiation. The results of NOËL and METHOT (1970) were less satisfactory: only 46% survived for 5 years though the longest survival time was 12 years. With these differences in mind, BLEHER et al. (1982) spoke of a 5-year survival rate of 35%–70% when total radiation of the CNS was applied (further references: TOKARS et al. 1979; CUMBERLIN et al. 1979).

Finally, we should mention the early results of M. LINDGREN (1953, 1958), to whom we owe one of the basic discussions of the radiation of brain tumors and the most exact data about dose tolerance. He reported on a medulloblastoma patient surviving 9 years when treated by surgery and subsequently by radiation. RICHMOND also as early as 1953 had reported in his series of children with medulloblastoma a survival period of 5 years in 43% after radiation. I personally have histologically classified a case of KAHN et al. (1955) with a 15-year survival.

When we report these early results, however, we have to admit that M. LINDGREN, for instance, obtained excellent survival rates but was also confronted with simultaneous delayed radionecrosis of both occipital lobes in some of his cases.

Craniopharyngioma. In the treatment of this tumor radiation by way of stereotactic implantation of radionuclides has been attempted by LEKSELL (1951) and later by STURM et al. (1982) and STEINER (1982).

In inoperable brain stem tumors MUNDINGER (1966; MUNDINGER and METZEL 1968) implanted iridium-192, as did also BOND et al. (1965) and KRAMER et al. (1961), who reported excellent results.

Metastases. Significant amelioration of symptoms and even a median survival of 6 months have been achieved in 70% of cases (GLANZMANN et al. 1976). NISCE et al. (1971) also held it worthwhile to irradiate in 560 cases, in 54% of which palliation was obtained. When the patients actually completed the planned course of total brain radiation (35 Gy), this occurred in even as high as 80%.

We ourselves saw dramatic amelioration with angiographic changes in a woman patient with a metastasis from a breast carcinoma. When we repeated the angiography after irradiation with 92 Gy over two frontal fields most of the "fistulous vessels" had disappeared (ZÜLCH 1969b, Fig. 2).

Meningioma. We have also illustrated (ZÜLCH 1969b, Fig. 4) delayed radionecrosis of the whole of the white matter of both frontal lobes in a case of olfactory meningioma with a survival of 5 years (Figs. 21, 22). The patient had not been operated on due to the particular circumstances of World War II. She died of intercurrent disease. In this case (ZÜLCH 1969b, Fig. 4) progress was noted of the delayed radionecrosis into the healthy tissue with early clinical manifestations. FUKUI et al. (1977a) tried radiation in meningiomas when they were highly vascularized, using 30–60 Gy (see also WARA et al. 1975).

Pinealoma/Germinoma. Excellent results obtained with radiation in the group of the two-cell pineal tumors (of the pinealoma or germinoma type) were reported by HORRAX and WYATT (1947). We could confirm these excellent results in an 8-year-old girl, whom we described (ZÜLCH 1969b, p. 96) broadly because of her "ectopic pinealoma". She was terribly emaciated and had a complete diencephalic and infundibular endocrine syndrome as well as ocular symptoms (ZÜLCH 1963c; Fig. 1; the weight of the patient at that time was 12.7 kg). The two-cell type of pinealoma was diagnosed with *certainty* by the shape of the cells found in the CSF (ZÜLCH 1969b, Fig. 1), which showed the same long processes with club-like endings as those seen in DEL RIO HORTEGA's excellent figures of the large cells of the pineal gland.

After radiation of 90 Gy there was a good recovery from the hypothalamic and midbrain symptoms and the ocular muscle paralyses also disappeared. She went to school and was active as a completely healthy individual, surviving 5 years overall.

Because of clinical recurrence she was given elsewhere a total dose of 235 Gy through four fields to the chiasmatic region. The child finally died with severe cerebellar signs, a progressing tetraparetic syndrome and, towards the end, quadrigeminal symptoms. We believe that the final phase may have been related to the growth of the primary pinealoma in the midbrain, which was not irradiated at all, rather than to delayed radionecrosis around the radiated ectopic pinealoma. Repeated pneumoencephalography 2 years and 3 months after the first irradiation disclosed that the metastasis in the chiasmatic region had completely disappeared. Autopsy permission was not obtained, but the case showed the excellent early results of radiation.

JENKIN et al. (1978) reported about 81% survival of 5 years if the patient was under 25 years. However, only 37% of the patients over that age survived so long.

Tumors at Particular Locations. Unclassified tumors in specific sites were radiated by PEIRCE (1964), who reported in mesencephalic tumors 45% survival over 3 years, 40% over 5 years, and finally 25% survival over 10 years. Corresponding figures for *pontine* tumors were 33% survival over 3 years, 33% over

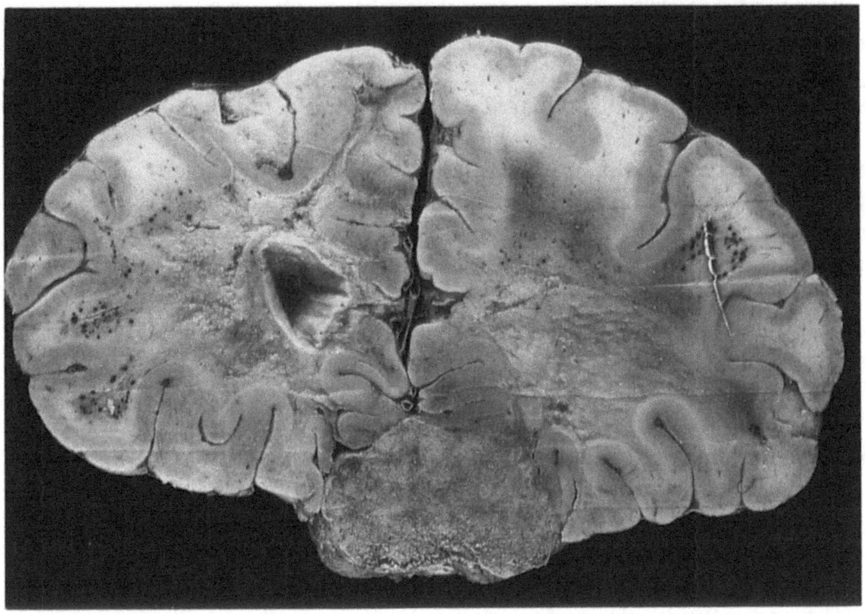

Fig. 21. Delayed radionecrosis in a case of olfactory meningioma not treated by surgery

5 years, and 23.8% over 10 years. Similar figures may be found for brain stem tumors in the paper by WHYTE et al. (1969).

Late (Delayed) Radiation Necrosis

This undesirable effect of radiation on normal brain tissue has received considerable attention during the second half of this century (SCHOLZ 1934; ZÜLCH 1951b, 1956, 1960b, c, 1963c, 1969b; ARNOLD et al. 1954; ZEMAN 1955, 1966; M. LINDGREN 1958; SCHOLZ et al. 1959; BOUCHARD 1966; LÖHR and VIETEN 1967; ZÜLCH and OESER 1974; OESER and ZÜLCH 1974; DI LORENZO et al. 1978).

Apparently, however, the first cases of late radiation necrosis in man were described by FISCHER and HOHLFELDER (1930), SCHOLZ and HSÜ (1938), KALBFLEISCH (1946), and PENNYBACKER and RUSSELL (1948).

We described late radiation damage of the brain (Figs. 21, 22) in 26 autopsies in detail in 1956 (p. 93ff.). In these cases the white matter appeared necrotic (Fig. 22) and asbestos like (GP, Fig. 318); the cortex usually being uninvolved unless in the "crossfire" of several "ports" of radiation, so that it would be exposed to an excessive dose as in EICKE's (1952) case.

We have tried to mimic these radiation sequelae in our institution by experiments with animals as did M. LINDGREN (1958). Satisfactory results were achieved (HARDER 1965) and even expanding space-occupying cysts were produced. As SCHOLZ had noted earlier we found para-amyloid lesions (ZÜLCH 1960c, d, 1963c). However, HARDER's experimental work demonstrated that quantitatively the para-amyloid change in the vessels remained less prominent,

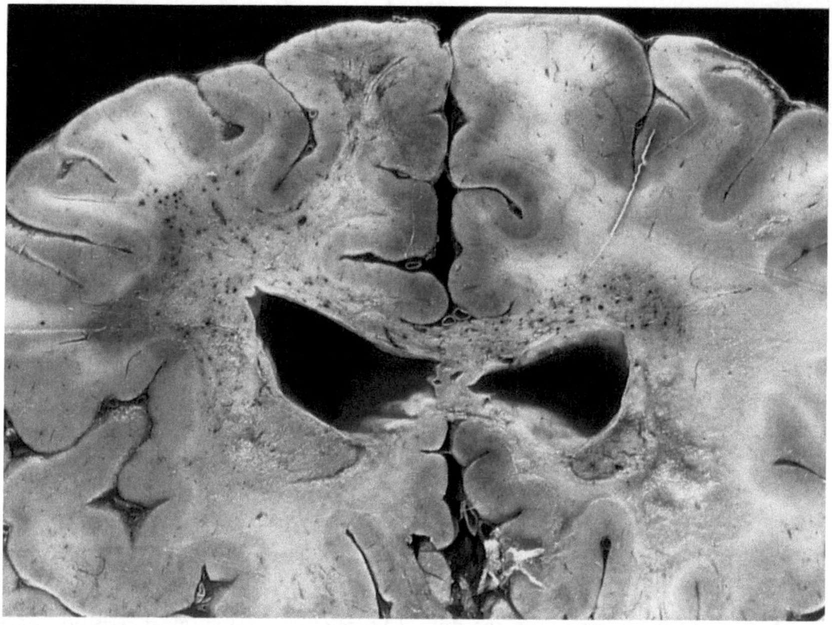

Fig. 22. Same case as Fig. 21; note that the white substance is demyelinated whereas the cortex is almost uninvolved. (ZÜLCH 1975a)

while in contrast the primary destruction of myelin sheaths and, particularly, an early, gross primary change in the glia were the outstanding features. These findings did not conform to SCHOLZ's conclusion that the primary change was increased vascular permeability, with the subsequent appearance of para-amyloid, half-moon-like structures. The ensuing ischemia produced secondary necrosis of the tissue and the vessels no longer remained patent to deliver oxygen and nutritive material. We also found the formation of multinucleated giant cells among the astroglia particularly significant; they almost mimicked the appearance of malignant tumors (ZÜLCH 1969b, Fig. 9).

We developed also the working hypothesis that an allergic autoimmune process occurred with primary damage to the myelin sheaths. MARKIEWICZ (1935) and BERG and M. LINDGREN (1958) had envisaged a similar process as the basic phenomenon. Curiously enough no radiation changes occurred in about one-fifth of the animals, a fact already noted by the aforementioned authors. Constitutional factors perhaps may first induce an autoimmune process which initiates the late radionecrosis. It is also interesting that in the experiments a variable latent period to the occurrence of delayed radionecrosis was evident. Such latent period is usually from the customary 7–9 months but can be as long as 5 years.

The white matter of the spinal cord is as radiosensitive and the late radiation changes are as prominent (KRISTENSSON et al. 1967) as in the brain. We have published two interesting cases which are both important because of the pathogenesis and the liability of the radiologist. However, the latter was denied in both cases (ZÜLCH and OESER 1974; OESER and ZÜLCH 1974).

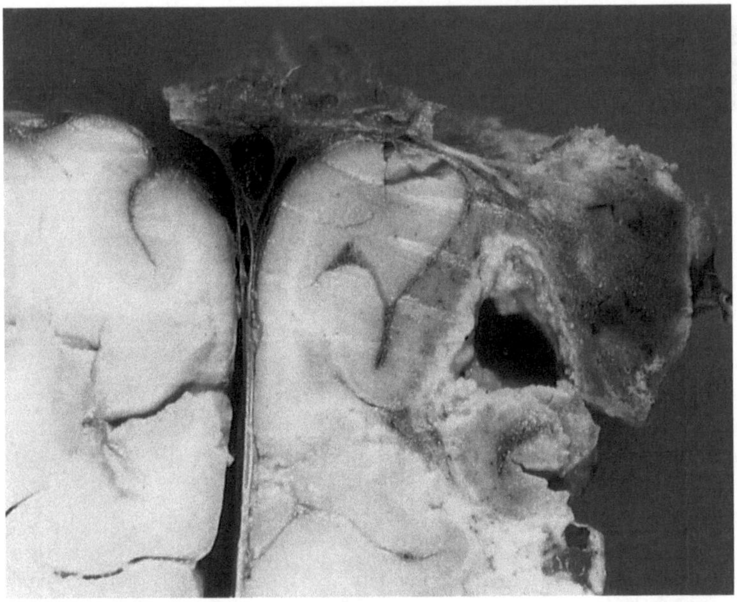

Fig. 23. Annular fibrosarcoma in the dura 7 years after total surgical resection of a cerebral extraventricular ependymoma in an adolescent. No recurrence was encountered. Radiation dose around 80 Gy (ZÜLCH 1975a)

We have described above the features of most cases of radionecrosis (Fig. 22; ZÜLCH 1960b, Figs. 2 and 5; GP, Fig. 318). In some, however, made a puzzling and disturbing observation, namely, that in some human cases (ZÜLCH 1956) a development was evident that made the necrotic tissue "grow" so that clinically it acted as a space occupying lesion (GP, Fig. 320) that was even operable.

This mimicking of either a recurrence or a second neoplasm has also been mentioned by other authors (EYSTER et al. 1974; MARTY and MINCKLER 1973).

Development of Radiation-Induced Tumors

In some rare cases malignancies (Fig. 23), usually of the fibrosarcomatous type (GP, Figs. 231, 232), developed in the radiated region (the first case apparently was reported by MANN et al. 1953). Other similar cases have been reported by TERRY et al. (1959), WENDE (1962), NÖTZLI and MALAMUD (1962), RUSSELL and RUBINSTEIN (1959/1977), and WALTZ and BROWNELL (1966: ten cases from the literature and two of their personal cases).

BERG and M. LINDGREN (1958) observed in their experimental work an osteosarcoma in the treated region when radiating normal rabbits during their experimental work.

Other types of tumors have been described such as a neurofibroma (DONOHUE et al. 1967) and astrocytoma (SOGG et al. 1978).

The observation of meningiomas in a region of external radiation of the scalp was very frequent. BELLER et al. (1972) saw 16 patients with meningiomas, which occurred after radiation for treatment of fungus infection of the scalp. Other radiation induced meningiomas have been reported by WAGA and HANDA

(1976: 12 years after radiation) and FEIRING and FOER (1968); meningiomas after medulloblastoma radiation see IACONO et al. (1981).

MODAN et al. (1974) pointed out the occurrence of both malignant and benign head and neck tumors particularly in brain, parotid gland and thyroid after radiation.

Further Reference: RAVENTOS et al. (1960).

Undesirable Effects of Ionizing Radiation: Increased Malignancy of Radiated Tumors

Foci of increased malignancy manifested by a higher number of mitoses than previously encountered in any other human tumor were observed in the vicinity of large necroses in two irradiated glioblastomas (ZÜLCH 1960b, Fig. 1a, b). Acceleration of growth was noted clinically and the explosive proliferation or irregular mitoses and other irregularities of cell architecture, histologically. It would appear that the number of mitoses was almost equal to that of the cells and was due to an increase in the rate of growth similar to that reported by NETSKY et al. (1956) following irradiation of cell cultures.

A similar experience from Tönnis' clinic in Berlin was reported before World War II. Prolongation of survival was attempted by the introduction of radium needles into highly malignant tumors (LORENZ 1949). It was perhaps scarcely a coincidence that in both these test cases the tumor growth was accelerated to a degree not previously encountered. Within 6 months, gigantic recurrent masses almost the size of a fist developed and were removed on six occasions by operation (ZÜLCH 1940b). Similar cases were published by WALTER and MÜLLER (1959) and WENDT and SIEDSCHLAG (1965).

Other Radiation Techniques

It is interesting that in tests of the effect of boron-neutron capture radiation, extensive radionecroses were encountered. There was "little or no improvement," and furthermore residual parts of the neoplasm "survived" in all instances (ASBURY et al. 1972).

Further References: SWEET and JAVID (1952), HATANAKA and SANO (1973), SHAW et al. (1978).

When we read the results of combined surgery and radio- and chemotherapy regimens (pp. 142ff., 150ff.), we see that not much has changed since the statements of POOL and KAMRIN (1966). They believed that among those patients surviving surgery and radiation treatment of intracerebral gliomas about 70% generally lived normally for some period of time. Of the remaining patients, 20% would be disabled but retained the capacity to care for themselves, and 10% would be totally incapacitated. Of patients with glioblastoma up to 70% survived therapy and had a *useful* postoperative survival for some time. Of those with an astrocytoma or ependymoma approximately 50% would even be able to resume their former occupation, while another 40% might not require further hospital care.

This earlier pessimistic outlook has not changed much even with combinations of all forms of available therapy.

9 Effects of Chemotherapy

Operative intervention is very often impossible because of the location of the tumor, the age and/or the general condition of the patient. Moreover, total removal, which might greatly influence the length of survival, is often technically impossible (JELSMA and BUCY 1969) so that a tumor which is biologically benign may behave as "clinically malignant" (see p. 32), especially if shunt operations are impossible.

In such cases of inoperable or only partially resectable tumors, and in cases of first or second recurrence, there remains the possibility of x-ray treatment (see p. 142) and/or chemotherapy. Radiotherapy plays an important role particularly in certain types of tumor. When using more modern technique delayed radiation necrosis can be avoided (M. LINDGREN 1958; ZÜLCH 1960b, 1963c, 1969b; BOUCHARD 1966). Often, however, when surgical intervention can only remove the brain tumor incompletely the addition of radio-/chemotherapy may be desirable. However, some problems remain particularly the concentration of the cytostatic effects of chemotherapy at the site of tumor growth, since most of the known active substances do not cross the blood-brain barrier and/or do not enter the CSF.

This has led to the direct injection of some of these substances such as methotrexate, intrathecally (WHITESIDE et al. 1958). This drug actually seems to be rather effective against meningeal tumor seedings. Other cytostatic agents, such as the vinca alkaloids (DEAN et al. 1967) and bleomycin (TAKEUCHI 1972), have also been reported to be effective although the side-effects, especially on hematopoiesis, often greatly limit their curative usefulness.

As mentioned above the following requirements are basic in the chemotherapy of brain tumors: (a) the compounds to be used must readily pass the blood-brain barrier and also enter the CSF, and (b) they should have minimal toxic side-effects. VICK et al. (1977) discussed the problematic issue of this concept in their editorial.

Considerable progress has been made in the last few years toward meeting these requirements. Treatment schedules have been established especially for neoplastic disease of the hematopoietic system; to this end a combination of the synchronizing and cytostatic effects of various substances is used. Indeed, chemical compounds interfering with the cell cycle at a defined stage may lead to synchronization in systemic neoplasia.

It is known that colchicin blocks cell division at the end of the metaphase by interfering with spindle formation and vincristine has also been shown to act as a synchronizing substance in both experimental and clinical tumor research. After the partial synchronization of cells, an alkylating agent, such as cyclophosphamide (Endoxan) or one of the nitrosourea compounds, can act in the S or G2 phase of the cell cycle.

Similar treatment strategies for brain tumors have been developed by POUILLART et al. (1975, 1976), which we have also used in our wards. This triple combination therapy consisted in adriamycin, VM 26 (epipodophyllotoxin), and BCNU/CCNU. The results obtained by POUILLART and also on our own wards were in some cases very satisfactory and in others almost ineffective (MENNEL et al. 1982). We were not able to determine the reason for these differences in outcome. Our attempts to clarify this in experiments will be reported below.

In pediatric oncology, however, a number of embryonal tumors have responded favorably to polychemotherapy. With medulloblastomas a favorable outcome has been achieved by using the "sandwich" principle, i.e., surgery – chemotherapy – radiotherapy. The drugs, to date, which have been effective in CNS tumors, are nitrosoureas, vincristine, procarbazine, methotrexate and VM 26 (NEIDHARDT 1982).

Earlier basic studies of the value of chemotherapy of brain tumor were reported by SHAPIRO and AUSMAN (1969), SHAPIRO et al. (1970), FEWER et al. (1972), and SLANSKY et al. (1974), and investigations of this kind continued by WALKER and WEISS (1975), C.B. WILSON (1976), HEISS et al. (1978), LEVIN et al. (1979), PAILLAS et al. (1979), and members of our team (MENNEL and SZYMAS 1978; PETROVICI and ILSEN 1978; ILSEN et al. 1982; and MENNEL et al. 1982).

Unfortunately we did not have the opportunity of investigating a larger series. However, we were able to study each single case very thoroughly employing all the available methods of clinical investigation, radiology, and later on, whenever possible, morphology. We were still unable to clarify the differences in response to administration of similar therapeutic regimens in apparently similar malignant gliomas. Our impressions after reviewing the different results cited in the literature were the following:

1. Heterogenity of the series, which included patients with as well as those without operation, some with subtotal and other with total removal of the tumor, and with differing "clinical malignancy," and last, but by no means least, the different grade of malignancy of the neoplasms.
2. Evaluation of the therapy can be made only by comparison with similar series from former times when either no therapy or surgery only was given. Moreover, modern technical developments in neurosurgery and anesthesiology, preoperative, intraoperative, and postoperative have to be considered (see FRANKEL and GERMAN 1958; JELSMA and BUCY 1969).
3. Another important problem was the difference in classification systems which has only recently been overcome by applying the WHO classification of tumors (see p. 16ff.).
4. The course of the tumor growth must be followed in vivo. This was difficult in former times when only radioisotope scintigraphy and angiography were available, whereas today serial CT scans can be made.
5. Different criteria were employed in the evaluation of therapy with different emphasis. Some investigators merely reported survival time, others the quality of social life of the patient, and still others the capability for work.

One additional problem not clarified up to now but prominent in our personal series, was that some of the patients, for instance, those with glioblastomas, were "good responders" to chemotherapy (even up to 20%), whereas the statistical results of chemotherapy in general appeared to be poor. Some of these patients, inspite of coming to the wards already with signs of increased intracranial pressure went back to work some months later. To separate these "good responders" from the general statistical results of outcome, one has to take the "median" for comparison (see papers of PETROVICI and ILSEN 1978; ILSEN et al. 1982, from our institute).

Experimental Attempts to Clarify the Effectiveness of Cytostatic Drugs

MENNEL and SZYMAS (1978) and TAMURA et al. (1979) were able to show that of the compounds used in the triple therapy of POUILLART et al. (1977), epipodophyllotoxin and adriamycin as a single agents were equally ineffective in a rat glioma model. The only strong cytostatic factor was the nitrosourea derivative lomustin. A further step was reported in 1979 by TAMURA et al., who stated that CCNU in a rat glioma model was highly effective and increased the life-span of tumor-bearing rats by 53%–86% when administering three doses of 40 mg/kg. A total quantity of CCNU amounting to less than 30 mg/kg was not effective. On the other hand, large dosages exceeding the LD_{10} proved to be toxic. There was a mild depression of platelets and white blood cells after a single dose of 40 mg/kg CCNU with recovery by the 6th day.

Histologically there was an increase in the extent of necrobiosis of the tumor tissue, ballooning of tumor cells with nuclear pyknosis, a lack of mitotic figures and sometimes microcystic changes appeared more frequently than in the controls (see also SWENBERG et al. 1975).

My successor HEISS (HEISS et al. 1978) verified the results with CCNU. He used a modified clinical program by combining CCNU, vincristine, methopterine and procarbazine, which increased the median postoperative survival time in malignant gliomas to 10.7 months. Other reports in the literature may add support to this outcome. REAGAN et al. (1976) found median survival of 6.6 months with CCNU alone, 11.6 months with radiotherapy alone, and 12 months with a combination of both. Their conclusion that CCNU was relatively ineffective was certainly paradoxical compared with the literature.

Returning to the experimental attempts, we based our model on the concept of KIRSCH et al. (1976), who had studied both normal and malignant glial cell kinetics. This was the target factor for models of "combination" therapy (such as the "triple"). From this source we got basic information about the cellular changes in the treatment of malignant brain tumor therapy. WILSON (1976) demonstrated the superiority of BCNU, but there was a minor augmentation in its effect when it was used in a combination. MENNEL et al. (1982) showed in a comparison of various treatment methods that the median survival time was longest in the cases where radiation and chemotherapy had been employed (CCNU; Fig. 1, p. 92; see also STEINBOK et al. 1979; M.D. WALKER et al. 1978).

Evaluation

At the end of these citations of data a few words of clarification and criticism may permit better understanding of the discrepancies, which are also seen in the experimental field:

1. Terminology: We have to watch carefully which terms are used, the "median", the "average" or "middle survival time".
2. There are differences in the methods of application of various chemotherapeutic agents (tumor model? species of experimental animal?). A careful reading of Sect. 3.2 and Sect. 3.7 will better explain this statement.
3. Different systems have been used for histologic classification: The use of the WHO system would help to avoid such discrepancies.
4. It is by no means yet clarified why chemotherapeutic agents like CCNU and others have different effects on different types of tumor, however, with the same grade of malignancy.
5. It is surprising to note the satisfactory response of some of the embryonal tumors to chemotherapy (medulloblastoma; NEIDHARDT 1982).

Conclusion. Apparently, the most radical removal of tumor tissue at operation (so far as it is possible and tolerable for the patient), radiotherapy, and several cycles of chemotherapy probably constitute the best treatment program for malignant tumors (grade IV). Whether such a combination is applicable in grade III tumors is dependent upon the kind of tumor. This program always leaves the possibility open that a patient may be a good "responder."

In the case of glioblastoma multiforme one can count on a postoperative survival after surgery alone of 2–4 months depending upon the "clinical malignancy," after chemotherapy of around 6–7 months, with radiotherapy 8–9 months, and with combined radio-/chemotherapy 10–14 months (for more information on chemotherapy in glioblastoma see also BATZDORF 1966). Clinical improvement during the first months may even allow the patient to return to work.

The basic account of the tumor growth in a glioblastoma has been given by WILSON (1976). He maintained that the neurosurgeon can remove 90% of a glioblastoma and at the same time establish an unequivocal diagnosis and reducing the mass from 100 g to about 10 g. Although a 90% reduction seems impressive, the residual tumor still contains 10 billion (10^{10}) cells. Radiotherapy will further reduce the number of cells but, even assuming a 99% kill, the residual mass of 100 mg still contains 100 million (10^8) cells. With optimal enhancement, the CNS has qualitatively similar but quantitatively less efficient immune mechanisms, so that the number of glioblastoma cells that can be rendered nonproliferative is probably less than 100000. In the population of remaining tumor cells, there may be only milligram amounts of residual tumor under optimal conditions, yet regrowth is inevitable while even one replicating tumor cell remains viable.

10 Tumor and Brain

10.1 Reactions of the Surrounding Tissue

The reactions of the surrounding brain can be divided into two types: *primary* reactions are direct changes in the morphologic and physico-chemical structure of the surrounding brain tissues, while *secondary* reactions are such sequelae as displacement and distortion of the brain produced by purely mechanical factors. The latter can lead to changes of the first type, as a result of constriction, herniation, circulatory inadequacy, or stasis accompanied by changes in brain volume.

The reaction of the part of the brain immediately adjacent to the tumor varies, depending on its nature and type of growth and its location. Infiltrating gliomas, like astrocytomas or oligodendrogliomas, may elicit minor reactions, with the tumor tissue merging imperceptibly with the almost uninvolved brain. In the case of oligodendrogliomas, zones of calcified capillaries occasionally overlie the tumor in the neighboring gyri (HBT, Fig. 33b). Reactive astrocytes are occasionally seen here and in the border zone of gangliocytomas (TÖNNIS and ZÜLCH 1939). They also occur between the papillae of the growth zone of ependymomas or surrounding metastatic carcinomas. The numerous vascular changes associated with glioblastomas have been described in the discussion of stroma (p. 126). The findings in the surrounding tissue of monstrocellular sarcomas are quite surprising, since away and within the normal brain neoplastic cells begin to detach themselves from the capillaries (HBT, Fig. 86c) which make a humoral "carcinogenic" factor progressing in the tissue very likely.

Phagocytic activity is observed particularly around glioblastomas, where rod cells appear at the margin of the necrosis and microglia proliferates (PENFIELD 1927). In malignant tumors especially, numerous vascular lesions have been observed at some distance from the tumor (small foci of demyelinization due to edema). The astrocytes, too, are thought to proliferate reactively at some distance from the tumor or in the zones of former edema.

Changes in the fluid content and the consistency of the tissue (brain edema, extra- and intracellular) are particularly prominent in malignant tumors, such as glioblastomas, metastases, and monstrocellular and other types of sarcomas. As long as there are no hemorrhages, the intracellular edema of the white matter in the immediate vicinity of the tumor, the lobe, or even the whole hemisphere, is most prominent. This increase in volume created clinical localization of small metastases extremely difficult before the advent of CT. Moreover, intracellular edema produces a considerable increase in volume which, adding to the volume of the tumor, can lead to a marked shift of intracranial structures and to symptoms of herniation with its dire consequences (see p. 128ff.). On the other hand, we have observed extracellular edema mainly in the vicinity of hemorrhages into the tumor and in the case of brain abscesses, when the increase in fluid volume can be so marked that the hemisphere is virtually "drowned" (ZÜLCH 1943; GP, Fig. 338).

Brain edema may also be very prominent after operation and trauma (see p. 163).

10.2 Brain Edema and Brain Swelling

Historical Note and Definition

Our discussions of mass lesions leading to displacement and distortion of intracranial contents and herniation have included brain edema in its various forms.

Brain edema is by definition an accumulation of water and other constituents – usually proteins – within the tissues, e.g., either *within* the cellular elements themselves or in the *extracellular* compartments. However, in contrast with the pathophysiology of edema in other organs, in the brain the distinction as to whether the fluid is located *within* or *between* the tissue elements plays an important role. Although well described already by ANTON (1904) and SCHMAUS (1901), a clear concept of the pathogenesis of edema in its various forms was not developed until REICHARDT in 1905 defined it as an increase in volume of the brain. He referred to the "dry" cut surface as "brain swelling," since histologically fluid could not be demonstrated. The phenomenon was observed mainly in psychiatric disorders such as catatonic schizophrenia and those associated with intoxications. If, on the contrary, the "cut surface" was wet and the "blood points flowing" and the presence of fluid in the free spaces between the tissue elements histologically confirmed, he called this condition "edema" (see also REICHARDT 1957).

There has been much discussion as to whether this distinction made by the German school between edema and swelling had any importance for neurosurgery and neuropathology. However, we were able to distinguish readily between the two conditions by normal histologic methods or special stains. Subsequently, ultrastructural studies and pathophysiologic metabolic experiments have confirmed again the validity of this dualistic concept (ZÜLCH 1940e, 1941c, 1943, 1951c; GABRYEL 1962; ZÜLCH and TZONOS 1964, 1965; HOSSMANN et al. 1965; SCHRÖDER and WECHSLER 1965; KLEIHUES et al. 1966; RIVERSON et al. 1966; KLATZO et al. 1967a; WECHSLER et al. 1967; ZÜLCH 1967b).

BAETHMANN (1978) has provided detailed review of modern findings and concepts.

Gross Pathology

Brain edema is a reaction of the surrounding brain to a pathologic process within the cranium or to one which effects the general metabolism of the body. Edema is a detrimental reaction due both to increase in volume and to the decomposition of brain tissue particularly when the fluid is: (a) rich in protein

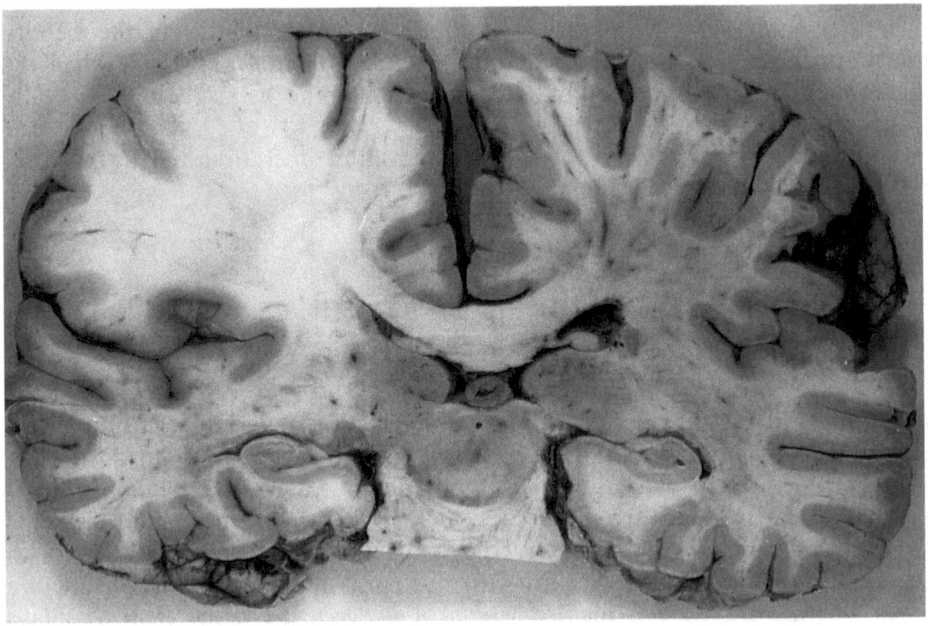

Fig. 24. Marked swelling of the right parietal white matter with lack of displacement to the opposite side. A case of frontal glioblastoma

and impairs oxygenation and nutrition, (b) it is of subacute or chronic duration, or (c) it leads to microcirculatory changes.

Brain "edema" can be recognized (Fig. 24) with the naked eye by the increase in volume of the brain tissue particularly when it is localized within the white matter (GP, Figs. 10 and 23), and in CT by inducing loss of tissue density. In the cut brain (ZÜLCH 1959b, Fig. 10) fluid runs out of the surface as described above. Brain edema may sometimes be colored greenish when it develops around melanoma metastases (ZÜLCH 1959b, Fig. 11) or brownish-black around hematomas.

Histologically brain edema may be recognized in light microscopy with the aid of Masson's trichrome stain – staining blue, when rich in proteins – and particularly well in ultramicroscopy because of its intra- or extracellular localization of the fluid (ZÜLCH 1941c, 1943).

Histologically, "brain swelling," as defined by REICHARDT (1905), corresponds to *intracellular* edema. The cut surface of the anatomical specimen is dry and sticky and the cross sections of the vessels remain clearly visible. The tissue is firm and sticky, although later, when more advanced, it becomes doughy, but it is typically dryer than in *extracellular* edema.

In *extracellular* edema the consistency is elastic and in more advanced cases with a protein-rich fluid it becomes more rubbery and after a longer duration, doughy.

The *distinction between "intra"- and "extracellular" edema* is always a crucial point in the discussion of the "various forms" of edema, or if you will, "the edemas." Final proof came through the tragic discovery of the sequelae of intoxication by TET (Triethyl-Tin). In this disorder the accumulation of fluid was entirely *intra*-cellular, corresponding to REICHARDT's definition of "Hirnschwellung".

On the other hand, the experimental results of our own team (Vienna Symposium 1965, see WECHSLER et al. 1967) and of KLATZO (1967) revealed morphologically and functionally convincing evidence regarding the pathogenesis of the *extra*cellular form of edema and its behavior. We shall continue below to describe our observations about the edemas, which we made from pathologic specimens obtained during neurosurgical procedures before the experimental era.

Historically, the development of new concepts went on rapidly. In 1940 we observed (ZÜLCH 1940e) that there was a *primary* intracellular edema with swelling of the myelin sheath and oligodendroglia, as well as of the astroglia with disintegration leading to "clasmatodendrosis" in toxic conditions. There was no fluid extracellularly (see the mention of "TET edema," above). One important new observation was that "grape-like" accumulation of vesicles in myelin sheaths (ZÜLCH 1967b, Fig. 3). Apart from "toxic" conditions, we observed a "hemodynamic" form of increase in water in the perivascular tissues created by permeation of the vascular wall and from there into the extracellular tissue compartments. From there the fluid was quickly sucked up by the tissue elements increased their volume (Quellung).

Histologic Changes. In the histologic end-stage there was no notable difference between a primary (toxic) intracellular uptake of water or a "secondary" uptake caused by a swelling of the tissue cells situated in the area of extracellular edema.

Further observations of the behavior of extracellular edema rich in proteins (stained by the Masson trichrome stain) revealed the *flow of the edema* along the myelin bundles of the white substance and occasionally throughout a hemisphere (ZÜLCH 1941c, Fig. 5). This could lead to "drowning" of the whole hemisphere, as may be seen in the case of a small purulent abscess or infected brain wound. This was later referred to by REULEN et al. (1977) as "bulk flow" (for details see p. 161).

Edema in the cortex (ZÜLCH 1943) was at that time not well substantiated by stains. We interpreted this as an indication that the fluid in the extracellular tissue compartment was immediately sucked up by the tight network of dendrites, axons, or processes of glia cells, leading to enlargement of the so-called Obersteiner spaces (see ZÜLCH 1943, Figs. 4, 5; 1967b, p. 96 and Fig. 7). I emphasized at that time that there were several forms of edema, an opinion in contradiction to that of various authorities, including GREENFIELD (1939). I came to this conclusion because the different states of intra- and extracellular fluid and the secondary uptake of intracellular edema could already be so easily demonstrated by light microscopy. The pericapillary and perivenous permeation and accumulation of the protein-rich fluid was *impressive* (ZÜLCH 1943, Figs. 10, 11, 12, 18, 19, 20, 25; 1967b, Figs. 6, 10), and the secondary "acidophilic swelling" of the oligodendroglia, resulting from a sucking up of edema fluid, were highly remarkable.

The many different conditions observed in internal medicine, neurosurgery, and neuropathology, which lead to edema, were listed in an invited paper presented to the German Neurological Congress (Zülch 1953c).

In summary, there are apparently different forms of *primary* and *secondary intracellular* edema, corresponding to Reichardt's "Hirnschwellung" (Klatzo's "cytotoxic" edema). Furthermore, *extracellular* edema was evident in brain wounds, around hemorrhages, brain infections, and obstruction of the venous outflow. The danger of destruction of myelin sheaths by protein-rich edema was emphasized. This occurs together with acidophilic change of the oligodendroglia and swelling and disintegration (clasmatodendrosis) of the astroglia (Zülch 1967b, Fig. 11). In edemas associated with inflammation or infection proliferation of the microglia and granulomatous changes of the vascular walls were noted. Furthermore, the chronology of edema in aseptic brain trauma (puncture wounds for ventriculography) was followed from the 5th hour to 20 hours, and for 3 days and more (Zülch 1971b).

It was demonstrated in glioblastomas and metastases that the brain edema was never stained by Masson's trichrome unless there were hemorrhages, and then only in their vicinity. By definition, this must have been intracellular edema. On the other hand, *extracellular* edema, which was stainable, occurred in all infections, in trauma as well as near any hemorrhages. The free flow of fluid (now called "bulk flow") was described in detail and depicted (see p. 161). Yet, these conclusions are apparently somewhat opposed to those made from recent results by K.-A. Hossmann and his associates (K.-A. Hossmann 1982).

While preparing for the Vienna Symposium in 1965 we developed models corresponding as nearly as possible to different processes in human pathology, such as:

1. Stab wound into the brain tissue
2. Blocking of the venous outflow
3. Local pressure (as in extracerebral tumors)
4. Local intoxications (by diphtheria toxin)
5. Microembolism of the vasculature.

In all of these cases extracellular fluid was observed in accordance with our expectations (see Wechsler et al. 1967; Zülch 1967b; and p. 156). All of these changes were investigated by both light and electron microscopy and illustrated.

In order to explain the pathogenesis of *primary intracellular* edema it was thought that in the process of providing nutrients for the neuron on the way from the blood through the blood-brain barrier into the astroglia and from there into the neuron, a disorder of metabolism and nutrition was induced (Zülch 1967b, Fig. 4). For *extracellular* edema transudation of the fluid (including proteins etc.) was presumed to take place through the cellular connections and bridges within the vascular wall after their destruction. It was thought that this was effected by a toxic (anoxic?) or mechanical (blowing-up) event within the vessel walls, whereby open channels were formed, which allowed the edema fluid to escape into the extracellular compartment. So-called *secondary intracellular edema was assumed to originate from sucking-up of the edema fluid by the local cellular elements, and in the extracellular compartment this meant particularly the swollen myelin sheaths and axons.*

The next decisive and exceedingly important step in the development of concepts regarding the various "edemas" came from the experimental field, and specifically from Klatzo's "cold induced edema" in the cat (KLATZO et al. 1967). He noted that from an area of acute necrosis of the cortex, edema seeped out into the underlying white matter and could be followed stepwise, particularly by fluorescence, and by tests of the blood-brain barrier until its final resolution. Since then this has been one of the standard experiments.

The pathogenesis of this cold-induced edema was defined by KLATZO as being "vasogenic," whereas such forms as TET edema were considered to be "cytotoxic."

However, in the final analysis, the pathogenesis still seems not to have been clarified completely. According to AARABI and LONG (1979), in cold induced edema the fluid must come out of the vascular walls of the frozen (necrotic?) cortex. If the injured brain was discarded or replaced in its bed immediately after induction of freezing or at 2, 4, or 8 hours after production of the lesion, the vasogenic brain edema was completely abolished and with or without replacement, the advancement of the edema was stopped. Therefore it appears that an intact vascular bed is necessary to produce the extracellular fluid component of brain edema and that no "edematogenic" factors exist within the brain which can influence either the production or the propagation of the increased extracellular fluid volume.

Further important information about pathogenesis of edemas has been published by K.-A. HOSSMANN and associates (HOSSMANN and SCHUIER 1979a, b; HOSSMANN et al. 1979; HOSSMANN and BLÖINK 1981; HOSSMANN 1982). This group made a real step forward when they demonstrated proteins in edema fluid in old paraffin embedded material (WILMES and HOSSMANN 1979). Not only were they able to show quite clearly the perivenous edema that I had described in the investigation with TZONOS (ZÜLCH and TZONOS 1964, 1965), but also the uptake of proteins in the cells, both in neurons and in astrocytes.

They then investigated the various types of edema in *stroke* and *tumor*. In stroke, they came to the conclusion that in the first 4 hours a metabolic edema occurred, which was intracellularly located and in the sense of Klatzo it was a cytotoxic form. At that period the blood-brain barrier was not yet involved. However, subsequently as a result of this metabolic change, the blood-brain barrier was opened and a delayed extracellular or vasogenic edema developed after stroke (HOSSMANN and SCHUIER 1979a).

A convincing model for experimental peritumorous edema resulted from the development of a technique by WECHSLER (1977) in our laboratory for injecting tumor cells from a clone grown in tissue culture. By stereotaxic injection each time a neoplasm, which fulfilled all the requirements, grew in the same place. After 2–3 weeks reactive signs of the peritumorous tissue were seen and there was apparently an immune rejection of the early growth of tumor. Four weeks after the injection the initial parts were already becoming necrotic. During that time typical peritumorous edema developed. The edema fluid was rich in protein, mainly confined to the white matter and characterized both by an increase in sodium and potassium (K.-A. HOSSMANN 1982). The blood-brain barrier was damaged only in the region of the lesion, that means *within* the tumor, while the blood-brain barrier in the edematous tissue remained intact. The spread of peritumorous edema seemed to be slower than that occurring after cold injury (where REULEN et al. 1977 had observed that Evans blue stained albumin travelled about 10 mm in 3 hours).

The main characteristics of cytotoxic (ischemic) edema were the break-down of the blood-brain barrier to serum proteins, the increase of sodium and the decrease of potassium in brain water. These factors were thought to have some importance (K.-A. HOSSMANN 1980) from the therapeutic point of view.

In this experimental tumor model the same decrease of edema was observed following corticosteroid administration as had been noted clinically. Vasogenic edema in experimental brain tumors could be demonstrated not only by fluorescence microscopy but also by cathodoluminescence (HÜRTER et al. 1981). For differential diagnosis of the type of edema the potassium level seemed to have great significance. Brain swelling (intracellular edema) associated with a decrease in potassium indicated that edema was at least partially of the cytotoxic type. Moreover, a disturbance of flow regulation and of vascular resistance in cerebral edema indicated a complicating cytotoxic component most probably due to intracranial hypertension and compression ischemia.

For precise evaluation of proteins introduced into the brain tissue with the edema, an immunochemical method developed for this purpose (BODSCH et al. 1982) allowed to follow the protein content in a timely relation. Impressive and at the same time appalling was the demonstration of the serum proteins in the edema fluid up to the last peritumorous convolution although Evans blue showed that the blood-brain barrier was intact and had been breached only within the tumor (K.-A. HOSSMANN 1982, Figs. 1, 2).

Investigations for extravasated proteins (edema) were made in specimens (SZYMAS and K.-A. HOSSMANN 1984a, b) from human malignant gliomas, based on a double layer immunofluorescence technique. Proteins were mainly located *extra*cellularly. *Intra*cerebral uptake was observed in some but not all tumor cells, in reactive astrocytes, and occasionally in oligodendrocytes and in neurons. The distribution of extravasated proteins corresponded precisely to that previously observed in transplantation tumors in cats (HOSSMANN et al. 1979) suggesting that the pathophysiology of human tumor edema is similar to that of experimental animals.

When these results are compared with our earlier findings one must recognize that "the immunochemical approach is much more sensitive than Masson's trichrome stain for edema fluid and probably even for smaller amounts of protein."

We should discuss here the further development of the microembolization experiments, which we had begun with TZONOS (1964) in order to promote further understanding of the mechanisms underlying edema formation.

At the Vienna Symposium we had already demonstrated that by blocking the great part of the cortical circulation with microspheres sized 37 µm, perivenous edema appeared in the depth of the white matter after 4 hours, and that this then seeped through the entire white matter and destroyed it. The debris was transported away by the scavenger cells during the following 3 weeks. Later experiments conducted in collaboration with TAMURA and SUGI using 15 ± 5 emboli of the Minnesota Company led to the same sequelae (see TAMURA and ZÜLCH 1978; SUGI et al. 1980). In these experiments the perivenous edema in the deep white matter, distant from the blocking of the vasculature, was the region of interest.

Also similar experiments performed with VISE et al. (1977) and SCHUIER et al. (1978) yielded new information about the early changes in the cortex. The blood-brain barrier was broken down for 4 hours, during which time edema developed around the capillaries and only later *after* 4 hours did it also develop around the deep veins. Edema fluid was seen in the neurons and astrocytes as well. After 4 hours the blood-brain barrier was tightened again and the animals died soon thereafter.

These experiments were performed in order to mimic the sequelae of fat and other microemboli in humans (ZÜLCH and TZONOS 1964, 1965).

Three mechanisms for the action of corticosteroids, which could improve the resolution in experimental edema, were discussed by MATSUOKA and K.-A. HOSSMANN (1981). One of the decisive factors, according to the authors, must be the uptake of serum proteins and water by the cellular elements. Furthermore it seemed possible that there was a permeation into the vessels again and a bulk-flow into the ventricles was considered as a third possibility.

It is our opinion that the first and second possibilities are probably the most important ones. Based on clinical observations (see also LANKSCH and KAZNER 1976) in edema caused by meningiomas, where it can be of a very high volume, the third possibility can be excluded by CT.

Our early findings and also the later investigations of KLATZO et al. (1980) tend to prove that the resolution of edema may be promoted by uptake of proteins into the intracellular compartment.

The Bulk Flow of the Edema Fluid. In my studies of the edema in brain wounds and brain infections (ZÜLCH 1943), I emphasized the rapid expansion of edema fluid in the white substance of one hemisphere, which may even cross the midline through the corpus callosum. I showed (GP, Fig. 356) that the stream apparently follows along the myelin sheaths of the nerve fiber bundles, such as the pyramidal and optic pathways, to the point where transverse structures, such as the pathways of association fibers, stopped the flow (ZÜLCH 1943, Fig. 9c). This was particularly impressive when the patient had been lying on this back.

REULEN (1977) was able to prove this "flowing" by demonstration of a streaming down of the edema fluid from the frozen necrotic cortex into the deep white matter, which is clearly substantiated by his pictures. The experimental array of AARABI and LONG (1979) proves likewise that edema fluid comes from the freezing lesion in the cortex and seeps downwards into the subcortical white matter and stops promptly when the "supply" from the frozen cortex is arrested. The volume of this perifocal localized edema may be considerable. For example, brain edema progressing in the first two days around a hemorrhage adds an additional mass effect, which is tought to have a volume of at least 50 cm^3 (COHEN and ARONSON 1968).

Edema in Infarction and Tumor. The edema can be far greater in volume following infarction when we have noticed surprising increases in volume and marked midline shift (see ZÜLCH 1981a, Fig. 142). This occurs particularly with infarction in the middle cerebral artery territory and was even more pronounced in cases of combined infarction of the anterior and middle cerebral arteries, where we have noted extreme cerebral edema on the third day. In some of these cases the extreme shift led to symptomatology pointing to the "wrong", i.e., *ipsilateral* side resulting from pressure against the opposite tentorial edge (Kernohan's notch) (ZÜLCH 1981a, Fig. 154a, b; GP, Figs. 353, 356, 360a, b).

We shall cite here an observation of more practical importance concerning perifocal edema adjacent to a sphenoid wing meningioma. I depicted it morphologically (GP, Fig. 212), calling it "a large cystic infarct." To date, I cannot decide whether this represented "edema necrosis" or was actually an infarct with cystic desintegration following mechanical blockade of the nutritional artery by the meningioma.

Edema in and around meningiomas is observed very commonly in CT and has been thoroughly investigated in 160 patients. The authors (STEVENS et al. 1983) mentioned the "tongue-like" or "flame-like" processes from the edema margin invading the internal and external capsules. They described the invasion of various parts of the white matter by these tongue-like processes in 70% of cases with severe edema and in only 41.2% with moderate edema. The corpus callosum and posterior limb of the internal capsule were involved when the lesions were in close proximity. In 88% of patients who developed edema the edema margin reached the ependymal surface. The aforementioned cysts appeared in 35% of cases with edema. The authors contended that the movement of edema fluid through the tissues from its site of formation mainly takes place by bulk flow. Apparently the flow was propagated by the ability of the extracellular spaces at the periphery of the edema to expand at low pressures. FENSTERMACHER and PATLAK (1976) and REULEN et al. (1978) suggested that perivascular spaces constitute preformed pathways for conduction of edema fluid. There are apparently transcerebral arteries and medullary veins extending from the cortex to a subependymal plexus (SORGO 1942; ZÜLCH et al. 1974b). These vascular cascades are most numerous in the white matter areas that are susceptible to edema. My observations in the Moya-Moya syndrome speak in favor of such a concept (see p. 459).

STEVENS et al. (1983) also investigated the rate of edema resolution after surgery. The time needed for clearance was 1–3 weeks if the edema was moderate or 4–8 weeks if it was severe. In the Klatzo model (KLATZO et al. 1967) the clearance rate ranged from 4 days to 1 month. From data of other authorities we have confirmation of our edema rates in astrocytomas and oligodendrogliomas, in which we found little edema perifocally (oligodendroglioma: Fig. 57; astrocytoma: GP, Fig. 87). In the cases with an anaplastic degeneration the edema was more pronounced, reaching its largest volume in glioblastomas, sarcomas, and metastases (e.g., glioblastoma: GP, Fig. 125, where in the centrum semiovale of both hemispheres there is pronounced edema in a case of butterfly glioblastoma of the anterior corpus callosum). In a temporomedial glioblastoma and in a temporolateral glioblastoma (GP, Figs. 121, 123) edema was considerable and of approximately equal amounts in both parietal lobes (see also Fig. 90).

Medulloblastomas are accompanied by hardly any edema (GP, Figs. 164–167), and this is true for all parts of the brain because the obstructive hydrocephalus counteracts edema formation.

Fibrosarcomas, like other sarcomas (GP, Fig. 230) and many other malignant tumors, induce considerable perifocal edema. The same is true, for metastases, where the edema volume may be out of all proportion to the small secondary malignancy inducing it (see Fig. 134).

Edema in Brain Trauma. Not only is closed or open brain trauma complicated by edema formation but the trauma consequent to operation also induces edema. It has been long known (see LÖHR and JACOBI 1933) that severe concussion is followed apparently by an increase in brain volume. Whether the loss of brain substance subsequent to demyelination is the direct consequence of edema or of the circulatory disorders following concussion has not yet been clarified. In any case one can assume that extracellular and partly perivenous edema occurs experimentally after severe concussion (shown by SATO et al. 1971). Open lesions of the skull, such as occur with brain wounds, particularly when infected, also lead to severe edema formation. We investigated this aspect of edema formation by a quasi-experiment of the needle lesion produced during ventriculography (see ZÜLCH 1943), in which I have constructed a cronicle for the perifocal alterations (see ZÜLCH 1971 b, p. 1520).

In severely infected brain wounds edema formation can be a vital complication (see ZÜLCH 1943, Figs. 7, 8, 9a, b). I have described how from a small wound in the temporal region severely infected protein-rich edema fluid has filled the entire hemisphere. Today, more rapid "cleaning" of the brain detritus and primary closure of the wound, supported by more effective antibiotic treatment, prevents such infections and consequently the edema. Moreover, the action of dexamethasone and other steroids may facilitate the suppression and later resolution of the edema (see AULICH et al. 1976, p. 135).

The early observation of neurosurgeons, obtained from operations and trauma, that edema formation started after 4–5 hours, was readily diagnosed after 20 hours and came to its height on the 4th day, was exactly coincidental with our later morphologic observations of human brains and our experimental work in this field.

Brain Edema: Correlations of Some Experimental Findings – Observations in Human Pathology

Certainly CT has permitted many new observations and promoted subsequent concepts in human neuropathology. However, some of the findings in light microscopy contradict the observations in experimental neuropathology. According to experimental evidence, the edema within a malignant glial tumor is induced by a disturbance of the blood-brain barrier in the center of the neoplasm. From there it flows outwards into the white matter. It is presumed to be extracellular, vasogenic edema, which diffuses by bulk flow into the surrounding white matter and spares the U fibers. Beyond the limits of the neoplastic tissue the blood-brain barrier is not disturbed.

Edema associated with human glioblastomas follows a similar, though not identical, mode of expansion. It flows into the corpus callosum and may even enter the contralateral hemisphere. However, it does not stain blue with Masson's trichrome as do all the other forms of extracellular/vasogenic edema.

It may have a few spots of stainable edema immediately adjacent to hemorrhages, which are not uncommon in glioblastomas. In CT the edema shows a "three-finger" pattern, which is an important diagnostic criterion for distinction from edemas of other pathogenesis, such as infarction.

However, the edema associated with infarction is, according to experimental evidence, cytotoxic in the early phase and also vasogenic in the second phase. It does not flow, however, and probably for that reason does not show the three finger pattern in CT. In experimental microembolism during the first hours the blood-brain barrier is open in the cortex and intracellular/cytotoxic edema arises, but this, however, does not "flow" and after 4 hours the blood-brain barrier is impermeable again. At this point extracellular edema fluid begins to transudate from the veins into the deep white matter while possibly some small amount of vasogenic edema fluid from the infarcted area may flow outwards. Therefore comparison between experimental and human findings in infarction is difficult. Even more difficult is the genesis of edema in meningiomas where it is very common according to CT. The three finger pattern characteristic for tumors is present, and it frequently stains with Massons's trichrome. Even if one believes that in malignant tumors edema comes *only from inside* the tumor, it is impossible to apply that concept to a meningioma, because edema fluid from *within* the tumor could never pass the thick collagenous capsule. It is highly likely, as postulated by Tönnis (1938), that it is a form of edema, which is entirely hemodynamic and subsequent to obstruction of large proximal veins with transudation from the smaller supplying venous channels and is hence extracellular (vasogenic).

These observations indicate that the neuropathology of the human and the experimental findings have to be once again critically investigated in order to permit reasonable correlations.

Conclusions: When the time of our early morphological studies of the edemas (1940–1953) is reviewed it seems remarkable what already was seen by conventional light microscopy and what concepts were derived at that time. The existence of two forms of edema *intracellular* (later "cytotoxic") and *extracellular* (later "vasogenic") was already proposed by Reichardt (1905). The occurrence of a third form, namely "secondary intracellular edema" by the taking up of extracellular fluid into the tissue elements was observed by us and confirmed for the first time. The "flow" of large amounts of protein-rich edema fluid in the brain was exactly described (later called "bulk flow") and the arrest by tight myelin fascicles such as the pyramidal pathway of this free flow within the hemisphere and the preservation of the U-fibers were clearly depicted. The resolution of edema was described as being due to either sucking up by the cells, or by reabsorption into the vessels, or by a flow along the veins and bundles into the CSF spaces. All of this was accomplished using light microscopy (Zülch 1943). *Cortical* edema, which was mainly intracellular, had already been described and depicted at that time, and the principal pathologic processes (Zülch 1967b, Table 1), leading to various forms of intracellular and extracellular edema, had been listed.

In our subsequent experimental studies for the Vienna Symposium we were able to mimic the basic forms of edema in the human and discuss the pathogenesis. These studies included the model of microembolism, which was later expanded and more recently reinvestigated (TAMURA and ZÜLCH 1978).

10.3 Increased Intracranial Pressure and its Consequences: Mechanical Distortion and Displacement of Intracranial Contents (Mass Movement and Herniation)

The increase in volume resulting from tumor growth leads to displacement of the adjacent brain parts. This is not the only space-consuming process associated with neoplasias, since reactive brain edema and swelling which occur with malignant tumors (p. 161 ff.) provide sometimes and even greater increase in volume than the actual bulk of tumor tissue itself. In addition, circulatory disturbances, which produce hyperemia and alteration in the cerebrospinal fluid pathways occur. This may lead to obstruction and local hydrocephalus of individual ventricles (i.e., hydrocephalus of the ipsilateral inferior horn, or the ventricle of the opposite side).

All of these processes take up space and this results in displacement of the brain. For a long time it was difficult to interpret such displacements, and they were called "hernias" (A. MEYER 1920). SPATZ and HASENJÄGER (1937) later correctly related them topographically to the cisterns (see LILIEQUIST 1956). The studies of TÖNNIS (1938) and of RIESSNER and ZÜLCH (1939), however, interpreted the nature of these hernias not as swelling of brain parts within the cisterns, but rather as a part of gross displacements of brain tissue into the reserve spaces of the cisterns. These hernias are, so to speak, only an "indicator" of the direction of the displacement process, by which the more advanced portions of the shifting brain suffer severe distortions as they are caught against the dural folds and sharp ridges of bone and thereby become more apparent. The cisterns are usually so located that they protect the brain from these sharp dural and bony edges by providing a fluid cushion, which permits a certain mobility of the brain parts lying in or around them.

The falx, for example, is covered by the interhemispheric cistern, the tentorium by the peripeduncular, ambient, and basal cisterns, and the sphenoid ridge by the cistern of the lateral fissure, all of which protect the brain from direct contact with these structures.

Following a local rise in volume the cisterns may become filled with brain as a part of the mechanically produced displacement process. This mechanism serves to compensate for the increase in volume by the mass lesion, since the cisterns must be considered as "reserve spaces" filled with movable CSF.

The direction of displacement of the brain is determined by the partitioning of the intracranial cavity, by the attachment of the brain at its base, and by the stresses and strains set up within the brain by the fiber tracts and blood vessels (see KAUTZKY, ZÜLCH et al. 1976, 1982). In summary, then displacement begins when the brain yields locally to the pressure of the enlarging mass. As this occurs, the adjacent portions of the ventricles are deformed and the reserve space in the neighboring cisterns and overlying sulci is used up and filled with brain tissue. The shift of the brain often exceeds the confines of the cisterns and indents the corresponding portion of the opposite hemisphere. The local increase in pressure does not confine itself to the *ipsilateral* hemisphere but may be transmitted to the opposite hemisphere by displacement of tissue between the edge of the falx and the base. Also pressure may be transmitted from the structures above the tentorium to those beneath it ("axial displacement").

General Rules for Displacement Due to Space-Occupying Lesions

The brain is completely surrounded by the bony skull and its closely adherent, tough, inner dural lining. This converts the enclosed space into a watertight chamber (Fig. 25), with the exception of the basally situated foramen magnum through which it communicates with the enclosed spinal subarachnoid space. In adults these structures combine to limit the brain from expanding. Consequently the intracranial volume cannot fluctuate. In addition the intracranial contents, consisting of blood, brain, and spinal fluid, are essentially noncompressible. These realities must be considered in the light of another fact, namely that a large number of pathologic states which affect the brain are mass-producing or expanding. When one takes into account all of these facts, one must accept that secondary local displacements within the cranial cavity are inevitable. In response to an expanding mass lesion, a compensatory reduction in the volume of the normal intracranial contents equal to that of the pathologic mass will be required in order to prevent an increase in intracranial pressure. Conversely, when the pathologic process leads to reduction in the volume of the cerebral tissues, as occurs in the atrophic states, a compensatory increase in another intracranial component will be required to fill the void (Fig. 25). The cranium, both vault and base, is rigid in adults, but it is elastic in children. Because of this, a sustained increase in intracranial pressure occurring in the early years of life is followed by secondary enlargement of the head.

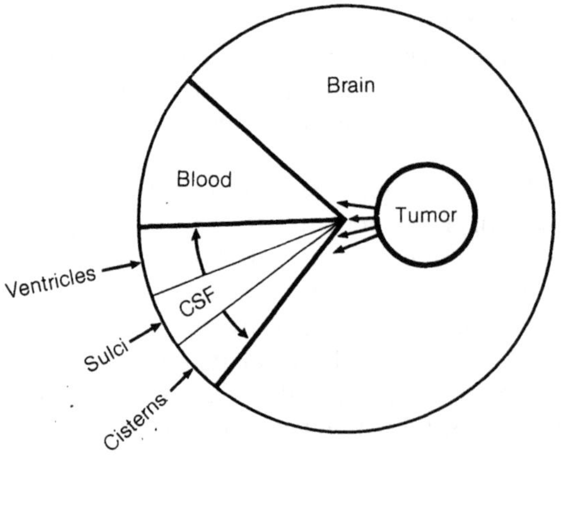

Fig. 25. The rigid, "watertight" skull is filled with brain, blood and CSF. When a tumor growth begins, a compensatory decrease in the volume of one of these components must occur to prevent a generalized increase in intracranial pressure. The first component to decrease in volume is the CSF (relative volumes are approximately correct). (Kautzky, Zülch et al. 1982)

Differentiation of such mass lesions as tumors, abscesses, acute suppuration in association with meningitis, granulomas, parasitic processes, intracerebral or extracerebral hemorrhages, empyemas, arachnoidal cysts, advancing radiation necrosis, hydrocephalus, or cerebral edema is not always possible, since all are expanding processes, which can lead to displacements and distortions of the intracranial contents. Therefore, the factor of greatest importance is the recognition of the displacement itself, rather than the precise pathologic process causing it, which is of a second order of importance. Moreover, the precise pathologic process associated with mass displacements, which accompany cerebral atrophies is not of primary concern, whether the atrophies follow trauma, inflammation, infarcts or other etiologies. The rules of mass displacement from whatever cause are fundamentally the same and vary only with the location, size, and rate of increase or decrease of various lesions.

Of the cerebral contents mentioned earlier the CSF lends itself most readily to displacement. For this reason, pathologic processes that are "mass producing" or "mass decreasing" will first be compensated for by changes in the volume of the spinal fluid spaces. Fluctuations in the volume of blood within the skull are of less importance in the compensatory process, but loss of autoregulation of blood flow and dilatation of cerebral vessels can also contribute adversely to the mass effect. The venous sinuses are incapable of much change, but other venous structures are easily compressed. Secondary atrophy of the cerebral tissues, as opposed to primary atrophy, may follow longstanding compression as a result of extracellular fluid extravasation or any other cause of cell destruction.

We have emphasized above that the rules, which govern displacement are dependent upon the fixed volume of the adult skull. The situation in *children* is fundamentally different. Since the sutures of a child's skull are still open, stretching of the dura and widening of the sutures can occur with a secondary increase in intracranial volume, often to grotesque proportions. Localized swelling of the skull can also occur particularly in association with underlying arachnoidal cysts, but less frequently from other causes, such as underlying tumors. On the other hand, since the normal infant skull expands in response to growth of the developing brain, failure of a part of the brain to develop may lead to underexpansion of the overlying skull when compared with the expected size and shape.

Every mass lesion initially exerts evenly distributed eccentric pressure on the surrounding tissues. Conversely, each atrophic process exerts an evenly distributed "pull" on its surrounding tissues. These forces, however, are opposed by other forces, the most significant of which is mechanical resistance caused by noncompliance of the cerebral tissues and by points of fixation to the surrounding membranes. Another opposing force is the hydrodynamic resistance of the ventricular fluid, which is being actively produced and which can resist compression deformity of the ventricular spaces. Yet another hydrodynamic force is produced by the arterial blood pressure as it maintains the patency of the intracranial arterial circulation. It is also of great significance that three principal cerebral arteries proceed in wide curves against which the pressure waves act, as it were, to stretch out the vessel. Because of the surrounding

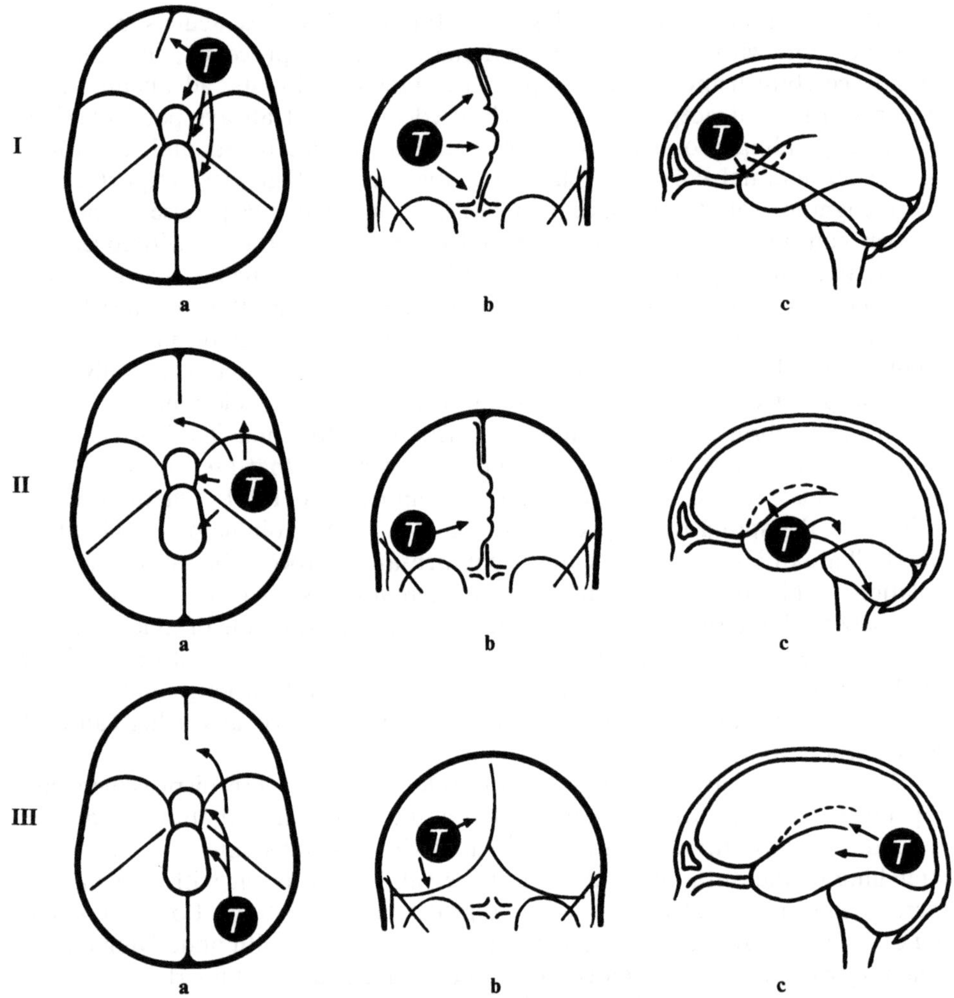

Fig. 26. Diagram of the important mass displacements caused by *I* frontal, *II* temporal, and *III* occipital tumors. *I* the mass effect of the frontal tumor displaces the falx obliquely, causes herniation of brain tissue over the sphenoid wing against the temporal lobe, and exerts pressure against the brain stem in an "axial" direction. *II* The temporal tumor causes herniations anteriorly toward the frontal lobe and elevates the sylvian fissure. The uncus is forced medially and inferiorly into the tentorial hiatus. Note that the falx is not affected by tumors in this area. *III* The occipital tumor, surrounded by rigid dural sheets forming a cone-shaped enclosure, can only displace tissue anteriorly in the direction of the open end of the cone until a point is reached where lateral displacements can take place. Elevation of the posterior sylvian fissure is also seen here. (KAUTZKY, ZÜLCH et al. 1982)

cerebral tissue, the vessel maintains its shape and in so doing forms a dynamic support or a sort of skeleton for the brain tissue that functions as long as the intraluminal pressure is adequate to maintain it.

In addition, the brain is supported by the CSF channels within which it is suspended within the skull, attached to its dural lining by loose connections of blood vessels, cranial nerves, and the pituitary stalk. Two thick dural folds,

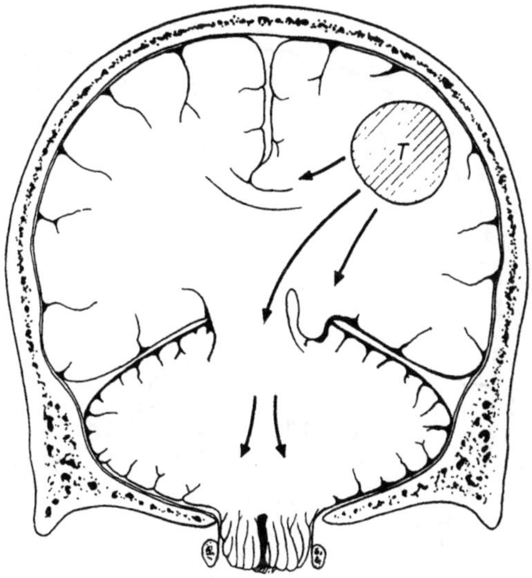

Fig. 27. Semischematic model of the mass displacements that accompany a parietal lobe tumor.
Above: The gyrus cinculi is pushed to the opposite side. *Middle:* Medial portions of the temporal lobe are forced through the tentorial hiatus as a hernia displacing the midbrain. *Below:* The brain stem is forced caudally and the cerebellar tonsils herniate into the foramen magnum. In the vicinity of the tumor, the convolutions are flattened. (KAUTZKY, ZÜLCH et al. 1982)

the falx and the tentorium, partition the intracranial space into three large compartments (GP, Fig. 3). Specific regions of the brain impinge upon them so that they act as support structures and as barriers to mass displacements, however, inferiorly the brain rests upon the base of the skull itself. The falx bisects the supratentorial region into right and left compartments, while the tentorium separates the infratentorial compartment, or posterior cranial fossa, from the supratentorial compartments. The supratentorial compartments are further partitioned into anterior and middle cranial fossas, the dividing line between them being the edge of the lesser wing of the sphenoid. For the sake of the discussion below, it is worth mentioning that the dural partitions are of far greater significance than the division into anterior and middle cranial fossas.

On each side of the falx are found the two cerebral hemispheres in their respective supratentorial compartments, which are joined below the inferior edge of the falx (Fig. 26). The brain contents of the posterior fossa are connected with the cerebral hemispheres by means of the midbrain, which passes through the relatively small tentorial hiatus (Figs. 26, 27). Although usually small, the actual size of the tentorial hiatus can vary considerably. These divisions of the intracranial space permit large mass displacements only in certain directions:

1. Within the confines of the compartment
2. From one supratentorial compartment to the other beneath the falx (Fig. 27)
3. Through the tentorial hiatus in the direction of the posterior cranial fossa (Fig. 27)
4. From the posterior cranial fossa superiorly through the tentorial hiatus (Fig. 28)
5. Through the foramen magnum into the spinal canal (Figs. 27, 28)

Even within the confines of these spaces, mass displacements are resisted and modified by means of the internal and external support structures of the brain. The external support structures hold the brain through attachments by means

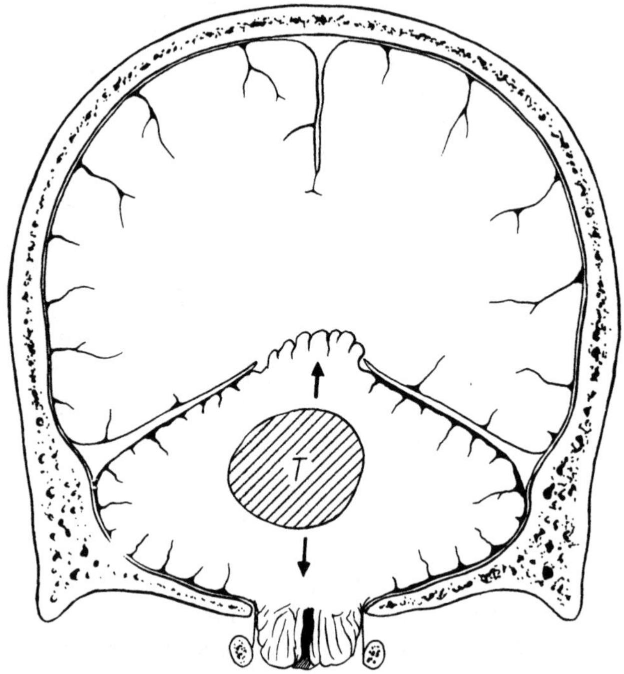

Fig. 28. Semischematic model showing mass displacement by a tumor in the posterior cranial fossa. Note the upward herniation through the tentorial hiatus and the downward herniation into the foramen magnum (cerebellar or tonsillar pressure cone). (KAUTZKY, ZÜLCH et al. 1982)

of veins, arteries, nerves, and the pituitary stalk to extracerebral structures, while the internal support structures consist mainly of the cerebral tissues themselves, particularly white matter pathways such as the internal capsule, corona radiata, association tracts, and cerebral peduncles. Although the CSF-producing ventricular system also acts as both a buttressing force and a safety valve in mass displacements, it is of much greater significance from the pathologic standpoint when blockage of the various CSF pathways results in noncommunicating hydrocephalus. This subject will be presented in greater detail in the next section.

Displacements Produced by Mass Lesions

Mechanisms of Localized and Generalized Increase in Intracranial Pressure

One can distinguish a definite temporal sequence in the evolution of mass lesions.

Phase I: In this phase a tumor squeezes spinal fluid from the subarachnoid spaces of the adjacent brain, flattens the convolutions against the inner surface of the skull, distorts the nearest ventricular cavity by compression and produces an initial displacement of the nearby arteries and veins (see upper part of Fig. 26). These changes all contribute to localized increase in intracranial pressure.

Phase II: As the volume of involved brain increases further, a point is reached where spinal fluid shifts can no longer accommodate the expanding mass. Moreover, localized cerebral edema (Fig. 24) contributes to the mass effect causing the localized increase in intracranial pressure to spread and ultimately to involve eventually the entire hemisphere. There will follow an attempt to accommodate the mass lesion by expansion into the fissures, cisterns, and ventricles to the greatest degree possible (upper part of Fig. 27). Further compensation requires the shifting of increasing quantities of brain tissue from one anatomical compartment to the other. Brain tissue will begin to herniate beneath the falx medially, as well as in an axial direction through the tentorial hiatus (Fig. 26/Ic). Because of impedance by the falx, which is tightly connected to the skull and only slightly movable at its lower edge, lateral displacement must take place predominantly in the open space below the falx. The lower edge of the falx changes its position only in response to local pressure from a large mass lesion in its immediate vicinity, usually after intense pressure over a long period of time. However, exceptions to this rule are rare, but they do occur. For example, an enormous infarct in the territories supplied by the anterior and middle cerebral arteries associated with extensive edema, can cause within a few days acute lateral displacement with slanting of the falx (Fig. 26; KAUTZKY, ZÜLCH et al. 1982, Figs. 13–15).

Mass displacement of the brain beneath the falx varies depending upon the site of origin of the mass. Masses originating in the frontal areas are most frequently associated with this kind (Fig. 26/Ib) of displacement, since the falx is shorter anteriorly and the free space beneath it is greater than that found posteriorly (Fig. 24) where the falx and splenium of the corpus callosum are in direct contact with one another (GP, Fig. 11). The falx also supports the corpus callosum posteriorly as well as adjacent cerebral tissues including the septum. It is only possible for parietal lobe displacements to shift beneath the falx and across the midline when the expanding lesion first displaces the corpus callosum from the lower posterior edge of the falx. Lateral mass displacement beneath the falx first requires displacement downwards, mediobasally, at least as far as the inferior margin of the falx itself (GP, Fig. 11). In parietal lesions the displaced structures cannot undergo the shift without displacement of the corpus callosum away from the posterior falx. One can identify a mass displacement in this region on angiograms by the shifting of the deep veins located there.

Whenever displacement causes brain tissue to cross the midline, secondary compression of the opposite hemisphere results. Axial herniations (Fig. 26/Ic) can also occur simultaneously through the tentorial hiatus into the posterior cranial fossa (GP, Figs. 1, 12). This is especially true with frontal mass lesions where the effects are oriented in a more longitudinal direction. Such axial herniations or transmissions of pressure can cause distortion and displacement of the midbrain, a process which can progress to involve the brainstem in a rostral-caudal fashion, eventually pressing on medial parts of the cerebellum, which in turn are pressed against the foramen magnum and into the spinal canal (Figs. 26, 27, 29, 30). In the latter case, the medulla oblongata, and particularly the adjacent cerebellar tonsils, are wedged down into the spinal canal, resulting

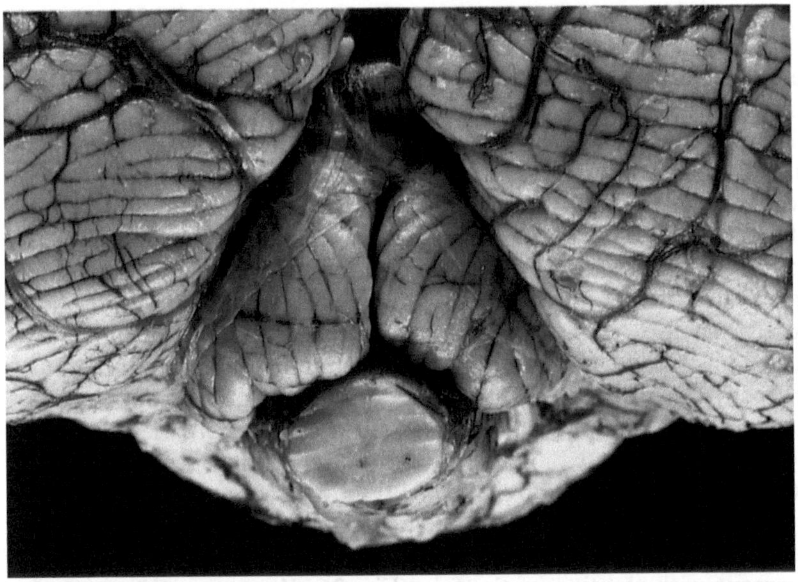

Fig. 29. Cerebellar pressure cone (IInd degree)

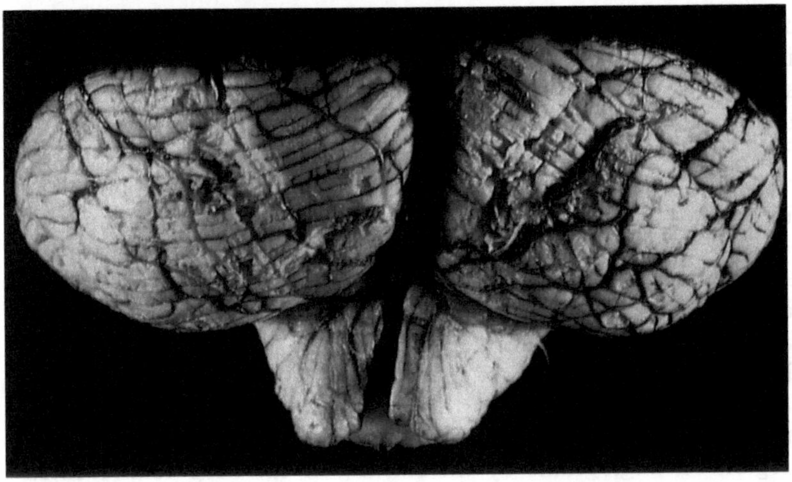

Fig. 30. Particularly prominent cerebellar pressure cone (IIIrd degree)

in the so-called "cerebellar or tonsillar pressure cone" (Figs. 3, 9/II, 10, and pp. 3–19, in KAUTZKY, ZÜLCH et al. 1982). In this manner, a localized intracranial pressure effect may spread to become generalized and may result in axial displacement in the direction of the posterior cranial fossa (TÖNNIS 1938, 1959; ZÜLCH 1951b, 1959b; ZÜLCH et al. 1974a; ZÜLCH 1981a).

We have subdivided the cerebellar pressure cone into three stages according to the severity:

1. Mark of a pressure groove on the tonsils
2. Caudal displacement of the tonsils (Fig. 29)
3. An elongated tonsillar cone (Fig. 30)

Herniations Into the Cisterns

In the preceding section the various phases of growth of a mass lesion were described. Local pressures may spread to involve an entire hemisphere and are transmitted to the opposite hemisphere, and eventually the contents of the posterior fossa are involved. In each phase the reserve spaces provided by the cisterns are systematically eliminated as brain tissue moves into them. These cisterns are portrayed in the conventional manner in Figs. 167, 168, 169, 173, and 174 in KAUTZKY, ZÜLCH et al. (1982), whereas Figs. 5, 6, and 7 correspond better to what is seen in CT. The mere presence of such a herniation is clearly indicative of a mass displacement. We now recognize the topography of herniations for each expanding process (RIESSNER and ZÜLCH 1939).

A detailed description of the cisterns has been published by LILIEQUIST (1956) and by KAUTZKY, ZÜLCH et al. (1982, p. 208).

The following herniations are of clinical importance:

1. Small hernias consisting of one or both gyri recti can be forced into the prechiasmatic portion of the chiasmatic cistern.
2. The uncinate gyrus and neighboring tissues can be displaced medially into the anterior portion of the ambient and crural cisterns.
3. Portions of the hippocampal gyrus and medial occipital cortex can be shifted into the posterior portion of the crural and ambient cisterns (Figs. 31, 32).
4. The uncinate plus the hippocampal gyrus and the medial occipital cortex as a unit can also be displaced into the entire interpeduncular and ambient cisterns ("total" temporal or transtentorial pressure cone) (Figs. 31, 32).
5. Anterior portions of the medial surface of the frontal and parietal lobes, especially the cingulate gyrus, can be displaced along with the adjacent corpus callosum under the falx toward the opposite side.
6. Expanding lesions in the posterior cranial fossa can lead to upward herniation of the anterior aspect of the cerebellum through the tentorial hiatus (Fig. 28).
7. An expanding lesion in the posterior cranial fossa can produce tonsillar herniations downwards into the foramen magnum (Figs. 29, 30). These are frequently asymmetrical.
8. Sometimes laterally situated cerebellopontine angle masses cause cerebellar herniation into the contralateral cerebellopontine angle.
9. Axial displacements of the lower brainstem in either direction, upwards or downwards, can effect the exiting cranial nerves, but the pathogenesis is not clear with respect to involvement of the 3rd or the 6th cranial nerves (ZÜLCH 1964b).

Herniations can be recognized by means of angiography (see ZÜLCH 1950c; Fig. 10: transtentorial pressure cone).

The three principal arteries of the brain lie within three large cisterns, namely, cisterna interhemispherica (anterior cerebral artery); cisterna lateralis (middle cerebral artery); and cisterna ambiens (posterior cerebral artery) (Fig. 32). A pronounced displacement or herniation of the brain into any one of these cisterns, can cause an infarct at certain sites. For example, a serious consequence of transtentorial herniation into the ambient cistern occurs when the posterior cerebral artery is pressed against the sharp edge of the tentorium and is so distorted as to produce a hemorrhagic infarct (Fig. 32) in the calcarine area

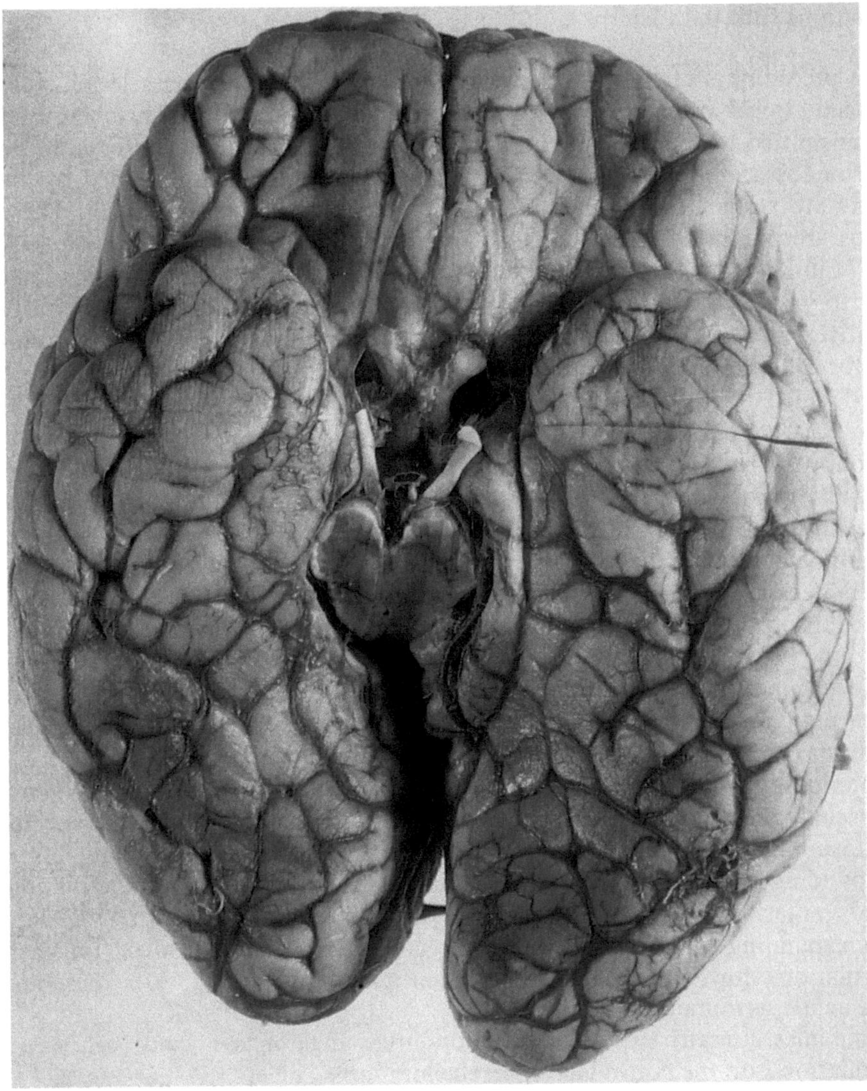

Fig. 31. Left-sided transtentorial temporal herniation whith shift of the midline to the opposite side

of the occipital lobe with homonymous hemianopia (RIESSNER and ZÜLCH 1939; ZÜLCH et al. 1974a).

In the case of chronic, generalized increased pressure tiny herniations of the brain may force themselves into small dehiscences of the dura at the base or into any burrholes which have been performed, as was formerly seen with ventricular punctures.

Special Patterns of Displacement Due to Expanding Lesions. By applying these fundamental rules of displacement to specific mass lesions one will observe

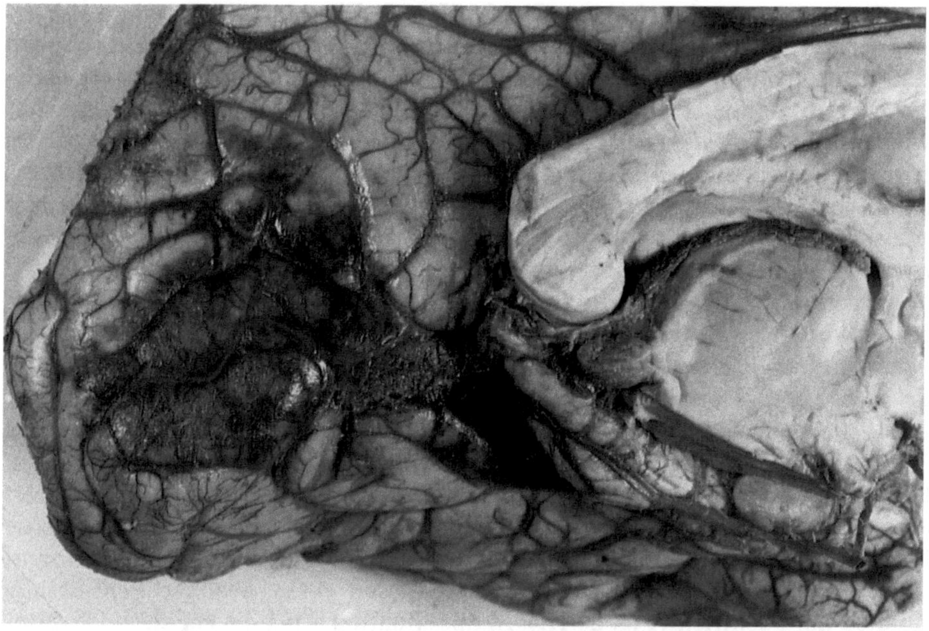

Fig. 32. Marked temporal pressure cone, which has displaced the posterior cerebral artery downwards and medially (seen also in the arteriograms). The artery is stretched over the sharp tentorial edge, which has resulted in a hemorrhagic infarction of the medial surface of the occipital lobe (ZÜLCH 1975a)

that a tumor located in the *frontal* region (Fig. 26/I) may result in an unobstructed side-to-side displacement of brain tissue into the anterior midline in the region of the septum pellucidum. *Axial* displacements from the frontal region toward the posterior fossa are also possible. This is the explanation for the appearance of a cerebellar pressure cone at the onset of an expanding lesion in the frontal lobe (Fig. 26/I); in contrast, *side-to-side* displacements rarely occur with such lesions further posteriorly in the region of the third ventricle or the posterior corpus callosum/quadrigeminal region (Fig. 26/II).

Parietal expanding lesions (Fig. 26) produce an initial displacement toward the base of the skull. At the base, the mass encounters large reserve spaces of the cisterns which can be filled. Displacements toward the frontal lobe and from there towards the opposite side are also possible. Towards the occipital region (Fig. 26/III) on the other hand, there is the cone-shaped tentorium and dura, which provide an obstruction to displacements. This is important in older persons because the occipital lobe is not affected by senile atrophy. As previously emphasized, in the case of a parietal space-occupying lesion a direct *side-to-side* shift is possible only if the corpus callosum has already been depressed. It has been mentioned earlier that this cannot occur in the early stages of a parietal shift because the falx lies directly above the splenium of the corpus callosum and acts as a barrier. In the more posterior parts of the brain (i.e., in the area of the cella media and around the posterior part of the third ventricle) displacement can occur only after depression of the corpus callosum.

Temporal expanding lesions (Fig. 26/II; GP, Figs. 18–20) move in a *side-to-side* direction, primarily displacing the third ventricle so that it becomes rounded due to its fixation at the infundibulum. The shift of the lower basal ganglia across the midline is possible because the distance below the falx is greater, whereas a *side-to-side* displacement in the superior posterior parts of the cranial cavity is initially limited. A temporal tumor presses forward against the frontal lobe above the lesser sphenoid wing. However, at the same time it also exerts pressure towards the posterior fossa by creating a hernia into the tentorial hiatus. This occurs first medially and then with a change of direction by 90° downwards towards the posterior fossa. Overall, this medial shift produces its greatest effect either anteriorly (GP, Fig. 26) or posteriorly (GP, Fig. 27), depending upon the location of the tumor within the middle fossa. In addition, an *axial* effect is produced primarily in a frontal direction (GP, Figs. 19, 20). Axial effects in a posterior direction are less common (Fig. 26/II).

In the early phase an *occipital* expanding lesion can only displace brain tissue anteriorly towards the temporal, parietal, and the frontal lobes. A shift across the midline occurs only after a preceding displacement of brain tissue forward as far as the middle or anterior parts of the corpus callosum or at the level of the septum pellucidum and to a lesser extent near the *more basally* situated third ventricle (Fig. 26/III). In this situation a *side-to-side* shift occasionally occurs quite far forward because an expanding lesion in the occipital lobe lies mainly above the temporal lobe in the parietofrontal axis.

In essence, all sorts of expanding lesions produce the *same* displacements. The nature of these depends, however, on the *volume* as much as on the *location* of the expanding lesion. The effective size of the displacing mass is ultimately determined by a combination of factors. These include not only the volume of the mass lesion itself (tumor, hemorrhage, etc.), but also secondary increases in adjacent *brain* volume due to infiltration of water. Tumor *type* may influence volume not only because tumors vary in their speed of growth, but also because certain lesions tend to be associated with more severe brain edema (glioblastoma, metastases; GP, Figs. 10, 23, as well as sarcomas and abscesses, GP, Fig. 338).

Development of Obstructive Hydrocephalus

The intracranial mass displacements described above have a profound effect upon the CSF pathways. It is well recognized that the major producer of CSF is the choroid plexus in each lateral ventricle, although additional contributions are made by the plexuses in the third and fourth ventricles (Fig. 33). From each lateral ventricle the CSF flows through the foramina of Monro into the third ventricle and then through the aqueduct of Sylvius to the fourth ventricle. From the fourth ventricle the CSF exits through the foramina of Luschka into both lateral recesses and through the foramen of Magendie into the cisterna magna and pontocerebellar cisterns. From the cisterna magna flow continues through the subarachnoid channels to the convexities of the cerebral hemispheres, from where the CSF is reabsorbed into the venous circulation through the arachnoidal granulations (Fig. 33). Although an additional quantity of CSF is probably formed by the vessels lying close to the ependymal and cortical surfaces, these contributions are of minor significance. There is also substantial

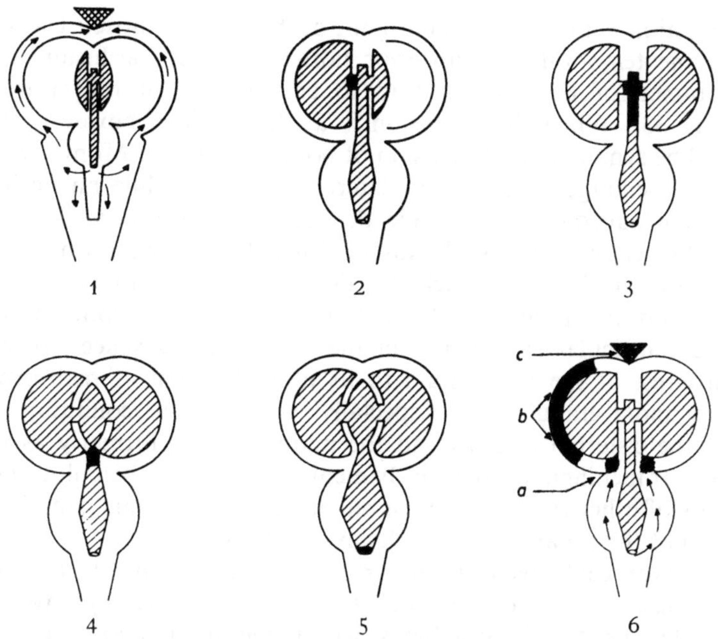

Fig. 33. The various forms of occlusive hydrocephalus and the typical sites for obstruction. *1*, schematic demonstration of the normal CSF circulation; *2*, unilateral obstruction of the foramen of Monro with asymmetrical hydrocephalus: *3*, bilateral obstruction of the foramina of Monro at the level of the third ventricle, producing symmetrical hydrocephalus of both lateral ventricles; *4*, obstruction at the level of the aqueduct producing hydrocephalus of the lateral and third ventricles; *5*, obstruction at the level of the foramen of Magendie producing proximal hydrocephalus of all four ventricles; *6*, obstruction of the subarachnoid spaces at midbrain level and over the cerebral convexity. The latter is also called "communicating hydrocephalus." *a*, ambient cisterns; *b*, sylvian fissure and subarachnoid spaces of the convexity; *c*, pacchionian granulations and sagittal sinus. (KAUTZKY, ZÜLCH et al. 1982)

evidence that edema fluid can pass through the white matter of the hemisphere and through the ependyma of the ventricles into the CSF.

It is generally accepted that most of the CSF is reabsorbed by means of the arachnoid granulations but additional reabsorption takes place along the entire subarachnoid space and through the ventricular walls. This pathway is confirmed by the absence of arachnoidal granulations in newborn infants, in whom they are not yet developed. Therefore the accompanying hydrocephalus is usually mild and of no clinical significance.

Regardless of the precise manner of reabsorption of the CSF, which is still the subject of debate, of greater significance for the present discussion is the fact that obstructions to the flow of spinal fluid from the ventricular system to its major point of reabsorption, the subarachnoid space over the cerebral convexities, *can occur through mass displacements and can in turn be mass producing when hydrocephalus ensues*. This situation may also result from scarring within the ventricles themselves, as long as the isolated portion of the ventricular system contains the choroid plexus. The hydrocephalus may be quite asymmetrical depending on the site of obstruction. For example, a mass that causes obstruction at the level of the trigone of the lateral ventricle leads to hydrocephalus of the temporal and posterior horns, while an occlusion at the level of the foramen of Monro will lead to enlargement of the entire lateral ventricle (Fig. 33). When the occlusion is at the midline, however, the hydrocephalus will be symmetrical. Occlusion of both foramina of Monro will lead to hydrocephalic enlargement of both lateral ventricles, while an occlusion at the level of the aqueduct will include the third ventricle as well. When the foramina of Magendie and Luschka are obstructed, the resultant hydrocephalus will also involve the fourth ventricle (for details see ZÜLCH 1940e).

Additional sites of obstruction to the flow of spinal fluid can be outside the ventricular system within the subarachnoid spaces, thereby blocking the progress of the spinal fluid to its ultimate point of reabsorption through the arachnoid granulations. Especially typical of this condition is the obliteration of the cisternal ring around the midbrain seen formerly as a complication of basilar meningitis, particularly medically treated tuberculous meningitis. Meningitis of other types, as well as subarachnoid bleeding, can also lead to obliteration of the subarachnoid pathways (GP, Fig. 361).

Hydrocephalus resulting from obstruction outside the ventricular system has been designated nonobstructive or "communicating" hydrocephalus, whereas that produced by a block within the ventricular system is referred to as "obstructive". Logically, however, both conditions should be considered obstructive.

The various sites of obstruction will now be compared with the major tumor "groups" or other processes causing them.

If an obstructive process develops within the ventricular system, or immediately adjacent to it, the resultant obstructive hydrocephalus may be considerably more severe than that caused by obstruction which occurs *outside the ventricular system*. Acoustic neurilemmomas of the cerebellopontine angle, for example, cause a fairly mild degree of hydrocephalus and even more remote expanding processes can cause a significant degree of secondary hydrocephalus when mass herniations of brain tissue lead to distortion and obstruction of the ventricular pathways at the level of the aqueduct of Sylvius or foramen of Magendie.

One or both of the foramina of Monro can become occluded when a sufficiently large mass in the cerebral hemisphere (glioblastoma, metastasis, abscess with significant brain edema) causes herniation beneath the falx and distortion of the contralateral hemisphere. In this fashion, cerebrospinal fluid accumulates proximal to the foramina of Monro, resulting in symmetrical enlargement of the lateral ventricles. Sometimes, however, the ventricle ipsilateral to the mass lesion is incapable of expansion due to localized pressure. Consequently, only the contralateral ventricle may enlarge, and its enlargement may only be moderate since the obstruction is usually not complete. Nonetheless, whatever degree of hydrocephalus develops, the addition of this secondary expanding process in one or both of the supratentorial compartments causes further increase in intracranial pressure with further mass herniations, particularly in an axial direction, with considerable danger of catastrophic consequences.

Without a sufficient knowledge and understanding of these mass movements, displacements, and shifts, which follow secondarily a space-occupying or scarring process, a CT scan of a brain tumor cannot be properly interpreted and the planning of an operation must take into consideration all of these factors for the result to be adequate.

All cases of hydrocephalus are completely reversible at first but only partly so later on. This can be explained by the initial expansion of the ventricles and the "inflation" of the brain, an expansion that takes place at the cost of the subarachnoid space. This space may disappear with the increase in intracranial pressure. If the increased pressure abates the size of the ventricles returns to normal and the subarachnoid spaces are reestablished. If the hydrocephalus persists it may no longer be reversible and the brain is compressed into a thin mantle, most dramatically exemplified by a paperthin third ventricular floor.

In addition to these well recognized processes, mention should be made of other hydrodynamic mechanisms which have been described more recently. Following occlusion of the aqueduct, the suprapineal recess can expand to the size of a chestnut (see below) and push its way under the tentorium against the superior cerebellar vermis. The brain substance may perforate at various places, most frequently through the medial wall of the trigone of the lateral ventricle, and the CSF may escape through the opening and form a subarachnoid cyst (GP, Fig. 362). This cyst may extend into the cisterna ambiens and then in the direction of the anterior lobe of the cerebellum. Even this rare mechanism does not, of itself, succeed in re-establishing a connection between the ventricles and subarachnoid space, thus resulting in a spontaneous relief of symptoms. This has to be accomplished surgically by a procedure such as ventriculocisternotomy, or ventriculoatrial shunt.

Symptoms of Intracranial Hypertension and Herniations

We have listed among others the symptoms of headache, vomiting, nausea, dizziness, altered personality, depression of consciousness, etc. in a chapter in the Handbook of Clinical Neurology (ZÜLCH et al. 1974a). These do not need further elaboration. However, the symptoms of "convulsions or fits" and "decerebration" should be discussed. These terms have been used to describe a type of seizure experienced by patients with raised intracranial pressure and distortion of the midbrain (Fig. 34). The "fits" are governed by the location of the mass lesion and may also be related to herniation occurring after a *local* rise in pressure. It is important to try to define exactly what this disorder really is. This depends on the historical background of the term "fit", notably JACKSON's (1906) account of "cerebellar fits." It has long been known that the phenomena involved are only superficially related to the convulsions associated with epilepsy. They are more likely to be clonic spasms in rhythmic sequence, manifested by extension of the extremities with the arms rotated inwards. The attacks have the same pathogenetic mechanism as that activated tonically in association with other signs of decerebration (see Pette's sign: when the skin over the sternum is pinched the extremities are extended and are rotated inwards).

JACKSON's original description (1906) was of peculiar "tetanoid" fits suffered by a child with a midline cerebellar tumor, who showed stretching of the legs, flexion of the arms with adduction of the upper arms, opisthotonus and extension of the neck. These features are typical of decerebration at a level above

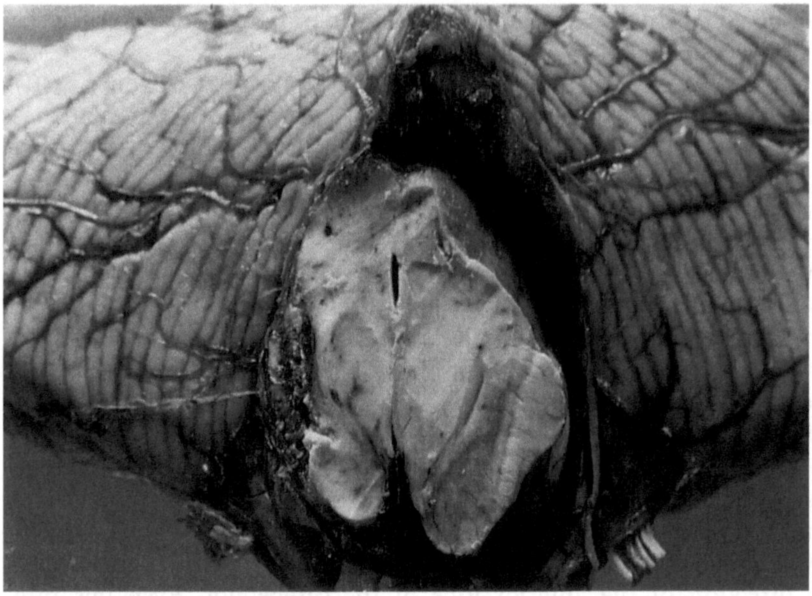

Fig. 34. Deformation of midbrain and adjacent cerebellum by a large temporal pressure cone. Note the notching and hemorrhage in the contralateral brain stem. (ZÜLCH 1975a)

the red nucleus (RIESSNER and ZÜLCH 1939; see STEWART and HOLMES 1904; MAGNUS and DE KLEIJN 1912).

Clinical Signs of Downward Transtentorial Herniation

This is of particular importance because it may lead to remote or misleading signs regarding the site of the causative lesion. Mydriasis with retention of a sluggish pupillary response to light develops rapidly after mild, transient miosis. Later, the mydriasis increases and the pupil becomes nonreactive. The nerves were formerly thought to be compressed at the edge of the clivus, the so-called "clivus edge syndrome", as suggested by FISCHER-BRÜGGE (1949, 1950, 1951). However, ZÜLCH (1959b) showed that these disorders actually arise from strangulation of the 3rd cranial nerve at two sites, most often at the "medial petroclinoid ligament", and less commonly at the point where the nerve passes between the posterior cerebral and superior cerebellar arteries. Another possible causative lesion is produced through stretching and tearing of the 3rd nerve by "axial displacement" of the midbrain (ZÜLCH 1951b, former edition).

It was described previously that during herniation the posterior cerebral artery may be strangulated. When this occurs there may be an ischemic infarction of the calcarine area (Fig. 32) of the occipital lobe (ZÜLCH 1959b; ZÜLCH et al. 1974a; GP, Figs. 31, 33, 34). ETHELBERG and JENSEN (1952) reported visual field disturbances, even to the point of total loss of vision, in 150 of 500 cases of cerebral tumor.

Other associated disorders are either a positive vestibulo-ocular sign and motor signs such as contralateral and/or ipsilateral hemiplegia. Hypothalamic and hypophyseal disturbances may also be observed. GROENEVELD and SCHALTENBRAND (1927) and KERNOHAN and WOLTMAN (1929) suggested that the motor abnormalities were due to transtentorial (or "temporal") herniation which forced the cerebral peduncle against the edge of the tentorial hiatus, thus "notching" it (GP, Figs. 37, 38).

Clinical Signs of Downward Cerebellar Herniation

The signs and symptoms of a tonsillar pressure cone resulting from downward cerebellar herniation were described by CUSHING (1917) and consist of arching of the neck and back, respiratory disturbances, changes in pulse rate, fear of death, loss of consciousness, areflexia, cardiac arrhythmias, "electric shocks" in the shoulders and limbs, as well as respiratory disorders. Paresthesiae, stiffness of the neck, fits of giddiness, hypotension and dysarthria have also been regarded as typical effects of cerebellar coning (RIESSNER and ZÜLCH 1939).

Tönnis was particularly interested in the sensory disorders accompanying cerebellar herniation, which may take the form of "rippling" paresthesiae, and which long precede disturbances of consciousness and of muscle tone. ZÜLCH (1964b) emphasized the possibility of misinterpreting these symptoms as "sensory Jacksonian fits with generalization".

The nuchal rigidity observed with tonsillar pressure cone has also been suggested as one of the cardinal features of transtentorial herniation, although this was not confirmed by RIESSNER and ZÜLCH (1939). They found neck stiffness only in conjunction with cerebellar and not with transtentorial herniation, which is in agreement with most authorities (WALKER 1969).

Autonomic signs such as alterations in pulse and respiration as well as Cushing's reflex and loss of consciousness may also be present.

Changes in cerebral circulation have also been encountered. Pulmonary edema and gastrointestinal disorders are among the last major signs to occur.

A more detailed discussion is given elsewhere (Handbook chapter of ZÜLCH et al. 1974a).

10.4 Cytology of the Cerebrospinal Fluid With Brain Tumors

When is it permissible to assume on the basis of CSF findings that tumor is present adjacent to the ventricular system or the subarachnoid space? This can be anticipated when tumor specific cells are found in the fluid.

After breaking into the subarachnoid space or through the ependymal wall, some neuroepithelial and mesodermal tumors may spread diffusely, as is usually the case with medulloblastomas and rarely with oligodendrogliomas. Other tumors such as ependymomas, choroid plexus papillomas, astrocytomas, and the majority of oligodendrogliomas tend to form circumscribed metastases (CAIRNS and RUSSELL 1931). Glioblastomas occasionally metastasize along the cerebrospinal fluid pathways (HASENJÄGER 1939b) and monstrocellular sarcomas may also spread in this fashion. We have seen diffuse metastases throughout the entire subarachnoid space associated with ependymomas, plexus papillomas, and oligodendrogliomas. This type of diffuse metastatic spread by these tumors is even more common following surgical intervention (GP, Figs. 70, 71, 72, 80, 82, 111, 112, 132, 237, 238, 239).

The sedimentation method of SAYK (1960) may provide not only proof of a neoplastic process near the cerebrospinal fluid channels, but in some cases it may also reveal the histologic characteristics of the lesion (see: the large cells resembling those of the pineal gland in a pinealoma described by RIVERSON and ZÜLCH 1979, Fig. 4). In the cases of CNS malignancy reported by SAYK and OLISCHER (see SAYK 1974) the percentage of positive diagnoses by cytologic examination for primary intracranial tumors was 14.1%, for metastatic tumors 30.4%; BISCHOFF (1961), on the other hand, reported a figure of 62.7%, and BOTS et al. (1964) found 50% in a smaller series. When one calculates separately the percentage of positive diagnoses for metastatic tumors, there is an increase to between 70 and 91%. BALHUIZEN et al. (1978) pointed out that increased intracranial pressure with obstruction of the cerebrospinal fluid pathways may hamper the detection of exfoliated tumor cells from the lumbar cerebrospinal fluid. The highest detection rate will understandably be in medulloblastomas which tend to shed cells and seed throughout the CSF. After surgery of medulloblastomas, the percentage of positive findings will increase remarkably. The percentage of positive findings will also depend upon whether smeared or embedded material (see pp. 200, 204) or sedimentation methods have been used. Secondary aseptic meningitis, with corresponding pleocytosis, is commonly a consequence of operation on epidermoids which contain fatty acids that constitute a strong meningeal or ependymal irritant (KRIEG 1936a; VERBIEST 1939). Pleocytosis can even develop spontaneously following rupture of epidermoids and teratomas (GAUPP 1942).

Further References: WIECZOREK (1964, 1965), WILKINS and ODOM (1966), BOTS et al. (1968a), DEN HARTOG JAGER (1969), RICH (1969), OEHMICHEN (1976).

New Techniques for Cytopathologic Diagnosis

New methods have been developed for better study of morphogenesis and organogenesis, such as culturing in a net of glass fibers (KAJIKAWA et al. 1973) or as well as particularly the culturing in "organ cultures", e.g., a culture in "sponge foam" has been used by RUBINSTEIN and HERMANN (1975). They also used the milipore filter platform of culture for various important problems.

SOROUR et al. (1975) were able to investigate the difference in infiltrative capacity of meningiomas and astrocytomas by using the "gel foam" method.

Excellent results were obtained with using the ultrastructural modification of scanning electron microscopy.

Recent developments in tissue culture have produced extremely useful cloning techniques. Clonal cell lines can be separated from tissue cultures and used for a variety of biologic investigations. PFEIFFER and WECHSLER (1972), for example, used the technique for identification of a Schwann cell clone controlled by a S-100 protein test. WECHSLER (1977) later discussed the different functions of glial and Schwann cells based on the behavior of such clones. STAVROU et al. (1980) also used an astroglial clone for therapeutic tests (for a detailed review see HERSCHMAN 1978).

11 Spontaneous Intra- and Extracranial Metastases of Brain Tumors in Man – Artificial Seeding

Metastasis of brain tumors *within* the CNS is common in a few groups of tumors and by specific routes. True metastasis of most groups of brain tumors to *other organs* is certainly uncommon. Acceptable descriptions, particularly for neuroepithelial tumors, are rare. Confirmed metastases have been demonstrated only in the following groups: pinealomas, sympathoblastomas and retinoblastomas, medulloblastomas of the cerebellum, glioblastomas, meningiomas and sarcomas, particularly of the monstrocellular type. Occasional cases of "artificial iatrogenic implantation" at the time of operation or shunting have been reported. Examples of these include oligodendroglioma of the galea, glioblastoma of the subcutaneous tissue, craniopharyngioma of the galea, etc. However, these "implantation metastases" only "vegetated" like a tissue culture and underwent no appreciable "autonomous" growth.

In cases of extracranial seeding of neuroepithelial blastomas the histologic characteristics have to be carefully examined, specific example being the differential diagnosis between a glioblastoma multiforme and a monstrocellular sarcoma, with which metastasis to the lungs is not uncommon.

The debate over these issues is exemplified by Maria MITTELBACH's case, which was first presented at the German Pathological Congress in 1934 and despite a renewed defense by her in 1935, not generally accepted. On the contrary, the detailed description appeared later and pointed more to the opposite direction, namely, a bronchogenic small cell carcinoma was said to have metastasized to the brain.

Frequency of Extracranial Metastasis of Primary Intracranial Tumors

PASQUIER et al. (1979) described 9 cases of primary brain tumors of which 7 had metastases within and 2 outside the brain. In addition they reviewed the published literature and found 248 cases of histologically confirmed, central nervous system tumors with metastasis outside of the nervous system. The secondary sites were encountered more frequently in adult males. The frequency of tumor type in descending order was gliomas (39.5%), meningeal tumors and sarcomas (28.2%), neuronal tumors (14.1%), lymphoma-microgliomas (12.5%), pineal tumors (4%), and melanomas (1.6%).

SLOWIK and BALOGH (1980) on the other hand, referred to GLASAUER and YUAN (1963), who in reviewing the literature found 89 cases, and to KRETSCHMER (1974b), who found 171 cases. Among the cases listed by KRETSCHMER the primary tumor type was glioblastoma multiforme in 43 instances. Since then more glioblastoma cases with extracranial metastases have been reported (see also WINKELMAN et al. 1952).

Metastasis or Multiplicity of Tumor Growth?

In the discussion of the so-called "multiple gliomas" it was pointed out (p. 112) that the question has not yet been settled in a number of cases whether one is confronted with an unrecognized form of metastasis or a multifocal origin is involved. Reference was made to four of our own cases of glioblastoma occurring in both the second and third frontal convolutions and coincidentally in the occipital lobe (GP, Fig. 134a, b). A direct connection by means of cellular bridges could not be demonstrated in these cases and because of the superficial position of the lesions, metastasis via CSF was seriously considered.

Still less clear was our case of monstrocellular sarcoma in a 40-year-old patient, who had a plum-sized tumor on one side between the lenticular nucleus and internal capsule, and on the other side a similar cherry-sized nodule situated in the white matter of the hemisphere, again without demonstrable connection by any cellular bridge. This problem, therefore, can only be elucidated by microscopic examination of similar cases.

In this chapter on metastases of primary brain tumors, it would be appropriate to enumerate the various forms of seeding at this point:

1. Diffuse or circumscribed spontaneous CNS metastases within the subarachnoid and/or ventricular spaces. Medulloblastomas, pinealoblastomas, and pinealomas/germinomas very frequently seed spontaneously within the CSF pathways (Figs. 82, 103, 104, 105; GP, Figs. 168, 169, 246).

This type of seeding is rare in oligodendrogliomas and ependymomas although diffuse seeding after operation is frequent (GP, Figs. 70–72, 112). In glioblastomas a peculiar form of seeding on the ventricular wall has been described (GP, Figs. 129a, b, 132).

The monstrocellular sarcomas may seed in both ways, intra- and extracranially. Intracranially they metastasize diffusely in a manner similar to medulloblastomas, and extracranially, they tend to seed into the lung (Zülch 1953; Gropp 1955; GP, Figs. 236, 237, 239).

2. Metastases to different parts of the body are observed with only a few tumors and in these only rarely:

a) Among these entities, mesodermal tumors such as the above-cited monstrocellular sarcomas, and perhaps somewhat more frequently, meningiomas may seed even after a long clinical course of the disease (Cushing's famous case of Dorothy May Russell; see Cushing and Eisenhardt 1938, p. 692; Zülch et al. 1954).

b) When metastasis of a glioblastoma is described the question always arises whether or not this diagnosis has been a misinterpretation of a monstrocellular sarcoma.

c) Not infrequently metastases occur with retinoblastomas, where seeding into the frontal bone is well known. Seeding can occur also in sympathoblastomas which are very similar biologically. Finally, a series of medulloblastomas has been described in which these tumors sent extracranial metastases to the pelvic bones and into the lower extremities and even to lymph nodes and liver (Haberich and Zülch 1959).

Pathogenesis: Route of Metastases

The only well recognized route of metastases of primary brain tumors is via the CSF. It has been clearly demonstrated that in addition to spread in the known direction of the CSF flow, counter-currents must exist. Medulloblastomas, for example, seed into the third ventricle, the infundibulum, and lateral ventricles (GP, Figs. 168, 169), pinealomas into the infundibulum (Fig. 82), and some glioblastomas "upstream" as well (GP, Figs. 132, 133). In general, metastases understandably select the dependent parts of the CSF channels around the cauda equina or the dense meshwork of arachnoid in the region of the posterior columns in a manner similar to meningitis.

Today, metastasis can be more satisfactorily diagnosed by CT (Ascherl et al. 1981) than it was formerly by air studies (Learmonth and Camp 1933).

We have mentioned that apart from spontaneous metastases along the CSF pathways, "artificial iatrogenic" seeding by mechanical implantation of blastoma tissue occurs after operation. Several mechanisms have been suggested to explain why spontaneous metastasis from primary intracranial, and particularly neuroepithelial tumors, into other parts of the body is so rare. Among these are (a) lack of lymphatic pathways from the intracranial cavity into the body; (b) the very rare occurrence of tumor cell invasion into a vein within a malignant glioma; (c) the difficulty in finding a suitable stroma in which to grow; and finally, (d) the host reactions (immunologic?) of the tissue against blastoma "germs".

The possibility of the propagation of cells through the blood stream may be important. Theoretically, it should be possible in glioblastomas that during necrosis veins are opened permitting the entrance of tumor cells into the blood stream. Zimmerman (1975) points to the fact that tumor cells have been observed in the blood of the sagittal sinus, however, he comes to the general conclusion that "extracranial metastases of human gliomas practically never occur".

We have seen on one occasion a medulloblastoma of the posterior fossa in which six months following surgery there had been metastasis to local lymph nodes in the neck. Whether this was hematogenous or by some unknown lymph channel is still unknown. In medulloblastomas it is not uncommon for the sacral portion of the pelvic bone to become a site of metastasis. Whether this occurs by the blastoma cells following the perineural sheaths along the sacral roots of the cauda equina is not clear. The same is true of retinoblastoma which may seed into the neighboring frontal bones; but why and by what route has not been determined. Perhaps, the answers will be forthcoming as a result of experimental seeding which is described on p. 188).

Atypical Sites of Metastasis

We noted once pinhead-sized metastases of a medulloblastoma developing beneath the ependyma. In the case reported by Hasenjäger (1939b) the spread of daughter tumors from a glioblastoma, which lay adjacent to the ventricle, occurred at defects in the ependyma and the tumor cells did not extend into the subependymal tissue, in contrast to the aforementioned medulloblastoma.

On the other hand, in a case of ependymoma (ZÜLCH 1940b) the seeding occurred over the ependymal surface and the blood vessels of the tumor stroma apparently had arisen from the shed-off tumor fragment itself. In the same case of ependymoma the metastatic neoplastic tissue had developed in the outer layer of the arachnoid of the cisterna magna where arteries had also developed (GP, Fig. 71), which would otherwise never have appeared in the external layer of a cistern. According to the view of HASENJÄGER (1939b) the blood vessels did not arise from the subependymal tissues purely in the capacity of stroma, but either grew out of this layer as a consequence of a neoplastic stimulus or arose from the shed-off tumor fragment itself.

In one of this experiments in our institute, KLEIHUES noted during the neoplastic transformation of ependymal cells that vascular stroma developed from the subependymal layer (personal demonstration).

Next, we want to refer to the difference in the specific conditions present in various tumor forms. We have cited in the former edition of this book those authors who had described dissemination of focal or less widespread extension of metastasis.

We want to emphasize, however, the concept of CAIRNS and RUSSELL (1931) that spontaneous metastasis of neuroepithelial tumors within the CSF channels is even more frequent than had been assumed. They found metastases 8 times in 22 consecutive cases of neuroepithelial tumors in which the spinal cord was carefully sectioned. If the spinal cord was sectioned routinely, metastases would probably be found more frequently in the region of the cauda equina and along the dorsal columns, where the cellular residues collect. OSTERTAG (1941) reported such metastases in 20% of the cases he examined.

The Special Seeding Trends of Various Intracranial Tumor Types

Meningiomas. These appear to metastasize only rarely to distant extracranial sites. According to the literature (see SALVATI 1981) only 56 well documented cases of metastatic meningioma have been reported since 1880. One of the famous cases is that of Dorothy May Russell (CUSHING and EISENHARDT 1938), in whom, after 17 operations, the tumor finally developed anaplasia in the form of a papillomatous type of meningioma, which seeded into the lung. KALM (1950) described a case of diffuse spread within the meninges in a 46-year-old patient with sarcomatous degeneration of a tentorial meningioma. I had the opportunity to study his histologic sections and can fully confirm his conclusions. ZÜLCH et al. (1954) had described a case of meningioma with a 22-year history, where death ultimately resulted from seeding, particularly to the lungs, where the metastasis weighed 1780 g. In this case tissue culture was made at the time of operation and a poor prognosis given. LORENZ (1940) had also described this tumor which, according to his interpretation, rested between sarcoma and meningioma and yet, the survival time was nonetheless 22 years.

One of the exceptional tumors of mesodermal origin was reported in a neonate with a meningioma of the angiomatous type that metastasized (HABERICH and ZÜLCH 1959) to numerous organs and the skin. A survey of metastatic meningiomas is reported by KARASICK and MULLAN in 1974.

One remark has to be made about descriptions of "multiple meningiomas in the dura" as, for example, SCHMINCKE's (1925) case of "implantation metastases" from bilateral cerebellopontine angle tumors. Since the latter were neurilemmomas, in all probability the dural tumors were the multiple fibroblastic meningiomas of von Recklinghausen's disease (or its forme fruste).

Monstrocellular Sarcoma and Other Sarcomas. Early in our experience (ZÜLCH 1953a; GP, Fig. 239ff.) we mentioned the propensity for extracranial metastasis of this type of tumor, particularly into the lungs. This was also confirmed by GROPP (1955). Another case of extracranial metastases of a primary intracerebral sarcoma was described by SHIMURA et al. (1980a).

Neuroepithelial Tumors

Medulloblastoma: In 1956 (p. 136), I reported two cases of metastasis from typical medulloblastoma. The first of these was in an 8-year-old boy with lesions in the vertebral column and pelvis and the second, a 12-year-old girl with metastases to the skin of the thigh. Because of these observations, I felt that WOHLWILL's (1930) report of metastasis from a medulloblastoma to the lymph nodes of the neck would have to be considered the first report of such a case. A 20-year-old patient of ours, reported earlier, with a very similar looking meningeal sarcomatosis did not have a medulloblastoma. At first, I had made a diagnosis of medulloblastoma on the basis of a small fragment of cerebellar tissue, in which only the leptomeninges were infiltrated with tumor. But I had left open the possibility of the sarcomatosis. Two years later, after intensive x-ray therapy, a tumor nodule, developed in the neck, close to the hairline. Three years postoperatively the patient died of a recurrence. At autopsy a fist-sized mass of tumor was found which extended from the operative site into the musculature of the neck and was attached to the superficial lymph nodes. Histologically a diagnosis of sarcomatosis of the meninges was verified.

Whereas the most frequent site of extracranial metastasis in medulloblastomas is the pelvic bones and the neighboring extremities, pulmonary metastasis from a cerebellar medulloblastoma was reported by KOMATSU et al. (1980). At that time they found 54 cases of extracranial metastases from medulloblastomas, only 8 of which had metastatic deposits in the lung. Today, the leptomeningeal spread, the ventricular spread, and also extracranial metastases can now be determined by CT enhanced by contrast medium (see M. SATO et al. 1980).

Glioblastoma Multiforme: Extracranial spreading from glioblastoma multiforme, after the diagnosis of monstrocellular sarcoma is excluded, has been reported by several authorities. Previously, it had been disputed for a long time by other authors, including ourselves. GLASAUER and YUAN (1963) searched the literature and found 89 cases of primary intracranial tumor seeding into other parts of the body. In the tabulation by KRETSCHMER the primary tumor was glioblastoma multiforme in 43 instances. Extracranial spreading of glioblastoma multiforme is also described by SLOWIK and BALOGH (1980). In a case reported by SHIMURA (1980b) the glial nature of the metastasis was confirmed by the ultramicroscopic demonstration of glial fibers in the metastatic lung tumor. This was probably the result of hematogenous seeding.

Other neuroepithelial tumors with extracranial metastases have been diagnosed as "cerebral neuroblastomas" (SAKAKI et al. 1981). These authors made a preliminary diagnosis of "ependymoma" and according to their Figs. 2 and 6 they were correct, particularly since this was a large cystic tumor in a 9-year-old girl. According to this evidence it will probably belong among the extraventricular ependymomas described by TÖNNIS and myself (1937) and later further described by us especially for their biological behavior (1940, and 1956). Anaplastic change occurs frequently in this sort of tumor. However, I have never seen in my very large series, much of which was sent in for consultation, any extracranial metastases in the form of seeding into the upper cervical lymph nodes bilaterally. This is understandable, probably because of the anaplastic change in the tumor which is apparent from their Fig. 6 in the work published by SAKAKI et al. (1981).

Whereas extracranial seeding is certainly extremely rare in ependymomas and oligodendrogliomas (KUMMER et al. 1977), diffuse spontaneous seeding of these tumors within the subarachnoid space is well documented (see GP, Fig. 111; BAILEY and BUCY 1929b; see also pp. 253, 268).

Experimental Seeding in Man. Transplantation of an anaplastic astrocytoma into the subcutaneous tissue in man has been successfully performed by BATTISTA et al. (1961). Histologically the tissue remained similar to the original brain tumor. The response of this transplant to x-ray therapy and chemotherapy could be studied, which yielded some information about the most effective form of therapy.

MITTS and E. WALKER (1964) transplanted glioblastoma cells in five patients and in two of them also normal brain tissue into the subcutaneous tissues. the latter transplants, namely normal brain tissue, did not take. Of the tumor transplants two of five showed evidence of growth and adhesion to the surrounding tissues. Reticulin fibers were a prominent picture. Malignant glial cells grew but were not as active as the reticulin producing cells. Any conclusions with respect to therapy were apparently not available.

Experimental Seeding in Animals. For diagnostic purposes GREENE (1951a, b) tried to determine the biologic malignancy of tumor cells by injecting them into the anterior chamber of the eye. If brought traumatically into the brain, it turned out to be a very good host for heterologous tissues, especially tumor tissue. However, GREENE preferred the eye because it was easier to determine the malignancy of an operated and transplanted human tumor with this site, since the eye remained accessible for continued observation. According to a personal communication from H. GREENE (1953), the transplants of such malignant tumors as glioblastoma "took" better in male than in female guinea pigs (see p. 79). Neuroepithelial tumors have been also transplanted into chick embryos for eight generations, as well as into the brains of rodents. However, in the chick embryos the tumor lost most of its characteristics and only regained them when transplanted back into the mice (COHN and ZIMMERMAN 1955). The transplantability of human malignant brain tumors has been tested by various attempts to produce an immunologic host defense reaction (see p. 80).

Experimental transplantation has been tried for comparison of the results with the findings in man. BALLINGER and SCHIMPFF (1979) showed in their model that cells of an experimental fibrosarcoma could be found in the capillaries after injection into the carotid artery. Metastatic tumors developed by the 5th day as proliferating nodules. The tumor cells then surrounded the capillaries and grew along and around these vessels. The blood brain barrier was broken down within these tumors. The proliferation of the capillary endothelium was occasionally remarkable when examined between 18 and 24 days after injection. Although this model is not fully applicable to *neuroepithelial* tumors, the very rare invasion of the venous system by tumor cells appears to be the main cause of the lack of neuroepithelial seeding into the body.

12 Postoperative Recurrence

Postoperative recurrence is described also in the chapter on postoperative survival and depends vastly on (a) the kind of tumor (the "grade" see p. 37), (b) the local operability, and (c) the adjunct therapy such as radiation and chemotherapy. The frequency of recurrence was expressed in my table, published in 1951 (see p. 39ff.), which now must be modified by the success of modern techniques of radiation and chemotherapy. Recurrence varies from extracerebral tumors, such as meningiomas and neurilemmomas, through very benign pilocytic astrocytoma (which may be "curable" by total removal) to highly malignant medulloblastoma, where surprisingly with radiation of the total neuraxis, 15 years or more postoperative survivals have been achieved. Finally, we have glioblastoma multiforme, in which the fatal outcome has only rarely changed appreciably. Additional information may be found in the appropriate sections.

Further References: NETSKY et al. (1960), ROTH and ELVIDGE (1960), JELSMA and BUCY (1969).

13 Methods of Pathological Study

13.1 Cytopathology

The techniques of studying the pathologic processes in the nervous system are only slightly different from those used in a general pathology department. In the latter, routine study is fairly simple and generally limited to the application of a few methods, whereas in neuropathology it may become more diversified. Selective demonstration of particular components of the CNS using specific staining methods is often necessary. These demands make the course of investigation longer and more difficult. To arrive at an opinion about the classification and grading of a tumor, we investigate by site, manner of growth, and type. Our study includes not only the cell type, to which too much attention was given in the former times, but the following as well: manner of growth and expansion, spread of the tumor cells, behavior toward the brain tissue; architecture formed by cell groupings; the degree of cellularity; life-span of individual cells; rate of growth (number of mitoses); formation of fibers; behavior of the stroma (free and associated with blood vessels); and regressive processes such as necrosis, fatty degeneration, calcification, mucoid degeneration, tendency to metastasize after surgery, recurrences, etc.

We try to classify a tumor after all of the foregoing points have been taken into account. Only those tumors will be classified together that agree in a majority of these characteristics. Identical or similar cells alone, with differences in other characteristics, do not constitute a decisive criterion for the classification of most tumour groups. It has been shown that no single criterion, such as a bipolar form of a cell, for instance, but rather the total sum of the above criteria list, is the decisive factor in a tumor's biologic behavior.

The purpose and value of such pathologic studies lies in the setting up of a *biologically uniform* system in which the tumor's classification and nomenclature indicate the prognosis and its probable behavior. Pathologic anatomy, in this regard, is a clinically applied science.

We begin specifically with a survey stain, which may be for the neuropathologist a hematoxylin and eosin or a cresylviolet stain. If the impressions obtained with the two stains agree, further detailed study with special methods such as impregnations may be superfluous unless there is a specific scientific interest. If they do not agree, we must employ special methods: gold and silver impregnations, silver stains for demonstration of reticulin fibers, Grinyo or Girolami's impregnation for special cell types, Masson's trichrome stain, or special stains for the pituitary tumors.

With few exceptions, the experienced investigator can recognize and adequately classify brain tumors on the basis of paraffin-embedded material stained with H & E, a routine method in general pathology. The specific diagnostic value of the different staining methods will be mentioned in subsequent discussion of individual tumor types.

13.2 Histochemistry

Histochemistry is the analysis of the tissue by chemical means. Basically any stain or even impregnation is a method that is relevant to this section. The reader is again referred to the comment made by Johannes MÜLLER (cited on p. 2) "that the essential criteria for a classification of tumors according to their intrinsic properties can be found only in the study of their chemical nature, their microscopical structure, and the manner and sequence of their development." However, with the development of chemical analytic methods and more detailed knowledge of the metabolism of living tissue, highly sophisticated data have been collected and are now available. Yet, even today when summarizing such data, we have to ask, to what purpose they can be used or how they enrich our knowledge. Naturally, with modern methods, we can analyze any chemical structure and the question we may desire, but again to what purpose?

Histochemistry of brain tumors is still at the stage of collecting data and classifying tumor cells and tumor tissue according to the results. By this method it is possible to gain new insight into many metabolic processes. After the initial stimulating paper by WOLF (1935) and more recent literature on the chemoarchitecture of the brain (ORTMANN 1961, 1964; FRIEDE 1966), the histochemistry of gliomas was reviewed by SPIGOLON and GULLOTTA (1961), LEHRER (1962), VIALE (1962), NASU and W. MÜLLER (1964), PERRIA et al. (1964). A summary of this work was presented at the International Symposium in Cologne 1961 (W. MÜLLER 1964). Apart from the more static methods of analysis by conventional histochemistry, the more dynamic technique of autoradiography had at this time been only rarely applied to the special problem of brain tumors (KISSEL et al. 1966).

Biochemistry of the brain has been left far behind in the different methods of investigation (see WOLLEMANN 1976). Histochemistry has tried to bridge the gap between morphology and biochemistry. It has the advantage of being capable of localizing enzymatic activity within specific intracellular structures thereby aiding in the chemical differentiation of normal and diseased organs. For elucidation of the dynamics of metabolic pathways, quantitative biochemical assays are essential. Furthermore in order to approach our goal of "molecular pathology," light and electron microscopy, must all be combined with histochemical and biochemical methods for the investigation of brain tumors.

The data known to date concerning the histochemical investigations of brain tumors would fill a volume in itself (see particularly SCHIFFER 1973). However, we would like to provide at least some of the data in order to show the direction of current investigations. For instance, a clear-cut difference in enzyme metabolism was found between astrocytomas and glioblastomas on the one hand, and oligodendrogliomas on the other, but the biologic significance of these observations is still not clear. MÜLLER and NASU (1960) found that the lipids in reticular parts of neurilemmomas were not of a regressive nature but rather there seemed to be a possibility that the Schwann cell produced "myelin building material". He also found that the pigment (MÜLLER 1962a) in this kind of tumor was not always hematogenous but could sometimes be of a lipopigmentous nature. LEHRER (1962) carried out the quantitative histochemical investigation of eight enzymes in human glial tumors and reported, that the β-glucuronidase showed consistent elevation that was most marked in malignant gliomas. Lactases were also significantly elevated.

UDVARHELYI et al. (1962) discussed the significance of DPN and TPN diaphorase, succinic dihydrogenase, alkaline phosphatase, and cytochrome oxidase, but to relate these findings to the rate of growth of a tumor still did not appear to be feasible. At best it might be said that oxidative enzymes (with the exception of DPN) were lower and alkaline phosphatase higher in highly vascular malignant tumors and that gliomas showed a low level of succinic dehydrogenase.

The investigations of LINDLAR (1970) demonstrated that the lipid contents of glioblastomas and giant cell tumors were different emphasizing the distinction between the giant cell (monstrocellular) sarcomas and giant cell glioblastomas. Other practical aspects were investigated by LINDLAR and BINGAS (1965) who found different histochemical contents in isomorphous and polymorphous oligodendrogliomas (oligodendrogliomas and anaplastic types, see pp. 246, 255). Also VAN VEELEN et al. (1977, 1979) pointed out some ways of defining malignancy according to the amount of alanine inhibition of pyruvate kinase present in gliomas and meningiomas. PERRIA and VIALE (1966) attempted to cast new light on the problem of cellular malignancy by histochemical studies. A greater degree of malignancy was also deduced by O'CONNOR and LAWS (1969) on the basis of changes in the histochemical staining of blood vessels within brain tumors, which led to either reduction or deletion of important energy-producing as well as energy-consuming processes within the endothelial cells.

NAKAMURA et al. (1973) investigated ATPase in nonglial tumors in which they found a higher activity and in the malignant glial tumors (medulloblastomas, glioblastomas) where they found a lower activity. The nucleic acids and proteins in cells of neuroectodermal tumors of different grades of malignancy were histochemically investigated by KHOMINSKY and BRODSKAYA (1973).

There are no doubt histochemical characteristics that indicate a greater degree of malignancy or a biologically more favorable behavior, but for routine work conventional methods, which were discussed on p. 27ff., will suffice. This statement is supported by SOBIN (1981, see also pp. 17, 197) who followed the work of the 24 groups preparing a classification of body tumors for the World Health Organization.

For the non-specialist most histochemical papers simply provide phenomenologic descriptions and not direct information on the growth and behavior of various tumor groups.

Further References: NACHLAS et al. (1957), MOORE and MCGREGOR (1965), HASS (1966), MOORE and PEREZ (1966), BENDA (1968), SNYDER et al. (1970), BRAND et al. (1971), LEHRER and MAKER (1971), S. SATO et al. (1971), STAVROU et al. (1971), PFEIFFER and WECHSLER (1972), HAGLID and STAVROU (1973), HAGLID et al. (1973), PICKEL et al. (1975), ENG and RUBINSTEIN (1978), PFREUNDSCHUH et al. (1978), ZOMZELY-NEURATH and WALKER (1980), RUBINSTEIN and BRUCHER (1981), HIRANO (1983).

13.3 Tissue Culture

The behavior of tumor cells in tissue culture has furnished important information concerning patterns of motion of individual cells and other growth characteristics of neuroepithelial neoplasms.

The early films made by Dorothy RUSSELL and BLAND (1933, 1934) were particularly instructive in showing type specificity not only of cells in their final stages of development but also in the patterns of movement occurring during their growth. Oligodendrogliomas and glioblastomas were clearly distinguishable, and the same was true for neurilemmomas and meningiomas. These factors were very important for differential diagnosis. Although the tumor cells had regressed developmentally during their migration, they kept considerable type specificity in their movements. Having reached their destination, they appeared to develop into their differentiated end-stage. The behavior of the stroma could not be evaluated so readily since the connective tissue cells multiplied quickly, because of their ready adaptability, and obscured the picture.

Meanwhile tissue cultures have been carried out on nearly all brain tumors (BUCKLEY 1929; KREDEL 1929; CANTI et al. 1935; COX and CRANAGE 1937; BLAND and RUSSELL 1938; MURRAY 1942; BENEDEK and JUBA 1943; KREMENTZ and GREENE 1953; COSTERO and POMERAT 1955c; DEREYMAEKER et al. 1958; LISS 1962; BRASSEUR et al. 1964; MANNWEILER and PALACIOS 1961; MANUELIDES 1965; CRAVIOTO et al. 1972; UNTERHARNSCHEIDT 1972; STAVROU et al. 1980).

Most of these investigations proved the stability of the Bailey/Cushing system of classification (like COSTERO 1962).

Excellent informations on tissue culture of brain tumors we owe to LUMSDEN (1951, 1955a, b, 1974) and particularly the basic monograph of KERSTING (1961), who summarized his extensive experience in 1968 at which time he had cultured 2000 tumors, 1200 of which were of neuroepithelial origin. He emphasized, in particular, that in tissue culture of human glioblastomas one never found divergent development into dissimilar cell types such as one was accustomed to find this in experimental mixed tumors in the mouse. From this method, he was also able to derive support for a precise cytologic classification. KERSTING furthermore pointed out that specific patterns of disorganization and reorganization of architecture had to be distinguished. These patterns appeared in cultures of pilocytic astrocytomas in the form of bundles, in oligodendrogliomas as satellite arrangements, in ependymomas as rosette-like structures, and in meningiomas as whorls. Such evidence of reorganization was never found in glioblastomas, however. This supported the concept that glioblastoma was separate type of tumor and did not develop from other primary tumors, as one could deduce from Kernohan's grading.

Tissue culture also permitted study of specific problems such as the derivation of medulloblastomas. KERSTING (1967) deduced from cultures that it originated from embryonic *mesenchyma* as an undifferentiated tumor inasmuch as there was no sign of glial or neuronal differentiation (see also GULLOTTA 1967b; p. 330). In tissue culture of glioblastomas FROELICH and LAPHAM (1965) found nuclear inclusions which corresponded to the eosinophilic inclusions seen in light microscopy. KREUTZBERG et al. (1965) showed an interesting enzymatic histochemical pattern of various transmitter agents in a ganglioneuroma. RUBINSTEIN and HERMAN (1975) were able do demonstrate precisely that there was fibrillogenesis both in glioblastomas and in ependymomas.

13.4 Electron Microscopy

The introduction of electron microscopy provided a new and valuable approach to the brain tumor problem. In this regard the pioneer work of FERNANDEZ-MORAN (1948) is particularly noteworthy. A few of the later more comprehensive studies deserve mention such as those of LUSE (1960, 1962), and RAIMONDI et al. (1962), as well as certain papers by LEVENTHAL (1959), GRUNER (1960), KEPES (1961 b), MANNWEILER and PALACIOS (1961), WECHSLER (1964), NYSTRÖM (1965), SOFFER et al. (1970), EBHARDT and CERVOS-NAVARRO (1981), CERVOS-NAVARRO and PEHLIVAN (1981), CERVOS-NAVARRO et al. (1981), and ZÜLCH (1981 c).

There are special advantages and disadvantages inherent in electron microscopic investigation. It is possible to investigate individual cell elements at high magnification almost without distortion artefact and with all the elements present being visible. Fine structural details of the nucleus, the cytoplasm and all the organelles, which were just grossly demonstrated in light microscopy, become recognizable. It is possible to make a distinction between cell types which previously had been thought to be very similar. One can depict organelles (Fig. 35)

a

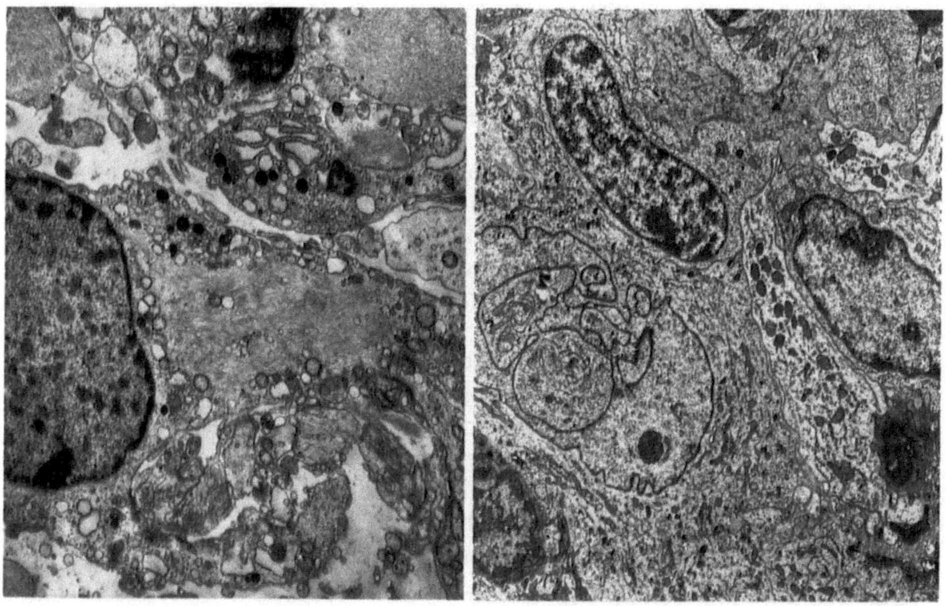

b

Fig. 35. a Astrocytoma (grade I): Tumor cells and processes containing considerable numbers of glial filaments with significant extracellular space. × 10000. **b** Anaplastic astrocytoma (grade III): Closely packed tumor cell with reduced number of glial filaments and pleomorphic nuclei and numerous mitochondria. × 6600. (Courtesy of Dr. SZYMÁS, Poznan, Poland)

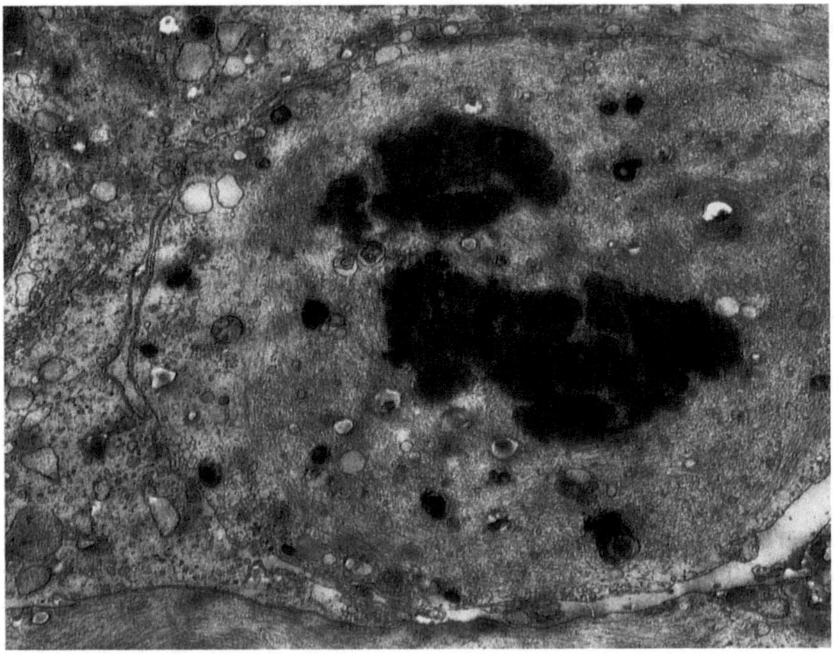

Fig. 36. Pilocytic astrocytoma (grade I): Rosenthal fiber with typical electron-dense aggregates associated with glial filaments. × 30000. (Courtesy of Dr. SZYMÁS, Poznan, Poland)

and chemical structures which can be shown only grossly by light microscopy and, perhaps, stained histochemically. Even biogenic amines, microdeposits of minerals (microcalcifications), artificial markers, secretion vesicles, granules, degeneration products, such like the "granulated bodies", and Rosenthal fibers (Fig. 36) in pilocytic astrocytomas can be investigated and more thoroughly analyzed. In addition, our knowledge of the extracellular space and all of the organelles within it has been clarified in detail. One can also understand better the mechanisms of fluid transport, edema, and the finer structure of the blood-brain barrier (Fig. 37) (see DUCKETT et al. 1978).

On the other hand, the use of ultrathin sections results in a fragmented picture of the whole. It would appear mandatory, therefore, to re-assemble the many fragments in a montage, while at the same time making comparison with the corresponding light microscopic sections. We must always be aware, that our vision when employing this method is in every sense of the word "tubular" since the electron microscope magnifies an area, which is only a minute part of the field of the light microscope. This obstacle can be partly overcome by using gross slices from the tip of a pyramid of the block and beginning study of the tissue with an anilin stained preparation. There is still a great danger that concepts may be developed which do not hold true later in the light of other morphologic methods.

It is interesting to note that electron microscopy initially seemed to simplify problems. RAIMONDI et al. (1962), in a review article arrived at the opinion that glial tumors schould be classified only as "gliomas" – benign and malignant

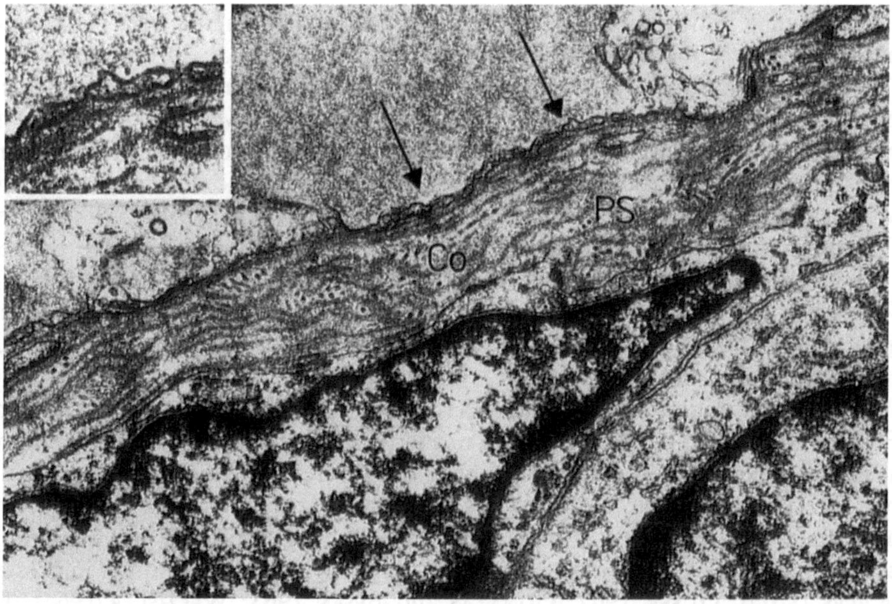

Fig. 37. Fenestrated endothelium (*arrows*) in the center of an astrocytoma (grade II). Enlarged pericapillary spaces (*PS*) contain collagene fibers (*Co*) and replicas of basal membranes causing distorted blood-brain barrier function. ×17500. *Insert* ×50800 (Courtesy of Dr. SZYMÁS, Poznan, Poland)

– since intracytoplasmic protofibrils were visible in most cells. One can also point to the idea, emphasized at the World Congress of Neuropathology in Munich 1961, that brain edema is always "intracellular". This impression was based on studies of *cortical* tissue, because white matter at that time could not be properly handled. Such concepts were in marked contrast to the light microscopic and even interference microscopic (GABRYEL 1962) evidence.

I believe, that in our review article (ZÜLCH and WECHSLER 1968) we came to the proper conclusion that electron microscopy would provide an enriching view only in special cases with special problems and that for *practical* purposes brain tumor diagnosis was better served by light microscopy. This was emphasized also by SOBIN (1981) (the general pathologist in charge of the WHO system of tumor classification) in a retrospective article on the excellent work performed by the study groups of scientists, employing mainly *light microscopic* methods.

We have compiled the known ultrastructural facts for most of the tumor groups in special articles in the second part of this book. Here, we shall merely mention some of the progress in knowledge such as the work on the oligodendroglia by LUSE (1960, 1962), MANNWEILER and PALACIOS (1961), and RAIMONDI et al. (1962) who directed attention in this tumor group to the particularly numerous mitochondria. According to CERVOS-NAVARRO and GULLOTTA (1961) and SPIGOLON and GULLOTTA (1961) glioblastomas contained occasional cells with abundant delicate intracellular fibrils similar to those seen in astrocyte. The majority of cells were, however, of a protoplasmic nature. In protoplasmic astrocytomas the pronounced interdigitation of protoplasmic processes was striking while in fibrillary astrocytomas intracellular filaments were very prominent. Therefore, the conclusion was reached that the glial fibrillae seen under the light microscope were composed of a countless number of very delicate intracellular elements. However, with ultrastructural investigation it was still not possible to distinguish definitely between normal and blastomatous astrocytes. In pilocytic astrocytomas, however, it was possible to obtain better insight into the regressive cellular elements (HOSSMANN and WECHSLER 1965) like Rosenthal fibers and "granular" bodies. "Furthermore, any resemblance between tumor cells and "embryonal spongioblasts" could be rejected (HOSSMANN and WECHSLER 1971b). Hence the naming in the WHO classification of a special group of "pilocytic astrocytomas", as proposed in the original work of PENFIELD (1931), turned out to be correct.

Many interesting side-problems have been solved by electron microscopy. For instance, ciliae have been shown not to be as numerous in plexus papillomas as in the cells of the ependyma, where they were seen packed closely beside one another with their blepharoplasts. Interesting details were found in meningotheliomatous meningiomas, where the interdigitation or dove-tailing of numerous cytoplasmic processes between neighboring cells was quite impressive (KEPES 1961b; GUSEK 1962; GONATAS and BESEN 1963; WECHSLER 1964). The findings in neurilemmomas were also of interest. There were numerous delicate cytoplasmic processes related to the tumor cells. The fine delicate fibrils were described as follows by LUSE (1962): "some are robust and have a pattern of longitudinally arranged fibrils with a cross banding of 1200 to 1400 Å," which is approximately twice that of collagen. The importance of this statement will be elaborated in Section 16.1 (on neurilemmomas). For these and other reasons HOSSMANN and WECHSLER (1971b) emphasized that electron microscopy was able to analyze the direction of differentiation of cells as "epithelial? glial/fibrillary? glial/protoplasmic? neuronal? mesenchymal? or vascular." This may help in problem cases.

WECHSLER started his ultrastructural studies in 1963 and analyzed, by combined light and electron microscopy, a series of 160 tumors comprising all tumors of the nervous system in our laboratory, operated upon by various neurosurgeons. His main goal was the correlation of light microscopy and ultrastructural findings (see also WECHSLER and HOSSMANN 1965a; WECHSLER and ZÜLCH 1968).

Some other questions were raised by POON et al. (1971), for instance:

1. Are gigantocellular neoplasms gliomas or sarcomas? (pp. 319, 408)
2. Are some tumors in the cerebellum sarcomas or "desmoblastic medulloblastomas"?
3. Which are the cells of origin of acoustic neurilemmomas? (p. 344)

Meanwhile, many investigations have highlighted these problems which have still not been completely clarified. WECHSLER and HOSSMANN (1965b) were able to distinguish Schwann cells from connective tissue elements since only the Schwann cells and their cellular derivatives were surrounded by both a cell membrane and a basement membrane. One interesting finding suggested that both cell types may be engaged in extracellular collagen synthesis, sometimes producing an unusual type of collagen, probably of a pathologic nature (long-spacing collagen). There seems to be little doubt now on the basis of electron microscopic evidence that neurilemmomas are Schwann cell tumors (LUSE 1960, 1962; PINEDA 1964b; WECHSLER and HOSSMANN 1965b; HILDING and HOUSE 1965).

One problem solvable by electron microscopy relates to the viral genesis of tumors. IKUTA and ZIMMERMAN (1965) observed in the early phase of tumor growth what they believed to be virus-like particles. However, HOSSMANN and WECHSLER (1971a) emphasized that in their series of more than 160 intracranial tumors from various neurosurgical centers, they had never detected virus or virus-like particles either in the nucleus or the cytoplasm of brain tumor cells. Only RAMSEY and KERNOHAN (1964) had seen in a circumscribed broadly investigated arachnoidal sarcoma an accumulation of round particles. Similar structures had been reported by HOSSMANN and WECHSLER (1971a) in a fibroma. Since than a large number of articles on that subject have been published.

One must conclude, however, that up to now electron microscopy has not yet delivered an incontrovertible argument for a viral genesis of intracranial tumors.

Can Electron Microscopy Provide Information About Anaplasia?

Authors had hoped to be able to assess the degree of cellular anaplasia by electron microscopy (HOSSMANN 1966) since BERNHARD (1961) had pointed to differences in the nucleoli of various types of benign or anaplastic cells.

In a study of WECHSLER (1963, personal communication), one of the problems which resulted was whether the criteria of cellular malignancy could be recognized better at the ultrastructural level, thereby basing the biologic evaluation of neoplastic growth on more reliable structural grounds. This question could only be answered positively to a minor degree. We will return to this subject later. There are certain characteristics pointing to the anaplastic nature of cells which have been discussed above (p. 27ff.). RAIMONDI et al. (1962) had already tried to tabulate the characteristic features of tumors and to assess prognosis of the more rapidly growing ones by characterizing (his Table 1) degeneration – nucleoli – ribosomes – endoplasmic reticulum – and mitochondria. All these were prominent features in rapidly growing tumors. On the other hand, intracytoplasmic pores and vesicles were seen in slowly growing neoplasms.

It is our opinion that the morphologic confirmation of anaplasia is possible with electron microscopy but more certain with light microscopy (see p. 29). The real value of the observed morphologic changes, however, is based on clinical experience and it is this element which allows the definition of "malignant" growth (see p. 31). We will return to this subject later.

In conclusion, we feel justified in making some statements about the value of EM for practical clinical diagnosis and classification of brain tumors:

1. Classification is still based mainly on light microscopy.
2. The rules of classification have gaps, where occasionally special methods like EM, histochemistry, or immunochemistry may be of some help, but where the problem may not be solved in near future, leaving some tumors "unclassified."

3. "Grading" is not defined by morphologic features alone but by the experience of the neurosurgeon and the correlation of morphology and postoperative survival time.
4. Anaplasia is more reliably defined by light than by electron microscopy at the moment.
5. A viral genesis is not supported for the majority of brain tumors by any of the methods available, including EM.

Further References: MÜLLER and OJAK (1960), FUKUMITSU (1964), HAGER (1964), ROBERTSON (1964), FRANÇOIS et al. (1965), MISUGI et al. (1967), TANI et al. (1969), RUBIN et al. (1969), BRUCHER et al. (1970), MATAKAS and CERVOS-NAVARRO (1970), GOEBEL and CRAVIOTO (1972), HIRANO et al. (1973), ERMEL and BRUCHER (1974), HASSOUN et al. (1975, 1981), BONIKOS et al. (1976), TOGA (1976), MAIR and ERDOHAZI (1978), ZÜLCH (1981).

13.5 Protein Analysis

We have described above the new and very sophisticated techniques of detecting in tumor cells specific proteins such as protein S-100, the protein 14-3-2, the GFA proteins (see ARMOND et al. 1980), α_2 glycoprotein, neurofilament protein, surface antigens, common glioma antigens, glioembryonic antigens, CGSA. However, to date these methods are available only in larger laboratories, and so time consuming that they are applied only to precise scientific problems.

13.6 Quick Diagnosis

13.6.1 Smear Technique

A safe method of rapid diagnosis consists of the supravital staining of crushed, squashed, or smeared preparations. A tiny piece of tissue is teased on to a slide with a dissecting needle and then covered with Loeffler's methylene blue (diluted 1:1 with distilled water), neutral red (1:10000), Alzheimer and Mann's methylene blue-eosin solution or stained with chlorazol black E. The cover glass is then pressed onto the tissue until it is only one cell-layer thick while being careful to avoid disturbing the tissue compositions. The excess stain is drawn off with filter paper and the section is adequately stained within a few minutes. An alternate method is to squash the tissue and smear it out with a slide, like a blood smear, and stain it appropriately. "Imprint cytology" is recommended by GERSTNER et al. (1977).

13.6.2 Quick Frozen Section

For rapid diagnosis during surgery (EISENHARDT and CUSHING 1930; BADT 1937; ZÜLCH 1937; RUSSELL 1939; MORRIS 1947; KAUTZKY 1951; KLATZO and McMILLAN 1952; see also p. 200) we use the following methods: A pea-sized piece of the most obviously neoplastic portion is selected from the specimen sent by the surgeon, if possible, from the growth zone. This is warmed in formalin until it begins to steam, but not allowed to boil. Starting with the first section from the freezing microtome (20 μm, or more if necessary) the slices are collected in warm formalin, then transferred into 1% aqueous cresyl violet solution, and again warmed for one minute. Then the sections are passed consecutively through distilled water and graded alcohol into 96% alcohol, where appropriate differentiation is carried out, depending on the thickness and cellularity of the sections. The sections are passed through absolute alcohol and then xylol, and mounted in Canada balsam. With skillful differentiation even thick sections (40 μm) can be sufficiently decolorized to obtain an excellent survey picture (the whole procedure takes about 8–10 min). Cryostatic sections can also be handled the same way.

Further References: KEPES (1971), BARNARD (1974), MEYERMANN and KLETTER (1976), KIESSLING et al. (1982).

Selection of Methods for Rapid Diagnosis

Needle Biopsy

1. If there is enough time, embedding in paraffin.
2. If diagnosis is required immediately, squash preparation.

Operative Specimen

Any freezing technique can be used; squash preparation is only necessary when the tissue cannot even be sectioned at 20–40 μm.

Other methods

In my experience, the use of the phase contrast method has no advantage over stained sections when a rapid diagnosis is needed (see KAUTZKY 1951; KAUTZKY and ZÜLCH 1955; KALM 1959).

14 Autopsy Techniques

14.1 General Introduction

We investigate the tumor by site, nature of growth and type. In detail, the following points have to be taken into account:
1. Manner of growth and spread of the tumor cells
2. Behavior toward the brain tissue
3. The "architecture"
4. The degree of cellularity
5. The life-span of the individual cells, e.g., degeneration forms
6. The formation of fibers
7. The behavior of the connective tissue

In order to classify a tumor, all of the foregoing points have to be taken into acount, and only those tumors will be classified together that agree in a majority of these characteristics. Identical or similar cells alone, with differences in other characteristics, do not constitute a decisive criterion for the classification (see Zülch 1958b; Table 7).

The purpose and value of pathologic studies lies in the establishment of a biologically uniform system in which the tumor's classification and nomenclature including its "grade" (see p. 31 ff.) indicate the prognosis of the affected patient. Pathologic anatomy, in this regard, is a clinical applied science, which in the routine can be restricted to very simple methods. Scientific analysis, on the other hand, may be very complex.

With few exceptions, the experienced investigator can recognize and adequately classify brain tumors on paraffin-imbedded material stained with H&E, a routine pathological method. It is on these methods that the volume of the WHO classification is based (Zülch 1979). The differential diagnostic value of the different staining methods will be mentioned in subsequent discussion of individual tumor types.

14.2 Fixation

Surgical Specimens. The tissue for investigation is usually obtained from craniotomy, less often from a needle biopsy – nowadays often stereotactic – or a smear. A recently described technique is "imprint cytology" performed by multiple touch from fresh tissue on glass slides (Gerstner et al. 1977). The fixative of choice is a 10% solution of formalin[1], except in the case of gliomas, when a piece of the specimen most likely to contain tumor – selected if possible from the marginal growth zone – may be fixed from the outset in Hortega's solution of formalin ammonium bromide. If immediate fixation in this solution is not possible, experience has shown that transfer after two to three days of formol fixation is still adequate.

When pituitary adenomas and gliomas are to be removed by suction, the surgeon should try to secure a solid fragment of the tumor for histologic study, removing it preferably with a sharp spoon. Immediate transfer of this tissue into formalin without delay is desirable, particularly with pituitary adenomas, in order to avoid the severe autolytic changes that take place in physiologic saline. A sterile dish of formalin, Bouin's or Susa's solution should be kept on the instrument table. For electron microscopy we process pieces of the specimen, each about 1 mm in diameter, and immerse them in 5% glutaraldehyde in 1/15 M phosphate buffer, pH 7.4; further processing them according to the laboratories instructions.

Autopsy Material. Removal of the brain should be carried out as soon as possible after death, preferably before the general autopsy.

When intracranial pressure is not increased a certain amount of preliminary fixation of the brain can be achieved by perfusing the subarachnoid space with formalin; this is done with two cannulas, one in the cisterna magna and the other inserted through the cribriform plate. However, this preliminary fixation should be called to the attention of the prosector, since a certain amount of this fluid can run down the esophagus and trachea into stomach and lungs, and can result in rather surprising, and at first inexplicable, changes in these organs.

When the intracranial pressure is raised, preliminary fixation is achieved by injecting the formalin into the blood vessels. Generally, in such cases, after injection of the carotid artery in the neck or after opening the skull and injecting the removed brain, only the region of the middle cerebral artery and a portion of the region supplied by the anterior cerebral artery are perfused. Injection of the innominate artery, left carotid and vertebral arteries after exposure by a collar-like incision from acromion to acromion is more reliable.

It is particularly difficult to preserve the form of the brain when there is a high degree of hydrocephalus, especially in children. In these cases the ventricular system can be filled with formalin soon after death, either through previous puncture sites or through the separated sutures. Good fixation can be achieved by exchanging the ventricular fluid for formalin – careful pressure upon the dilated lateral ventricles forces out the CSF and on release the fixative is drawn in by a natural sucking effect of the ventricles. After removal the brain must be carefully protected from any contact with water (because of Nissl's "water artifacts"), and after external inspection and description it should be fixed in ample quantities of formalin with the shape maintained as adequately as possible. The formalin *should be changed without fail after 3–5 days*. Brain-cutting

[1] Actually, such a solution contains 4% formaldehyde. This is prepared by diluting the 40% (concentrated) formol solution 1:10 with physiologic saline.

and other procedures – without any significant distortion of the shape of the brain – cannot be carried out until after at least 8 days of fixation.

The shape of the brain is best preserved by hanging it loosely in a sling of gauze, while at the same time supporting it, base up, with a thread under the basilar artery. Hanging it by a thread alone often results in distortion of the pons.

If poor fixation of the deeper portions of the brain is suspected, the floor of the third ventricle can be slit open, unless pathologic changes in this region are anticipated. This is particularly recommended when there is a high degree of obstructive hydrocephalus with blocking of the aqueduct or beyond.

With autopsy material, blocks of tissue from the deeper lying portions can be transferred to formalin ammonium bromide even after as little as 6–10 days and adequate results achieved with metal impregnations.

14.3 Brain Cutting

The opening up of the brain after the fashion of VIRCHOW and ZENKER destroys the regional relationships of the different parts and consequently should have no place in neuropathology. Today, in many neuropathology departments horizontal slicing is preferred for comparison with computed tomograms. Formerly, frontal sections were generally preferred but the method selected should be dictated by the peculiarities of the case.

At the time of brain cutting, one should record the external form and any alterations in it (for example, through local pressure), changes due to fixation, the character of the leptomeninges and blood vessels at the base and over the convexity, the pattern of the gyri and sulci, and changes in the regions of the cisterns.

The descriptions of the sections should include the position, extent, growth, color, and consistency of the lesion and the adjacent brain, displacement of the brain with possible enlargement of the white matter from edema, herniations, changes in position and form of the ventricles, metastases etc.

14.4 Routine Histologic Examination

Embedding Methods

There are three ways of handling the material: supravital squash preparations, routine or cryostatic frozen sections, and sections of embedded material.

Frozen Sections: Frozen sections can be prepared after as little as 24–36 hours of fixation. One advantage of these methods is that embedding is not necessary; others are better preservation of the tissue, particularly lessening of shrinkage artifacts, such as are seen in paraffin or paraplast embedding (which can otherwise be avoided only with time-consuming celloidin embedding), opportunity to study lipid substances, and better application of some of the metal impregnation methods. Among the disadvantages of these methods is difficulty of cutting soft, disintegrating tissue due to necrosis or fatty degeneration, etc.). Some of these disadvantages can be avoided by using gelatin embedding.

Gelatin Embedding: A method used only rarely with tumors since anilin stains work poorly here. It may be necessary to demonstrate fatty degeneration, lipid content, etc.

Plastic or Paraffin Embedding: With paraffin or paraplast embedding each specimen can be quickly and reliably sectioned – into especially thin sections – and stained with most methods. The disadvantages of the method include the high degree of shrinkage in material with a considerable water content (so that the fibers pull apart and spaces are formed around nerve cells and blood vessels), the fact that the sections come apart if cut very thin and the fact that such material is not suitable for all metal impregnation techniques (Foot, Tibor Pap, Grinyo, Bodian methods; see ROMEIS 1968).

Celloidin Embedding: Celloidin embedding was previously the only method that allowed the preparation of large sections, cut through complete hemispheres. However, this is now possible when using paraffin methods. It is the method of choice when the original technique of Nissl is to be used. Celloidin embedding lends itself particularly well to study of the growth and spread of a tumor and of the reaction of the surrounding tissue. The different components of the tissue can be selectively studied in successive sections (staining of cells, axons, myelinated fibers, glial fibers, connective tissue, or metallic impregnations). Celloidin embedding preserves the tissue best when it is softened or has a high fluid content. It is the method of choice in the study of alterations by brain edema under preferably "vital" conditions. The particular disadvantage of this method is the length of time necessary for embedding, the appreciable thickness of the sections (30–40 μm) and the less satisfactory demonstration of the external form of the cells when compared with paraffin material.

14.5 Selection of Stains for Special Tissues

Nuclei: The details of nuclear structure are shown best by H&E and cresyl violet staining of paraffin or frozen sections. Good results can also be obtained with other aniline dye methods.

Glia: The most beautiful demonstration of astrocytes is accomplished with Cajal's gold sublimate method, particularly with initial fixation in formalin ammonium bromide. If the latter fixation is used only secondarily, warming the frozen sections in formalin ammonium bromide solution before the actual staining is recommended. Hortega's methods are well described in CALVO's monograph (1954). Good results are also obtained with PTAH. More precise demonstration of the glial fibrillae can be accomplished with GFA protein antibody staining.

When there is special interest in degenerative processes, the microglia in the marginal zone of the tumor can be impregnated using Hortega's method. However, the method is very sensitive and demands that instructions be carefully followed.

Oligodendroglia can be demonstrated by Grinyo's method. The results, however, are not always reliable. For routine diagnosis of tumors, even for oligodendrogliomas, this method is often unneccessary since most tumors can be identified in H&E stains. For diagnosis of polymorphic oligodendrogliomas, and for differential diagnosis, however, it is extremely valuable.

If the metallic methods are not possible, Mallory's phosphotungstic acid and hematoxylin stain for glial fibers can be used on frozen sections as a substitute. However, the results are only really satisfactory after primary or early fixation in Müller's solution. The glial fibers can also be fairly well shown by using Heidenhain's stain on paraffin-embedded material. The Golgi method can also be used to reveal single tumor cells in their entirety.

Parenchyma: Methods for demonstrating axis cylinders are well known (particularly Bodian's method). Myelin stains can be performed after any method of embedding, including paraffin embedding (where, however, additional staining of glial fibers has to be taken into consideration), or the frozen technique of Spielmeyer.

Fats and Lipids: Fatty or lipid breakdown products can be recognized most clearly and simply with Sudan black or Scarlet red staining (fat Ponceau), but earlier stages of breakdown can be detected with myelin stains.

Summary

We use *frozen sections* for quick diagnosis, for demonstration of cells and nuclei, metachromatic substances (using cresyl violet), axis cylinders and myelin sheaths, glial fibers, microglia, oligodendroglia and fat. Frozen sections usually suffice for a quick survey of the material. It is impossible to work with softened tissue, and in such cases paraffin, paraplast, or celloidin embedding may be substituted.

Paraffin sections are currently used for basic routine work. They are especially suitable for the preparation of thin sections of cellular adenomas, for the rapid survey of larger blocks than those which can be handled as frozen sections, and for the processing of soft, disintegrating material. The basic methods are survey stains (H&E, cresyl violet, van Gieson), Mallory's PTAH, myelin sheath stains (Heidenhain), axons (Bodian) and connective tissue impregnations (Perdrau, Tibor-Pap, Foot, Gomori) or stains (Masson, van Gieson). For routine investigations of pituitary adenomas we recommend, in addition to H&E, Masson's trichrome stain (with its brilliant demonstration of acidophilic and basophilic cells), or the more difficult techniques of ethyl violet-orange G, neutral violet, and fuchsin red (see also pp. 462, 463).

Celloidin material is suitable for the preparation of large blocks when time is not a factor, and for serial and interval sections. The natural structure of the tissue is best preserved with this method of embedding.

Modern Protein Analysis

For more specific analysis of protein structure we apply the following methods:
1. Intracellular antigens for protein S-100, 14-3-2 glial fibrillary acid protein (α_2-glycoprotein, neurofilament protein)
2. Cell surface antigens

These methods may prove the nature and derivation of various cells in tumors and may also provide some indications as to the malignancy. Many of the methods are still in the development stage. This field of highly sophisticated research is discussed in modern pathology literature.

14.6 Selection of Stains for Particular Tumor Groups

Cells in the Cerebrospinal Fluid: For the study of tumor cells in the CSF the sediment can be embedded according to either Alzheimer's or the sedimentation methods (SAYK 1960; BISCHOFF 1961), or the material can be smeared on a slide.

Astrocytomas: Classically, demonstration of tumor cells is accomplished with the gold sublimate method; however, identification is generally sufficiently accurate with aniline stains. Astrocytes are also stained by Mallory's PTAH method.

Pilocytic Astrocytomas: Tumor cells are best demonstrated with H&E, and even better with the gold sublimate method; Rosenthal fibers and "granular bodies" are shown up with Heidenhain's stain, tumor architecture and the beginnings of mucoid degeneration with metachromatic cresyl violet.

Oligodendrogliomas: The classic honeycomb architecture is best seen after paraffin embedding and H&E staining, but also is visible to some extent on frozen sections. Mucoid degeneration shows up particularly well with metachromatic cresyl violet, and calcification with hematoxylin stains. The polymorphic regions should be impregnated with specific methods (Grinyo).

Ependymomas: The best demonstration of the architecture (perivascular zones free of nuclei) is achieved with cresyl violet staining of frozen or embedded material. The radiating patterns are best recognized with H&E or Masson's trichrome stain, blepharoplasts are visible in Heidenhain's hematoxylin and in ethyl violet-orange G as well as in silver impregnations.

Plexus Papillomas: H&E and cresyl violet on paraffin-embedded material provide the best demonstration of these tumors.

Pineal Cell Tumors: The best identification of these is also achieved with H&E stains on paraffin-embedded material, also Girolami's impregnation and PAS stain.

Gangliocytomas: The prerequisite for reliable cell type identification is the Nissl method, or its modification with cresyl violet. It is recommended that the sections be left overnight in an incubator in 70% alcohol. Reticulin fiber impregnation shows up the content of connective tissue, demonstration of axons with Bodian's method.

Glioblastomas: Histologic diagnosis is possible with routine chromatic stains. More "mature" cell forms and pre-existing glia can be demonstrated with gold sublimate or PTAH, and fatty degeneration with Scarlet-red while the extent of connective tissue with its abundant vascular component appears particularly clearly with reticulin fiber methods.

Medulloblastomas: Histologic diagnosis can be made on the basis of an aniline stain. Reticulin methods demonstrate the content of leptomeningeal connective tissue engulfed by this type of tumor or its desmoplastic variants.

Neurilemmomas: The architecture shows up best on routine chromatic stains and fatty degeneration is brought out with Scarlet-red. Silver methods show the absence of free reticulin fibers (which may be important in the differential diagnosis between these tumors and fibroblastic meningiomas) but they impregnate the fine "specific" fibers. After paraffin embedding and H&E staining the architecture may be reminiscent of oligodendrogliomas (because of fatty degeneration).

Meningiomas: Meningiomas can be recognized with any aniline stain. The subtypes can be distinguished best by using silver-reticulin methods, if the architecture in aniline stained sections is not already sufficiently characteristic.

Sarcomas: In addition to routine chromatic stains, a prerequisite for study of all sarcomas is the demonstration of connective tissue according to reticulin fiber methods (Perdrau, Tibor-Pap, Foot, or Gomori). This applies particularly to differentiation of monstrocellular sarcomas from glioblastomas.

Haemangioblastomas: The network-like architecture (angioreticulum) can be demonstrated well enough with chromatic methods. The connective tissue network of the blood vessels appears best with reticulin fiber methods, and fatty degeneration occurring in some of these tumors with appropriate fat stains.

Germinomas: H&E stain, PAS stain, and/or Girolami's method

Craniopharyngiomas: Decalcification is usually unnecessary. H&E stains should be used.

Epidermoid Cysts: An attempt should be made to obtain the capsular portions of the crumbly, scaly material for embedding. This is done by squashing the material with a pair of forceps so that ultimately only a delicate membrane of capsule remains. Then embed in paraffin.

Dermoid Cysts and Teratomas: Embedding in paraffin and staining with H&E, or according to van Gieson or Masson, give the best demonstration.

Vascular Malformations: Embedding in paraffin or celloidin (preferable because the blood remains in the vessels) and routine chromatic stains, or connective tissue stains, and metal impregnations.

Pituitary Adenomas: Thin paraffin sections should be prepared. Recognition of subgroups is generally possible on H&E stains, but progressive staining methods and special techniques are desirable (Masson's trichrome, ethyl violet-orange G, neutral violet-acid fuchsin, Heidenhain's hematoxylin, Azan, Gomori's chrome-alum-hematoxylin and phloxine, etc.).

Chordomas, Chondromas, Osteomas, and Lipomas: These tumors can be identified after paraffin embedding and routine chromatic staining. Lipomas can also be studied with fat stains on frozen sections. Osteomas usually have to be decalcified before embedding.

Adenoid Cystic Carcinomas: H&E stain should be used.

Metastatic Tumors: H&E stains on paraffin sections should be prepared.

Unclassified Tumors: If it is not possible at first to classify a tumor using routine methods, special stains must be employed in order to reach a diagnosis. In addition to routine chromatic stains, metallic impregnation methods that demonstrate the shape of the cell should be tried. A determination should also be made of the formation of fibers by the cells, the content of connective tissue, the type of regressive processes present, if any, and the reaction of the connective tissue to them. Characterization of the tissue type should be attempted on the basis of these observations.

Parasites: H&E and van Gieson's stain should be used in paraffin sections.

Granulomas: H&E, Azan, and reticulin fiber methods can all be used in paraffin sections.

Histochemical Methods: Although histochemical methods can be very useful in the scientific investigation of tumors, their diagnostic value up to now has not been significant. Consequently, we have not included them here and the reader is referred to specialist books on the subject.

15 Tumors of Neuroepithelial Tissue

15.1 Astrocytic Tumors

15.1.1 Astrocytomas

Synonyms in the older literature: Glioma durum, spider cell glioma, „Pinselzellgliom," star cell glioma, astroma, amoeboid cell glioma

Introduction

Viewing the different brain tumor classifications it becomes apparent that this large group of tumors is composed of many subtypes, which differ in macroscopic and microscopic features and which up to the present were insufficiently defined. In the WHO classification (p. 18), however, terminology and subclassification appear to be very logical. This classification is based upon the predominant cell type but also includes mixed and anaplastic forms. Correspondingly and logically, the terminology is based on the most frequent cell types, from which stem the names *fibrillary, protoplasmic*, and *gemistocytic* astrocytoma; ("gemistocytic" is derived from Greek, and not from the German *gemästete* (fattened) glia). The *pilocytic* astrocytoma – formerly called polar spongioblastoma – forms a distinct separate entity. Also included in the group of astrocytic tumors are the *subependymal giant cell* forms, which frequently occur as ventricular tumors of tuberous sclerosis, and the ill-defined – and rare – *astroblastomas*. Finally, an *anaplastic* (malignant) form of astrocytoma is listed. A tumor with mixed cell population will be described as a *mixed oligoastrocytoma* in the oligodendroglial tumor series (see p. 254). We have *not* included the highly malignant *astrocytoma IV* of Kernohan's classification in the astrocytoma group (see glioblastoma, p. 307 ff.).

Historical Note and Definition

The astrocytomas were precisely described by VIRCHOW (1863–1865) as the "glioma durum" and as early as around 1840 were among the first glial tumors to be recognized. Other terms include "spider-cell glioma" (T. SIMON 1874), "astroma" (M. VON LENHOSSEK 1895), "amoeboid giant cell glioma" (O. LOTMAR 1918), "fibrillary" and "protoplasmic astrocytomas" and "astroblastoma" (BAILEY and CUSHING 1926), "afibrillary" and "gigantocellular astrocytomas" (ROUSSY and OBERLING 1932), and the "piloid," "gemistocytic," and "diffuse astrocytomas" (PENFIELD 1932b). The history of the astrocytomas reflects that of gliomas in general.

H.J. SCHERER (1933, 1935) and DE BUSSCHER and SCHERER (1942) published a series of studies on astrocytomas (see also p. 13, historical development of classification).

Astrocytomas of the "juvenile type" (p. 222) are now included in the group of pilocytic astrocytomas, together with the polar spongioblastomas of the older nomenclature.

Epidemiology (Age – Sex – Frequency – Site)

Age: Astrocytomas occur predominantly in middle age, the peak incidence falling around 34–45 years (Fig. 9a). Our youngest patient was 4 years old, the oldest 67. A congenital fibrillary astrocytoma was observed by ROTHMAN et al. (1979).

Sex: In our series the male/female ratio was about 1.3:1.

Frequency: In our series of 9000 tumors astrocytomas proper occurred for 6.6%, as against 9.8% in CUSHING's (1932, 1935) series. Astrocytomas make up between one-quarter and one-third of all gliomas (see Table 2 in FINKEMEYER et al. 1975).

All the data in the literature have to be reviewed, and corrected, where appropriate, since the pilocytic astrocytomas have usually been included and the term *astrocytoma IV* (see p. 15) is often used for glioblastoma multiforme.

Site: Astrocytomas (GP, Figs. 84–101) lie predominantly over the convexity of the brain and we recognize the following types: *frontodorsal* astrocytomas of the first and second frontal convolutions (Fig. 38), which grow deep in the direction of the anterior horn and often contain a large cyst (Fig. 14, no. 2); *frontomedial* astrocytomas that extend into the white matter from the frontal pole along the first frontal convolution and the medial gyri (Fig. 39), often infiltrating and expanding the septum; *frontolateral* astrocytomas (Fig. 14, no. 9) in the laterobasal convolutions directly under the third frontal gyrus, with spread into the frontal white matter and occasional formation of a large cyst before the frontal horn, a fingerlike extension usually reaching into the white matter of the insula; *diffuse* (frontal?) astrocytomas of the entire (frontal?) white matter, which may grow across the corpus callosum to the opposite side. There are, furthermore, astrocytomas of the temporal poles (Fig. 14, no. 23) that grow in an *occipital* direction through the white matter or penetrate into the basal region of the frontal lobes and medially into the basal ganglia; *parieto-lateral* astrocytomas (Fig. 14, no. 20; Fig. 40), precentral or postcentral, with spread in the direction of the ventricular wall, and frequently with large cysts; *parasagittal* tumor growing through the parietal lobe and often reaching the medial surface (Fig. 41) of the brain (parietomedial astrocytomas); astrocytomas of the *thalamus*, often bilateral (Fig. 14, no. 51); astrocytomas of the *midbrain*, and astrocytomas of the *pons*, where they produce a nodular surface (whereas they can be circumscribed or diffuse when growing deep inside). Finally astrocytomas of the *spinal cord* are not uncommon. A breakdown by regions usually

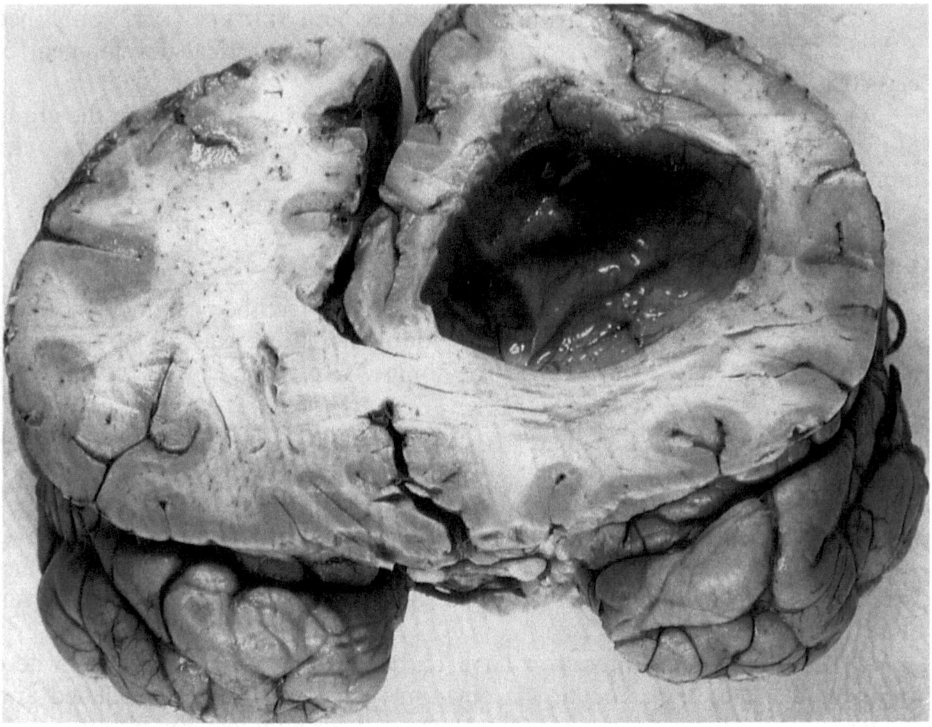

Fig. 38. Huge cyst in a frontodorsal gigantocellular astrocytoma. Considerable mass shifting has occurred. (ZÜLCH 1975a)

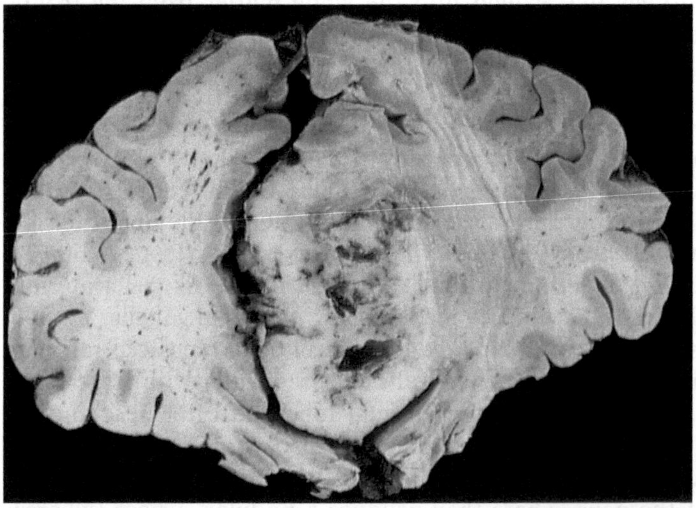

Fig. 39. Typical frontomedial astrocytoma. Note the multiple small cysts which are a frequent occurrence in such tumors. (ZÜLCH 1975a)

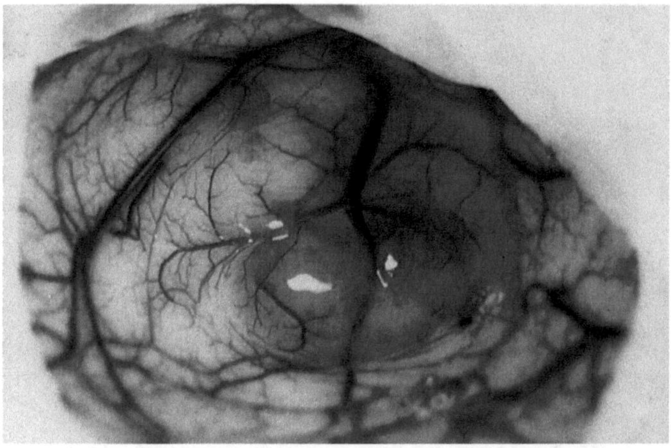

Fig. 40. Cystic astrocytoma of the precentral region (parietolateral astrocytoma). Picture taken at operation

shows that frontal astrocytomas are most common, followed by temporal and centroparietal astrocytomas, with only sporadic occurrences in other regions.

Gross Pathology

Astrocytomas are – depending on their subtype – often sharply circumscribed, firm, whitish tumors (Fig. 40), sometimes even cartilaginous (Fig. 41) in consistency, that grow superficially either diffusely or like a mushroom (Fig. 41). Degeneration into small and large cysts (Figs. 38, 39) often takes place when growing deep inside, in which case their consistency is softer. The protoplasmic and gemistocytic astrocytomas are also usually softer and sometimes somewhat gelatinous.

Astrocytomas vary from apple (Fig. 41) to chestnut size (Fig. 40). They may grow diffusely (25.8% of those reported by ELVIDGE and MARTINEZ-COLL 1956), predominantly at temporal sites. CLAVERIA et al. (1977) claim to have found more than 30% of the supratentorial astrocytomas to be calcified in adults (how many were actually oligodendrogliomas?) (see also PEDERSEN et al. 1981).

Histologic Appearance

At present we distinguish three histologic subtypes (HBT, Figs. 19–27) fibrillary, protoplasmic, and gemistocytic astrocytomas. Of these types fibrillary forms are the most common, protoplasmic the least, while the gemistocytic astrocytomas fall in the middle. Gemistocytic forms occur more often in the frontal lobes, the protoplasmic in the temporal lobes, and the fibrillary in both, with about the same freuquency. Astrocytomas usually consist mainly of one of the recognized types, but pure forms are actually not too frequent. Whether gemistocytic astrocytomas can develop from fibrillary and protoplasmic types,

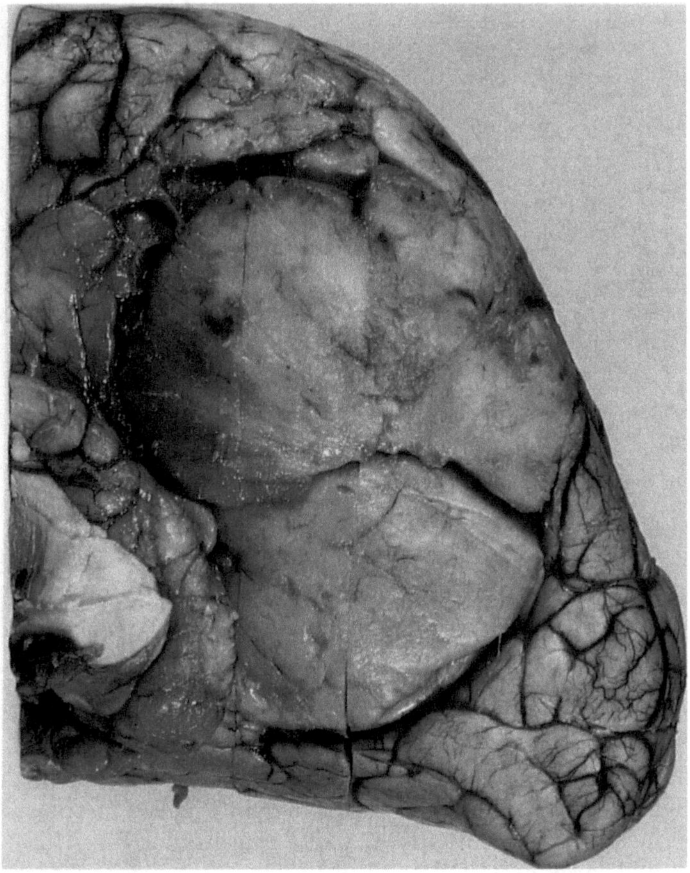

Fig. 41. Medial view of fibrillary astrocytoma. Note the knotty, hard appearance of this apparently well-circumscribed tumor. However, a more malignant portion was found to have traversed the corpus callosum to the opposite hemisphere. A tentorial pressure cone is readily apparent adjacent to the left inferolateral border of the tumor (cf. Fig. 92a). (ZÜLCH 1975a)

perhaps by a process of dedifferentiation, has not been clarified (GLUSZCZ 1972; RUSSELL and RUBINSTEIN 1977). The circumscribed astrocytomas grow by infiltration at the margin, but there is also considerable cell proliferation in the center, so that they grow by expansion as well. The rarer diffuse forms permeate the brain substance uniformly and expand it only slightly, so that they can be distinguished from brain swelling at first only by their firmer consistency (see ELVIDGE and MARTINEZ-COLL 1956).

The cells of all astrocytomas generally have medium-sized, round or kidney-shaped nuclei with a moderate amount of chromatin (Fig. 42). The fibrillary astrocytomas are characterized by their abundance of intracytoplasmatic glia fibrils (Figs. 42, 43), which can be demonstrated by special techniques (see pp. 200, 205). The protoplasmic astrocytomas have only very few or no glial fibers within the cell processes and may show a more abundant cytoplasm than the fibrillary type.

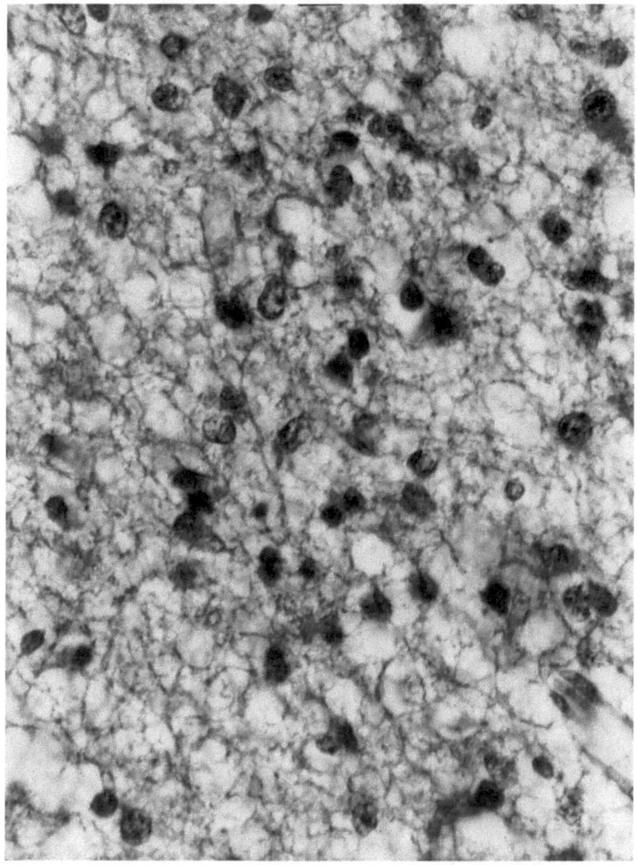

Fig. 42. Typical fibrillary astrocytoma

The gemistocytic astrocytomas (Fig. 44b) consist mainly of *cytoplasma rich* plump cells with eccentric nuclei, which are commonly hyperchromatic (pyknotic) forming usually fibrils (Fig. 45a).

The definition of the protoplasmic type (Fig. 44a) is still somewhat unclear. There are large cell astrocytomas, which with aniline stains may appear as gemistocytic and yet have no fibrils seen with gold sublimate impregnation (HBT, Fig. 21d). On the other hand, there is a clear distinction between the small cell type astrocytomas, which may either be rich in fibrils and correspond to the fibrillary type or be poor in fibrils and correspond to the protoplasmic type. The subtype is determined by the predominant cell type. How firm the consistency of astrocytomas is depends on the amount of intracytoplasmatic fibrils. The cellularity of most astrocytomas is not pronounced. The cells are uniformly distributed, and mitoses – an indication of rapid growth – are extremely rare in all types. The size of the cell body varies as described above.

Vessels are rare in the fibrillary types and consist usually only of capillaries. In some of the protoplasmic and gemistocytic tumors the vessels may be more numerous and sometimes show perivascular lymphocytic cuffing (TAKEUCHI and

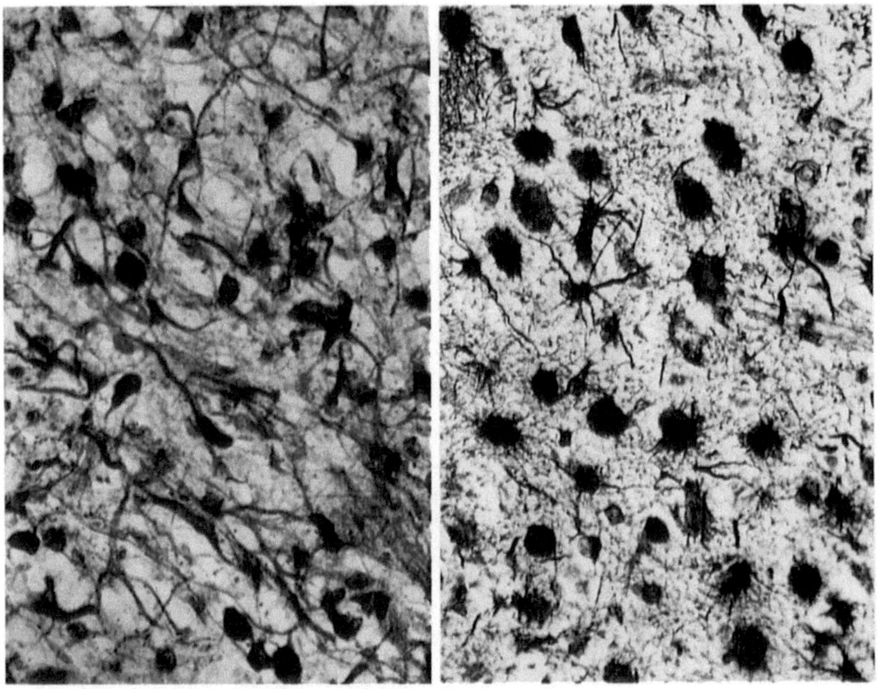

a b

Fig. 43a, b. Fiber formation: gold sublimate, ×220. **a** Unusually heavy fiber formation; **b** Slight fiber formation compared with **a**

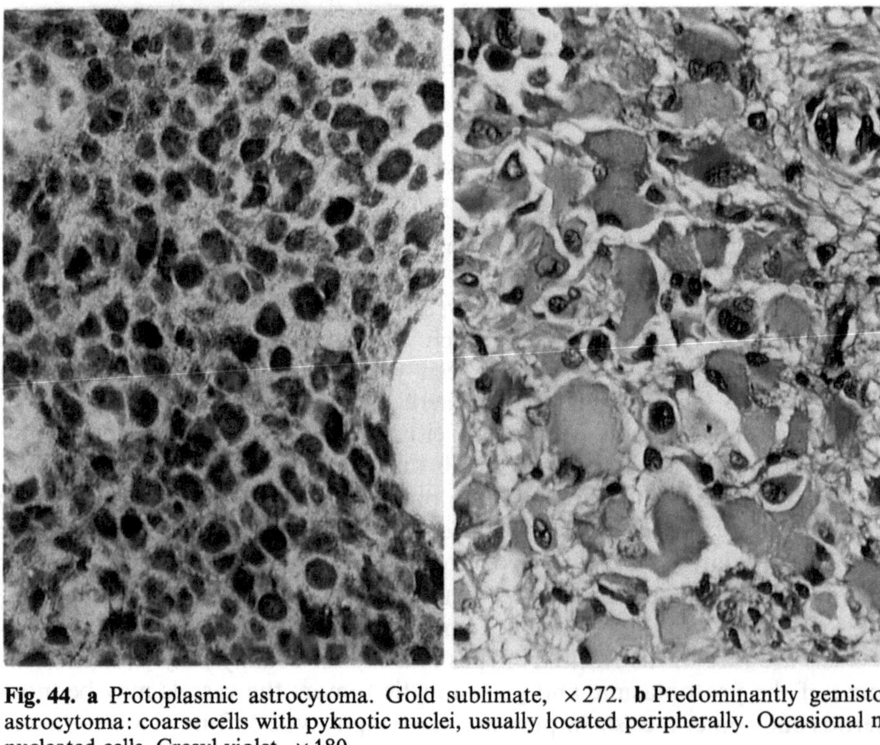

a b

Fig. 44. a Protoplasmic astrocytoma. Gold sublimate, ×272. **b** Predominantly gemistocytic astrocytoma: coarse cells with pyknotic nuclei, usually located peripherally. Occasional multinucleated cells. Cresyl violet, ×180

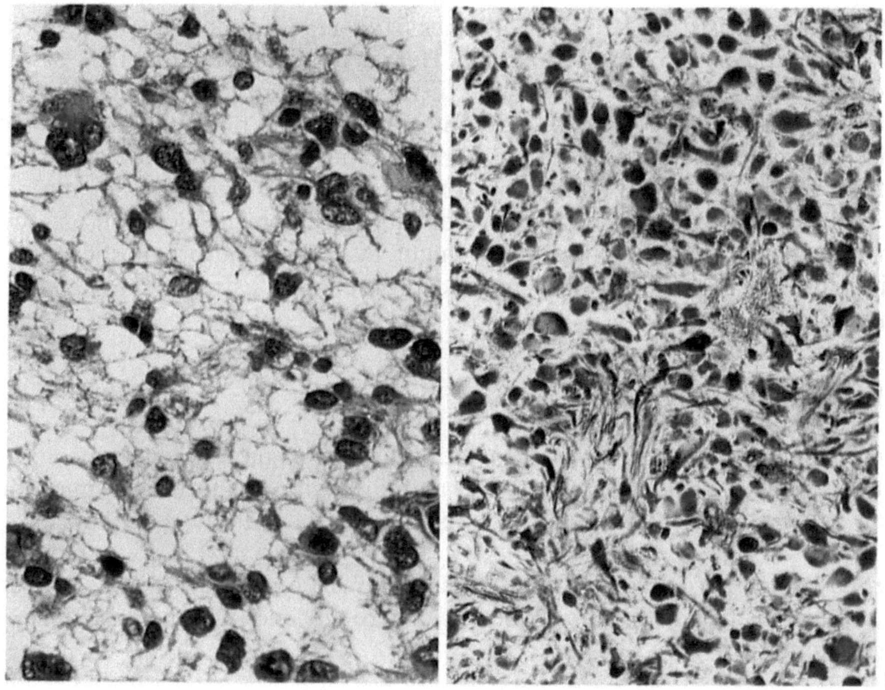

Fig. 45. a Typical nuclear shapes in a fibrillary astrocytoma (aniline stain): roundish or oval nuclei with a prominent chromatin network. Occasionally the nucleus is somewhat vesicular and a nucleolus stands out clearly, particularly in the case of fibrillary forms. Various forms of regressive changes, in particular mucoid transformation up to cyst formation in fibrillary and protoplasmic astrocytomas occur. Single, multinucleated cells can be recognized. H&E, ×312. b Typical pattern of an "astroblastoma." Coarse, large-bodied cells, usually with short processes, lie radially around the blood vessels. Gold sublimate, ×108

BARNARD 1976). In the gemistocytic astrocytoma vessels may be "coiled, tortuous and reduplicated" (ZÜLCH 1956, Fig. 156a, b). (For reference to the complex vascular stroma of astrocytomas, see p. 125.)

All astrocytomas, with the exception of the diffuse type, show an early tendency toward mucoid transformation with resulting cyst formation (Fig. 38). The fibrillary and gemistocytic astrocytomas tend to form large solitary or multiple cysts more frequently. Tumors with a system of small cystic cavities are frequently so-called astroblastomas (Fig. 45b) (see, however, the definition of astroblastoma, p. 18).

Calcification is rare, and necrosis is almost always absent in the more benign forms. Hemorrhage into the tumor substance is unknown; the presence of fat is limited to single gitter cells found mostly around blood vessels. Cartilage formation is extremely rare (KEPES et al. 1984).

Tissue Culture

This topic is dealt with briefly by reference to recent studies following the earlier experiments by KREDEL (1928, 1929), RUSSELL and BLAND (1933, 1934), COX and CRANAGE (1937), COSTERO and POMERAT (1955c), DEREYMAKER et al.

(1958), and LUMSDEN (1971, 1974). KERSTING (1961) reported on cultures of 37 astrocytomas, 33 of them successful. He was of the opinion that the classification eventually adopted was in agreement with the original separation made by BAILEY and CUSHING (1926, 1930) into fibrillary and protoplasmic astrocytomas. His cases included 10 of the fibrillary and 19 of the protoplasmic type. Moreover, he concluded that astrocytomas are not – like glial tumors in general – basically mixed neoplasms with secondary development along an astrocytic or oligodendrocytic direction. He thought that from the prognostic point of view the subdivision into fibrillary and protoplasmic astrocytomas was of no importance.

Electron Microscopy

Fibrillary Astrocytoma: Heterochromatin was located on the nuclear membrane. The surrounding cytoplasm was scanty and filled with rough endoplasmic reticulum, polyribosomes, mitochondria, a few lysosomes and fine glial filaments.

Protoplasmic Astrocytoma: The cytoplasm showed only a few surrounding delicate glial filaments, free ribosomes, and a rough endoplasmic reticulum and mitochondria.

Gemistocytic Astrocytoma: Coarse heterochromatin cytoplasm was filled with many ribosomes, rosettes, rough endoplasmic reticulum, mitochondria, and numerous fine glial filaments.

Intracytoplasmic protogliofibrils were found as in all astrocytomas, but varied in abundancy and distribution.

KERSTING (1968) pointed out the difference in structure and proliferation between the protoplasmic and the fibrillary astrocytomas compared with the anaplastic astrocytoma.

Histochemistry

Aldolase isozymes appear to have a higher activity in astrocytomas than in other gliomas (KUMANISHI et al. 1970). A high activity of oxydative enzymes (LDH, NADH) has been described, and also high phosphorylase and alkaline phosphatase (NASU and MÜLLER 1964) in tumor astrocytes.

Immunology

Immunologically specific tumor-associated surface antigens have been described in astrocytomas (COAKHAM and LAKSHMI 1975). These may be of great importance in the future for immunologic therapy. Tryptin-labile surface coat material seems to be associated with a higher degree of malignancy, i.e., seen in the anaplastic forms (SHERBET and LAKSHMI 1974a). It is also anticipated that implantation with corresponding reactions will allow better assessment of the malignancy of astrocytomas (SHERBET and LAKSHMI 1974b).

Differential Diagnosis

At operation, numerous large fistulous vessels filled with arterial blood and an abundancy of necrosis in the depths suggest *glioblastoma*. In biopsy and autopsy specimens glioblastomas are characterized by a variegated appearance, with hemorrhages, necrosis, and fatty degeneration, and by the proliferated and engorged blood vessels of bizarre formations (see HBT, Figs. 45–49). Further features (see p. 319) that should suggest a glioblastoma are (a) multinucleation, pleomorphism, and disorganized pattern of cells, with lack of abundant glial fiber formation, the presence of mitoses, and other signs of rapid growth; (b) wild proliferation of the vascular stroma and formation of fistular and sinusoidal vessels and of vascular loops with frequent formation of glomeruli, and occurrence of thrombosis; (c) destruction of the tissue by necrosis commonly bounded by barriers of proliferated blood vessels and gitter cells; (d) absence of calcification; and (e) massive infiltration of arachnoid spaces [but see descriptions of oligodendroglioma (p. 244) and pilocytic astrocytoma (p. 226)].

Features suggesting *astrocytoma* are (a) relatively sparse cells, orderly cell structure and pattern, formation of glial fibers (apart from the protoplasmic type), and absence of mitoses; (b) relative preservation of local elements (neurons) in invaded tissue; (c) few blood vessels, usually of the capillary type with uniform structure in distribution without evidence of endothelial proliferation; (d) absence of necrosis and fatty degeneration with preferential tendency towards mucoid degeneration and cyst formation; (e) complete lack of diffuse spread by the CSF. It can be more difficult, however, to distinguish between gemistocytic astrocytomas and large cell glioblastoma multiforme if the amount of tissue is meager. Nonetheless, sometimes the negative outcome of metallic impregnation by gold sublimate helps to distinguish the large protoplasmic cells of glioblastoma from the fibrillary gemistocytic astrocytoma. In any case the cluster of the features of glioblastoma multiforme, described in detail above, will satisfy in the distinction in most cases.

The distinction from *oligodendroglioma* occasionally presents difficulties, though this decision is less important at operation since both tumors are "semi-benign gliomas" (grade II). Oligodendrogliomas can sometimes be recognized macro- and microscopically by the firm cortical wart-like masses, which can be either seen or palpated as hardenings with the fingers. Astrocytomas have more circumscribed firmness. Moreover, oligodendrogliomas not infrequently grow into the leptomeninges, where they have the shape of a mushroom (see Fig. 58), and sometimes adhere to the dura (see Fig. 57), giving them the appearance of meningiomas at first. They quite often undergo calcification, which can sometimes be detected on roentgenologic examination or, more frequently, by histological tests, palpation or touching by an instrument, but most frequently by CT examination. After fixation the surface of oligodendrogliomas is velvety, finely granular, rather rough, and grayish pink; the cut surface of an astrocytoma is evenly distended, whereas an oligodendroglioma tends to infiltrate the cortex and enlarge convolutions in a garland-like fashion, so that they appear "hypertrophic." On histologic examination it may be difficult to distinguish an oligodendroglioma from an astrocytoma if mucoid degeneration has occurred.

Oligodendrogliomas are usually highly cellular, while astrocytomas are rather poor in cells. Of astrocytomas it can be said as a rule of thumb that the cell nuclei lie at the intersection of the cytoplasmic network, whereas in the oligodendroglioma the lymphocyte-like nuclei lie inside the center of the vacuoles (honeycomb pattern). Glial fibers are more common in astrocytomas. Pseudoneuronophagia (see p. 251; HBT, Fig. 34) is more frequently seen in oligodendrogliomas. – Routine metallic impregnations do not usually show up the oligodendroglia cells, whereas in fibrillary and gemistocytic astrocytomas the cellular elements are well impregnated. On the other hand Grinyo impregnation shows up the oligodendroglial elements distinctly. However, "transitional" cells positive in gold sublimate impregnation do occur (see HBT, Fig. 29c, d).

It is not especially rare for a real mixture of elements of both oligodendroglia and astrocytes to occur in one tumor. In view of this, the WHO classification includes a "mixed" variety under the name of *oligo-astrocytoma* (see p. 254).

Biologic Behavior (Grading), Metastasis, and Recurrence

The biological behavior of most of the astrocytomas is expressed by their qualification as "semibenign", which designation means grade II (see p. 31). Comparison of the various data concerning survival is difficult because the subtypes were not differentiated in most series and no account was taken of "clinical malignancy" (see p. 32).

Moreover, the grade has to be converted when a three-grade scale is applied, as has been done by RINGERTZ (1950), VORREITH et al. (1963), SCHRÖDER et al. (1968a, b), and SCHIFFER and FABIANI (1970). The real problem, however, is a different one: pilocytic astrocytoma may have been included in their grade I series, although they tried to distinguish the "Bergstrand tumor" as a special entity. – Therefore we will refrain from presenting too many different figures and state the general data of SCHRÖDER et al. (1970), who used the RINGERTZ classification: by this method they defined the median postoperative survival with astrocytomas corresponding to our grade II as 42 months and that with anaplastic astrocytomas (grade III; see p. 236) as 22 months.

Other data allowed the conclusion that the mean postoperative survival of patients with astrocytomas was 63 months and that after 3 years 57% were still alive (RINGERTZ 1950). The 5-year survival rose from 19% (LEIBEL et al. 1975) to more than 30% (WITTHAUT 1959) with additional radiation. However, the survival rate also depended heavily on histologic type, only 1 out of 11 patients with a gemistocytic tumor in the series of LEIBEL et al. (1975) passing the 5-year-mark, or only 1 of 24 patients according to ELVIDGE and MARTINEZ-COLL (1956). Hemispheric supratentorial astrocytomas in children tend to be more benign (MERCURI et al. 1981), especially when pilocytic and cystic (see p. 224).

It must be strongly emphasized that before comparison these data have to be adjusted for the extent of operative resection. This has not always been considered. Moreover, to date the survival rates depend very heavily on whether any additional chemo/radiotherapy has been given (see pp. 142, 150).

Multicentric (SOLOMON et al. 1969) astrocytomas in cerebrum and cerebellum must be distinguished from gliomatosis cerebri (see p. 341). Congenital astrocytomas are extremely rare (ROTHMANN et al. 1979).

Very often a small biopsy does not show whether the tissue consists of reactive astrocytes (which have an intensely eosinophilic enlarged cytoplasm, with processes very distinctly seen even with H&E) or the marginal zone of an astrocytoma. This can also distort statistical data. Further survival data are given elsewhere (p. 34ff.). The possibility of *anaplasia* is discussed in Sect. 15.1.5.

Metastasis is almost unknown. *Recurrence* is inevitable if excision is only partial (see also "Anaplastic Astrocytomas," p. 236).

Clinical Course

Some of the small fibrillary astrocytomas characteristically manifest themselves early by focal seizures. Other larger ones, particularly those growing in the frontal lobes, tend to show mental symptoms as a predominant feature. Signs of increased intracranial pressure are almost invariably present.

Further References: BAILEY and BUCY (1930a), BERGSTRAND (1932a, b, 1933), SCHERER (1933, 1935), ALPERS and ROWE (1937), WAGGONER and LÖWENBERG (1937), DE BUSSCHER and SCHERER (1942), TELTSCHAROW and ZÜLCH (1948), DUFFELL et al. (1963), ZÜLCH and WECHSLER (1968), GULLOTTA and FLIEDNER (1972), SIPE et al. (1973), STAGE and STEIN (1974), COAKHAM and LAKSHMI (1975), COSTERO et al. (1979), DUFFY (1983).

15.1.2 Pilocytic Astrocytomas

Synonyms: Polar spongioblastoma, astrocytoma of "juvenile type." Synonyms in the older literature: Gliomyxoma, myxosarcoma, fusicellular oligodendrocytoma, central neurinoma, gliome muqueux

Introduction

This special group of astrocytoma-like tumors has been clearly described under various names. The World Health Organization prefers the designation pilocytic/piloid astrocytoma, which was coined by PENFIELD.

Historical Note and Definition

Pilocytic astrocytomas were described in the BAILEY/CUSHING classification (1926) as polar spongioblastomas. This idea was derived from the similarity of the cellular elements with the spongioblastic cell of evolution. The name "spongioblastoma" appears to have been first used by KAUFMANN (1902), and reappears later in the writings of RIBBERT (1918) and GLOBUS and STRAUSS (1925). At first, however, this name was applied to ependymoma-like tumors (RIBBERT 1918) or even to medulloblastomas in the early attempts at classification by BAILEY and CUSHING (1925). To make the confusion in terminology complete, even glioblastoma multiforme was for a while called spongioblastoma multiforme.

The term "piloid" (pilocytic) astrocytoma is found in PENFIELD's nomenclature (1931). Its pattern was later well defined by BAILEY and EISENHARDT (1932). It corresponds to the "astrocytoma of the juvenile type" of KAGAN (1958), RUBINSTEIN (1972), RUSSELL and RUBINSTEIN (1977), and to BERGSTRAND'S (1932a, b, 1937) gliocytoma embryonale.

Position of the Pilocytic Astrocytoma in the System of Glial Tumors

From the very beginning there were difficulties with classification of gliomas of this type (see ZÜLCH 1937b, 1939a). They occurred as relatively benign tumors in young persons, arising in the cerebellum, brain stem, third ventricle, and optic tracts. Their tissue was composed of well-fibrillated uni- and bipolar cells, which formed intersecting bundles like "waves of hair" (BERGSTRAND 1932a, b, 1937). But in BAILEY's pedigree of neuroepithelial cells and the corresponding tumors spongioblasts were high up near the immature types and two classes higher than the fibrillary astrocytomas, although clinically more benign than the latter. This discrepancy was seen again when BERGSTRAND (1937), on the basis of impressive impregnations, separated the "so-called cerebellar astrocytomas" from the other cerebral astrocytic tumors. ZÜLCH (1937b, 1939a, 1940a, 1949b, 1956, 1959a, 1968) was able to show that this group of Bergstrand's was the same as the one that BAILEY and CUSHING (1926, 1930) had described as polar spongioblastoma and PENFIELD (1932b) as piloid astrocytoma.

Analysis of Bailey's material made it evident that this group of cerebellar tumors, clinically and biologically described in so masterfully a way as a *single entity* by CUSHING (1931), was later artificially separated into *two histological groups* of "piloid astrocytomas" and "polar spongioblastomas", according as whether most of the existing cell forms were more like astrocytes or more like spongioblasts. The tumor contained a mixture of cells with various forms, as shown in the impregnations reported by BERGSTRAND (1937). Therefore, ZÜLCH (1937b) came to the conclusion that this was a single tumor entity and that, histologically, biologically, and topographically they were "midline tumors", always occurring near the ventricular wall. He was able to point out a resemblance to the tissue of the subependymal zone during chronic inflammation (OPALSKI 1934), when the bulk of its Rosenthal's fibers are gathered in the resulting scar. The Rosenthal fibers had been seen in the spongioblastomas as the only tumor in the glioma group. This idea was consistent with that proposed by RINGERTZ and NORDENSTAM (1951).

On the other hand, numerous scientists based their groupings on the elongated either bipolar or multipolar cells that they called pilocytic or piloid astrocytes (PENFIELD 1931; KERNOHAN and SAYRE 1952; HENSCHEN 1955; RUSSELL 1955; RUSSELL and RUBINSTEIN 1977). There was one risk: the pilocytic appearance might occasionally be explained as a secondary architecture imposed on the cells by adaption to the structure of their environment, especially when the tumor was infiltrating the white matter of the optic tract or corpus callosum.

Apart from this, there is a genuine pilocytic growth, independent of environmental influences, and the hair-like wavy fibrillary processes are unmistakably seen in these tumors. The reason why the name "spongioblastoma" seemed inappropriate for this entity had been stressed from the beginning by ZÜLCH (1939a, 1956, 1965a, 1967a) and by RUBINSTEIN (1964) and RUSSELL and RUBINSTEIN (1977), among others. *Biologically* these tumors are definitely very benign and slow growing, while the term spongioblastoma implies a primitive tumor of high malignancy (see p. 340).

Even the "central neurinomas" (JOSEPHY 1924) and the "infundibulomas" (GLOBUS 1942) of the older literature belong to this entity, now defined as pilocytic astrocytoma. In the classification scheme of Santander it was termed "isomorphous glioma" (see OBRADOR ALCALDE and SANZ IBANEZ 1955).

"Cerebellar Astrocytoma"

The first examples of pilocytic astrocytoma in the cerebellum were described long ago by HILDEBRANDT (1906), Fedor KRAUSE (1908, color table IV; 1911), and LANDAU (1911). Because of the similarity of the tumor cells with those of the developing nervous system, BERGSTRAND (1932a, b, 1933) preferred for some time to call them "gliocytoma embryonale," but he changed his mind in 1937, and defined them as teratoid growths. They occur not too infrequently as a component of von Recklinghausen's neurofibromatosis.

With all due respect for Bergstrand, the term "Bergstrand's tumor" (KUHLENDAHL et al. 1975) should nonetheless definitely be avoided since the name of an author is not a suitable designation of a new tumor.

This group of tumors, located near the midline and – as we will see – sufficiently well characterized by its celltype and architecture and by its degeneration forms, such as Rosenthal fibers and granular bodies (ZÜLCH 1940a, 1959a), has finally been reclassified by the World Health Organization as *pilocytic astrocytoma* (ZÜLCH 1979).

In the WHO classification the term of *spongioblastoma* is reserved for the "primitive polar spongioblastoma" as defined by RUSSELL and CAIRNS (1947a), RUBINSTEIN (1964, 1972), and RUSSELL and RUBINSTEIN (1977). But these tumors are very rare and entirely different (see p. 340).

Epidemiology (Age – Sex – Frequency – Site)

Age: Pilocytic astrocytomas occur predominantly in the young. They are the most frequent tumors of the cerebellum and particularly the optic chiasmal region, in childhood and adolescence. The peak incidence lies between the ages of 3 and 7 years (Fig. 9b). Our youngest patient was 8 months old, the oldest 60 years. The youngest patient successfully operated upon was 8 months old. The peak incidence for cerebellar pilocytic astrocytomas lies between 8 and 15 years (Fig. 9b).

Sex: There might be a slight female preponderance: 134 of our cases in the tumor series of 4000 were males and 158 females, which means a ratio of 9:11.

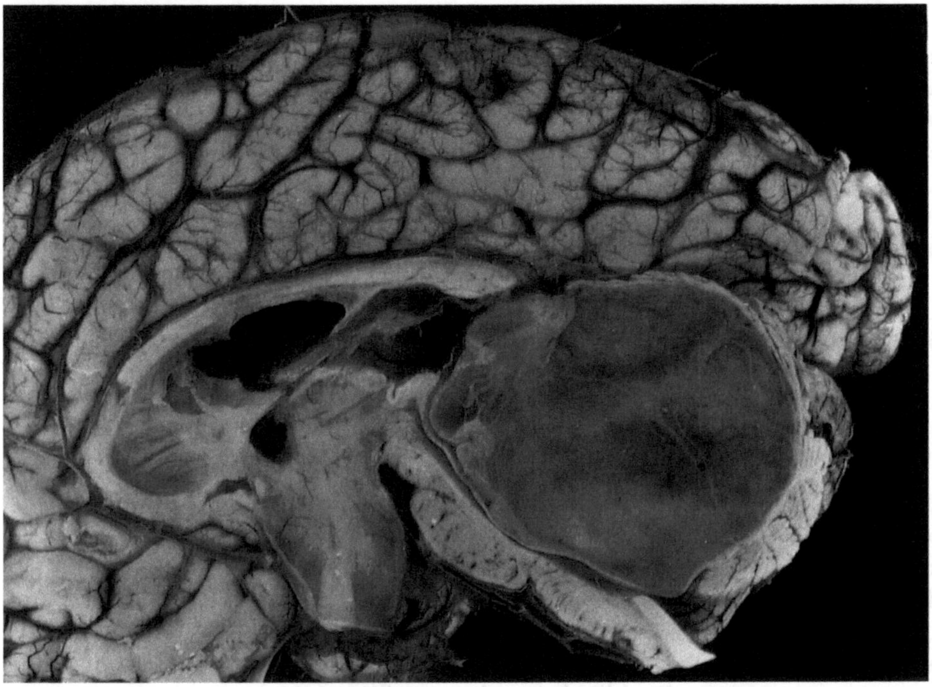

Fig. 46. Enormous cystic pilocytic astrocytoma of the midline cerebellum. Note the small mural nodule on the anterior superior cyst wall and the secondary hydrocephalus of the third ventricle (patient 18 months old). (ZÜLCH 1975a)

However, in a later series of 9000 tumors 270 were found in male and 268 in female patients, giving a sex ratio of 1:1.

Frequency: These tumors account for 6% of the total of our personal series of 9000 tumors. In Cushing's series 6.1% were pilocytic forms of astrocytomas with an incidence of *cerebellar* pilocytic astrocytomas of 5%. Of our series of 4000 intracranial tumors 187 (4.7%) were pilocytic astrocytomas of the cerebellum. They made up about one-third of the cerebellar gliomas in the series of KERNOHAN and SAYRE (1952) (around 8% of gliomas of all ages are in the cerebellum). The pilocytic astrocytomas form 30% of the gliomas in children.

Site (Figs. 46, 47; GP, Figs. 143, 145–159): The bulk of pilocytic astrocytomas usually lie around the midline and they commonly occur singly. They occur above the chiasmal region down to the hypothalamus (GP, Figs. 148–150), in the chiasm itself, or in the optic fascicles. They may fill the third ventricle and extend through the foramen of Monro into the lateral ventricles (GP, Fig. 150). Rarely they grow in the outer wall of the lateral ventricles as large hemispheric (GP, Fig. 151) tumors (like ependymomas of the cerebral hemispheres; see p. 262), in which case they can reach the size of a fist. They grow to the size of a pea in the aqueduct (GP, Fig. 152), of a walnut in the quadrigeminal plate (GP, Fig. 153), and of a plum in the fourth ventricle (GP, Fig. 147),

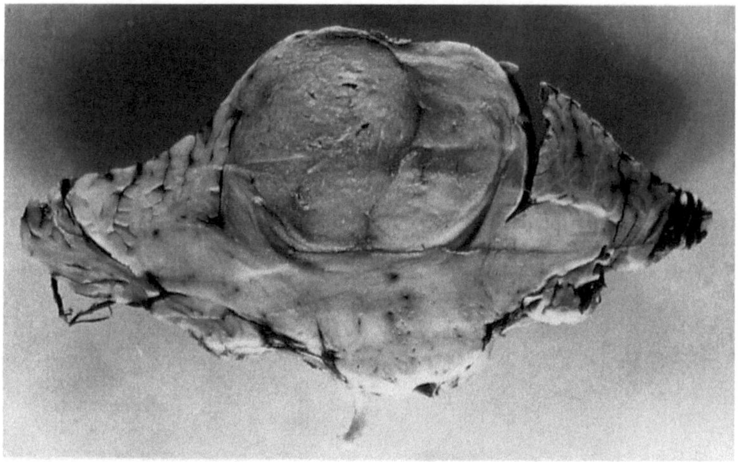

Fig. 47. Circumscribed pilocytic astrocytoma in the anterior superior vermis with distortion of adjacent midbrain. (ZÜLCH 1975a)

originating from the ventricular floor. In the cerebellum they are larger, very commonly becoming as large as a walnut or a tangerine, or even larger (Figs. 46, 47; GP, Figs. 143, 145, 146). In the cerebellum they occur in the midline but frequently expand into one or the other hemisphere. Finally, they grow in the pons and medulla oblongata and as thick as a pencil or thicker in the central portion of the posterior columns of the spinal cord and are commonly cystic in this position (GP, Fig. 159), where they have been often misinterpreted as syringomyelia.

Gross Pathology

Pilocytic astrocytomas are well-circumscribed tumors varying in size (Figs. 46, 47, 48); they are grayish pink and appear translucent, while they have a tough, elastic, firm, or occasionally mucoid consistency. Often they degenerate into small or large cysts (Figs. 46, 47). Occasionally there are small hemorrhages in the tumor tissue (see VINCENT et al. 1980) or the cyst wall shows remnants of brownish discoloration (Fig. 48). In the cerebellum the predilection site for pilocytic astrocytomas is the vermis (Figs. 47, 48), where they are well demarcated from the cerebellum and can sometimes be separated from the cerebellar folia – where the correct plane of dissection can easily be found – like an onion from its skin (Fig. 48) because they can apparently be almost encapsulated (GP, Fig. 146).

Pilocytic astrocytomas grow mainly by expansion, although they infiltrate at the margin (Fig. 49b). Cysts are present in most cases (Figs. 46, 48) and in the cerebellum (GP, Fig. 145) they may extend far into the hemispheres. When the cerebellar pilocytic astrocytoma is undergoing mucoid degegneration and becoming softer it can still be distinguished from a medulloblastoma, because of the latter's soft granular structure. Occasionally the cerebellar forms show calcareous portions visible in the x-rays.

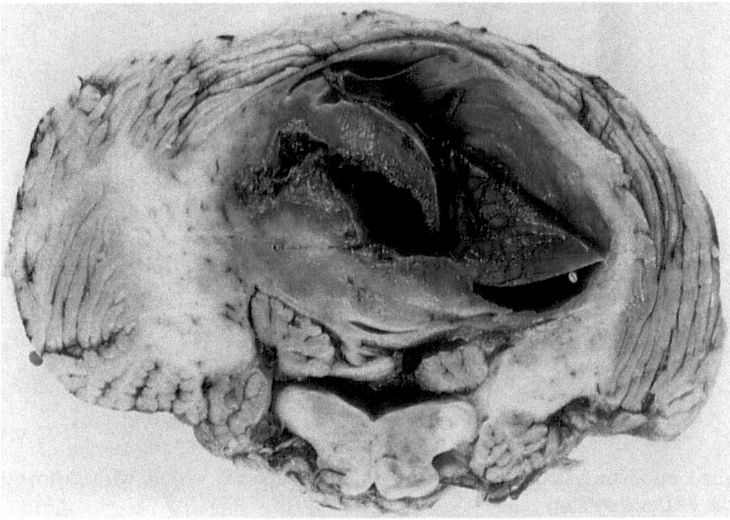

Fig. 48. Huge cystic pilocytic astrocytoma of right cerebellar hemisphere. Mural nodule visible at left lower corner of cyst

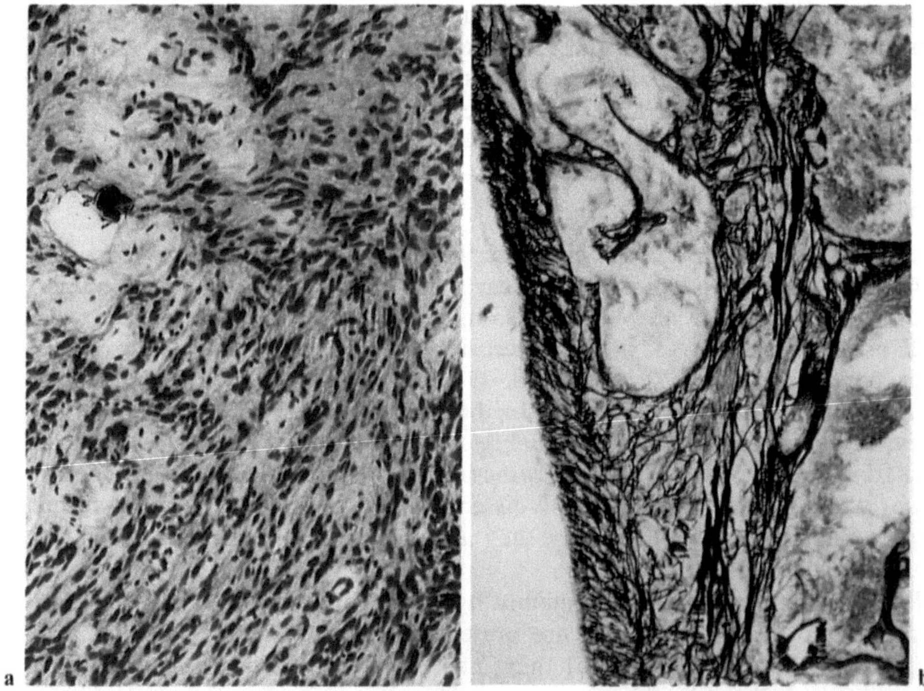

Fig. 49. a The typical architecture of a pilocytic astrocytoma shows the oblong cells arranged in long streams; they may tend to form parallel bundles. Cresyl violet, ×120. **b** Local invasion of the subarachnoid space accompanied by a moderate fibroblastic meningeal reaction. Tibor Pap, ×96

a
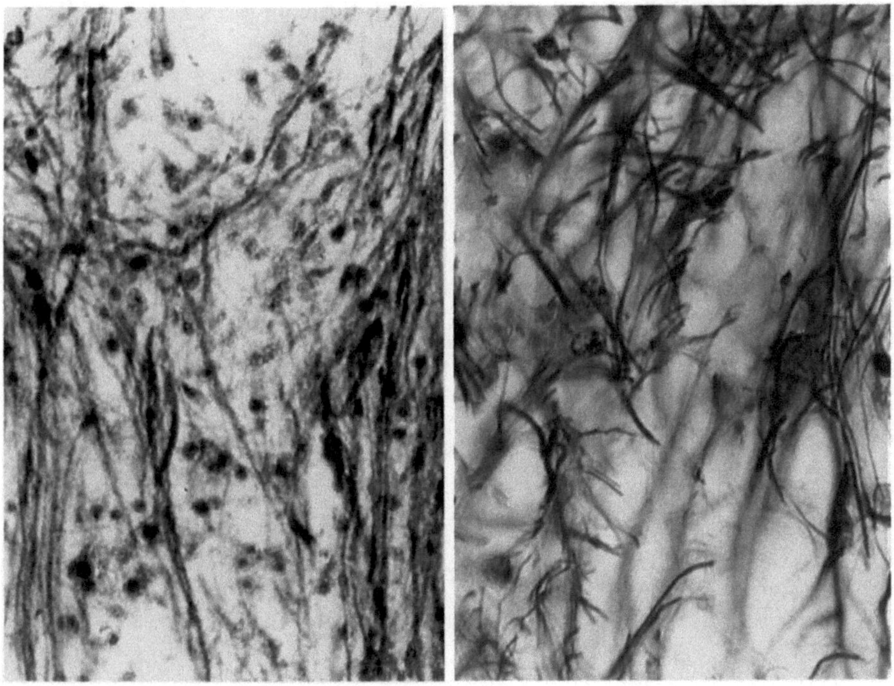
b

Fig. 50. a Impregnation reveals more astrocyte-like cells with long fibrils are revealed in some parts, and in others more bipolar cells, which have their processes arranged in narrow wavy bands. These patterns are clearly different from those of the cerebral astrocytoma. Gold sublimate, ×288. **b** Wire-thin glial fibers revealed in paraffin-embedded material from a pilocytic astrocytoma. Heidenhain's iron hematoxylin, ×576

Histologic Appearance

Pilocytic astrocytomas are moderately cellular tumors (HBT, Figs. 52–59) whose strongly fibrillated elements are oriented in streams and whorls (see Fig. 49a), as is sometimes observed in a neurilemmoma. There are no true palisades, however. The tumor cells are uniform, elongated, fusiform or worm-shaped uni- and bipolar cells, which have been variously described as "pilocytic," "piloid," or "hair-like" and "spongioblast-like" (Fig. 50a). There are also some with one long and many short processes, which seem to be like astrocytes. The streams and whorls of cells interdigitate or join in parallel or wavy bands, or form other patterns. The cell processes can be like corkscrews or gathered together like a braid of hair, or even form parallel bundles (particularly when invading the arachnoidal space). They form numerous PTAH-positive glial fibers (Fig. 50b) and have oval or elongated nuclei with a moderate amount of chromatin.

Mitoses do not occur, and growth is therefore very slow. The stroma is irregular, consisting of infrequent vessels that are sometimes clustered together like an angioma (HBT, Fig. 56). Not infrequently they develop reactively in the form of vascular coils along the margin of a cyst or an area of mucoid degeneration. Blood vessels coils also develop within the tumor inside the adven-

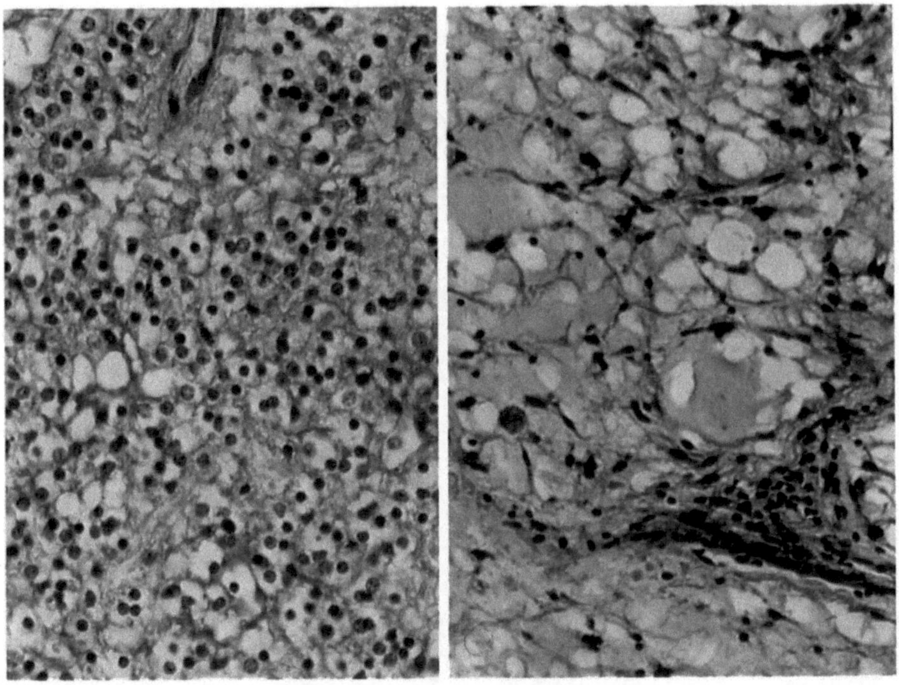

a b

Fig. 51. a In the course of mucoid transformation of the otherwise typical pilocytic astrocytoma of the cerebellum the honeycomb architecture of an oligodendroglioma can be simulated. Cresyl violet, ×272. **b** The mucoid transformation of a pilocytic astrocytoma of the cerebellum leads to the formation of a network with single pyknotic nuclei between the tissue bridges. Frequently cystic formation is found in the pilocytic astrocytoma, with coil-like, proliferated blood vessels lying at the border of the cyst. H&E, ×140

titial spaces, but this should not be considered as a phenomenon of anaplasia (see p. 124, and HBT, Fig. 56). The stroma has a marked tendency to hyalinization. A feature that is important for differential diagnosis is the occurrence of oligodendroglioma-like architectures (honeycomb pattern; Fig. 51a) due to mucoid changes of single tumor cells; moreover, the whole tumor can undergo mucoid degeneration and form microcysts harboring large amounts of protein-rich fluid, which is strongly eosinophilic (Fig. 51b). These parts, however, do not prove that the tumor is a "protoplasmic" form. Cuffs of cells persist around blood vessels during this process of mucoid degeneration, because of better nourishment. This may produce a pseudopapillary architecture similar to that seen in some ependymomas. Fatty degeneration is hardly ever seen, while microcalcification occurs early – though rarely – in the tumor proper or in the surrounding brain tissue.

Pilocytic astrocytomas regularly contain Rosenthal's fibers (see regressive processes, p. 140). These seem to be a typical degenerative form of glial fibers seen in the subependymal glia (Fig. 52a).

Because of the marked morphological resemblance between the elements of the subependymal glia (Opalski 1934), where in chronic inflammatory prolif-

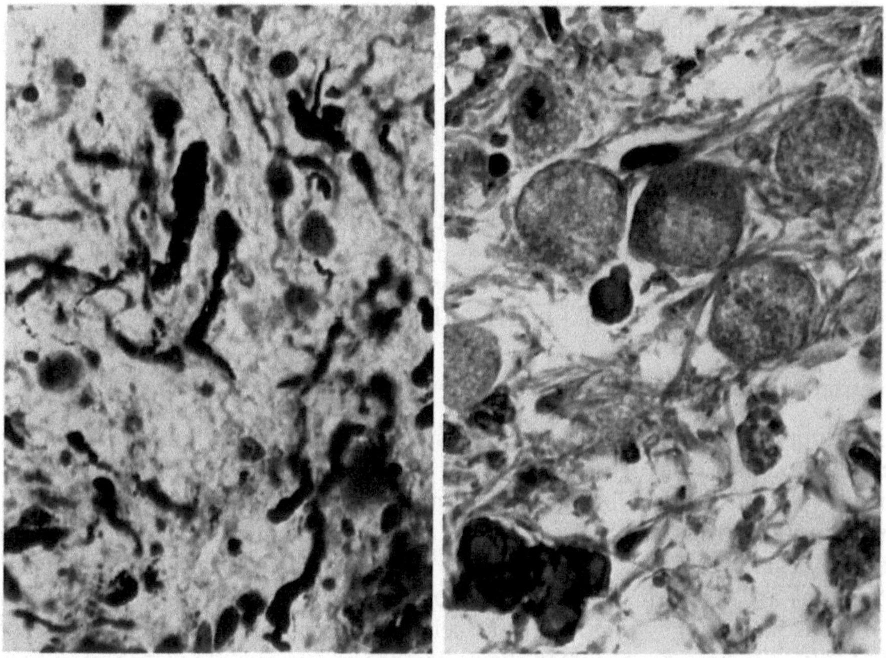

a b

Fig. 52. **a** Heidenhain's stain clearly reveals the sausage-shaped formations, which occasionally consist of single fragments tapering off like tails; Hortega's IVth variant. ×288. **b** Pilocytic astrocytoma exhibiting several "granular bodies." A calcareous deposit is encountered. H&E, ×500

eration Rosenthal's fibers are common, it seemed legitimate to assume that the "germ of origin" of the pilocytic astrocytomas was the subependymal glia. The fact that practically all pilocytic astrocytomas (including those of the optic fascicles, which embryogenetically are the optic vesicle of the lateral ventricle) grow near the subependymal glia also supports this assumption.

Rosenthal fibers were first discovered in a pilocytic astrocytoma in 1906 by HILDEBRANDT (unstained slide). ROSENTHAL himself (1898) had described them around a spinal ependymoma as a "glittery formation in the form of little bulbs or wavy sausages with one thick and one pointed end." Even then, he interpreted them as a "degeneration from glia fibers."

Rosenthal fibers (see HBT, Fig. 58) have been more carefully studied with modern techniques, but our old ideas about them (ZÜLCH 1937b) have basically been confirmed. They are also found in very many other – though rare – diseases (GRCEVIC and YATES 1957; OGASAWARA 1966, Table 1).

According to the findings observed by light microscopy (ZÜLCH 1940a) and histochemistry (DIEZEL and ROTTMANN 1958; FOTAKIS 1961b), by tissue culture (GULLOTTA and KREUTZBERG 1963), and by electron microscopy (RAIMONDI et al. 1962; K.-A. HOSSMANN and WECHSLER 1965: Figs. 10–14; SCHLOTE 1967), the Rosenthal fibers are, in fact, regressive products of extremely fibrillar tumor cells (see ZÜLCH and WECHSLER 1968, Figs. 11 and 12), especially in the region of the peripheral cell processes.

Together with the Rosenthal fibers, another characteristic structure is seen in these tumors, the so-called "granular bodies" (Zülch 1940a, Fig. 15a; HBT, Fig. 59). These are also products of the tumor cell, as shown by EM (Zülch and Wechsler 1968, Figs. 12 and 13), but the formation is due to a completely different regressive process (Fig. 52b).

While the Rosenthal fibers appear as products of the processes of the tumor cells that have undergone degeneration, the granular bodies are formed by gradual inclusion and augmentation of osmiophilic particles varying in size and structure, which in advanced stages conglomerate and finally fill up the swollen cell processes of a tumor cell (see K.-A. Hossmann and Wechsler 1965).

Electron Microscopy

According to EM findings pilocytic astrocytomas are extremely fibrillar, as already noted in the light microscope. At the subcellular level, therefore, a certain relationship to fibrillary astrocytomas cannot be denied (K.-A. Hossmann and Wechsler 1965, Figs. 10–14). Neither the mitochondria nor the cytoplasmic organelles for protein synthesis (free ribosomes, granular endoplasmic reticulum) are very conspicuous. Gullotta (1971) gave a detailed description of the EM picture of spongioblast-like cells and Rosenthal fibers, as did Schlote (1966, 1967), who also discussed their presence in various other disease entities.

Tissue Culture

In tissue culture (Kersting 1961, 1968), granular disintegration of the processes (Rosenthal fibers) and total cells (granular bodies) are also observed, but without signs of birefringency. Birefringency is observed as a primary phenomenon particularly in cell processes that have undergone little or no degeneration (Gluszcz et al. 1971). The spongioblast-like cells more frequently show condensation and thickening of the cell processes and glial filaments than the astrocytes. This degenerative process may end in the formation of Rosenthal fibers (Gullotta 1973).

Russell and Bland (1933, 1934) and Lumsden (1971) supported the interpretation of these tumors as astrocytomas on the basis of their results in tissue culture, while Kersting (1961), examining 11 cases of so-called cerebellar astrocytoma, came to the opinion that these tumors cannot be equated with the usual astrocytomas of the cerebral hemispheres.

Histochemistry

Histochemically the astrocyte-like cells contain oxidative enzymes with the highest degree of positive reactions, whereas the fusiform cells are less positive. The Rosenthal fibers, in contrast, are negative. The glial fibers are highly positive for phosphorylase, whereas Rosenthal fibers again are negative. The presence of hydrolytic enzymes is very marked in the tumor cells; in Rosenthal fibers they are absent. The Rosenthal fibers, on the other hand, are highly osmiophilic (Nasu and Müller 1964; Hanefeld 1967; Gullotta and Fliedner 1972), contain no carbohydrates and lipids, and can be stained only by protein-positive methods (Diezel and Rottmann 1958).

Differential Diagnosis

We have repeatedly emphasized the differentiation of these tumors from other astrocytomas (a) because so many biologic characteristics, such as site, age, predilection, differ from those of other astrocytomas; (b) because the histopathology, with its very distinctive cell types and its specific degenerative changes, such as Rosenthal fibers (ZÜLCH 1937b) and the so-called granular bodies (ZÜLCH 1940a, 1959a) distinguish these two groups; and (c) because the biological behavior is very benign. In this respect we are also impressed particularly by the surprisingly long course reported in the literature, for example, by BAILEY et al. (1939) and BUCY and GUSTAFSON (1939) (for details see p. 37ff.). This separation has now been accepted in the WHO classification.

Biologic Behavior (Grading), Metastasis, and Recurrence

Biologically pilocytic astrocytomas are the most benign group of all gliomas (grade I). After radical excision a cure or an extremely long survival can be expected (Tables 4, 5; see, however, anaplastic transformation, p. 239). Unfortunately, they are very often located in unfavorable sites for surgery, e.g., hypothalamus and midbrain, which means that they rather frequently have the characteristics of a "clinically malignant" tumor (see p. 32) unless shunt operations are performed [see recent attempts at multivariate analysis by LEVITON et al. (1978)].

According to a recent report published by KITAOKA et al. (1980), the long-term results are better in children than in adults. In the series of MILTZ and THAL (1978) a 10-year life expectancy was computed for 90%; and a 20-year life expectancy for 85%. Yet, KEPES et al. (1980) reported a case with invasion of musculature and soft tissues; with 17 months' survival after almost total resection and radiation; this case seems to be unique (see also p. 239).

Metastases: No metastases of pilocytic astrocytomas have been observed. We have seen general seeding in a cerebellar (protoplasmic) astrocytoma (ZÜLCH 1956, p. 174), but this was not one of the pilocytic type (see, however, SHAPIRO and SHULMAN 1976).

Recurrences: Recurrence is possible after any subtotal operations, but commonly arises only after a long time (see above BUDKA 1975; KLEINMAN et al. 1978: 48 years). If a cyst has only been emptied at operation a solid tumor may grow after many years of symptom free life (BAILEY et al. 1948).

In conclusion, it can be stated that the pilocytic astrocytoma is the only glioma in which a cure represented by survival for 20–40 years or a life without recurrence is commonly observed (GEISSINGER and BUCY 1971, for cerebellar forms; SCHISANO et al. 1963; GJERRIS and KLINKEN 1978, for other forms in this group).

Pilocytic Astrocytomas of the Optic Fascicle and Chiasm

Pilocytic astrocytomas can occur in the retina (ZÜLCH and NOVER 1960); in the optic nerve, either in its orbital portion alone, and particularly near the optic foramen, or on both sides of the optic foramen in the shape of an hourglass; or finally, they can grow predominantly in front of the chiasm, in the form of a pyramid, or in the chiasm itself (GP, Figs. 148–150). Thus, three gross forms can be distinguished: (a) intracanalicular, (b) intracranial, and (c) diffuse. In the latter form the chiasm is pressed into a flat band at the base of the tumor (Fig. 14, No. 39; GP, Fig. 149). Usually there is a transition to the hypothalamic forms. By virtue of the definite parallel arrangement of the nerve fibers in the optic pathways, the architecture and the cell forms of the tumor change and may be forced to orient themselves more longitudinally than in any other form of pilocytic astrocytoma (see architecture, p. 118). Mucoid degeneration with cyst formation also occurs. The pilocytic astrocytomas may balloon up the arachnoid sheath of the optic nerve by cell infiltration (see p. 552). The tumors of the optic system are usually hard and less elastic. The nerve and its mesodermal septa are diffusely infiltrated by tumor cells. Anaplastic malignant transformation is rare, as in most other pilocytic astrocytomas, particularly in middle aged patients (HOYT and BAGHDASSARIAN 1969; HOYT et al. 1973; A.M. HAMILTON et al. 1973; HARPER and STEWARTWYNNE 1978; BORIT and RICHARDSON 1982). Depending on their site, these tumors are surgically accessible either through the orbit or by a combined intracranial and orbital approach (LÖHLEIN and TÖNNIS 1949; see also OXENHANDLER and SAYERS 1978). Radiation is of little value except in the pontine location. Growth is very slow and prognosis is good (HOYT and BAGHDASSARIAN 1969; HEISKANEN et al. 1978). Usually they occur as a part of the picture of von Recklinghausen's neurofibromatosis or a forme fruste of this disease (with café-au-lait patches, etc.) (BUSCH and CHRISTENSEN 1937).

Clinical Course

The fully developed syndrome of the cerebellar form consists in early vomiting, headaches, loss of weight, rigidity, stiffness of the neck, and incoordination of gaze and nystagmus. Furthermore, there may be a cerebellar ataxia of the extremities etc. Tumors at other sites cause their own specific clinical manifestations.

Further References: MARTIN and CUSHING (1923), VERHOEFF (1932), HARE and WOLF (1934), RUSSELL and BLAND 1934), LUNDBERG (1937), ECHOLS (1938), DAVIS (1940), BUCY (1942), RETTELBACH and SCHUTZBACH (1942), BÜRKI (1944), FOWLER and MATSON (1957), KIM (1958), ZÜLCH and MACHTWEY (1958), GOL (1961, 1962), LUSE (1961 a), TYM (1961), SCHLOTE (1964, 1966, 1975), MCCORMICK et al. (1967), ZÜLCH (1968), HERNDON et al. (1970), GEISSINGER and BUCY (1971), MYLES and MURPHY (1973), BIEMOND (1974), GESSAGA and ANZIL (1975), T.W. SMITH et al. (1975), GJERRIS et al. (1976), MARTUZA et al. (1977).

15.1.3 Subependymal Giant Cell Astrocytomas (Ventricular Tumors of Tuberous Sclerosis)

Synonyms: Tumors in Bourneville's disease

Introduction

The ventricular tumor in tuberous sclerosis is listed as a special entity within the astrocytoma group as the subependymal giant cell astrocytoma.

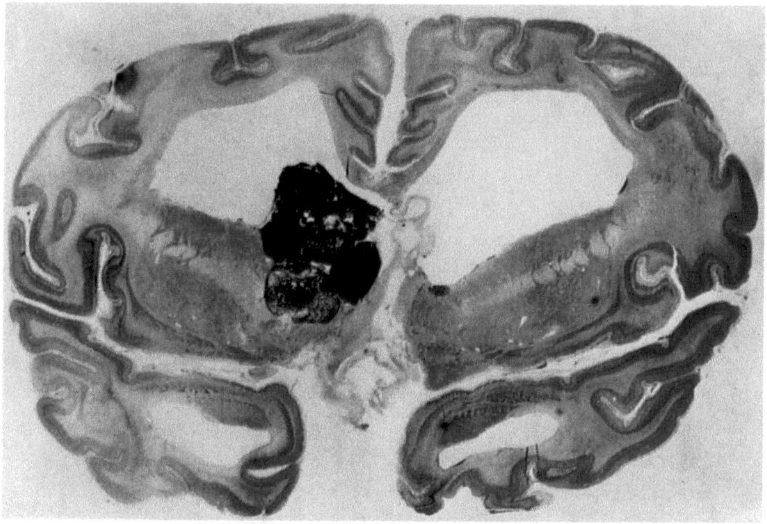

Fig. 53. Subependymal giant cell astrocytoma (ventricular tumor of tuberous sclerosis) arising from the medial part of the floor of the lateral ventricle

Historical Note and Definition

Tuberous sclerosis was first described by von RECKLINGHAUSEN (1863) and was recognized as a pathologic entity by BOURNEVILLE (1880). STENDER and ZÜLCH (1943) emphasized the existence of formes frustes of the syndrome without the traditional clinical triad (see also HALMAGYI et al. 1979).

SCHOB (1930), GAGEL (1942), and DONEGANI et al. (1972) have described the group in chapters written for handbooks.

Gross Pathology

The subependymal giant cell astrocytomas correspond to the ventricular tumors of tuberous sclerosis. They lie predominantly near the foramen of Monro (Fig. 53), into which they may grow and occlude (ZÜLCH 1956, Fig. 4; HBT, Fig. 15a–d; GP, Fig. 78). They arise predominantly from the medial part of the floor of the lateral ventricle (STENDER and ZÜLCH 1943; GP, Fig. 79).

Histologic Appearance

Microscopical examination reveals that they are composed of giant cells radiating out around blood vessels (HBT, Fig. 15). Their nuclei may be "ganglioid", i.e., with a clear center and a large nucleolus. Sometimes they are fusiform and arranged in long streams. Their cells are not infrequently polynuclear. They always form glial fibrils and tend to calcification. Their pattern is so characteristic (Fig. 54) that the diagnosis of tuberous sclerosis can be made from the tumor histologic appearance alone.

In addition to a large mass occupying the ventricle there may be multiple smaller nodules along the ependymal surface.

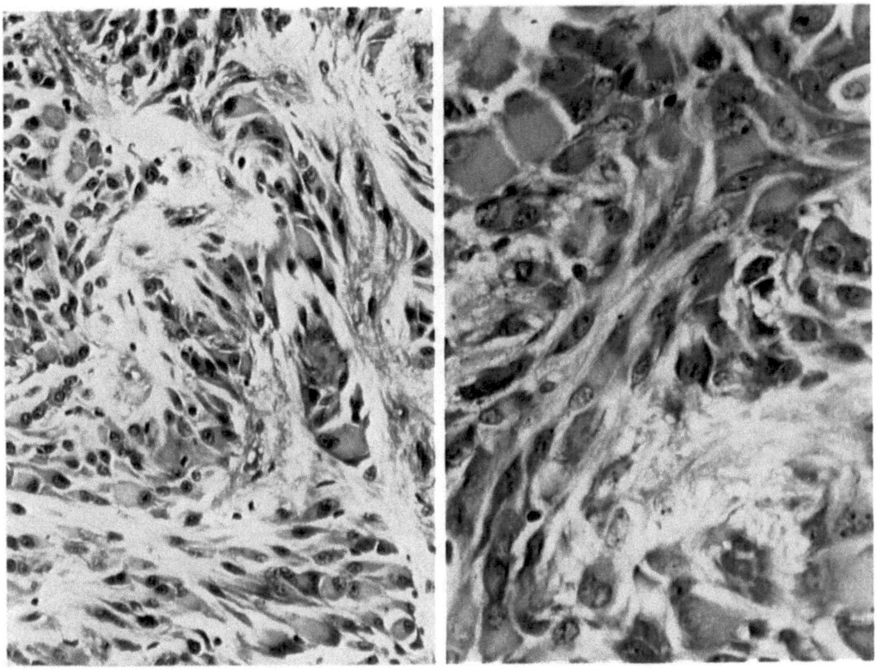

a b

Fig. 54. a Typical arrangement of spindle-shaped cells with abundant cytoplasm in lines interrupted by vessels. The vessels are surrounded by nucleus-free zones. H&E, ×160. **b** Very large cells with vesicular nuclei and large nucleoli are, in general, radially oriented to the vessels. Cresyl violet, ×272

Clinically it may be emphasized that the ventricular tumors occur in about half the cases as a forme fruste of tuberous sclerosis, i.e., without the typical triad: adenoma sebaceum, seizures, and mental deterioration.

Differential Diagnosis

The case of HALMAGIY et al. (1979) is not convincing if the brain cortex has not been sufficiently examined, as in the cases of STENDER and ZÜLCH (1943); histologically, namely even in the forme fruste cases one observes the typical cortical "tuberi", or at least cellular malformations and dysplasias with formation of giant cells, are observed. Electron microscopy reveals thick fibrils, which correspond to the filaments in astrocytes (SIMA and ROBERTSON 1979).

Radiologically these tumors are easily recognized and must be distinguished from the ventricular ependymoma (KAUTZKY and ZÜLCH 1955, Fig. 58). Their biologic behavior is benign (grade I).

Cure by operation can be expected with modern neurosurgical techniques (but see STENDER and ZÜLCH 1943; HOLANDA and HOLANDA 1980).

Further References: BIELSCHOWSKY (1924), MEDUNA (1930), GLOBUS et al. (1932), DRETLER (1938), ROSS and DICKERSON (1943), JERVIS (1954), BRUGGER (1955a), PEROT et al. (1966), KAPP et al. (1967), COOPER (1971), BROWN (1975), MEDLEY et al. (1976), LEE and GAWLER (1978).

15.1.4 Astroblastomas

Synonyms: None

Introduction

In BAILEY and CUSHING's (1926, 1930) histogenetic classification the "astroblast" was defined as a maturation stage between the immature spongioblast and the astrocyte, and tumors apparently consisting of such cells were classified accordingly. Astroblastic tumors as defined according to Hortega's classification, for instance, were very different. In the WHO classification the various definitions of *astroblastomas* are enumerated and the use of the term recommended only with strong reservations.

Historical Note and Definition

Astroblastomas have a very different definition in the published literature (BAILEY and BUCY 1930a). Therefore, when astroblastomas are mentioned in papers or statistics their histologic pattern must first be analyzed, since this name has been given a variety of benign and malignant gliomas (ZÜLCH 1939a, 1959a). In the papers of DEL RIO HORTEGA (1932, 1944b, 1945, 1962), for instance, three different types of tumors are found under this name (optic glioma, ependymoma, astroblastoma proper).

In our own discussions of this group (TELTSCHAROW and ZÜLCH 1948; ZÜLCH 1951b) we have counted only the truly "astrocytic" type of astroblastoma (HBT, Fig. 24), which we have discussed and described in detail in the publications cited. LIST (1936), DAVIS et al. (1950), and LUND (1952) discussed the significance of astroblastomas for the whole astrocytoma group.

The rather extensive report on our experience with glioblastomas published in 1959a should be recalled. In this we described the differential diagnosis between so-called astroblastomas, polymorphous (anaplastic) oligodendrogliomas, and monstrocellular sarcomas. We pointed out in particular that "astroblastic cells and patterns" or "astroblastic formations" quite frequently occurred in true glioblastomas (ZÜLCH 1959a, Figs. 13 and 14). There was a good reason, therefore, not to retain astroblastomas as a group, and I was of the opinion that this classification of tumors ought to disappear and the various types be distributed between the glioblastomas and astrocytomas if they contain "astroblastic patterns."

(In no circumstances must the word "blastoma" be used to indicate anaplasia and higher malignancy, as it often is by general pathologists.)

At this point we should like simply to state that the WHO classification group was reluctant to base a group on the existence of "astroblastic perivascular arrangement" in some, though rare astrocytomas and stating that the diagnosis of astroblastoma "should be restricted to pure growth of this type" (Fig. 45b; HBT, Fig. 50b). This statement corresponds to my earlier definition, formulated in collaboration with TELTSCHAROW (1948; see also ZÜLCH 1951b, 1959a).

For this term to be applied, the basic architectural pattern has to be present with a perivascular arrangement of cells having stout processes radiating around central vessels (HBT, Fig. 23). Such astroblastomas are rich in intracytoplasmatic glial fibers, while mitoses are rare or absent (HBT, Figs. 23 and 24). They tend to liquefaction of the tumor cells, remote from the "nourishing" vessel, which leads ultimately to the formation of microcysts. These astroblastic formations may appear in the marginal zone as a curious pattern of cells radiating around the blood vessels (ZÜLCH 1956, Fig. 153a, c; HBT, Fig. 23a, c). Astroblastomas, when properly defined as tumor rich in glial fibrils, seem to have biologic behavior similar to other astrocytomas; some authors admittedly believe that they may be more highly malignant, but probably this applies to tumors with different histologic pattern. Therefore, the World Health Organization left the problem open and merely discussed a grading with stages II, III, and IV.

Differential Diagnosis

The histological characteristics have been described above. Careful distinction from some ependymomas is necessary, which also have perivascular cell formations resembling those of the true astroblastoma in some respects. However, the latter are easily impregnated by gold sublimate (CAJAL's impregnation, see HBT, Fig. 24a, b), which is rarely the case with ependymomas. Moreover, between these formations the cells resemble stout astrocytes (HBT, Fig. 8) in astroblastoma, whereas in ependymomas these cells are quite different (see p. 71).

15.1.5 Anaplastic (Malignant) Astrocytomas

Synonym: Malignant astrocytoma

Introduction

The definition of the World Health Organization considers anaplasia in any of the recognized subtypes as a precondition for classification of the tumor as malignant anaplastic astrocytoma, even if anaplasia occurs only focally. Thus it is distinguished from glioblastomas by the amount of anaplasia. Any astrocytoma can become malignant during further development. The histologic features of anaplasia are discussed elsewhere in this volume (p. 27ff.).

Historical Note and Definition

In a study conducted in collaboration with TELTSCHAROW (1948), in a selected series of 55 astrocytomas – which included only cases that could be examined on large blocks – we found anaplastic foci in 6 instances (around 10%) and classified them as "malignant" astrocytomas. In one of our autopsy cases it was possible to demonstrate the coexistence of a circumscribed, firm astrocytoma (Fig. 41; GP, Fig. 95) the size of a small fist (Fig. 41) and adjacent to it diffuse spread throughout the brain. While the histological picture in the circumscribed firm part was that of a benign acellular fibrous astrocytoma (HBT, Fig. 27a, b), the pattern in the regions of diffuse spread – where necrosis was also present – was clearly that of a gigantocellular pleomorphic glioblastoma, with marked involvement of blood vessels.

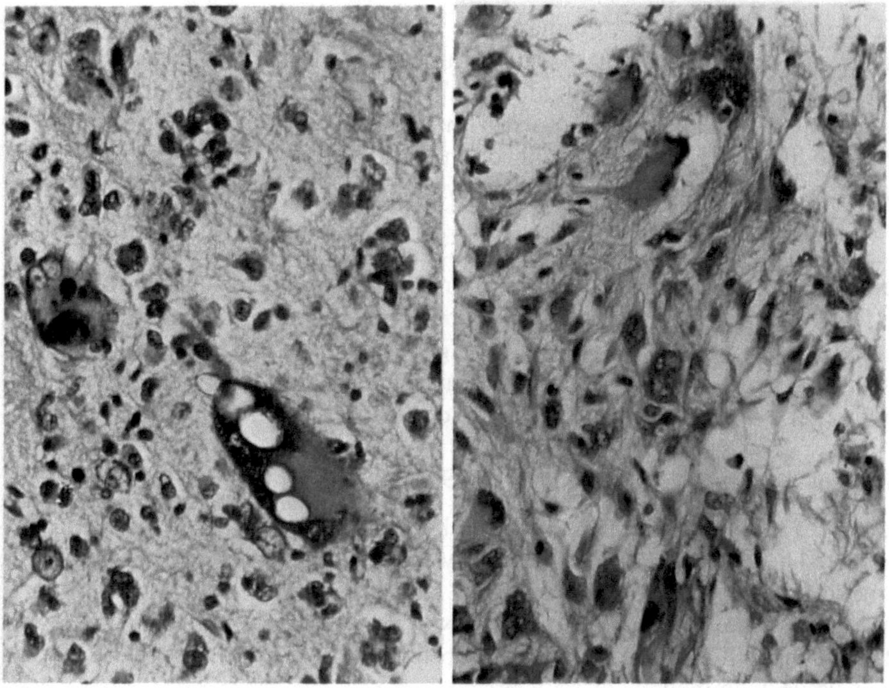

a b

Fig. 55 a, b. In the anaplastic portion of this tumor there are large-bodied, highly polymorphic cells: some cells have several very active ("ganglioid") nuclei. H&E, ×270 (**a**) and ×220 (**b**)

The more malignant portion in this case had quite obviously arisen, at a later stage, from its benign mate. Previously part of the calvarium had been eroded by the local pressure of the circumscribed hard portion, certainly a very rare occurrence, which substantiated very slow growth.

This thinning effect of a hard circumscribed tumor had already been seen by BRUNS, in the case of a right frontal glioma (1897, p. 87; see also BARRER et al. 1980) and curiously also in an oligodendroglioma.

K.-A. HOSSMANN (1964) in our laboratory later determined the frequency of malignant transformation of 24 cases (23%) among 104 supratentorial astrocytomas. Two types were observed: (a) local transformation; and (b) ubiquitous progressive changes seen in alternate examinations. The survival time in patients with anaplastic astrocytomas was 30 months or more. Furthermore, he also attempted to analyze and differentiate the signs of malignancy by electron microscopy.

Such malignant dedifferentiation of astrocytomas (Fig. 55 a, b) was already emphasized by H.J. SCHERER (1940 a) and many other authors (see FINKEMEYER et al. 1975, p. 15 ff.). KERSTING (1973), on the basis of tissue cultures, found that considerable dedifferentiation had taken place between first and second operations. However, DAVIS et al. (1950) and TUCKER et al. (1955) did not accept the concept of spontaneous malignant change in astrocytomas.

Discussing the position of anaplastic astrocytomas, ESCALONA-ZAPATA and DIEZ-NAU (1981) believed that tissue culture revealed glioblastomas and astrocytomas as essentially astrocytic tumors, but that the first showed more dedifferentiation. Astrocytomas usually ended with a reticular arrangement of multipolar astrocytic-like cells after passing through a shorter bipolar phase with a radial arrangement. With increasing malignancy the phase of bipolarity became longer; it persisted the longest in glioblastomas.

In summary, FINKEMEYER et al. (1975) assumed that (a) there may be malignant changes in recurrences; (b) some astrocytomas may have anaplastic properties from the beginning; (c) only exceptionally is anaplasia in astrocytomas the preliminary stage to the growth of glioblastoma; and (d) there is still no final answer as to whether therapeutic measures induce anaplasia in primarily benign astrocytomas (see also BINGAS and SCHULZE 1964).

Epidemiology (Age – Sex – Frequency – Site)

There is no difference in age, sex, or site between ordinary and anaplastic astrocytomas. There may be higher frequency in thalamic forms (GP, Fig. 99). The frequency has been variously reported as between 10% (TELTSCHAROW and ZÜLCH 1948) and 23% (K.-A. HOSSMANN 1964). It depends upon the source of the material (normal series versus biopsies sent in for opinion) and the quantity of tissue examined.

Gross Pathology

Macroscopic examination of anaplastic astrocytoma may show small foci with necrosis (and cysts) and perhaps even small hemorrhages. These changes are not infrequently seen in thalamic astrocytomas (GP, Fig. 99).

Histologic Appearance

The microscopic characteristics of anaplasia correspond to the pattern of glioblastoma multiforme (see p. 312).

Electron Microscopy

In EM fewer fibrils are found in anaplastic foci (ZÜLCH and WECHSLER 1968); moreover, according to HESS (1978), surface microprojections and coated vesicles are frequently observed.

Tissue Culture

LUMSDEN (1971, 1974) observed that in more malignant astrocytomas the cell processes were shorter and branch less.

Histochemistry

Histochemically, glycolytic enzymes are relatively highly represented in the astrocytic tumor group (LEHRER 1962; NASU and MÜLLER 1964; PERRIA et al. 1964). Differences between anaplastic astrocytomas and oligodendrogliomas are said to be noticeable (KUMANISHI et al. 1970, Fig. 1). The method of VAN VEELEN also reveals a far less pronounced inhibition pattern of pyruvate kinase by alanine in the anaplastic forms of astrocytoma (VAN VEELEN et al. 1979; for his method see p. 193).

More detailed data on the spectrum of enzymes in astrocytomas and glioblastomas versus malignant astrocytomas have been published by O'CONNOR and LAWS (1963) and VIALE and IBBA (1964); and a basic report appears in the monograph of SCHIFFER and FABIANI (1975).

Differential Diagnosis

Information on differential diagnosis is given elsewhere in this volume (p. 219).

Biologic Behavior (Grading), Metastasis, and Recurrence

The poorer prognosis of anaplastic astrocytomas is expressed by the shift to grade III (see p. 31 ff.). Detailed data have been reported by FINKEMEYER et al. (1975). Metastases are definitely rare in cases not treated by surgery, but have been reported in the literature (RUBINSTEIN 1967). Recurrences must be expected in all cases of subtotal excision. The value of radiation for the prevention of recurrence is discussed by WEIR (1973) and WEIR et al. (1976). Radical resection definitely prolongs the survival time (STAGE and STEIN 1974). Combined radio-/chemotherapy has been discussed by SEILER et al. (1978).

I have reported the outcome of radiation with 80 Gy in a case of astrocytoma: destruction in the form of delayed radionecrosis was found in the center, whereas the marginal growth was not suppressed (ZÜLCH 1960c).

Clinical Course

The clinical syndrome does not much differ – apart from rapid progress – from that seen with ordinary astrocytomas, since anaplastic astrocytomas are either rapidly growing primary forms or, more commonly, recurrences.

Further References: ESCALONA-ZAPATA (1966), LEHRER et al. (1967), KAWANO et al. (1977).

Anaplastic Pilocytic Astrocytomas

At the Colorado Springs Meeting in 1958a I described a case of the polymorphous malignant tumor of this type and referred to HENSCHEN (1955). Our tumor showed the typical architecture of bipolar cells, with many Rosenthal fibers and granular bodies, but appeared to be somewhat atypical in that it showed hypercellularity and cellular polymorphism and a relatively high incidence of mitoses. We assumed therefore there were anaplastic changes in this pilocytic astrocytoma, with a shift from grade I to grade III in our scale of malignancy.

With regard to histology, however, we want to emphasize that the pathogenesis of "multinuclear polymorphism" and "atypicality" of the cells has to be analyzed, because they often occur in pilocytic astrocytomas as a consequence

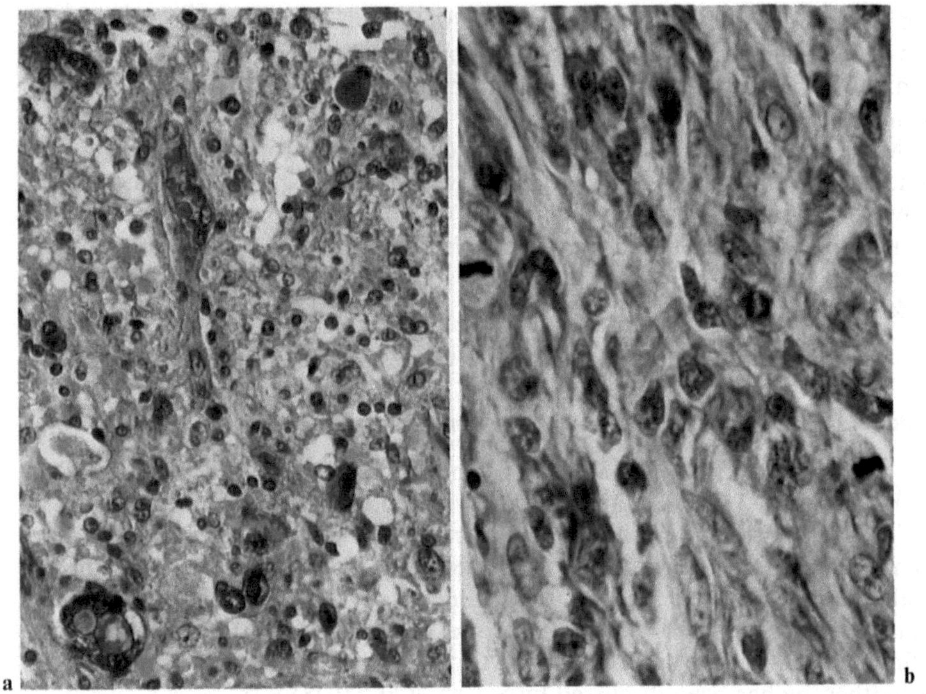

Fig. 56a, b. Pilocytic astrocytoma containing areas of anaplasia. Note the polymorphous polynuclear cells and mitoses. **a** H&E ×312; **b** PAS, ×500

of a *degenerative* process, in which is coalescence after incipient liquefaction (HBT, Fig. 54d). If they are "genuine" (Fig. 56a, b), however, and if in addition necroses and mitoses occur and glomerulus formation of the vessels is found at sites far distant from necroses or cysts, the tumor has to be classified as an anaplastic form (ZÜLCH 1958a). Meanwhile, numerous cases of such anaplastic tumors have been reported [BERNELL et al. 1972; SCOTT and BALLANTINE 1973; BUDKA 1975 (after 28 years; KLEINMAN et al. 1978) (after 48 years); AUER et al. 1981].

15.2 Oligodendroglial Tumors

15.2.1 Oligodendrogliomas

Synonyms: Oligodendroblastoma, oligodendrocytoma; in the older literature: diffuse glioma, round cell sarcoma, sarcoma angiolithicum, gliome à petites cellules rondes

Introduction

The new WHO classification, in addition to the oligodendroglioma proper, lists a mixed variant (*mixed oligo-astrocytoma*) and the *anaplastic (malignant)* forms.

Historical Note and Definition

The oligodendrogliomas as a tumor type were first predicted in 1924 by BAILEY (BAILEY and HILLER 1924) and later actually discovered and described in more detail by BAILEY and CUSHING in 1926 and in 1929b by BAILEY and BUCY. A large number of typical descriptions have appeared since then, though with little success as far as definition of the limits of this group is concerned, in which atypical cases are still controversial. This is proved by the differing percentages of oligodendrogliomas in the large series studied by CUSHING (1932), GAGEL (1938, Foerster's patients), BAILEY (see KÖRNYEY 1937), and KERNOHAN and SAYRE (1952) and in our own 9000 cases (ZÜLCH 1975a). Meanwhile, figures in more recent publications are gradually becoming more comparable. We therefore made attempts in 1941a, 1955a, and again 1956 to define the limits of this group, and once more in particular to specify a "polymorphous" (anaplastic, malignant) variant. H.J. SCHERER (DE BUSSCHER and SCHERER 1942) also tried to reclassify oligodendrogliomas and astrocytomas and, as suggested by COOPER (1935), to define oligoastrocytomas.

Numerous cases published in the older literature can still be recognized as oligodendrogliomas (MERZBACHER and UYEDA 1910; LANDAU 1910; BIELSCHOWSKY 1915; ORZECHOWSKI and KULIGOWSKI 1933; BODECHTEL 1934; SCHEINKER 1938a; BENEDEK and JUBA 1941b; DONAT 1944; WEIL and ROSENBLUM 1952; and even KLEBS in Prague already in 1877). However, the "fusiform oligodendrogliomas" of ROUSSY and OBERLING (1932), DEL RIO HORTEGA (1932, 1944) and BUSCH and CHRISTENSEN (1937) correspond to pilocytic astrocytomas (formerly referred to as polar spongioblastomas).

Epidemiology (Age – Sex – Frequency – Site)

Age: The oligodendrogliomas are tumors of the middle decades, with the peak incidence between 35 and 40 years (Fig. 9c). Only the oligodendrogliomas of the thalamus are found mostly in younger patients. Our youngest patient with an oligodendroglioma was 3, the oldest 68. An oligodendroglioma in a neonate was reported by KOEPPEN and CASSIDY (1981).

Sex: In our series of 9000 cases 484 oligodendrogliomas were in male (56.3%) and 375 in female (43.7%) patients, which means a male preponderance of around 5:4.

Frequency: The incidence figures vary from 1.3% (CUSHING 1935) through 1.6% (GAGEL 1938; Foerster's series), 2.7% (WEIR and ELVIDGE 1968), 5% (KERNOHAN and SAYRE 1952), up to 9.6% in our own series of 9000 cases (ZÜLCH 1975a). The average of all the percentages given by different authors combined is around 4%. This is probably too low, but higher frequency rates will be found in subsequent publications based on the modern classification.

Of the *glial* tumors, the oligodendrogliomas made up 18.8% of cases in our series (1975a) (6000 cases of intracranial tumors), 5% of RUSSELL and RUBINSTEIN's material (1977), and 8% of BARNARD's cases 1974).

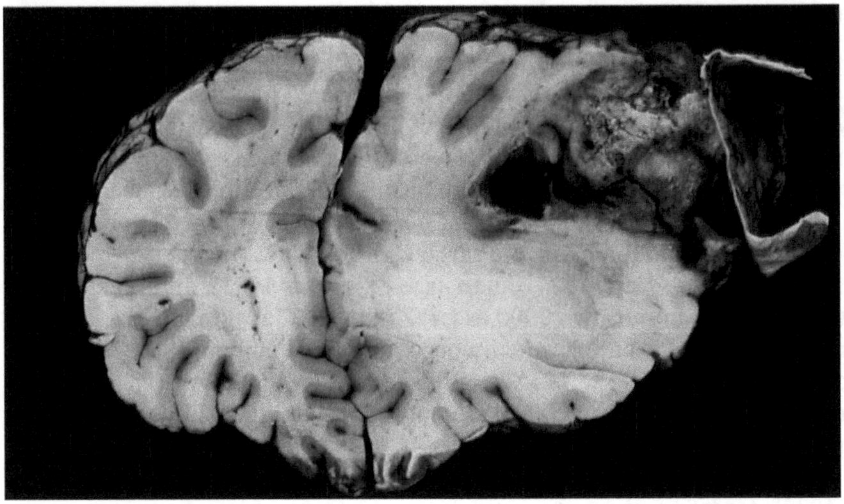

Fig. 57. Frontolateral oligodendroglioma which has broken through to the cortical surface, assuming the form of a mushroom, and adhering widely to the dura. A pigmented cyst is seen in the depths of the tumor, as are some fresh hemorrhages and perifocal edema (ZÜLCH 1975a)

Among the 1322 spinal cord tumors KERNOHAN (1971; SLOOFF et al. 1964) found 8 oligodendrogliomas.

Site: It has been possible to work out different subgroups of oligodendrogliomas according to their typical location. They lie most frequently at the base of the second and third *frontal* convolutions (Fig. 57) (frontolateral, Fig. 14, no. 8). These tumors can reach the size of an egg and invade the convolutions above the Sylvian fissure and the underlying white matter; they sometimes have the shape of a mushroom (Fig. 57).

A similar subtype lies more caudally in the *parietal* gyri (parietolateral oligodendroglioma) and again is often similar to a mushroom in shape (Fig. 58). In this location it may also spread subcortically or extend into the first temporal convolution. There are also *parasagittal* oligodendrogliomas, located in the frontal gyri (Fig. 60) bordering the sagittal fissure (frontomedial oligodendroglioma; Fig. 14, no. 13; GP, Fig. 106), and genuine oligodendrogliomas of the *corpus callosum*, either at the rostral end – where they also infiltrate the septum – or growing into the splenium corporis callosi (Fig. 14, no. 43). In the *temporal lobe* they infiltrate the gyri of the temporal pole (temporal oligodendrogliomas; Fig. 14, no. 24), from where they can extend into the frontobasal or temporomedial (hippocampal) regions. In the occipital lobes they lie medially or occupy the whole of the cortex. The location of each of these in our series of 9000 cases was: frontal 38%, temporal 35%, parietal 17%, occipital 7%, deep seated 3%.

A very frequent site (although mostly in children) is the *thalamus* (Fig. 14, no. 49), which can be expanded to the size of a small fist (oligodendrogliomas of the brain stem), and from where the tumors sometimes extend into the neigh-

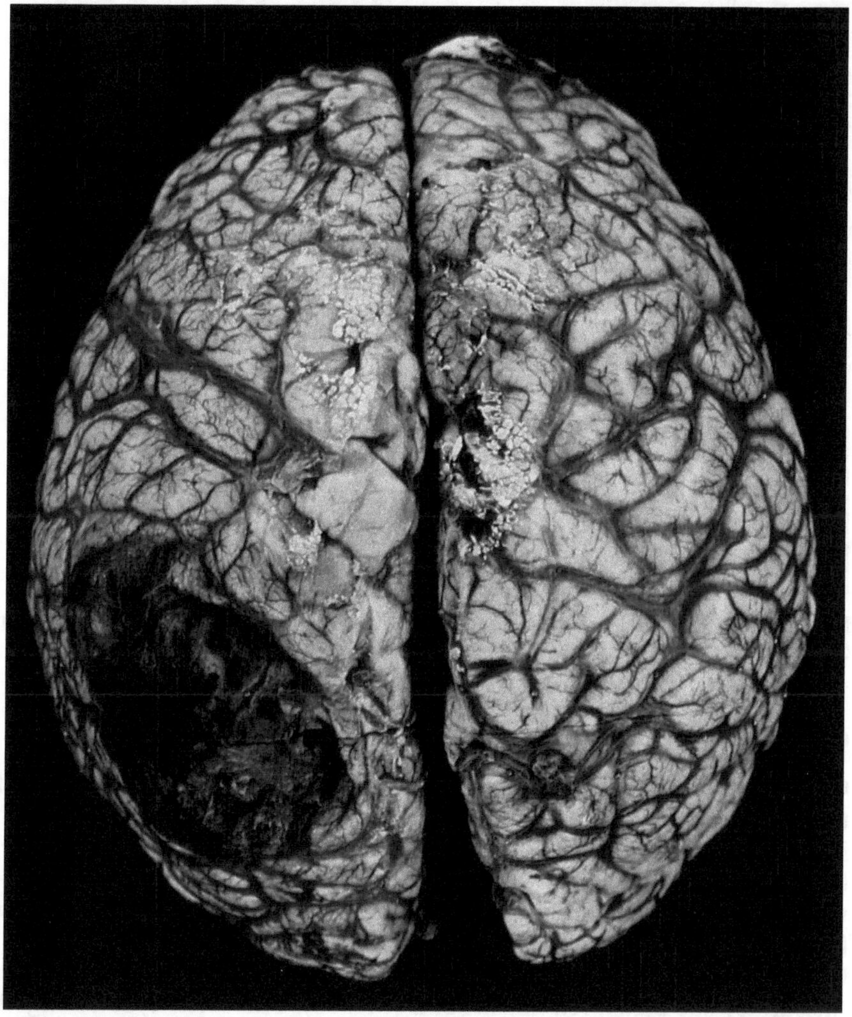

Fig. 58. Large mushroom-like parietolateral oligodendroglioma with fresh hemorrhage within the tumor (Zülch 1975a)

boring midbrain. Finally, oligodendrogliomas rarely occur in the *spinal cord*, and apparently extremely seldom in the *cerebellum* (only one case of our own). In the last two of these locations they must not be confused with pilocytic astrocytomas undergoing mucinous degeneration (see p. 228). This is important because regressive changes in pilocytic astrocytomas frequently give rise to architectural patterns confusingly similar to those of oligodendrogliomas (see Fig. 51 a). Conversely, oligodendrogliomas can contain spindle cell parts similar to those in pilocytic astrocytomas (HBT, Figs. 30a, 38d).

It has still to be determined whether some of the reported cases of "midline oligodendroglioma" might not be misinterpretations of ependymomas of foramen of Monro with their somewhat atypical cell pattern (GP, Figs. 54, 55, 74a; Sakai et al. 1980).

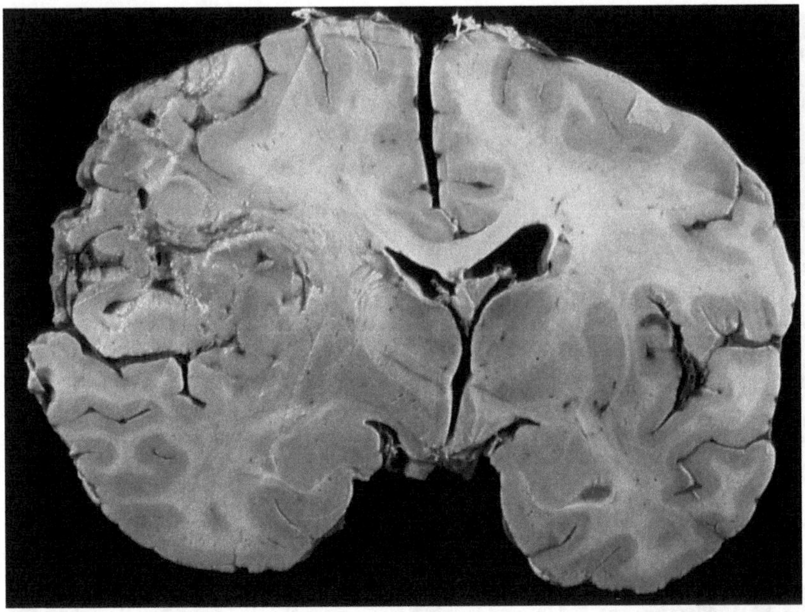

Fig. 59. Frontolateral oligodendroglioma also invading the insular gyri: Moderate contralateral displacement is evident. Note the "hypertrophy" of the convolutions (ZÜLCH 1975a)

Gross Pathology

Oligodendrogliomas (GP, Figs. 102–112) can often be specifically identified by their surface and manner of spread. They expand the cortex diffusely, making it appear "hypertrophic" (Figs. 59, 60), while the underlying white matter shows large and small mucinous cysts and even necroses (Garland pattern). Small wart-like hard nodules sometimes occur in the cortex and can be recognized by the surgeon on finger palpation or visual examination. When the tumor breaks through the leptomeninges, it forms large lumps that project beyond the surface like bluish red mushrooms (Fig. 58). This latter type of oligodendroglioma tend to adhere to the dura (Figs. 57, 66a) and are often first mistaken for meningiomas (Fig. 57). To the surgeon they appear either firm or moderately so, grayish or the color of raw meat; they may be friable or calcified, and occasionally small areas of necrosis are present. After formalin fixation oligodendrogliomas can be recognized by the cut surface of the cross section, which is grayish pink and velvety. Occasionally large or small calcified granules can be felt, which make a grating sound when cut with the knife (see also information on differential diagnosis from astrocytomas, p. 219).

Histologic Appearance

Typically oligodendrogliomas (HBT, Figs. 28–41) have a very uniform structure: there are closely packed, chromatin-rich, round cells with almost no or scanty cytoplasm, as in normal oligodendroglias. The nuclei are round or oval (Fig. 61a, b), the cytoplasm clear, and the cell membranes very well defined.

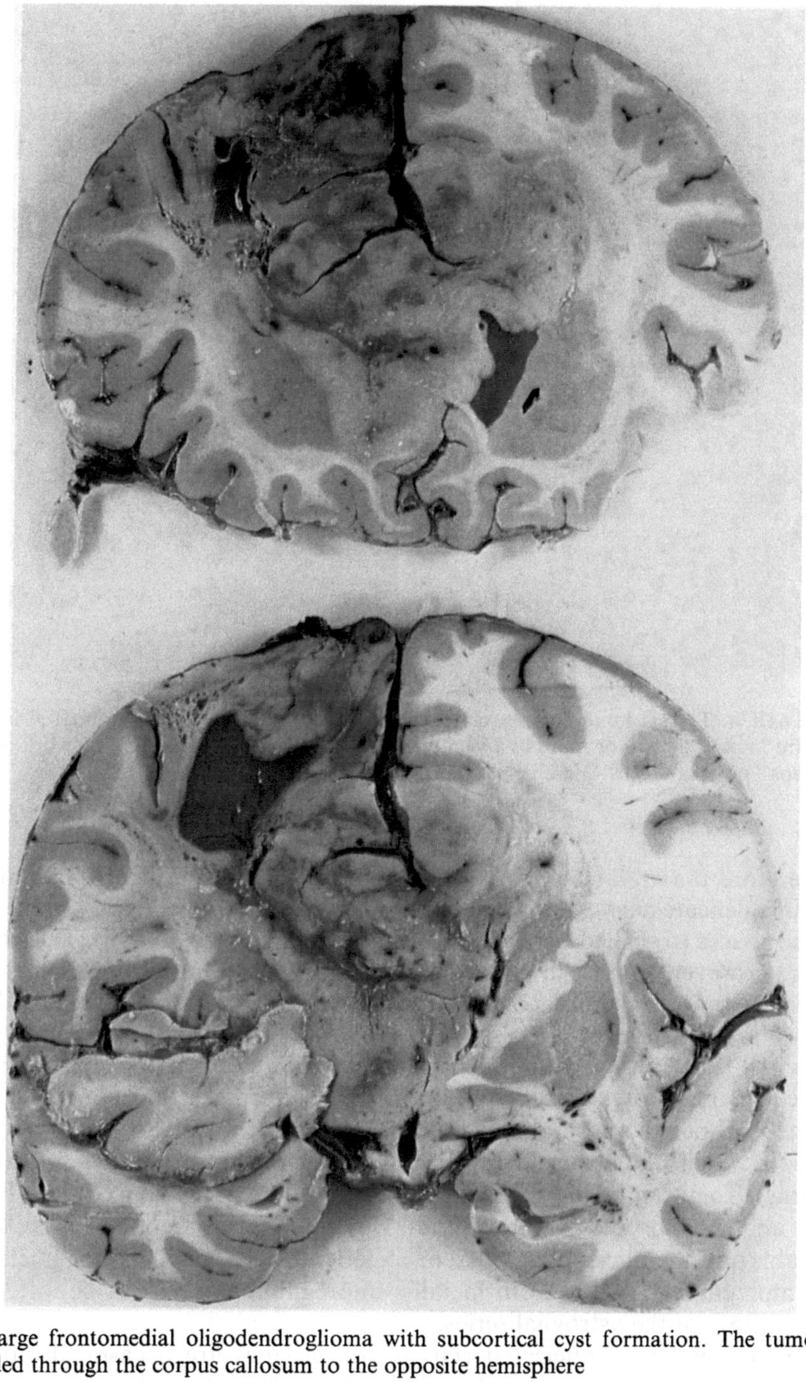

Fig. 60. Large frontomedial oligodendroglioma with subcortical cyst formation. The tumor has extended through the corpus callosum to the opposite hemisphere

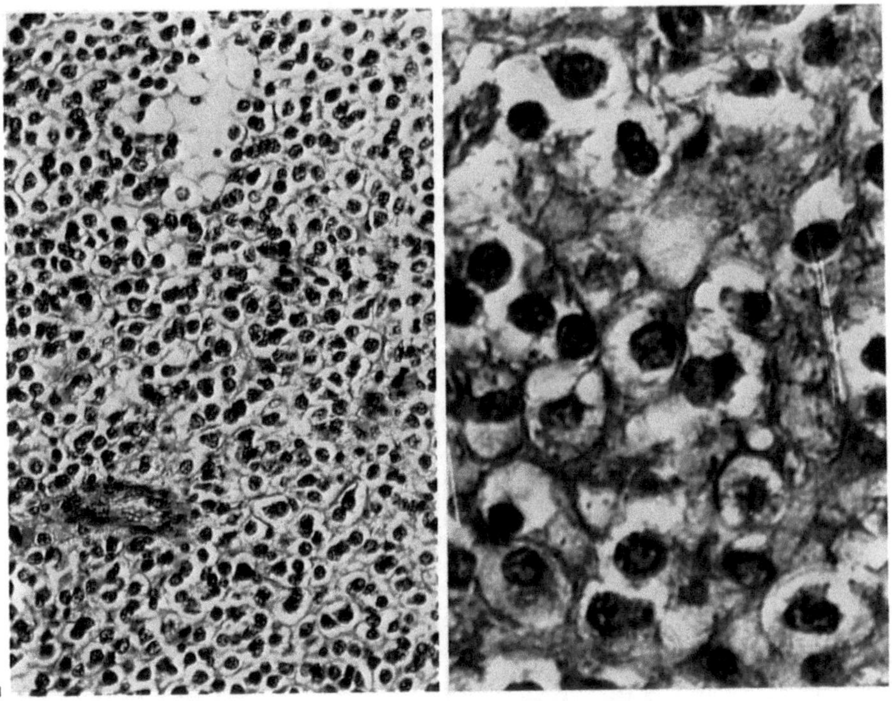

a b

Fig. 61 a, b. Typical honeycomb architecture of an oligodendroglioma embedded in paraffin: "bare" nuclei lie two or more in a vacuole. The pattern is compared to a network of "honeycombs" or "plant cells." H&E, ×160 (**a**) and ×616 (**b**)

Therefore the architectures of this tumors are very characteristic: Bare nuclei lie in a delicate network formed by small compartments of lightly stained vacuolated spaces (so-called honeycomb architecture; see Fig. 61 a, b). This characteristic, however, often shows up only after paraffin embedding. Sometimes the cells show a certain resemblance to plant cells. In occasional regions they may be (Fig. 62a) more spindle shaped (HBT, Figs. 30a and 38d; see Escalona-Zapata 1981), although the vacuolated pattern described above is strongly indicated in these cases also. In addition, there are parts that contain carpets of large PAS-positive eosinophilic cells (HBT, Fig. 29b; see also Escalona-Zapata 1981), which show considerable similarity to plump astrocytes (transitional forms). They can be impregnated with gold sublimate (Fig. 62b), but have very few and short processes, if any at all. Here the typical architecture is still recognizable and the nucleus is typical of oligodendroglia, in which the nuclei appear unimpregnated (Fig. 63b) in metallic impregnations and can be differentiated from those of the astroglial series.

Giant and multinucleated cells of all varieties are occasionally observed; but if they form the majority they may indicate (Fig. 64a) the "anaplastic ("polymorphous"), malignant variant (see p. 255ff.). The blood vessels consist of capillaries (Fig. 65a), which are liberally distributed throughout the tumor. The vessel walls tend to undergo hyalinization or mucinous infiltration. Typical

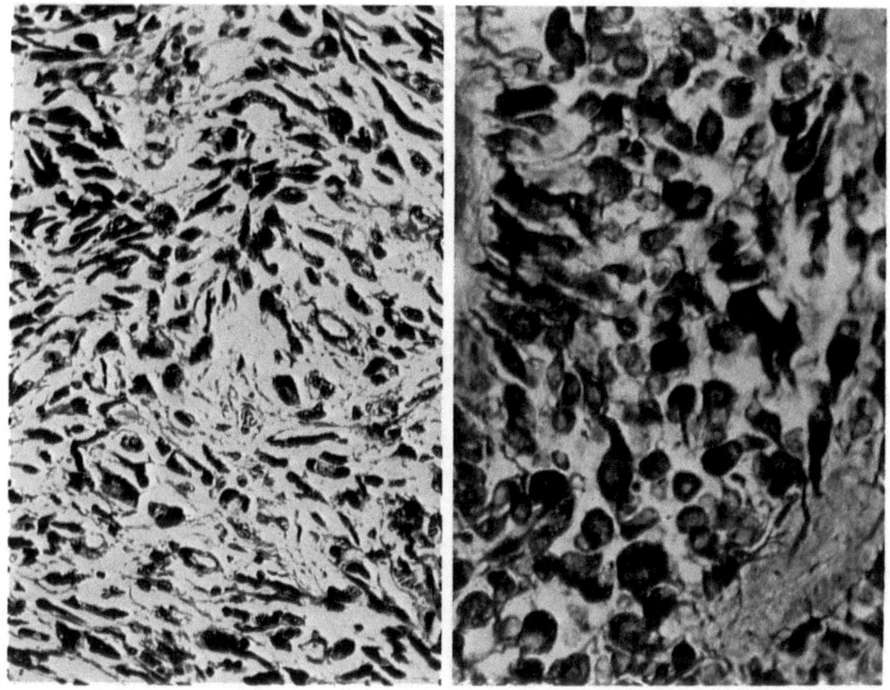
a b

Fig. 62. a Spindle-cell variants of an oligodendroglioma, in which the typical honeycomb architecture is still recognizable. H&E, ×168. **b** In the same oligodendroglioma, bizarre spherical, unipolar or astroblast-like cells are found on impregnation, but the nucleus is not impregnated and appears as a clear space. Gold sublimate, ×216

networks of vascular coils may arise around small areas of necrosis. The vessel walls often appear (Fig. 65a) calcified (HBT, Fig. 36), and patches of calcifications also lie free in the tumor tissue, being visible radiologically in up to 30% of cases. Positive CT findings are more frequent. The blood vessels may break easily, so that various sized hemorrhages are not rare ("apoplectic glioma"). Oligodendrogliomas have a tendency to undergo mucoid and cystic degeneration in either small or large areas. On the other hand, fatty degeneration is uncommon. The remnants of engulfed cerebral parenchyma – ganglion cells, myelinated fibers, glia – may persist for a long time. The tumor cells can accumulate around nerve cells ("pseudo-satellitosis") (Fig. 66b) in the growth zone (HBT, Fig. 35), since there is a general trend to grow from the white matter toward the cortex (HBT, Fig. 34). The adjacent brain, even if it is tumorfree, may show calcification due to calcium encrustation of capillaries (Fig. 65a) similar to that seen in the Sturge-Weber syndrome (HBT, Fig. 35b). Furthermore, abundant calcareous deposits are found within the tumor tissue itself or the vessels. The oligodendrogliomas are often sharply separated from the surrounding brain. They can invade the arachnoid (Fig. 66a) spaces and distend them with mushroom-shaped growths (Figs. 57, 58), from there proceeding to grow towards the pachymeninges (Fig. 57), to which they sometimes adhere (see p. 130). In the marginal zone there are often vessels showing small round cell ("lymphoid")

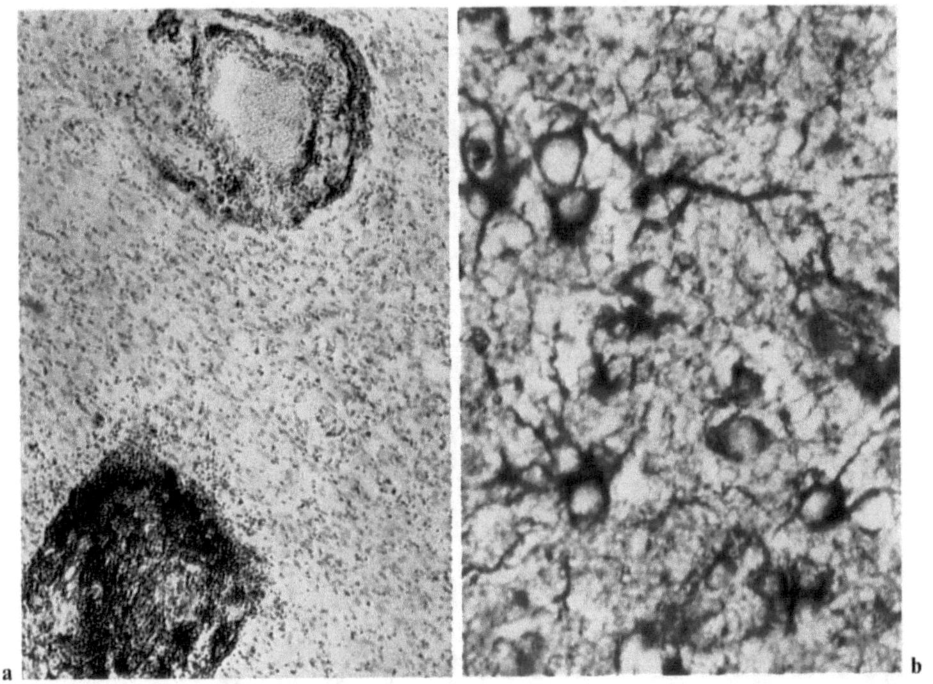

Fig. 63. a "Lymphoid" infiltration of an oligodendroglioma within the marginal zone. Cresyl violet, ×92. b On impregnation of the tumor cells by special methods the nuclei obviously do not become impregnated. Grynio's method, ×500

(Fig. 63a) infiltrations, which may be genuine tumor cells or real lymphocytes indicating an immunologic process. Typical mitoses are common. The rate of growth of these tumors is quite variable and depends on the general composition of the tumor (see Sect. 15.2.3).

Electron Microscopy

MANNWEILER and PALACIOS (1961) examined the cell types of various oligodendrogliomas by EM and were able to distinguish four distinct forms. ROBERTSON and VOGEL (1962) recognized three types of laminar structures and explained them by the apparent capacity to form sheaths and sheath-like structures through concentric lamination of several processes, as did BOUTEILLE et al. (1965) and ZÜLCH and WECHSLER (1968). These authors mentioned the tendency to form "myelin figures." Crystalline structures (RAIMONDI 1966) and aggregates of cylindrical particles have also been observed in oligodendrogliomas (TANI et al. 1969; HORMES 1974), as have intranuclear rodlets (VASQUEZ and CERVOS-NAVARRO 1969; CERVOS-NAVARRO et al. 1981; CERVOS-NAVARRO and PEHLIVAN 1981).

In electron micrographs, isomorphous oligodendrogliomas have round or oval nuclei with large amounts of endochromatin, similar to normal oligoglia. The tumor cells have a moderately developed endoplasmic reticulum (microtu-

a 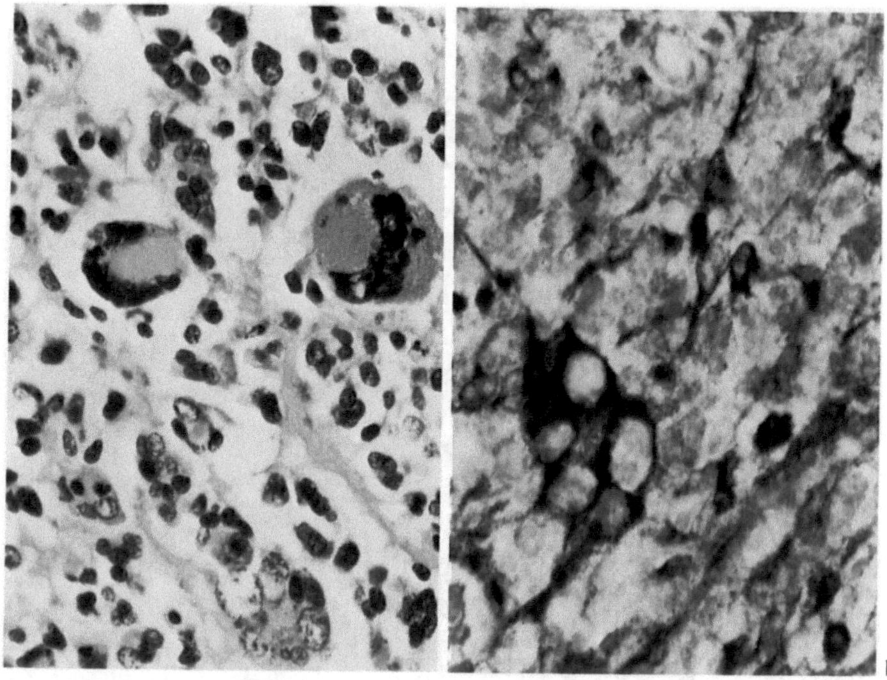 b

Fig. 64. a Langhans' type of giant cells with marginal, hyperchromatic nuclei occur quite frequently in anaplastic oligodendrogliomas. H&E, ×212. **b** The final proof of the oligodendroglioma nature is dependent upon the typical basic architecture and silver staining (Grinyo's method). Multinucleated elements are also seen in anaplastic forms, which possess the distinct features of oligodendroglia cells. ×262

buli), a small Golgi apparatus, and a variable number of mitochondria. Tumor cells can also form processes.

It is of interest that neoplastic oligodendrocytes do not produce glial filaments or that at least this capacity seems to be minimal, especially compared with astrocytomas. In this respect our EM observations (HOSSMANN and WECHSLER 1971 b) are in close agreement with the findings of LUSE (1960). On the other hand, RAIMONDI (1966) thinks that neoplastic oligodendrocytes have a cytoplasm occupied almost entirely by protogliofibrils (lipid-like material and crystalline structures). According to LUSE (1960), a distinctive feature of neoplastic oligodendrocytes is the "megamitochondria," while the cytoplasm is often crowded with mitochondria of the usual size which are increased in number. Some cells may contain huge mitochondria, but these are most often of the polymorphous type. A recent excellent EM study has been performed by SZYMAS et al. (1980), based on 22 cases. They discussed the viral nature of the polymorphous Langhans type of tumor cells. In the problem of oligodendrogliomas of the spinal cord, the possibility of a mucous degeneration (Fig. 51 a) of the far more common pilocytic astrocytomas (with their "spongioblastic, astroblastic and astrocytic elements"; GARCIA and LEMMI 1970) must be very carefully considered.

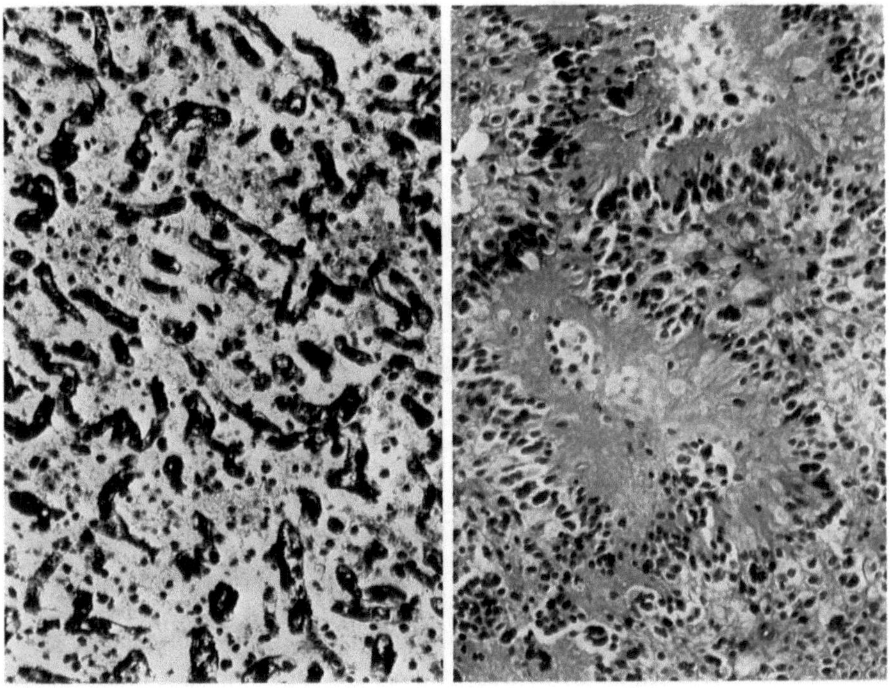

a b

Fig. 65. a Calcification of capillary network within an infiltration zone. Gold sublimate, ×229. **b** Anaplastic oligodendroglioma: in addition to the type of oligodendroglioma that is anaplastic as a result of the dysmorphism of the *cells* there is another type, in which the *tissue* architecture is polymorphic. In this latter type, necrotic areas appear and evoke a stromal proliferation, so that characteristics of the glioblastoma become noticeable. H&E, ×125

Tissue Culture

KERSTING (1968) has observed that the tissue culture is not quite as uniform as the histologic picture of the tumor might suggest. He points out that the outgrowing cells are never purely oligodendrocytic but include neoplastic astrocytes (see Sect. 15.2.2). It is of interest that many nuclei in the multinucleated giant cells are quite normal in shape and size, as also observed in normal oligodendrocytes (see also MIYAKE 1979).

Histochemistry

Histochemical examination reveal a relatively low oxidase activity compared with the astrocytomas (NASU and MÜLLER 1964). As shown by BINGAS (1972), the various enzyme histochemical patterns offer additional ways of differentiating anaplastic (polymorphous) tumors from isomorphic gliomas. This is particularly true for oligodendrogliomas. STAVROU et al. (1972) described higher LDH activity in pleomorphous (anaplastic) oligodendrogliomas than in the isomorphous type, in which, however, LDH was also present.

Pleomorphous (anaplastic) oligodendrogliomas are characterized by type K_4 and hybrid K_3M pyruvate kinase. In isomorphous types, besides K_4 and K_3M,

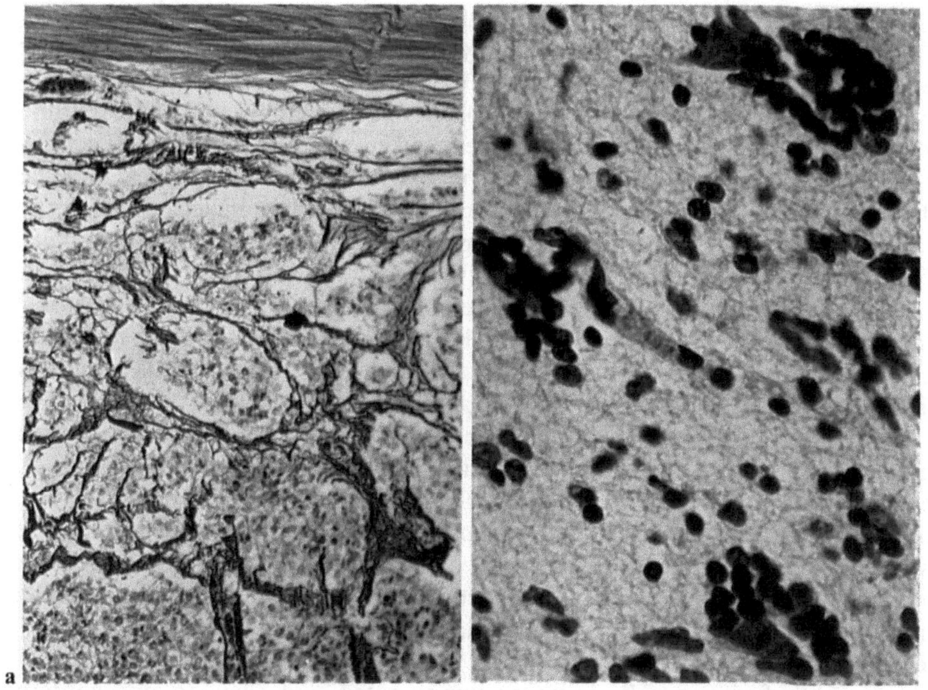

Fig. 66. a Local invasion of the leptomeninges by an oligodendroglioma, causing marked adhesion to the dura. Silver impregnation, ×108. **b** In the marginal zone of an oligodendroglioma the tumor cells tend to accumulate around the ganglion cells (pseudosatellitosis). Cresyl violet, ×108

subunit M_4 is also present. Residual activity of pyruvate kinase in the presence of alanine is also higher in isomorphous than in anaplastic tumors (Van Veelen et al. 1978, 1979).

Differential Diagnosis

The differential diagnosis of oligodendrogliomas from other glial tumors is sometimes difficult. The recognition of oligodendroglial cells is usually based on the observation of a typical pattern, which is a honeycomb or plant cell architecture, forming a system of small vacuoles with a lymphoid nucleus at the center. Differential diagnosis from astrocytic tumors has already been discussed (p. 219; see also Juhasz 1942).

Distinction of oligodendrogliomas in their *anaplastic* form from glioblastomas can also be difficult, and will be discussed below (p. 319). Impregnation and other methods are obligatory for the recognition of many oligodendrogliomas, particularly those of the anaplastic type. In our laboratory a method developed by K. Meller (1963) and later the Grinyo impregnation method (1968) have proved very valuable. Only very "wet" tissue, which is undergoing mucinous degeneration, gives a negative result. Calvo (1964), at the Cologne

Symposium on Classification, stated "that not all neoplastic oligodendrocytes are impregnated. Some of them show only a narrow ring of cytoplasm or appear as "naked" nuclei. This may be due to absence of argentophilia in some immature cells or result from the fact that many oligodendrocytes show a definite polarization of the cytoplasm; this can be so pronounced that following sectioning the nucleus and the cytoplasm are in two different sections (levels). The oligodendrocytes can be recognized by the clear rounded nucleus and heavily stained cytoplasm. Sometimes the cytoplasm is abundant and angular, with a few thin expansions in which corkscrew formations and a few branches can be distinguished, but they never produce vascular feet." Even in the very few cases where a large proportion of the cells are impregnated with gold sublimate – the transitional forms (HBT, Figs. 29c, d and 30d) – the nucleus remained unstained as a clear spot within the cytoplasm.

Differential diagnosis from pilocytic astrocytomas is more difficult when the histologic pattern of oligodendrogliomas shows its well-known variant, i.e., the presence of large cytoplasm-rich cells that can be misinterpreted (HBT, Fig. 29b) as gemistocytic astrocytes or [particularly important for the pilocytic astrocytoma (HBT, Fig. 30a)] when it consists of long fusiform cells (which, however, always show a basic honeycomb-type pattern). If Rosenthal fibers or granulated bodies occur it is easy to diagnose a pilocytic astrocytoma. Metallic impregnations can also help, since the cytoplasm of these oligodendrogliomas with fusiform cells is never impregnated and they do not contain fibers.

We have already referred to the variability of the histologic picture in oligodendrogliomas. The "mixed forms" should be examined for typical architectures, in either one large or several smaller sections. Differentiation from an astrocytoma that has undergone mucoid degeneration is frequently possible if the following rule of thumb which relates to the delicate cystic network found in both types of tumors; the nuclei in astrocytomas lie at the intersections, whereas those in the oligodendroglioma lie within the network's small compartments. In its "large cell" portion, an oligodendroglioma is similar to an astrocytoma. However, in an oligodendroglioma the nuclei have a vacuolated halo and remain recognizable as light spots in gold sublimate and other metallic preparations (HBT, Fig. 29). Calcification cannot be considered a mandatory characteristic of oligodendroglioma, since in our experience only a small percentage (20%) of these tumors show calcification histologically, but its presence always supports this diagnosis. It must be admitted that the histologic differential diagnosis between oligodendroglioma and astrocytoma can be one of the most difficult, but it is not of great importance because of the similar biologic behavior and the occurrence of mixed forms.

Confusion should not occur with acoustic neurilemmomas – simply because of the architecture or similarity with regions showing fatty degeneration – or with chordomas in the H&E preparation.

Finally, ependymomas, particularly those in the region of the foramen of Monro, may have a cellular pattern or architecture very similar to that of some oligodendrogliomas, especially when the wide nucleus-free mantle around the blood vessel, which is typical for ependymomas, is not apparent.

Biologic Behavior (Grading), Metastasis, and Recurrence

Oligodendrogliomas belong to the comparatively benign gliomas, i.e., grade II, or for the anaplastic forms to grade III. Extensive operative removal followed by radio-/chemotherapy sometimes results in improvement for a period of 3–5 or even up to 20 or 30 years (FREEMAN and FEIGIN 1963: 35 years; ROBERTS and GERMAN 1966, 1969; WEIR and ELVIDGE 1968), and under certain circumstances complete lobectomy can bring about a cure. On the other hand, the multifocal tumor distribution can mean in the long term that the prognosis is hopeless.

ZÜLCH (1955a, 1960a) noted a longer history and longer survival with the isomorphic than of the anaplastic (polymorphic) oligodendrogliomas (see also the case histories in ZÜLCH 1941a).

BINGAS (1966, 1970), distinguishing isomorphous and polymorphous (anaplastic) oligodendrogliomas on a histochemical basis, found for the former a postoperative survival of 54 months, and for the polymorphous (anaplastic) type, of only 26 months. The result after radiation have been discussed by SHELINE et al. (1964).

The growth of oligodendrogliomas is probably very slow. However, the exceptional case of a congenital tumor has been described by KOEPPEN and CASSIDY (1981).

Metastasis: (a) *Spontaneous* metastasis via the CSF probably occurs (GP, Fig. 111; ZÜLCH 1941a, 1956) ("oligodendrogliomatosis": BEST 1963b; see also BECK and RUSSELL 1942; BLUMENFELD and GARDNER 1945). (b) Seeding into the scalp after *surgery* was observed by CAIRNS and RUSSELL (1931) and BRAUN and TZONOS (1968). (c) *Extracranial* metastases to other parts of the body (skeleton, lung, lymph node, liver, kidney, etc.) has also been described (JAMES and PAGEL 1951; O'BRIEN et al. 1968; SPATARO and SACKS 1968).

Probably a similar route of extracranial metastasis occurs to that known for medulloblastomas: seeding over the meninges and along the spinal roots it invades the vertebral bodies (JELLINGER et al. 1969) or other adjacent bones.

Recurrence: After partial excision all oligodendrogliomas recur in 1–3 years (ZÜLCH 1960a). Recurrence is possible even if the resection seemed extensive or seemed complete. However, such oligodendrogliomas can grow in multiple foci (ZÜLCH 1941a, Fig. 18), which may be connected by thin bridges of neoplastic cells. Wide resection of whole lobes gives the best therapeutic results (SHELINE et al. 1964).

Clinical Course

Clinical histories can be very long (ZÜLCH 1941a) and earlier patients were sometimes sent to hospital from an asylum after a long history of seizures (AEBI and KRAUS-RUPPERT 1978; history of 22 years). The diffuse permeation of the cortex by the tumor with preservation of the neurons may explain the tendency to focal seizures. Since this tumor occupies only a moderate amount of space and the tendency to brain edema is only slight, raised intracranial pressure does not occur until late in the course. Massive hemorrhages into oligodendrogliomas that are frequently seen can be explained by the hyalinization of the blood vessels and their pronounced calcification (HBT, Fig. 36). The growth of the oligodendroglioma is very slow in the majority of cases, and the diagnosis may be difficult, as in one of our cases (see SCHUIER 1976): in spite of EEG, pneumoencephalography, and angiography in a patient with focal seizures no tumor was recognized. Since the seizures were well controlled the patient did not return for 8 years. At that time a temporal lobe tumor was diagnosed and partly excised and irradiated. Half a year later the tumor recurred, consisting then in a single focus of the highest degree of anaplastic change we have ever seen in any tumor (see p. 123). On the other hand, even connatal tumors have been described (KOEPPEN and CASSIDY 1981).

Further References: KWAN and ALPERS (1931), MARTIN (1931) GREENFIELD and ROBERTSON (1933), LÖWENBERG and WAGGONER (1939), EARNEST et al. (1950), REYMOND and RINGERTZ (1950), HORRAX and WU (1951), TROWBRIDGE and FRENCH (1952b), LISS (1961), ZÜLCH and WOOLF (1964), MANSUY et al. (1967, 1975), BARNARD (1968), BESTLE (1969), SCHRÖDER et al. (1970), KERNOHAN (1971), ZÜLCH and MENNEL (1974), ZANDER and KHAMLICHI (1978).

15.2.2 Mixed Oligo–Astrocytomas

Synonym: Oligodendroglioma with astrocytic admixture

Introduction

It must be noted here that the diagnosis of mixed oligo-astrocytoma depends on the proportion of astrocytes defined in the tumor. In the WHO classification this subgroup of oligodendrogliomas has been included to deal with the many cases where the percentage of astrocytes admixed to the majority of oligodendroglia elements is particularly high.

Historical Note and Definition

These mixed tumors were first given the name of oligo-astrocytoma by COOPER (1935) and DE BUSSCHER and SCHERER (1942). However, Bailey (BAILEY and HILLER 1924; BAILEY and BUCY 1929b) emphasized the "transitional" cells with a mixture of characteristics of oligodendroglia and astroglia, and in my detailed discussion of oligodendroglioma (ZÜLCH 1941a) I dealt with this particular problem. Furthermore, I illustrated larger, eosinophilic cytoplasm-rich cells, which are impregnated by gold sublimate (HBT, Fig. 29). The clear perinuclear halo clearly demonstrated the oligodendroglial nature of these transitional cells, however.

The definition of this group is based on the recognition of the types of cells (HART et al. 1974). Distinction remains difficult insofar as the ratio of astroglia and oligodendroglia that might be present has never been defined. The preponderance dictates which term is applied.

An oligodendroglioma can often be differentiated from an astrocytoma that has undergone mucoid degeneration by application of the general rule that in relation to the delicate cystic network that can be found in both types, the nuclei in the astrocytoma lie at the intersections, whereas those in the oligodendroglioma lie within the network's small compartments. In its large cell portion the oligodendroglioma may be similar to the gemistocytic astrocytoma. Histological differential diagnosis between oligodendroglioma and astrocytoma and the "compromise diagnosis" of oligoastrocytoma can admittedly be one of the most difficult, if only small tissue samples are available. From the biological standpoint, however, this distinction is not of great importance.

Gross Pathology

No particular characteristics are known that distinguish the appearance to the naked eye from that of an ordinary oligodendroglioma.

Histologic Appearance

The microscopical picture has been sufficiently described above in the definition of the tumor.

Biologic Behavior (Grading), Metastasis, and Recurrences

No difference is known in the biological behavior of the oligo-astrocytoma; these tumors are graded II. Nor do the tumor's tendency to metastasize or recur and its clinical course differ.

In summary, the diagnosis of oligo-astrocytoma seems legitimate when an admixture of unusually abundant elements of astroglia is recognized, which may be either separated into distinct areas or intermingled.

15.2.3 Anaplastic (Malignant) Oligodendrogliomas

Synonym: Polymorphous oligodendroglioma

Introduction

The not uncommon malignant forms of oligodendroglioma are grouped in the new WHO classification as anaplastic oligodendrogliomas.

Historical Note and Definition

Even in my first detailed report on the oligodendroglioma (Zülch 1941a) I pointed out the various forms of anaplasia and discussed the possible malignancy of this tumor. In 1955a, at the World Congress of Neuropathology in London, and again in 1964a, I described the "polymorphous" type of oligodendrogliomas. I was also able to show statistically that these polymorphous oligodendrogliomas were more malignant (with regard to history and survival time) than the isomorphic type of oligodendroglioma (Zülch 1960a, p. 254; Zülch and Woolf 1964). These ideas (Zülch 1956, Fig. 20b, 1959a) have since been supported (Barnard 1968) and confirmed. Thus, metallic impregnations revealed the characteristics of oligodendroglia with a multinuclear appearance in the majority of tumor cells (HBT, Fig. 39), and the basic honeycomb architecture usually remained identifiable (ZÜLCH and WECHSLER 1968).

This fact explains many reports in the literature of "glioblastomas" with fairly long histories and unusually long postoperative survival (e.g., WEIL and ROSENBLUM 1952). The risk of misinterpretation as glioblastoma multiforme is high.

Epidemiology (Age – Sex – Frequency – Site)

Age: The age curve shows a slow rise from 3 years up to 70 years, being markedly higher between the ages of 30 and 70 than during any other period.

Sex: The male: female ratio was 5:4.

Frequency: These polymorphous types may occur with a frequency of about 1 to 20 isomorphous tumors.

Site: In our own collection of 10000 cases, F. HOLANDA (personal communication) determined the gross site as frontal lobe in 37.2%, temporal lobe in 34%, parietal lobe in 16.3%, and occipital lobe in 7% of cases; the rest in other locations.

Gross Pathology

There can be some fairly small foci of necrosis and new formation of vessels; otherwise there does not seem to be much difference, as seen by the naked eye, in the anaplastic forms. This must be confirmed histologically (see MANSUY et al. 1975).

Histologic Appearance

Histologically these tumors are very interesting, having a variegated cellular picture, though we have also seen peculiar giant cells rich in cytoplasm which may grow like "glia rasen" (e.g., as continuous plasmatic cellular growth) (HBT, Figs. 37a, 40a). Often cells have a "ganglioid" nucleus, and a mixture of a cell-rich section with small round cells and very large-bodied polymorphic cells still with a honeycomb architecture may be seen. However, the classic pattern of anaplastic oligodendrogliomas may show a preponderance of one of the two forms of anaplasia or polymorphism. They occur usually in isolation but, more rarely, also in combination: (a) Signs of a *cellular* polymorphism (HBT, Figs. 39, 40), increasing cell density, many typical and atypical mitoses, and giant cells, usually of a hyperchromatic polynuclear character, may be observed, sometimes in increased numbers, in addition to the basic honeycomb architecture of cells. The Langhans type of giant cells (Fig. 64a, b) with marginal hyperchromatic nuclei are the typical cell type, rarely the Sternberg type; sometimes the nature of a glioma depends upon the typical basic architecture and the metallic impregnations (e.g., Meller's or Grinyo's method), which reveal these giant cells with the distinct features of oligodendroglia although they are multinuclear (HBT, Figs. 39a–d, 40a–b, 41b–d). (b) The second type of anaplasia ("*tissular*") takes the form typical of glioblastoma multiforme, namely of necrosis (Fig. 65b), vascular proliferation, and irregular formation of stroma, particularly of the vessels; here the lacunar and sinusoidal vessel types, similar to the processes in glioblastoma multiforme, can be observed (HBT, Fig. 40c).

Electron Microscopy

In the EM picture of the anaplastic type the most prominent feature is a greater cellular diversity. The anaplastic tumor cells may have a fine structure with the characteristics for immature cells and can show quite pronounced irregularities in the nuclear structure and in the cytoplasm. Of particular interest is the occurrence of multiple hypertrophic nucleoli within the karyoplasm of the giant cells. Together with a large amount of free ribosomes and an increased number of mitochondria this is a sign of an exaggerated cell metabolism due to quick proliferation or other activities. Ribosomes, Golgi apparatus, and sometimes a centriole may be noted (ZÜLCH and WECHSLER 1968; ZÜLCH 1981c; see also the data p. 248). We have never seen the crystalloid inclusions and rodlets reported by RAIMONDI et al. (1962). TOGA (1976) has given a detailed description.

Tissue Culture and Histochemistry

No particularly informative data about the anaplasia in oligodendrogliomas were revealed by tissue culture or histochemistry, except in the investigations of BINGAS (1966, 1970), STAVROU et al. (1972), and VAN VEELEN et al. (1979, p. 4264).

Differential Diagnosis

Apart from observation of the characteristics of anaplasia summarized above, impregnation seems to be obligatory for the recognition of anaplastic oligodendrogliomas. Otherwise differential diagnosis is similar to that in other oligodendrogliomas.

Biologic Behavior (Grading), Metastasis, and Recurrence

Anaplastic transformation can arise very abruptly, as in a case published from our laboratory (SCHUIER 1976): here 6 months after operation anaplasia had developed that had so completely changed the architecture of the cells that they could hardly be referred to as cells any longer, being merely an accumulation of disorderly nuclear chromatin almost devoid of cytoplasm. In this case the history went back more than 8 years.

The two forms of polymorphism described above do not show any difference in survival times as far as we have observed. This distinction has also been adopted by CERVOS-NAVARRO et al. (1981). The general survival time is definitely shorter in the anaplastic forms and may be only 1 or 2 years after radical operation (ZÜLCH 1960a, Fig. 254). Therefore these anaplastic oligodendrogliomas are classed as grade III for malignancy.

BINGAS (1966, 1970) distinguished isomorphous and polymorphous oligodendrogliomas on a histochemical basis (see p. 250). His patients with isomorphous oligodendrogliomas had a postoperative survival of 54 months, and those with polymorphous (anaplastic) oligodendrogliomas, of 26 months. The results after radiation have been reported by SHELINE et al. (1964). The recognition of higher malignancy in tumors has been discussed by VAN VEELEN et al. (1979).

Recurrence

Recurrence is more common than in the normal form of oligodendrogliomas. A particular trend to intra- or extracranial metastasis has not been yet described.

Clinical Course

Anaplasia is most frequently seen in recurrences, which in such cases appear only a short time after the first operation (see our case p. 257).

In one of our cases with recurrences we noted a curious pattern of large tumor cells in "epithelial" growth (ZÜLCH 1941a, HBT, Fig. 37c, d) in an otherwise typical oligodendroglioma. The advancing tumor cells had nest- and cone-shaped structures in the marginal zone with a certain resemblance to (corneal?) cancer, although the oligodendroglioma was originally typical.

15.3 Ependymal and Choroid Plexus Tumors

15.3.1 Ependymomas

Synonyms: Ependymoblastoma, ependymoglioma; in the older literature: adenoglioma, glioependymoma, ependymoepithelioma, blastoma ependymale, Pfeilerzellgliom, occasionally these were also described as "neuroepitheliomas" or gangliosarcomas

Introduction

In the WHO classification the ependymal tumors appear either as *ependymomas* or as *choroid plexus papillomas*. The ependymomas can be subdivided according to the prevalent pattern (papillary, myxopapillary) or to their location (subependymoma). Their differentiation from the neuroepitheliomas is discussed below (p. 270). A malignant form of the ependymoma is listed as *anaplastic ependymoma.*

Historical Note and Definition

The first description of the ependymal tumors is found in VIRCHOW's book (1863/65) and other publications. MUTHMANN and SAUERBECK (1903) related the ependymomas to the ependyma as the tissue of origin, in a similar way to MALLORY (1902) with his demonstration of blepharoplasts in both tissues. The ependymomas and ependymoblastomas were set apart as a distinct group by BAILEY and CUSHING (1926, 1930). ROUSSY and OBERLING (1932) distinguished ependymomas, and also ependymoblastomas, ependymocytomas, and ependymogliomas. KERNOHAN and FLETCHER-KERNOHAN (1936) recognized epithelial, myxopapillary, and cellular types. Many true ependymomas have been described in the general pathological literature, for instance as "neuroepitheliomas" (BESOLD 1896; ROSENTHAL 1898; STORCH 1899; ROMAN 1913; RIBBERT 1918; MARBURG 1921).

The subdivision into ependymomas and ependymoblastomas was abandoned long ago by BAILEY (1932a), and only in experimental tumors is the term ependymoblastoma still in use (transplantable ependymoblastoma; ZIMMERMAN 1961; RUBIN et al. 1968). I have emphasized that the ependymomas of the cerebral hemispheres in children are biologically more unfavorable than other ependymomas. They differ in their rate of growth, as measured by the number of mitoses (ZÜLCH 1940b). Although otherwise they cannot be distinguished morphologically, they are in contrast very typical representatives (HBT, Figs. 6, 7a) of the ependymoma pattern.

Furthermore, I have noted that the ependymomas around the foramen of Monro (ZÜLCH and SCHMID 1955) and the third ventricle show the common typical architecture (nucleus-free spaces around the blood vessels) to a lesser extent than the others, and that ependymal tubules occur more frequently in the ependymomas located near the aqueduct, the fourth ventricle, and the spinal cord. However, I have been *unable to discover a biological difference between these last subtypes* (ZÜLCH 1956).

KERNOHAN et al. (1949) proposed a morphological subdivision into four "grades," while at the same time abandoning his previous definition (KERNOHAN and FLETCHER-KERNOHAN 1935), which included the plexus papillomas. His present grade 1 shows a structure similar to the one we have described in the ependymomas around the foramen of Monro; yet, in this respect this type is somewhat atypical of ependymomas. His grades 2 and 3 correspond to the classic description of ependymomas. In his illustrations and descriptions we cannot find any difference between them, except perhaps the presence of mitoses in grade 3, which might make them correspond to "our" extraventricular ependymomas of the cerebral hemispheres. His grade 4 seems to be extremely rare; I have seen this pattern on accasion in recurrences and described it as a stage of dedifferentiation (HBT, Fig. 13a, c; ZÜLCH 1940b; ZÜLCH and KLEINSASSER 1957). KERNOHAN et al. (1949) also include the medulloepitheliomas in grade 4, which now form a separate group in the WHO classification (see p. 338). Their grading concept raised some basic problems insofar as it was based on the presupposition that all graded subgroups had the same basic histological pattern though with different degrees of anaplasia. However, this is not true for the ependymomas, as shown above. On the contrary, subgroups with identical patterns are (a) the extraventricular cerebral forms (grade 2); and (b) the intraspinal ependymoma (grade 1), but these differ only in that mitoses occur in the former. However, another grade 1 subgroup has a completely different architecture, namely the ependymoma of the foramen of Monro and also the trabecular/papillary and the papillary types, which are both grade 1.

This confirms our assertion that grades should not be determined primarily by the histology but by the biological behavior of a particular histological subgroup according to clinical experience (see pp. 31, 32). It is interesting to

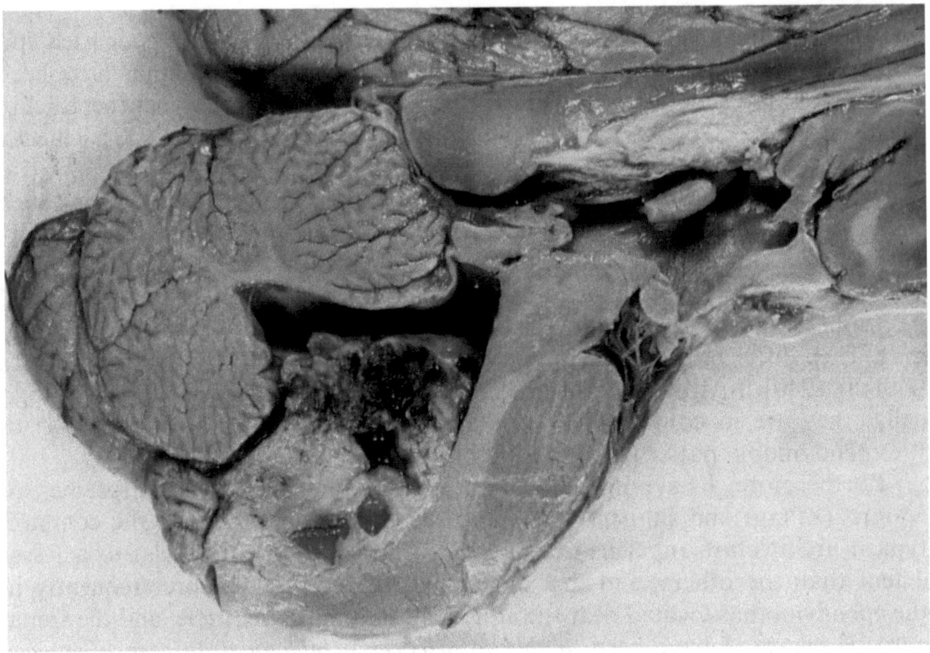

Fig. 67. Typical ependymoma of the fourth ventricle, with a small process extending into the cisterna magna. Small cysts and hemorrhages can be seen. The anterior portion of the fourth ventricle is markedly dilated. (ZÜLCH 1975a)

know that ROSENTHAL'S (1898) description of the Rosenthal fibers is part of his report of a spinal "neuroepithelioma," i.e., an ependymoma.

Detailed descriptions have been published by SAXER (1902), BITTORF (1904), GOLD (1924), FINCHER and COON (1929), VON HASSELBACH (1931), RINKE (1933), FOERSTER and GAGEL (1934b, 1936), ANTONI (1936b), GAGEL (1938), ZÜLCH (1940b, 1955b, 1956, 1960a), KRICHEFF et al. (1964), FOKES and EARLE (1969), ARENDT and SENITZ (1972), and DOHRMANN et al. (1976b).

Epidemiology (Age – Sex – Frequency – Site)

Age: The ependymomas of the cerebral hemispheres (TÖNNIS and ZÜLCH 1937) occur predominantly in childhood and adolescence, incidence peaking at around 8 and 15 years. The other groups show a predilection for the age group 11–40 years (Fig. 9d). Our youngest patient was 7 months of age, the oldest 81 years.

Sex: In all our patients with ependymomas the male:female ratio was 6:4.

Frequency: Ependymomas of the cerebral hemispheres are the most common hemispheral gliomas of childhood. The spinal ependymomas account for 60% of all gliomas in the spinal cord according to KERNOHAN and SAYRE (1952). Overall, 4.3% of all intracranial tumors in our series of 9000 cases were ependymomas. The corresponding figure in CUSHING'S (1932) material was 1.3% and

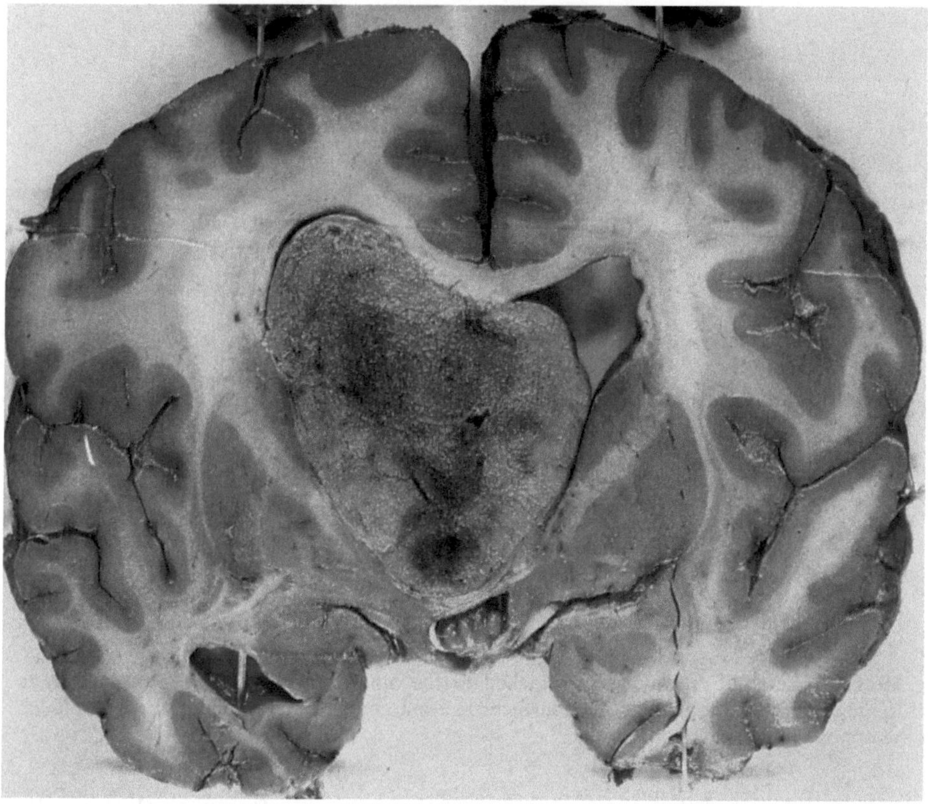

Fig. 68. Ependymoma of the foramen of Monro with hemorrhages into the tumor. Ipsilateral occlusion of the foramen of Monro and contralateral stenosis; hydrocephalic enlargement of third ventricle

that in Olivecrona's (RINGERTZ and REYMOND 1949), 6.3%. Ependymomas made up 9.1% of all *gliomas* at the Mayo Clinic (SVIEN et al. 1953).

Site: Ependymomas occur predominantly in the vicinity of the ependyma. The sites (Figs. 67, 68; GP, Figs. 54–61, 63–72) in declining order of frequency are: fourth ventricle, lateral ventricles, third ventricle, aqueduct, spinal cord, cauda equina, extraventricular hemisphere. The extraventricular ependymomas of the *cerebral hemispheres* reach the size of a small fist and may lie in any lobe, with a predilection for the temporo-parieto-occipital junction (Fig. 69). They lie up against the lateral ventricle (particularly at the trigone) and from there can grow out and push against the overlying cortex (GP, Figs. 64–66), particularly the supramarginal and angular gyri. They may occasionally even reach the cortex (Fig. 14, no. 30, Fig. 69). These large ependymomas have a lobulated and tufted surface (Fig. 69) resembling a placenta or cauliflower (Fig. 67; GP, Fig. 69). The danger of tearing off these tufts during operation is considerable. The ependymomas in the *fourth ventricle* are usually the size of a plum (Fig. 14, no. 71, Fig. 67; and are attached firmly to the posterior

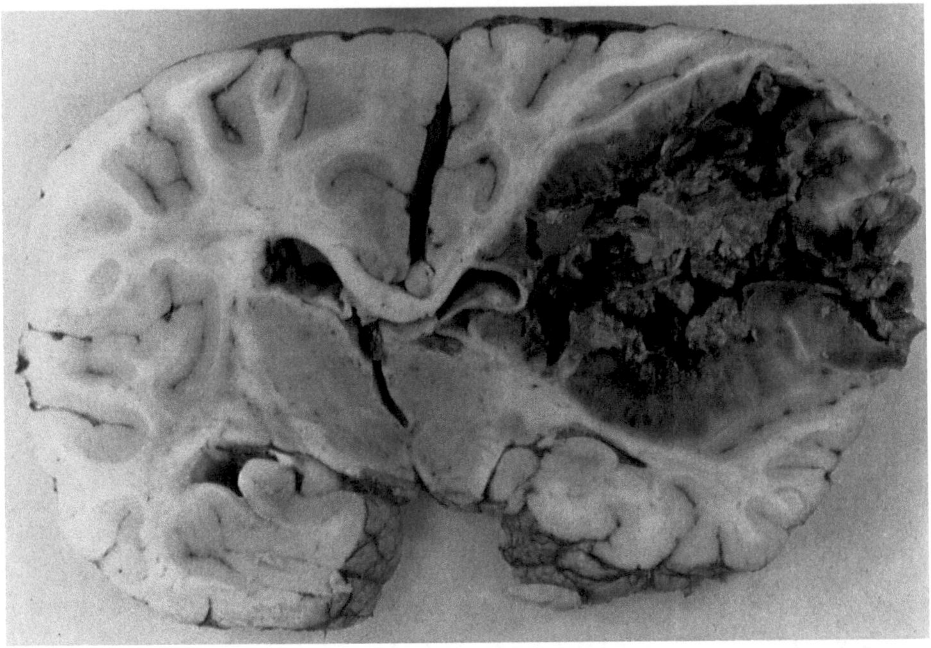

Fig. 69. Large cerebral ependymoma attached to the outer wall of the trigone. Large cysts within the tumor and a lobulated outer surface are apparent, as is the secondary hydrocephalus on the opposite side

part of the floor of the ventricle (Fig. 67). A process often extends into the cisterna magna or the lateral recesses (GP, Figs. 58–60), the former occasionally reaching down to the midcervical cord (down to C5 in one of our cases). Less frequently, ependymomas lie in the *lateral ventricle* (Fig. 68) at and over the foramen of Monro (Fig. 14, no. 54, Fig. 68; GP, Figs. 55–56) or in the *third ventricle* (ZÜLCH 1960) rostral and dorsal to the *quadrigeminal plate* (Fig. 14, no. 56) and finally – though rarely – in the *cerebellopontine angle* (GP, Fig. 58) or actually in the aqueduct. In the *spinal cord* they appear either in the shape of a pencil, extending over several segments, in the region of the posterior columns, or as large reddish-white gelatinous tumors in the region of the *cauda* and on the *filum terminale* where they may reach a length of 9–11 cm.

The cerebral forms frequently contain a large cyst (Fig. 69), are commonly rostrally placed (GP, Figs. 64, 65), and tend to be calcified. In the spinal cord there is often a cavity above and/or below the tumor, resembling syringomyelia and corresponding to the cyst formation of the cerebral forms. Its elongated shape conforms to the longitudinal orientation of the spinal cord tracts.

Heredity: A congenital and familial case has been reported by SATO et al. (1982).

Gross Pathology

Ependymomas are reddish, nodular, and lobulated, often resembling a placenta or cauliflower (GP, Fig. 69, see above), and they adjust themselves in form

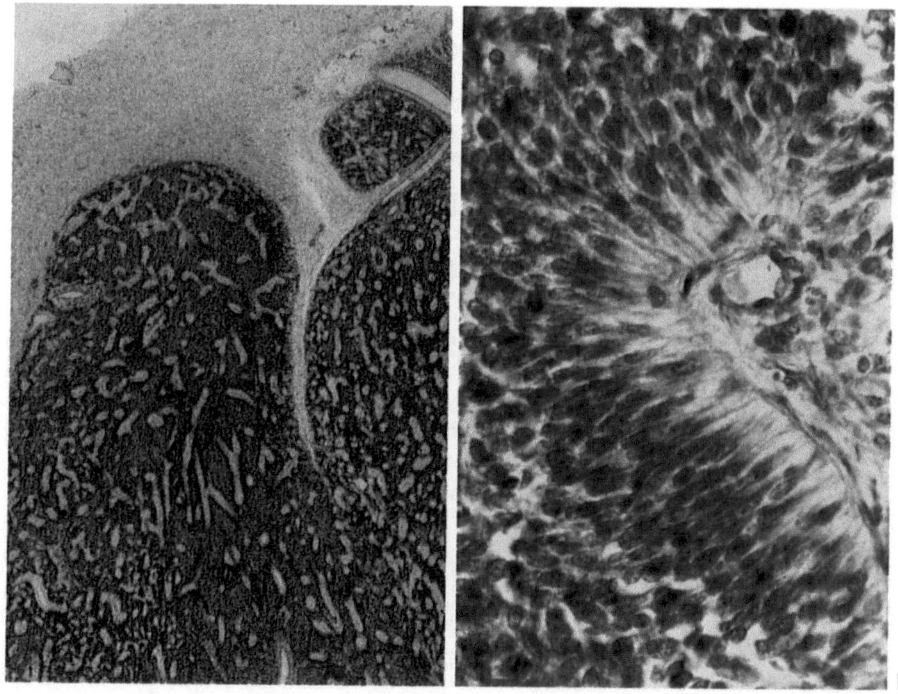

a b

Fig. 70. a Typical architecture of an ependymoma. Numerous blood vessels with nucleus-free cuffs give the tumor its peculiar appearance (leopard skin). The expanding growth against the cerebral cortex is clearly discernible. Cresyl violet, ×14.5. **b** The same architecture at a higher magnification. Cresyl violet, ×272

and size to their surroundings. The benign forms grow towards the neighboring tissue purely by expansion. It has been shown that the histopathology of ependymomas varies with the localization (ZÜLCH and SCHMID 1955; ZÜLCH 1956; ZÜLCH and KLEINSASSER 1957). Therefore, the histology has to be described separately for the various forms, and only a general characterization is given at the beginning of this chapter.

Histologic Appearance

Generally, ependymomas are characterized by a perivascular (HBT, Fig. 7) radial formation of cells (crown-like patterns, see Fig. 70b), and not infrequently they contain ependymal rosettes or canals (Figs. 20b, 72a). They are uniformly isomorphic, very cellular tumors with densely packed cells. The typical architecture is a uniform distribution of cells with an equally uniform arrangement of blood vessels between the masses of tumor cells. Nucleus-free mantles form cuff-like spaces around the vessels (when only a nuclear stain is used the section takes on a spotted leopard-skin (HBT, Fig. 6) pattern; Fig. 70a). These nuclear-free mantles around the vessels contain coarse or finer cell processes, which attach themselves to the vessel walls [these processes are sometimes even seen with H&E stains (Fig. 71a) and earlier led Bailey to call this particular form ependymoblastoma (BAILEY and CUSHING 1926, 1930)]. Otherwise, they can

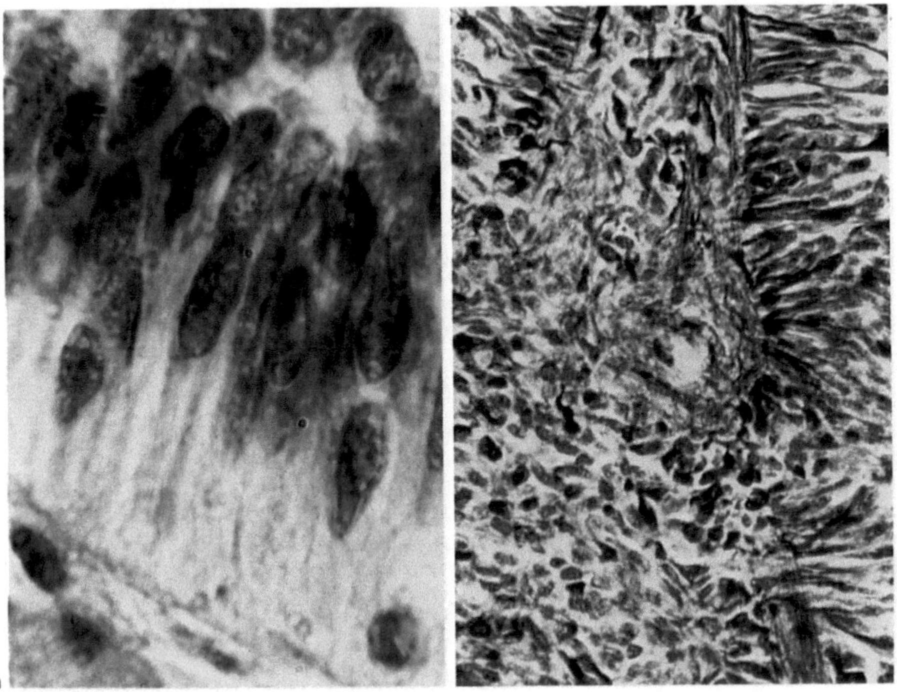

a b

Fig. 71. a Magnification of the cell processes in the nucleus-free zones. H&E, ×1400. **b** The vascular processes of the cells are often *well* demonstrated with gold sublimate. ×312

be demonstrated (HBT, Fig. 8) only by special stains, e.g., PTHA, gold impregnations of Cajal (Fig. 71b), Mallory's stain; they correspond to the "gliovascular systems" (Del Rio Hortega 1932, 1962; Costero 1962; Polak 1966); occasionally single rosettes (Fig. 72a) may be noted, particularly in those tumors below the level of the aqueduct (HBT, Fig. 10a). This characteristic is of absolutely no significance in the biological evaluation of these tumors, however, and should under no circumstances lead to the obsolete diagnosis of neuroepithelioma.

Generally the cells are poor in cytoplasm. The nuclei (Fig. 71a) have abundant chromatin and are round or oval. Mitoses occur almost exclusively in the extraventricular cerebral forms, which are therefore conceived as "anaplastic" by some authors. With special stains blepharoplasts can be demonstrated (however, they are visible only with oil immersion), particularly along the luminal margin of the cells forming rosettes and canals.

The intima of the blood vessels tends to proliferate with closures of the lumen (this in contrast to some descriptions in the literature). This results in the tendency to undergo regressive changes, including cyst formation. Only rarely is there necrosis and fatty degeneration. Not so rarely massive formations of calcareous deposits have been seen in cerebral extraventricular forms.

As already emphasized, particularly in a paper published in collaboration with Kleinsasser (Zülch and Kleinsasser 1957), the histology (HBT, Fig. 12)

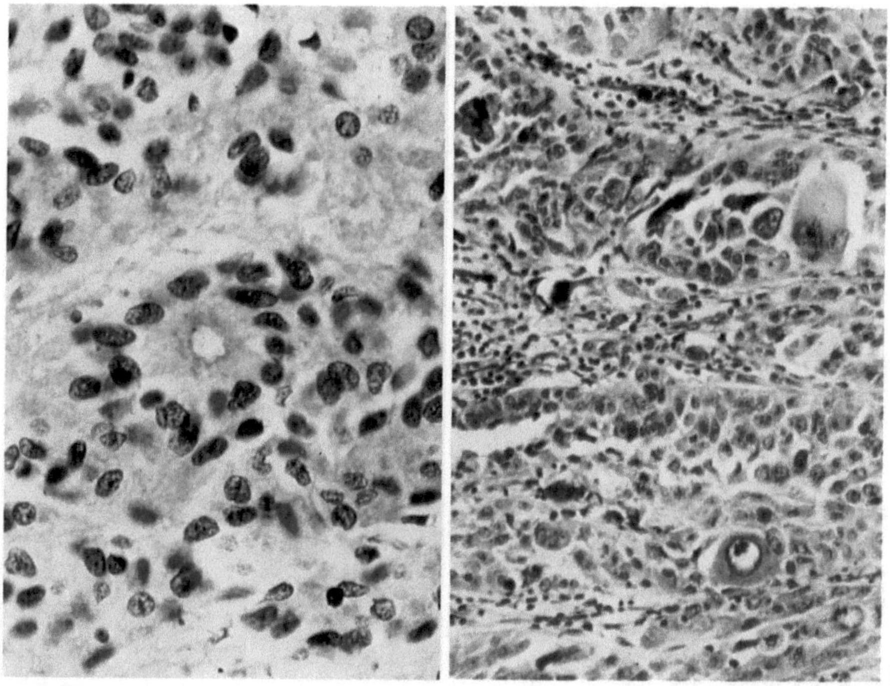

a b

Fig. 72. a True "rosette" in an otherwise typical ependymoma. H&E, ×272. **b** Anaplastic ependymoma of considerable cellularity composed of polymorphous cells, but with typical ependymal features also. Note the polynuclear, polymorphous cells. Cresyl violet, ×175

and the biological behavior of the ependymomas varies depending on their localization.

The last-cited paper describes a particular study of 75 cases among 210 ependymomas of our collection for whom large sections were available, and in it we have made the following statements:

Ependymomas of the Fourth Ventricle: Only a few of these tumors had mitotic activity, but otherwise they showed the pattern typical for the ependymomas. However, it must be emphasized that if a tongue-like process extended from such a tumor into the cisterna magna atrophy of the cellular elements took place (Fig. 73), which finally led to an architecture corresponding to that of the subependymomas (as described on page 273). GIAMPALMO (1937) had also alluded to this.

Spinal Ependymomas: Ependymal canals were very common, but mitoses never occurred.

Cerebral Ependymomas: A very typical architecture was prominent; occasionally ependymal canals occurred, and frequent mitotic activity was seen as stated above (sometimes variations of the typical pattern of these ependymomas were observed, as I have described for instance in 1956, Figs. 221–226).

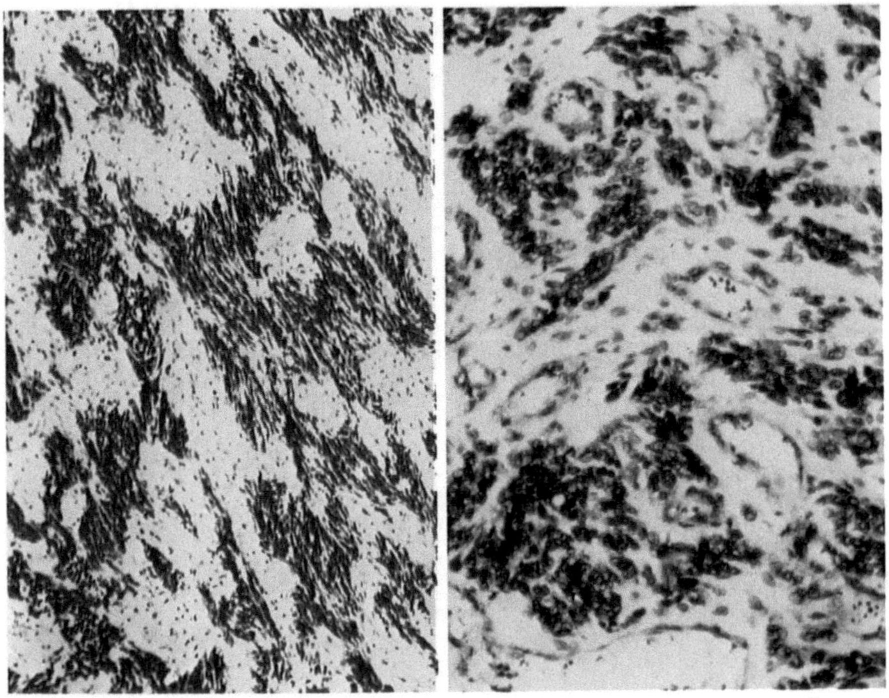

Fig. 73. **a** Distinct enlargement of the nucleus-free, perivascular zones. Cresyl violet, ×120. **b** The typical architecture of the ependymoma is hardly recognizable, because the tumor parenchyma is limited to a few bands and the nucleus-free spaces have expanded further. Cresyl violet, ×200

Ependymomas of the Foramen of Monro: These tumors deviated very markedly from the characteristic pattern (Fig. 74a). Cells were small and the nuclei lymphoid; no particular architecture was seen; there were very few capillaries and no patterns of nuclei-free mantles around the vessels; and no crown-like patterns characterized this type (see also KERNOHAN et al. 1949). Ependymomas of the *cauda equina* are described on p. 270).

Electron Microscopy

Neoplastic ependymal cells have desmosomes at some points of intercellular contact; especially adjacent to free surfaces, cilia and microvilli can be detected. Within the tumor cells single or multiple blepharoplasts may be identified, as derivatives of the centriole (LUSE 1960, 1962). Moreover, numerous cell processes can be detected, with varying degrees of synthesis of glial filaments. Between the more epithelium-like cells there are tumor cells with the same characteristics as those of the protoplasmic or fibrillary astrocytes. Here the electron micrograph may suggest that cells of the ependyma must be regarded as the tumor matrix (see also HIRANO et al. 1975a, b; HIRANO 1978). Usually the cytoplasm contains organelles and glycogen granules. Most of the cells have no ependymal specialization such as cilia or microtubules. Features characteristic of primitive

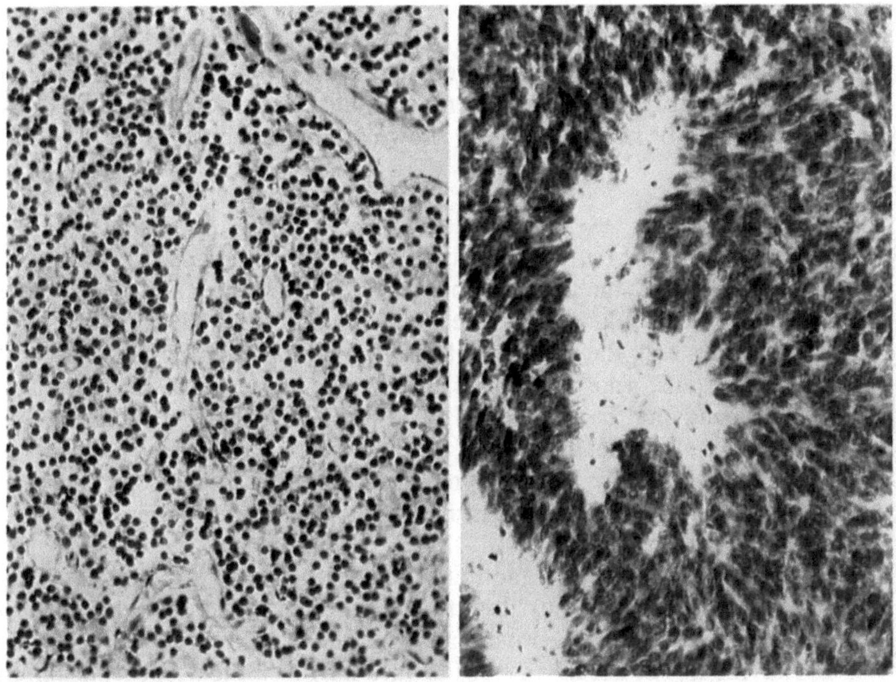

a b

Fig. 74. a Typical architecture of an ependymoma of the foramen of Monro. Nucleus-free zones around the vessels are missing. Cresyl violet, ×112. **b** Ependymoma of the fourth ventricle. In the dense areas there is a tendency to form pseudoresettes which are considered characteristic for the medulloblastoma. Cresyl violet, ×180

ependymal glia have been described by FRIEDE and POLLAK (1978), and were also reminiscent of pilocytic astrocytomas.

Tissue Culture

The findings in tissue culture are in good agreement with the above description of the ependymomas. COSTERO and POMERAT (1955a, b), COSTERO (1962), and LUMSDEN (1971) emphasized the capacity of the neoplastic cells to form gliofibrils both in vivo and in vitro. The cells migrate into the culture without becoming disorganized; only some of them have a tendency to transform themselves into astrocyte-like cells. In KERSTING'S (1968) series of tissue culture the cells demonstrated a more epithelial character; of 16 ependymomas cultivated in vitro, 13 (4th ventricle, spinal cord, cauda equina) presented the same typical epithelium-like proliferation with a tendency to form rosettes. Only three cases of intramedullary tumors have shown any differences from this picture, and these had features more similar to those of the pilocytic astrocytomas of the cerebellum. In the early stages of development ependymomas, especially the well-differentiated ones, have a tendency to form cellular columns and rings (LISS 1972) or even to undergo normal ependymal growth (BATZDORF and POKRESS 1968).

Histochemistry

By histochemical methods oxidative enzymes in the tumor cells are demonstrated as well as acid phosphatase, the latter particularly in the regressive parts. Cholinesterase seems to be more frequently shown as acetylcholinesterase (TOGA 1976).

Differential Diagnosis

The ependymomas of the fourth ventricles can be distinguished from medulloblastomas grossly by the harder consistency of the former and the noninvasive growth, and microscopically by the absence of mitoses (in this location) and the architecture, e.g., the presence of nucleus-free cuffs and crown-like patterns around the vessels, and commonly also by the presence of true rosettes (see Fig. 72a), ependymal canals (see HBT, Fig. 13b), and finally blepharoplasts; only exceptionally pseudorosettes are encountered in true ependymomas (Fig. 74b). Occasionally in ependymomas, regressive processes can cause the cells to swell, so that the tissue assumes the typical appearance of an oligodendroglioma.

It may be that KERNOHAN and FLETCHER-KERNOHAN (1935) did not recognize the *secondary* nature of this alteration of the tissue and falsely conceived a *primary* kinship between ependymomas and oligodendrogliomas.

Ependymomas of the foramen of Monro may lack the usual typical architecture and be somewhat similar to oligodendrogliomas (Fig. 74a) without being specifically impregnated. The papillary type, occurring usually in the cerebellopontine angle (Fig. 75a), may be mistaken for a choroid plexus papilloma (see p. 269). KLEIHUES (1965) was able to show a very curious "composition" of a tumor consisting of both ependymoma and sarcoma tissue. A similar mixed tumor was described by ZÜLCH (1940b, Figs. 9, 10), which had characteristics of an ependymoma and of a pilocytic astrocytoma at the same time. Mixed tumors do actually occur (GP, Fig. 63).

Biologic Behavior (Grading), Metastasis, and Recurrence

As expressed in grades, the ependymomas proper, including the myxopapillary types, correspond to grade I (see p. 272), and the anaplastic forms to grade II or III (see p. 275). Total removal in some of these cases involves quite a degree of risk, because of the firm adherence of the tumor to the ventricular floor, where the caudal cranial nerve nuclei of the fourth ventricle are very close. Partial excision with a subsequent chemo-/radiotherapy may be the method of choice for these particular tumors. Following total removal of the tumors the 5-year survival rate is 50%; following subtotal removal, 25%; and after biopsy only, 16.6% (OI and RAIMONDI 1980).

Other ependymomas are also difficult to treat surgically, e.g., ependymoma of the foramen of Monro or of the mesencephalic region, or ependymoma in the aqueduct. The ependymomas of the spinal cord – often with large cysts – and of the cauda equina apparently have a fairly favorable prognosis after total excision. Recent results obtained in children have been published by OI and RAIMONDI (1980).

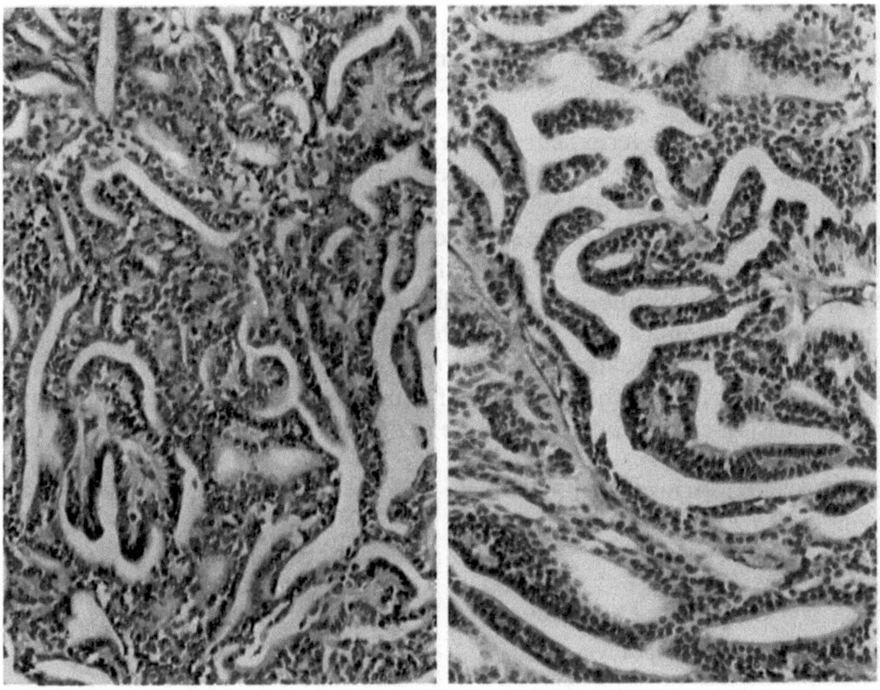

a b

Fig. 75a, b. Papillary trabecular variant of ependymoma which occurs only in the lateral recess of the cerebellopontine angle. H&E, ×125 (**a**) and ×220 (**b**)

Metastases occur spontaneously only occasionally, but are not uncommon after operation on the hemispheral forms (the whole CSF system may be involved with nodules and plaques; WERNER 1939; ZÜLCH 1940b). In the hemispheral forms, recurrences even after "total removal" are frequent; not so in other ependymomas. In the literature many cases of extracranial metastasis have been described, which, however, need further study (PERRIN 1958; HESSELVIK and TYGSTRUP 1965; RAPAPORT and RUBEN 1974; SUREN 1974).

The recurrence of the extraventricular cerebral forms is not so rare even after so-called total removal, because of the friability of the lobulated tissue some tumor pieces may escape removal. They are commonly anaplastic (grade III to IV; HBT, Fig. 13a) and have been called "embryonic" (FOWLER 1968) when primary, as in one of our cases.

Clinical Course

The "cerebral" extraventricular forms occurring during childhood often remain clinically silent for long periods in spite of excessive growth with cyst formation. Ependymomas of the fourth ventricle can also have a long history and after decompression run a benign course over many years (woman of 25 years of age: ZÜLCH 1956, p. 30).

Further References: HILDEBRANDT (1906), ELSCHNIG (1913), HIRSCH and ELLIOT (1925), NAESLUND (1926), HARDMAN and JEFFERSON (1938), BENEDEK and JUBA (1943), RAUCH (1944), SEI-

FARTH (1948), DOERNBACH (1949), RINGERTZ and REYMOND (1949), MATTOS PIMENTA and MAFFEI (1950), LÜTHY and IRSIGLER (1952), ZONDEK (1952), TÖNNIS and BORCK (1953), RUBINSTEIN (1970), MINAUF et al. (1970), SHUMAN et al. (1975), AFRA et al. (1981).

Neuroepitheliomas: The term neuroepithelioma was used earlier by neuropathologists, e.g., WINTERSTEINER (1897: neuroepithelioma retinae), ROSENTHAL (1898: spinal case), STORCH (1899), RIBBERT (1918), MARBURG (1921), ROUSSY and OBERLING (1931), and BAILEY himself (1932), who emphasized that these tumors occur most frequently in the retina and rarely in the brain and spinal cord. Whereas actually the neuroepithelioma in the retina could be discussed instead of the retinoblastoma, most of the other cases cited above were typical ependymomas with ependymal canals or even real rosettes; however, this observation should not lead to the diagnosis of neuroepithelioma (see p. 118). Details of this discussion can be found elsewhere (ZÜLCH 1939a, p. 330–332).

Further References: BITTORF (1904), NAESLUND (1926), BUCY and MUNCIE (1929), GRINKER (1932), GLOBUS and CARES (1953).

15.3.1.1 Myxopapillary Ependymomas

Synonym: Mucopapillary ependymoma

Introduction

Within the main group of the ependymal tumors the special form of *myxopapillary ependymomas* is included in the WHO classification.

Historical Note and Definition

KERNOHAN and FLETCHER-KERNOHAN (1935) and FOERSTER and GAGEL (1936) have described this subgroup of ependymomas and emphasized that its particular histological pattern occurs virtually exclusively at the filum terminale. The papillary architecture is very conspicuous and the tumor has a clear tendency to mucinous-hyaline degeneration of the vessel walls (mucopapillary forms) and to cell destruction between the papillae.

Epidemiology (Age – Sex – Frequency – Site)

There is some preference for the younger decades, but no sex predominance. The localization is, as already emphasized, the region of the cauda equina, and probably these tumors stem from the filum terminale. There are many papers describing an "extraspinal" localization in the sacrum (MORANTZ et al. 1979).

Gross Pathology

FOERSTER and GAGEL (1936) have given an excellent description in their basic paper: these tumors can be 6–12 cm long; they are shaped like a small finger and have a rather lobulated surface (see also WATT 1968; VAN DUINEN 1976).

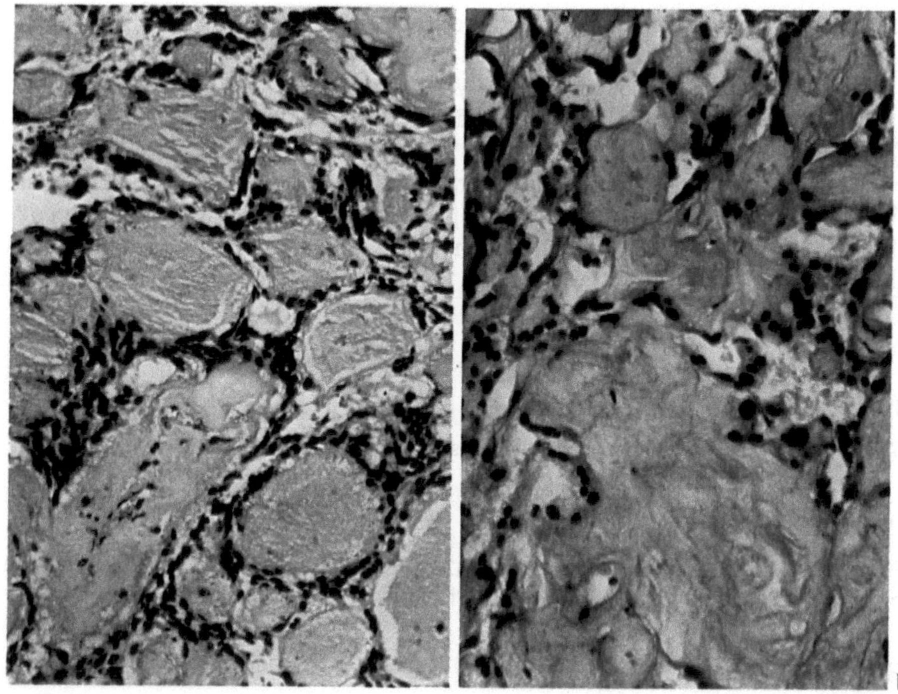

a b

Fig. 76. a Ependymoma of the filum terminale with marked regressive mucoid changes. H&E, ×136. **b** Sections showing even more markedly regressive changes. H&E, ×136

Histologic Appearance

The papillary architecture of this tumor is rarely seen and the diagnosis is not made very early. After a period of growth, i.e., by the time of clinical manifestation, the final stage is commonly reached, when only swollen acellular hyaline (HBT, Fig. 10c, d), fingerlike, processes covered with a single cell layer can be distinguished (FOERSTER and GAGEL 1936). These are remnants of a former core with a papillary wreath of tumor cells. Then the former ringlike papillary architecture around the vessels is completely blurred (Fig. 76). Single ganglion cells may occur (RAWLINSON et al. 1973) as we have also noted. Since these tumors are originally highly vascular and their capsule very thin, subarachnoid hemorrhage is possible.

Electron Microscopy

The EM structure has been discussed by RAWLINSON et al. (1973) and WOLFF et al. (1972).

Biologic Behavior (Grading), Metastasis, and Recurrence

Radical removal, if appropriate combined with radiotherapy, is indicated, and there is usually a long benign course or even cure (SCOTT 1974). However, metastases infiltrating in the CSF and even extravertebrally (RUBINSTEIN and LOGAN 1970) have been observed even after total excision.

The biological behavior is generally benign (grade I), although subcutaneous sacrococcygeal cases with extraspinal delayed metastases (?) have been observed (M. WOLFF et al. 1972).

The true nature of the primary extraspinal ependymomas has not been clarified. MORANTZ et al. (1979) have apparently observed an incidence peak in the age group 21–30 and localization in the soft tissue (ANDERSON 1966) of the pelvis and also in the os sacrum or the postsacral region (NICOLA et al. 1976).

15.3.1.2 Papillary Ependymomas

Synonyms: Papillary trabecular ependymomas

Introduction

Although this papillary (trabecular) form is very rare, a special subgroup has been included for it in the WHO classification.

Historical Note and Definition

This tumor was first mentioned and depicted by ALEXANDER (1937), and it was portrayed in the atlas of brain tumors by KERNOHAN and SAYRE (1952, Figs. 45, 46). We have described such tumors in a basic article on the ependymomas of various histological patterns with Kleinsasser (ZÜLCH and KLEINSASSER 1957) as the "papillary trabecular" form of ependymoma (Fig. 75a, b; see also SCHARRER and HEIMING 1974).

Epidemiology (Age – Sex – Frequency – Site)

These tumors are too rare for any data on their epidemiology to have been collected. They are, however, almost exclusively located in the cerebellopontine angle.

Gross Pathology

Again, there are no particular characteristics known for these tumors.

Histologic Appearance

This tumor is characterized by a mixture of genuine papillae of an ependymal tissue and a trabecular communication between these papillae (Fig. 75), so that a differential diagnosis from choroid plexus papilloma is sometimes difficult. However, the basic point is that the trabeculae connect the papillae directly, which means that the basic papillary architecture is blurred. There is no basement membrane separating the tumor cells from the central vascular connective tissue stroma.

Biologic Behavior (Grading), Metastasis, and Recurrence

It has already been mentioned that the tumor is so rare that few biological data are available. There is nothing to suggest metastasis or a particularly malignant behavior of this tumor.

15.3.1.3 Subependymomas

Synonym: Subependymal glomerate astrocytoma

Introduction

The WHO classification includes a group for subependymomas, which corresponds to the tumor type described by SCHEINKER (1945).

Historical Note and Definition

SCHEINKER (1945) described such tumors as a separate category, which appeared as small, sometimes pendulous masses in the ventricles and were usually asymptomatic. He also discussed the typical histology.

However, the same histological pattern had been already described by GIAMPALMO (1937) when he showed that ependymomas can lose their architecture and much of their cellularity, while at the same time an increase of fibrils and atrophy takes place when there is pressure on the tumor.

He saw this picture in the ependymoma lobules extending into the cisterna magna (ZÜLCH 1956, Fig. 229a–d; Fig. 73). There the cells have largely disappeared, leaving a mass that can be characterized as rich in fibers and poor in cells. This change is probably associated with the pressure on the tissue protruding into the foramen magnum (see also GANDOLFI et al. 1981).

Gross Pathology

Subependymomas (GP, Fig. 160) generally reach a size of 1 or 2 cm, but can be much larger (48 cases reported in 1978 by SCHEITAUER). They are whitish, hard, sometimes somewhat lobulated masses. Only in a minority of cases do they become so large, i.e., larger than a hazelnut or walnut, that an operation is necessary (SLOWIK et al. 1979).

Histologic Appearance

Histologically the architecture of these tumors is highly conspicuous by the mixture of nests of ependymal cells situated in a mass of fibrillary substance. Not uncommonly microcysts are seen (see also FU et al. 1974).

This histological pattern also resembles the small ependymal granulations that occasionally occur as incidental findings after chronic inflammations within the CSF space (so-called ependymitis granularis) associated with chronic meningitis, particularly earlier after syphilitic infections.

Differential Diagnosis

The differential diagnosis from parts of ependymomas that have probably been subjected to chronic pressure has been mentioned above (see GIAMPALMO 1937).

Biologic Behavior (Grading), Metastasis, and Recurrence

Subependymoma is a benign tumor (grade I) and following complete surgical removal recurrences are unlikely. Metastasis is unknown.

Tumors producing symptoms may be located in the region of the fourth ventricles (GANDOLFI et al. 1981), the walls of the lateral ventricles, near the septum pellucidum (GP, Fig. 160), and on the spinal cord (see SLOWIK et al. 1979).

Clinical Course

In a mass of the lateral ventricle bleeding has been observed (CHANGARIS et al. 1981), which led to a typical subarachnoid hemorrhage. The occurrence of such tumors in identical twins with simultaneous clinical manifestations has been described by CLARENBACH et al. (1979).

15.3.2 Anaplastic Ependymomas

Synonyms: Malignant ependymomas, ependymoblastomas

Introduction

The WHO classification includes a grouping for the anaplastic form of the ependymoma. It embraces the many forms of malignant ependymomas described in the literature.

Historical Note and Definition

The anaplastic ependymomas were discussed by BAILEY and CUSHING (1926, 1930) in their first description under the term of ependymoblastoma, a form of ependymoma characterized by easily visible perivascular processes forming a "Strahlenkrone" (crown of rays). However, BAILEY (1932a) rightly discarded this concept of malignancy as not corresponding to the facts.

At this point the problem of "ependymoblastoma" has to be discussed in more detail. In the English-speaking countries the name "blastoma" is given to a tumor to characterize its malignancy. Since this particular tumor is not malignant the term has been withdrawn. In experimental neuro-oncology only, ZIMMERMAN used the term of ependymoblastoma for a tumor cultivated in tissue culture for many generations (RUBIN et al. 1968).

We described malignant ependymomas in 1940b (Fig. 77) and later in 1956, particularly in the group of cerebral extraventricular ependymomas but also in some fourth ventricle ependymomas that were in transition to medulloblastoma-like tumors (HBT, Fig. 13c; GP, Fig. 63) and beginning to infiltrate the floor of the fourth ventricle.

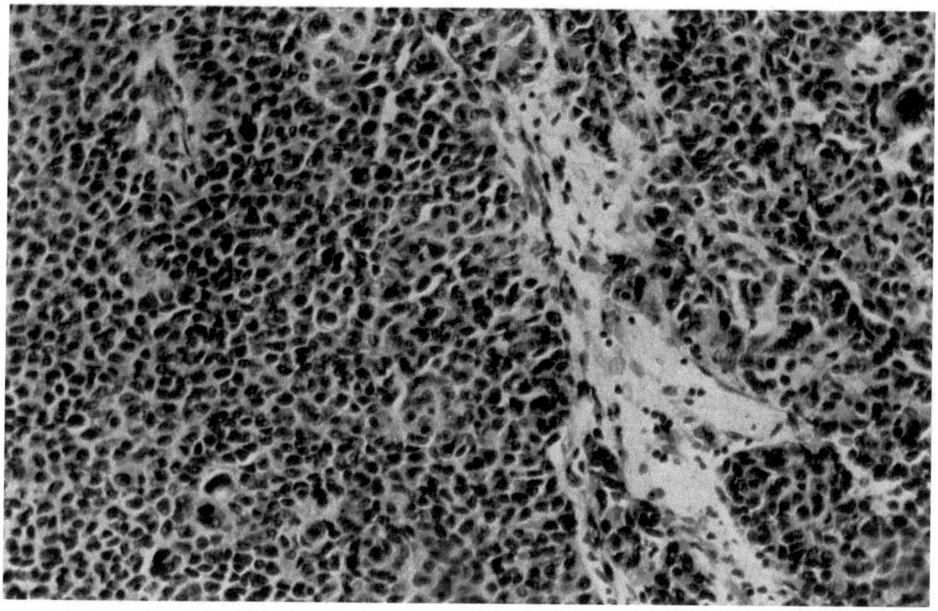

Fig. 77. Unusually compact layer (epithelial sheet) of cells in a recurring cerebral ependymoma. Rare giant cells. Nissl, × 700

As already mentioned, the large cystic (and not infrequently also calcified) extraventricular ependymomas occurring in youth and childhood definitely seem to have a worse prognosis (GP, Figs. 64, 65). Whether glioblastomas with a certain histological resemblance to ependymomas have really originated from this tumor type is still open to discussion (RINGERTZ 1950). Histologically the anaplastic type is characterized by an (Fig. 77) epithelium-like arrangement of the large cells, high mitotic activity, or complete loss of the highly organized pattern of the ependymoma (HBT, Fig. 6) and a disorderly arrangement of the stroma. In some cases metastasis to the arachnoidal space may even be encountered (HBT, Fig. 13d).

Such tumors can even be primary ependymomas with the typical architecture (HBT, Fig. 7) in which the high mitotic activity suggests that they are in anaplastic transformation but the original ependymoma pattern is preserved. Occasionally anaplastic giant cells are encountered (Fig. 72b).

Biologic Behavior (Grading), Metastasis, and Recurrence

It seems to be a general rule that extraventricular ependymomas in young patients have a poorer prognosis than those in adults, according to the WHO grading (KRICHEFF et al. 1964; PHILLIPS et al. 1964; SHUMAN et al. 1975; DOHRMANN et al. 1976b). Some of these extraventricular tumors even seem to be congenital (LUYENDYJK and STAAL 1964; SHUMAN et al. 1975). We have observed a very highly anaplastic form of such an extraventricular ependymoma in a boy aged 2 years.

Therefore SHUMAN et al. (1975) have formulated a very grim prognosis for all childhood ependymomas and suggested careful excision and radiation with 45 Gy over a 60-day period. LIU et al. (1976) were of the opinion that the biological behavior of an ependymoma could be predicted to a large extent from the degree of cytological differentiation. Unfortunately they included "ependymoblastomas located in the supratentorial region," which have a histological picture that is actually not convincing evidence for their inclusion in this classification.

Spontaneous metastases occur only occasionally (HBT, Fig. 13d) but are not uncommon after operation of the extraventricular hemispheric forms. In these cases the whole of the CSF system may be filled with nodules and plaques of tumor tissue (ZÜLCH 1940b; GP, Figs. 70–72; MÜLLER/Halle 1940). In the literature many cases of extracranial metastasis have been described, which, however, sometimes need further study (for references see PERRIN 1958; HESSELVIK and TYGSTRUP 1965; SCHIEFER 1969; RAPAPORT and RUBEN 1974; SUREN 1974).

In the case of anaplastic hemispheric tumors recurrences are not infrequent even after so-called total removal, but this is not true for other ependymomas (ZÜLCH 1940b).

15.3.3 Choroid Plexus Papillomas

Synonyms: Plexus papilloma; in the older literature: epithelioma, carcinoma, or adenoma of the choroid plexus, choroid epithelioma, choroid papilloma

Introduction

Under the general heading of Ependymal Tumors the choroid plexus papillomas are a special group in the WHO classification.

Historical Note and Definition

The papillary tumors of the choroidal epithelium have often been described as single cases in the classic literature, particularly in connection with attempts to differentiate them from ependymal tumors (STUDNICKA 1900; SAXER 1902; VONWILLER 1911; ASKANAZY 1914; AGDUHR 1922; etc.). In the neurosurgical literature only a few comprehensive studies have appeared between the first successful operation by PERTHES (1919) and the present (DAVIS and CUSHING 1925; VAN WAGENEN 1930; BOHM and STRANG 1961); nonetheless, they furnish us with an almost exhaustive account of the subject. I am convinced that many cases, especially those described in the older literature, were not true choroid plexus papillomas (e.g., LE BLANC 1868; BIELSCHOWSKY and UNGER 1906; VAN BOUWDIJK-BASTIAANSE 1914) but were actually cancer metastases (see also p. 496).

Epidemiology (Age – Sex – Frequency – Site)

Age: The choroid plexus papillomas occur particularly in the first 10 years of life: in fact this tumor probably appears earlier than any other tumor (45%

with signs in the first year: LAURENCE 1974). There are cases in the literature that are either directly congenital or in which the first symptoms appeared in the early years of life (VAN WAGENEN 1930; BRAUNSTEIN and MARTIN 1952; EISENBERG et al. 1974). Our youngest patient was 2 years old, our oldest 16.

Sex: In our former series – also particularly in the very early years of life – there were equal numbers of male and female patients with choroid plexus papilloma. In the series of BOHM and STRANG (1961; cases from the literature) 70% were female, and the series of LAURENCE (1974) contained 81 male versus 68 female patients.

BOHM and STRANG (1961) collected 143 cases from the literature; they were, however, perhaps not very critically selected. In my earlier (unpublished) attempts I found only 56 undoubted cases of choroid plexus papillomas in the literature published between 1833 and 1941, and there the statistical data were not consistent with those of BOHM and STRANG (1961), for instance with regard to site.

Frequency: In our series of 9000 cases the choroid plexus papillomas accounted for 0.6%; in CUSHING'S series (1932 and 1935), 0.6%; in the series of BOHM and STRANG (1961), 0.4%. According to MATSON and CROFTON (1960) the frequency in children *below* 12 years is 3.9%.

Site: Choroid plexus papillomas are understandably confined to the parts of the ventricles that contain choroid plexus, and occur equally on the right and on the left. However, they have certain preferential locations. In order of frequency they occur: (a) in the lateral ventricles (sometimes reaching the size of a fist: diameter 7 cm), in the trigone, where they may completely obliterate the lumen and expand all the way out to the cortex or to the temporal horn; large cysts can occur next to the tumor; (b) in the fourth ventricle (the size of a plum), where they expand its lumen; (c) in the third ventricle (Fig. 78), where they reach the size of a chestnut, and (d) in the cerebellopontine angle, where they are the size of a cherry (DAVIS and CUSHING 1925; MORELLO and MIGLIAVACCA 1964; DEVADIGA et al. 1969; HAMMOCK et al. 1976).

In the statistics of cases from the literature collected by BOHM and STRANG (1961) there were 32% situated in the lateral ventricle, 60% in the fourth ventricle, and 8% in the third ventricle. In my own collection of literature cases 38% were in the fourth ventricle, 35.5% in the lateral ventricle, 12.7% in the third ventricle, and 3.8% in the cerebellopontine angle. More detailed data are given by LAURENCE (1974, p. 556).

Bilateral locations occur (PLATH 1884; CUSHING 1925, Fig. 6, associated with hypersecreting hydrocephalus). Separate choroid plexus papillomas at various sites in the same patient were described by LAURENCE (1974).

Gross Pathology

The choroid plexus papillomas are well demarcated from the surrounding tissue, but tufts of tumor may be forced by pressure into the cerebral substance. They

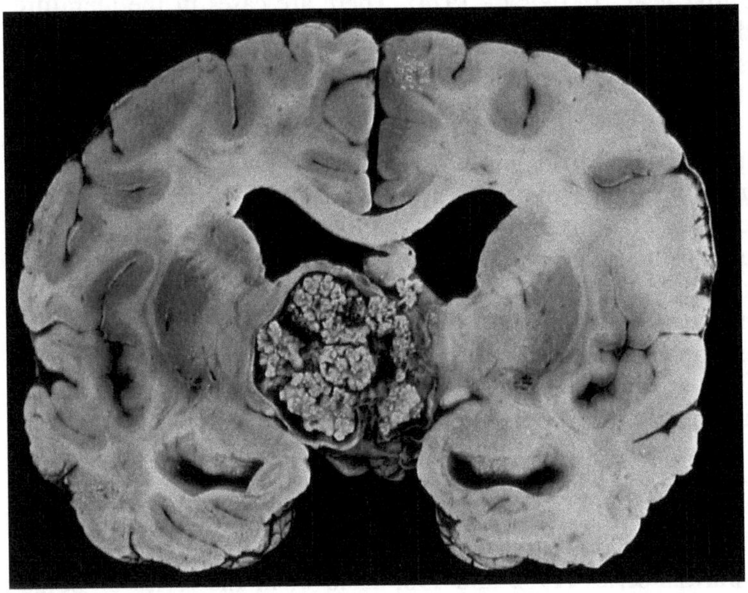

Fig. 78. Large choroid plexus papilloma of the third ventricle. Secondary obstructive hydrocephalus. (ZÜLCH 1975a)

are pinkish gray, have a fine or coarsely tufted surface, and even though they have a certain general firmness, are tender and friable and tear easily. On occasion they are highly calcified (BERTHA and SORGO 1940; SORGO 1940, Figs. 36, 37). In the case of choroid plexus papillomas within the ventricle obstructive hydrocephalus will arise (Fig. 78).

In choroid plexus papillomas that are congenital or arise in early youth hypersecretion with subsequent hydrocephalus may occur (CUSHING 1925, Fig. 6; BRAUNSTEIN and MARTIN 1952; LAURENCE 1974; EISENBERG et al. 1974; GHATAK and MCWHORTER 1976; GUDEMAN et al. 1979: bilateral).

In a specimen at the Royal Children's Hospital, London, I was shown (see also LAURENCE 1974, p. 567) a "hydrocephalus externus," i.e., a child's brain where all the fissures of the Sylvian arteries and also the cisternae were enlarged. This was apparently the way by which the hypersecreted CSF passed from the base to the sagittal sinus, where the "external" CSF was under pressure due to insufficient resorption.

Histologic Appearance

Histologically the tumors have a papillary structure (Fig. 79) with a single layer of epithelium of different heights (more columnar than cuboidal or flat). The choroid plexus papillomas, then, somehow duplicate the normal structure of the choroid plexus, although the cells covering the tufts of stroma are more frequently columnar than in a normal plexus of the aged. It is more similar to the form of the plexus epithelium in the first years of life (HBT, Fig. 16a–d).

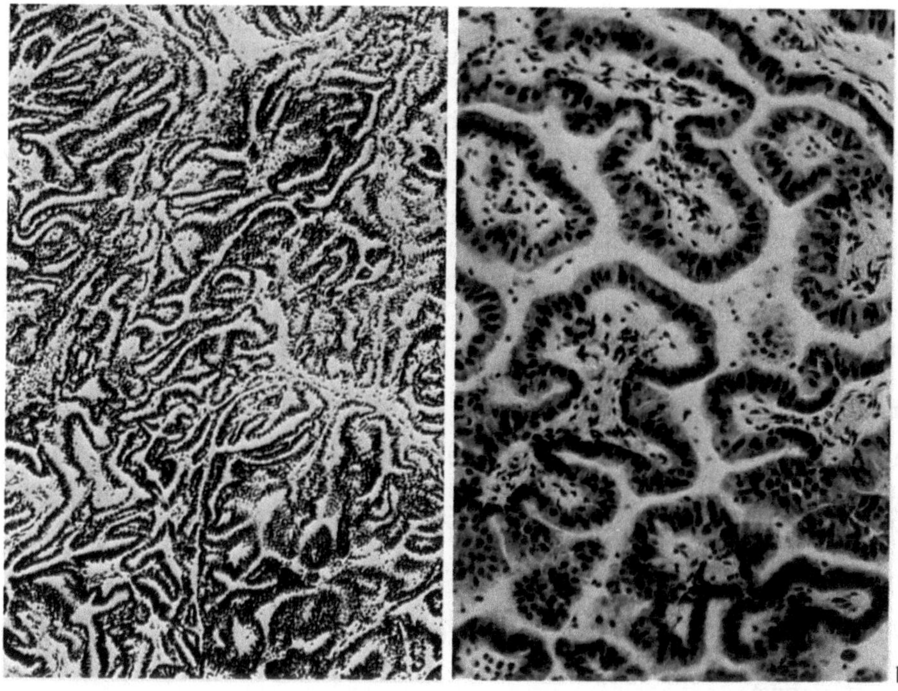

a b

Fig. 79. a Distinct formation of papillae with a central stroma. The papilla is surrounded by the parietal cells in a regular formation. Cresyl violet, ×25. **b** Higher magnification allows a more distinct view of the papillae. Most contain a capillary vessel. The epithelial cells are pavement-shaped or cylindrical. Cresyl violet, ×112

The cells often contain small cytoplasmic granules visible even in the Nissl stain. No cilia or blepharoplasts are seen in light microscopy. Mitoses are infrequent or absent. The connective tissue stroma shows edematous mucoid and hyaline changes, being therefore often widened, and occasionally contains calcified foci in the form of laminated spheres or psammoma bodies (highly positive in the x-ray and CT). There is no tendency to other regressive changes.

Electron Microscopy

The EM shows the apical-basal polarity of the columnar cells. Apical borders are irregular owing to the occurrence of numerous microvilli; well-developed cilia can also be identified, this in contrast to light microscopy. The lateral surfaces of the cells have numerous interdigitating cytoplasmic projections as well as apical tight junctions (see also Wakai et al. 1979). The basal poles are characterized by the occurrence of many mitochondria, cytoplasmic invaginations, and large amounts of pinocytic vesicles; the tumor cell is finally outlined by a continuous basal lamina. Cytoplasmic glycogen may be seen only in childhood choroid plexus papilloma as described by Carter et al. (1972). These authors also found differences among their three cases, for example in the organelle population.

Navas and Battifora (1978) described ultrastructural lipid droplets, filamentous material, and cytoplasmic inclusions (Bondi's "silver bodies"?). Bastian (1971) saw electrodense particles, which do not exist in normal choroid plexus. The stroma consisted of fibroblasts, collagen fibers, and fenestrated capillaries. It was virtually identical with that of the normal human choroid plexus (Shuangshoti and Netsky 1966a; Carter et al. 1972).

Ghatak and McWhorter (1976) suggested that the morphological difference from normal choroid plexus in the case of choroid plexus papilloma is the presence of tubular bodies in the endothelium and of well-developed pericytes; this provides strong evidence for CSF production by choroid plexus papillomas.

Tissue Culture

In tissue culture it is almost impossible to distinguish between ependymomas and choroid plexus papillomas according to Kersting (1968), because both grow in lawn-like formations (Unterharnscheidt 1972).

Histochemistry

With appropriate stains the choroid plexus papillomas show many PAS-positive substances (Navas and Battifora 1978; see also "acinar mucous cells," Davis and Fox 1970).

Differential Diagnosis

Choroid plexus papillomas can be distinguished even by gross inspection from the coarsely lobulated but firmer ependymomas, by their more even surface and the delicately tufted, friable structure. Histologically, when their cells are markedly compressed, they are often mistaken for papillary ependymomas (see p. 269). Distinction of a tumor from simple cystic hypertrophy of the plexus, particularly around the glomus, is not difficult. Apparently lectin binding may help in differential diagnosis (W. Müller et al. 1980). Choroid plexus papillomas must, however, be distinguished from xanthomas of the plexus (Zülch 1956, Figs. 359, 360d; see also Wolf et al. 1950; Hu and Friede 1967; Kepes 1970).

Even in a study of the classical literature one is faced with the problem of eliminating all cases of metastasis of a cancer elsewhere in the body. There are many cases where it is easy to make this differential diagnosis. However, if no primary malignancy in the body is found, this does not justify definition of the cerebral tumor as a primary (anaplastic choroid plexus papilloma). Even at autopsies a considerable percentage of small primary carcinomas is missed (e.g., in the thyroid gland). Ceruminal malignant adenomas near the meatus acusticus may at first sight look similar in the H&E stain (see below, p. 283).

Biologic Behavior (Grading), Metastasis, and Recurrence

The ordinary plexus papilloma belongs to grade I in the WHO classification, the anaplastic forms to grades III and IV (see below).

Complete removal of plexus papillomas – which is difficult, however, since the tumor itself is so friable – can result in a permanent cure (NORLÉN 1950; but see also GUIDETTI and SPALLONE 1981, who give a worse prognosis). Small fragments can easily tear off and be liberated, and may lead to the artificial seeding of tumor "transplants." However, in some cases even normal papillomas are liable to diffuse widespread involvement of the external CSF pathway from a ventricular papilloma without any intervention [GP, Fig. 82; ZÜLCH 1938b, 1956, Figs. 247c, 248, 249: Here we have portrayed metastases of a choroid plexus papilloma of the left trigone into the cerebellopontine angle (cherry-sized) and parabulbar (bean-sized) (GP, Fig. 80)].

These cases, however, have to be distinguished from the rare multiple (?) choroid plexus papillomas. A CT scan can give the preoperative diagnosis if the pedicle is depicted (VEIGA-PIRES et al. 1978).

Clinical Course

In younger patients progressive hydrocephalus is not uncommon, usually with rapid development. Sometimes hemorrhages develop. Neurological signs such as hemiparesis may develop. Finally, papilledema may be present, associated with any other tumors signs, e.g., headache and vomiting. Such signs may indicate that oversecretion or obstruction of CSF has already developed. Reactions after ventricular or lumbar punctures can be disastrous.

"*Villous hypertrophy of the choroid plexus*" is a term coined by DAVIS (1924) for a condition portrayed by CUSHING (1925, Fig. 6), manifesting diffuse gross enlargement of both lateral ventricle choroid plexuses (for details see LAURENCE 1974, p. 588ff.).

Further References: WALKER and HORRAX (1947), RINGERTZ and REYMOND (1949), ZANDER (1949), KERNOHAN and SAYRE (1952), SKALA (1956), SEARS and BURNETT (1961), MORELLO and MIGLIAVACCA (1964), SZEGEDY and HUSZAR (1966), TAPTAS and ANDREADIS (1966), LEWIS (1967), NASSAR and MOUNT (1968).

15.3.4 Anaplastic Choroid Plexus Papillomas

Synonym: Choroid plexus carcinomas

Introduction

For the anaplastic (malignant) cases of choroid plexus papilloma a special subgroup is included in the WHO classification.

Historical Note and Definition

Disregarding the cases of metastases of body tumors falsely interpreted as cancer of the choroid plexus, an anaplastic dedifferentiation definitely occurs in choroid plexus papillomas (see LAURENCE 1974: 38 certain cases, 14 less certain). We had the opportunity of seeing personally the slides of two such anaplastic examples reported in the literature, namely those of CARDAUNS (1957) and VAN HOYTEMA and WINCKEL (1957).

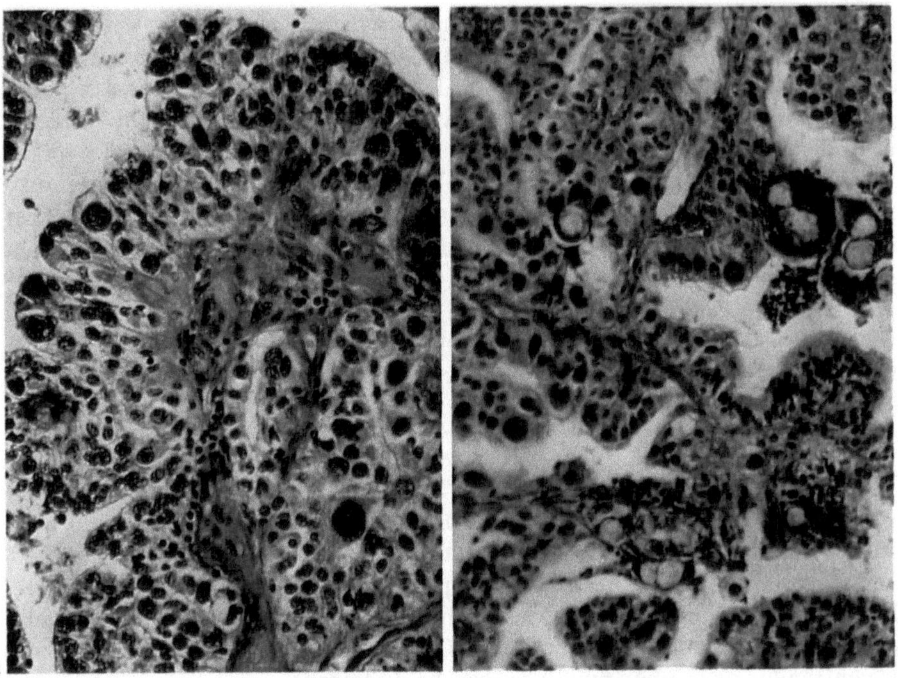

Fig. 80a, b. Anaplastic choroid plexus papilloma. The papillary type of basic architecture is present in other locations of the same tumor. Psammoma bodies are visible. In some locations the epithelium is even more irregular and in places the papillary structure is not retained, the epithelial cells and polymorphic giant cells being interspersed. H&E, ×125 (**a**) and ×200 (**b**)

Epidemiology (Age – Sex – Frequency – Site)

Since malignant choroid plexus papillomas are so rare, the epidemiology (preferential age, sex, site, etc.) has not been clarified.

Gross Pathology

The malignant forms have no particular characteristics in gross pathology.

Histologic Appearance

In the anaplastic cases the papillomatous structure is only partly preserved, and in parts it is completely blurred by a disorganized growth (HBT, Fig. 17a, b). Isolated papillae with almost normal structure are still seen and even some with psammoma bodies (Fig. 80) (appearing calcified in the CT). A few giant cells and mitoses may already be present, however. The architecture and epithelial pattern can nonetheless give a definite indication of the anaplastic transformation of the original choroid plexus papilloma.

Differential Diagnosis

Melanomatous tumors of the plexus have been described by Beatty (1972: later metastasizing) and similarly by Lana-Peixoto et al. (1977: no primary melanoma). A pigmented papilloma has been described by BOESEL and SUHAN (1979).

Ceruminal malignant adenomas invading the petrous bone around the cerebellopontine angle and advancing toward the brain can mimic a choroid plexus papilloma (see KLEINSASSER and SCHARFETTER 1957; SATO et al. 1973b).

As demonstrated (ZÜLCH 1938b) above (p. 281), choroid plexus papillomas, though histologically benign, can seed in solid gross tumors or metastasize diffusely (Figs. 80, 82). In either case clinical malignancy can result, with a fatal outcome for the patient.

Biologic Behavior (Grading)

The anaplastic forms correspond to grade III and IV.

Further References: VINKEN and SLOOFF (1965), P. LEWIS (1967), SHUANGSHOTI et al. (1971), RUBINSTEIN (1972), DOHRMANN and COLLIAS (1975), KIDA et al. (1978), CASENTINI et al. (1979), GULLOTTA and DEMELO (1979), VALLADARES et al. (1980).

15.4 Pineal Cell Tumors

15.4.1 Pineocytomas

Synonyms: Pinealocytoma, spongioblastoma of the pineal gland

Introduction

This term is used in the WHO classification to characterize an uncommon tumor composed of isomorphous pineal cells.

Historical Note and Definition

The reader is referred to the extensive discussion on classification of the pineal tumors on pp. 20, 286ff., and 414ff. The WHO classification has taken account of these controversial ideas in describing two groups that are apparently well defined. In a very different system of terminology HORRAX and BAILEY (1925, 1928) used the term of "spongioblastoma," which was not adequate because of the possibility of confusion with the genuine spongioblastomas (which are now termed *pilocytic astrocytomas*). Even the name pinealoma of spongioblastic type cannot be recommended. Pineocytoma according to the WHO definition has tumor cells with polar processes radiating toward the vascular stroma, and in specific silver impregnation for pineal parenchymal cell typical cells processes with club-like expansions at their tips may be seen, as originally described by DEL RIO-HORTEGA (1932). It is an *isomorphic* tumor (Fig. 81) with a certain weakly papillary pattern due to the above-mentioned orientation of the cells toward the vessels. This tumor type in the pineal region with an isomorphous or one-cell pattern is definitely rare. We were able to examine a tumor of this histological type thoroughly, which, however, did not infiltrate into the surrounding area; the tumor was of chestnut size.

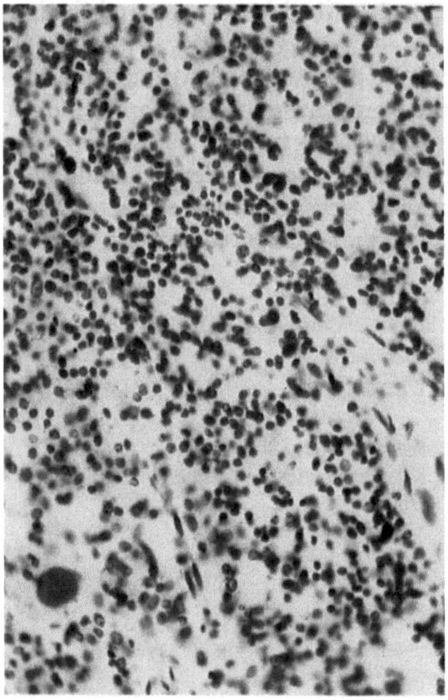

Fig. 81. Isomorphic type of pinealoma. The cells are medium sized and round or oval. Only single, somewhat large, hyperchromatic nuclei can be seen. Small lymphoid cells are lacking. Nissl, ×224

Epidemiology (Age – Sex – Frequency – Site)

Since up to now the tumors in the pineal region have not been sharply differentiated details of the frequency of these apparently rare tumors and their preferences with regard to age and sex have not been published.

Gross Pathology

Our well studied case was well delimited and did not show the typical infiltration of the adjacent tissue of some two cell tumors.

Histologic Appearance

The main characteristic is the isomorphous nature of the tumor cells, which show a certain papillary pattern. There is apparently no rapid growth, which would be reflected in mitoses. The tumor is very rich in cells, while the stroma is sparse. In summary, the main point is that the two-cell pattern is lacking and the cells are isomorphous, of medium size, and round or oval.

We have seen good examples in the paper of HORRAX and BAILEY (1928, case 5) and in the description of VAN WAGENEN (1931), in Fig. 55 of BENNETT (1946) and our own histological figure (ZÜLCH 1956, Fig. 253d).

Differential Diagnosis

It is important to distinguish this tumor from the two-cell pattern type of tumor and from pinealoblastoma. The latter is characterized by the typical picture of the medulloblastoma (see p. 327). It has the same cellularity, has isomorphous, particularly beet-shaped cells, with a tendency to form Homer Wright pseudorosettes.

Biologic Behavior (Grading), Metastasis, and Recurrence

In the WHO classification these tumors correspond to grades I–III, but none of the details and characteristics of this group can be specified with adequate precision, since this tumor is rare and most papers do not differentiate between pineocytoma and germinoma/pinealoma. According to our own observations pineocytoma must be more benign, since it probably does not infiltrate.

Further References: WURTMAN et al. (1964), RAMSEY (1965), CRAVIOTO and DART (1973), TABUCHI et al. (1973), KAWAGUCHI et al. (1975).

15.4.2 Pineoblastomas

Synonyms: Pinealoblastoma, medulloblastoma of the pineal gland

Introduction

This is a rare and highly cellular tumor, consisting of poorly differentiated cells resembling those of medulloblastoma. In the WHO classification it is listed as a special entity.

Historical Note and Definition

Among the vast number of papers on tumors of the pineal gland very few deal with this particular type, which, however, can be adequately characterized by the name of "medulloblastoma of the pineal gland", a name which I have suggested in addition to pinealoblastoma. The nature of the tumor is expressed best by this term.

Epidemiology (Age – Sex – Frequency – Site)

There is little information concerning this tumor group, but it can be characterized very well morphologically.

Gross Pathology

These are usually medium sized tumors, which can occur in the quadrigeminal region, where they reach a fairly large size; they infiltrate the surrounding tissue and appear as whitish or gray, friable, soft masses, displacing the midbrain downward and the pons caudally and sometimes extending to the foramen of Monro in the cephalad direction (see GP, Figs. 245, 246).

Histologic Appearance

The tumor resembles medulloblastoma so closely that no special description is required.

Differential Diagnosis

All details of the differential diagnosis are discussed in Sect. 15.4.1.

Biologic Behavior (Grading), Metastasis, and Recurrence

The tumor corresponds to grade IV, and behaves similarly to the medulloblastomas with regard to seeding via the CSF. It seems to be highly sensitive to radiation. Details about survival times are not available.

Further References: DE GIROLAMI and ZVAIGZNE (1973), NIELSEN and WILSON (1975), DE GIROLAMI (1977), GLASBERG et al. (1979), HERRICK and RUBINSTEIN (1978, 1979), KLINE et al. (1979), STEFANKO and MANSCHOT (1979), BORIT et al. (1980), KOIDE et al. (1980).

15.4.3 Pinealomas

Synonym: In recent times germinoma

Introduction

The WHO classification includes as entity only the germinoma as a prototype of the two-cell-pattern tumor, and in addition the pineocytoma and the pinealoblastoma (see p. 20).

The "pinealoma" of KRABBE (1916, 1923) has been abandoned as a separate entity, since most pathologists in the English-speaking world have adopted the concept by FRIEDMAN (1947) that this two-cell-type tumor actually corresponds to germinoma of the testis. For a detailed discussion see p. 414ff. In Europe and Japan the name of pinealoma is still in use for certain patterns.

Historical Note and Definition

The first case of pineal tumor is said by FUKUO (1914) to have been described by BLAUE (1800). VIRCHOW knew about the pathology of the pineal gland, yet only with the publications of WEIGERT (1875), OGLE (1898), OESTREICH and SLAWYK (1899), BAILEY and JELLIFFE (1911), and the detailed papers of MARBURG (1909, 1913), KRABBE (1916, 1923), ASKANAZY (1921), HALDEMAN (1927), BENDA (1932a), and particularly BERBLINGER (1922, 1926, 1930, 1944) was interest in pineal gland tumors aroused (see also later DE GIROLAMI and SCHMIEDECK 1973).

KRABBE (1916, 1923) coined the term pinealoma, while BERBLINGER (1922, 1926, 1930) preferred the "more correct" name of "pinealocytoma." An excellent review of the historical development and the then current state of knowledge about tumors of the pineal region was given by RINGERTZ et al. (1954), based on knowledge of 65 cases including 38 pinealomas (11 undifferentiated) and 11 teratomas. These authors subdivide the pineal tumors into undifferentiated and germinal types, and further, into ordinary two-cell-pattern types and finally the tumors with the pattern of the mature pineal gland. This apparently was the first use of the term two-cell-pattern tumor, now in common use.

In the discussion of germinomas I have mentioned the importance of Dorothy RUSSELL's (1944) idea that pinealomas are actually "immature teratomas," also that of FRIEDMANN and PLAUT (1935) and FRIEDMAN (1947) about the nature of germinomas and also the extensive description and analysis of KALM and MAGUN's case (1950) so excellently illustrated.

HERRICK and RUBINSTEIN (1979) distinguish amongst the pineal tumors the pineoblastomas histologically similar to medulloblastomas and the pineocytomas of which some show a more advanced differentiation of their elements towards astrocytes or ganglion cells or towards both.

I have discussed previously (p. 283) the arguments as to why a *dualistic* concept of the nature of the two-cell-pattern tumor is legitimate and asserted that germinomas and pinealomas exist as separate entities. I shall enumerate my arguments again at this point.

1. There is a difference in histologic appearance, particularly in germinomas, which commonly contain large, sometimes multinucleated, cells and the two-cell pattern is not as prominent as in pinealomas.
2. In our material the pinealomas were impregnated by Girolami's method and were PAS negative, whereas the opposite was true for the germinomas: they were PAS positive and Girolami impregnation negative.
3. SANO (1983a, 1985) reported a convincing observation of a difference in the fine architectural pattern of the cells between pinealoma and germinoma (see p. 414ff.).
4. MATSUTANI et al. (1975; see also MATSUTANI 1976) proved that immunologically the large cells of the two-cell-pattern tumor were derivates of the pineal parenchyma cells (see BARGMANN 1943).
5. Cells in the spinal fluid of patients with pinealomas had exactly the same cell pattern as was described by DEL RIO HORTEGA (see ZÜLCH 1963c, Fig. 1; and RIVERSON and ZÜLCH 1979, Figs. 3, 4).
6. GLOBUS and SILBERT (1931) drew attention to the similarity between pineal tumor cell patterns and the developing pineal gland.
7. The small lymphoid cells, according to KALM and MAGUN, are immature tumor cells, a concept shared also by Dorothy RUSSELL (1944) and FRIEDMAN (1947) (small maturating cells).
8. Ectopic tumors probably can be but are not necessarily primary tumors. Observations definitely show the seeding of a pineal tumor via the CSF into the pituitary stalk (see Fig. 82; and the case of KALM and MAGUN 1950, where this is demonstrated on large celloidin sections).
9. Pineal tumors of the germinoma/pinealoma type are frequently heavily calcified, and testicular tumors are not.
10. SANO (1985) emphasized again the dualistic concept and was of the opinion, that 20% of the "ectopic" type were also of true pineal origin.

The pinealoma described in this chapter, then, corresponds to the pinealoma of KRABBE (1923), with the histological characteristics defined above.

Our own classification, which is similar to that suggested by MAHAIM (1953), has the following groupings:

1. Teratoma
2. Germinoma (two-cell-pattern tumor)
3. Pineocytoma (one-cell-pattern tumor)
4. Pineoblastoma (medulloblastoma-like tumor)
5. Pinealoma (two-cell-pattern tumor)

Epidemiology (Age – Sex – Frequency – Site)

Age: The majority of the tumors of the pineal parenchyma make their clinical appearance between 11 and 30 years of age, but some also occur before the age of 10, and up to and beyond the age of 40. Our youngest patient was $1^1/_2$ years old, our oldest 74.

Sex: Patients with pinealomas are predominantly male (in our series 12.5:1; in an earlier review of 53 cases of the literature, only 9 were found in female patients, i.e., a ratio of about 5:1).

Frequency: Since up to now no distinction has been made between pinealomas in the strictly defined sense and germinomas, we must use the figures provided for germinomas. The percentage of these tumors in published neurosurgical series in the west is between 0.5% and 0.7%; the percentage in the Japanese and Chinese statistics is definitely higher, with 4%–5%.

From personal communications the figures I have obtained were similar [HANDA/Kyoto: 48 cases among 2250 intracranial tumors, i.e., 2.1%; KITAMURA/Fukuoka: annual incidence of around 4%; KATSURA et al. (1959): 3.1%; ARAKI and MATSUMOTO (1969): 5.4%; KALUMPAHETI et al. (1978) in Thailand: 4.14%]. During a recent visit to China I received similar reports of the incidence of these tumors.

Site: The pinealomas lie in the region of the quadrigeminal plate and usually displace this structure downwards, the posterior third of the corpus callosum upward, the thalami laterally while penetrating the caudal portion of the third ventricle. Eventually they may press the superior vermis downward and force themselves beneath the tentorium. They range in size from that of a hazelnut to that of a chestnut and grow mainly by expansion except for infiltration in the marginal zone.

Gross Pathology

The color of pinealomas is grayish pink, their consistency tough and hard, and sometimes friable if the tumors are calcified. Isolated small cysts may occur in the tumor substance (Fig. 82). Occasionally the pineal gland is still recognizable, being rather well demarcated from the tumor and displaced caudally (GP, Figs. 243, 244; see also DE GIROLAMI 1977).

Pinealomas can also have a suprasellar localization (so-called "ectopic" type). We have shown (Fig. 82) that this may be consequence of seeding, as in the case reported by KALM and MAGUN (1950: large celloidin sections). When these tumors occur in the supraoptic location they are particularly likely to infiltrate the optic chiasm (LEBLANC et al. 1976; see also our clinical experience p. 292).

Histologic Appearance

There is a typical juxtaposition of large clear cells (Fig. 83a) with large nuclei and small lymphoid elements arranged in bands and strands so that large cells

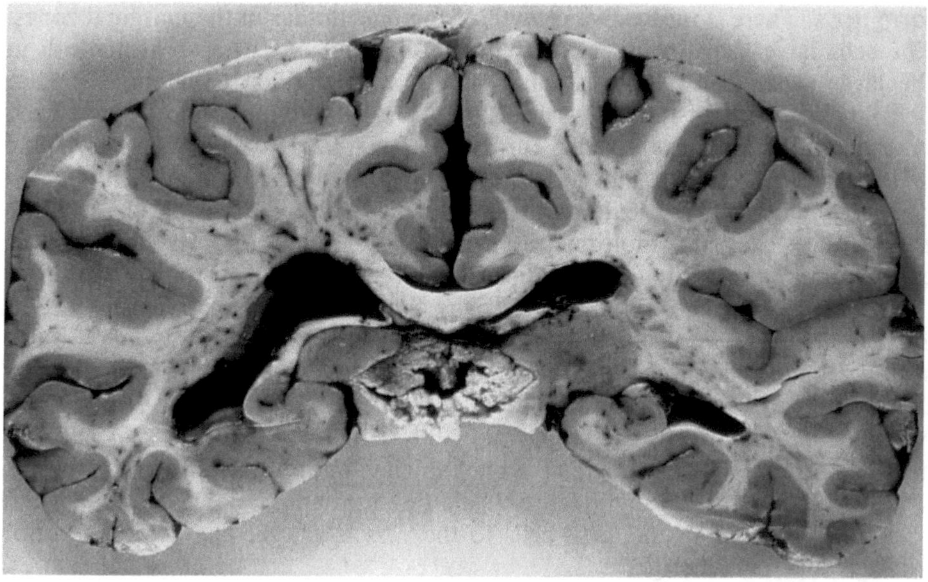

Fig. 82. Typical two-cell pinealoma with metastasis via the spinal fluid to the infundibular recess (see GP, Fig. 242 above, *arrow*)

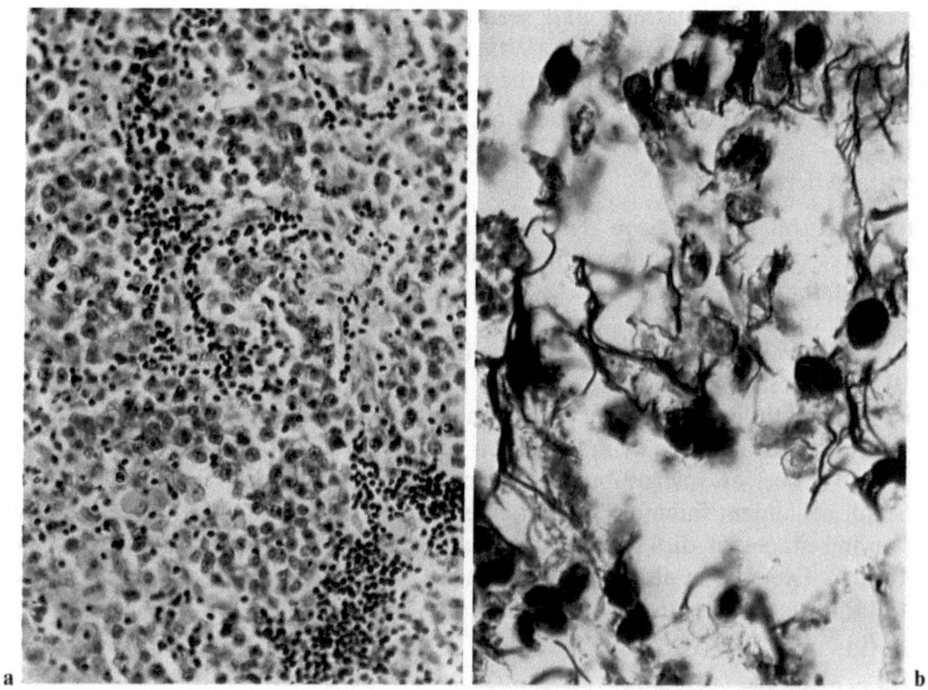

Fig. 83. a Typical juxtaposition of the large clear cells and the small "lymphoid" elements in the anisomorphic pinealoma. Cresyl violet, ×144. **b** Demonstration of fine and coarse processes in the larger cells of a "two-cell" pineal tumor. Girolami's impregnation, ×500

form nests. There is infiltrative growth of the pinealomas in the marginal zones. The cells have a distinctive nuclear membrane and one or several nucleoli in the large cells; there are commonly small vacuoles filled with lipoid (hyalin or colloid droplets of PAPPENHEIMER 1910). The small lymphoid cells have been interpreted as immature juvenile forms (UEMURA 1917) or a preliminary stage of the large cells (KALM and MAGUN 1950). KALM and MAGUN saw the small lymphoid elements particularly in perivenous accumulations in the seeding zones; giant cells and multinuclear elements do not occur. The tendency to calcification has already been mentioned.

The large cells can be impregnated by the technique of DE GIROLAMI and ZVAIGZNE (1973). With this method long processes with clubbed ends are observed (Fig. 83b), resembling those seen in DEL RIO HORTEGA's pictures of the pineal parenchymal cells. Blood vessels usually following the strands and bands of lymphoid cells are seen within the network. Small areas of necrosis may be present, but other regressive phenomena are unknown. NAKAZATO et al. (1978) have described ganglioneuroblastic differentiation. For SANO (1985) the particular relations of the large cells to the vessels are the characteristic proof for a genuine pineal origin.

Histochemistry

The demonstration of melatonin-synthesizing enzymes (SAT and HIOMT) and the occurrence of melatonin and serotonin within the tumor tissue support the diagnosis of a true pinealoma (WURTMAN et al. 1964; WURTMAN and KAMMER 1966; SCHMIDEK 1977), since these are found in the normal pineal gland (CRAVIOTO and DART 1973).

Electron Microscopy

Ultrastructural studies have described a variegated ensemble of cells within the tumors; three different specific cell types have been observed:

1. Undifferentiated large cells
2. Differentiated large cells
   a) Cells similar to the pineal primordium
   b) Cells similar to the pineal bud
   c) Cells with features of the pineal photoreceptor cells in lower vertebrates
   d) Cells with features of mammalian pineal parenchymal cells (club-shaped cell processes, microtubules, and smooth endoplasmic reticulum)
3. Small cells identifiable as lymphocytes and plasma cells; plasma cells show varying stages of differentiation (RAMSEY 1965; HOSSMANN and WECHSLER 1971a; TABUCHI et al. 1973; MATSUTANI et al. 1975; NIELSEN and WILSON 1975; KURUMADO and MORI 1976; MARKESBERY et al. 1976; MATSUTANI 1976)

Differential Diagnosis

Differentiation from the germinomas is important and can be achieved on the basis of various characteristics that we have already mentioned:

1. A less pronounced two-cell pattern
2. The occurrence of giant cells
3. The negative reaction with De Girolami's impregnation and the positive PAS stain

Distinction histologically from other tumors in the mesencephalic region, such as ependymomas, is relatively easy.

Biological Behavior (Grading), Metastasis, and Recurrence

Since the germinomas correspond to grade I–III the same applies to the pinealomas; nonetheless a distinction has been made in some large series. According to SANO (1976, 1983a), both pinealoma and germinoma are radiosensitive. Inasmuch as there is no operative mortality in SANO's series these tumors should be treated surgically. His Table 8 shows, surprisingly, that the survival time for pinealoma versus germinoma cases treated by direct operation and postoperative irradiation is different. Of the 20 patients with pinealoma only 66.9% survived for 10 years, whereas of the 22 germinoma patients 85.6% survived this long. This difference must be discussed again with reference to other larger series, since it does not correspond to the biological expectation, but may be a consequence of the high radiosensitivity of the intracranial germinomas and those in the testis.

Metastasis to other parts of the body has been reported for all the pineal tumors (TOMPKINS et al. 1950; KAWAGUCHI et al. 1975; BORDEN et al. 1973).

Clinical Course

Since in other series the patients had received shunts and radiation therapy comparison is not yet possible.

The best form of *radiation* has not been clarified; reports on radiation have been published by HORRAX and WYATT (1947, with excellent results), PERTUISET et al. (1976), ISHII et al. (1976), and SUNG et al. (1978).

It is of interest to note that the pioneer operations for tumors in the pineal region (details see ZÜLCH 1981) were performed by OPPENHEIM and F. KRAUSE in 1913 (probably a meningioma in the tentorial notch) and by Otfrid FOERSTER in 1928.

TÖNNIS was able to remove two teratomas (1935; WEBER 1939) and the descriptions of successful removals by PEET (1929), SACHS (1931), VAN WAGENEN (1931), and HARRIS and CAIRNS (1932) opened the way for routine removal of pineal and quadrigeminal region tumors.

Further References: HORRAX (1947, 1949, 1950), MÜLLER and WOHLFART (1947), HENSCHEN (1955), KAGEYAMA and BELSKY (1961), ARSENI et al. (1968), BOOKALLIL (1975), YONEMASU et al. (1975)

15.4.4 Suprasellar (Ectopic) Pinealomas/Germinomas

It still remains a problem – and we have discussed it above under *Site* (RIVERSON et al. 1973) – whether large suprasellar tumors with the two-cell pattern are primaries in that location or metastases from a primary tumor in the quadrigeminal region, which may be very small, as in our own case (ZÜLCH 1963c). These suprasellar germinomas/pinealomas have been well described by HORRAX and WYATT (1947) with respect to their typical location and clinical syndrome.

In the English-speaking world the suprasellar tumor is usually classified as a primary germinoma in the infundibular region. The other possibility, i.e., a seeding, has been shown in Fig. 251 in ZÜLCH 1956, in GP, Fig. 242 above, and finally in the pneumogram of our case in 1963 (Figs. 2 and 3). These cases must be taken as proof that seeding actually occurs. This is particularly well demonstrated in the case reported by KALM and MAGUN (1950).

On the other hand, WARZOK and ARNOLD (1972) believe they have proven that in their case the pineal gland was normal. DAYAN et al. (1966) refer to a "multifocal" pineal and "simultaneous" suprasellar tumor. SANO (1985) holds that only four-fifths of the suprasellar tumors are true germinomas.

The interesting case of FAN and AGBATA (1976) showed, in addition to suprasellar tumor, an accumulation of connective tissue in the pineal gland infiltrated by "lymphocytic" cells. The latter corresponded to the small tumor cells, and also a few large epithelioid cells were also encountered, which were identical with the suprasellar elements. It is difficult to decide where the primary actually originated, particularly, it seems, when the suprasellar tumor considerably outgrows a smaller pineal tumor (as in our clinical case; ZÜLCH 1963c).

The symptomatology is usually attributable predominantly that of the infundibular tumor and a well-known syndrome of inanition and diabetes insipidus and/or hyperphagia, endocrinological signs etc. may be present.

Other ectopic localizations are also known (see p. 414ff.): we have seen a typical two-cell-pattern tumor in the occipital cortex, which was successfully removed by operation (see ZÜLCH 1956, p. 355; KLEINSASSER and KLOSS 1958, Fig. 3). The patient had already survived for 14 years by the day of our check.

15.5 Neuronal Tumors

(Synonyms in the older literature: Ganglioneuroma, glioneuroblastoma, neuroastrocytoma, ganglioglioma, true neuroma, Purkinjeoma, Lhermitte-Duclos disease, ganglioneurome myélinique diffuse de l'écorce cérébelleuse; diffuse hypertrophy of the cerebellum)

Introduction

Among the neuronal tumors the WHO classification distinguishes the following five groups:

1. *Gangliocytomas* from mature ganglion cells
2. *Gangliogliomas*, the same tumor with an admixture of glial elements
3. *Ganglioneuroblastomas*, a mixed form from neurons of different levels of maturation from undifferentiated neuroblasts onward
4. *Anaplastic* forms of 1–3
5. *Neuroblastomas*, consisting only of undifferentiated neuronal cells

Historical Note and Definition

True gangliocytomas were first described by VIRCHOW (1863/65) in the sympathetic system and the subsequent cases observed by LORETZ (1870) and MANASSE (1896) followed. Most cases, however, were published only after the advent of the Nissl stain for ganglion cells. A decisive step forward was made with the "system of neuromas" devised by PICK and BIELSCHOWSKY (1911):

Neuroblastomas – Undifferentiated
Ganglioneuromas – Differentiating and differentiated
Ganglioglioneuromas – Differentiated, containing glia

In this area our knowledge has been enriched particularly by SCHMINCKE (1909/10, 1914), HERXHEIMER (1913), BIELSCHOWSKY and HENNEBERG (1928), COURVILLE (1930), CHRISTENSEN (1937), and above all, FOERSTER and GAGEL (1932a, b, 1933a, b).

In spite of these reports there is a considerable lack of clarity regarding the classification and interpretation of the variants of this group, however.

Gangliocytomas of the cerebral hemispheres and brainstem are fundamentally different from tumors of the same name in the cerebellum and peripheral nervous system. The first group, despite a large number of case reports, is still difficult to characterize. Biologically the individual cases show little uniformity, especially since they are apt to lie in inaccessible sites deep in the brain. However, the group located in the mediobasal temporal lobe, described by TÖNNIS and ZÜLCH (1939), differs from the others and is also readily amenable to surgical treatment.

One can subclassify ganglion cell tumors by particular names (e.g., "ganglio-glio-neuroma etc.) according to the content of glia, axis cylinders, and myelinated fibers. The typical gangliocytomas of the cerebellum, which are almost hamartomatous (Lhermitte-Duclos type), comprise a rare but definite subtype. Gangliocytomas most often contain immature cells, and those of the sympathetics, i.e., ganglioneuroblastomas are well known to general surgeons as predominantly benign tumors most commonly encountered in the thorax. The anaplastic (malignant) neuroblastomas (sympathoblastomas) of the adrenals and of the sympathetics have some resemblance. The gangliogliomas have been differentiated by WORCESTER (see Table 1 in COURVILLE 1931, for the older literature), and were described in detail by COURVILLE (1931). Excellent reports of single cases have been published by FOERSTER et al. (1933a, b, c).

The term of ganglio*neuroma* is incorrect (STALEY et al. 1967), since neuroma is a proliferative scarring in or on a peripheral nerve.

It seems important, however, apart from a histological classification, to distinguish three different types depending upon *location*:

1. Cerebral hemispheres, brain stem, and spinal cord
2. Cerebellum
3. Sympathetic trunk

As H.J. SCHERER (1934) pointed out correctly, in recording a diagnosis of gangliocytoma, special care must be taken not to misinterpret pre-existing ganglion cells, particularly in the region of the "nuclei" around the third ventricle, where neurons are densely accumulated. The demonstration of ganglion cells actually infiltrating the leptomeninges will prevent mistakes of this kind.

I have separated from the gangliocytomas and defined as (monstrocellular) sarcomas certain tumors that were first described in 1910 and 1914 by SCHMINCKE (p. 408). The term "ganglioglioma" is found in the literature, and this also leads to an erroneous interpretation of these tumors, which belong to the sarcomas as I hope to prove (see p. 410).

Epidemiology (Age – Sex – Frequency – Site)

Age: Since all neuronal tumors are rare it is difficult to determine their age incidence accurately. There is a definite predilection for the first 30 years of life. TÖNNIS and ZÜLCH (1939) described a series of operable tumors of the mediobasal temporal lobe, observed earlier already (but misinterpreted) previously by SCHÄR and CHRISTENSEN (1939). These patients had long histories; the average age at onset of symptoms was 11 years and the average age at operation was 19. The youngest patient of our entire group was 5 years old, the oldest 52 years. Gangliocytomas of the sympathetics are also found predominantly in childhood and adolescence.

Sex: The sex ratio seems to show a male preponderance of 6:4. Gangliocytomas of the sympathetics are thought to occur more often in women than in men.

Frequency: The neuronal tumors are rare. Of our 9000 cases 38 were gangliocytomas, i.e., 0.4%.

Site: In declining order of frequency the preferential sites for these tumors are as follows:

1. Cerebral hemispheres (particularly the medial part of the temporal lobe, where they form large cysts and calcifications and show a marked tendency to nodular growth within the leptomeninges).
2. Tuber cinereum and third ventricle (where they reach the size of a plum or a chestnut).
3. Pons and medulla oblongata (which they may invade diffusely).
4. Cerebellum (where they form dysplastic/hyperplastic-looking cerebellar folia within a circumscribed "neoplastic" region, particularly in the anterior lobe; Lhermitte-Duclos type).
5. Sympathetics (where a tough tumor with a partly necrotic interior may grow by expansion and vary in size from that of a chestnut to that of a child's head). The order of frequency within the sympathetic nervous system is lumbar, thoracic, and cervical. For tumors of the nonchromaffin ganglia see the section on glomus tumors (p. 474).

Gross Pathology

Most of these tumors are recognized as an enlargement of the infiltrated area (GP, Fig. 53). The surface may be nodular, with warts and lobules rising above the surface. The center may be cystic.

Histologic Appearance

The different forms (see above) must be defined separately; however, it is of fundamental importance to decide whether the cells under consideration are really ganglion cells at all and, if so, whether they are of neoplastic origin. The mere finding of a ganglion-like (ganglioid) vesicular nucleus with a large nucleolus is not enough. This can also be found in sarcomas (see Monstrocellular Sarcoma, HBT, Fig. 84b–d), carcinomas, proliferating connective tissue, and freshly reactive astrocytes. One can only be certain about such a diagnosis when there is definite Nissl substance in the cytoplasm or the tedious and difficult Golgi method positively (FERRER et al. 1979) demonstrates a neuron. This demonstration is only rarely possible with other "specific" methods for neurons.

1. When the *neuronal nature* of a neoplastic cell has been definitely established a more positive interpretation of *immature* precursor forms seems justified. Neurofibrillae, however, can only be rarely demonstrated in or at neuronal neoplastic cells.
2. The next step is to make certain of the *neoplastic nature* of the ganglion cells. Care should be exercised not to confuse a neuronal tumor with a gliomatous one invading a region of abundant nerve cells – for example, one of the large vegetative nuclei of the hypothalamus. The normal anatomy has to be kept in mind and the possibility that the cells are entrapped and have pre-existed there has to be excluded. Particularly noteworthy in neuronal tumors is the local abundance of reticulin fibers (Fig. 84a) in some of them, the cells often lying in groups and acini within small compartments of connective tissue (HBT, Fig. 3a, b). This latter situation is usually due to invasion and nodular growth of these tumors into and within the neighboring leptomeninges (HBT, Fig. 3c, d), as is particularly apparent in basal temporal forms, or it can be a malformated character of the region.
3. Finally, lymphoid infiltrates around blood vessels, such as are frequently seen in oligodendrogliomas, can often be observed in the marginal zone of the tumor. Their true nature (neuroblasts?) has not yet been ascertained. In an EM study ROBERTSON et al. (1964) found small cells with morphologic properties suggestive of immature nerve cells.

15.5.1 Gangliocytomas

Gangliocytomas of the cerebral hemispheres (see TÖNNIS and ZÜLCH 1939) can contain mature nerve cells (Fig. 85a, b), frequently neuroblast-like immature stages (Fig. 85b), and occasionally newly formed myelin sheaths; the mature neurons vary in size and form (Figs. 84b, 85; HBT, Fig. 2) and are accumulated in nests (HBT, Fig. 3), this being particularly characteristic for the basal temporal form. The neurons lie in acini encased by connective tissue stroma – mostly of the leptomeninges – and in some cases multinuclear nerve cells even occur. The presence of axons may be difficult to assess and they must be thoroughly differentiated from reticular fibers. Calcification is most uncommon in the tumor

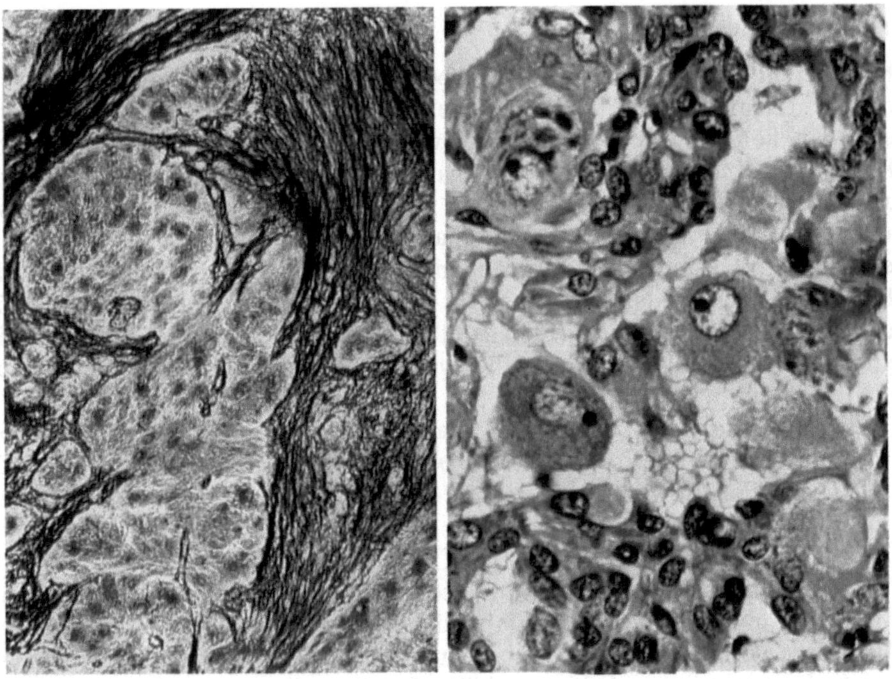

a b

Fig. 84. a Gangliocytoma: the extensive connective tissue with blood vessels leaves individual islands free, in which the ganglion cells are located. Silver impregnation, × 120. **b** Ganglioneuroblastoma: the tumor is composed of a complete spectrum of cells, from immature neuroblasts to mature ganglion cells. Gallocyanin, × 500

and the adjacent parts of the brain, except in the basal temporal tumors, where it may be radiologically characteristic (see TÖNNIS and ZÜLCH 1939, Fig. 8).

These gangliocytomas may be hard and they are frequently cystic in the basal temporal region (GP, Fig. 51). When infiltrating other parts of the brain they may be softer. In the mature forms their growth seems to be very slow; mitotic activity is very rare except in occasional anaplastic forms (see below p. 299).

Gangliocytomas of the *peripheral nerves* (HBT, Fig. 5a–d) may have parts which are medulloblastoma-like or consist of neuroblasts and many mitoses (HBT, Fig. 5a); or they may contain parts with mature ganglion cells (HBT, Fig. 5b, c), sometimes dysplastic and multinucleated; or finally, in the sympathetic there may be an admixture of undifferentiated cells, neuroblasts, and mature ganglion cells (HBT, Fig. 5d).

The *cerebellar* forms (Lhermitte-Duclos type) have a particularly characteristic appearance (Fig. 86) with large ganglion cells, corresponding to the Purkinje cell layer (GESSAGA 1980: total number in the literature 42 cases). However, it must be emphasized that other forms also exist in the cerebellum (see PROBST et al. 1979).

In the gangliocytomas of the *sympathetics* the mature forms consist principally of well-formed ganglion cells of the sympathetic type and a few less mature

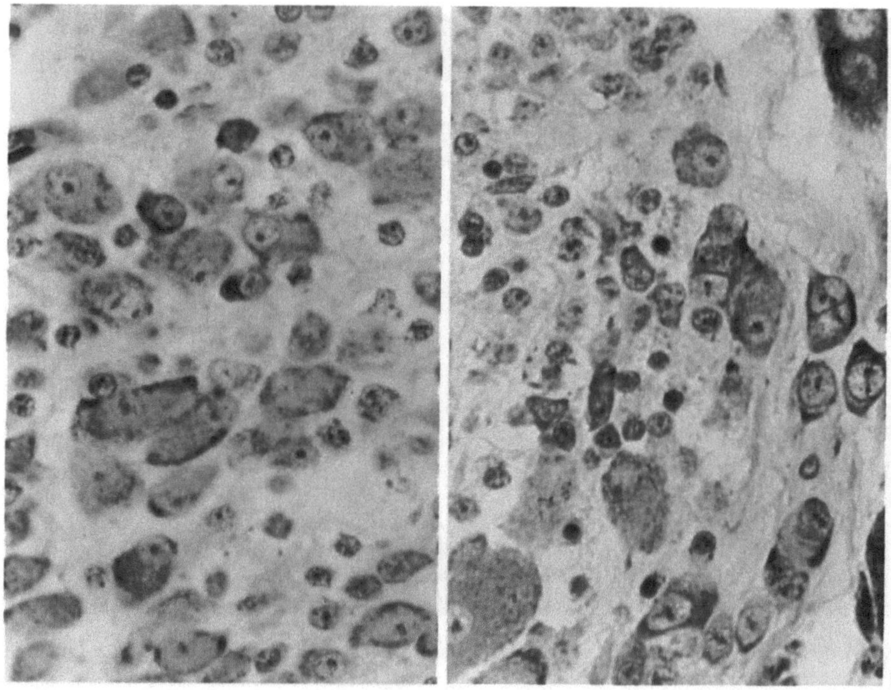

a b

Fig. 85a, b. Various patterns of the tumor cells in a gangliocytoma. Many cells have typical Nissl bodies and in between them lie the spindle or lymphoid cells of the interstitial tissue. In others the Nissl substance is present only as a fine powder. In other microphotographs "ganglioid" nuclei only are recognized, while the true nature of the cells can only be determined with certainty from other positions of the tumor. In the literature these cells are designated as "neuroblasts." Cresyl violet, × 500

representatives, which are encased in a thick network of axons and Schwann cells. The infundibular hamartoma-like tumors show axonal and dendritic reactions, bullous vacuolations, etc., as well as pleomorphic "blastomatoid astrocytes" (BEDWELL and LINDENBERG 1961; see p. 447).

Electron Microscopy

Three cell types can be found: (a) Large, well-differentiated neurons and their processes, varying in size and form. These neurons contain abundant mitochondria, lipid bodies, coarse bundles of neurofilaments and microtubules near the periphery of the cell membrane, branches of rough endoplasmic reticulum, and small areas of polyribosomes. Cell processes consist of numerous dendrites and less frequent axons. Clear and dense core vesicles and synapses also are frequently observed. Large nuclei with up to three or more macronucleoli have been seen. (b) Small cells, probably immature nerve cells. (c) Fibroblasts within a dense collagenous stroma.

Further References: ROBERTSON and HETHERINGTON (1964), ROBERTSON et al. (1964), LERMAN et al. (1972), PRITCHETT and KING (1978), FERRER et al. (1979).

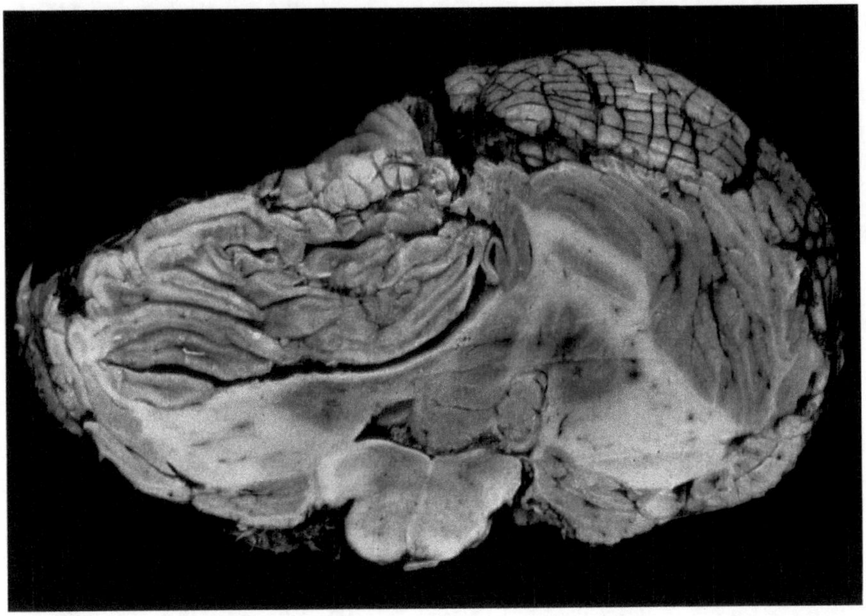

Fig. 86. A dysplastic variant of the gangliocytomas in the cerebellum (type: Lhermitte-Duclos)

Tissue Culture

The tumor is characterized in tissue culture by a very slow migration and a moderate number of highly dendritic cells (LUMSDEN 1971, 1974), but the potential of the cells for growth is low and their survival time is surprisingly short.

15.5.2 Gangliogliomas

It is thought that gangliogliomas are located in the temporal, parieto-occipital, or frontal lobe, the cerebellum, and the spinal cord (HENRY et al. 1978). They may be cystic and the neoplastic tissue only represented by a nodule. Histologically most of their cellular elements may resemble the pilocytic astrocytomas and are mixed with dysmorphic neurons. If they become anaplastic the malignant transformation is thought to involve the glial elements.

By electron microscopy three main cell types can be identified:

1. Well-differentiated ganglion cells.
2. Glia cells, corresponding to pilocytic astrocytes, the processes being filled with filaments. Rosenthal's fibers and granular bodies are also seen.
3. Mesenchymal cells adjacent to abundant collagen fibrils.

Tissue Culture

In addition to numerous neurites a proliferation of elongated bipolar glial cells corresponding to spongioblasts (GULLOTTA et al. 1970) has also been identified in tissue culture of this tumor type.

Further References: LEE and GLASAUER (1968), GULLOTTA et al. (1970), RUBINSTEIN and HERMAN (1972), PROBST et al. (1979), JOHANNSSON et al. (1981), NASS and WHELAN (1981).

15.5.3 Ganglioneuroblastomas

This entity contains a complete spectrum of neuronal cells of different levels of maturation (Fig. 84b) in transition from neuroblasts into mature neurons but the neuroblasts still forming the majority (see also Fig. 1 in DURITY et al. 1968).

Further Reference: GULLOTTA et al. (1973), who studied the neuronal cells by electron microscopy and enzyme-histochemistry and also the maturation in tissue culture.

15.5.4 Anaplastic (Malignant) Gangliocytomas/Gangliogliomas

Introduction

In the WHO classification a special entity is listed for gangliocytomas and gangliogliomas with areas of anaplasia. Neuroblastomas are not included in this class (see p. 301).

Historical Note and Definition

Reports of such tumors in the literature are scarce. But we must mention here the paper of TÖNNIS and ZÜLCH (1939) and ZÜLCH (1940).

We have observed a case of an 18-year-old boy with a tumor (ZÜLCH 1940) consisting of large dysplastic multinucleated ganglion cells (Fig. 87) which generally looked mature (HBT, Fig. 4a–d) in spite of the mitoses. The biologic behavior was that of glioblastoma multiforme, with death 1 year after operation.

When other signs of anaplasia including multinuclearity, a macroscopical resemblance to glioblastoma multiforme (GP, Fig. 52), and abundant mitoses occur in gangliocytomas and gangliogliomas, the tumors must be classified as *anaplastic* (KERNOHAN et al. 1932; TÖNNIS and ZÜLCH 1939; COURVILLE and ABBOTT 1955; RUSSELL and RUBINSTEIN 1962). However, this is rare. Furthermore, there are case reports in the literature from JENTZER and FATZER (1937), who described an anaplastic tumor in "ganglioneurofibromatosis" of autonomic nerves in the abdominal cavity, and another by STALEY et al. (1967), who also reported on ganglioneuromas (including several large EM pictures, of abdominal malignant tumors).

Biologic Behavior (Grading), Metastasis, Recurrence, and Prognosis

Postoperative recurrences are known even for the basal temporal forms, which, biologically, are quite benign (metastasis has only ever been described in one case). Due to the lack of experience, the question of recurrences cannot be answered with sufficient certainty, since the biologic behavior of the different

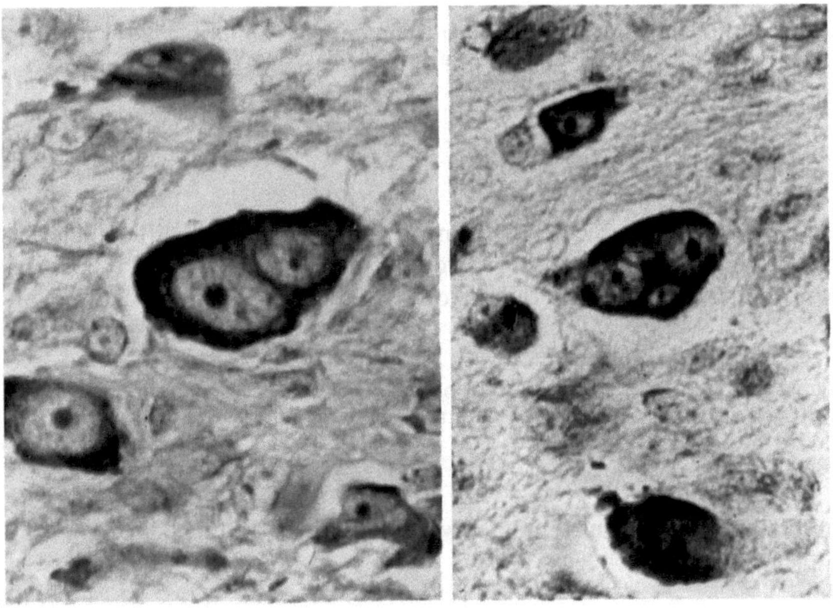

a b

Fig. 87 a, b. Multinucleated ganglion cells from a malignant gangliocytoma. All the cells are "mature". Biologically, the tumor behaved like a glioblastoma. Cresyl violet, ×648

forms of neuronal cell tumors has not been evaluated with any degree of reliability. SCHÄR and CHRISTENSEN (1939) and TÖNNIS and ZÜLCH (1939) reported the good prognosis of the group we identified as the "basal temporal gangliocytomas of the young." The operability of these lesions was emphasized further by DIBA et al. (1979). However, data recorded in the series of gangliocytomas of HENRY et al. (1978) put postoperative survival at 7 years.

In the *WHO classification* gangliocytomas have a probable biologic behavior assigning them to grade I, gangliogliomas to grade I and II, ganglioneuroblastomas to grade III, and anaplastic neuronal tumors to grade III or IV.

The neuronal cell tumors of the cerebrum and cerebellum may be readily operable and therefore of importance to neurosurgeons. Mature neuronal tumors of the sympathetic nervous system are often seen by the thoracic surgeons; they can easily be totally resected and do not recur. On the other hand, immature neuroblastomas of the sympathetics have a tendency to metastasize (also into the bone) and to recur.

Fourty-four years after successful resection of a gangliocytoma the growth of a second tumor, a meningioma, was noted in one of our cases by WALDBAUER (Erlangen, personal communication).

Clinical Course

The clinical course is determined by the site of the tumor and the slow growth so that a 4- to 6-year history of seizures may be noted with the more benign types.

Special Sites of Gangliocytomas

The *cerebellar* – hamartomatous – type (LHERMITTE and DUCLOS 1920) shows enlargement of the folia, leading eventually to obstructive hydrocephalus (GESSAGA 1980: 42 cases including two personal cases). Apart from this very particular type "typical" cerebellar gangliocytomas/gangliogliomas (PROBST et al. 1979; MØRK et al. 1979) also occur, which are easily identifiable by their neurons and nonmyelinated axons, and also by their glial, particularly pilocytic, elements.

The *infundibular* gangliocytomas (hamartomas) have given particular attention because of their typical symptomatology, including pubertas praecox (p. 447) (DRIGGS and SPATZ 1939; J.E. MEYER 1948; LANGE-COSACK 1951; SCHMIDT et al. 1958; for further references see BEDWELL and LINDENBERG 1961). However, there are other dissimilar gangliocytomas of the third ventricular and the infundibular region (genuine blastomas) which also have typical symptom clusters (diabetes insipidus, inanition and/or hyperphagia and sometimes somnolence etc.; see OSTERTAG 1936a, Fig. 118; BEAL et al. 1981).

Further References: MARCHAND (1907), ROBERTSON (1915a, b), OLIVECRONA (1919), BIELSCHOWSKY (1925), BIELSCHOWSKY and SIMON (1930), ALPERS and GRANT (1931), BAILEY (1932a), TÖPPICH (1936), AMSTAD (1937), WOLF and MORTON (1937), LICHTENSTEIN and ZEITLIN (1937), HEINLEIN and FALKENBERG (1939), SCHÖPE (1942), DE HAENE et al. (1953), COURVILLE (1958), LIST et al. (1958), BRUCHER and VAN DEN BERGH (1959), HALLERVORDEN (1959), CHRISTIAN (1961), COOK et al. (1962), RUSSELL and RUBINSTEIN (1962), DAUM et al. (1967), AMBLER et al. (1969), DOM and BRUCHER (1969), STEFANI and MEHRALIN (1971), RUBINSTEIN and HERMAN (1972), LEECH et al. (1977), DIBA et al. (1979).

15.5.5 Neuroblastomas – Retinoblastomas – Sympathoblastomas

Neuroblastomas

This is a tumor located in the intracranial compartment which, when it occurs peripherally either along the sympathetic system or in the adrenal gland, is referred to as sympathoblastoma.

Introduction

The WHO classification includes a separate entity among the neuronal tumors for neuroblastomas. The retinoblastomas and sympathoblastomas are added because of their resemblance. These tumors although controversial and difficult to interpret will be described here because of acceptance as a special entity by the WHO classification.

Historical Note and Definition

I discussed the definition and classification of a possible entity of neuroblastomas in detail as long ago as 1939. Nonetheless I disregarded this group for a long while, and rejected it again in 1956, where I referred to the fact that the neuroblastomas reported in the literature were so different in type that it would be not appropriate to form a single group of neuroblastomas. The "neuroblastomas" of the Hortega school are medulloblastomas (see p. 324).

KERNOHAN et al. (1932), in their classic work on neuronal tumors, had already defined neuroblastomas as an entity. A general description was attempted by HORTEN and RUBINSTEIN (1976) with reference to a series of 35 primary cerebral neuroblastomas. They distinguished three variants of this group, which they thought to be the largest single group of supratentorial neuroepithelial neoplasms in children, all of whom were referred to them from outside sources because of diagnostic difficulties. Their definition is only grossly clarified, however. May be that some of them were little differentiated "extraventricular ependymomas" (see p. 69).

Epidemiology (Age – Sex – Site)

Age: Most of the tumors arise in the first 3 years, and they are exceptional in adults.

Sex: The sexes are apparently equally involved.

Site: There is no special predilection and a cerebral and a cerebellar localization have been described (DURITY et al. 1968; SHIN et al. 1978).

Gross Pathology

There are no particular characteristics for this cerebral tumor group.

Histologic Appearance

These are highly cellular tumors consisting of small or even medium-sized dark lymphoid elements. The formation of pseudorosettes (Homer Wright) makes the diagnosis easier. Otherwise, attempts to differentiate the cells by impregnation are necessary, where caps and short slender plasmatic processes may be visible and sometimes even axons can be demonstrated by specific methods. They are closely packed and show a high degree of mitotic activity (ESCALONA-ZAPATA 1972, Fig. 4). Some of these tumors may be rich in reticular tissue, as are some of the gangliocytomas. – By employing techniques developed in recent years one can substantiate the diagnosis by the demonstration of catecholamines.

The neuroblastic precursors of neurons are naturally difficult to identify. It is easier when – as in some of our cerebral neuroblastomas – the nuclei show neuronal properties, e.g., vesicular structure with one or several nucleoli. However, the neuroblastomas sometimes resemble medulloblastomas so closely that they can hardly be distinguished.

The *electron microscopical* and *biochemical* studies may determine the neuroblastic nature precisely (dense core vesicles etc.) of the tumor.

Further References: EYRE-BROOK and HEWER (1962), KNUDSON and AMROMIN (1966), DALFORNO and GIGLIARDI (1968, for all neuronal tumors), LAERUM et al. (1978).

Differential Diagnosis

The problem of what sort of ganglion cell tumors should be included in the group of neuronal tumors is important, and has been solved in a preliminary fashion by the WHO classification. We have emphasized above (p. 292ff.) that considerable attention should be maintained before classifying a tumor as being of neuronal origin.

It is necessary to differentiate neuroblastomas from reticulosarcomas and other undifferentiated sarcomas, from medulloblastomas (which are extremely rare in the supratentorial space), and from oligodendrogliomas. [I emphasized years ago that ORZECHOWSKY and KULIGOWSKI's case (1933) was an oligodendroglioma.]

Biologic Behavior (Grading), Metastasis, and Recurrence

Neuroblastomas tend to grow rapidly and correspond histologically to grade IV. Metastasis may occur and recurrence is usual if the tumor is not totally removed and irradiated postoperatively.

Neuroblastomas may undergo spontaneous regression, or they may mature to ganglioneuroblastomas, gangliocytomas, or even to tumor patterns resembling neurofibromas or neurilemmomas, as has been emphasized in the literature. Cases of *familial* neuroblastoma tend to develop at an earlier ages. Yet most are diagnosed before the patients are 1 year old. Long-term survivors frequently have other tumors develop subsequently.

Further References: KNUDSON and AMROMIN (1966), MILLER and RAMSDEN (1966), JELLINGER et al. (1970a), HENRIQUEZ et al. (1973), AZARELLI et al. (1977), BIEDLER et al. (1978), RHODES et al. (1978), ROMANSKY et al. (1978), STRONG (1978), BOUDOURESQUES et al. (1980).

Retinoblastoma

Introduction

Retinoblastomas are malignant tumors composed of cells of the neural crest, arising from the retina in infants and young children; they are rarely congenital and rarely occur after the age of 5 years. Their elements are similar to the primitive ependymal cells and to the photoreceptors (Ts'O et al. 1969, 1970). EM studies revealing the occurrence of microtubules tend to confirm these similarities (ALBERT et al. 1970).

Historical Note and Definition

VIRCHOW (1863/65, II, p. 150) was of the opinion that these neoplasms might be related to brain tumors and were probably gliomas. However, the investigations by FLEXNER (1891) and WINTERSTEINER (1897: Wintersteiner's rosettes) suggested that they might be connected with the layer of the photoreceptors. FISCHER (1918: neuroblastoma) and MAWAS and DE AUTREVAUX (1930: retinocytoma) introduced the modern definitions. In BAILEY and CUSHING'S (1926, 1930) opinion, these tumors could be related to neuroepitheliomas based on the observation of the true rosettes that apparently consisted of primitive unipolar spongioblasts. GRINKER'S (1932) subdivision into the three groups of medulloepitheliomas, retinoblastomas, and neuroepitheliomas is only partly valid, because the formation of medulloepithelial cavities during tumor growth is probably artificial (see ZÜLCH 1956, Fig. 74c), moreover the separation of the more primitive forms into retinoblastomas and neuroepitheliomas depending on whether or not true rosettes occurred divides a tumor group with identical biological behavior throughout artificially into two subgroups with neither clinical nor biological significance (see also the EM investigations of BIERRING et al. 1967).

Epidemiology (Age – Sex – Frequency – Site)

Age: The preferential age period is in the 2nd to 4th years, with a peak in the 3rd year. The nonhereditary cases occur at a later age and are usually only unilateral.

Sex: A suggested preference for the male sex has not been confirmed.

Frequency: Retinoblastomas are rare tumors. Among 12000 patients with ocular disease at the University of Basel only one had retinoblastoma. JENSEN and MILLER (1971) estimated that there were 11 new cases per year per 1 million of population. MERRIAM (1950) figured the frequency of 0.001%–0.053% of all patients with ocular disease. The incidence of these tumors was reported as 1:18000 live births in the United States of America (see STRONG 1978).

Hereditary cases (VÖTISCH 1980) are common (40%). Familial occurrence was observed in one series of 84 patients with glioma retinae, in which 5 of the women who later married all had babies with retinoblastoma (see GEIGY, Folia ophthalmologica, Basel). There is little racial or geographical variation.

Site: These tumors, as implicit in the name, occur exclusively in the retina.

Gross Pathology

These are grayish, soft, brittle tumors, which can force the eye ball to protrude out of the orbita.

Histologic Appearance

The elements may be round or spindle shaped, or even polygonal, with a predominance of round cells. The nuclei are very rich in chromatin and in impregnation very fine cell processes are sometimes visible (see also MARCHESANI 1930). The number of mitoses and corresponding rapidity of growth is far greater than with medulloblastomas. The cells are arranged in bands and garlands but when they invade the vitreous body perivascular cell wreaths seem to prevail. Because of the very low vascularity of this part of the eye the tumor tends very early to become necrotic and only the perivascular portions are preserved.

Some canals and tubules may appear from the retina epithelium during the disorderly growth of the tumor, which must be distinguished from the true genuine (smaller) rosettes (Fig. 160) of the tumor tissue (HBT, Fig. 18a, b). There are many controversial opinions on the histology of this tumor, and particularly about the formation of the rosettes. The medullary epithelial canals (ZÜLCH 1956, Fig. 74c) must be distinguished (ZÜLCH 1956, p. 142) from other different types of rosettes, particularly those of various sizes. True rosettes and pseudorosettes were also the subject of discussion by GULLOTTA and LANZA (1965). POPOFF and ELLSWORTH (1971) reported that they found cilia with a "9+0" pattern. In spite of ultrastructure with the occurrence of microtubules the derivation is still not yet quite clear (are they primitive glia cells? neuroblasts? multipotential cells? photoreceptor elements?; see TS'O et al. 1969, 1970). The rosettes have been discussed with MEYER-SCHWICKERATH (1947), who investigated them on reconstruction and differentiated a ball and a bowl type. During this discussion I presented the opinion that true rosettes in the retinoblastomas (MARCHESANI 1930) and the true rosette in the ependymoma (ZÜLCH 1956, Fig. 231a) seemed to me entirely different structures and patterns (see also WIEDERSHEIM and HERZOG 1952, Fig. 10).

Electron Microscopy

EM studies have been reported by ALLEN et al. (1962), ALBERT et al. (1970), and POPOFF and ELLSWORTH (1971).

Biologic Behavior (Grading), Metastasis, and Recurrence

Retinoblastomas are highly malignant tumors (grade IV) with a tendency to metastasize to distant sites. WINTERSTEINER (1897) gave the targets of this seeding with the following order of declining frequency: brain and meninges, skull and face, regional lymph nodes, carotis, skeleton, liver, spinal cord, kidneys. PAARMANN (1952) encountered diffuse metastases along the hematogenous or lymphogenous pathway in three of seven cases and also found rosettes in the metastases, but this is rare. Recurrence must be expected after partial excision. Modern treatment consists in surgical excision, which is easier than for any other sort of similar "neuroblastic" tumor because of the early occurrence of visual symptoms and growth outside the skull. Therefore, a 5-year survival rate of 90% is recorded for cases diagnosed and treated by appropriate surgery while the tumor is still localized (DEVESA 1975). The mortality rate in black children is said to be 2.5 times that in white children (JENSEN and MILLER 1971).

The preferred surgical technique described by F. and A. PINTO (1959) is a combined intracranial and orbital operation.

Sympathoblastoma

Synonym: Neuroblastoma of the sympathetic chain

Introduction

The sympathoblastomas are by definition closely related to the neuroblastomas.

Historical Note and Definition

The sympathoblastomas were first defined as round cell or lymphosarcomas or hemorrhagic sarcomas, and then correctly described as originating from the sympathetic chain or the adrenals. The term neuroblastoma was used by WRIGHT (1910).

Like BAILEY (1932a) I pointed out early that most immature sympathoblastomas are very similar in malignancy and morphological pattern to the retinoblastomas and the medulloblastomas, and tried to combine these tumors and the pineoblastomas into a single group of medulloblastomas (of cerebellum, pineal gland, retina, respectively). However, this suggestion has never been generally accepted. The histology has been well studied by BIELSCHOWSKY (1932).

Epidemiology (Age – Sex – Frequency – Site)

Age: These tumors occur in all age groups; probably one-third occur in the first 2 years of life, and an additional 10%–15% are said to occur in older children. However, more than 50% are between 14–65 years (ORF 1972; MACKAY et al. 1976; DOSIK et al. 1978).

Sex: There is apparently no sex predilection.

Frequency: The frequency of sympathoblastomas in large series can be characterized by the following data. Among 223 malignancies in children (HOCH 1951) 87 were nervous system tumors, and of these 14 were sympathoblastomas. In a series of 16816 necropsies performed in Zürich between 1942 and 1951 only 15 were sympathoblastomas (DIETRICH 1952). BRONSON (1953) described 30 cases of sympathoblastoma in an aged population.

Gross Pathology

These are tumors the size of a walnut up to that of a child's head. Their consistency is soft and the outer surface often nodular. There is a connective tissue capsule with septa running through the interior. The cut surface may be whitish and yellowish or grayish pink or even grayish. Necrosis, yellowish fatty degeneration and earlier hemorrhages with a brown color are visible. The tumors all infiltrate the neighborhood and invade blood and lymph vessels agressively.

Histologic Appearance

For the classic description of sympathoblastomas we are indebted to BIELSCHOWSKY (1932). The histology of the sympathoblastoma is similar to that of neuroblastomas, but maturation and formation of higher stages and even of genuine neurons is far more common.

We find a closely packed tumor tissue containing lymphoid, dark, undifferentiated cells, (more highly developed) neuroblasts, and in some cases, genuine neurons. Fibers in these tumors, when they may occur be reticular tissue or axons. Differential diagnosis can be made only with the aid of specific impregnations. Glial elements are probably not present; these are thought to be distinctive when seen in tissue culture (MURRAY and STOUT 1947, 1948). For differential diagnosis the tests for secretion of catecholamines (MASON et al. 1957; CIESIELSKY-TRESKA et al. 1975) should be undertaken in order to differentiate this type of tumor from others. KLEINSASSER and MONTELEONE (1957) showed that sympathoblastomas are always positive for catecholamines, while Ewing's sarcomas are negative.

Biologic Behavior (Grading), Metastasis, and Recurrence

The biologic behavior is highly malignant (grade IV) and metastases are common. In adult patients the average survival in one study was only 11 months (Dosik et al. 1978; vast list of references). Surgical therapy plus radiation and particularly chemotherapy are strongly indicated. Metastases to skull, skeleton, lung, and liver, have all been described (Dietrich 1952), and the average age of the patients in these cases was 24.7 months while survival after the first manifestation of symptoms is only 5 months. Chemotherapy is now effective in about 80%–90% of cases (Bachmann 1979). Seeding into the leptomeninges has been described by Carrillo and Oribe (1939) and Biedler et al. (1978). Encephalopathy due to occult neuroblastomas can occur (Berg et al. 1974).

Other factors that must be borne in mind are the spontaneous regressions in children in the early years of life (Bachmann 1979: 10%; see also Buffoni 1955; Lo Schiavo and Amici 1971), and the clinical development of spontaneous cures in children with congenital sympathoblastoma with subcutaneous seeding and metastasis to the liver. There are small "sympathoblastomas in situ" (Beckwith and Perrin 1963), which are microscopic in size and have absolutely no metastases.

15.6 Poorly Differentiated and Embryonal Tumors

15.6.1 Glioblastomas

Synonyms in the older literature: Spongioblastoma multiforme, polymorphic glioma, gliosarcoma, "buntes Gliom"; most cases of "glioma teleangiectaticum" and "glioma apoplecticum" in the older literature belong to this group

Introduction

Glioblastomas are tumors with little cell differentiation, and as such described in the WHO classification with two variants, (a) *glioblastoma with sarcomatous component* (mixed glioblastoma and sarcoma) and (b) *giant cell glioblastoma.* This latter group is characterized by its bizarre (monstrous) cells, which some authors consider to be of glial, others of mesodermal, origin (see p. 408 ff.).

Historical Note and Definition

The malignant glioblastomas were recognized by Virchow (1863/65) as gliomatous tumors and can be found in each of the earlier classifications of brain tumors under the name of "variegated" ("bunt") or "hemorrhagic" gliomas or as "glioma apoplecticum" and "teleangiectaticum." Some were also classed under the term of "gliosarcoma" (for details see pp. 5, 322). Around the turn of the century a widespread controversy arose over the nature of this apparently neuroepithelial tumor type. Beginning with the name of the tumor itself the argument was directed to the question of possible sarcomatous components within the tumor. This controversy can be considered settled, since it has been possible (a) to separate true sarcomas from those tumors previously considered glioblastomas (see monstrocellular sarcomas, p. 407), and (b) to describe a special form of glioblastoma in which a sarcomatous component is apparent.

The modern histogenetic approach began with STRAUSS and GLOBUS (1918; GLOBUS and STRAUSS 1925), who deserve credit for the first precise description of this group, and with BAILEY and CUSHING (1926). The name of the tumor was then changed from "spongioblastoma multiforme" to "glioblastoma multiforme" (BAILEY and CUSHING 1926, p. 95). MANUELIDIS and SOLITARE (1971) mention that the term "glioblastoma" was probably used for the first time by MALLORY (1914) and is a final stage of the maturation line of RIBBERT (1918) (see p. 7). Glioblastomas appear in the works of ROUSSY and OBERLING (1932) as polymorphic gliomas are included in DEL RIO-HORTEGA's (1932, 1962) classification along with the "isomorphic" gliomas; KERNOHAN et al. (1949) considered that grade 4 and some grade 3 astrocytomas corresponded to glioblastomas.

Three histological subtypes of the malignant glioblastoma are well defined: round cell (globuliform), fusiform, and multiform variants. It has been definitely confirmed, however, that despite marked cytologic differences the biologic behavior of immature glial tumors is quite uniform. The "ensemble" evidenced by the common histologic features of fatty degeneration, necrosis, hemorrhage, and pronounced connective tissue reaction and proliferation, and particular the vascular changes with formation of large fistulous vessels, may be common to all three subgroups.

Other subgroups, proposed by BUSCH and CHRISTENSEN (1947a) and DAVIS et al. (1949), have not been accepted. Macroscopically the subgroups are not different nor well defined by the names used in the terminology of these authors.

Epidemiology (Age – Sex – Frequency – Site)

Age: The incidence of glioblastomas in various age groups is well known. They occur very rarely in the young (DOHRMANN et al. 1976a: 8.8% in children in a series of 488). They become more frequent after the age of 30 and have a definite peak around the ages of 45–65 (Fig. 9e, p. 88), being the typical gliomas of middle age and senescence. Our youngest patient was 7, and the oldest 78 years.

MÜLLER (1973) emphasized that in his series of tumors sited in the caudal brain stem, children of 6–15 years were particularly strongly represented; children were also strikingly often affected by glioblastomas of the cerebellum in the series of FRESH et al. (1976). However, clear and sharp definitions of this entity of glioblastoma multiforme are necessary for such unusual statements.

Sex: Our series of 9000 tumors included 674 male and 419 female patients with glioblastomas, i.e., male:female ratio of 6:4.

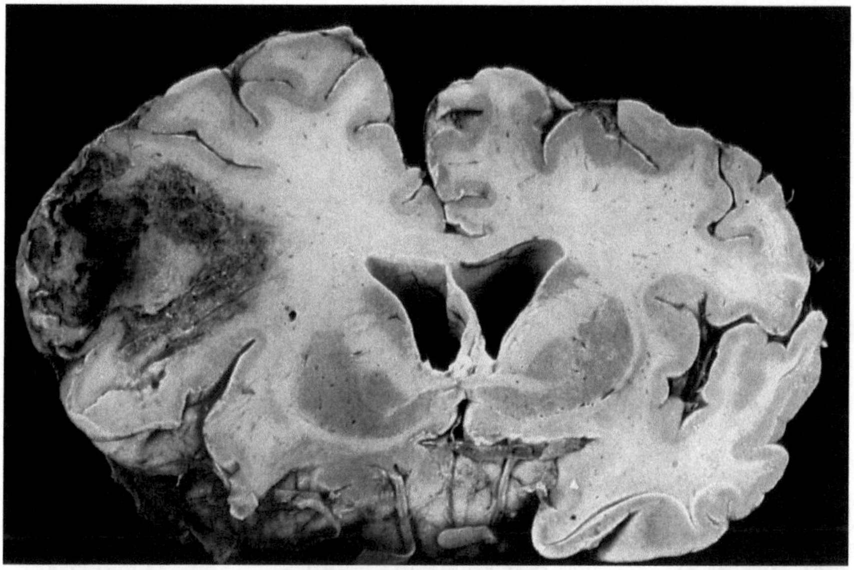

Fig. 88. Frontolateral glioblastoma with moderate brain swelling and minimal shift of the midline structures. Variegated patterns of necrosis can be seen within the tumor mass. (ZÜLCH 1975a)

Frequency: Glioblastomas constituted 12.2% of all our intracranial tumors in the series of 9000 cases. In the series of BAILEY and CUSHING (CUSHING 1932/1935) they represented 10.3%; in FOERSTER's material (see GAGEL 1938) 15%; and in that of DAVIS et al. (1949), 29.5%. In the series of MANUELIDIS and SOLITARE (1971) glioblastomas accounted for 17.5% of all intracranial tumors.

The highest frequency was found in the series of ELSBERG and GLOBUS (1929) and in the series of BENNETT (1946) with 22.9% (with the latter one has to consider the male preponderance since it was a "military" series).

Site: For glioblastomas it is now possible to point out specific sites of preference (p. 104). They occur in a *lateral frontal* position (Fig. 88, the size of a hen's egg), in the *third frontal* convolution (Fig. 14, no. 7), where they involve the subcortical white matter; in *dorsal frontal* locations (Fig. 14, no. 3; GP, Fig. 114) in the first and second convolutions reaching to the tip of the anterior horn (GP, Fig. 115); and in *frontal basal* locations (Fig. 14, no. 15) in the gyrus rectus and the adjacent lateral basal convolutions, from where they occasionally spread through the corpus callosum to the opposite side. Further caudally they are found in *lateral parietal* locations (Fig. 14, no. 21, Fig. 89), extending subcortically from the foot of the third frontal convolution through the middle and inferior parts of the pre- and postcentral gyri into the inferior part of the parietal lobe. In the *dorsal parietal* region (Fig. 14, no. 18; GP, Figs. 117–119), also subcortically located, they originate at the foot of the first and second frontal convolutions, extending through the superior third of the pre- and post-

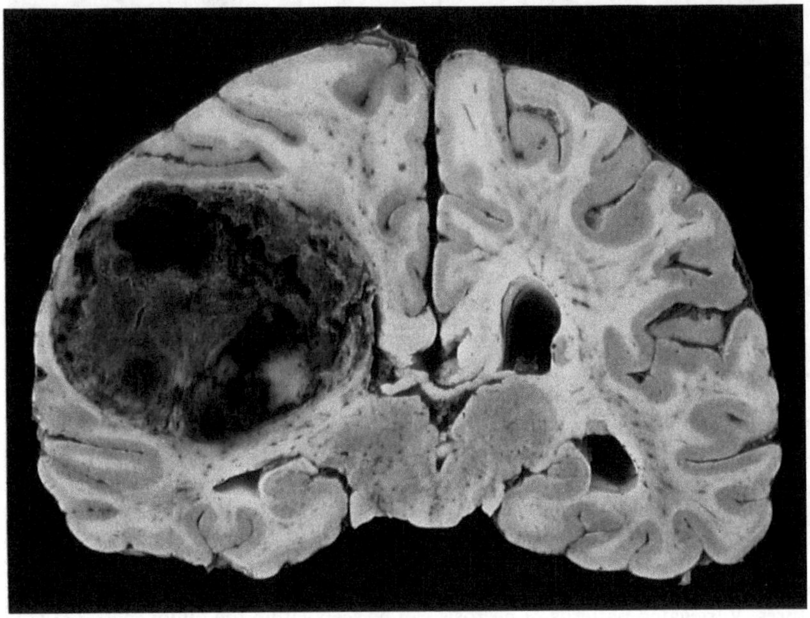

Fig. 89. Parietolateral glioblastoma with only slight midline shift. The falx has cut through the splenium of the corpus callosum. (ZÜLCH 1975a)

central gyri into the superior parietal lobe. In the *temporal* lobe we recognize (a) *lateral* temporal (Fig. 14, no. 25) and (b) *medial* temporal (Fig. 14, no. 26) glioblastomas. The lateral temporal (GP, Figs. 121, 122) forms extend from the temporal tip through the first and second convolutions and through the whole of the white matter of the lobe. The medial convolutions (GP, Fig. 123) remain tumor free in this instance. They are particularly affected in the medial temporal glioblastomas. The main bulk of the tumor lies in the adjacent white matter, with extensions spreading to the pole and the occipital lobe. Glioblastomas of the *occipital* lobe have either *lateral occipital* (GP, Fig. 124a, b) or *basal occipital* positions, and can grow across to the opposite side through the splenium of the corpus callosum. These types, however, have not been very clearly characterized. Certain glioblastomas loop from the frontal into the temporal lobe. They may spread in a *butterfly pattern* (Fig. 14, nos. 41, 42) from the corpus callosum (GP, Figs. 125, 126) deep into the white matter on both sides as *anterior* (Fig. 90) or *posterior callosal* ("butterfly") (Fig. 14, no. 42) glioblastomas. Alternately, they may infiltrate the white matter on one side only, as a glioblastoma of the anterior (Fig. 14, no. 45, Fig. 91) or posterior (GP, Fig. 128) *callosal radiation* (Fig. 14, no. 46), or finally, grow along the *fornix* (Fig. 14, no. 48; GP, Fig. 129), particularly in its frontal, parietal, or temporal sections. Glioblastomas are also found in the *thalamus* (Fig. 14, nos. 50, 52; GP, Fig. 130), but rarely in the region of the *quadrigeminal* plate (Fig. 14, no. 57; GP, Fig. 131) and only exceptionally in the *pons* and the *spinal cord.* Likewise they have been confirmed in the *cerebellum* only exceptionally (DOHRMANN and DUNSMORE 1975). Generally speaking, glioblastomas spread subcorti-

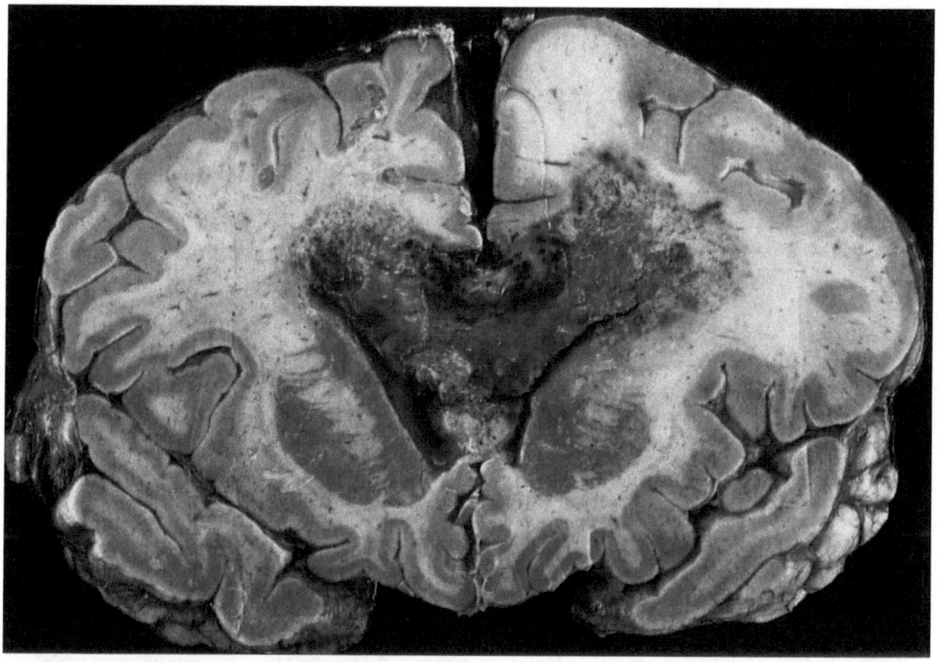

Fig. 90. Typical bilateral glioblastoma of anterior corpus callosum and left-sided white matter ("butterfly" distribution); considerable adjacent brain swelling

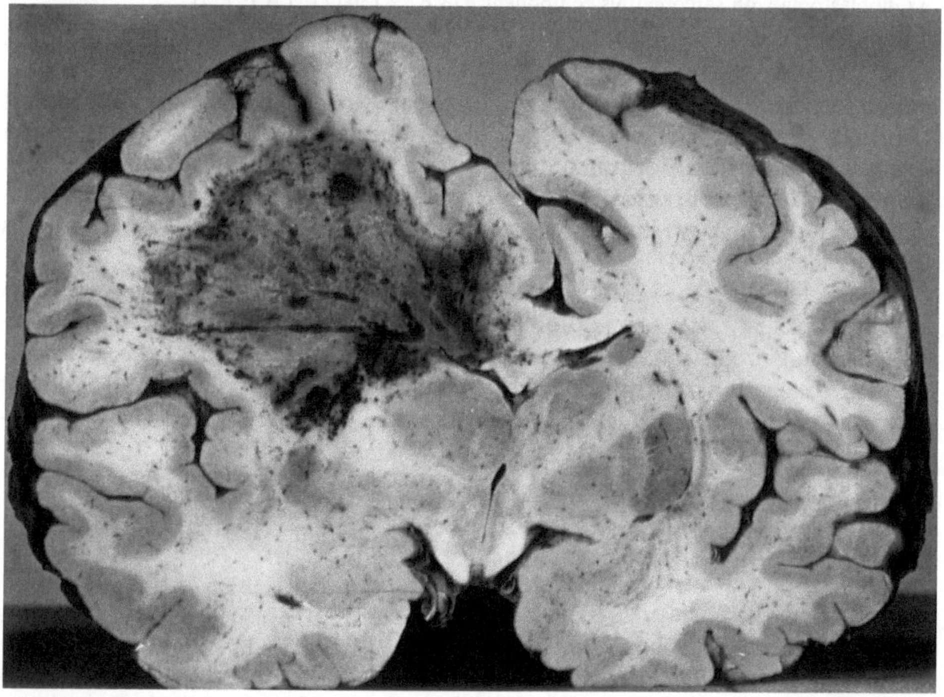

Fig. 91. Typical glioblastoma of the rostral radiation of the corpus callosum with considerable mass displacement to the opposite side. (ZÜLCH 1975a)

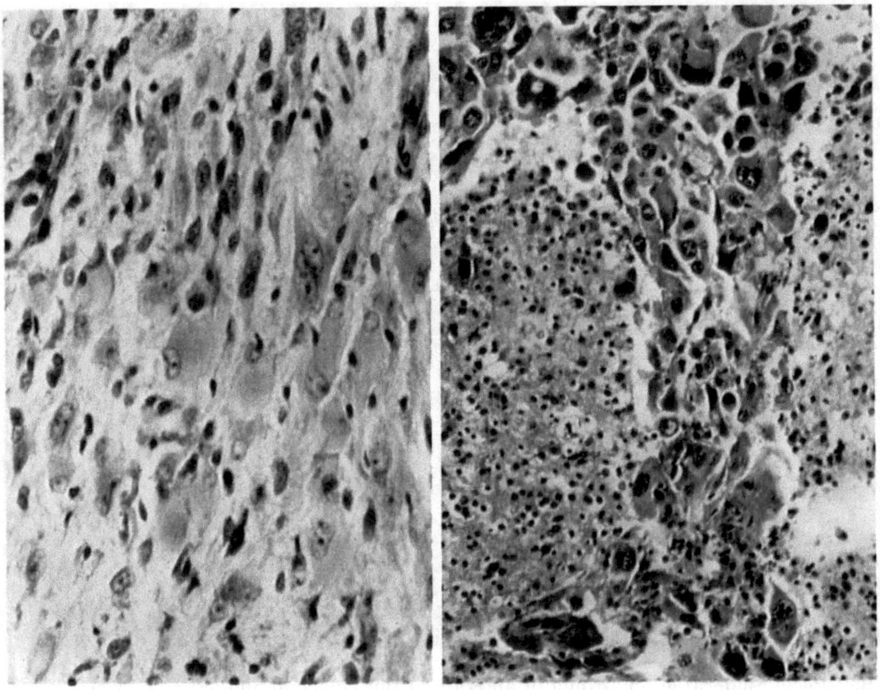

a b

Fig. 92. a Anaplastic degeneration of hard fibrillary astrocytoma (cf. Fig. 41). H&E, ×224. **b** Glioblastoma with sarcomatous component. H&E, ×130 (ZÜLCH 1975a)

cally. On frontal sections they may appear wedge shaped, like an infarct (Fig. 91). But they can also – especially in the temporal and occipital region – assume a cylindrical form and extend along the long axis of the lobe (Fig. 89). The almost "photographic" similarity possible between two tumors has been explained by their origin from certain "trouble spots" beside the ventricles (OSTERTAG 1936b, 1941).

It is interesting that the two malignant neuroepithelial tumors have almost mutually exclusive sites: medulloblastomas occur almost exclusively in the cerebellum, the glioblastomas almost exclusively in the other parts of the neuroepithelium. Exceptions to this rule are very rare. The two tumors are also almost mutually exclusive with regard to age incidence, but they have male predominance in common (see p. 93).

Gross Pathology

The variegated color which all glioblastomas, despite their cytological variations, have in common is explained by the necroses (Figs. 88–91 (gray), fatty degenerations (yellow, ochre yellow), and hemorrhages (Fig. 89) in various stages (brown to red) (GP, Figs. 119, 120). These different colored regions with their "geographic borders" alternate in the depths of the tumor with nondegenerated

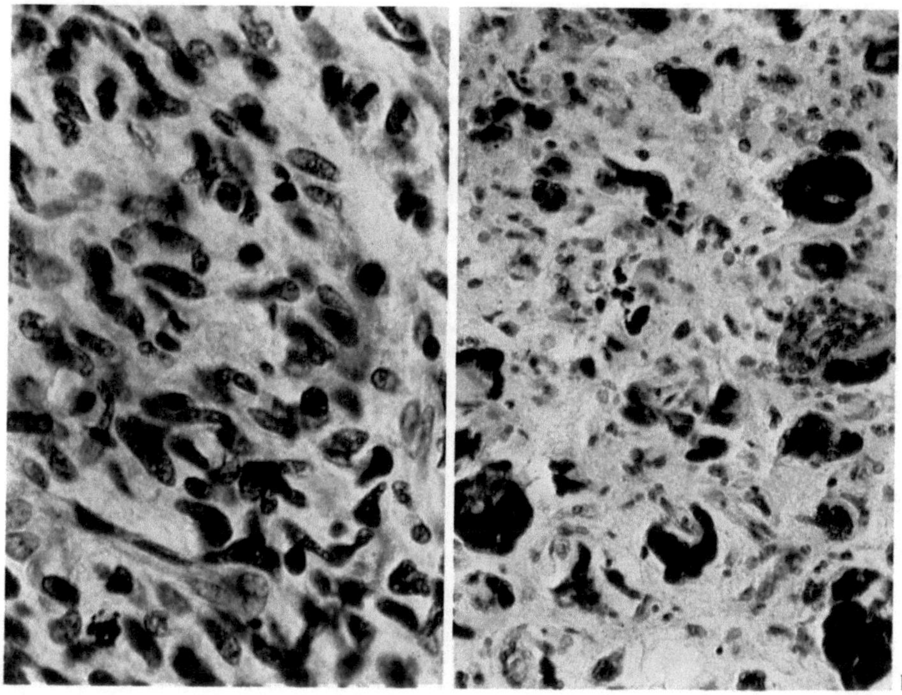

a b

Fig. 93. a Typical glioblastoma multiforme. Spindle cell glioblastoma with occasional giant cells and numerous mitoses. Cresyl violet, ×180. **b** Pronounced multiform glioblastoma with hyperchromatic giant cells and multinucleated cell complexes. Cresyl violet, ×180

marginal zones, which appear white, yellowish, and glassy. Occasionally, glioblastomas resemble a "necrotizing inflammation" (GP, Figs. 132, 135, 138). The tumor frequently cannot be differentiated from the surface of the brain, since it grows in the white matter and the convolutions only appear widened and flattened and the necroses are revealed only when the brain is cut. Dilated blood vessels, sometimes with lumina as wide as knitting needles (GP, Figs. 135, 136), surround many of the tumors or their peripheral zones. Only occasional vessels are thrombosed. They represent the surrounding "fistulous" or "lacunar" (Fig. 91) vessels and form a specifically recognizable pattern in arteriograms (usually in the parietal region: Kautzky 1948). Taken as a group, the glioblastomas are often more circumscribed than other gliomas.

Cases where gliomatous and sarcomatous tissue occurs in a mixture will been mentioned below (p. 322). Formerly they were interpreted as malignant gliomas with an extensive stroma, their genuinely mixed nature is now acknowledged by many authors (Rubinstein 1956; Mayo and Barron 1966; Simon 1970; Tsubokawa and Richardson 1975; Lalitha and Rubinstein 1979). This mixed variant of glioblastoma (Fig. 92b) has been listed as a separate entity in the WHO classification.

It is interesting to point out that a genuine sarcoma has been known to develop from a transplant of hyperplastic stroma from a glioblastoma (Greene and Harvey 1968).

a 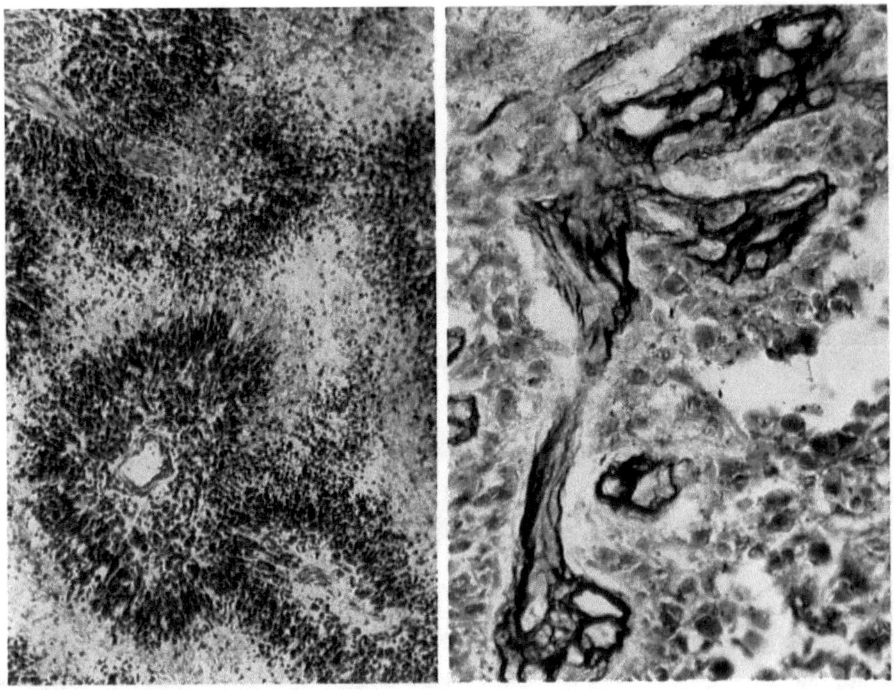 b

Fig. 94. a Band-like necroses in a glioblastoma. Pseudopalisading of the neighboring cells. Cuffs of cells are best preserved around the vessels. Cresyl violet, ×96. **b** Coil and loop formation of blood vessels in a typical glioblastoma. Silver impregnation, ×112

Histologic Appearance

The recognized subtypes of glioblastoma proper include the small round cell, the spindle cell (Fig. 93a), and the large cell (Fig. 93b) pleomorphic types (HBT, Figs. 42–44), depending on which cell type predominates. The most common is the spindle cell/fusiform element (Fig. 93a). On the whole, glioblastomas tend to grow along the fiber tracts or the vascular pathways, and occasionally have a streaming architectural pattern similar to that of pilocytic astrocytomas. Regressive changes result in architectural patterns, such as perivascular cell cuffs (Fig. 94a; HBT Fig. 50a) or pseudopalisading around necrosis (Fig. 95a). Reactive processes lead to "different" histological patterns, such as vascular proliferation (Figs. 94b, 96a) leading to dense networks of blood vessels (HBT, Fig. 45). Glioblastomas seem to grow outward toward the cortex. They occasionally penetrate and engulf the leptomeninges (but rarely form wart-like structures like oligodendrogliomas). The surrounding brain sometimes shows progressive astrocytic gliosis. – Sometimes astroblast-like elements may be encountered (Fig. 95b).

Tumor cells of the three subtypes afore mentioned produce scarcely any glial fibers visible in light microscopy; however, glial fibers are often demonstrated by electron microscopy. Scattered giant cells (Fig. 96b) naturally occur most often in the multiform type, however, also may occur in the fusiform

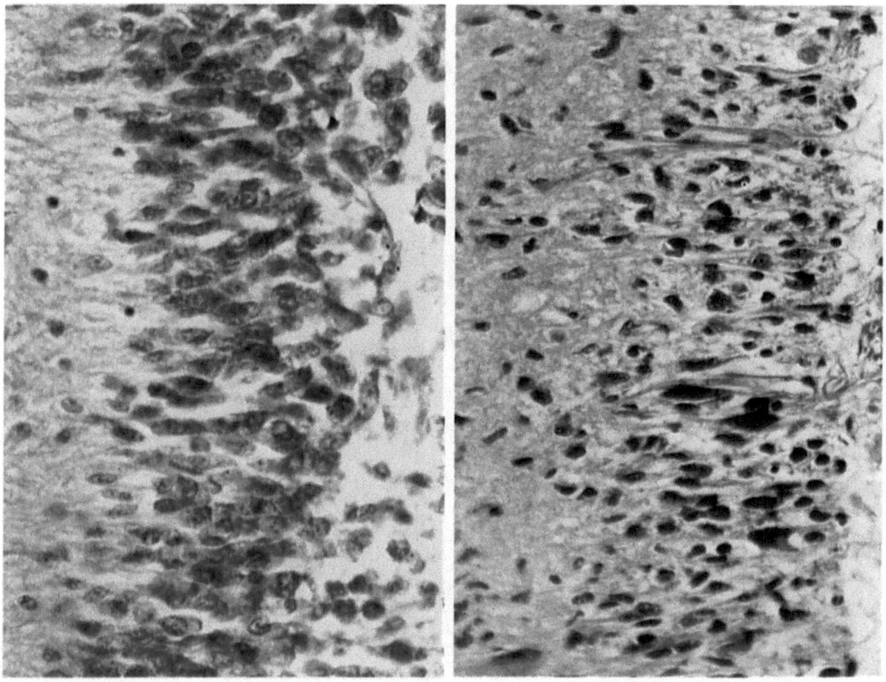

a b

Fig. 95. a Pseudopalisading of nuclei at the border of a band-like necrosis. Cresyl violet, ×256. **b** Astroblast-like elements in a multiform glioblastoma situated radially to the vessel lumen. H&E, ×212

type. The rarest are the round cell glioblastomas, which can occasionally arise from oligodendrogliomas. The speed of growth in all of these types is accelerated with a corresponding number of mitoses (Fig. 97). The connective tissue stroma in glioblastomas is very prominent (HBT, Figs. 45, 46). Large lacunar or fistulous vessels (HBT, Fig. 47) of predominantly venous type lie in the mantle zone of the tumor or in the immediately adjacent brain (GP, Figs. 135, 136). In the marginal zones there are numerous vascular coils and loops, which as part of reactive processes occur with great frequency and regularity along the margin of necroses (HBT, Fig. 49). We can distinguish a number of different forms of vascular reaction:

(a) capillary network (HBT, Fig. 46a); (b) barriers of usually glomerular vessels (Fig. 96a) around the margin of necrosis (HBT, Fig. 50c); (c) proliferation of the intima and adventitia of the endogenous blood vessels (HBT, Fig. 50d); (d) large, reconstituted blood vessels with endovascular proliferation (HBT, Fig. 47c); (e) remnants of larger vessels with outgrowth of fibroblasts from their walls (HBT, Fig. 48d); and (f) ectatic medium-sized to large blood vessels, endogenous or newly formed, which have fistulous dilatations and can form lacunar sinusoids (HBT, Fig. 47).

These arteriovenous fistulae or shunts give rise to *early veins*, i.e., the early filling of veins with light red, oxygen-rich blood, or the early appearance of venous channels in the angiogram. The blood vessels within the tumor have

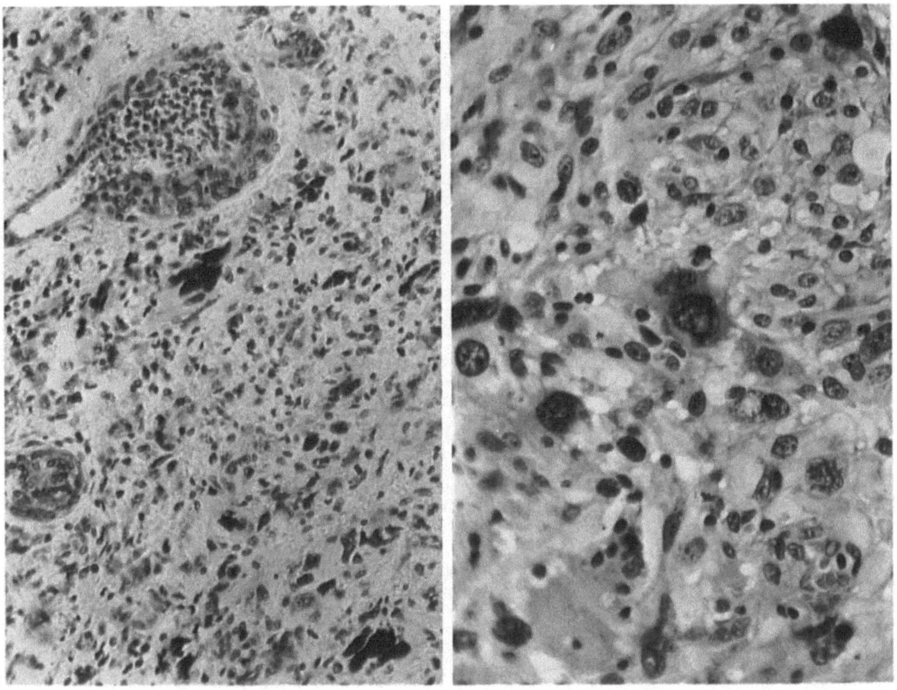

Fig. 96. a Hyperchromatic multinucleated cells, atypical, in many cases giant, mitoses and proliferations of vessel walls. Cresyl violet, ×84. **b** Mixture of multinucleated giant cells and smaller elements. H&E, ×240

a pronounced tendency to thrombotic occlusion (HBT, Fig. 47d). Whole regions of the tumor undergo (ischemic?) regressive fatty degeneration (HBT, Fig. 51) or acute necrosis. An early striking feature is the presence of layers of compound granular corpuscles at the margins of necrotic areas (HBT, Fig. 51c). The connective tissue forms part of the blood vessels and is also involved in the reparative organization of the necrotic regions by the formation of collagenous or reticulin fiber scars. Cyst formation is rare, and calcification exceptional. The excessive proliferation of the blood vessel walls and the high degree of ectasia of the giant lacunar vessels seem to be responsible for the fragility of the blood vessel walls (HBT, Fig. 47d) and the consequent occurrence of small and large hemorrhages. Glioblastomas spread almost purely by infiltration (contiguity), and rarely by seeding (SALAZAR and RUBIN 1976, see also p. 320). The permeated tissues and the tumor undergo necrosis rapidly.

Electron Microscopy

The work of RUBINSTEIN et al. (1973) noted the development of a progressive increase in glial filaments associated with an increase of free ribosomes and granular endoplasmic reticulum, which are apparently characteristic of the astrocytic series into which astrocytoma and glioblastoma may develop in tissue culture. Electron microscopy has revealed that the difference between glioblasto-

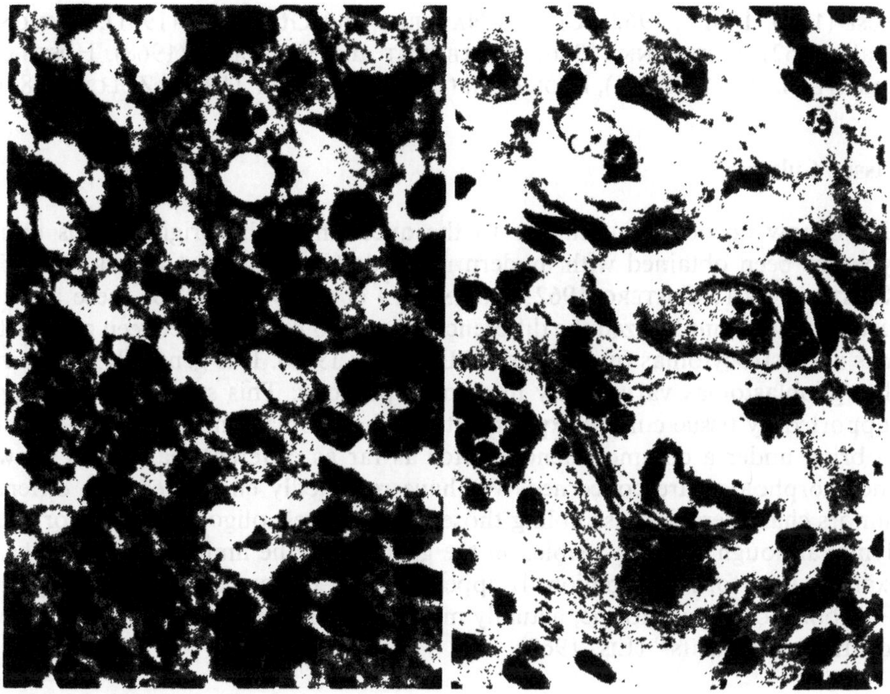

Fig. 97 a, b. Glioblastoma. Enormous number of atypical mitoses, in many cases highly atypical (after radium radiation). Cresyl violet, × 504

mas and isomorphous astrocytomas can be expressed partly by a higher degree of cellular variability and anaplasia (see CERVOS-NAVARRO and GULLOTTA 1961; TOGA 1976). Under the EM glioblastomas present an extremely cellular polymorphism (POON et al. 1971). The differentiation pattern of the cell varies from case to case, and within one tumor from region to region. The tumor cells have an irregular outline and have nuclei that are irregular in size and in chromatin distribution. The neoplastic cells in glioblastoma contain an increased or decreased number of normal or atypical mitochondria. While the Golgi apparatus is only rarely seen there are often many ribosomes frequently associated with the endoplasmic reticulum (ZÜLCH and WECHSLER 1968).

Some of the tumor cells and their processes contain numerous delicate intracytoplasmic glial filaments. This is evidence of astrocytic differentiation. Apart from protoplasmic and fibrillary tumor cells there are also transitional forms of polymorphous, immature, and anaplastic tumor cells. The latter are characterized by a cytoplasm with abundant free ribosomes, a minute Golgi apparatus, a decreased endoplasmic reticulum, and a low number of mitochondria, while the nuclei are iso- or polymorphous. TANI and AMETANI (1971) detected "curious characteristic stacks" of membranes on EM examination of some human glioblastomas; TANI et al. (1970) also found virus-like particles in EM preparations of glioma cultures, similarly to those reported by Dorothy RUSSELL (1932) and ROBERTSON and MACLEAN (1965) in light microscopy. For further details see

LUSE (1960, 1961 b, 1962), CERVOS-NAVARRO and GULLOTTA (1961), RAIMONDI et al. (1962), HOSSMANN (1966), SEHRBUNDT and SCHRÖDER (1968), HOSSMANN and WECHSLER (1971 a, b), POON et al. (1971), TANI et al. (1972), ZÜLCH (1981 c).

Tissue Culture

Up to now no definitive answer to the question of the origin of this tumor type has been obtained with modern methods (COSTERO and POMERAT 1955c; KERSTING 1961; COSTERO 1962; RUBINSTEIN et al. 1973). All of these authors just cited have emphasized the difference in in vitro behavior between glioblastomas and astrocytomas (in contrast to LUMSDEN 1963). It is generally recognized that glioblastomas vary widely in cytomorphology. This statement is strongly supported by tissue culture experiments: "The glioblastomas are most difficult to bring under a common denominator as far as different features of growth and morphology are concerned. We have repeatedly encountered in different tumors characteristics resembling those of astrocytes, oligodendroglia, or ependyma, although it is impossible, on the grounds of the limited number of cases examined, to form an opinion. It appears that a tumor classified histologically as glioblastoma multiforme, actually may arise from one or more of the abovementioned elements" (LISS 1962).

Histochemistry

Histochemical methods have already shown the significant difference between isomorphous astrocytomas and glioblastomas (LEHRER 1962; NASU and MÜLLER 1964; PERRIA et al. 1964). Nonetheless, the basic problem, concerning the transformation of an isomorphous astrocytoma into a glioblastoma multiforme, cannot be resolved objectively by these methods. Enzyme histochemistry of human glioblastomas demonstrates semiquantitative differences in the enzyme activity of the tumor cells, with special reference to the oxidoreductases. This variation in intracellular enzyme location is particularly striking in the polymorphous type of glioblastomas. In comparison with other isomorphous gliomas, such as oligodendrogliomas and astrocytomas, glioblastomas have relatively high levels of oxidative enzymes. This seems also to be a particular characteristic of the giant cells and proliferating vessels (NASU and MÜLLER 1964; KREUTZBERG et al. 1966). Other methods of defining malignancy in glial tumors have been discussed by VAN VEELEN et al. (1979; see p. 192ff.).

HANEFELD (1965, 1967) found higher glycoxidase activity in malignant than in benign tumors. In the giant cells of glioblastomas particularly he showed highly positive reactions for DPNH-D. NASU and MÜLLER (1964) depicted the alkaline and acid phosphatase and several oxidative enzymes as well as phosphoroxylase in a large series of gliomas. They felt that they had defined the specific activities of the blastoma cells and their pathologic vessels (see also the work of STAVROU et al. 1972 on LDH, and TAPER et al. 1971 on DNAse and RNAse).

Differential Diagnosis

Identification of this tumor is easy on sectioning of the fixed brain. The variegated color and the numerous necrotic areas allow a clear, early diagnosis. Histological differentiation from astrocytoma (Fig. 92a) and oligodendroglioma is more difficult if only a biopsy or the marginal zone can be studied. Oligodendroglioma is nearly always more highly cellular than the glioblastoma. The way to distinguish these three tumors from one another has already been presented in some detail in Sect. 15.1.1 (p. 219). At operation the surgeon will often recognize the true nature of the tumor when he encounters necrosis deep inside the tumor or when he recognizes the characteristic fistulous blood vessels containing arterial blood. However, he might already have deduced the malignant nature of these neoplasms from the presence of *early veins* or the pathologic vessels in the angiogram, that occur in 50%–80% of cases, or finally, *abundant edema*, *necroses*, and *hemorrhages* revealed by the CT scan.

Occasionally it is difficult to distinguish glioblastoma from monstrocellular sarcoma (see p. 410). Grossly, the latter does not usually appear so variegated, and cyst formation is more prominent than in glioblastoma. Necrosis is rare, and the tissue is fibrous and "asbestos-like."

Histologically, the disproportionately huge monster cells, the presence of spindle and monster cell regions side by side, and the isolated presence of generally hyperchromatic giant cells adjacent to capillaries in the surrounding normal brain all support a diagnosis of sarcoma. Large vessels that can be demonstrated by arteriography are more frequent in glioblastoma. Vascular budding of the capillaries in the marginal zone but outside the tumor indicate a monstrocellular sarcoma. In many cases differentiation is possible only after use of the reticulin stain. In sarcoma this reveals abundant production of fibers between the spindle-shaped cells, whereas in glioblastoma – in the regions that have not yet undergone regressive changes – the reticulin fibers are confined to the blood vessels. An exceptionally large proportion of mesodermal stroma is found in the glioblastoma with a sarcomatous component (see p. 322).

In all doubtful cases silver impregnations must be used. Biologically, however, there is little to distinguish the three kinds of glioblastoma; they all have similarly high malignancy (see pp. 39, 40).

Biologic Behavior (Grading), Metastasis, and Recurrences

The clinical picture of glioblastoma can be explained by the tumors' great rapidity of growth (accounting for short clinical histories) and the sometimes tremendous expansion of the tumor with concomitant edema formation. It causes increased intracranial pressure. Hemorrhages and thromboses of large vessels are responsible for the tendency to "apoplectiform" episodes. The particularly high degree of brain edema in the adjacent white matter, which often spreads to involve the entire hemisphere, is responsible for the early signs of raised intracranial pressure and herniation. A meningeal syndrome may be produced by a glioblastoma following the spillage of blood and lipid products (from tumor necroses and malignant cells) into the CNS (BERNAT 1976).

In the WHO classification all tumors classified as glioblastomas correspond to grade IV.

Metastasis: Metastasis takes place by way of the CSF (small ependymal nodules or implants along the ventricles, which can reach the size of a cherry (GP, Figs. 132, 133), but is never as diffuse as in the case of medulloblastomas; SPATZ 1938). They are reported to have the ability to spread by other pathways in addition, however (WISIOL et al. 1962; MOORE and EISINGER 1963). How rare cases of multifocal glioblastomas grow without no connecting bridges is not clearly understood (e.g., tumors in both the second and the third frontal convolutions and in the occipital lobe simultaneous as we have seen in four of our own cases; see GP, Fig. 134).

Many reports in the literature describe extracranial metastases. The young age of most of such patients with extracranial metastases consider two possible sources of error: (a) whether the diagnosis was correct; and (b) whether the tumor is not rather a monstrocellular sarcoma, with which extracranial metastases would be more commonly seen (GRAMPA and BAROLDI 1958; LEY et al. 1961: patients of 22 and 28 years; NIGOGOSYAN et al. 1962; WISIOL et al. 1962: patient of 31 years; MANUELIDIS and SOLITARE 1971; EL GINDI et al. 1973: young patients; KRETSCHMER 1974b: listing of 42 cases and extensive literature; YAO et al. 1975).

Recurrence: Even after radical excision all glioblastomas recur within a short time and chemo-/radiotherapy (pp. 142, 150) has not basically changed this fact. This leads me to call glioblastoma the "real cancer of the brain," a disease rather than a tumor (ZÜLCH 1969a).

Clinical Course

Short preoperative histories and postoperative survivals characterize the average course of glioblastomas. The postoperative survival was defined at 9–15 months before the introduction of modern forms of nonsurgical therapy. Apoplectiform episodes, seizures, raised intracranial pressure, and herniation have often been seen in the clinical course of such tumors (see above, p. 139).

In recent years the prognosis of glioblastomas has been changed slightly by the introduction of combined radio-/chemotherapy, but not dramatically (GULLOTTA and BETTAG 1967; WEIR 1973; TAKEUCHI and HOSHINO 1975; YAMASHITA and GILLINGHAM 1975; POUILLART et al. 1976; BRISMAN et al. 1976; ILSEN et al. 1982).

The average postoperative survival, which used in favorable cases to be 9–15 months (JELSMA and BUCY 1969), is occasionally increased now to 18–24 months, or even longer in cases where the diagnosis of glioblastoma is precisely correct and may depend from surgery, location and rapidity of growth.

Special Forms of Radiation: As long ago as 1954, KLAR et al. (cobalt radiation) reported survival times of 3–4 years in cases where I had checked the histological diagnosis. On the other hand, SHAW et al. (1978) deny that fast neutron irradiation is effective.

All these discussions depend on a correct diagnosis and on the factors affecting survival time (TAKEUCHI and HOSHINO 1977). SCHRÖDER et al. (1968a, b) had cases of glioblastoma with surprisingly long survival times (as also PALMA et al. 1978) when lymphocytes in the tumor – perhaps by way of immune reactions? – apparently induced longer preoperative histories and postoperative survival times.

Origin of Glioblastomas

The origin of glioblastomas, like that of most glial tumors, has not yet been clarified. *Heredity* has been suggested for rare cases by ZÜLCH (1951), who reported two brothers with parietal glioblastomas in their sixties, and by KOCH and MIDDENDORF (1960), who reported three sisters aged 50–54 years, all with glioblastomas. Whether morphological investigations will provide any information in the future (e.g., LAPHAM 1959) is uncertain. Dorothy RUSSELL (1932) reported on nuclear inclusions suggestive of viral activity. This has been put in doubt, however, since ROBERTSON and MACLEAN (1965), for instance, showed that in glioblastomas there were protoplasmic inclusions in nuclear folds. – There are also observations of glioblastomas in the scars after leucotomy (HEYCK 1954) or a brain wound (NOETZEL 1953; see p. 74).

Particular importance in the composition of the glioblastoma must be attached to the sometimes excessive proportion of mesodermal stroma (see Sect. 15.6.1.1).

It is not yet clear why these vessels are not formed in other highly malignant tumors as medulloblastomas, yet in many metastases (as well as in gastric carcinomas and in osteosarcomas; see p. 127; ZÜLCH 1959a).

By chance we observed the formation of such vessels around a small intracerebral metastasis from a glioblastoma that was not yet necrotic (see GP, Fig. 133). But why such obscure secondary formations were regularly induced is still not known. When I called glioblastoma the cancer of the brain and almost more of a disease than a real neoplasm (Symposium Cologne 1961: ZÜLCH and WOOLF 1964) my intention was to characterize the common features of these glial tumors, in which either the cells (multiforme) or the stroma (mixed forms) are predominant in different cases.

Glioblastoma is a tumor that must be defined as having a primary origin and growth. Only atypical forms would arise from a typical fibrillary astrocytoma with very slow growth (Fig. 41; GP, Fig. 95; HBT, Fig. 27). The most extraordinary and impressive feature of this group is that it has hardly ever yet been possible to induce it by the usual chemical carcinogens in the hundreds and thousands of attempts made in various laboratories throughout the world (p. 54).

Further References: BERGSTRAND (1933), HASENJÄGER (1938, 1939a), NETSKY et al. (1950), PERRIA and SACCHI (1950), KERNOHAN and SAYRE (1952), SCHIEFER and UDVARHELYI (1954), STORRING and DUGUID (1954), UDVARHELYI et al. (1955), TÖNNIS and WALTER (1959), ROTH and ELVIDGE (1960), GRACE et al. (1961), LEY et al. (1961), MATSUKADO et al. (1961), JELSMA and BUCY (1967, 1969), SCHRÖDER et al. (1968a, b), ZÜLCH (1969a), RUBINSTEIN et al. (1973), SIPE et al. (1973), DOHRMAN and DUNSMORE (1975).

15.6.1.1 Glioblastomas With Sarcomatous Component

Synonym: Mixed glioblastoma and sarcoma

Introduction

This is a tumor belonging to the group of glioblastoma multiforme which contains a sarcomatous component, originating through malignant transformation of hyperplastic vascular elements.

Historical Note and Definition

The term gliosarcoma (see p. 5) was coined early in the development of pathology, but certainly for two different types of tumor: (a) very highly cellular, undifferentiated tumors such as medulloblastoma, oligodendroglioma or even some meningiomas; and (b) tumors we would now classify as glioblastoma multiforme, particularly if the amount of stroma was pronounced (see p. 126; Stroebe 1895; Storch 1899; Borst 1902a).

The entity listed in the WHO classification was excellently described by H.H. Meyer (1937). He published very instructive illustrations of glioblastomas with a component of very firm, apparently sarcomatous stroma, in which vascular proliferation was also prominent: for these reasons it is considered a "mixed" tumor. Feigin and Gross (1955), Feigin et al. (1958), and Rubinstein (1956) have given good descriptions of such cases.

In this context we would also mention the concept of Spatz (1938) regarding the significance of abundant vascular formations in glioblastoma ("gliosarcoma"). This particular feature of glioblastoma (Russell and Rubinstein 1977) presents an interesting problem for general neuro-oncology, namely the comparison of gliosarcomatous mixed tumors in man with experimental brain tumors (Zimmerman and Arnold 1940; Zimmerman 1962, 1967; B. Schiefer 1958, 1964; Greene and Harvey 1968).

In our series of experimental tumors (B. Schiefer 1958, 1964) we induced an oligodendroglioma with a sarcomatous component by cells developing and swarming out from the vessels, ultimately forming monster cells.

Gross Pathology

Macroscopically the hard consistency of some parts of the tumor is conspicuous and this malignant mesodermal component may even predominate in some cases.

Histologic Appearance

Microscopically, apart from the typical glioblastomatous pattern a network of reticulin and even collagenous fibers may prevail, and hyperplastic vascular elements may be formed.

Electron Microscopy

EM seems to be helpful in the distinction of gliomatous and sarcomatous parts of the tumors (Hossmann 1966); the high resolution power of the EM may make it possible to recognize and identify single traces of extracellular collagen.

Biologic Behavior (Grading)

All tumors classified as glioblastoma correspond histologically to grade IV in the WHO classification.

Further References: RUBINSTEIN (1956), MAYO and BARRON (1966), SIMON (1970), PEÑA and FELTER (1973), TSUBOKAWA and RICHARDSON (1975), MORANTZ et al. (1976), LALITHA and RUBINSTEIN (1979).

15.6.1.2 Giant Cell Glioblastomas

Synonyms: See also "Monstrocellular Sarcoma", p. 407

Introduction

The WHO classification includes this subgroup of glioblastoma for a form having a predominance of bizarre (monster) giant cells with many nuclei, frequently showing an abundant reticulin network in their stroma. However, the same entity has actually been interpreted by other authorities as a monstrocellular type of sarcoma (see p. 407; my first descriptions: ZÜLCH 1940b, 1953a; SEITZ and KALM 1958; BRUCHER 1962; KERNOHAN and UIHLEIN 1962; BINGAS 1964a).

Historical Note and Definition

As defined by the WHO, the tumor is typically granular in consistency and more definitely circumscribed than the usual glioblastoma, is often cystic, and showing no age and sex preference. In vitro the monstrocellular sarcoma behaves morphologically very differently from other tumors of the glioblastoma group (KERSTING 1961; KREUTZBERG et al. 1966). *Histochemically* there are more similarities than differences between glioblastomas and monstrocellular sarcomas.

In analyzing tumor cells it is sometimes difficult to decide whether an element is of glial or mesodermal origin, but this cannot be proven except by identification of typical glial or collagen fibrils, which can be provided by special stains or impregnations or by EM examination. Therefore, it is of interest that monstrocellular sarcomas consist to varying degrees of cells with discrete intracytoplasmic filaments. These filaments also can be detected in glial cells, in the cells in meningiomas (KEPES 1961a, b; RAIMONDI et al. 1962; YOSHIDA et al. 1962; HIZAWA and WECHSLER 1966: fibrosarcomas), and within reactive Schwann cells (BLÜMCKE 1965; BLÜMCKE and NIEDORF 1966). It is understandable therefore that KERNOHAN and UIHLEIN (1962) classified this entity as a subtype of fibrosarcoma, viz. giant cell fibrosarcoma or monstrocellular sarcoma. Their Figs. 5 and 6 illustrate an intracerebral fibrosarcoma and a typical monstrocellular sarcoma of the brain. The EM observations obtained from two monstrocellular sarcomas revealed the anaplastic nature of the tumor cells *and their* mesodermal character (their Fig. 7).

From the standpoint of EM it is still open to discussion whether (a) there is a particular type of giant cell glioblastoma that is different from monstrocellular sarcoma; and (b) monstrocellular sarcoma may also contain a certain amount of a glial component.

My personal opinion is that there are two types: a typical glioblastoma with very large giant cells that nonetheless do not have the "monstrous" character of the sarcoma cells, and the sarcoma with its very typical, gigantic cells up to 400 μm in size (SCHMINCKE 1914), which is of mesodermal character. Tissue cultures support the assumption that these sarcomas arise from the adventitia of the cerebral blood vessels. Typical giant cells are seen in the vicinity of the tumor in "free" tissue, swarming out from blood vessels with pathologic hull cells. This acounts for the inclusion of monstrocellular sarcoma in the group of "tumors of the blood vessels."

Further References: HADFIELD and SILVERBERG (1972), ARJONA et al. (1978), TANI et al. (1978); see also p. 407 "Monstrocellular Sarcoma."

15.6.2 Medulloblastomas

Synonyms in the older literature: Glioma sarcomatodes, isomorphic glioblastoma, neuroblastoma, granuloblastoma, embryonic neurogliocytoma, neurospongioma, spheroblastoma. Many tumors previously described as "meningeal sarcoma" also belong in this group

Introduction

The very well-characterized and well-known medulloblastoma is included in the WHO classification with two variants; desmoplastic medulloblastoma, with a substantial component of fibrous connective tissue; and medullomyoblastoma, which is characterized by the occurrence of striated or nonstriated muscle cells.

Historical Note and Definition

Medulloblastomas were first described as an entity under this name in 1925 by BAILEY and CUSHING, although pathologists had previously known and already described them as "glioma sarcomatodes," "meningeal sarcoma," "diffuse sarcomatosis of the meninges", and "spongioblastoma" (KAUFMANN 1902). The symptomatology and biologic behavior of medulloblastoma were outlined in CUSHING'S study (1930). At present, we regard the medulloblastoma as a neuroepithelial tumor. The idea of NISHII (1929) and GULLOTTA (1967a, b), that it is a sarcoma, is no longer accepted. Most "medulloblastomas" of the cerebral hemispheres have turned out on close investigation to be tumors of another type, often oligodendrogliomas. HORTEGA'S group tends to interpret medulloblastomas as neuroblastomas (POLAK 1967) with "neuroblastic" and "spongioblastic" differentiation. My own first detailed investigation on this group (ZÜLCH 1940c) defined both its nature and its growth.

Epidemiology (Age – Sex – Frequency – Site)

Age: Medulloblastomas are well known as the malignant cerebellar tumors of childhood and adolescence. The peak incidence falls between the ages of 7 and 12 years (Fig. 9f). However, occasional cases occur as early as the first weeks of life (see PAPADAKIS et al. 1971) and as late as the fourth decade.

In the Memorial Sloan-Kettering Cancer Center series (see ALLEN and EPSTEIN 1982) the younger groups had a higher incidence of primary seeding. The idea that all patients above 20 years of age have tumors of a desmoplastic nature in the cerebellar hemispheres has been shown to be false by MÜLLER et al. (1978).

Our youngest patient was 6 months old, the oldest 53 years. The average age of patients with cerebellar medulloblastomas was 7.5 years in the series of INGRAHAM and MATSON (1954) and 13.8 years in the patients of RINGERTZ and TOLA (1950).

Sex: According to CUSHING (1932, 1935), boys are affected 3 times more frequently than girls. In a series of 4000 brain tumors we had 159 patients with medulloblastomas and performed a demographical analysis. Of these 114 were males and 47 females, a ratio of around 2.5:1. In our series of 9000 cases the ratio was only 7:3, and in the series of MÜLLER et al. (1978), only around 8:5. These discrepancies are not yet explained.

Frequency: The medulloblastomas make up 20% of all brain tumors of childhood and adolescence, but only 8.8% of tumors occurring after 20 years of age. In our series of 9000 tumors they comprised 4.2%, in CUSHING'S series (1932, 1935) 4.3%, in the series of RINGERTZ and TOLA (1950) 6.5% of the *total.* In a series reported by KEITH et al. (1949) they accounted for 20.1% of brain tumors in children; in a collection of 1792 *gliomas* reported on by various authors 10% belonged to the medulloblastoma group.

Site: Most medulloblastomas lie in the inferior cerebellar vermis, into which they spread from the roof of the fourth ventricle, and they can reach the size of a tangerine (Fig. 98). From this site they expand in all directions, but infrequently (1 out of 6 cases) do they have with their main part in one hemisphere (Fig. 99). This proportion is higher in patients over 15 years of age (see above). The fourth ventricle is filled with the tumor projecting down from above and is usually enlarged, while the vermis is compressed into a thin lamella on the upper surface of the tumor. With further growth, tongues of tumor (GP, Fig. 163) may push between the cerebellar tonsils into the cisterna magna, as in the case of the ependymomas, or less commonly extend into the cerebellopontine angle. Medulloblastomas also occur, though rarely, in the pons. Medulloblastomas in the supratentorial space are exceedingly rare and their classification requires particular care, when they are reported in this location.

Heredity: Of special interest is Cushing's experience with identical twins with medulloblastomas (see LEAVITT 1928). I know of a similar observation (see GRIEPENTROG and PAULY 1957; BICKERSTAFF et al. 1967: in brothers). There are also isolated case reports in identical twins (KOCH 1964).

Gross Pathology

Grossly, the medulloblastoma often appears (GP, Figs. 165, 166) well circumscribed. However, at its margin it invades diffusely the surrounding tissue (GP,

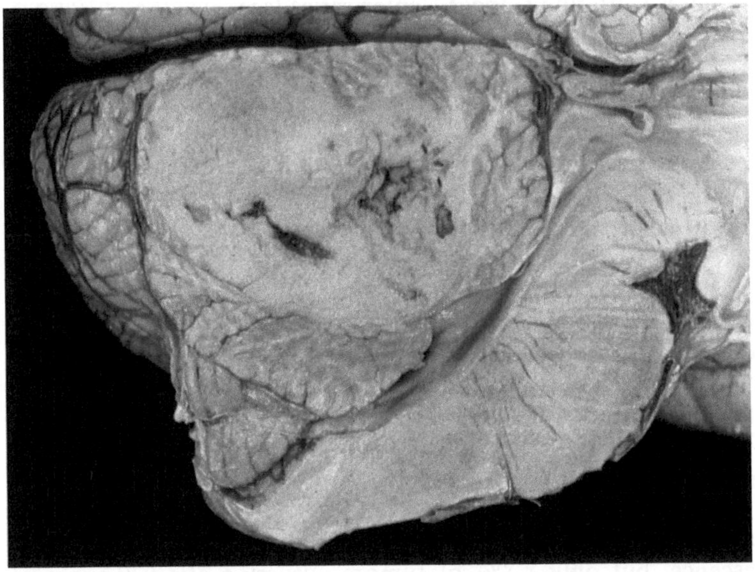

Fig. 98. Typical medulloblastoma situated in the lower vermis with extension into the 4th ventricle and infiltration of its floor. Secondary occlusive hydrocephalus with dilatation of the 3rd ventricle, the floor of which is paper-thin. (ZÜLCH 1975a)

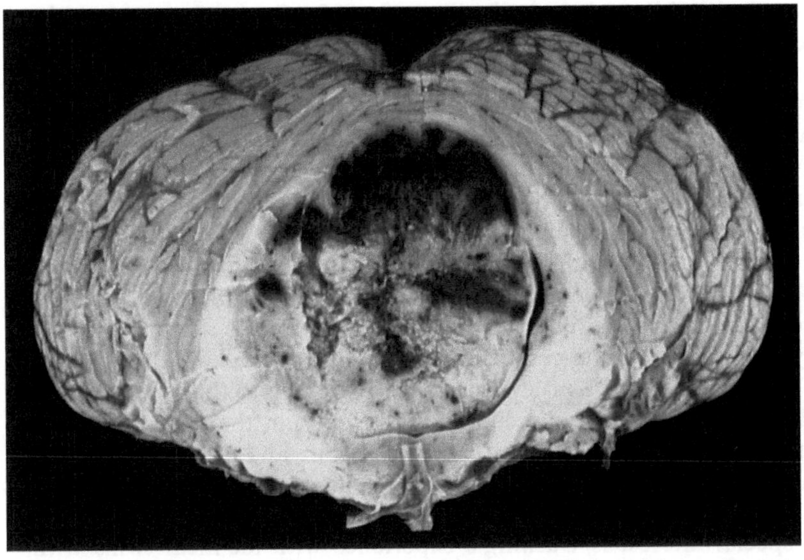

Fig. 99. Medulloblastoma arising from the roof of the 4th ventricle on the right. Hemorrhage into the tumor mass followed attempts at surgical excision. Note sharp demarcation of tumor from surrounding cerebellar tissue. (ZÜLCH 1975a)

Fig. 162). The cerebellar folia with their leptomeninges are thus engulfed in the tumor mass, and therefore include the local neuronal tissues. Medulloblastomas are grayish pink, since they are not very vascular; their consistency is soft and granular, becoming firmer only when a large amount of connective

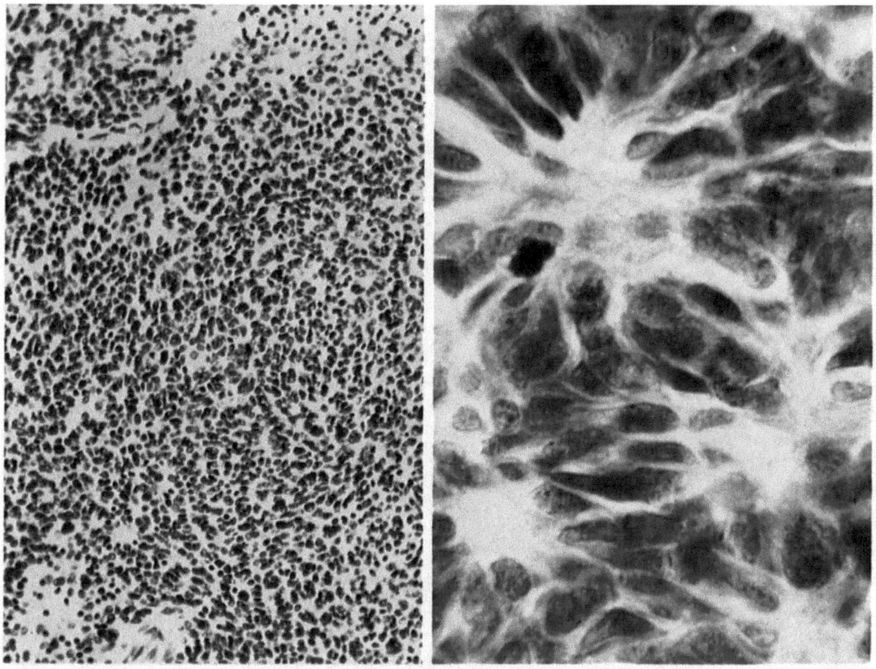

a b

Fig. 100. a General view of a typical medulloblastoma: The cells lie very densely packed in a typical architecture, in particular, pseudorosettes. Cresyl violet, ×84. **b** A "classical" pseudorosette formation is further accentuated by the turnip-shaped appearance of the tumor cells. Cresyl violet, ×780

tissue has been included (see Sect. 15.6.2.1). Occasionally they can appear partly (GP, Fig. 166) encapsulated, for instance when one wall is formed by the roof of the ventricle.

Histologic Appearance

Histologically medulloblastomas consist of closely packed (Fig. 100), isomorphic, elongated cells with round or oval nuclei, or of beet- or carrot-shaped cells in an orderly arrangement, often (HBT, Fig. 61b) in concentric patterns (pseudorosettes, see Figs. 100a, b, 101a) or clustering in islands. True rosettes do not occur (see pp. 118, 265). Here and there a comb-like pattern (HBT, Fig. 62b) may be observed. Occasionally the nuclei are rather vesicular (HBT, Fig. 61a) and neuron-like, which might have been responsible for the idea of Del Rio Hortega (1932, 1962) and his school that the cells were "neuroblasts." The rate of growth is very rapid. Numerous typical mitoses can be found even though many cells have only a short life-span (disintegration of nuclei). The remnants of degenerated nuclei must be distinguished from mitoses which often stain more lightly (HBT, Fig. 63b). The elongated tumor cells (Fig. 100b) have to be differentiated from the dark, round, "granule cells" of the invaded cerebellum. I regard most of the mature ganglion cells and astrocytes that occasionally occur in these tumors as remnants of the pre-existing infiltrated tissue

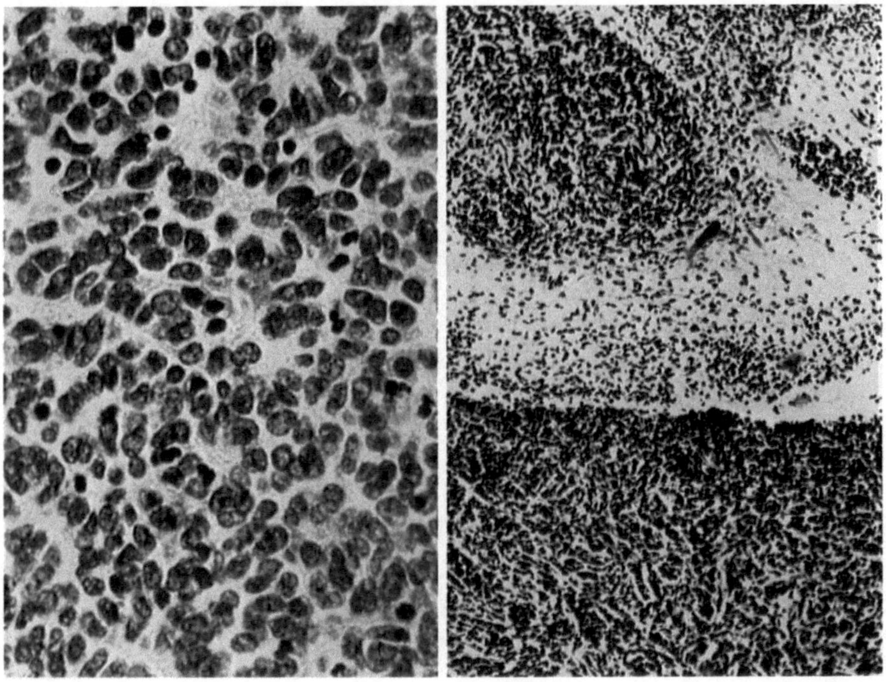

a b

Fig. 101. a Typical cell arrangement in a medulloblastoma with pseudorosettes and many mitoses. Cresyl violet, ×230. **b** On low magnification the infiltration of the arachnoidea is demonstrated (*bottom*), while one recognizes a cerebellar lobule still containing some Purkinje cells (*top*). The molecular layer is thinly infiltrated and the granular layer densely permeated. Cresyl violet, ×78

(Fig. 101b). Some authors consider the medulloblastoma cell is multipotent (and compare it with the "indifferent cells" of SCHAPER 1897). Medulloblastomas show little tendency to degeneration. Small areas of necrosis (HBT, Fig. 63d) or fatty degeneration occur only occasionally, and then usually in the center of the tumor. Calcification and cyst formation are exceptional. Any blood vessels are predominantly capillaries and are sparse. The tumor cells form neither glial nor reticulin fibers. The reticulin fiber network (Fig. 102a) that may be present comes from the engulfed leptomeninges (different: see also Sect. 15.6.2.1). Hemorrhages do not occur in this tumor. Melanin formation has been rarely described. In one of our cases the medosermal stroma was transformed into a sarcomatous tissue with monster cells (see TZONOS and BRUNNGRABER 1963a). In their expansion the tumor cells prefer to follow the course of blood vessels, resulting in intermittent perivascular spread in the marginal zone (HBT, Fig. 65d). On breaking into the leptomeninges (Fig. 101b), the tumor assumes different architectures: the cells arrange themselves into single rows (Fig. 102a) between the "arachnoidal meshes" (HBT, Fig. 62a, c); a similarity to the architecture of some carcinomas may be seen (Fig. 102a). From there the cells proliferate beneath the pia and spread into the neighboring cerebellar folia (HBT, Fig. 65a), occasionally in the above-mentioned comb-like pattern of infiltration between the dendrites (Fig. 102b) of the Purkinje cells.

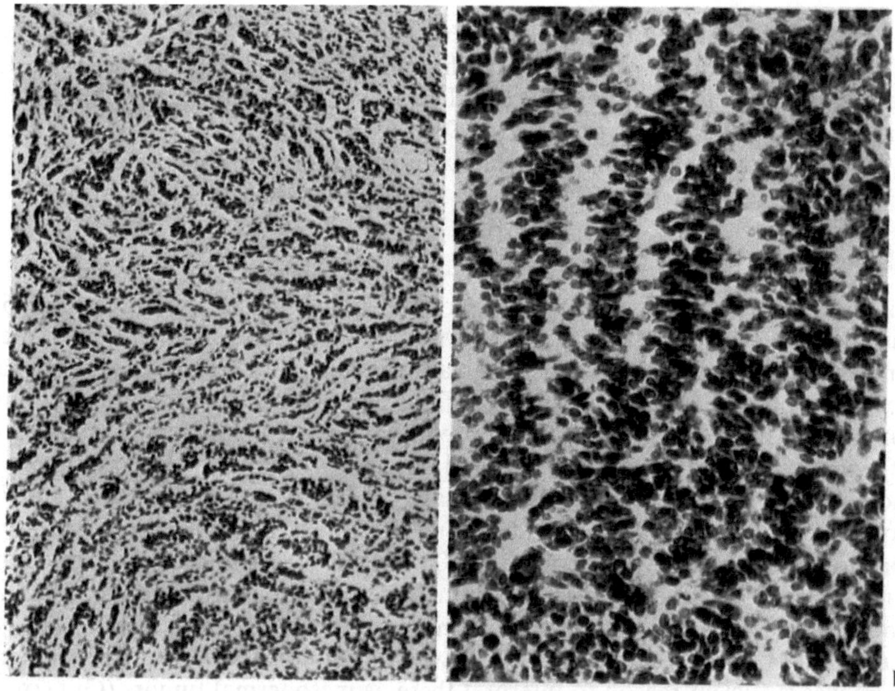

a b

Fig. 102. a The action of the arachnoidal meshes in shaping the tumor cells of a medulloblastoma can be perceived here in that the cells are all placed in narrow bands. Cresyl violet, ×84. **b** Occasionally, on infiltration of the cerebellar cortex, a "comb" formation occurs between the dendrites of the Purkinje cells. Cresyl violet, ×272

Electron Microscopy

So far EM has provided no evidence of a mesodermal origin of medulloblastoma. According to RAIMONDI et al. (1962) and RAIMONDI (1966), medulloblastomas consist of "two distinct types of neoplastic cells." One of these has the characteristics of neurons, and the other, those of glial cells. LUSE (1960, 1962) was not able to distinguish different cell types, and mentions the relative uniformity of the tumor cells as a prominent feature of this type of tumor. She feels, however, that there may be a morphologic similarity between the tumor cells and their neural progenitors, which she sees as the cells of the "external granular layer" of the immature cerebellum [as already suggested earlier by MARBURG (1931, 1934)]. In fact, there are many similarities in the fine structure of the embryonic granular cells of the cerebellum in normal chicken embryos (MUGNAINI and FORSTRØNEN 1967) and the tumor cells of medulloblastomas. According to our findings (ZÜLCH and WECHSLER 1968) in EM pictures, the fine structure of tumor cells of medulloblastomas is rather uniform and is typical of very immature and/or undifferentiated cells. We are not convinced that a neuroblastic differentiation can be substantiated by ultrastructural studies; some glial differentiation with an intraplasmatic synthesis of glial filaments has sometimes been demonstrable.

ESCOUROLLE and POIRIER (1967) were also unable to detect any indication of a double potentiality and were of the opinion that this was a neuroblastic tumor with some glial supporting cells. The "immature" undifferentiated nature was also supported by ISHIDA et al. (1964a). CERVOS-NAVARRO and MATAKAS (1970) could not find any relationship with either gliomas or normal neuroglia in the EM (see also LYSER 1975; WAGA 1965; VOIGT 1968; PEARL et al. 1979).

Tissue Culture

Tissue culture was first investigated on by KREDEL (1929) and BLAND (1936), but the results were controversial. KERSTING (1961) emphasized that they offered "no indication that medulloblastomas are similar or homologous to what has been interpreted as neuroblastomas by the Spanish school of Hortega." The tumor cells have a unique nuclear morphology in vitro, which is characteristic of primitive or undifferentiated cells and different from that of embryonic spongioblast or immature astrocytes. The later observations of KERSTING (1967), however, were interpreted as indications of a *mesodermal* origin, a concept meanwhile proposed by his co-worker GULLOTTA (1966, 1967a, b). GULLOTTA tried to show in several papers that the interpretation of the tumor cells as undifferentiated neuroepithelial cells [in the sense of SCHAPER (1897) and of KERSHMAN ("indifferent cells," 1938)] was inadequate. Moreover, he thought there was sufficient reason to interpret these as mesodermal tumors (GULLOTTA and KERSTING 1972).

LUMSDEN (1963), however, regards the medulloblastoma cells as "only a special type of *neuroblast* or as a special type of primitive and otherwise undifferentiated cell with a precocious and intense fiber-forming capacity." Therefore, in his opinion the medulloblastomas behave in vitro like primitive *neuronal* tumors. According to LISS (1962) the in vitro behavior of medulloblastomas shows particular features. "The tendency of outgrowth to curve and form a closed ring is similar to the behavior observed in undifferentiated neuroepithelial elements from embryonic retina".

In analyzing the arguments of the authors cited above we feel that there is not yet sufficient new material available to change the old interpretation, particularly since the predilection for the posterior fossa and the close morphological and biological correlation to the pineo-, retino-, and sympathicoblastomas (ZÜLCH 1951b, 1965a) provide so much support for the traditional interpretation, as also does the observation that the *intracranial sarcomas* are the only tumor group with no age, site, or sex predilections, which are so pronounced in the medulloblastomas.

RUBINSTEIN et al. (1974) reported a tumor with some characteristics of astrocytoma and medulloblastoma, which according to them had differentiated in that direction, e.g., had matured; BAILEY and CUSHING had considered this possible as long ago as 1926. In 1978 HERMAN and RUBINSTEIN even observed a glial and neuroblastic differentiation.

Histochemistry

Histochemical examination has revealed the typical pattern in medulloblastomas, with no cholinesterase (VIALE and IBBA 1964) and butylcholinesterase and coincident high activity of diaphorases and LDH. On the other hand, activity of GDH and MAO is very low, as is that of NADH and succinodehydrogenase. Both alkaline phosphatase and acid phosphatase were negative. The tumor cells of the medulloblastoma have a low rate of oxygen consumption, which is consistent with the apparently low cytochrome oxidase activity in these tumors. On the other hand, their high lactate levels suggest that they have a high rate of anaerobic glycolysis (LEHRER 1962; NASU and MÜLLER 1964; PERRIA et al. 1964; MÜLLER 1967; VAN VEELEN et al. 1978).

Differential Diagnosis

Medulloblastomas can be differentiated from pilocytic astrocytomas of the cerebellum by the naked eye. The astrocytomas frequently have a definite capsule and peel off from the surrounding brain tissue. They are firm and elastic. Histologically they possess glial fibers in considerable quantities when they are relatively acellular, showing the formation of Rosenthal fibers and granular bodies. Mitoses and perivascular infiltration in the marginal zone are always suggestive of medulloblastoma. Ependymomas of the fourth ventricle are harder, smoother, and more nodular, and can be separated easily from the overlying brain. They generally grow from the posterior portion of the floor of the fourth ventricle, and though they have a similarly high cellularity they can be differentiated histologically on the basis of its characteristic architecture: perivascular spaces free of nuclei and a lack of mitoses, which occur only exceptionally. Angioblastomas usually lie in the cerebellar hemispheres, are highly vascular, and often have large cysts; they generally occur in older age groups; they can be easily differentiated histologically by the vascular network. The tumor cells often have fibrillary processes oriented radially towards the vessel. True primary diffuse sarcomatosis of the meninges sometimes cannot be distinguished *locally* from metastases of a medulloblastoma into the subarachnoid space. In sarcomatosis, however, large circumscribed tumors are absent. Sometimes the differential diagnosis between medulloblastoma seeding in the spinal fluid spaces and meningeal sarcomatosis or carcinomatosis can be difficult during life (SCHOLZ 1973). It should be relatively easy to recognize the rare variety of melanotic medulloblastoma (BOESEL et al. 1978).

Biologic Behavior (Grading), Metastasis, and Recurrence

The WHO classification grades the medulloblastoma as IV and as "a risk" for recurrence. The survival period used to be an average of 8–15 months after the onset of symptoms before chemotherapy and modern radiation of the entire neuraxis were added to surgical therapy (QUEST et al. 1978). After operation alone survival seldom exceeds the above period very much. Since the introduction of systematic chemotherapy and radiation, ARON (1971) has published a series of 22 cases with a 5-year survival rate of 46% and a 10-year survival rate of 35% (see also SMITH et al. 1973; NOËL and MÉTHOT 1970; BROWN et al. 1977). SMITH et al. (1961) reported a 5-year survival rate of 40% after radiotherapy, while BLOOM et al. (1969) recorded 32% survival after 5 years and 26% after 10 years.

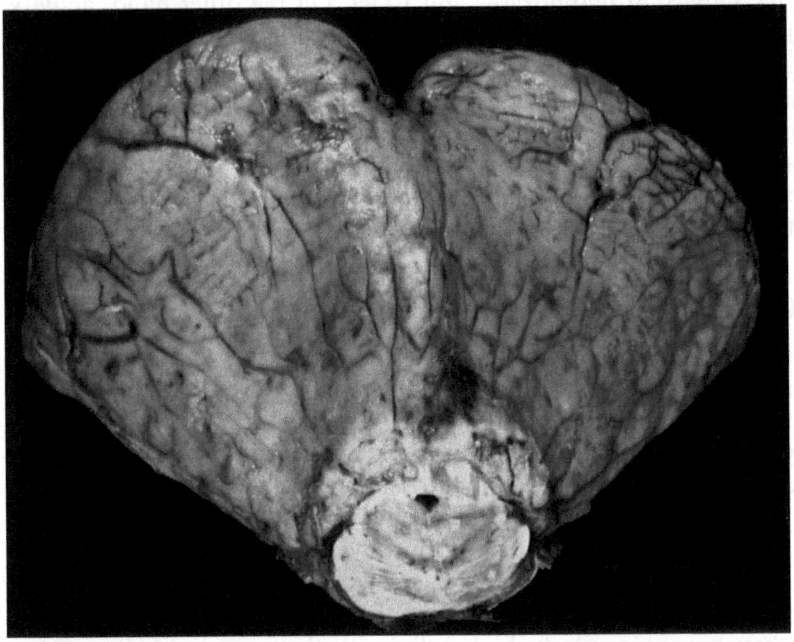

Fig. 103. Diffuse metastases of a medulloblastoma in the leptomeninges of the dorsal surface of the cerebellum

CHATTY and EARL (1971) have made an excellent study of 201 cases of medulloblastomas. In adults the prognosis was better than in children (around 50 months versus around 11 months). Curiously, the survival time seemed to be worse (21 months) in boys than in girls (31 months). For tumors, located in the hemispheres the postoperative survival was defined at 47 months, but for midline medulloblastomas it was only 17 months. Histological differentiation to the neuronal or glial side was of no consequence for predicting survival as had been suggested earlier (BLOOM et al. 1969). In the study conducted at the Memorial Sloan-Kettering Cancer Center (see ALLEN and EPSTEIN 1982) the average age of the patients who had a primary seeding was considerably lower than that of the rest of the series.

Metastasis: Upon reaching the open subarachnoid space the cells can be carried either with or against the CSF current, and seed out (GP, Figs. 168–169) in the form of buttons, plaques, or nodules, or diffusely like frosting [the area may involve aqueduct, infundibulum, floor of the lateral ventricles, dorsal surface of the cerebellum or spinal cord (Figs. 103–105), cauda equina, or the leptomeninges over the hemispheres, where the tumor molds itself into the sulci and cisterns].

Extracranial Metastases: I have observed three cases of metastasis of cerebellar medulloblastomas to other organs (see BUCHMANN and ZÜLCH 1959). Usually metastases occur in the pelvic or other bones (DEBNAM and STAPLE 1973), the

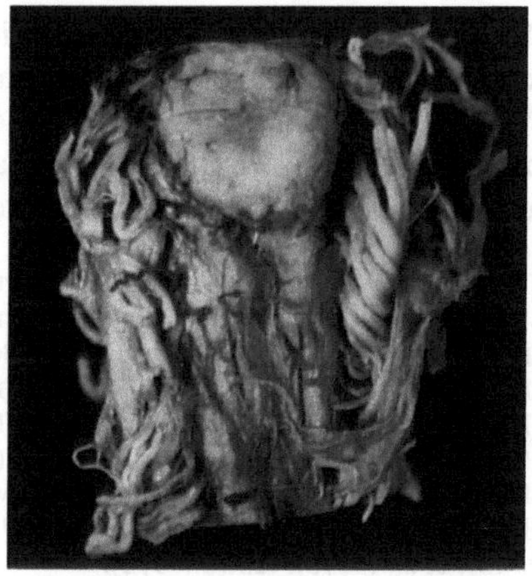

Fig. 104. Nodular metastasis of a medulloblastoma to the dorsal surface of the cervical cord. This particular tumor was most unusual in that it was calcified. (ZÜLCH 1975a)

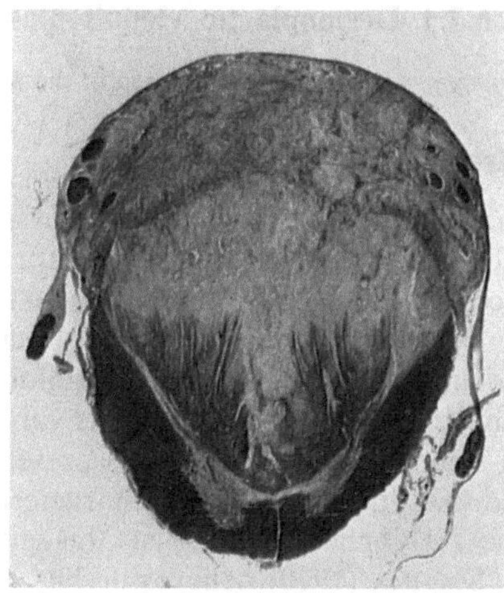

Fig. 105. Half-moon shaped metastasis of a medulloblastoma over the dorsal surface of the spinal cord

lymph nodes (cervical region, personal observation), or other tissues (see also LEWIS et al. 1973 and their reported literature cases; BRUTSCHIN and CULVER 1973; also RUBINSTEIN 1959; SCHNITZLER et al. 1978). The tendency to metastasize is considerable, and yet survival times of 10 years or more have been described after modern chemotherapy and radiation of the entire neuraxis.

Clinical Course

Non surgical therapy, when expanded by the introduction of chemotherapy, which can also be applied intrathecally (WILSON 1970), and TEM (CRUE et al. 1967), has successfully prolonged postoperative survival, particularly when radiation has also been applied postoperatively to the whole neuraxis (D.G. HARDY et al. 1978; VENES et al. 1979).

The rapid growth of the medulloblastoma explains its short clinical history. The clinical picture is a combination of the cerebellar symptoms and signs of general increased intracranial pressure, principally by aqueduct obstruction.

As this tumor often lies in the midline, symptoms of the vermis and anterior lobe of the cerebellum predominate. Spinal metastases account for the early signs of posterior column and cauda equina involvement (loss of reflexes, root pain in the distribution of the cauda). In cases with severely increased intracranial pressures paresis of the 6th nerve can occur, in some cases on both sides.

Further References: MASSON and DREYFUSS (1925), WOHLWILL (1930), ROUSSY et al. (1931), STEVENSON and ECHLIN (1934), RAAF and KERNOHAN (1944), SPITZ et al. (1947), RINGERTZ (1955), BENNINGTON and JONES (1962), BOFIN and EBELS (1963), RUBINSTEIN and NORTHFIELD (1964), DEXTER and HOWELL (1965), WAGA (1965), WORLD FEDERATION OF NEUROLOGY (1966), HOPE-STONE (1970), MISUGI and LISS (1970), POLLICE and MARZULLO (1970), RUBINSTEIN (1970, 1972), GRUSKIEWICZ et al. (1972), BEST (1973), SMITH et al. (1973), SUNG et al. (1973), LINS (1974), OLIVERA-RABIELA et al. (1974), MÜLLER and SCHÄFER (1974), HASSOUN et al. (1975), HOFFMAN et al. (1976), ARNOLD et al. (1978), BOESEL et al. (1978), GUTJAHR and VOTH (1978), ISHIDA et al. (1978), KLUG (1978).

15.6.2.1 Desmoplastic Medulloblastomas

Synonym: Circumscribed sarcoma of the arachnoid of the cerebellum

Introduction

This specific type of tumor was first described by FOERSTER and GAGEL (1939), and the description has been confirmed in the literature many times (for references see RUBINSTEIN and NORTHFIELD 1964). However, RUBINSTEIN and NORTHFIELD (1964; RUBINSTEIN 1972) were of the opinion that these were tumors showing a transition from medulloblastomas infiltrating the arachnoidal space (Fig. 103) into the desmoplastic variant, in which the identical pattern of reticulin-free islands and lobules is present (Fig. 106a, b) (as described by FOERSTER and GAGEL 1939) which is characteristic for the arachnoidal cerebellar sarcoma. The WHO classification lists this entity as *desmoplastic medulloblastoma*.

SOEJIMA (1970) believes he has confirmed the accuracy of this by EM. The large amount of connective tissue within the tumor seems to justify the term desmoplastic.

Historical Note and Definition

Discussion about the nature of the tumor may not yet be over, since many of its characteristics – as FOERSTER and GAGEL (1939) have emphasized – are very *atypical* of medulloblastomas, e.g., age group affected, location, histology, and prognosis (see also SOEJIMA et al. 1973; BERGHORN 1982), which are all so specific in medulloblastoma. Nonetheless, regardless of how this entity is interpreted and named, there can be no doubt that it exists in the form FOERSTER and GAGEL (1939) originally described it.

Gross Pathology

These are highly circumscribed nodular tumors (Fig. 107), usually sited in the hemispheres and often spreading over the *surface* of the cerebellum like a mushroom but not adherent to the dura. They are more frequently situated laterally

a 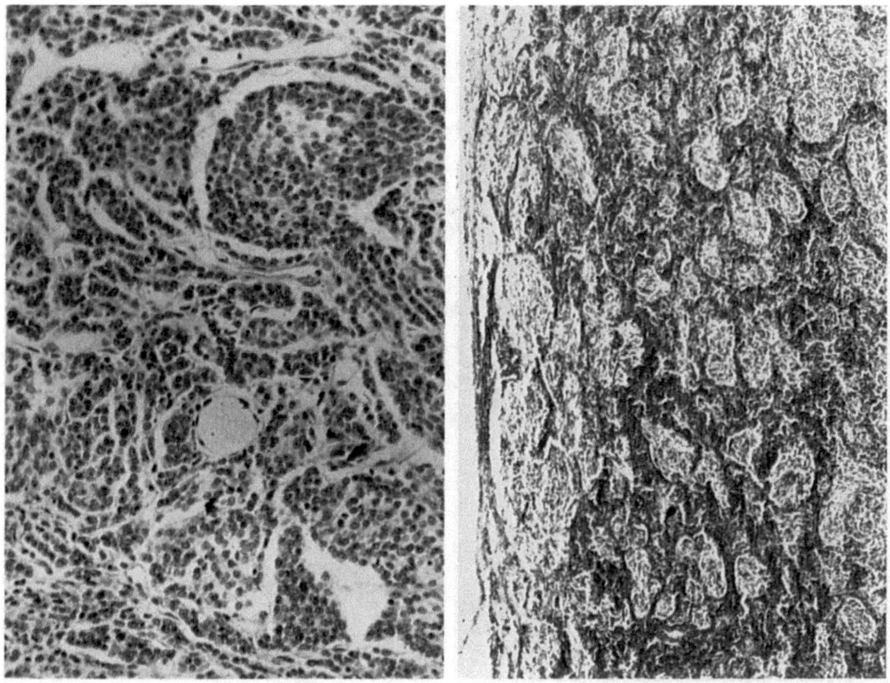 b

Fig. 106a, b. Medulloblastoma. Invasion of the arachnoid; "pale" islands are noticed in the leptomeningeal masses. H&E, × 136 (**a**) and × 50 (**b**)

or directly in the cerebellar hemispheres, where they can look like metastases at first sight.

Histologic Appearance

Histologically these tumors are characterized by the coexistence of islands of large light-staining pale cells (Figs. 106b, 108), without any connective tissue; furthermore of streams of dark, round, or beet-shaped cells around these islands. These are situated in a dense network of reticulin fibers permeating the whole tumor, and this is seen in places where the leptomeninges could not have been engulfed. We have seen several cases corresponding to this description in our series (see SCHRÖDER and PLOGSTIES 1966); the most recent was apparently congenital, the patient first being seen early in the second year of life.

Electron Microscopy

Several EM (HIZAWA and WECHSLER 1966; BRUCHER et al. 1971) and combined ultrastructural and tissue culture studies (GULLOTTA and KERSTING 1973; MENA and GARCIA 1978) have been published.

Differential Diagnosis

The typical architectural pattern makes it easy to differentiate between this type and the ordinary medulloblastoma.

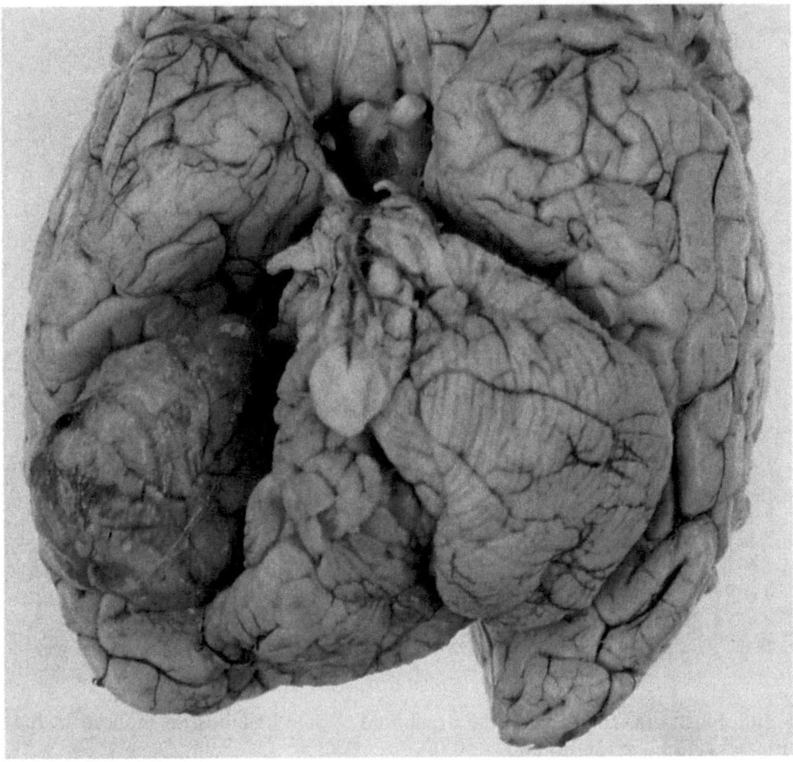

Fig. 107. "Desmoplastic" medulloblastoma (otherwise known as "cerebellar arachnoidal sarcoma") located in the right hemisphere and sharply demarcated from surrounding brain. (ZÜLCH 1975a)

Biologic Behavior (Grading), Metastasis, and Recurrence

In the WHO classification these tumors are graded IV, but even FOERSTER and GAGEL (1939) emphasized that the survival period may be better than that of ordinary medulloblastomas. The median survival time of this group has been defined by CHATTY and EARLE (1971) as 51 months. The better prognosis for these than for ordinary medulloblastomas was suggested earlier by BERGER and ELVIDGE (1963). MÜLLER et al. (1978) conducted a basic study on the correlations between this kind of tumor and the ordinary medulloblastoma. These authors determined from their series of 327 cases of medulloblastomas that 22.7% of the patients were older than 15 years. In 55 of cases (16.8%) the tumor was located in the hemispheres (in this study there were 30 male patients, as against 25 female patients). Beyond the 15 years age level a lateral localization was encountered in 41.9% of cases, while during childhood this occurred only in 9.5% (highly significant difference). Of 272 histologically classified medulloblastomas 57 were desmoplastic (38 male:19 female patients). There was a higher frequency of hemispheric location in adolescent and adult patients.

a 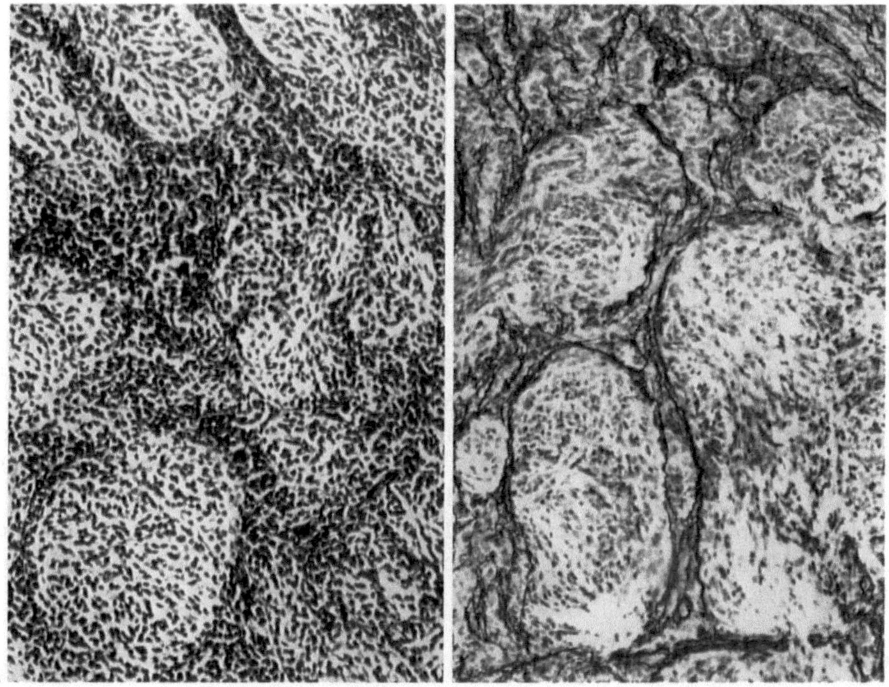 b

Fig. 108. a "Desmoplastic" medulloblastoma (otherwise known as "arachnoidal cerebellar sarcoma"). Typical architecture with "pale" islets containing few cells lying within the highly cellular tissue of the tumor. H&E, ×128. **b** Similar architecture seen following silver impregnation: there is hardly any fiber production within the cells although such fibers are present in abundance in the tumor. Silver impregnation, nuclear stain, ×96

15.6.2.2 Medullomyoblastomas

Introduction

These tumors resemble typical medulloblastomas but may include cellular features of nonstriated or striated muscles. This group is a separate entity in the WHO classification.

Historical Note and Definition

Striated muscle fibers have been reported in cases published by MARINESCO and GOLDSTEIN (1933), GAGEL (1938), BOFIN and EBELS (1963), BOELLARD (1964), MISUGI and LISS (1970), LEWIS (1973), FELIX et al. (1976), and STAHLBERGER and FRIEDE (1977). The combination of medulloblastomatous, rhabdomyosarcomatous, and melanotic patterns has been described by DUINKERKE et al. (1981).

I have observed a typical example with nonstriated muscle fibers originating from the vessels in a medulloblastoma in a 5-year old boy (ZÜLCH 1941b). These cells were different from the medulloblastoma tumor cells.

Epidemiology

The epidemiology is not different from that of other medulloblastomas.

Gross Pathology

These tumors are similar to other medulloblastomas in gross appearance.

Histologic Appearance

The origin of these striated or nonstriated muscle cells is thought to be either the vessel walls or the leptomeningeal stroma. In our case (ZÜLCH 1941 b) we observed the muscle cells swarming out from the vessels. Occasionally myogenic giant cells are observed (BOELLARD 1964), as also in other medulloblastomas (TZONOS and BRUNNGRABER 1963 a). ZÜLCH (1941 b) emphasized that the myogenic fibers are derived directly from the vessels, that is to say, that medulloblastoma and myoblastoma cells are derived from different cell lines.

Myogenic elements can be easily identified from the undifferentiated elements. No comparable structures are seen in the medulloblastoma component (STAHLBERGER and FRIEDE 1977).

Biologic Behavior (Grading), Metastasis, and Recurrence

It is probable that these medulloblastomas are very similar to the other types in these aspects (i.e., grade IV).

15.6.3 Medulloepitheliomas

Introduction

Medulloepithelioma of the WHO classification is a very rare embryonal tumor with features resembling those of the primitive neural plate. Therefore the cells are undifferentiated, medium or large, columnar or cylindrical, with a resemblance to primitive neural or medullary epithelium.

Historical Note and Definition

Medulloepithelioma made up the group that was highest up in the scheme of development in Bailey's original pedigree of neuroepithelial cell development. He probably introduced it principally for theoretical reasons. He made particular reference to the tumor described by EMANUEL (1900) in the retina. BAILEY combined the medulloepitheliomas and the neuroepitheliomas in one group even as long ago as 1932 a.

In the earlier editions of this textbook and in the very detailed discussion in the *Handbuch der Neurochirurgie* (ZÜLCH 1956) I suggested to omit both, medulloepithelioma and neuroepithelioma, because of their extreme rarity and the poor definition. In 1954 I discussed most of the cases of the older literature (pp. 332–334) of which some were merely ordinary ependymomas (see also "neuroepithelioma", p. 21).

However, I had to change my ideas after seing the case reported by IKUTA (Niigata, Japan) (GP, Fig. 83, which I had by courtesy of the author permission to reproduce). In this case (see HBT, Fig. 14b, c) Bailey's original idea had actually been realized. Furthermore, MENNEL (1974) was able to induce tumors with the exact pattern by the experimental method.

A review of the literature, however, will probably reveal that some of the cases (as stated in my early critical interpretation; 1956) do not fit into this group of rare tumors, e.g., those of GREENFIELD (1934) and of LOLOVA et al. (1972). Therefore, the critical evaluation detailed in the case of T. SATO et al. (1980) is especially commendable in the face of so much discussion, particularly that of MABON et al. (1950), and Dorothy Russell's concept of rejection (see RUSSELL 1960; RUSSELL and RUBINSTEIN 1977).

Epidemiology (Age – Site)

Age: Mostly children or juvenile patients are compromised. It seems likely that some such tumors may even be congenital.

Site: Most of the probable cases have occurred in the supratentorial space with a predilection for the temporal lobe (see GP, pp. 67–68). A cerebellar localization would be rare (BEST 1974).

Gross Pathology

The tumors are well delimited, probably not very invasive, and are soft and containing necroses and even hemorrhages.

Histologic Appearance

The characteristic elements are tubules or strands, bands, or cords of cylindrical or columnar epithelium, and not just normal ependymal rosettes (p. 265). There is high degree of mitotic activity, and some cells may have matured to higher stages (neuronal, DECK 1969). An epithelium resembling that of the medullary plate, with an internal and external limiting membrane and a connective tissue stroma, is characteristic.

Differential Diagnosis

Since these tumors have no cilia and no blepharoplasts, differential diagnosis against anaplastic ependymoma and choroid plexus papilloma is possible. Moreover, metastases of adenocarcinoma have to be considered (see also neuroepithelioma, p. 21).

Biologic Behavior (Grading), Metastasis, and Recurrence

These tumors appear to be highly malignant (grade IV), and most cases reported in the literature ended rapidly in death. Malignant extracranial metastases have been described (VAN EPPS et al. 1967).

Treatment

Surgery and radiation must be attempted.

Further References: TREIP (1957), RUBINSTEIN (1970, Fig. 134), JELLINGER (1972), KARCH and URICH (1972, who collected 9 cases of the literature), GULLOTTA and ENTZIAN (1975).

15.6.4 Primitive Polar Spongioblastomas

Introduction

The *primitive polar spongioblastoma* of the WHO classification must be clearly distinguished from the "polar spongioblastoma" of BAILEY and CUSHING (1926, 1930), which is now listed as pilocytic astrocytoma (Sect. 15.1.2).

Primitive polar spongioblastoma is an extremely rare tumor composed of unipolar or bipolar cells with delicate processes that form a remarkable pronounced palisading pattern.

Historical Note and Definition

The primitive polar spongioblastoma was described originally by RUSSELL and CAIRNS (1947), and the name was coined by RUBINSTEIN (1964) at a time when the group of polar spongioblastomas according to Bailey's definition was still present in most classifications. The difficulty in the naming of glial tumors has been discussed at great length by ZÜLCH (1939a) in a paper written in honor of CUSHING'S 70th birthday (see also ZÜLCH 1968). The heart of the problem was that in the classifications of BAILEY and CUSHING (1926, 1930) and PENFIELD (1931, 1932b) the term polar spongioblastoma was applied to a group for which the name was by no means adequate. This has been discussed on many occasions (see Symposium on Classification in Bilbao 1955: OBRADOR-ALCALDE and SANZ IBANEZ 1955; and Symposium on Classification in Cologne 1961: ZÜLCH and WOOLF 1964). But since the renaming of this "old" polar spongioblastoma as pilocytic astrocytoma (see p. 221) because its name was never satisfactory, the name of the primitive polar spongioblastoma currently under discussion and defined by RUSSELL and RUBINSTEIN seems to be adequate.

As long ago as 1939a I had discussed the position of the spongioblast in the system of development of the neuroepithelial cells, and it may be necessary to determine whether comparison of the cellular elements of this tumor with those of the spongioblast of the developmental system is legitimate, particularly since this tumor group seems to be extremely rare. There are hardly any tumor descriptions in the literature that correspond to the original cases of RUSSELL and CAIRNS, described in detail by RUBINSTEIN and presented at the Cologne Symposium 1961.

I saw the slides of these cases and in our own vast collection I found only one case, which I had first depicted in 1940 (Fig. 9), later in 1956 as Fig. 78c, and in HBT as Fig. 54c. Although histologically our case would be quite consistent, apart from the lack of mitoses: it was a large cystic tumor at the outer edge of the ventricular system in a youth and it had demonstrated no signs of malignancy.

Moreover, the case of DUCKETT and WILSON (1964) was also not consistent with the case of RUSSELL and CAIRNS (1947b).

In Cologne in 1961 (see ZÜLCH and WOOLF 1964) RUBINSTEIN had pointed out again that on purely theoretical grounds a polar spongioblastoma must be composed of cells similar to the migrating polar spongioblasts observed during the development of the nervous system. Such a tumor would then presumably have a malignant biological behavior dependant upon the rapidity of its growth.

Epidemiology (Age – Site)

Age: These tumors arise most often before the age of 20.

Site: They are probably located near the third or fourth ventricle.

Gross Pathology

These are well-demarcated tumors, often attached to the ventricular wall and are invasive locally.

Histologic Appearance

Primitive polar spongioblastomas have a compact pattern of palisading cells separated by delicate vascular stroma without proliferation. Neuroglial fibers may be present, and occasionally the elements may show some differentiation in which the microscopical picture is identical with that of a benign cerebellar astrocytoma.

Differential Diagnosis

Medulloblastoma and pilocytic astrocytoma must be taken account of in the differential diagnosis.

Biologic Behavior (Grading), Metastasis, and Recurrence

Up to now there is very little experience to draw on with these tumors, which seem to metastasize widely throughout the cerebrospinal leptomeninges. Consequently the prognosis is very poor.

15.6.5 Gliomatosis Cerebri

Synonyms: Diffuse gliomatosis, glioblastosis, central diffuse schwannosis, astrocytosis

Introduction

In the large group of diffuse gliomas one rare entity is observed, which is characterized by a diffuse blastomatous growth of glia cells in one or both hemispheres. In such cases, these glial cells have undergone neoplastic transformation with variable degrees of differentiation. The cells may resemble spongioblasts, astrocytes, or oligodendroglia and foci of glioblastoma multiforme.

To allow better distinction of similar entities I have recommended that differentiation of (a) diffuse gliomas, e.g., astrocytomas or oligodendrogliomas; (b) multicentric gliomas; and (c) diffuse gliomatosis. In the WHO classification diffuse gliomatosis features as *gliomatosis cerebri.*

Historical Note and Definition

Literature cases such as those of SCHWARTZ and KLAUER (1927) and NEVIN (1938) gave rise to the discussion of this group, and many other cases allowed a general definition, yet with differences in defining the cellular elements present, e.g., gliomatosis, central diffuse schwannosis.

Epidemiology (Age – Site)

Age: Middle-aged people are perhaps most often affected.

Site: Gliomatosis cerebri can involve the deep white matter of the cerebral hemispheres or the cerebellum (SCHEINKER and EVANS 1943), the medulla oblongata (FINKEMEYER and TZONOS 1965; SARHADDI et al. 1973), and the spinal cord (MOORE 1954; RYZKOW 1959) or there can be diffuse involvement of the cerebrum, cerebellum, brain stem, cranial nerves, and spinal cord.

Gross Pathology

Diffuse enlargement of the brain stem and central white substance of the hemispheres etc. (all involved parts) with gross preservation of the original form is typical. There may be small foci of necroses and hemorrhages, associated with anaplastic transformation.

Histologic Appearance

Histologically the elements are different. Some of them may resemble Schwann cells (central diffuse schwannosis of FOERSTER and GAGEL 1934a), while others look like undifferentiated bipolar spongioblastic cells (gliomatosis) or oligodendroglial or astrocytic forms. Adaption of the cells to the local architecture of the fibers is typical hence most elements are long bipolar cells. Some more polymorphous cells even resemble cells in glioblastoma multiforme (glioblastosis, SCHEINKER 1936, 1938b; HALLERVORDEN 1938; NEVIN 1938; KAUTZKY 1939; SCHEINKER and EVANS 1943; MOORE 1954; SEITZ and KALM 1957).

If there are focal condensations of the cells transition to "multicentric glioma" may be under way.

Further References: BEBIN and TYTUS (1956), DUNN and KERNOHAN (1957), KAHLE (1957), BANGERT and ORTHNER (1959), WÜNSCHER and LEHMANN (1960), COUCH and WEISS (1974).

A note on meningeal gliomatosis or blastomatous meningitis (REYMOND 1953) must be added here, with especial reference to the terminology.

Meningeal Gliosis – Astrocytosis of the Cerebellar Arachnoid

SCHMINCKE (1924) and OBERLING (1922, 1943) described cases of a pilocytic astrocytoma-like tumor of the cerebellum and optic nerve, in which extension into the meninges exceeded that of the primary tumor. In our large collection we have never seen cases in which such an additional classification would be necessary. Only one case of diffuse spread into the meninges and under the pia could justifiably have been called "gliomatosis of the meninges." However, most of this tumor had undergone mucoid degeneration and it rather resembled a protoplasmic astrocytoma. It remained unclassified. O.T. BAILEY (1936), WALKER (1941), and ABBOTT and GLASS (1955) have described leptomeningeal gliomas related to the astrocytoma group. They were derived from glial rests. Meningeal "gliomatosis" or "blastomatous meningitis" should also be critically considered (REYMOND 1953) in such cases.

16 Tumors of Nerve Sheath Cells

16.1 Neurilemmomas

Synonyms: Schwannoma, neurinoma; in the older literature: perineural fibroblastoma, chitoneuroma, gliofibroma, peripheral glioma, acoustic neuroma

Introduction

As the many synonyms demonstrate, *neurilemmomas* are one of the entities that were known and investigated early on, and they are therefore well defined and discussed in the WHO classification. The term has been chosen as a compromise between "schwannoma," which is frequently used in the Americas and "neurinoma," which is still the most common term in Europe.

Historical Note and Definition

Neurilemmomas had already been described at the beginning of the 19th century, but VIRCHOW (1863/65) was the first to recognize them for what they were. The considerable contributions of von RECKLINGHAUSEN (1882), MALLORY (1904/05), VEROCAY (1908), ANTONI (1920, 1936), and PENFIELD (1932b) have not yet fully clarified the nature of neurilemmomas. However, Antoni's subdivision into types with A and B architectures is a classic work. There is still opposition to the predominant concept of a derivation from the Schwann cells (mesodermal cells as against an ectodermal origin?). The argument hinges on the interpretation of (a) the behavior in tissue culture; (b) nature of the silver-impregnated fibers; (c) modern protein chemistry; and finally (d) experiments, for instance of HARRISON (1904).

The interpretation of this tumor as a glioma no longer warrants any serious consideration. The "central neurinomas" of the older literature were most probably pilocytic astrocytomas with a particularly marked tendency to rhythmic cell patterns.

Pathogenesis

As emphasized above, the real nature of the neurilemmomas has not been definitely decided. The American school of MALLORY (1904/05) and PENFIELD (1932b) referred to them as "perineural" fibroblastomas, while the classical European scientists VEROCAY (1908) and ANTONI (1920) thought they originated from the neuroectodermal Schwann cells, basing this opinion particularly on the classic experiments of HARRISON (1904).

The silver-stained fibers found in neurilemmomas must not be mistaken for common reticular fibers, as will be emphasized below and has been largely discussed in an earlier paper (ZÜLCH and MILHAUD 1960). The evidence supplied by tissue culture is summarized on page 344. The contradictory data will also be summarized.

New results have been obtained in experimental tumor research with N-nitrosoureas administered by the transplacental route and in other forms of resorptive carcinogenesis (see various papers by MENNEL and ZÜLCH 1971 b, MENNEL 1972). In these circumstances the neurilemmoma is a particularly frequently induced tumor. Of the experimental neurilemmomas, those of the trigeminal nerve are the most frequent (30%), the tumors of the great plexuses in the cervical–brachial and lumbar region next, and finally all other types. There is a close similarity in the experimental tumors with the fibrillary and reticular structures, i.e., architectures A and B (pp. 349, 351), of human neurilemmomas. However, less differentiated structures are seen with small islands of uncharacteristic round cells in addition.

Anaplastic forms (anaplastic neurilemmomas and neurosarcomas) among the experimental tumors are less uniform and sometimes difficult to identify. However, in most cases a continuous transition from neurilemmomas into malignant anaplastic forms is recognizable, since the various characteristics of the neurilemmomas are occasionally seen in the anaplastic forms. Yet, their appearance in large series of these experimental neurilemmomas supports the concept of their derivation from the typical neurilemmoma.

One feature that has not yet been sufficiently clarified is the occurrence of so-called "intramedullary neurilemmomas or neurofibromas."

STAEMMLER (1939) and later SCHOEPE (1951) described miniature neurilemmomas in the spinal cord roots. Vascular bundles with a mixture of myelin sheaths were identified in the pia and in the spinal cord itself. Whereas in this particular case it seems possible that this was a germ of a spinal root neurilemmoma; in other instances tumors classified as intracerebral and intramedullary neurilemmomas or neurofibromas have probably in fact been pilocytic astrocytomas (see LU et al. 1963, Fig. 1 c, d).

In the observations cited the zone around the entering or exiting spinal roots may show excessive accumulation of Schwann cells and even small neurilemmoma-like formations. Some authors believe that such Schwann cells enter the neural tissue along the pathways of penetrating vessels and form the matrix for neurilemmomas within the brain or spinal cord (SCOTT and BENTZ 1962; RUSSELL and RUBINSTEIN 1977).

Epidemiology (Age – Sex – Frequency – Site)

Age: Solitary neurilemmomas occur particularly in the middle and later decades of life, with a peak around 35–40 years (5th decade, GERMAN 1961 b) (see p. 89), and are only rarely seen in childhood (LAHA and HUESTIS 1975). Our youngest patient was 11 years old, the oldest 67. In later life they can also occur as incidental finding in the region of the cauda equina (GP, Fig. 176) and are often asymptomatic.

Sex: In our patients the sex ratio was 2:1 with a female preponderance [similarly, 61% female patients in the series of POIRIER and ESCOUROLLE (1970)].

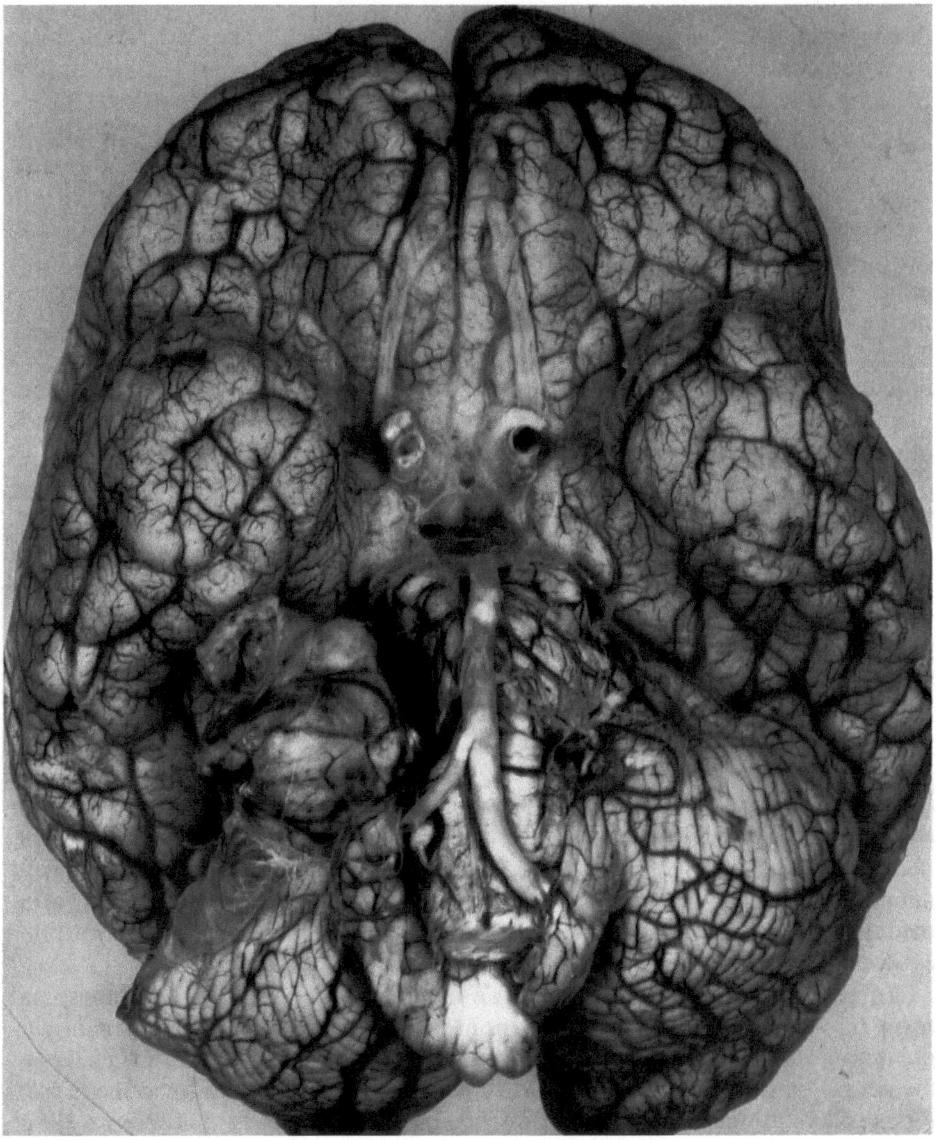

Fig. 109. Large acoustic neurilemmoma with a small arachnoid cyst located in its posterior portion in a nonsurgical specimen. A marked cerebellar pressure cone had occurred, with mass shifting from right to left. Arteriosclerosis of the vertebrobasilar system is seen. (ZÜLCH 1975a)

Frequency: Neurilemmomas accounted for 6.8% of all the brain tumors in our series of 9000 cases; 8.7% in CUSHING's (1932) series, and of OLIVECRONA's (1967, p. 11) 6169 tumors 7.6% were neurilemmomas. POIRIER and ESCOUROLLE (1970) reported a proportion of 5.6% neurilemmomas in their series. Among the spinal tumors 25% are usually neurilemmomas (ZÜLCH 1980b).

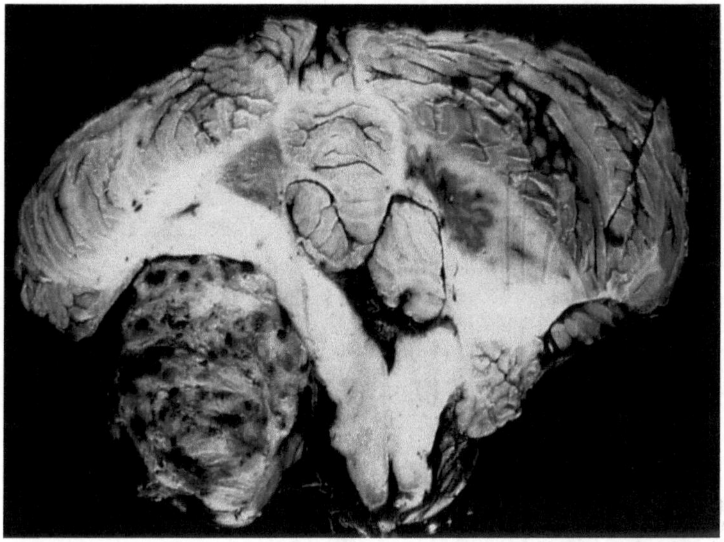

Fig. 110. Large neurilemmoma of the cerebellopontine angle, with marked shift of the pons and medulla. Postoperative state

Site: Neurilemmomas occur most frequently in the vestibular part of the 8th cranial nerve. The tumors can be as big as hazel- or chestnuts (Fig. 109) in the cerebellopontine angle, but with modern otologic and neuroradiologic diagnostic techniques they are often found when they are considerably smaller ("minimal tumors"). During growth they can force the cerebellum (Fig. 110) both up- and downward [forming superior and inferior cerebellar pressure cone (Fig. 109); see p. 170]. The caudal end of the tumor is often the site of one or more arachnoidal, space-occupying cysts (Fig. 109). As a result of pressure or disturbances in circulation small areas of softening may develop in the neighboring pons. Bilateral acoustic neurilemmomas occasionally occur and are looked upon as a forme fruste of von Recklinghausen's neurofibromatosis.

Rarely neurilemmomas occur on the other cranial nerves, most frequently the 5th (Krayenbühl 1936; Baker and A. Bailey 1952; Loew and Tönnis 1954; Basauri and Asenjo 1967; Olivecrona 1967). Sometimes they are very small (Levinthal and Bentson 1976). Massive extracranial extension may destroy the middle fossa (Yamada et al. 1980).

Rare sites are trochlear nerve: King (1976), Boggan et al. (1979), Ho (1981); facial nerve: Money and Halliday (1965), Isamat et al. (1975); vagus nerve: Bailey and Sanchez (1946); spinal accessory nerve: Pou-Serradell et al. (1978); hypoglossal nerve: Morelli (1966), Ignelzy and Bucy (1967), Fujiwara et al. (1980); and infraorbital nerve: Kahl (1973).

In addition, they are encountered more rarely at other locations of the cranial base, e.g., a curious frontal tumor (Ulrich et al. 1978; Auer et al. 1982); in the foramen lacerum posterius (Ruberti and Carteri 1961); the jugular foramen (Ishiyama et al. 1975; Martinez et al. 1981); below the orbita (Kahl 1973); and in the gastrointestinal tract (Pross et al. 1972).

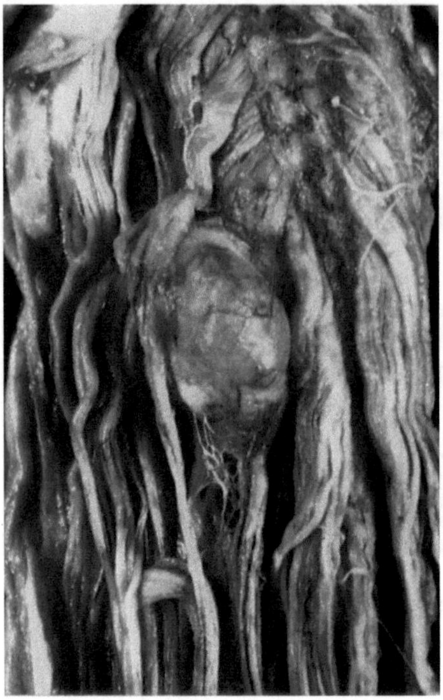

Fig. 111. Small neurilemmoma of the cauda equina (incidental finding)

Neurilemmomas are among the most common tumors found in the *spinal canal.* They may be distributed over one or more segments and are attached to the posterior roots or cauda equina (Fig. 111); they can be finger-shaped if large, or they may resemble a lima bean. Dumbbell forms are not uncommon and arise when the tumor grows through an intervertebral foramen, particularly in the thoracic or cervical segments. These tumors are sometimes accompanied by a large segmental artery, which may be inadvertently divided and lead to subsequent neurologic – spinal – deficits. Spinal neurilemmomas quite often show mucoid degeneration and cyst formation, occasionally with varying degrees of hemorrhage into the cysts (see clinical course, p. 354). Spinal neurilemmomas can be located intra- or extradurally (distinction in x-ray: DANZIGER et al. 1975). A particular group occurs in the upper cervical segments (C 2/3, FIELDS et al. 1972).

In von Recklinghausen's disease neurilemmomas can be present on every cranial, spinal, or peripheral nerve (gastrointestinal tract; PROSS et al. 1972). Solitary neurilemmomas of peripheral nerves are rare (see Sect. 16.3).

Gross Pathology

Neurilemmomas are moderately smooth, well-encapsulated tumors, often with a finely nodular appearance (Fig. 109). The arachnoid capsule contains the feed branches of the vascular supply. The color of the tumor varies from reddish gray or yellow to deep yellow and/or to a translucent gray. The consistency also varies, depending on the extent of regressive changes – particularly fatty

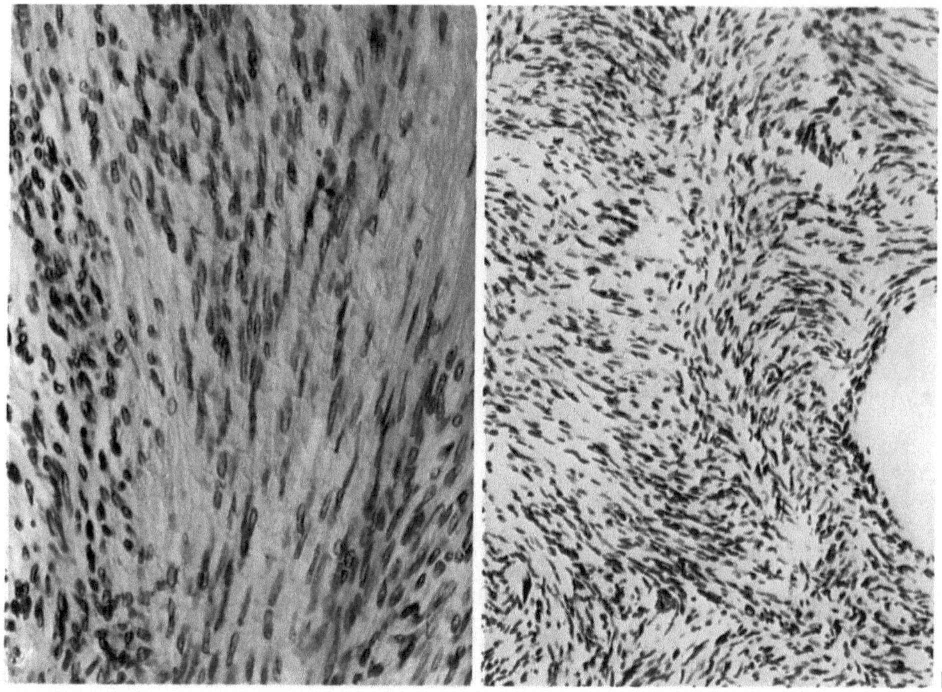
a b

Fig. 112. a Arrangement of the tumor cells in long streams. Cresyl violet, ×284. **b** Retroversion and whorl formation. Cresyl violet, ×108

degeneration – that have taken place. The tumor may be hard and fibrous or rubbery in the marginal zone close to the capsule, but friable and softer in its center, so that intracapsular curettage can be easily accomplished. Cystic degeneration is common in the large spinal tumors, but rare in the cerebellopontine type. Here the tumor usually starts to growth within the internal auditory meatus and later enlarges it by erosion of the bone (GP, Fig. 177). Their size is different small (even minimal when intracanalicular), medium, large, or giant (Kasantikul et al. 1980).

Histologic Appearance

Histologically, two architectures are recognized in the neurilemmomas, viz.: Antoni's (1920) fibrillary and reticular types (A and B). Type A is composed of cells of moderate density, which appear to be arranged in a syncytium and show such typical patterns as streams, loops, and palisades (Figs. 112, 113). Otherwise the nuclei are like rods (Fig. 114a) or cigarettes in shape and contain a medium amount of chromatin. The spinal forms are particularly likely to show the classic palisading of nuclei (Fig. 113).

Antoni's type B is loosely reticular, less cellular, and shows hyalinization and fatty degeneration as a result of regressive changes (Fig. 115a, b). This very distinct tendency to tissue disintegration mainly by lipid degeneration is a unique characteristic of this tumor, otherwise found only in phagocytic cells

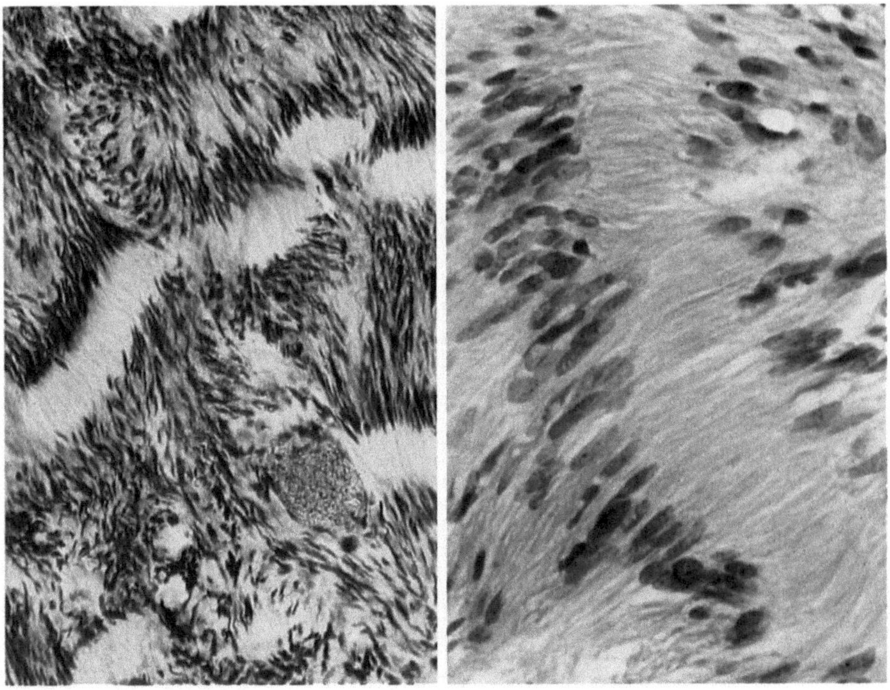

Fig. 113. a Very pronounced palisading of the nuclei in a spinal neurilemmoma. Cresyl violet, ×134. **b** Typical palisading in an acoustic neurilemmoma. H&E, ×522

after myelin destruction. This characteristic has not been observed in any mesodermal tumor. The fatty degeneration can readily be recognized histologically and in areas of severe change the architecture is altered by the inclusion of lipids so that grossly it is similar to that of an oligodendroglioma. This fatty degeneration is present to such a degree that superficial observation in an H&E section one immediately thinks of this tumor (Fig. 115). In addition, there is a type of hyaline change, without genuine mesodermal hyaline appearance. It is noteworthy that there is a tendency to liquefaction and cyst formation in all these tumors, but is more pronounced in tumors of the spinal canal than in those which are intracranial. The formation of huge cysts is especially evident in the large neurilemmomas on the nerve roots of the cauda equina. The reason for the difference in the tendency to form lipid deposits in the intracranial tumors and liquefaction with the formation of mucoid substances in the tumors of the spinal canal (formation of cysts) is not yet clear. Possibly it is caused by differences in local pressure.

The palisading of tumor cells is not a feature exclusively of neurilemmomas (Krumbein 1925, Lauche 1925). It has been observed in certain myomas and even occurs in normal organs with smooth musculature, such as the pylorus.

The silver impregnation method makes it possible to demonstrate fine fibrils (Fig. 115b), which are probably not of the nature of connective tissue, however. Mallory (1904/05) and Penfield (1932b) assumed that they were collagenous.

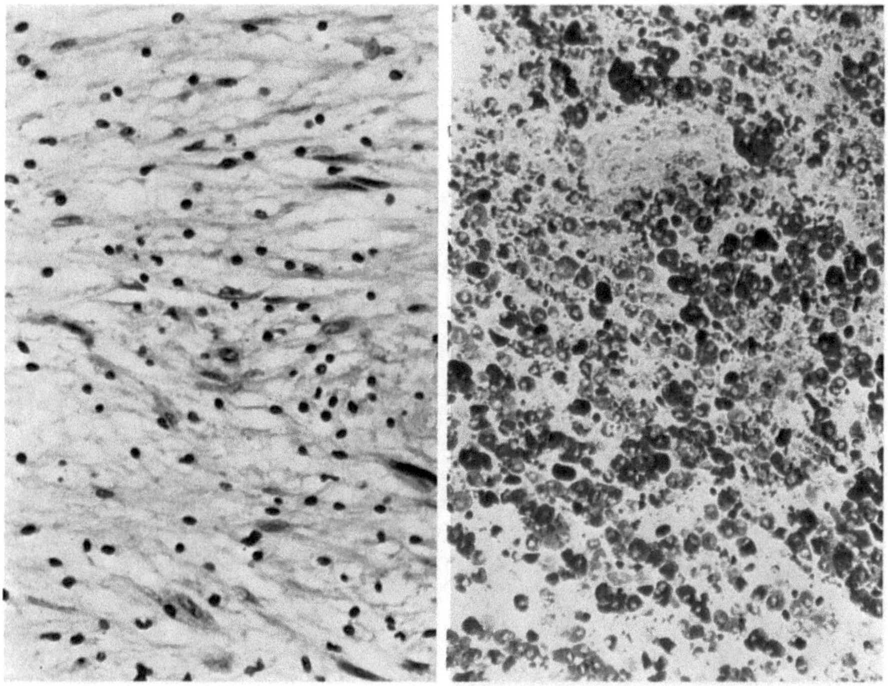

a b

Fig. 114. a Hyalinization and fatty degeneration of fibrillary sections. Cresyl violet, ×120. **b** Region with total fatty degeneration of the cells where, in the cell body (demonstrated in the print), the clear vacuole of the nucleus is spared. Scarlet, ×128

A detailed study conducted in collaboration with MILHAUD (see ZÜLCH 1951b, 1956, 1965a; ZÜLCH and MILHAUD 1960) has demonstrated clearly that neurilemmoma cells are surrounded by a membranous envelope in which fiber-like condensations or even small fibers of the kind observed in normal Schwann cells occur. Neurilemmoma fibers are flimsy, lie on the external surface of each cell, and often zig-zag in a saw-like fashion. They are more slender than mesodermal fibers and different in thickness. The fibers in neurofibromas will be discussed below (p. 355). Nerve fibers can be occasionally found stretched over the capsule of a neurilemmoma, but are not found within the tumor. True reticulin fibers are found in the marginal zone and apparently originate from the covering arachnoidal connective tissue.

Blood vessels are more numerous in the marginal zone and their walls have a tendency toward hyalinization. Occasionally they accumulate to such an extent that they resemble a cavernoma (see also KASANTIKUL and NETSKY 1979). The growth of neurilemmomas is slow, and mitoses are never seen.

Electron Microscopy

EM studies on these fibers by RAIMONDI and BECKMAN (1967) prompted the conclusion that the tumors belong to the fibroblastic and not to the Schwann cell series. Other studies by WECHSLER and HOSSMANN (1965b) concluded that

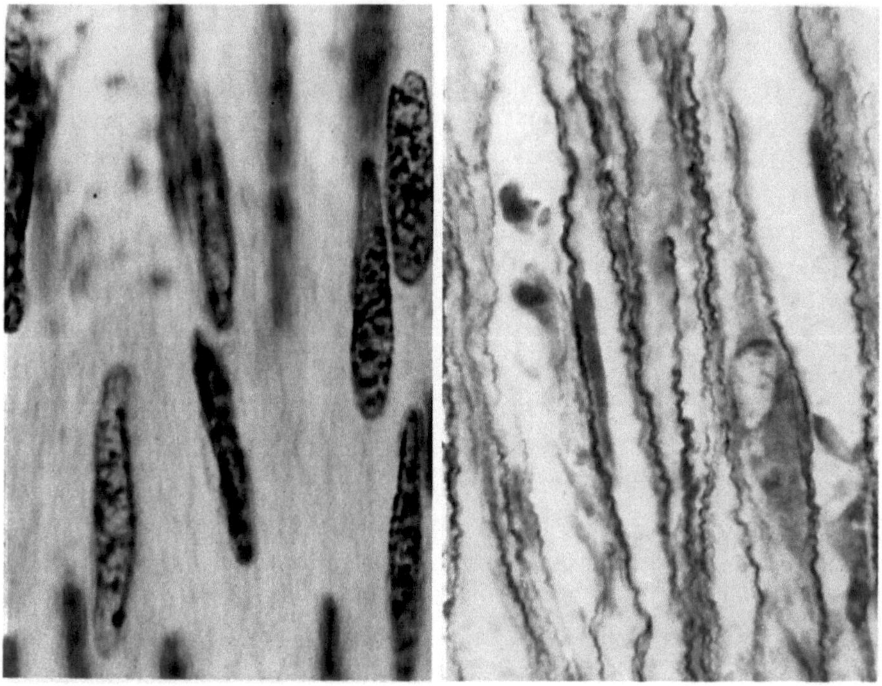

a b

Fig. 115. **a** Typical rod-shaped nuclei. Cresyl violet, ×1040. **b** Fine saw-like silver fibers spinning around the spindle cells in an acoustic neurilemmoma. Perdrau's silver impregnation, ×1054

the fibers were of Schwann cell origin. PINEDA (1964b, 1965) found a variety of configurations and concluded that Schwann cells produced collagenous fibers, an opinion also held by POIRIER and ESCOUROLLE (1967). WAGGENER (1966) was of the opinion that neurofibroma cells resemble nonneoplastic Schwann cells. He found extremely thin processes in the Antoni A type and globular structures with many organelles, and osmiophilic material in Antoni B (see also HILDING and HOUSE 1965; CERVOS-NAVARRO and MATAKAS 1968; CRAVIOTO 1969; FEIGIN 1971; TOGA 1976). Other EM investigations (GRUNER 1960; LUSE 1962) revealed differences in fiber structures between neurilemmoma fibers and collagen fibers, although the findings did not seem conclusive. Finally, JUNQUEIRA et al. (1981) observed thin, weakly bifringent, argyrophilic fibers formed by thin collagen structures. One must conclude that the results are still controversial.

Tissue Culture

Tissue culture results suggested a neuroectodermal origin of neurilemmomas from the Schwann cell. Particular attention should be drawn to the work of KERSTING and FINKEMEYER (1958) and KERSTING (1961), who were able to eliminate mesodermal fibroblasts in tissue culture by the use of trypsin and were still able to grow a typical neurilemmoma culture with all its very specific cellular characteristics. This appears to provide convincing proof of the tumor's neuroectodermal origin. On the other hand, differences between neurilemmomas and neurofibromas can be shown in tissue culture (CRAVIOTO and LOCKWOOD 1969; KUBO et al. 1976). CRAVIOTO found four different types of cells, (a) amoeboid microglia-like cells, (b) slender spindle-shaped cells, (c) racket-shaped cells, and (d) large kite-shaped cells, the first two being of Schwann cell character, the third undetermined, and the fourth fibroblastic. DASTUR et al. (1967) saw phagocytic Schwann cells with melanin granules (see also MANDYBUR 1974).

Histochemistry

Histochemistry has not provided convincing evidence regarding the nature of neurilemmomas. W. MÜLLER and NASU (1960; W. MÜLLER 1965) found alkaline lipids. Moreover, they assumed that the lipids were not the product of a degenerative process but reflected the capacity of the nerve sheath cells to produce lipids. The oxidative activity was different in the A and B type cells, as was the cholinesterase reaction. The fatty substances, according to HEGEDUS (1962), were similar to those which occur in myelin decomposition.

Differential Diagnosis

Neurilemmomas of the cerebellopontine angle and the spinal canal can be macroscopically differentiated from meningiomas or ependymomas. Histologic differentiation from fibroblastic meningiomas is occasionally difficult. The mixture of fibrillary and reticular tissue suggests a neurilemmoma, but the demonstration of true reticulin fibers (see above) makes this unlikely. The possibility of confusion with oligodendroglioma and chordomas, particularly in paraffin-embedded material stained with H&E, has been discussed above. Differentiation of this tumor from tumors of the glomus jugulare is not difficult.

Biologic Behavior (Grading), Metastasis, and Recurrence

Neurilemmomas are among the most frequent benign slow-growing groups of intracranial and intraspinal tumors. From OLIVECRONA's observations we know that some of them can even stop growing (see MINKOWSKI 1969: a clinical course of 32 years). Recurrence depends largely on the type of operation performed (intracapsular, subtotal, or total). Ordinarily recurrence will occur late and after incomplete removal, and a second operation is often rewarding. Total removal results in permanent cure.

Operative mortality has decreased from around 35% in the 1920s (see GERMAN 1961 b) to 8.3% (ZLOTNIK et al. 1979, Minsk/Russia); in the last 10 years these authors have not had a single death. KASANTIKUL et al. (1980) had a zero mortality rate in a series of 103 patients. Microtumors can now be diagnosed and resected with no mortality while still in the meatus.

In the WHO classification neurilemmomas correspond to grade I, as do the neurofibromas. The anaplastic (malignant) counterparts, i.e., the neurofibrosarcoma or neurogenic sarcoma correspond to grades III and IV. The serious nature of these tumors is often not recognized (QUICK and CUTLER 1927). The treatment is radical excision and radiation or even amputation of the extremities.

But even after amputation 50% may develop pulmonary metastases. The worst prognosis is that of neurosarcomas in the thigh.

Clinical Course

Paraplegia can occur in cases of spinal neurilemmomas, following hemorrhage into a cyst within the tumor (see KRAYENBÜHL and LÜTHY 1947). We have observed a similar case. After hemorrhages into cysts, rarely subarachnoid bleeding occurs (GLEESON et al. 1978; BOJSEN-MØLLER and SPAUN 1978; BABA et al. 1980).

HOLLIN et al. (1978) have observed that these tumors are sometimes mobile in the spinal canal (discrepancy between myelographic location and that found on surgery). Differential diagnosis between neurilemmomas and meningiomas can be difficult (MÖLLER et al. 1978; NUMAGUCHI et al. 1980). Intracanalicular neurilemmomas can be detected by CT or NMR alone (SCHUBIGER et al. 1978; see also HATAM et al. 1978) and by contrast radiography.

Further References: MENNEL and BÜCHELER (1974b), CERVOS-NAVARRO et al. (1968).

16.2 Anaplastic (Malignant) Neurilemmomas

The malignant counterpart of the neurilemmoma is characterized by the anaplastic features, such as increased cellularity and an excessive number of mitotic figures, but without any coordinated changes in the mesodermal component, particularly the vessels.

There is some confusion in the terminology because a distinction was made earlier between "malignant neurinomas" and "neurogenic sarcomas" (FOOT 1949). Some pathologists, however, have assumed that both types are "neurogenic sarcomas" (STEWART and COPELAND 1931; GESCHICKTER 1935). The characteristical neurogenic sarcomas contain multinucleated and large giant cells, which are irregular in size (MASERITZ 1942). They can appear as primary malignancies or as anaplastic changes in pre-existing neurofibromas, when they resemble fibrosarcomas, at which stage the amount of fibrils is becoming conspicuous.

The problems of terminology and definition have been discussed in detail by MENNEL and ZÜLCH (1971b). They arrived at the opinion that it was desirable to distinguish between anaplastic neurilemmomas (see above) and neurosarcomas. The latter should be classified with the true sarcomas. This was particularly recommended on the basis of the results obtained in the series of experiments performed by MENNEL 1972). Of the five clinical cases of MENNEL and ZÜLCH (1971b) two were classified as malignant neurilemmomas, two as true neurosarcomas, and the last one as a medulloblastoma – or neuroblastoma-like tumor of the peripheral nerve. HEDEMAN et al. (1978) reported two cases of malignant neurilemmomas involving the Gasserian ganglion. Similarly LIWNICZ (1979) reported two bilateral trigeminal "neurofibrosarcomas." We have personally observed a Gasserian ganglion tumor with a history of several years in an elephant (HBT, Fig. 83d) which turned out to be a neurosarcoma.

If all the characteristics are considered, classification as an anaplastic neurilemmoma depends on increase in cellularity, loss of specific differentiation, high number of mitoses, multinuclearity, pleomorphism, giant cell formation, and excess of fibrils; these dictate the classification of the tumors as anaplastic neurilemmomas. Their malignancy has been discussed above with the neurilemmomas.

16.3 Neurofibromas

Tumors of the neurilemmoma-type involving the peripheral nerves (neurofibromas) commonly occur in von Recklinghausen's disease. In such tumors the content of connective tissue is far greater than in intracranial and spinal neurilemmomas, since the perineural connective tissue has undergone pronounced reactive proliferation.

These tumors are still classified with the neuroectodermal neoplasms, for the same reasons that a scirrhus carcinoma does not become a sarcoma simply because the stroma shows excessive proliferation (for EM investigations see POIRIER et al. 1968).

It is an old tradition to call these solitary neurilemmomas of the peripheral nerves "neuro*fibromas*," because they provoke the formation of such an abundant amount of collagenous fibrous stroma. Histologically they are a mixture of Schwann cells and fibroblasts with loosely arranged collagen fibers (Fig. 116)

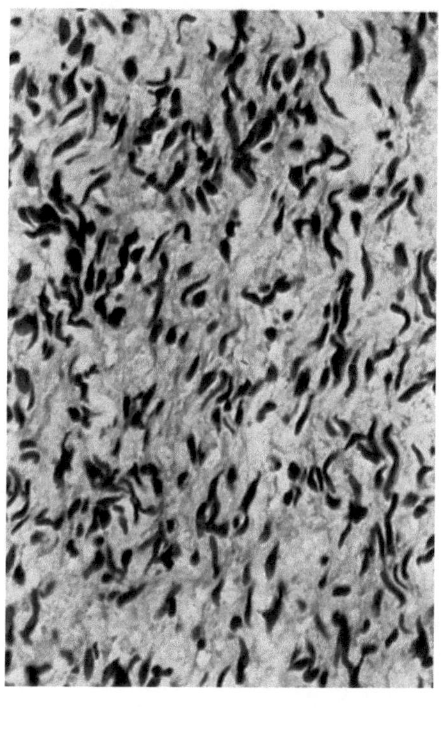

Fig. 116. Rare variants of peripheral neurofibromas: The cells are longer and twisted or kinked. Cresyl violet, ×336

and some *mucoid material.* These tumors have wavy architectures and have fascicular structures; they commonly contain axons.

"Plexiform" types were described by GAGEL (1936), and were recently reported in the cauda equina by SCHUMACHER et al. (1978).

16.4 Anaplastic (Malignant) Neurofibromas

Synonyms: Neurofibrosarcoma, neurogenic sarcoma

Anaplastic neurofibroma are malignant counterparts of the neurofibromas. This complication of transformation into a sarcoma is frequently encountered in von Recklinghausen's disease, but may also occur in an isolated case. In von Recklinghausen's disease the anaplastic transformation of the peripheral neurofibroma is not rare, but we do not have any idea what factor in these hamartoblastomatoses (phakomatoses) might activate the "inactive" malformation into a tumor-like growth, and in particular why it later becomes anaplastic. Since the transformation originates predominantly in the mesodermal part, the assumption of a *"sarcomatous"* change seems legitimate. The definition of the anaplastic form (neurosarcoma) is discussed elsewhere (p. 354; STEWART and COPELAND 1931; BUSCH and CHRISTENSEN 1947b; LIWNICZ 1979) and regarding neurosarcomas in patients without von Recklinghausen's disease by STEWART and COPELAND (1931), MURPHY et al. (1952), TASKIRAN and YENERMEN (1957), D'AGOSTINO et al. (1963b), and BEHRENDT and SCHULTRICH (1963).

Further References: Von KAHLDEN (1895), STAEMMLER (1939), SCHOEPE (1951), SCOTT and BENTZ (1962), MCCORMICK (1964), GIBSON et al. (1966), ADELMAN and ARONSON (1972), LILIEQUIST et al. (1972), HORI (1973), FEIGIN (1975), PRAKASH et al. (1980).

17 Tumors of Meningeal and Related Tissues

17.1 Meningiomas

Synonyms in the older literature: Fungus durae matris, psammoma, fibroma, sarcoma, endothelioma, exothelioma, or mesothelioma of the dura mater, meningeal fibroendothelioma, meningeal or arachnoidal fibroblastoma, meningothelioma, arachnothelioma, leptomeningioma, etc.

Introduction

The meningiomas are the most important types of mesodermal tumors. Macroscopically uniform, they can be subdivided histologically into 3 (ZÜLCH 1951 b), 10, or 22 (BAILEY and BUCY 1931; CUSHING and EISENHARDT 1938) subtypes. Biologically, as Cushing himself admitted (CUSHING and EISENHARDT 1938), this subdivision has no great significance. The WHO classification has compromised on 9 histological subtypes.

Historical Note and Definition

In all probability, meningiomas are the brain tumors that have been known longest. Because of the occasional production of grotesque cranial deformities, they had attracted the interest of doctors (ANDERSON 1879) and laymen alike even before the advent of classic pathological anatomy (see also CUSHING and EISENHARDT's monograph 1938; e.g., the case of KAUFMANN et al. cited in this volume).

A series of excellent reports began with that of LOUIS (1774), followed by those of CRUVEILHIER (1829/35), LEBERT (1851), and ROKITANSKY (1855/56), ending with one from VIRCHOW (1863/65), who produced the first precise descriptions of the sarcomas and endotheliomas of the dura and the psammomas, which he studied more extensively (VIRCHOW 1900).

GOLGI's (1869) concept of "endothelioma" started the controversy over the origin of the meningioma from the dural endothelium, which subsequently also involved BIZZOZERO and BOZZOLO (1874) and MARBURG (1935). The question seems now to have been settled, largely because of the findings of M.B. SCHMIDT (1902) and FERNER (1940), i.e., the derivation of this tumor from the arachnoidal granulations. However, only the collection of large numbers of these meningeal tumors in certain North American clinics has allowed the final classification of their tissue type, localization, and clinical symptomatology. This information resulted from the investigations of MALLORY (1920), BAILEY and CUSHING (1926), and their co-workers, and was finally set down in a comprehensive book by CUSHING and EISENHARDT (1938). In the German literature,

ESSBACH's (1943) monograph treated the subject thoroughly from the anatomicopathological point of view. However, even up to a relatively short time ago there were two opposing points of view, one group attempting to relate the meningioma to the arachnoidal endothelium and the other, to the fibrous connective tissue ("meningeal fibroblastoma"; PENFIELD 1932b). On the other hand, attempts to prove the neuroectodermal origin of meningiomas (OBERLING 1922) failed to find acceptance, although this point was taken up again by DIEZEL (1954).

Epidemiology (Age – Sex – Frequency – Site)

Age: The meningiomas show a clear predilection for the middle and later decades of life (Fig. 9h). They begin to become more frequent in the 21–30 age group, a fact that is useful in differential diagnosis (e.g., in the prechiasmal region, where craniopharyngiomas occur preferentially around the second decade, pituitary adenomas around the third decade, and tuberculum sellae meningiomas thereafter). However, the age incidence of meningiomas is variable, depending on whether the material to be studied comes from a neurosurgical clinic, a pathology institute, or a mental hospital, where many meningiomas have been discovered as asymptomatic incidental findings. In our collection, made up of material from mixed sources, the peak incidence lay around the age of 45 to 55 years (Fig. 9h). The average age of CUSHING's (1932, 1935) patients was 46.6 years for both sexes together: the average of the male patients alone was 52, and that of the female patients 42.9. Our youngest patient had a congenital tumor (HABERICH and ZÜLCH 1959; cf. MENDIRATTA et al. 1967). PENDL (1975) emphasized the occurrence of meningiomas in childhood and youth (15 years). Our oldest patient was 86. The youngest case in CUSHING's series seems to have been a 5-year-old child with a spinal meningioma.

Sex: There is a striking female preponderance of meningiomas, which in some localizations is overwhelming. In our 9000 cases series the overall female:male ratio was 9:5. In the malignant form there was a reverse preponderance of 3:2. In a statistical survey of sphenoidal ridge meningiomas 97% were in female patients (KIENECKER et al. 1975). The female:male ratio for the spinal meningiomas was also extreme [20:1 (LAPRESLE et al. 1952) and 3.6:1 (HOSSMANN and ZÜLCH 1966)]. This ratio, however, changes with the selection criteria of the series considered. In psammomatous meningiomas at all levels the ratio was 10:1 and in the thoracic spine, 20:1, as in the series of LAPRESLE et al. (1952). In multiple meningiomas the female:male ratio was 12:3 (SCHARRER and BRUNNGRABER 1974).

Frequency: Of our 9000 patients, 1492 had meningiomas, i.e., 16.6%: 532 were found in male and 960 in female patients. In CUSHING's (1932, 1935) material the meningiomas accounted for 16.6%. OLIVECRONA (1947) had 3256 cases, of which 608 (=18.7%) were meningiomas. ESSBACH (1943) summarized several sets of statistics relating together to 6116 intracranial tumors, 14.3% of which were meningiomas; of 888 *spinal* tumors, however, 32% were meningiomas,

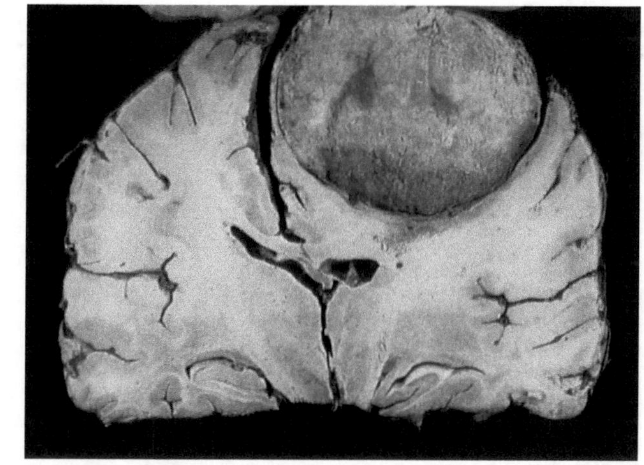

Fig. 117. Section through an apple-sized meningioma of the middle third of the sagittal sinus. Note marked distortion of the adjacent brain and ventricular system. (ZÜLCH 1975a)

a figure that was slightly lower at the Mayo Clinic (25.9%). Data about malignant meningiomas are given in Sect. 17.1.9.

Site: The increased incidence of meningiomas in certain key localizations has long been recognized, and corresponds to the distribution of the arachnoidal granulations (BAILEY 1933, Fig. 66; 1951). Arranged in order of frequency we have the following groups [basically following CUSHING and EISENHARDT'S (1938) groupings and with only slight changes and additions]:

1. Meningiomas of the *sagittal sinus* or parasagittal region (Fig. 14, nos. 1, 4; GP, Fig. 180) (of the anterior, middle (Fig. 117) and posterior thirds (Fig. 118) of the sagittal sinus; OLIVECRONA 1934; HOESSLY and OLIVECRONA 1955) can reach the size of a tangerine or an apple (GP, Figs. 183–185), and usually lie in the angle formed by the falx, the sinus, and the dura of the convexity (GP, Fig. 181). They are most frequent in the middle third of the sinus, less common in the anterior third, and rare in the posterior third. The overlying bone is often infiltrated by the tumor or hyperplastically thickened (hyperostosis) (GP, Fig. 218). They can occur bilaterally (GP, Fig. 187), and in these cases the sinus is commonly invaded and not infrequently occluded. More details about the gross pathology are given elsewhere (GP, p. 115 ff.).
2. Meningiomas of the *falx* can be distinguished from the parasagittal meningiomas (Fig. 14, nos. 5, 6; GP, Figs. 188–190) by their broad attachment to the falx (they usually extend bilaterally) and their mantle of brain tissue toward the top. Their attachment is therefore distant from the sinus. Most of them are in front of the central fissure.
3. Meningiomas of the *convexity* (Fig. 14, nos. 11, 19; Fig. 119; GP, Fig. 192) differ from the foregoing types in their lack of relationship to the falx or sinus. They are distributed over the whole of the convexity, the majority of convexity meningiomas lying anterior to the fissure of Rolando. In these cases we also find local or diffuse hyperostosis with or without actual infiltration of the bone.

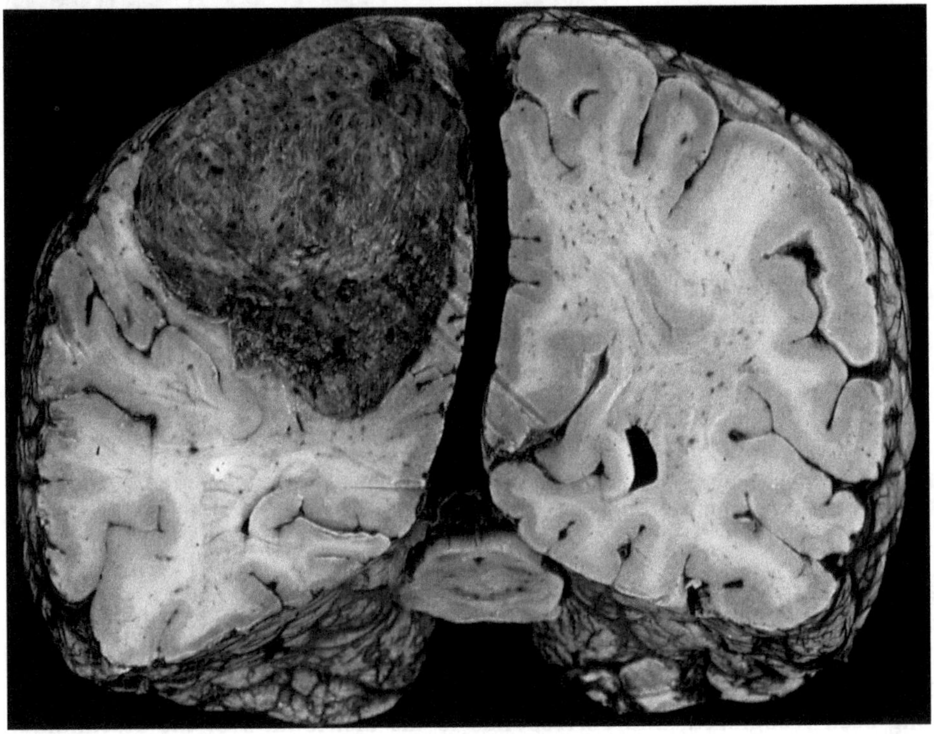

Fig. 118. Anterior view of a meningioma of the posterior third of the sagittal sinus. (ZÜLCH 1975a)

It is not rare for such tumors to be sited in the third frontal convolution (Fig. 119; GP, Fig. 192) (frontolateral meningioma, ECTORS and ACHSLOGH 1959, R.C. BEHREND 1962). In these circumstances they tend to press the contralateral peduncle against the edge of the tentorium and produce homolateral symptoms (GROENEVELD and SCHALTENBRAND 1927; see KERNOHAN'S "notch," KERNOHAN and WOLTMAN 1929; F3 meningiomas, BEHREND 1962).

4. Meningiomas of the *olfactory groove* (Fig. 14, nos. 14, 31; Fig. 120) or of the *cribriform plate* lie on the lateral or medial floor of the anterior fossa (GP, Figs. 193, 194). They reach the size of a tangerine, are hemispherical in shape, and displace the brain upward. They may extend in the posterior direction to the optic nerve and the chiasm (Fig. 120), depressing them and pushing them backward. They can straddle the falx. Meningiomas also occur in the paranasal (frontal, sphenoid) sinuses (LEE et al. 1979).

5. Meningiomas of the *tuberculum sellae* (Fig. 14, nos. 32, 35) (suprasellar or prechiasmal meningiomas; GP, Fig. 195) lie in the midline, posterior to those of the olfactory groove. They are usually the size of a cherry or a tangerine, definitely smaller than the olfactory meningiomas (because of the early optic or chiasmal symptomatology). They often have a finely nodular surface, and they displace the chiasm, the carotids and adjacent structures upward. Small tumors spread out along the sheaths of the optic nerves (see below, pp. 365, 552).

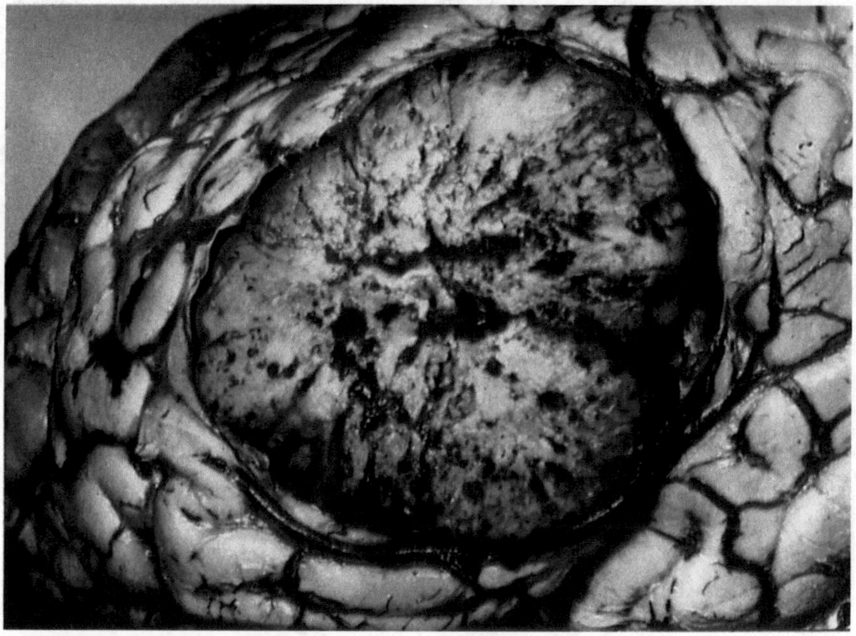

Fig. 119. Large frontolateral meningioma, in its typical location in the third frontal convolution. Such a meningioma commonly results in mass shifting with a resultant involvement of the contralateral cerebral peduncle ("tentorial notch"). (ZÜLCH 1975a)

6. Meningiomas of the *sphenoid ridge* and the *Sylvian fissure* lie along the sphenoid ridge (Fig. 14, nos. 28, 29; GP, Figs. 197, 198), being round or flat like a plaque or carpet. They vary in extent and may grow into either the anterior or the middle fossa. The structures at the base arteries (cranial nerves) can be surrounded by the tumor carpet-like outgrowth. More than any other type, these meningiomas tend to produce hyperostosis of the sphenoid (GP, Figs. 218, 219) wings and of the whole base of the skull. Meningiomas lying more laterally around the sylvian fissure (Fig. 14, no. 22) merge with the group over the convexity (GP, Fig. 199). In this type, frequently growing en plaque, some portions of the tumor occasionally interdigitate with the brain.

The lateral sphenoid wing (pterion) tumor may invade the ridge (hyperostosis, see above) or, in rare cases, the bones of the convexity and the temporal muscle (ZÜLCH 1956, Fig. 310b), vessels and nerves being unaffected. Their average frequency is thought to be around 17% (POLAK 1966).

7. Meningiomas of the *temporal fossa and Meckel's cave* lie beneath the temporal lobe at the base. They are spherical, and are positioned between the meningiomas of the sphenoid anteriorly, the cerebellopontine angle meningiomas posteriorly, and Meckel's cave meningioma medially (PINTO 1958, KREBS et al. 1932). Micromeningiomas of the cavum Meckeli have been also described (KIRCHHOFF 1975).

8. Meningiomas of the *cerebellopontine angle* lie along the medial portion of the petrous pyramid (Fig. 14, no. 62; GP, Figs. 200–203, 205), i.e., in the posteri-

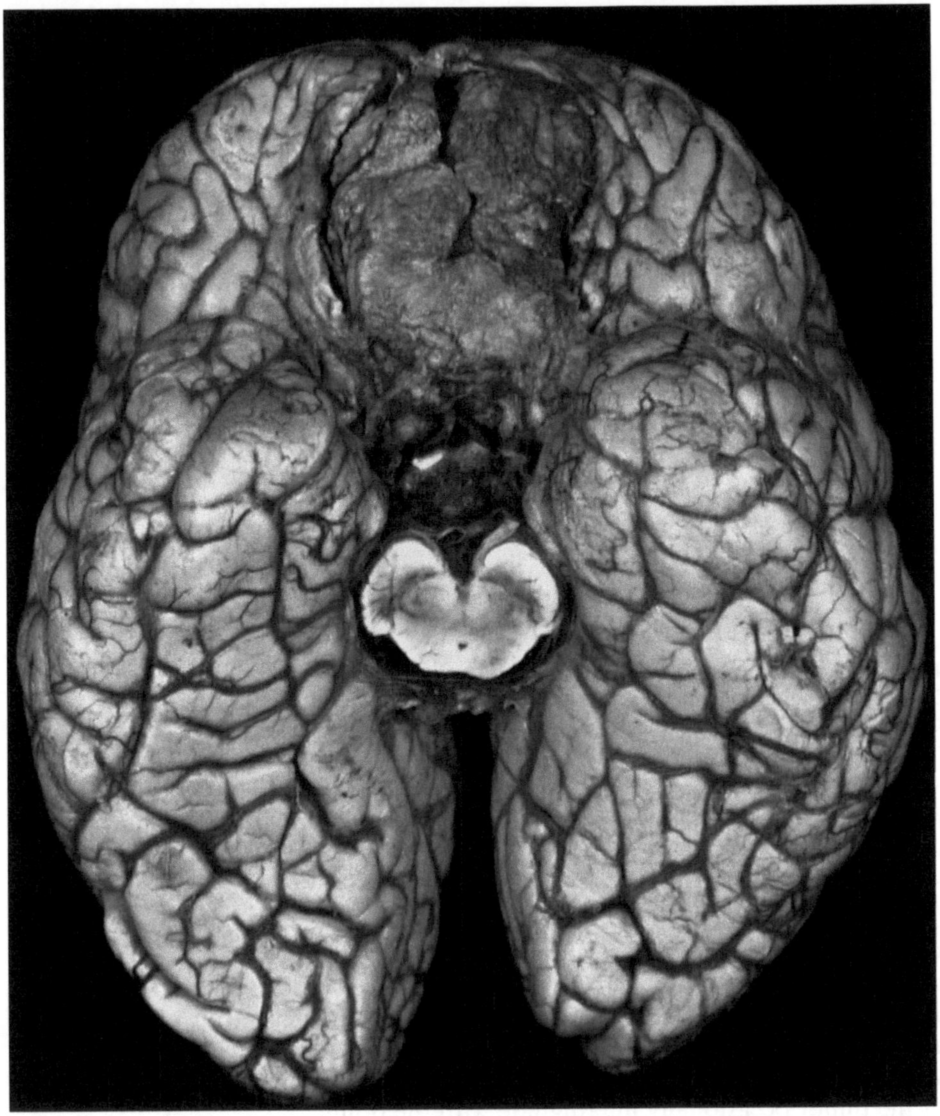

Fig. 120. Large midline olfactory groove meningioma

or fossa (VALAVANIS et al. 1981). They can resemble the acoustic neurilemmoma in size and extension. However, they do not enlarge the internal acoustic meatus.

Some tumors of the petrous region may extend to the neck or grow as dumbbell tumors (BALSYS and NORTON 1980) (GP, Fig. 196).

9. Meningiomas of the *tentorium (peritorcular meningioma)* (Fig. 14, nos. 65, 66) – and of the *cerebellar convexity* either grow supratentorially (expanding beneath the temporal or occipital lobes) or infratentorially (Fig. 121) (over the surface of the cerebellum). They amount to 10% of all tumors of the posterior fossa (BLAGOWESCHTSCHENSKAJA 1952). CASTELLANO and RUGGIERO (1953) have

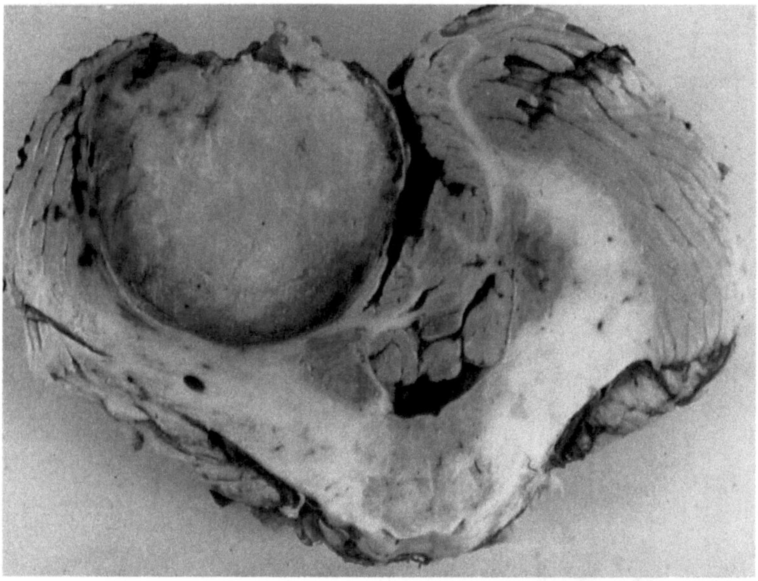

Fig. 121. Tentorial meningioma extending into the posterior fossa (so-called peritorcular meningioma)

distinguished five different locations in these tumors. On the cerebellar convexity they occur preponderantly in middle-aged women (KENDALL and SHAH 1972). In general they are most frequent around the torcular herophili (confluens sinuum).

10. Meningiomas of the *lateral ventricle* occur as egg-shaped tumors (1.5%, FORNARI et al. 1981) that can reach the size of a fist (KOBAYASHI et al. 1971) and lie mainly in the trigonal region (Fig. 14, no. 53), where they are firmly attached to the choroid plexus (see BORCHERS 1910; youngest case VASSILOUTHIS and AMBROSE 1978: 22 months; portrayed by CT: MANI et al. 1978). Meningiomas of the velum interpositum project into the third ventricle (HEPPNER 1954, 1955; MARKWALDER et al. 1979; SUGA et al. 1971; ITO et al. 1981). They are extremely rare in the fourth ventricle (see Figs. 2, 8, BURGER and VOGEL 1976).

11. Meningiomas of the *clivus* or *craniospinal* meningiomas, including meningiomas of the *foramen magnum*, proceed from the lateral or medial clivus (GP, Fig. 204) toward the temporal lobe, anterior surface of the cerebellum, or pontine region, and may send a tongue of tumor down into the foramen (Fig. 14, no. 75) (RESNIKOFF and CARDENAS 1964) or the spinal canal (see below). According to the volume of tumor tissue they can be called either *craniospinal* (GP, Fig. 207) or *spinocranial* (CHERRINGTON and SCHNECK 1966); they can also be dumbbell shaped (BITO et al. 1974). Some are located just around the foramen magnum (STEIN et al. 1963; RESNIKOFF and CARDENAS 1964).

12. Meningiomas in the *hiatus tentorii* are rare (Fig. 14, no. 60). They occur near the great cerebral vein, extending (GP, Fig. 208) over the quadrigeminal region (Fedor KRAUSE: his first case successfully operated on in the quadrigeminal region, cited by ZÜLCH 1981; see OPPENHEIM and KRAUSE 1913; later

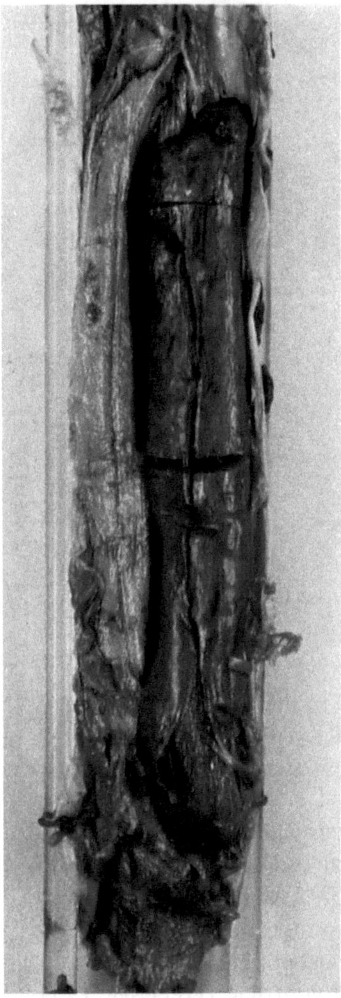

Fig. 122. Unusually long fingerlike meningioma extending over approximately ten spinal segments. (ZÜLCH 1975a)

ARAKI'S two cases, 1937; see also ZEITLIN 1935; SCHNABEL and WUTTKE 1960; SACHS et al. 1962; PAPO and SALVOLINI 1974).

13. *Spinal* meningiomas (or meningiomas of the *spinal cord)* are the size of beans or acorns (GP, Fig. 209), occasionally finger-shaped (GP, Fig. 110), and extend over several segments (Fig. 122). They are most common in the thoracic region (HOSSMANN and ZÜLCH 1966) and most extensive in the cervical or caudal regions. They are firmly attached to the dura, usually dorsolaterally but occasionally elsewhere, and this may allow their distinction from neurilemmomas. Curiously, they tend to have a high frequency in women and a preference for the 5th or 6th decade, when they occur in the thoracic segments. These tumors are exceptionally calcified. Parts of such meningiomas are outside the dura (SINGH et al. 1968; WAGA et al. 1970; CALOGERO and MOOSSY 1972; SATO et al. 1973a; HAMADA et al. 1977).

14. Meningiomas at *rare localization:* some meningiomas are situated in the orbita, near the optic nerve (SHUANGSHOTI 1973), or encasing the optic fascicle (bilateral: HIRST et al. 1979), while others occur within the orbital roof (FINKEMEYER and PFINGST 1966), or at the trigeminal sheath (KREBS et al. 1932).
15. Meningiomas can grow *extracalvarially* (SIEGEL and ANDERSON 1966) and have even been reported in the oral cavity (SUZUKI et al. 1967, Table 1); the cutis (see SUZUKI et al. 1967, Table 2) or subcutis; the scalp and neck; and beside the vertebral column (LOPEZ et al. 1974).
16. *Multiple* meningiomas (*meningiomatosis*): on rare occasions meningiomas are multiple (GP, Fig. 215), ranging in size from that of a cherry stone to that of an apple; any sizes over this range can be encountered and there may be as many as 100 (KHOMINSKY 1958; see also FRAENKEL and HUNT 1903). The incidence of multiple meningiomas is between 1%, and 2% (ECHOLS 1941; LUYENDIJK 1954; LEVIN et al. 1964; SCHARRER and BRUNNGRABER 1974; ABTAHI 1975; NAHSER et al. 1981). They are often associated with acoustic nerve tumors, or other neurilemmomas and neurofibromas in von Recklinghausen's neurofibromatosis (see HARBITZ 1935; GIRARD et al. 1977). Some authors apply the term "meningeal meningiomatosis" to these multiple tumors. Others use this term for the primary "diffuse," usually sarcomatous tumors in the subarachnoid space (see BLACK and KERNOHAN 1950).

Gross Pathology (Size and Form)

The fresh operative specimen is dark red, with lighter translucent parts; the cut section is coarsely fibrous, and cysts are found only rarely. The angioblastic types can sometimes be recognized by the coarse vascular meshwork on the cut surface. Meningiomas range in size from a pinhead to the size of a man's fist, depending on the location and type of growth. The giant type is discussed elsewhere (GP, p. 114 and Figs. 179, 180, 190). Their form can be spherical, hemispherical, or conical, or they can grow en plaque (Fig. 123), flat or like a carpet, particularly in the temporal fossa (GP, Fig. 179). Occasionally both types of growth are combined, a conical tumor growing out of a flat one. A local hyperostosis (spicula) can induce a corresponding impression, an umbilication, in the tumor. When meningiomas straddle a bony ridge such as the sphenoid wing, falx or petrous ridge, a corresponding saddle-shaped impression results (GP, Fig. 178). If growth takes place in two directions, as it does in tumors of the tentorium, a dumbbell form develops (GP, Fig. 196). The weight of the meningiomas is mostly between 50 and 300 g (giant variants see GP, p. 114), or may be even heavier (600 g: WINKELBAUER 1930; 1300 g, circumference 48 cm, actual size 18 × 14 × 9 cm: KERSCHNER 1928; 1890 g: BALAPARAMESWARA et al. 1971; see GP, Fig. 217).

Meningiomas are smoothly encapsulated (Figs. 122, 124), or coarsely or finely nodular. The consistency varies, depending on the size, the amount of degeneration (hyalinization, liquefaction, microcyst formation), formation of fibers and cartilage, fatty tissue, or calcification, and is described as rubbery or hard. At the site of dural attachment, where the connective tissue of the meninges radiates into the tumor, meningiomas are often harder than in other

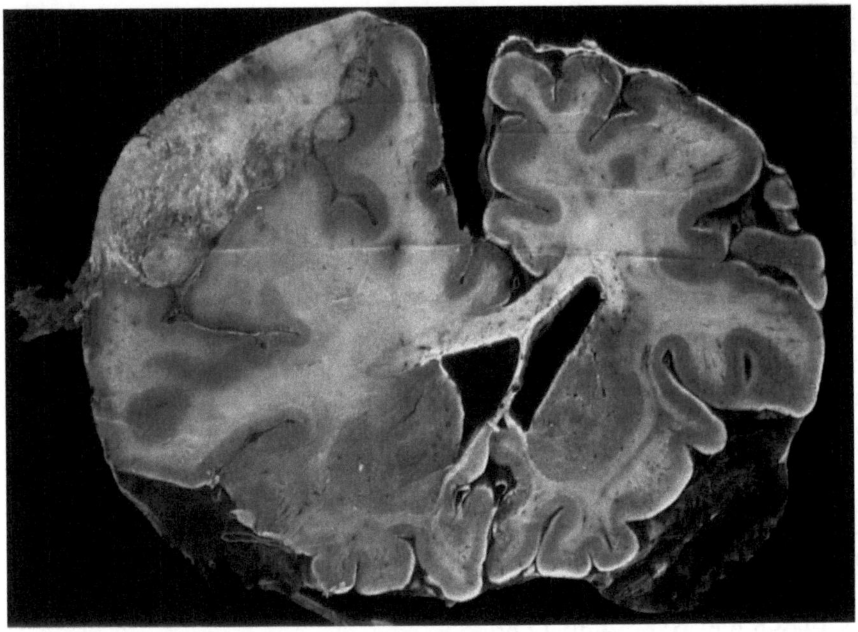

Fig. 123. Flat meningioma of the convexity extending with nodules

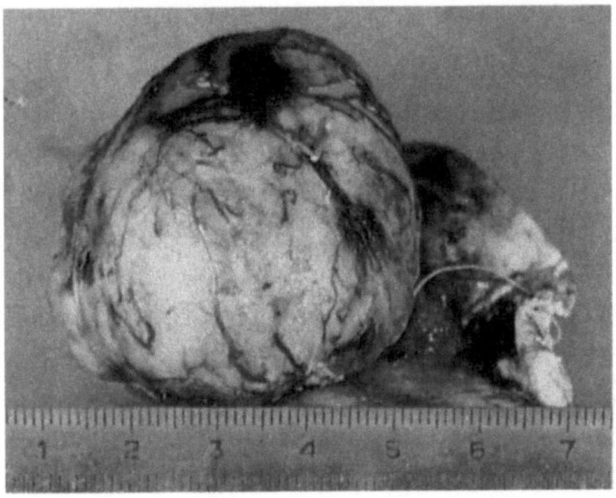

Fig. 124. Typical spherical meningioma with a richly vascular capsule

regions. The brain substance adjacent to the meningioma can either be pushed aside and compressed or both softened and edematous, as now very commonly shown by CT. It may even have undergone cystic degeneration. The occurrence of massive hemorrhage in meningiomas is extremely rare (KLEINMAN et al. 1979); cyst formation is also rare (BECKER et al. 1979; IWANAGA et al. 1980). An association with arteriovenous malformations or aneurysms has been described but its causal correlation is still obscure. Cerebral infarction after involvement of the carotid or middle cerebral artery has been recognized. The vascular supply most often comes only from the dural vessels, but in rare (more malignant) cases can also arise from internal carotid branches (for pathology see also TEDESCHI et al. 1981 a).

Histologic Appearance

Meningiomas behave differently according to the structure with which they are in contact. Generally they only displace the brain (Fig. 123) and spinal cord but on rare occasions they interdigitate by means of finger-like processes, most commonly in the temporal region. The dura and the sinus are infiltrated almost consistently, which explains the tumor's firm adherence to these surfaces. The overlying bone is also quite frequently invaded and parts of the tumor extend without interruption along the Haversian canals (see below). This usually results in hyperplastic bony overgrowth, accounting for the protuberances and projections on the skull. Occasionally large parts of the base of the skull become hypertrophic because of overlying tumor growth en plaque. However, there are also many instances of bony hyperplasia without actual tumor cell infiltration. The disproportion in size between the paper-thin tumor, consisting only of a few rows of cells, and the enormously thickened bone in these cases may be grotesque. Sometimes meningiomas can even infiltrate the temporal muscle or present in the neck (BALSYS and NORTON 1980).

The meningiomas with hyperostosis compress the brain more markedly than do osteomas proper (ECHLIN 1934). These hyperostotic changes can reach enormous sizes, as in the case of ROEMER (1896), where the circumference of the skull was 90 cm and the size of the tumor 14 × 12.5 × 11 cm (WHITE et al. 1950). OEHLECKER (1952) took away bone 3.5 cm thick (see also ROWBOTHAM 1939; ESSBACH 1943; FREEDMAN and FORSTER 1948). According to CUSHING and EISENHARDT (1938) hyperostotic phenomena may occur in 25% of meningiomas. This is explained partly by the osteoblastic potential properties of the original cells.

Meningiomas contain no elastic fibers (KLOSE 1961), but may have abundant reticular fibers, particularly in the fibromatous type. Some meningiomas are tremendously pleomorphous (see CUSHING and EISENHARDT 1938: type IV, 2, and MARCOS 1954), but in these cases the malignancy is not increased.

As suggested by the old terms of endothelioma, fibroma, and psammoma, subgroups were distinguished from the beginning (BAILEY and BUCY 1931: 9 subgroups) and this culminated in the subclassification of CUSHING and EISENHARDT (1938) with 22 different subentities.

GARRIDO and KEPES (1978), on the basis of 1300 meningiomas, were of the opinion that a subdivision into meningotheliomatous, fibroblastic, hemangiopericytic, and transitional meningiomas was sufficient. MASSON (1970) introduced a "humid type" which was said to be characterized by secretory activity seen in the EM picture (CHOUX et al. 1975).

The very detailed subdivision of CUSHING and EISENHARDT (1938) is certainly not clinically relevant. However, for clinical purposes the entities used in the new WHO classification seem to be practical (ZÜLCH 1979):

1. Meningotheliomatous meningiomas (endotheliomatous)
2. Fibrous (fibroblastic) meningiomas
3. Transitional (mixed) meningiomas
4. Psammomatous meningiomas

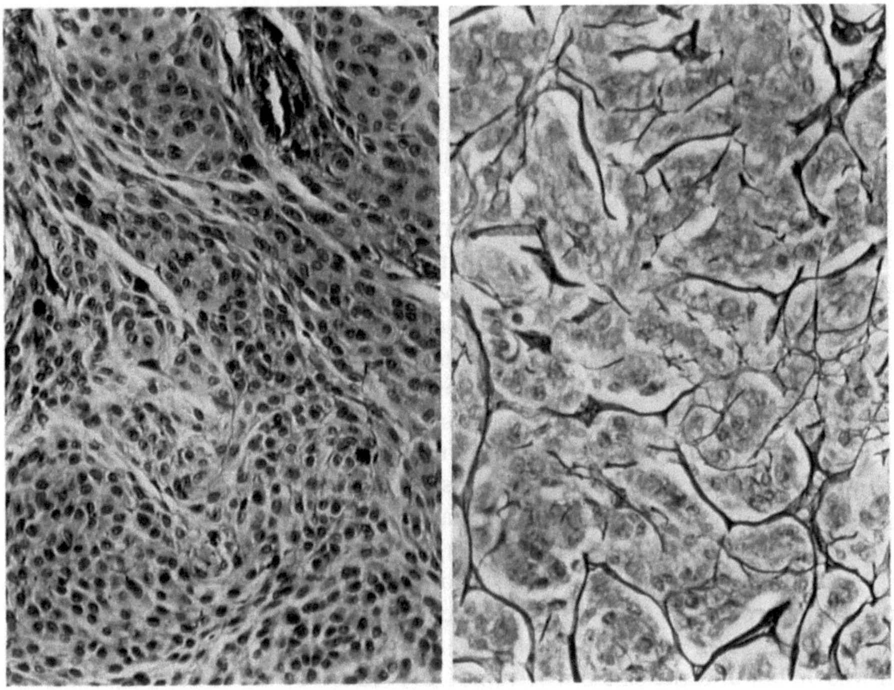

a b

Fig. 125. a In the meningotheliomatous meningioma whorls are not prominent and a tendency to form solid masses of cells prevails. H&E, ×272. **b** Silver impregnation shows the stroma between the islands of cells. Silver impregnation, ×312

5. a) Angiomatous meningiomas
   b) Hemangioblastic meningiomas
   c) Hemangiopericytic meningiomas
6. Papillary meningiomas
7. "Anaplastic" meningiomas (malignant de-differentiated)

17.1.1 Meningotheliomatous Meningiomas

The meningotheliomatous meningiomas include all those that form densely cellular tissue consisting of large meningothelial cells, sometimes without, but more frequently with, an interstitial tissue dividing the cell masses into islands, nests (HBT, Fig. 73), and other cell groups (Fig. 125). A feature characteristic of this form is its similarity to the nests of normal (arachnoidal) meningothelium. The cells usually form a syncytium; they are large and they are distributed uniformly, diffusely, or in long streams. The interstitial tissue is sparse, being limited to a few vessels and fibers, and separates the individual cell groups from each other (Fig. 125b). Silver impregnation methods allow particularly reliable identification of this form (Fig. 125b), as the reticulin fibers are confined to the stroma. The cell nests quite frequently show a subdivision with a concentric (HBT, Fig. 74), cellular arrangement (like onion skin) into rings, whorls

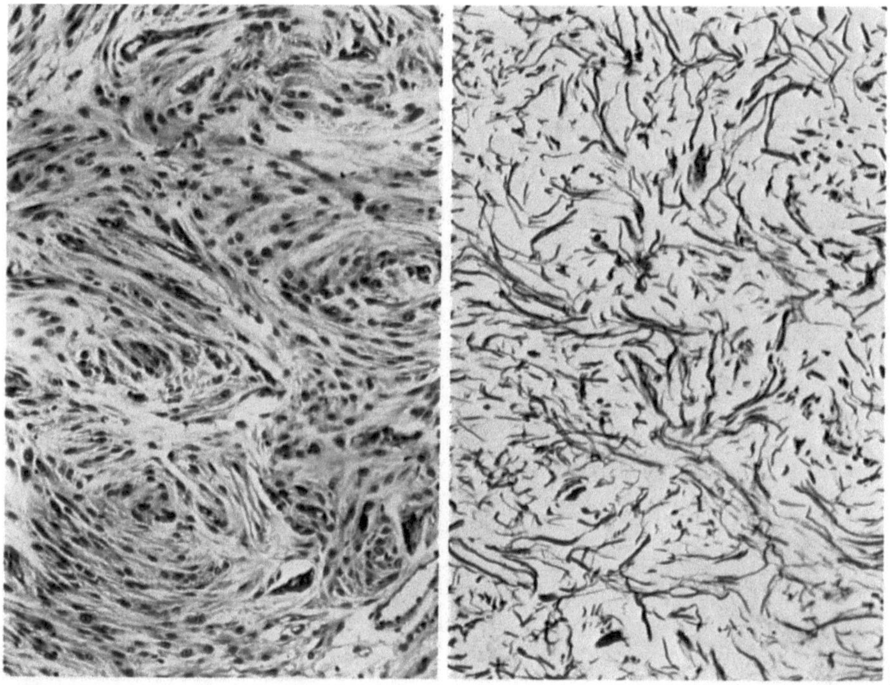

Fig. 126. a Predominantly cellular form of fibrous meningioma where spindle shaped cells predominate. Cresyl violet, ×125. **b** Tight feltwork of silver fibers in fibrous meningioma. Silver impregnation, ×120

(Fig. 128), or other patterns in which psammoma bodies develop (see below). Some of the cells show *cytoplasmic invaginations* (Bonis 1961) and folded nuclei, so that pseudoinclusions are mimicked. There are PAS-positive inclusions, which, it is thought, may be glycogen (see Font and Croxatto 1980).

17.1.2 Fibrous (Fibroblastic) Meningiomas

The fibroblastic meningiomas include most of the spindle-shaped (Fig. 126a) cell tumors and are somewhat similar to a fibroma. The long spindle-shaped cells (HBT, Fig. 75) lie in streams and whorls, and sometimes palisade-like formations are seen. Around the capillaries there are loop-shaped formations and concentric layers of cells, which bear a certain resemblance to the similar formations of the first group, where the central capillary, however, is missing. Parallel and interlacing bundles of cells with abundant pericellular collagen (Fig. 126b) and reticulin are highly characteristic. Metal impregnation reveals a dense network of true reticulin fibers between the cells, which is the best means of differentiating these tumors from neurilemmoma (HBT, Figs. 70, 71), where the type of silver-impregnated fibers is different (p. 352). Calcifications are spear and club shaped. Syncytial areas and the tendency to form whorls and psammoma bodies are less common.

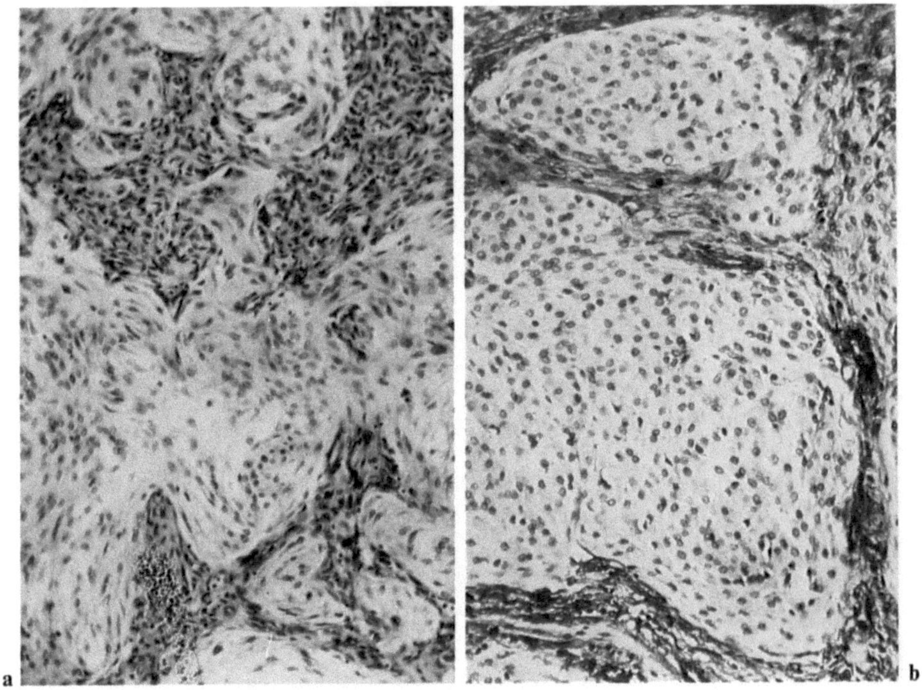

Fig. 127a, b. In the transitional meningioma a mixture of cells with syncytial and fibroblastic features predominates. Cresyl violet, ×120

17.1.3 Transitional (Mixed) Meningiomas

This form of meningiomas is composed of a mixture (Fig. 127) between the main architectural types, and therefore deserves the name "transitional." Such tumors have syncytial and fibroblastic patterns, and even have a tendency to form concentric whorls with hyaline cores or psammoma bodies.

17.1.4 Psammomatous Meningiomas

When psammoma bodies are very definitely the predominant feature (Fig. 128) and the meningotheliomatous parts are only present in small nests, meningiomas can be called psammomatous (HBT, Fig. 74). They occur most often at the – thoracic – spinal cord (p. 532ff.) or, at the base of the skull, particularly when clinically silent, as with slow-growing tumors. Their content of calcospherites can be so high as to appear on a plane x-ray.

Biological Behavior (Grading) of 17.1.1–4

In the WHO classification all these are graded I.

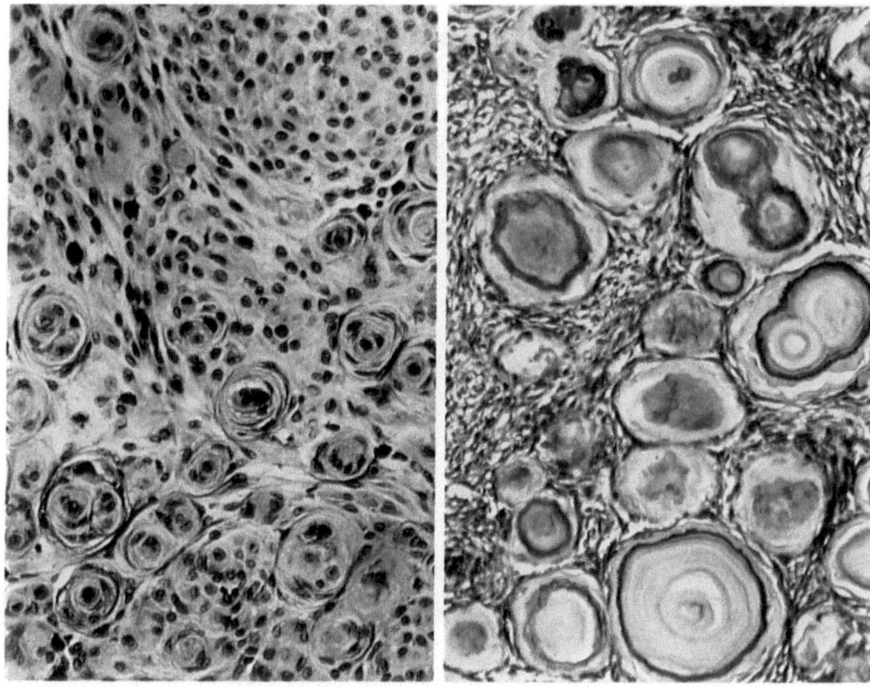

a b

Fig. 128a, b. Meningotheliomatous meningioma with a pronounced tendency towards the formation of concentric whorls, hyalinization and calcium deposits (psammoma bodies). This extreme calcification is especially frequent in spinal meningiomas of the thoracic region. H&E, ×272 (**a**) and ×136 (**b**)

17.1.5 Angiomatous Meningiomas

The WHO classification includes three subgroups of particularly high vascularized meningiomas:
a) Angiomatous meningioma
b) Hemangioblastic meningioma
c) Hemangiopericytic meningioma

Age: The average age of patients with the hemangioblastic variant was 47 years, and that of patients with the hemangiopericytic variant, 40 years.

Sex: No divergent data distinguished these from other meningiomas.

Site: No preferential site is known for these subgroups.

Details of the particularly vascular variants of meningiomas have been published by BAILEY et al. (1928), BERGSTRAND and OLIVECRONA (1935), CUSHING and EISENHARDT (1938), COURVILLE and ABBOTT (1940), STOUT and MURRAY (1942), RAMSEY (1966), PALACIOS and AZAR-KIA (1975), HORTEN et al. (1977).

An *angiomatous* meningioma (Fig. 129a) consists of tissue with a considerable content of large and small vascular channels (HBT, Fig. 78a) of venous

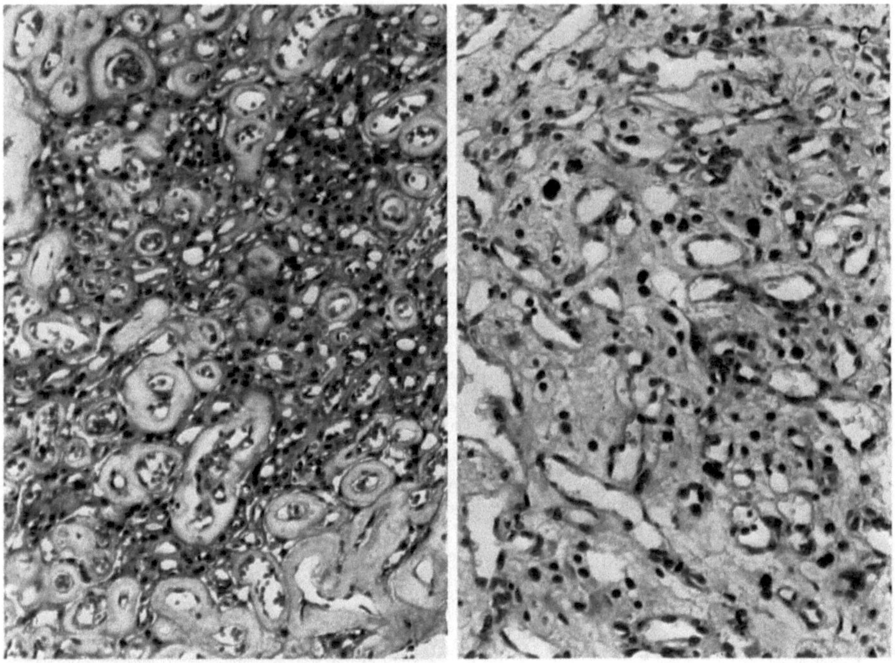

Fig. 129. **a** Angiomatous meningioma. Cresyl violet, ×150. **b** Hemangioblastic meningioma. H&E, ×175

and capillary type arranged in a network, interspersed with large lining cells or nests of meningotheliomatous (Fig. 130a) or fibrous meningioma. The endothelium of the vessels is a single layer.

Hemangioblastic meningiomas (Fig. 129b) are a second form with a particular vascular structure: This form bears some relation to the capillary hemangioblastoma (HBT, Fig. 78c), and histological distinction between the two is frequently not possible. However, the meningiomas are always well encapsulated, and they grow by expansion, in contrast to the infiltrating angioblastoma in the posterior fossa and elsewhere. The hemangioblastic structure is best revealed by silver impregnation. Despite their benign biological behavior, a few examples of this type present the histological picture of a pleomorphic tumor (Fig. 130b) with atypical cells, hyperchromasias, etc. These, however, are secondary regressive processes and are in no way indications of malignancy. This last variant represents transition to the meningotheliomatous type, which corresponds to type IV,2 of Cushing and Eisenhardt (1938; see also Marcos 1954).

Pitkethly et al. (1970) have made a study of 1900 meningiomas, 81 of which, i.e., 4.3%, were hemangioblastic or hemangiopericytic. In the WHO classification the angiomatous and angioblastic meningiomas are grouped under grade I.

Hemangiopericytic meningiomas are rare meningiomas (Fig. 131); they are indistinguishable from the hemangiopericytomas elsewhere in the body (a detailed discussion of the histology has been given by Fabiani et al. 1980).

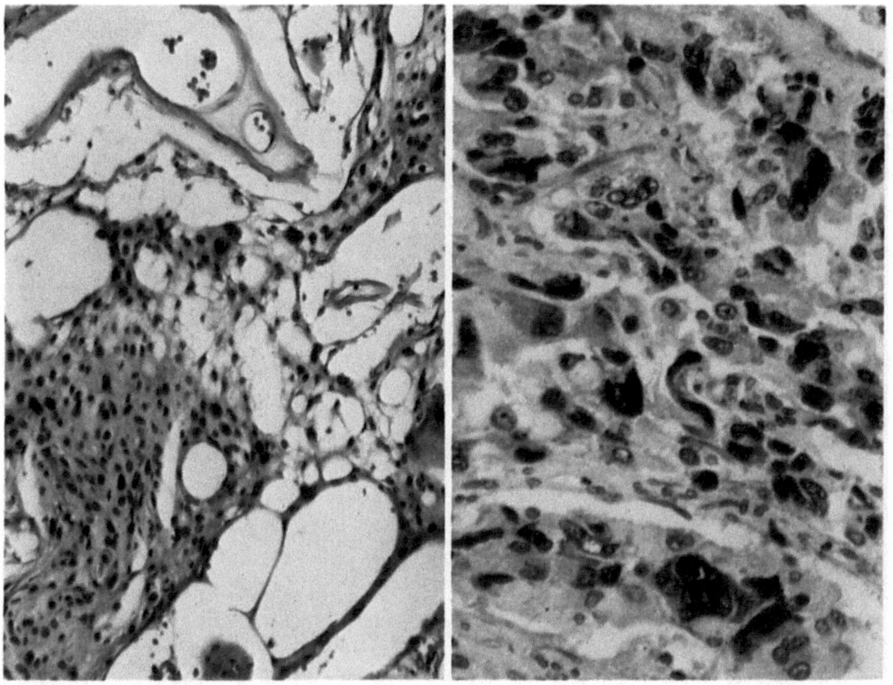

a b

Fig. 130. a Angiomatous meningioma: The large number of blood vessels in an angioma-like arrangement is characteristic of this tumor. Between the blood vessels, however, there are nests of cells showing the typical structure of a meningotheliomatous meningioma. H&E, ×120. **b** In some (probably angioblastic) meningiomas giant cells with bizarre single or multiple nuclei may be encountered. Cresyl violet, ×154

It is interesting to see that the prognosis of the hemangiopericytic type is definitely worse than that of the other meningiomas. In the WHO classification they are classed as grade II. Recurrences are 3 times more common for the hemangiopericytic than for the hemangioblastic type. Metastases have almost only been observed with the hemangiopericytic type. GLASAUER and YUAN (1963) collected 35 meningiomas with extracranial metastases. All were of the hemangiopericytic type. Our own strange case, with a history of 22 years and an ultimate 1780-g metastasis to the lung, was also of the hemangiopericytic type (HBT 77a shows the final state of this tumor; see also ZÜLCH et al. 1954).

17.1.6 Papillary Meningiomas

Occasionally in meningiomas papillary patterns prevail. A typical example has been described by CUSHING and EISENHARDT (1938) in the famous case of their patient Dorothy May Russell, in whom ultimately (17th operation) a papillary meningioma was found as a metastasis to the lung. Thus, they usually show biologically malignant behavior (LUDWIN et al. 1975) and correspond to grades II and/or III (see also STEFANKO and MACKAY 1981).

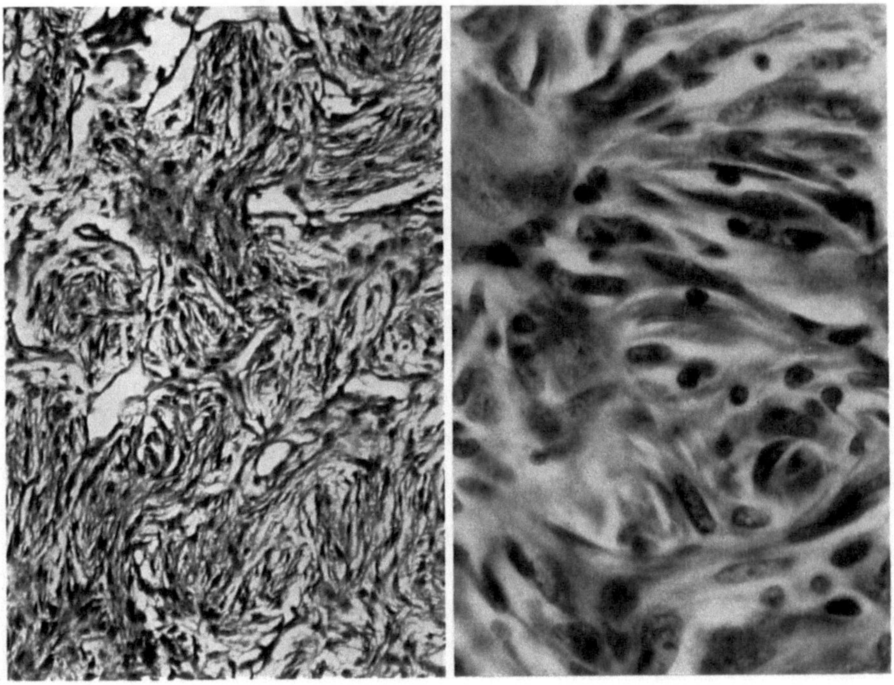
a b

Fig. 131 a, b. The hemangiopericytic forms grossly resemble meningiomas, but are microscopically indistinguishable from other hemangiopericytomas. H&E, ×125 (**a**) and ×500 (**b**)

Other variants: Beside these main types, in rare instances fatty, cartilagenous, or bony tissue is formed *within* the tumor. These cases have been characterized by the addition of one of the words "lipo-" (Fig. 132a), "chondro-," or "osteoblastic," as in BAILEY and BUCY's (1931) subdivision. However, some of these formations are produced during regressive phenomena (HBT, Fig. 76). The most prominent of the regressive phenomena is the tendency to hyalinization of the interstitial tissue and the blood vessel walls. In the fibromatous type, particularly, we find broad hyalinized strands of tissue, to a degree that the architecture is lost. Calcification in the form of concentric psammoma bodies or spear-shaped or plaque-like deposits has been described above, but it can lead to complete calcification of the whole tumor, allowing it to be demonstrated roentgenologically (intracranially and in the vertebral column). Highly pleomorphous cells may be formed even in meningiomas with slow growth (MARCOS 1954, from our institute).

Fatty degeneration, though, is less apparent but can occur diffusely in scattered cells and fibroblastic types or in the center of the cell islands in the meningotheliomatous type (HBT, Fig. 76). A few meningiomas tend to be "humid" and undergo diffuse mucoid degeneration with resulting small or large cysts (IWANAGA et al. 1980). This can be recognized by CT (BECKER et al. 1979). Hemorrhages into the tumor are extremely rare.

During growth single cases can extend to an excessive degree, both intra- and extracranially (GP, Fig. 217) (see BRUGGER 1955b, from our institute).

A very remarkable variant is the *melanoblastic* meningioma (Fig. 132b),

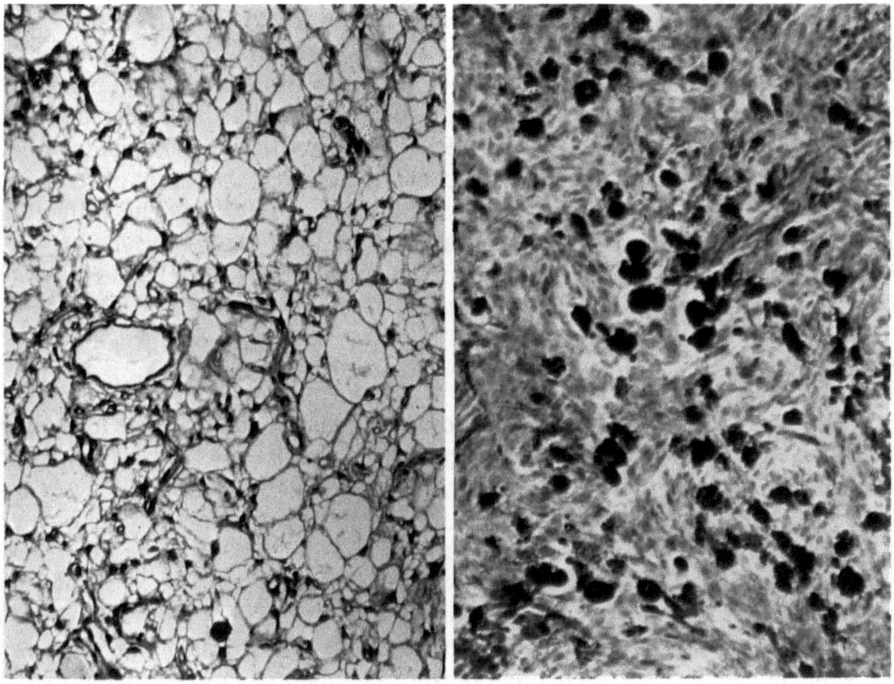

a b

Fig. 132. a Rare lipoblastic meningioma. H&E, ×125. **b** Meningioma containing melanotic cells, an exceptionally rare form. Carmine, ×125

which is well recognized and occurs both in the cranial cavity and in the spinal canal (KEEGAN and MULLAN 1962; TZONOS and BRUNNGRABER 1963b; TURNBULL and TOM 1963; ABBOTT et al. 1968; LIMAS and TIO 1972; TITRUD 1973). These meningiomas are well encapsulated, like the other forms, and must be strictly differentiated from the rare primary melanomas (p. 391) and from melanosis (HAFERKAMP and RISOPATRON 1955; ERBSLÖH 1956). Amelanotic cells can be recognized in all melanin-bearing tumors by the nuclear vacuoles, which are encased by a mantle of chromatin (APITZ 1937).

Metastasis of carcinoma to meningioma has been observed (SAVOIARDO and LODRINI 1980). HOPE and SYMON (1978) give a good reference list.

In summary, up to now hardly any fundamental progress in our knowledge of the pathogenesis or the biological behavior of the meningiomas has been achieved with modern methods; however, the most important statements will be reported.

Electron Microscopy

There are abundant descriptions of the EM picture, but only very few points of importance for the determination of growth of the types (CASTAIGNE et al. 1966a) or for differential diagnosis (GONATAS and BESEN 1963; ISHIDA et al. 1964b; NAPOLITANO et al. 1964; CERVOS-NAVARRO 1967, 1971; CERVOS-NAVARRO and VASQUEZ 1969; TANI and HIGASHI 1972; TANI et al. 1974; TOGA 1976).

The absence of basement membranes is a recognized feature (WOYKE et al. 1971). In the endothelial cells in meningiomas more filaments, mitochondria and large electron-dense granules are seen, and also tubular bodies (OSUGI et al. 1977). Cilia in meningothelial and fibroblastic meningiomas have been described by CERVOS-NAVARRO and VASQUEZ (1966). Pinocytotic vesicles and glycogen granules in the cortex adjacent to the meningiomas have been observed by KOIZUMI et al. (1973) and also by CASTAIGNE et al. (1966a). The differential diagnosis of the angiomatous variants rests on light microscopy, i.e., gross characteristics, whereas EM histology may not show many differences (CERVOS-NAVARRO 1971; ERMEL 1974; POPOFF et al. 1974; TEDESCHI et al. 1981b).

Tissue Culture

The early studies of KERSTING (1961) show that genuine architectures like whorls were formed even from a one-cell culture. Apparently several cells have even been known to fuse into a single syncytial complex (KERSTING 1961; see also SIPE 1976). A striking resemblance was found between cultures of meningiomas of fetal leptomeninges and of fetal dura, on the one side, and the culture of fetal mesenchyma on the other (BLAND and RUSSELL 1938). Cells with two or three nuclei were not common (COSTERO et al. 1955a, b; KERSTING 1961; LISS 1972). It is interesting, however, that tissue culture also did not reveal any valid distinction between angioblastic meningioma and hemangiopericytoma (MÜLLER and MEALEY 1971).

Histochemistry

Histochemically one indication of an existing anaplasia may be found in the absence of alkaline phosphatase activity, which is high in intensive calcified cases and totally absent in malignant cases. In such cases increasing acid phosphatase levels can be observed and the activity of esterase and oxidative enzymes is higher (NASU 1964; BINGAS and GRUMME 1971). Rapidly growing meningiomas are rich in glycogen (LIPCINA 1952).

Immunochemistry

Immunochemistry has lately yielded the first results: the amount of antibodies that reacted with meningioma-associated antigens was highest in meningioma patients (WINTERS and RICH 1975).

Chromosome Studies

Chromosome studies of the meningioma have been performed, but with little informative conclusions (ZANG 1970; ZANKL and ZANG 1972).

Endocrinology

From the endocrinologic viewpoint it is interesting that the estrogen receptor level is high. A connection with the high frequency of meningiomas in women has been discussed (DONNELL et al. 1979).

Differential Diagnosis

Early in the operation the surgeon may mistake an oligodendroglioma attached to the dura (p. 242), or more rarely also a metastatic tumor, a tuberculoma, or a gumma, adherent to the dura, for a meningioma. However, the nature of the tumor usually becomes apparent during the operation owing to the absence of encapsulation. In the cerebellopontine angle, or in the spinal canal, meningiomas are sometimes difficult to differentiate from neurilemmomas (unless they are calcified on x-ray, which is only rarely demonstrable in the spinal forms).

Histology

Histological differentiation between meningiomas and neurilemmomas is also sometimes difficult, particularly with the fibromatous form of meningiomas. The spindle-shaped nuclei of the neurilemmoma, its true palisading, the coexistence of such different tissue types as A and B, and its pronounced tendency to undergo fatty degeneration all support the diagnosis of neurilemmoma, while any calcification suggests a meningioma, Only the meningiomas form concentric whorls (HBT, Fig. 74) and show a dense intercellular network of true reticulin fibers (HBT, Fig. 75b); the neurilemmomas possess delicate "specific" argyrophil (see p. 352) fibers (HBT, Figs. 70, 71; ZÜLCH and MILHAUD 1960, pp. 545–547). The meningiomas must sometimes also be distinguished from the tumors of the glomus jugulare; there may be a certain similarity between the pattern of the latter tumors and the meningotheliomatous variety of meningiomas (for discussion of their specific impregnation trends see pp. 206, 207). The hemangioblastic and hemangiopericytic meningiomas histologically resemble the corresponding tumors elsewhere in the body so much that a differential diagnosis can be made only from the gross appearance (capsule, etc.). Modern methods seem to put more emphasis on the reticular character.

Biologic Behavior (Grading), Metastasis, and Recurrence[1]

The meningiomas and the neurilemmomas are the most benign extracerebral tumors. They are classed as grade I (with the exception of the hemangiopericytic type, which corresponds to grades II and III). When surgery is indicated the prognosis for patients with meningiomas is certainly better than for those with any other brain tumor. Total removal commonly leads to a permanent cure. With recurrences, a further operation is usually successful. Chemotherapy and radiation are of no great value.

Meningiomas rarely metastasize. In a few cases, spread via the CSF (KALM 1950) or via the blood stream to other organs (see p. 183ff.) has been described.

If total removal is successful – sometimes this has to include surrounding structures such as sinus, dura, or bone, into which the tumor is growing – recurrence is unlikely. En-bloc operation of lateral ventricle meningioma entails a higher mortality (FORNARI 1981). It is difficult to decide whether the hyperplas-

[1] For information on metastasis and recurrence see also Sect. 17.1.7.

tic bone is really infiltrated by the neoplasm or not, and it is therefore often preferable to excise. CUSHING and EISENHARDT (1938) themselves had numerous recurrences, as is apparent from the fact that 522 operations were performed in 282 patients with meningiomas. If the "totality" of the operation is graded (5 groups, SIMPSON 1957) the likelihood of recurrence can be determined; this is definitely higher in the anaplastic types. Meningotheliomatous forms are said to recur earlier than the fibroblastic forms (CROMPTON and GAUTIER-SMITH 1970). The recurrence rate in the angiomatous forms is discussed on p. 371 ff.; for an extensive description see HOPE and SYMON (1978).

Clinical Course

Meningiomas, because of their slow expansive growth, can remain clinically asymptomatic for a long time, when growing in silent areas. In other regions, however (e.g., the parasagittal type), seizures may give an early indication of the tumor growth (PENFIELD et al. 1940; PENFIELD and WARD 1948; FLYGER 1956). Sometimes, however, they can reach an enormous size while clinically producing few and mild symptoms, especially in the frontal lobes (GP, Figs. 189, 190).

WOOD et al. (1957) emphasized that among 300 neoplasms not discovered until autopsy, there were 100 cases of meningioma, 16% of which were multiple. According to BARROWS and HARTER (1962), meningiomas with tentorial attachment are particularly likely to escape clinical diagnosis.

The history of the diseases can often extend over many years before symptoms of increased intracranial pressure set in. A history with an apoplectiform onset is unusual (EL-BANHAWY and WALTER 1962; GORAN et al. 1965), although subarachnoidal hemorrhage may occur (ROSENBERG et al. 1975; V.R. SMITH et al. 1975) or intracranial hematomas (MODESTI et al. 1976) may even arise. The expansive growth leads to specific patterns of cerebral vessel displacement on the arteriogram and the demonstration of arteries belonging to the external circulation is not infrequent. Sometimes a diffuse network of capillaries within the tumor is recognized. Because of the slow displacement of the adjacent brain, obstruction of the CSF pathways is less frequent than with tumors that arise from the brain substance proper. The ventricles in cases of meningioma can be rather small. However, a perifocal edema is far more frequent, as we now know from CT observations. The significance of the bony changes seen on x-rays, viz. vascularization and erosion, formation of hyperostosis or spiculae and enlarged bony channels of the A. meningica (MCLEAN 1936a), may help in diagnosis of this specific tumor type. Calcification of a spherical tumor to the point where it is roentgenologically visible is specific. The abundance of blood vessels in certain meningiomas is so great that in the venous phase of the arteriogram the tumor appears "stained." In rare cases the outer vascular system of sinusoid vessels may lead to the roentgenological appearance of early veins (ZÜLCH et al. 1973) even in benign types. Their growth into the dura sinuses and Haversian channels has been mentioned, as has their invasion of the temporal muscle (CUSHING and EISENHARDT 1938; NAGER 1964), which we have also noted. Growth into the brain, with strands along the vessels, sometimes makes complete removal difficult.

Experimental Meningiomas

As ZÜLCH and MENNEL (1971a) stated in their report on experiments with resorptive carcinogens, almost no true benign meningiomas have been found experimentally. Tumors in the meninges have been almost exclusively malignant meningeal sarcomas, which, however, were not very numerous in these experiments. In contrast, these sarcomas were regularly induced by *topical* application of carcinogenic carbohydrates and in *viral* carcinogenesis in the CNS.

Neuro-oncogenic viruses, as already emphasized, almost regularly produce very malignant tumors of the meninges. One of the most recent results is that of OGAWA (personal communication; see also OHMORI 1965), who used adenovirus 12.

Meningiomas in the human are the only neoplasm for which external initiating factors are not so uncommon. They have definitely been observed to follow local skull injuries (p. 72ff.). However, in recent decades it has been noted that meningiomas are significantly more frequent in patients formerly subjected to x-irradiation to the skin of the head than in other populations (p. 148). The general problem of tumorigenesis (see p. 41 ff.) has not yet been clarified.

We have emphasized on p. 94 the significance of the sex difference in incidence of the benign (here the meningiomas) and malignant tumor groups, which is particularly apalling and indicates some initiating factor for the meningiomas. SMITH et al. (1978) and BURGER and VOGEL (1976) came to the opinion that a difference of such a magnitude as 1:10 between the two sexes must have a significance relevance to the pathogenesis.

We have observed a case where the tumor consisted of two parts: a fibromatous central core and a fairly nicely separated plaque of meningotheliomatous tissue, as if an arachnoidal granulation had begun to undergo neoplastic growth. Yet even this observation does not elucidate the process of the triggering of neoplastic growth.

According to all observations (gross appearance, light and electron microscopy, tissue culture, immunochemistry, etc.), the meningiomas seem to originate from the tissue of the pia, the arachnoidal granulations and the blood vessels, the periosteum, the bone, or the dura. These contain all the ingredients essential for the growth of the various components of meningiomas (GLOBUS 1937). CUSHING (1925) emphasized the parallel in the number and site of the arachnoidal granulations and the number and site of meningiomas.

Further References: RIBBERT (1910a), AOYAGI and KYUNO (1912), LEARMONTH (1927), BUCKLEY and EISENHARDT (1929), FRAZIER and ALPERS (1933), BERGSTRAND and OLIVECRONA (1935), ARLT (1936), WOLF and COWEN (1936), GLOBUS (1937), KALBFLEISCH and GREBE (1937), BLAND and RUSSELL (1938), TÖNNIS (1938, 1948), O.T. BAILEY (1940), COURVILLE and ABBOTT (1941, 1942), ECHOLS (1941), MAJERSZKY-SANTHA (1943), RUSSELL (1950), NOETZEL (1951), PETERS (1951), TÖNNIS and SCHÜRMANN (1951), CASTELLANO et al. (1952), LAPRESLE et al. (1952), ZÜLCH (1956, 1962a), SCHNABEL and WUTTKE (1960), EL-BANHAWY et al. (1963), STEIN et al. (1963), NYSTRÖM (1965), CHERRINGTON and SCHNECK (1966), GUIOT and DEROME (1966), HOSSMANN and ZÜLCH (1966), BAKEY and CARES (1972), ZÜLCH and MENNEL (1974).

17.1.7 Anaplastic (Malignant) Meningiomas

Introduction

Anaplastic (malignant) meningiomas form a special subgroup in the WHO classification. The prerequisite for inclusion in this subgroup is that the common anaplastic features (p. 27) are recognized, but a frank fibrosarcoma has not yet developed.

Historical Note and Definition

Malignant meningiomas have been described many times in the literature (ZÜLCH and MENNEL 1975). They are thought to be rare and are most commonly hemangiopericytic in nature (THOMAS et al. 1981). In a special count of our series of 9000 tumors, we found that 1492, i.e., 16.6%, were meningiomas. In our series a particular study was made of the malignancy of this tumor type in a group of 624 cases, 57 (9.1%), of which were malignant (ZÜLCH and MENNEL 1975; see also TURNER et al. 1942: 10% of 370 cases). A particularly well-known example is the case mentioned under papillary meningiomas: the tumor operated on 17 times in the patient Dorothy May Russell (see CUSHING and EISENHARDT 1938). This tumor ultimately had a complete architectural and cellular transformation and had metastasized to the lung. We have described several cases (ZÜLCH 1956) with an extraordinary anaplasia (ZÜLCH and MENNEL 1975), and we have, for instance, reported a corresponding case (ZÜLCH et al. 1954).

Epidemiology (Age – Sex – Frequency – Site)

Age: The age incidence of 567 benign and 57 malignant tumors was almost identical and corresponded to Fig. 9h. The age curve shows clearly that malignant meningiomas are quite different than sarcomas. Sarcomas in the CNS have no age peak.

Sex: The female: male distribution of meningiomas was approximately 9:5 for the whole group of 624 tumors of all grades of malignancy. However, in the malignant forms of this tumor there was a reverse preponderance of the male sex, with a ratio of 3:2. This was apparently consistent with a general trend in pathology of intracranial tumors, i.e., that some malignant tumors are more common in male patients (see p. 94).

Frequency: TURNER et al. (1942) reported a frequency of 10%, ZÜLCH and MENNEL (1975), of 9.1%.

Site: Spinal meningiomas are less commonly malignant (ZÜLCH and MENNEL 1975). In contrast malignant forms were more frequent among tumors in the cranial cavity, particularly in the frontal regions (ZÜLCH and MENNEL 1975).

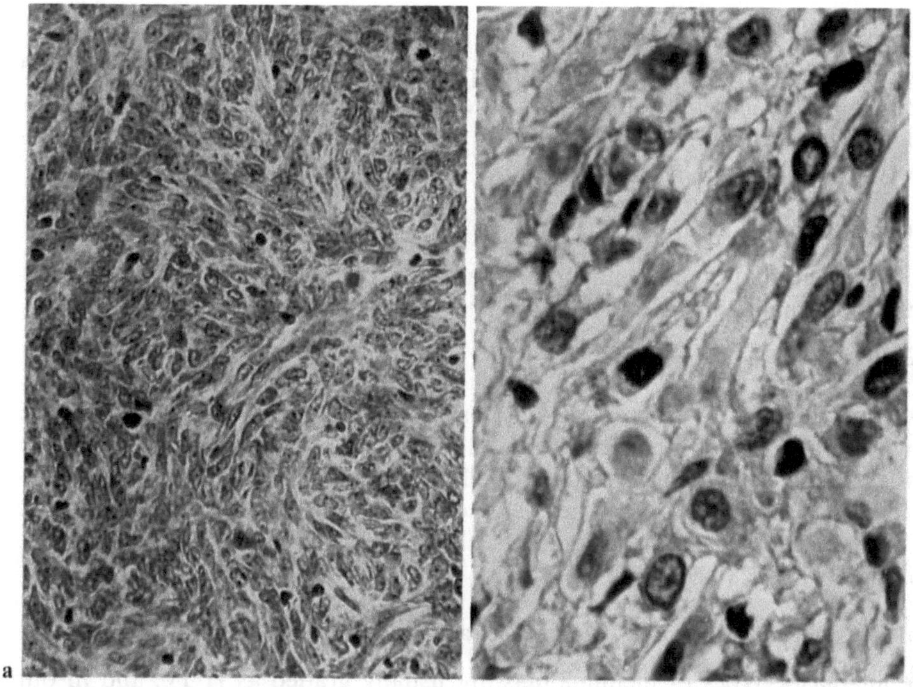

Fig. 133. **a** Malignant meningioma with metastasis to the lung and various organs after a total of 22 years of growth. Cresyl violet, ×272. **b** Rapidly growing meningiomas with mitoses. They are usually of the fibroma-like type. Cell columns and whorls are clearly seen: the nuclei are quite vesicular and have large nucleoli, and numerous mitoses can be seen. H&E, ×1040

Gross Pathology

Anaplastic meningiomas usually possess a sort of capsule, which is not, however, comparable to the tough collagenous capsule of the benign meningiomas (GP, Fig. 216, which was a special type of anaplastic tumor). The cells are clearly demarcated from the brain tissue but may invade it along the vessels (ZÜLCH 1956, p. 425).

Histologic Appearance

The criteria of malignancy are: high number of mitoses (Fig. 133), especially atypical ones, pleomorphism, and increased cellularity when combined with the former; poor differentiation; necroses with pseudopalisading; infiltration of the brain tissue; CNS and/or extracranial metastases.

Most of the anaplastic meningiomas are either fibromatous or hemangiopericytic. The form of the frequent mitoses (HBT, Fig. 77a–d) – typical or atypical – seems to be an index of malignancy. If the number of the atypical is equal to that of the typical forms higher malignancy can be assumed.

Histochemistry

Histochemically the absence of alkaline phosphotase suggests malignancy; acid phosphatase is increased and more oxidative enzymes occur in the presence of a malignant meningioma. Rapid growth is also connected with a high glycogen content (LIPCINA 1952).

Chromosome Studies

Chromosome analysis of meningiomas has not provided any informative conclusions about malignancy (ZANG 1970; ZANKL and ZANG 1972).

Differential Diagnosis

The most important differential diagnosis is distinction from fibrosarcomas, which are also clearly connected with the dura mater. Histologically these are seen as fibromatous tumors with high cellularity, polymitotic growth, and moderate prominence of stroma, whereas pleomorphism is *not* a prominent feature of the typical fibrosarcoma. It grows along the perivascular spaces into the brain (HBT, Fig. 83a).

Biologic Behavior (Grading), Metastasis, and Recurrence

The anaplastic types of meningiomas are usually graded as II–IV, and in our investigation of 57 cases we classed 32 as grade II; 20 as grade III; and only 5 as grade IV (ZÜLCH and MENNEL 1975). A particular feature of the anaplastic meningioma is extracranial metastasis. Again we cite CUSHING and EISENHARDT (1938: case of Dorothy May Russell, in whom metastasis to the lung took place after the 17th operation). We have described a similar case (GP, Fig. 216) with late metastasis to the lung after 22 years of growth. However, in this case it had been suspected from the first that the tumor was malignant. The weight of the metastasis in the lung was 1780 g (ZÜLCH et al. 1954; Fig. 133a).

There are many cases in the literature of extracranial metastases: a congenital metastasis was reported by HABERICH and ZÜLCH (1959) in a neonate who died on the 7th day of life. There were metastases to thyroid, thymus, heart, liver, pancreas, stomach, colon and skin. Further cases of metastases have been reported by GESSAGA (1968: skeletal muscle), GORDON and MALONEY (1965: thyroid), STEINKE and EDER (1964), JESTICO and LANTOS (1976: pancreas, kidney), KEPES et al. (1971: cervical nodes and scalp), LAYMON and BECKER (1949: vertebrae, sacrum, ribs, clavicle, mediastinum), and MEREDITH and BELTER (1959); see also FENYES and SLOWIK (1972), GULLOTTA and WÜLLENWEBER (1968), KOLLMANNSBERGER et al. (1975), KINOMOTO et al. (1982).

In summary, it is only possible to state, with SHUANGSHOTI et al. (1970), that the four most common sites of extracranial metastases of meningiomas are: lung, liver, pleura, and lymph nodes.

17.1.8 Melanocytic Meningiomas

Melanocytic meningiomas are rare (KEEGAN and MULLAN 1962, with references; TZONOS and BRUNNGRABER 1963b; TURNBULL and TOM 1963; TITRUD 1973), and they seem to involve a less benign prognosis than other meningiomas (Fig. 132b). Ultrastructural observations suggest an origin of the tumor from the leptomeningeal melanoblasts (LIMAS and TIO 1972).

Further References: PISCOL and HOFFMANN (1961), ABBOTT et al. (1968).

17.2 Meningeal Sarcomas

Synonyms: Medulloblastoma, oligodendroglioma, meningioma, and glioblastoma have all been called sarcomas in the older literature

Introduction

Sarcomas were sometimes listed in older statistics as making up 30%–40% of brain tumors, owing to inadequate definition and classification. Recently they have accounted for only a few percent of the intracranial and spinal tumors in large series. Some special entities are contained in the WHO classification.

Historical Note and Definition

According to general pathology the sarcoma is a malignant tumor of the mesodermal tissue, and for such tumors the term is still appropriate. However, in such a very specialized classification as this we have to distinguish various types of such tumors (see p. 22). The WHO classification includes three types of meningeal sarcomas:

1. Fibrosarcoma
2. Polymorphic cell sarcoma
3. Primary meningeal sarcomatosis

Apart from these particular entities a certain number of other tumors have been recognized and described in recent decades, e.g.,

4. *Circumscribed arachnoidal sarcoma* (see also Sect. 15.6.2.1)
5. *Rhabdomyosarcoma/osteosarcoma* (see Sect. 17.2.5)
6. *Monstrocellular sarcoma* as a tumor of the blood vessels (see Sect. 15.6.1.2)
7. *Reticulum cell sarcoma* (for this see Chap. 18)
8. *Periadventitial diffuse sarcomatosis*, corresponding also to the term "microglioma" (see "lymphomas", Chap. 18)
9. *Sarcomas mixed with glioblastomas* (see Sect. 15.6.1.1)
10. *Sarcomas of a special tissue type*, such as chondrosarcoma (see Sect. 24.4) and liposarcoma (see Sect. 24.5)

These entities will be described in more detail below, after some remarks about the sarcomas in general (which are understandably a very inhomogeneous group). The descriptions of the separate entities, however, will be very specific.

Other Classifications. There have always been a great many of different classification systems for the sarcomas. In the first edition of this book (ZÜLCH 1951b) and in 1974 (ZÜLCH and MENNEL) we distinguished (a) the "diffusely growing" and (b) the "circumscribed" sarcomas. In the first group "primary meningeal sarcomatosis" and "primary adventitial diffuse sarcomatosis" were distinguished. Amongst the circumscribed sarcomas, fibrosarcoma of the dura, monstrocellular sarcoma and circumscribed arachnoidal cerebellar sarcoma – if as such classified – figure as entities. Finally, reticulum cell sarcoma (reticular sarcoma) and various other malignant lymphomas were listed.

For our own classification we drew particularly on the suggestions of HSÜ (1940), of NEUBUERGER and GREEN (1946), and finally of ABBOTT and KERNOHAN (1943). Other similar classifications can be found in the work of NICHOLS and WAGNER (1952), LIU and SELBACH (1953), OLIVERAS DE LA RIVA (1955), ZAPATA (1963), ZÜLCH and BINGAS (1963), BINGAS (1964a), BRUCHER (1964), RUBINSTEIN (1971), MENA and GARCIA (1978), and KISHIKAWA et al. (1981).

Epidemiology (Age – Sex – Frequency – Site)

Age: It is difficult to define the predilection age for sarcomas, as there are so many types and all age groups are affected. Some forms, on the other hand, occur mostly in infants and children (CHRISTENSEN et al. 1961), and occur even in the first year of life. The age curve for monstrocellular sarcoma shows that there is no predilection age for this entity.

Sex: There is probably no sex preponderance and it appears that there is not even any male preponderance in the group of reticulum cell sarcomas.

Frequency: The frequency of all groups of sarcomas together may be around 3% (KERNOHAN and UIHLEIN 1962, in a series of about 8000 tumors). Our own figures were similar, but steadily increased over the years, from 1.9% in the series of 4000 to 4.3% in the series of 9000. However, the latter percentage may be somewhat distorted by the influx of questionable cases sent in for an opinion from other sources. We believe that the average frequency may be between 2.5% and 3%. However, because of differences in the definition criteria it will remain always arbitrary.

Site: The sarcomas occur with no specific site preference, as we have always emphasized in our former publications except that by definition: the meningeal sarcomas are localized in the meninges and the periadventitial sarcomas around the vessels. The ratio supratentorial to infratentorial sarcomas is 3:1 (KERNOHAN and UIHLEIN 1962: 28% in the cerebellum). Yet this corresponds almost to the volume of the brain mass in these compartments.

The origin may be the connective tissue of the dura (fibrosarcoma), the hull cells of the leptomeninges (meningeal sarcomatosis), the perivascular sheath (reticulum cell sarcoma, periadventitial sarcoma), or other mesodermal tissues. Ultrastructure and tissue culture of sarcomas have been reported by GULLOTTA and KERSTING (1973) and MENA and GARCIA (1978).

After these general remarks the most prominent entities will be described in detail.

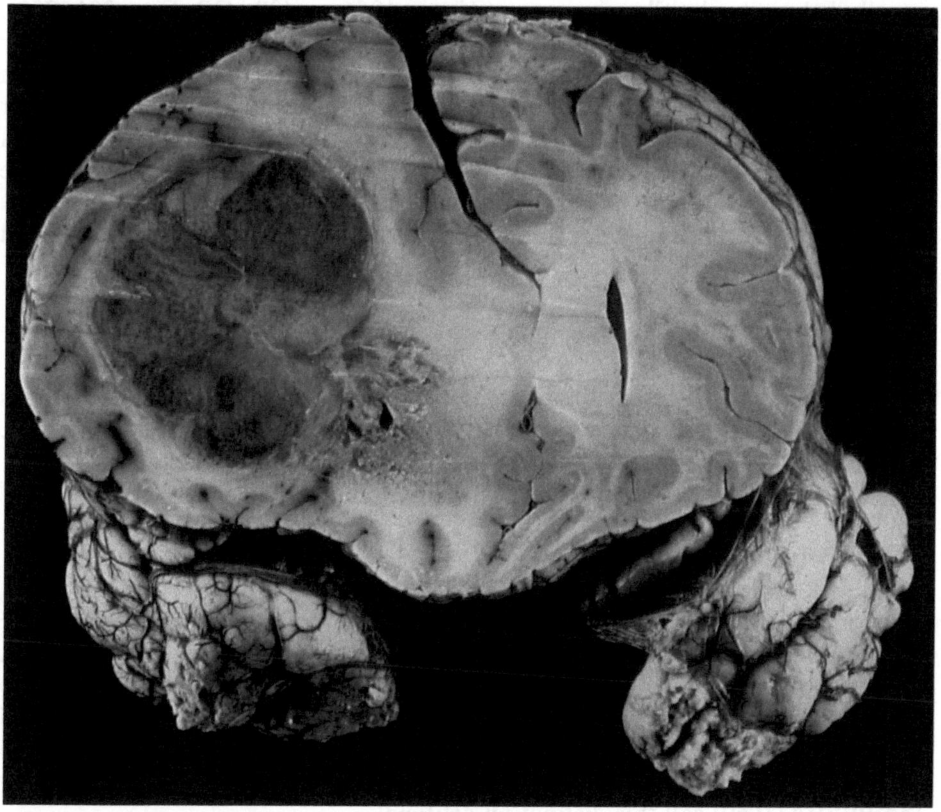

Fig. 134. Large right frontal fibrosarcoma of the dura

17.2.1 Fibrosarcomas

Fibrosarcomas grow both inside and outside the dura (GP, Figs. 229, 230), but they tend to infiltrate the adjacent brain tissue despite their fairly circumscribed appearance (Fig. 134). They can provoke massive edema. The main feature distinguishing them from the meningioma, which they resemble, is the lack of a definite capsule. They can have the same firm consistency as a meningioma (due to the great amount of fibers), so that macroscopic distinction may not be possible at first sight. Sometimes they show small areas of ossification (GREENDYKE 1965; see also BINGAS 1965; MANSFIELD 1977; CHAUDHARI et al. 1978: of the scalp).

Occasionally they occur intracerebrally (BRUCHER et al. 1971). Familial sarcomas have been observed (four cases of fibrosarcoma in two families: GAINER et al. 1975). EM studies have been conducted in our laboratory (HIZAWA and WECHSLER 1966; BRUCHER et al. 1971).

It is still a matter of debate whether the so-called giant cell fibrosarcoma reported by HITSELBERGER et al. (1961) is not actually a monstrocellular sarcoma. Sarcomas can occur as a late result of massive radiation therapy and usually belong to the fibrosarcomas (ZÜLCH 1956, p. 492; GP, Figs. 231, 232). In a girl aged 15 years a cerebral extraventricular ependymoma had been totally removed and radiation (approximately 50 Gy) given to the operation field. Seven years later a ring-like fibrosarcoma (GP, Fig. 231) began to grow in the scar tissue. At autopsy there was not a vestige of the primary ependymoma (ZÜLCH 1956, Figs. 356b, 357). Other cases have been reported by WENDE (1962: average manifestation 6–8 years), WALTZ and BROWNELL (1966: 19 years), RUBINSTEIN (1972, Fig. 205: 18 years after radiation), SCHRANTZ and ARAOZ (1972), and SIEBEN et al. (1980).

Differential Diagnosis

It is necessary to distinguish sarcomas from meningiomas, although there is no indication that they arise as an anaplastic variant from a pre-existing tumor. There is no preferred localization as in the case of meningiomas.

17.2.2 Polymorphic Cell Sarcomas

There are usually superficial infiltrating tumors composed of more protoplasmic than fibrillary small or medium-sized mesenchymal cells (CHRISTENSEN and LARA 1953). The spindle cells may show variations in size and shape and develop some polymorphism (Fig. 135a). It seems necessary to distinguish spindle cell sarcomas from this rare type of sarcoma, which was also extremely rare in our series (total number of sarcomas 283 among 9000 cases), since GRUMME and BINGAS (1969) call this distinction artificial.

17.2.3 Primary Meningeal Sarcomatosis (Diffuse Sarcomatosis of the Meninges)

This is a diffuse sort of sarcoma of the leptomeninges, which are clouded and give the appearance of meningitis. The cisterns may be thickened and filled with a whitish tumor mass (Fig. 136; see also ZÜLCH 1956, Figs. 338, 339, 340c, d, 356b). Single small nodules may occur as a diffuse seeding, but no large circumscribed tumors are found. Patients are usually young or middle aged. (For references see: BRONFMAN and REUMONT 1947; GRIEPENTROG 1952; SCHEIDEGGER 1954; ZÜLCH 1956, p. 469; KOSTKA and DRAHOZAL 1973; BUDKA et al. 1975).

According to their published pictures the "meningeal meningomatosis" of BLACK and KERNOHAN (1950) probably belongs to this entity. But a *true* diffuse meningomatosis, i.e., formation of hundreds of meningiomas (GP, Fig. 215) does also exist. The term "meningeal meningomatosis" was certainly misleading because it suggested that true seeding of a meningioma had occurred in the leptomeningeal spaces. Furthermore, the cells of diffuse sarcomatosis do not resemble those of meningiomas. A multicentric origin has been discussed by ONOFRIO et al. (1962), but it seems not to be very likely in spite of a sometimes

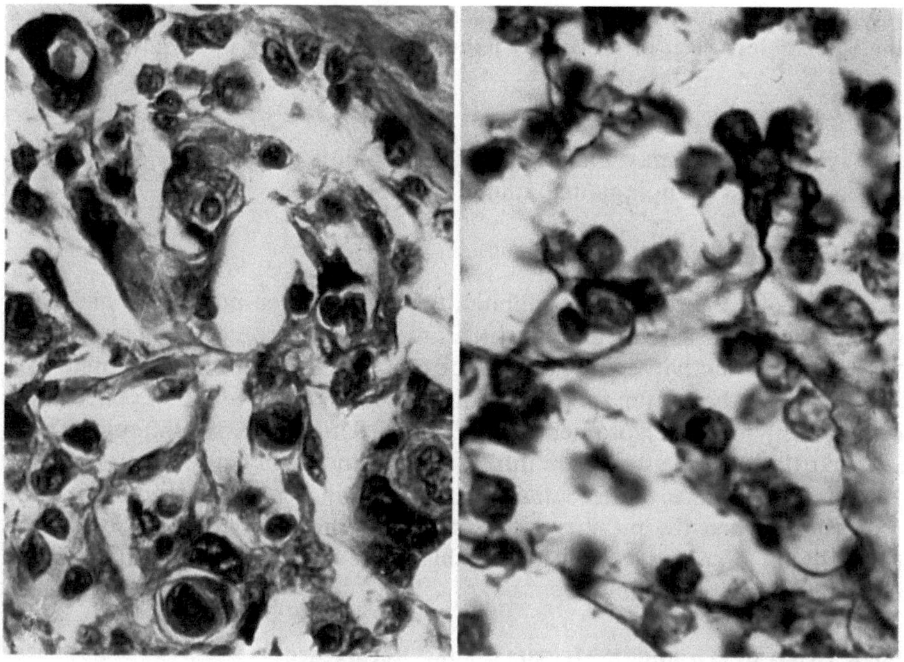

a b

Fig. 135. a Spindle cells with variations in size and shape and some polymorphism are encountered in the polymorphous cell sarcoma. H&E, ×500. **b** Tumor cells on fibers like "buds on a pussy willow twig." Perdrau's method, ×500

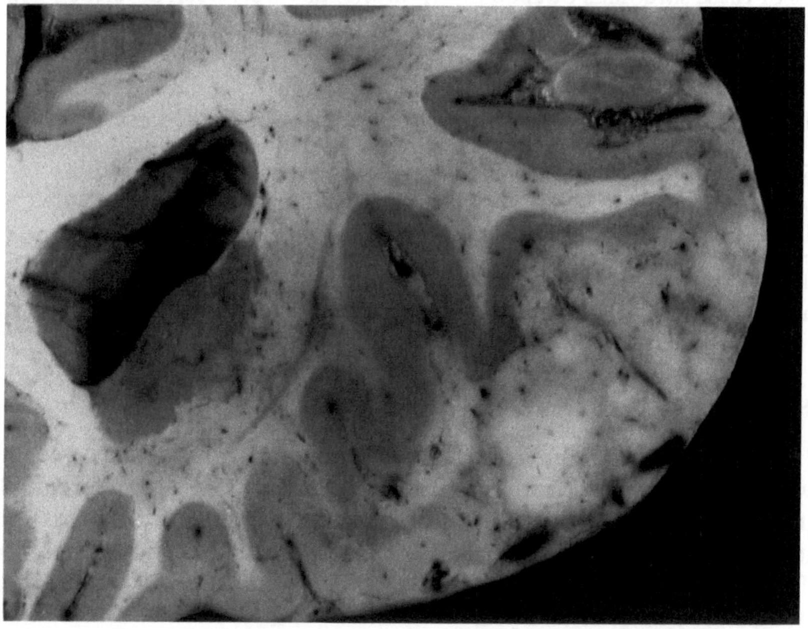

Fig. 136. Diffuse infiltration of the leptomeninges forming thick plaques in diffuse sarcomatosis. (ZÜLCH 1975a)

patchy tumor-like distribution. Experimental sarcomatosis in the leptomeninges of the chicken has been produced by Rous viruses (SIEGLER and PIENTA 1962).

Clinical Course

Clinically the picture may mimic chronic meningitis (HUFFMANN et al. 1967), and even the gross pathology may mimic this process.

Histologic Appearance

Histologically the elements are lymphoid, fusiform or even polygonal, and have only scarce cytoplasm and nuclei which are rich in chromatin. They show a very high mitotic activity. The network of reticular fibers in the leptomeninges is increased and the tumor follows all the vessels (HBT, Fig. 82c), penetrating into the brain from the leptomeninges (ZÜLCH 1956, Figs. 339, 340c, d). Thus, the first cortical layers usually are infiltrated and there may even be an invasion of the white substance. Differential diagnosis from medulloblastoma is sometimes difficult when the primary circumscribed tumor has not been identified. The possibility of a very small medulloblastoma with extraordinary primary seeding must also be considered.

Biologic Behavior (Grading), Metastasis, and Recurrence

This tumor is graded in the WHO system as IV. BUCY (1962) was of the opinion that biologically the behavior is more favorable than that of medulloblastoma, but this is contradicted by our own observations (ZÜLCH 1956, p. 479). Metastasis of these sarcomas outside the cranium has rarely been described (BENNINGTON and JONES 1962). Recurrence on the other side is regular.

17.2.4 Circumscribed Arachnoidal Sarcomas of the Cerebellum

Synonym: Desmoplastic medulloblastoma? see Sect. 15.6.2.1

Introduction

The WHO classification defines this entity according to RUBINSTEIN's scheme as a "desmoplastic medulloblastoma." However, scientific discussion of its nature continues.

Historical Note and Definition

In 1939 FOERSTER and GAGEL described a tumor entity of the cerebellum, which was sharply circumscribed and had a nodular surface, was preferentially situated in the dorsal or lateral surface of the hemispheres, and on gross examination it resembled a metastasis. It had a hard consistency and had no firm capsule. The authors had observed four cases, all in patients aged 22–25 years; the history was short: 6 months to 1 year.

RUBINSTEIN and NORTHFIELD (1964) and OLVERA RABIELA et al. (1974) considered that this tumor was a "desmoplastic" variant of medulloblastoma, and the WHO classification has followed their lead (pp. 334, 388). Other cases are described by MARQUARDT (1941, Fig. 1, pale islands surrounded by strands), NEUBUERGER and GREEN (1946), and LANGHEIM et al. (1962, Fig. 10); the case of SOEJIMA et al. (1973) was probably a medulloblastoma. There does not seem to be any doubt that this entity exists, even if its nature is still under discussion.

Epidemiology (Age – Sex – Frequency – Site)

The mean age seems to be higher than in the case of ordinary medulloblastomas, neither sex is preferentially represented, and the frequency is deduced when the ratio between the desmoplastic type and the ordinary type of medulloblastoma is defined.

Gross Pathology

As has been emphasized, this entity is easily recognized by its hard consistency and sharp delineation, and finally by its site at the surface in the cerebellar hemisphere. It can resemble a metastasis (GP, Fig. 240) in these features. Connection with the dura does not occur, nor is there an intimate connection with the cerebellar tissue; this means that they can be easily removed with the fingers and a clear separation from the normal tissue is possible (Fig. 107).

Histologic Appearance

The specific architecture or pattern differs significantly from that of medulloblastoma. It is characterized by rows and loose pale islands of cells, in which the nuclei are larger and paler than in the other parts, where they are small and dark. There is no differentiation into neural or gliogenic cells. The loose pale islands are free of reticular network, which is otherwise present in considerable quantities between the islands (Figs. 106, 108).

In these tumors virus-like particles have been observed by RAMSEY and KERNOHAN (1964). On the other hand, POLLICE and MARZULLO (1970) called the pale or glomerular areas, which are free of reticulum, "inconstant" (Fig. 108). SCHRÖDER and PLOGSTIES (1966) had quite a different idea, and though that his entity was related to the meningotheliomatous meningiomas (their Figs. 1–4). The case reported by SOEJIMA et al. (1973) seems more likely to be a medulloblastoma than a sarcoma of the cerebellum. RUBINSTEIN and NORTHFIELD (1964) noted transitional forms with characteristics of both groups.

Differential Diagnosis

The architectural pattern is so pronounced that differential diagnosis is easy. Regions with large amounts of silver impregnated fibers are only seen in the normal cerebellum if parts of the leptomeninges are invaded and encased in the tumor (see Figs. 101b, 102a). The other differential diagnostic points have already been emphasized: namely higher age, location in the hemispheres, sharp delineation, hard consistency.

Though a member of the WHO's classification group, which has not accepted the arachnoidal sarcoma as a separate entity but instead the *desmoplastic medul-*

loblastoma, I feel that a solution to this problem has still to be reached. The differences between the entity described by FOERSTER and GAGEL (1939) and the typical normal medulloblastomas are so great that the likelihood of a sarcomatous nature does not seem to me to be as remote as is sometimes emphasized.

17.2.5 Rhabdomyosarcomas

Synonym: Embryonal sarcoma

Rhabdomyosarcomas are uncommon in the brain. Such tumors with the presence of striated muscle fibers have been recorded in the CNS as highly exceptional. Their elements are derived from the mesenchyma, in contrast to medulloblastoma (p. 324ff.). They have been found in the supratentorial space (in frontal lobe, with the size of a golf ball: MIN et al. 1975; in middle fossa: TAKEMI et al. 1977; near falx: YAGISHITA et al. 1979; in the pineal region: MARSDEN 1974), and also in the posterior fossa (LEGIER and WELLS 1967; LOPEZ DE FARIA 1957; SHUANGSHOTI et al. 1968).

Aberrant differentiation of mesenchyma to striated muscle has been considered a mechanism of pathogenesis. A mixture of elements of the neural germ layer and a rhabdomyosarcoma has been described by HOLIMON and ROSENBLUM (1971), and because of this mixture a "teratomatous" nature has been discussed. A melanotic rhabdomyomedulloblastoma has been described by DUINKERKE et al. (1981).

The tumor is thought to be highly malignant.

Further References: PASQUIER et al. (1975), MATSUKADO et al. (1975).

17.3 Xanthomatous Tumors: Fibroxanthoma – Xanthosarcoma (Malignant Fibroxanthoma)

Introduction

The xanthomas are composed of mono- or multinucleated giant cells with morphological features resembling histiocytes. The giant cells are similar to the Touton-type giant cells and they may adopt pinwheel or "storey-form" patterns of spindle-shaped tumor cells. They also contain foamy cells, which include birefringent lipids.

Historical Note and Definition

These extremely rare tumors were first described by KEPES et al. (1973), occurring in boys in the first two decades. They were sited in the temporal region and one was leptomeningeal, yet later reclassified as xanthoastrocytomas (KEPES et al. 1979b).

The necessity of differentiating this group from other giant cell sarcomas or fibromas may be derived from the trend to differentiation of the giant cell tumors of glial and mesodermal derivation (JÄNISCH et al. 1976), and particularly to separate the various types of giant cell sarcomas (lipo-, rhabdomyo-, xantho-sarcomas, etc.).

Histiocytes occur in the more benign groups of lymphomas such as the reticulum cell sarcomas of the plexus choroideus.

More recent research on the xanthomatous tumors has demonstrated by fluorescence and immunoperoxidase techniques glial fibrillary protein in some of these tumors (KEPES 1979a; KEPES and RUBINSTEIN 1981). These authorities therefore classify some of these tumors as a variant of astrocytomas, namely "pleomorphic meningocerebral xanthoastrocytomas" (instead of fibrous xanthomas). These are according to their experience gliomas of young subjects with a relatively favorable prognosis.

The survival of some of the cases reported has been long; in one case there was an early recurrence, but the second operation was successful. There was also one case where malignant transformation had taken place (xanthosarcoma), and anaplastic cells of various sizes, round cells, and giant cells were found. We had a case of this kind in our own collection.

Differential diagnosis from glial tumors is sometimes difficult, as is differentiation of the sarcomatous variant from monstrocellular sarcoma (ZÜLCH 1953a) and the giant cell fibrosarcoma (HITSELBERGER et al. 1961).

Further References: KEMPSON and MCGAVRAN (1964), CARILLO et al. (1975), KEPES et al. (1978), TERAO et al. (1978).

17.4 Primary Melanotic Tumors: Melanomas and Meningeal Melanomatosis

Introduction

By definition, the melanoma is a primary tumor in the CNS and arises from a focal site in the meninges, whereas meningeal melanomatosis spreads diffusely in the subarachnoid space.

Historical Note and Definition

The existence of primary melanotic tumors of the brain was first emphasized by VIRCHOW (1859).

Primary melanoblastomas in the brain are related to the chromatophores of the leptomeninges as their tissue of origin; however, the pigment of the tumors must satisfy the staining criteria of the pathologist, and the primary nature of these tumors must be assured by excluding the presence of a primary melanoma elsewhere in the body.

Epidemiology (Age – Sex – Frequency – Site)

Age and Sex: The mean age is considered to be around 50 years and there is probably a male preponderance.

Frequency: Primary melanomas of the CNS are rare. Their relative frequency can be deduced from the fact that only 100 definite cases were known in 1972, including the 9 cases encountered in Sweden in a 10-year period, according to BERGDAHL et al. (1972). Since then 186 cases of the circumscribed type (BOJSEN-MØLLER 1977), and 101 cases of diffuse melanomatosis (FOX et al. 1964) have already been collected.

Site: These tumors can be sited anywhere in the supratentorial space, and there is apparently no local preponderance (ARNVIG and CHRISTENSEN 1939; BERGDAHL et al. 1972: 10 personal cases; BOJSEN-MØLLER 1977). Primary circumscribed melanomas also occur in the cerebellum (FOWLER and SIMPSON 1962; HAHN et al. 1976; PASQUIER et al. 1978), in the choroid plexus (BEATTY 1972), in the pituitary (SCHOLZ and SIU 1976), in the spinal cord (DE BLASI 1930; KING et al. 1952; HIRANO and CARTON 1960; CLIFFORD et al. 1968; YAMAMOTO et al. 1975), and in the pineal gland (ARLANT et al. 1977).

Primary *diffuse melanomatosis* (ERBSLÖH 1956) occurs particularly in youth and middle age, but is rare. *Macroscopically* in such cases the melanomatous neoplasia spreads diffusely in the subarachnoid space. The leptomeninges appear thickened and smokey gray or dark brown in appearance. Occasionally lentil-sized nodules are present. Sometimes only a histologic study will reveal the true source of the grayish discoloration of the leptomeninges.

Histologic Appearance

The histologic picture is very uniform. The melanin-containing cells are either multipolar, or more rounded or elongated. Some of the cells may be amelanotic (see APITZ 1937). These tumors penetrate into the nervous tissue along the blood vessels (Virchow-Robin spaces) and produce only slight reactions in the infiltrated tissue (ERBSLÖH 1956). Primary melanomas spread diffusely throughout the CSF spaces and even encase the nerve roots, but they do not metastasize to other organs. An ultrastructural and biochemical study has been published by ARAOZ and MOORE (1979).

Patients with such tumors in the cerebrum have a shorter postoperative survival (2 years) than those with spinal tumors, survival up to three years being possible in the latter cases (PISCOL and HOFFMANN 1961; BERGDAHL et al. 1972).

HAFERKAMP and RISOPATRON (1955) seem to have seen a more benign primary melanomatosis, with a sometimes patchy infiltration. But in this case the melanin was also found in neurons and glia cells as well as spreading diffusely in the meninges. The basic discussions on melanin pigment published by H. JACOB (1934) and VOLLAND (1954) should be consulted.

Since there are more melanocytes in the leptomeninges of the Javanese than of other peoples it may be that *there* are entirely benign non-neoplastic melanomas of the meninges. On the other hand, the neurocutaneous form of melanoblastosis (TOURAINE 1949) may be the basis of *malignant* melanomas.

Differential Diagnosis

The most important step is the exclusion of a primary extracranial melanoma, which occurs most frequently in the skin or the eye. Occasionally a small cutaneous melanoma has been excised years before without the patient's being aware of this.

CT diagnosis has been discussed by CRISP and THOMPSON (1981) and HOLTÅS and CRONQVIST (1981).

Information on other melanin-containing tumors, such as meningiomas, can be found on p. 382.

Details of the significance of the melanotic tumors are given elsewhere in detail (ZÜLCH 1956, p. 493 ff.).

Further References: LENCE (1937), GIBSON et al. (1957), CACUDI and CAZZATO (1960), PAPPENHEIM and BHATTACHARJI (1962), OLISCHER and SCHRÖTER (1963), FOX et al. (1964), TVETEN (1965), TOLNAI et al. (1966), MINAUF and SUMMER (1972), ENGELHARDT and LANG (1977), SILBERT et al. (1978), STEINBERG et al. (1978), PAL et al. (1979), FLASCHKA and POPPER (1981), GÖSSINGER (1983).

17.5 Others

Fibromas

Only a few cases of true intracerebral fibroma remain once fibromatous meningiomas have been eliminated (ZÜLCH 1956, p. 467 ff.). However, there are some tumors with no connection to the dura, which nonetheless deserve clearly the name fibroma. Various degenerative processes, such as hyalinization, calcification, chondromyxoid changes (RAMANI 1974), mucoid degeneration, and ossification (KAMISASA et al. 1973), have been excellently described. Our own first case, a tumor in a 14-year-old boy – described by MEYER and SCHELLER (1937) – had most of these changes; it was presented at the Annual Meeting of the Society of British Neurological Surgeons in 1937 in Berlin (see ZÜLCH 1956, Fig. 337a, b). Other cases have been described by ALPERS et al. (1932), BAKER and ADAMS (1937), as well as by PETIT-DUTAILLIS and BERTRAND (1932), KOOS et al. (1971: 11-month-old infant), and LLENA et al. (1975).

EM studies have been conducted in our own laboratory (BRUCHER et al. 1971) and by HIRANO et al. (1975d).

The "elastoma" of EBELS and GO (1974) seems to have been unique.

18 Primary Malignant Lymphomas

Synonyms: Reticulum cell sarcoma/microglioma, reticulosarcoma, microgliomatosis, adventitial diffuse sarcoma, Ewing sarcoma, Hodgkin sarcoma, non-Hodgkin sarcoma etc.

Introduction

The WHO histological typing system for tumors of the CNS includes a category for primary malignant lymphomas, which embraces all the tumors previously cited in the list of synonyms above. The arguments for the integration of all these subgroups into the main group will not be discussed here and can be found in the appropriate textbooks (K. LENNERT 1978).

Experimental lymphocyte research and immunology have introduced revolutionary concepts into the new classification. There are still two schools of thought regarding this topic (see RAPAPORT 1966, 1974; and the book of LENNERT 1978, cited above). Of these two very different concepts, the so-called Kiel classification of LENNERT is more generally accepted throughout the world.

A discussion of the details of the classification of the lymphomas is not of any great importance for our present purpose. Individual entities, such as reticulum cell sarcoma/microglioma, adventitial diffuse sarcoma, and the Hodgkin's and non-Hodgkin's tumors will be described and the more common spinal epidural reticulum sarcoma (lymphosarcoma) will be reported in more detail because of surgical interest. Apparently also histiocytosis X, especially in the hypothalamus, is counted by some authorities as a lymphoma, but in this volume it is described as a type of granuloma.

The Kiel classification of malignant lymphomas (other than Hodgkin's disease) is so highly sophisticated that for the practical purposes of neurosurgery, neurology, and neuroradiology we suggest the following neuropathologic classification:

Primary tumors of the lymphoreticular system

1. Reticulum cell sarcomas
2. Adventitial sarcomas
3. Hodgkin's disease
4. Plasmocytomas
5. Hypothalamic granulomas (histiocytosis X)

Secondary tumors of the lymphoreticular system (metastatic and invasive)

1. Reticulum cell sarcomas
2. Hodgkin's disease
3. Plasmocytomas
4. Leukemias

The attempt to combine the individual entities cited above in one group – as the WHO classification has also done – is based on the assumption that lymphoreticular tissue is the "mother germ" of this large number of variants. The entities, such as lymphosarcoma, mycosis fungoides, plasmocytoma, reticulosarcoma, unclassified malignant lymphoma, morbus Hodgkin, eosinophilic granuloma, and plasmocytoma, will not all be described here for practical reasons (see also VUIA 1975).

The latest development in research on systemic and local neoplasms of the reticuloendothelial and lymphatic systems led to the notion that lymphocytes and plasma cells are not derived from reticulum cells and that these cells are not obligate end-cells, but transform into larger blast cells. It was also thought that most cases of supposed reticular sarcoma are actually immunoblastic lymphomas and, finally, it is evident that a more definite classification of the non-Hodgkin's lymphomas according to their immunological properties would be a considerable advance in therapy and prognosis.

The Kiel classification (LENNERT 1978) may represent a real step forward in understanding the pathogenesis of leukemias and lymphomas of both low-grade and high-grade malignancy, and may be very helpful in the classification of these entities and the development of appropriate forms of therapy. However, it does not seem to be any available advantage for the neurosurgical cases, if the mass lesion under discussion is not part of a *systemic* disease. For this reason we will therefore retain the "traditional" and well-known entities, most of which we include in this group of "malignant lymphomas."

18.1 Primary Tumors of the Lymphoreticular System

18.1.1 Reticulum Cell Sarcomas

Introduction

This entity is mentioned as a subgroup of malignant lymphomas in the WHO classification. The category of reticulum cell sarcoma (or retothelsarcoma) was conceived by ROULET (1930) and RÖSSLE (1939).

Dorothy RUSSELL et al. (1948) described proliferations of the microglia and compared them with the sarcomas derived from the primitive reticulum cell (see above). Later, in RUSSELL's monograph with RUBINSTEIN (1977), the view was expressed that the tumor elements arose from dedifferentiation of more mature forms. A more detailed discussion of these problems has been published by KERNOHAN and UIHLEIN (1962). RUBINSTEIN (1971) finds the term reticulum cell sarcoma/microglioma as an acceptable compromise that satisfies the two alternative points of view.

Epidemiology (Age – Sex – Frequency – Site)

Sex and Age: The series of NISHIURA et al. (1980) contained more male than female patients and the highest frequency was observed in the 5th to 7th decades. The frequency was difficult to assess in our series of 9000 tumors (ZÜLCH and MENNEL 1974). We observed 80 cases (i.e., 0.98%) including 51 intracerebral or intraspinal tumors. BURSTEIN et al. (1963) reported 242 sarcomas of the brain,

5 of which they classified as microgliomas, 6 as Hodgkin's sarcomas, and 26 as reticulum cell sarcomas. There is an exception to the general rule on age: the epidural reticular sarcomas of the spinal canal have a definite peak in the age curve around the 20th year (BINGAS and ZÜLCH 1964, Fig. 1).

Site: There does not seem to be any preferential location apart from the group of epidural spinal tumors (BUCY 1962; BUCY and JERVA 1962; BINGAS and ZÜLCH 1964; COUTINHO and ZÜLCH 1974). Figure 2 of BINGAS and ZÜLCH (1964) shows the preferred site in the epidural space of the middle and lower thoracic spine.

Gross Pathology

These tumors have a dark brownish surface, are of a soft consistency, and merge into the adjacent tissue. Sometimes they are very firm, in which case they may contain fresh necroses and then they have a granular surface.

Histologic Appearance

The tumors are very highly cellular. Some of the nuclei are clear and contain quite large nucleoli, while others are dark. There are more protoplasmic and also more fibrillary types, where in silver impregnations (Fig. 135b) the nuclei appear sited on the fibrils "like the buds on a willow-twig" (RÖSSLE 1939).

Furthermore, there is a pattern of infiltrating perivascular small cells that can aggregate and form dense complexes. This perivascular pattern may be found even in the solid, deeper part of the tumor where the cells have large dark nuclei, scant cytoplasm, and are ill defined. Sometimes the associated nuclei are pleomorphic. The ultrastructural findings have been reported by HORVAT et al. (1969).

Ewing's Sarcoma

VIRCHOW (1863–65) apparently coined the terms of lymphoma and lymphosarcoma for tumors of the lymphoid tissue. In the Anglo-Saxon literature EWING was apparently the first to recognize it as an entity (1913/14), and he described it in his "*Neoplastic Diseases*" (1928).

There is no doubt that RÖSSLE (1939) persisted for a long time in use of the term "retothelsarcoma" (instead reticular sarcoma) for such tumors of the lymph nodes, which were described in detail by his co-worker F. ROULET (1930, 1932, 1953).

Cases of neurosurgical importance have been described by BINGAS (1964c) and by GRUMME and BINGAS (1969). They emphasized the well-known experience that Ewing's sarcoma was highly sensitive to radiation and that survival times of 5–10 years were not exceptional.

Biologic Behavior (Grading), Metastasis, and Recurrence

Most of these sarcomas are malignant, with survival of only months or 1–2 years, with some exceptions (GRUMME and BINGAS 1969: 5–10 years; GARCIA-BENGOCHEA and COLLINS 1969: 6½ years).

The strikingly better prognosis is well-known for the epidural spinal reticulosarcomas, particularly after operation followed by radiation (LEFEVRE et al. 1956). On the other hand, a good response to immune suppressive therapy can be achieved (MOSER et al. 1972). Metastases hardly visible to the naked eye may occur (JÄNISCH et al. 1973; see also CHO et al. 1974).

Differential Diagnosis

The more diffuse types of reticular sarcoma have to be differentiated particularly in sparsely cellular regions, from the lymph cell infiltrates of encephalitic conditions, disseminated leukoencephalitides, etc. (VAN GEHUCHTEN and BRUCHER 1960). Apparently EM does not help in the distinction according to ISHIDA (1973, 1975), who found indifferent cells without any significant difference from cells elsewhere in the body, while histochemistry reveals a high content of glycoproteins in the PAS-positive substance (MILLER and RAMSDEN 1963). The usefulness of tissue culture has been emphasized by GAZSO and SLOWIK (1975).

Further References: BURSTEIN et al. (1963), BINGAS (1964c), ADAMS and JACKSON (1966), CASTAIGNE et al. (1966b), SAMUELSSON et al. (1966), VUIA and MEHRAEIN (1971), SCHAUMBURG et al. (1972), BARNARD and SCOTT (1975), KUMANISHI et al. (1975), LENNERT (1975), ZIMMERMAN (1975).

18.1.2 Adventitial Sarcomas

This entity is cited under the malignant lymphomas in the WHO classification. KÖRNYEY (1934), who first categorized this particular type, considered it to be a reticular form of tumor propagating in and around the vascular sheaths (see SCHALTENBRAND and BAILEY 1928). It was somewhat similar to the former pathologic entity of "perithelioma." The perivascular infiltrations can flow together to form compact tumors, although globally they may mimic a diffuse encephalitis of the white cerebral matter. The lesion also must be distinguished from primary meningeal sarcomatosis (see p. 386) in that it restricts itself to infiltration around the *intracerebral* vessels, while the leptomeninges are not involved primarily (see BAILEY 1929). However, they may be infiltrated secondarily in exceptional instances by growth from inside outward. To what extent this entity might also be correlated with "microgliomas" (D. RUSSELL et al. 1948) or to "microgliomatosis" (ADAMS 1970, 1975) must remain open (see KERSHMAN 1939).

The aforementioned authors themselves place microglia or microgliomatosis as very close to the reticulum cell sarcoma. Nevertheless, the final definition of the germ cells of microglia is still incomplete (see also BINGAS and ZÜLCH 1966; SCHAUMBURG et al. 1972; HIRANO 1975).

Differential diagnosis from glioblastomas must be made grossly by the looser tissue texture and the pronounced infiltration around cerebral vessels in the mantle zone of adventitial sarcomas (KÖRNYEY 1934). It may be difficult, however, in the more highly reticular cases of "histiocytic granulomatous encephalitis," a problem discussed in detail by WILKE (1950, 1955).

We believe that we can differentiate the groups of adventitial sarcoma and reticulohistiocytic granulomatous encephalitis on histologic grounds. The adventitial sarcoma is characterized by its ubiquitous location; its composition of lymphocytes, histiocytes, few reactive glial elements; the severe destruction of single cells; perivascular accumulation; and frequent mitoses (BINGAS and ZÜLCH 1964).

18.1.3 Hodgkin's Disease

Synonyms: Hodgkin's granuloma, granulosarcoma

For many years there has been discussion as to whether primary Hodgkin's disease occurs in the brain (see SCHÖPE 1938). KERNOHAN and UIHLEIN (1962) reported 8 cases of Hodgkin sarcoma out of 40 cases of reticulosarcoma. However, parts of the central nervous system, such as the leptomeninges, may be involved as part of systemic Hodgkin's disease.

Further References: FEIN and NEWILL (1954), THIES et al. (1961), BIRAN and HERISHIANU (1972).

18.1.4 Plasmocytomas

We have seen 13 examples of plasmocytoma that arose apparently as primary tumors in the brain and involving particularly the dura or the hypothalamus (FRENCH 1947; HERMANN 1963). The histologic picture is typical.

Further References: THEUNISSEN (1978).

18.1.5 Histiocytosis X

Granulomatous tissue has been encountered particularly in the infundibular region (BERNARD and AGUILAR 1969; KEPES and KEPES 1969).

Histologically this is a granulomatous reaction characterized by histiocytes, plasma cells, and reactive glial elements, usually of the astrocytic type, and also with the formation of reticulin fibers. The differential diagnosis from other conditions has been discussed by MOOSSY and WILSON (1967).

Further References: SPARLING and ADAMS (1946), BATSON (1955), DEN HARTOG et al. (1960), LJUNGDAHL et al. (1965), WEINER et al. (1966), TRUELLE et al. (1976), TRIMBLE (1973), KENNERDELL et al. (1974), ISHIDA (1975), KEPES and KEPES (1975), JELLINGER and RADASZKIEWICZ (1975).

General discussions of classification of the lymphomas can be found elsewhere (JELLINGER et al. 1975; MATHÉ et al. 1976).

18.1.6 Eosinophilic Granuloma (of Bone)

This type of mass lesion is well-known to the neurosurgeon (FINZI 1929) because of its radiologic and surgical importance (OTANI and EHRLICH 1940; LICHTENSTEIN and JAFFEE 1940; BECK 1943; OSBORNE et al. 1944; ESCALONA and BAEZ 1963; IZAWA et al. 1976).

It is a tumor-like lesion that grows exclusively outside the dura in the skull, with a predilection for the frontal region and without much compression of the underlying brain. Histologically it consists of reticular cells in a fibrous network, intermingled with dense infiltration by eosinophilic leukocytes.

The lesion is very radiosensitive. Surgical removal and subsequent radiation is the treatment of choice and the prognosis is very good.

18.1.7 Burkitt's Lymphoma (African Lymphoma)

This lymphoma will rarely be of any neurosurgical importance, since the CNS is not commonly compromised. GAWISH (1976: Zambia) and MAGRATH et al. (1974: 6 patients) have published interesting reports.

19 Tumors of Blood Vessel Origin

19.1 Hemangioblastomas

Synonyms: Angioblastomas, capillary hemangioblastomas, cerebellar hemangioendotheliomas, Lindau's cysts/disease/tumor, angiomatosis of the CNS; in the older literature: cerebellar angiomas, epithelial angiomas, angioreticulomas

Introduction

Since Arved LINDAU first coined the term hemangioblastoma in 1926, this entity has been so well described that it was introduced without argument into the WHO classification as the main representative of the *blood vessel tumors of the brain.*

With regard to terminology:

1. Hemangioblastoma (or Lindau's tumor) is a single or multiple brain tumor
2. Lindau's syndrome comprises the hemangioblastic brain tumor plus cysts in both pancreas and kidney
3. Lindau's disease: isolated cerebellar angioblastomas, which must be hereditary
4. Von Hippel's disease is hereditary angiomatosis of the retina
5. Von Hippel-Lindau disease is a *hereditary* association of retinal angiomas and cerebellar angioblastomas (see also GP, Figs. 220–226).

Historical Note and Definition

During a study of cerebellar cysts in 1926 LINDAU found that a number of them contained hemangiomatous mural nodules and that they were often associated with small angiomas of the retina (the so-called retinal angiomatosis of von Hippel). Lindau named this combined syndrome of retinal and cerebellar angiomas "angiomatosis of the nervous system." In rare instances this is hereditary. This story is partly reproduced in "Neurological Classics 39" by WILKINS and BRODY (1971).

Since then the name von Hippel-Lindau's disease has become generally accepted for the *hereditary* forms of this combined lesion of the retina and cerebellum (MCKCRAIG et al. 1941; BONEBRAKE and SIQUEIRA 1964; CORNELL et al. 1979: 5 members of a family).

OPPENHEIM and KRAUSE (1913b) reported on the partial excision of a lymphangiosarcoma plexiforme in the cerebellar vermis.

BERBLINGER (1928) had previously noticed a relationship between spinal hemangioblastomas and cysts of the pancreas, as well as with hypernephromas. Later an association with facial hypertrophy was reported (FURUKAWA et al.

1973). ROUSSY and OBERLING (1930), on the other hand, emphasized the connection between hemangioblastoma and the reticuloendothelial system ("angioreticuloma").

The name "angioma of the cerebellum" should be avoided because of the danger of misinterpretation. BAILEY (1932a) had rejected the idea of considering certain tumors of this group as "angiogliomas" (ROUSSY and OBERLING 1930), while the "angioglioma" of BERGSTRAND et al. (1936) was simply a highly vascular tumor belonging to the pilocytic astrocytoma group. The "angioglioma" of SCHEINKER (1938a) was an oligodendroglioma, and the "angiogliomas" of KOELLA (1947) were not convincing as a homogeneous group.

Heredity

The occurrence of this "disease" in many organs, and its multiplicity indicate that there is a defect in the "anlage" of the mesoderm, particularly of the vasculature. For detailed studies we are indebted to many authors (BRADFORD 1948; MCKCRAIG and HORRAX 1949; TONNING et al. 1952; ADAMS 1953). VAN DER HOEVE (1933) classified von Hippel-Lindau disease with the phakomatoses (see hamartoblastomatoses, p. 63; PENNYBACKER 1954).

Epidemiology (Age – Sex – Frequency – Site)

Age: The preferential age curve shows definitely peaks for hemangioblastomas between 35 and 45 years with the curve beginning to rise even more steeply at 20, and trailing off between 50 and 60 (Fig. 9i). The average age in CRAMER and KINSEY's series (1952) was 31 years. Our own youngest patient was 16 years old [TOMASELLO et al. 1980 reported a parieto-occipital case in a 10-year-old patient, and a patient of LEU and RÜTTNER (1973) was 1.5 years old]; our oldest patient was aged 69.

Sex: In our 9000-case series, 41 patients were male and 19 female. The male:female ratio has continued to be 2:1. No sex preference was found by LEU and RÜTTNER (1973), however.

Frequency: Hemangioblastomas comprised 1.2% of intracranial tumors in CUSHING's series (1932) and 1.3% in our series.

Site: Hemangioblastomas are usually restricted to the mesencephalon and the spinal cord. Only sporadic cases have been described in the cerebral hemispheres (ROCHAT 1931; KELLER 1933; KAUTZKY and VIERDT 1953; BRASSEUR 1961; MORELLO and BIANCHI 1963; GEILE and MOGHAREI 1965; RIVERA and CHASON 1966; HOFF and BRONSON 1968; NELLER et al. 1969: statistical data!; MCDONNELL and POLLOCK 1978).

More rarely hemangioblastomas occur either in the intradural space, presumably arising outside the medulla in the pia (WISOFF et al. 1978), or in the epidural space (BRONFMAN and ECTORS 1949). If there are *multiple* tumors in the supra- and infratentorial region the histology must be studied with great care (LÖWENTHAL 1950). Caution is necessary, as in the cases reported by ISHWAR et al.

(1971), where the tumor was "attached" to the falx. (This may have been a hemangioblastic meningioma. In such cases it would be important to know whether the tumor was encapsulated. See "Differential Diagnosis".) JEFFREYS (1974) critically reviewed the cases in the literature.

The *preferential* sites for hemangioblastomas, then, are

1. Cerebellar hemispheres and vermis
2. Roof of the fourth ventricle (area postrema)
3. Spinal cord
4. Rarely the cerebrum.

In the *cerebellar* hemispheres one usually finds such tumors near the cortex (GP, Figs. 225, 226) and they are less often solid (OKAWARA 1973) than cystic (Fig. 137). The cysts may be as big as a chestnut, but are sometimes as large as a child's fist. They are usually many times larger than the solid parts (GP, Figs. 221, 222). Occasionally blue mural nodules the size of cherry stones are found due to their vascularity, but often only after a prolonged search. The cysts are usually unilocular, only rarely multilocular (GP, Fig. 223), and large clusters of cysts are almost never encountered.

The hemangioblastomas of the second group lie between the cerebellar tonsils and the exit from the *fourth ventricle* at the calamus scriptorius (Fig. 138), in such a way that the underlying cysts interdigitate firmly with the floor of the fourth ventricle (GP, Fig. 224); at first sight, therefore, they may be mistaken for large tumors of the medulla or as ependymomas. In rare cases a tongue of tumor may reach down to the level of the upper cervical segments (see also WALKER et al. 1952; GUERIN et al. 1974).

Multiple hemangioblastomas can occur as in our case of a 31-year-old man who had five tumors in the cerebellum and spinal cord (see also the cases of BROWNE et al. 1976, who found a combination in 33%): it is probably a multiplicity of tumors that is responsible for the sudden appearance of so-called recurrences.

The third preferential site is the *spinal cord*. In this position hemangioblastomas very often form large longitudinal cysts (BROWNE et al. 1976: in 2/3 of cases). If cystic they are frequently mistaken for syringomyelia.

The full-blown syndrome can include cysts in the kidney and pancreas, and also angiomas in the retina.

In the *brain* they are encountered occasionally as large, frequently cystic tumors.

Gross Pathology

Hemangioblastomas are bluish red (like a cherry) to brownish red, well-circumscribed tumors (GP, Figs. 225, 226), usually with large cysts; the interior of which may be brown owing to hemorrhages. The cyst fluid coagulates spontaneously upon cooling, and is yellowish or brownish black. The consistency of the mural nodule is soft and elastic. The solid tumors can be as large as a chestnut, cysts as large as child's fist; the tumors are often covered with tortuous cortical vessels. These tumor may be within the confines of the cerebellum

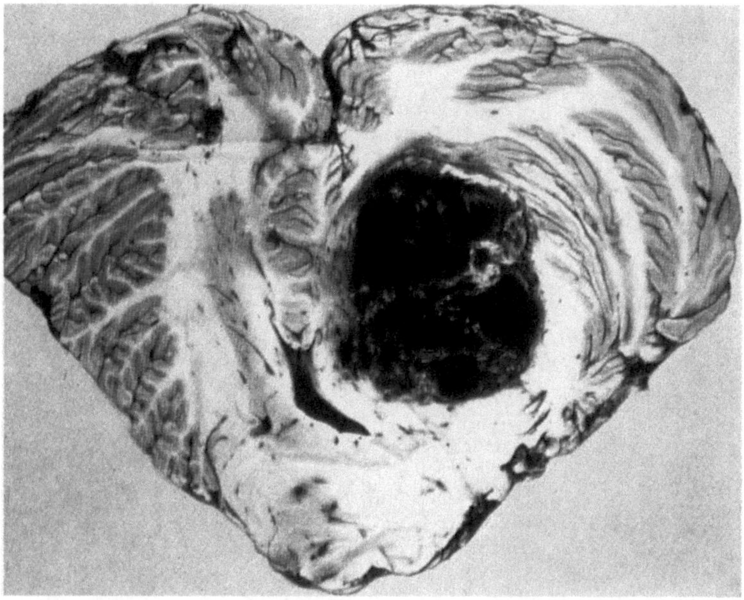

Fig. 137. Circumscribed, partly cystic angioblastoma with intrinsic hemorrhage. A marked shift of the 4th ventricle has occurred. (ZÜLCH 1975a)

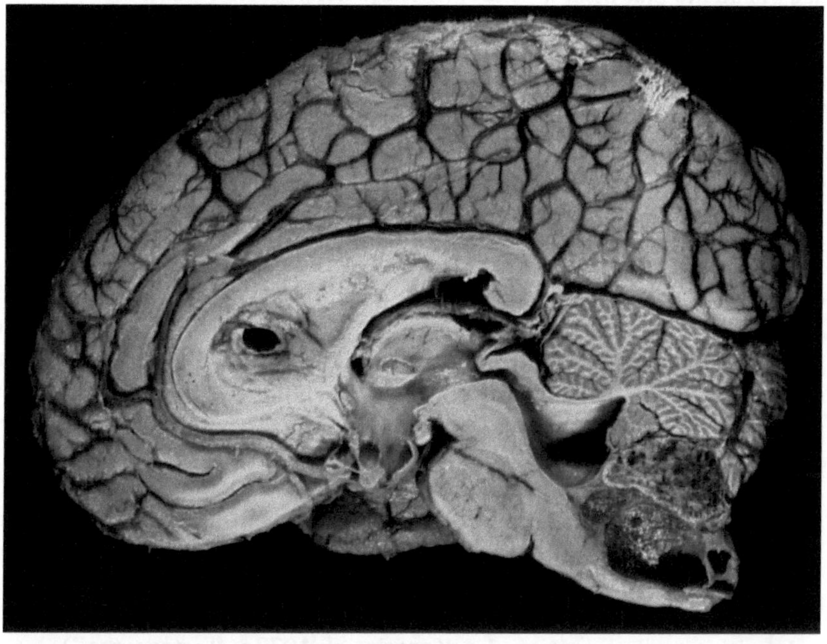

Fig. 138. Plum-sized angioblastoma at the caudal end of the 4th ventricle (area postrema). Two cysts have developed within the tumor and have markedly flattened the medulla oblongata

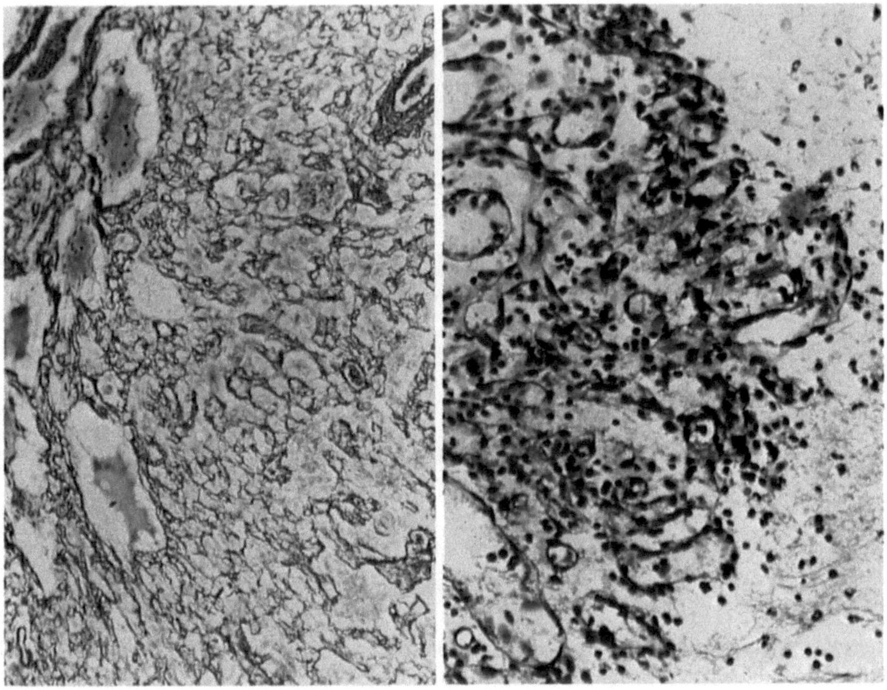

Fig. 139. a Capillary network, well demonstrated by impregnation: small cysts are recognizable, a few lined with connective tissue. **b** The hemangioblastoma (Lindau) lacks encapsulation and "infiltrates" the tissue in spite of its benign nature. Cresyl violet, ×136

(GP, Fig. 22), or outside, like an extracerebral tumor. At the caudal end of the fourth ventricle it may resemble an ependymoma (see Fig. 67; GP, Fig. 224).

Histologic Appearance

The solid part of a hemangioblastoma (GP, Figs. 225–226) is formed by dense networks of capillaries (Fig. 139) or large cavernous vessels (HBT, Fig. 78c, d), whose walls are covered with lining cells (interstitial cells) (Fig. 140a). These stromal cells have a clear cytoplasm. In certain types, the interstitial cells predominate and form broad epithelial bands, or nests, which are separated by capillaries. While the interstitial cells are usually small, elongated or triangular elements, the epithelioid cells can sometimes be large and give rise to the possibility of misinterpretation as "angiogliomas."

The large epithelioid cells (Fig. 140b) have a pronounced tendency to accumulate fat (pseudoxanthoma cells with birefringent lipids) caused by infiltration rather than by degeneration. Sometimes even giant cells occur (LINDAU 1926, Fig. 60).

The gliovascular nature of some cell complexes (JUNG 1935) must be accepted only with reservations (see also KEPES et al. 1979a, "astrocytes").

The walls of the capillary network sonsist of endothelium and a meshwork of abundant reticulin fibers. Numerous mast cells are often found between

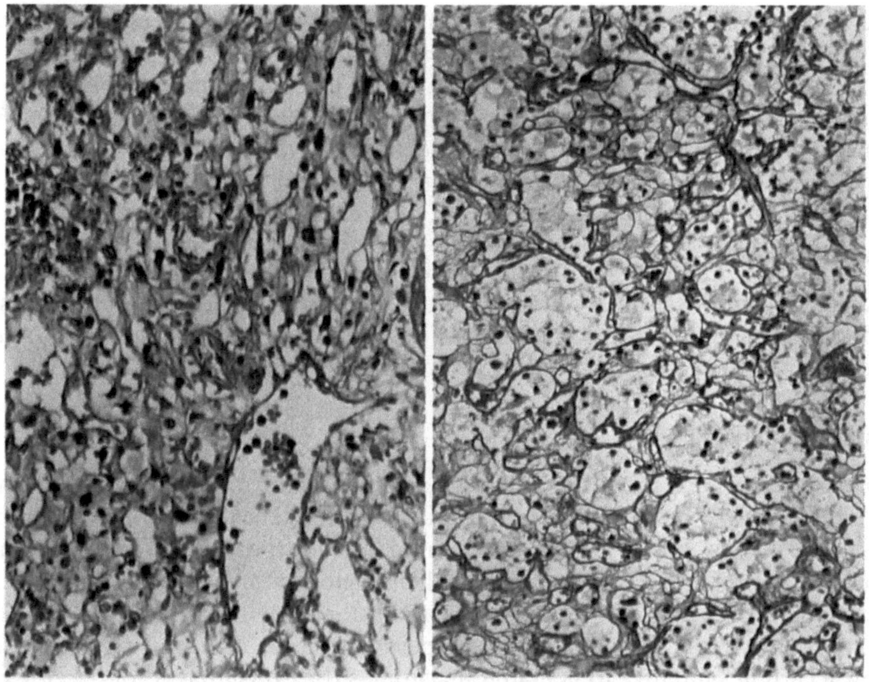

a b

Fig. 140. **a** The hemangioblastoma (Lindau) is characterized by a network of capillaries, larger blood vessels and, in between, the so-called intermediate cells. Occasionally these cells have a hyperchromatic nucleus. The intermediate cells are frequently loaded with lipoid substances. H&E, ×150. **b** In some areas the intermediate cells of the hemangioblastoma appear in a syncytial arrangement. Although the nuclei are hyperchromatic the benign character of the growth is not altered. Silver impregnation, ×125

the blood vessels. Growth seems generally slow, and mitoses do not occur. In the growth zone the tumor advances into the adjacent nervous tissue by infiltration with capillary loops (Fig. 139b). Hemangioblastomas also grow into the leptomeninges and infiltrate them. Lastly, they can even invade the dura, muscles, and skin – at least after operation (PENNYBACKER 1954). Noteworthy among the regressive changes are hyalinization and mucinous degeneration of the connective tissue with the occurrence of mast cells (see regressive processes, Chap. 7).

How the giant cysts so characteristic of this tumor develop is not clear. Secondary transudation into small primarily degenerative cysts probably plays some role. Macrophages containing old blood pigment often lie within the vessel walls. Calcification is never seen.

Electron Microscopy

In EM the cells are characterized by numerous intracytoplasmic fibrils, dilated endoplasmic reticulum with dense granular material, lipid bodies and unusually myelin forms, by "Zwischenzellen" (intervascular intermediate cells, see above) and mast cells. The extracellular spaces are filled with a protein-rich exudate or with collagen fibrils and the capillaries with pericytes.

Whether the intervascular intermediate cells are of vascular origin or belong to the reticular system (CANCILLA and ZIMMERMAN 1965; CASTAIGNE et al. 1968; ISHWAR et al. 1971) is still a matter of debate (CERVOS-NAVARRO 1971; KAWAMURA et al. 1973; SPENCE and RUBINSTEIN 1975).

Tissue Culture

Such investigations have been reported only rarely (see CRAMER and KINSEY 1952; BRASSEUR 1961; KERSTING 1961; SPENCE and RUBINSTEIN 1975). *Histochemically* nothing particularly characteristic has been reported.

Differential Diagnosis

Pilocytic cerebellar astrocytomas can be distinguished from hemangioblastomas by the naked eye, by their firmer and tougher consistency, by their low number of blood vessels, and by their preferential midline position. The two tumor types tend to differ with respect to age, hemangioblastomas in childhood being exceptional. Formation of large cysts is about the same in both.

Metastatic clear cell carcinomas (hypernephromas) may on first inspection show a certain similarity to hemangioblastomas (brownish red color, etc.). Even histologically the epithelial forms of the angioblastomas bear a certain resemblance in architecture to some hypernephromas, as was pointed out by Lindau (see, e.g., HUECK 1937, Fig. 714).

One of our own cases resembled this picture so much that a diagnosis of metastatic clear cell carcinoma was made, and accepted by an experienced general pathologist. The diagnosis had to be revised when the patient survived for many years without any signs of a primary renal tumor.

After surgical exposure hemangioblastomas can sometimes be easily identified by the overlying arteries and particularly veins in the leptomeninges. Furthermore, for differential diagnosis against hemangioblastic meningiomas it seems important to check that the hemangioblastoma is *not encapsulated*, because meningiomas with the same histology can be encountered (see BORCHERS 1910; BAILEY and FORD 1942; ISHWAR et al. 1971; and p. 372).

Biologic Behavior (Grading), Metastasis, and Recurrence

Prognostically the hemangioblastomas should be listed among the benign intracranial tumors (grade I), even though they infiltrate the nervous parenchyma during growth. Anaplastic (malignant) degeneration does not occur. Solid tumors are said to have a less favorable prognosis, as have the more pleomorphic and undifferentiated forms. The tumor is moderately x-ray sensitive. Total removal results in a permanent cure (KRAYENBÜHL and YASARGIL 1958), but recurrence should be expected if the cyst has merely been opened (IIZUKA 1969). It is often difficult at a second operation to decide when one is dealing with a recurrence whether it is a new tumor or a mass overlooked at the first operation, since multiple tumors are not uncommon (see LEVIN 1936; PENNYBACKER 1954).

No case of metastasis has so far been recorded. The rare concomitant occurrence of renal carcinomas should stimulate appropriate clinical investigation.

Clinical Course

The clinical symptoms are accounted for by location of the tumor in the cerebellum and, in particular, by its tendency to form large cysts, which may fill up progressively by transudation and then produce signs of marked displacement of the intracranial contents (especially of the cerebellar tonsils). This may produce ventricular obstruction and recurrent attacks of acute hydrocephalus and herniation.

Our own case (GP, Figs. 225, 226, hemangioblastoma of the cerebellar tonsil) intermittently compromised the vertebrobasilar system (confirmed by angiography).

Clinically hemangioblastomas are (OKA et al. 1982; good reference list) not infrequently associated with polycythemia (polyglobulia, erythropoesis), which may disappear after operation. If this is present it may give an indication of the tumor type before operation (WALKER 1945; BRODY and RODRIGUEZ 1961; BOIVIN et al. 1965; PALMER 1972; ANDRIOLI and SCANARINI 1979). Vertebral angiography may even reveal multiple tumors (DAVID et al. 1966).

Sometimes familial cases occur with a relatively high incidence, as in the Hudson Valley/USA (GOODMAN et al. 1964), where out of 200 members of a family 10% had cataracts or Lindau's disease. According to a large-scale investigation by OERTELT (1970) around 5% of angioblastomas are familial.

Further References: TANNENBERG (1924), SCHUBACK (1927), CUSHING and BAILEY (1928a), MÖLLER (1929, 1944), VINCENT et al. (1930), KUFS (1932), BERNHUBER (1935: reference to old cases!), LOTMAR (1935), PUTSCHAR (1935), DAVISON et al. (1936), MENNENGA (1936), URBAN (1936), ZEITLIN (1942), CORRADINI and BROWDER (1948), PERLMUTTER et al. (1950), OLIVECRONA (1952), SILVER and HENNIGAR (1952), UMBACH (1954), STEIN et al. (1960), DAUM and LE BEAU (1963), ISFORT and SUNDER-PLASSMANN (1965), DAVID et al. (1966), LEGRE et al. (1968), PALMER (1972), OKAWARA (1973), GOODBODY and GAMLEN (1974).

Angioendotheliosis (Neoplastic)

Whether this disease entity (PFLEGER and TAPPEINER 1959) has any relation to the group of hemangioblastomas must be doubted. It presents as a malignant, i.e., neoplastic transformation of endothelial cells within vessels of all sizes. Hence the vascular lumina may be occluded and secondary microinfarcts can arise. It is a rapidly progressive disease (DOLMAN et al. 1979; ANSBACHER et al. 1981). Some authors believe it is more likely that small vessels are plugged with malignant cells of an unrecognized carcinoma than that a malignant transformation had taken place (see also HUSAIN et al. 1979).

19.2 Monstrocellular Sarcomas

Synonym: Giant cell glioblastoma, see Sect. 15.6.1.2; in the older literature: ganglioglioneuroma, ganglioneuroma, spongioblastoma multiforme ganglioides, spongioastroblastoma, spongioneuroblastoma, retothelial sarcoma (reticulosarcoma)

Introduction

Monstrocellular sarcoma is a tumor entity that appears in the WHO classification under two terms: (a) *giant cell glioblastoma* or (b) *monstrocellular type of sarcoma*. Although the description is complete in this section it can count only as a critical summary for the "glial" entity (see Sect. 15.6.1.2).

Historical Note and Definition

The discussion on the position of the monstrocellular sarcoma in the system of intracranial tumors has continued since they were first described by SCHMINCKE (1909/10). However, they were separated from the nerve cell tumors (SCHMINCKE 1914) and from glioblastomas (FOERSTER and GAGEL 1931) by my investigation of 1939a, which led me to discuss its sarcomatous nature in 1940b. In 1948 I demonstrated 22 cases, and defined them as an entity which was thereafter broadly described in 1953a under the term of "monstrocellular sarcoma." The epithet "monstrous" was first used by CUSHING and EISENHARDT (1938) in another relation.

A comparison with certain giant cell tumors (e.g., sarcomas of the vertebral column misdiagnosed by H.J. SCHERER 1933) comes to mind at once, as does the parallel with a benign cousin, the "giant cell epulis," which was earlier thought to have originated from vascular buds. Some authors are still not convinced of the mesodermal origin of these monstrocellular tumors, interpreting them as "giant cell glioblastomas" or "monstrocellular astrocytomas" (LYNN et al. 1968), though KERNOHAN and UIHLEIN (1962) preferred the term of "giant cell fibrosarcoma." KUBO et al. (1974) were in favor of the term *monstrocellular sarcoma*, since neither EM nor tissue culture revealed a difference between glial filaments and tonofibrils.

After all these discussions and new investigations I am still of the opinion that the monstrous character of the cells, which sometimes attain a size of 0.5 mm and are thus visible to the naked eye, merits a special designation under this chosen name. Moreover, the very abundant formation of reticular silver fibers and the frequent origin of these monster cells far distant from the tumor in the marginal capillaries also indicate a mesodermal character, as do its free invasion of the dura and its not infrequent trend to metastasize extracranially; and finally there is absence of a predilection for age and site. This is a characteristic of sarcomas and not of glioblastomas.

Epidemiology (Age – Sex – Frequency – Site)

Age: These tumors have been described in patients of all age groups, i.e., there is no preferential age (our youngest patient was 5, our oldest 80 years old; see BINGAS 1964b). WITTE (1979) found an uneven age curve in our series with an early peak in youth: 20% of patients with monstrocellular tumors were below 20 years of age, as against 2% with glioblastomas.

Sex: There is a male predominance (5:3) in our series of 9000 cases, a similar ratio to that for the glioblastomas (6:4).

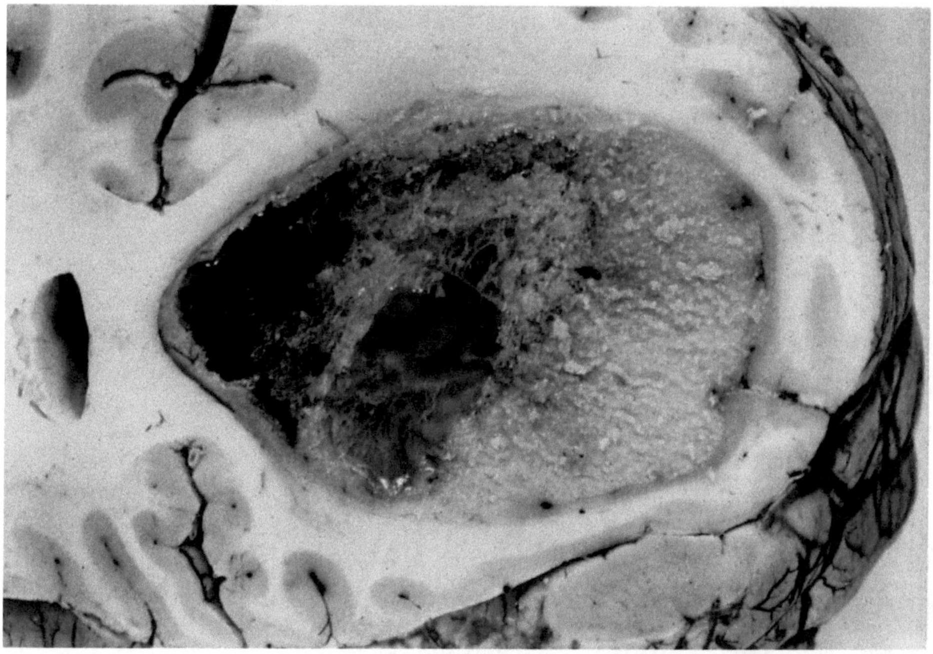

Fig. 141. Egg-sized, well-circumscribed monstrocellular sarcoma with formation of a large cyst. Note the cut surface, which typically resembles asbestos. (ZÜLCH 1975a)

Frequency: Since these tumors are frequently encountered in large collections of tumors with the diagnosis of "giant cell glioblastoma" it is not yet possible to determine their true frequency. Our early figures (BINGAS 1964b) suggest that the frequency is between 0.7% and 1.3% of all intracranial tumors (WITTE 1979). GLUSZCZ (1970) gave a similar figure: 1.4%. We suspect that about 1 monstrocellular sarcoma occurs for every 20 glioblastomas.

Site: Monstrocellular sarcomas have no preferential site, like all the other sarcomas. They are found in all sections of the brain, with a certain accumulation around the brain stem (Figs. 141, 142; GP, Figs. 234, 235, 237–239). In a detailed study of our series of 71 cases WITTE (1979) found an even distribution throughout the brain.

Gross Pathology

These tumors may be fairly well delineated (Fig. 141; GP, Fig. 238), and occasionally they resemble metastases (GP, Figs. 238, 239). They are fleshy tumors (Fig. 141) with a finely tufted, fibrous cut surface looking rather like asbestos (GP, Figs. 234–239). The variegated color of typical glioblastoma is not seen (GP, Fig. 235), since the sarcoma is a uniform grayish pink neoplasm. Necroses, fatty degeneration, and hemorrhagic foci seen in glioblastoma are not very evident. There are none of the fistulous vessels so characteristic of glioblastomas. They are frequently cystic (Fig. 142): multiple quite small cysts occurred in

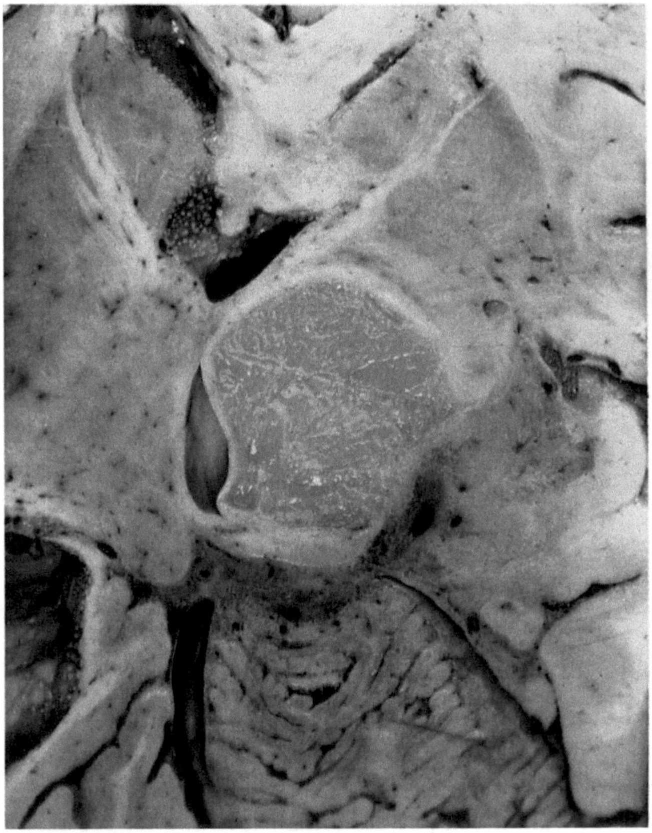

Fig. 142. Monstrocellular sarcoma of the thalamus, which has extensively invaded the leptomeninges of the adjacent basal cisterns. (ZÜLCH 1975a)

one-third of our cases. Their consistency is firmer than that of the brain itself and may often be tough and hard, due to the abundance of reticulin fibers. They may infiltrate and rupture the dura (infiltration noted in 10 of 71 cases, penetration in 4; GP, Fig. 239). Infiltration of the meninges is common.

Histologic Appearance

These sarcomas are characterized by a wide variety (HBT, Fig. 84) in histologic picture, but two architectural patterns predominate: (a) In the periphery there are regions containing fibrous spindle cells, densely arranged (Fig. 143a) in streams (HBT, Fig. 86a); and (b) in the center there are areas of giant tumor cells with extremely bizarre and fantastic forms (HBT, Fig. 85a–d) "which, because of their form and size, cannot be compared to anything else in the human body" (SCHMINCKE 1909/10, 1914). Both types can occur simultaneously. The monster cells are atypical in every conceivable way: they can assume almost any shape and any size up to 400–500 μm, i.e., they are visible to the naked eye. There are single giant nuclei or multinucleated masses (HBT, Fig. 85c, d).

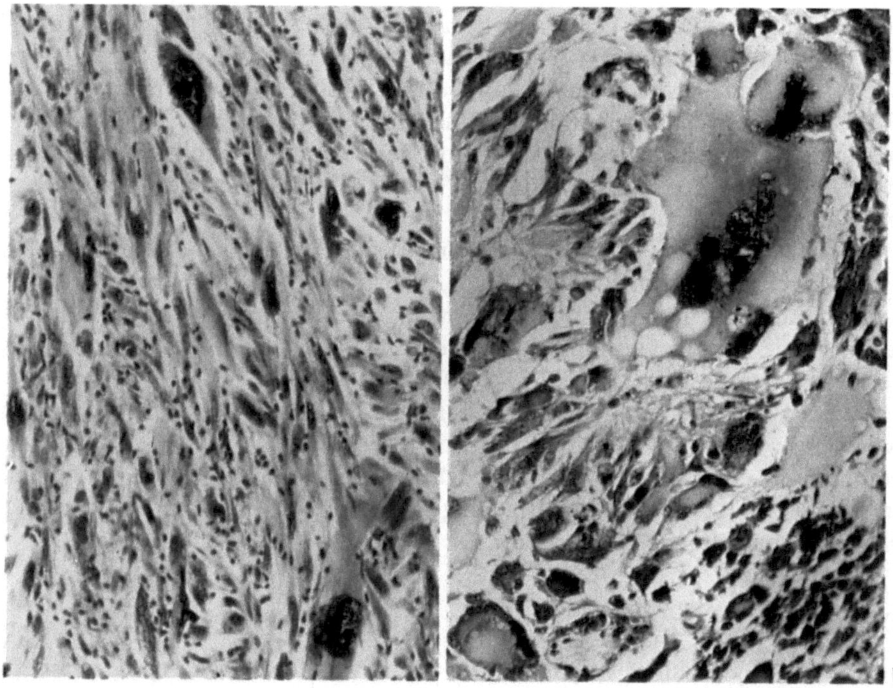

a b

Fig. 143. a Polymorphous cells of monstrocellular sarcoma. Cresyl violet, ×112. **b** A monster cell with countless nuclear components of all sizes. These components were formerly described as "inclusion bodies," "bird's-eye inclusion," etc. Some nuclei have distinct nuclear vacuoles. Cresyl violet, ×128

They may contain as many as 50–80 inclusion bodies in a single cell (HBT, Fig. 85c), giving the so-called bird's eye patterns (Fig. 143b) (a central core surrounded by a halo). There are intranuclear vacuoles, lobulation of the nuclei, hyperchromasia of nuclei, neurone-like patterns of nucleus (HBT, Fig. 84b, c, d), and also ghost cells with no nuclei. Mitotic figures (HBT, Fig. 85a) may also be grotesquely abnormal (details given by ALTMANN 1961). In their earlier stages the spindle cells resemble fibroblasts.

HITSELBERGER et al. (1961) observed 27 cases of giant cell fibrosarcoma, which they characterized by stating that in some parts they could be distinguished from ordinary fibrosarcomas by the presence of anaplastic giant cells. But this is a well-known feature of our tumor group (see above). Attempts to demonstrate neuronal or glial elements were unsuccessful.

Occasionally lymphoid infiltrates (HBT, Fig. 86b) are found in the marginal zone. Between these various types of cells a dense network of reticulin fibers is usually formed even in the center of the tumor, but not always in and between the monster cells. In the growth zone the tumor not infrequently spreads by way of vascular buds (HBT, Fig. 87a, b). Large hyperchromatic tumor cells seem to detach themselves from the adventitia of these vessels (HBT, Figs. 84a, 86c), and are found lying singly in brain tissue that has so far scarcely been infiltrated; hence our assumption that they are "vascular" tumors. On the other hand, the tumor cells may lie in dense rings, with abundant reticulin fiber formation around the blood vessels (HBT, Fig. 87c, d). Regressive processes are seen in the form of fatty degeneration of the tumor cells, or of the formation of small necrotic foci and particularly of cysts. There have been no reports of fistulous vessels and shunts (not even after radiological examination; see KAUTZKY, ZÜLCH et al. 1976, 1982), which are very characteristic of glioblastomas.

NOETZEL and HAUPTMANN (1964) have called attention to the resemblance to liposarcomas in other body organs. KEPES et al. (1973) published cases of xanthosarcomas that are actually somewhat similar to the monstrocellular variant in some features, although they are basically different (see, however, their change in classification Sect. 17.3, p. 391).

We have never seen calcification in these tumors. Vascular overgrowth, which is so prominent in glioblastomas, particularly at the edge of necroses, is much less significant. The monstrocellular sarcomas seem to have a tendency to diffuse spread into the leptomeninges; this trend is uncharacteristic of the glioblastomas, though it can occur.

Electron Microscopy

Several authors, such as LYNN et al. (1968), have refused to accept the sarcomatous nature of these tumors, since in light and electron microscopy differentiation between the monster cells and monstrous astrocytes did not seem possible. HADFIELD and SILVERBERG (1972) probably had a majority of cases of particularly polymorphous glioblastomas in their studies, following which they declined – correctly – a sarcomatous nature. BECKER et al. (1967) and HASSOUN et al. (1973) depicted typical glial filaments in EM. However, the true nature of their tumors is not sufficiently clear. Moreover, the literature has emphasized the difficulty of distinguishing glia filaments and mesenchymal tonofibrils in EM (KUBO et al. 1974) despite the high enough number of collagen fibers to justify calling the tumor sarcoma. MOGHIMI (1965) also accepted the sarcomatous nature.

Tissue Culture

KUBO et al. (1974) were not able to grow fibroblasts together with the tumor cells although collagen fibers were cultivated. GULLOTTA (1964) apparently recognizes the entity of monstrocellular sarcoma.

Histochemistry

Histochemistry did not reveal any specific characteristics of these tumors.

Differential Diagnosis

Differential diagnosis of this tumor against glioblastoma is discussed on Sect. 19.2.

Biologic Behavior (Grading), Metastasis, and Recurrence

As far as we can tell from the observations we have collected over more than 30 years, this is a highly malignant, rapidly growing tumor (grade IV in the WHO classification), however, with a somewhat better prognosis in some instances. It may characteristically infiltrate the dura (GP, Fig. 239) and can penetrate it; extracranial seeding is also not uncommon; none of these events is characteristic of glioblastomas. We noted postoperative survival of 2.5 years in a case, where the tumor was clearly circumscribed. BINGAS (1964b) found one case with a 7-year survival in our series. The postoperative mortality – investigated in our series of 71 tumors by WITTE (1979) – differed somewhat between the two groups: after 6 months 60% of our patients with monstrocellular sarcomas were still living, as against 30% of the patients with glioblastoma. Therefore, the prognosis seems to be better in some instances than for glioblastomas (GARCIA-BENGOCHEA and COLLINS 1969).

Differential diagnosis from glioblastomas is not difficult if the histological characteristics described above are observed.

Recurrence is early when only partial resection is achieved, but it also occurs after supposedly total excision. We have observed metastases in extracranial organs, e.g., heart and lung, and also diffuse intracranial seeding after radiation (GP, Figs. 237, 239).

GROPP (1955) observed a small metastatic nodule in the heart in the case of a "glioma", which he considered most likely to be a monstrocellular sarcoma.

Clinical Course

There are no particular events associated with the clinical course of this group (see WITTE 1979).

Further References: PAUL (1926), WÄTJEN (1930), ALPERS (1931), FOOT and COHEN (1933), H.J. SCHERER (1933, 1935), SEITZ and KALM (1958), BRUCHER (1962), GLOWACKI and SELOSSE (1965), BECKER et al. (1967), SHUANGSHOTI and NETSKY (1971), ROESSMAN and WEISS (1972).

20 Germ Cell Tumors

20.1 Germinomas

Synonym: Dysgerminomas

Introduction

The WHO classification has followed the trend of the English-speaking countries in defining the two-cell-type pattern pineal tumors as *germinomas*.

Historical Note and Definition

The parenchymal tumors of the pineal region were first interpreted as "pinealomas" (KRABBE 1923) when they had a two-cell-type pattern; however, in a discussion Dorothy RUSSELL (1944, 1954b) pointed out the relationship between the pinealoma and immature teratomas. FRIEDMAN (1947) came to the conclusion that most pineal tumors had the histological pattern of germinoma (seminoma of the testis) and therefore all had to be considered as such. The direction these discussions took was determined by histological factors, such as the teratoid character and the similarity of the histological pattern (DIXON and MOORE 1952; HERTIG and GORE 1961; PIERCE 1966).

In the last decade most general pathologists have accepted the identity of the two-cell-type pineal tumor with the germinoma of testis, whereas most neurosurgeons, particularly in Europe, still retain the old term, pinealoma. SCHMIDEK (1977) has reviewed the problems extensively in a monograph. ZÜLCH (1969b) showed that in his clinical case the CSF seed was identical with the type of cell described by DEL RIO HORTEGA (1932) as the pineal parenchyma cell (pp. 20, 283, 287), and RIVERSON and ZÜLCH (1979) emphasized the coexistence of two types of two-cell-type pattern tumors, one derived from the pineal parenchyma and the other corresponding to the germinoma.

JÄNISCH et al. (1976) also found it difficult to distinguish between germinomas (Fig. 144) and true pinealomas. Meanwhile, on the basis of a very extensive and detailed study of 48 personal cases, SANO (1983a) has perpetuated this duality and has further enlarged on this problem (1985).

The World Health Organization, however, has only kept one group, namely the germinomas, for two-cell-type tumors of the pineal region. The other tumors of the pineal parenchyma are designated pineocytoma and pinealoblastoma (see p. 20).

My opinion since 1951 (see ZÜLCH 1951b, 1956) has been that until this scientific problem has been clarified the existence of two types of two-cell-pattern

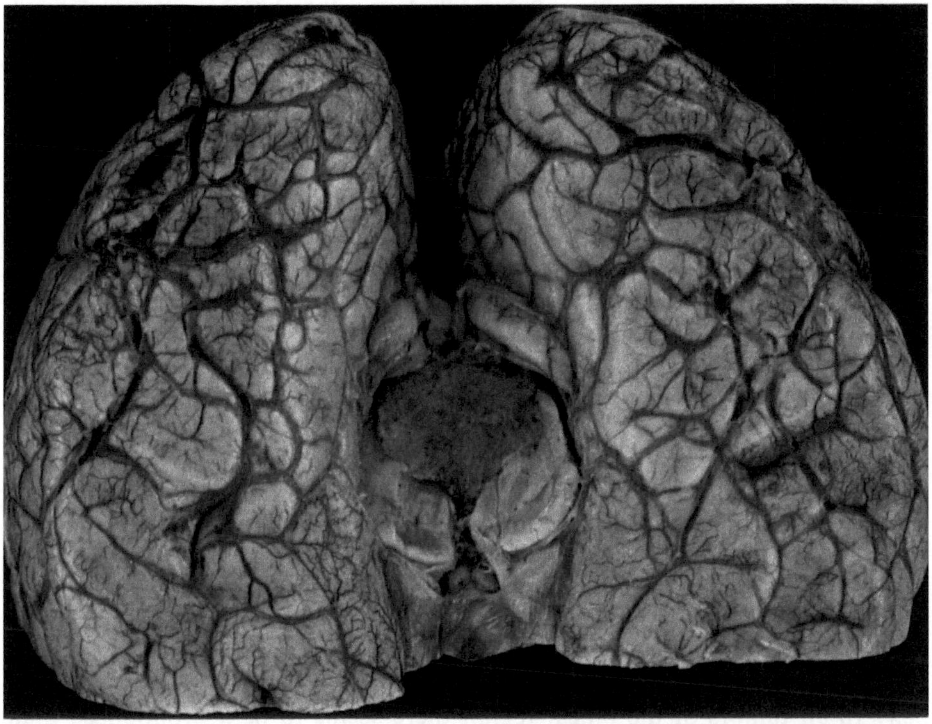

Fig. 144. Germinoma with remarkable deformation of the midbrain. Two small tentorial hernias

tumors has to be accepted, and it is left to each scientist to decide which concept he wants to adopt.

Our personal definition and differentiation of two-cell pinealoma in the sense of Krabbe (1923) and two-cell germinoma in the sense of Friedman (1947) during the discussion of the WHO working group were as follows: since in our series of 104 tumors we found by histological examinations that most pinealomas were impregnated by the Di Girolami method and were negative for PAS stain and in contrast germinomas were all positive for PAS stain and negative for Di Girolami's impregnation, the dualistic concept was logical.

Our further arguments for the duality of the two-cell pineal tumors have been given on pp. 283, 287 in the description of the pinealoma. We were supported in our dualistic concept by Matsutani's statement (personal communication, and Matsutani et al. 1975, Matsutani 1976) that some of the two-cell pinealomas were derived from the pineal parenchyma, as proven by immunohistological methods.

Relatively recently, Sano (1983a) reported on his series of 48 cases, 26 of which were located in the pineal region, 11 at suprasellar, and 9 at other sites. Histologically he found that there were actually two types of two-cell pattern tumors, i.e., the old pinealoma of Krabbe (1923), and the germinoma of Friedman (1947). Histologically he found an intimate proximity of cells of the pinealoma type to sinusoid vessels as the tumor's stroma. The "capillaries

[are] often found in the midst of the cell clusters"... "Contrarywise the cells of the seminiferous tubules in the seminoma have no interrelationship with blood vessels"... "There is no evidence of tumor cells [in the seminoma] of an attaching to the capillaries"... "Tumor cells in seminoma are somewhat larger than those of pineal origin tumor"... [Therefore,] "they can be divided into two groups pinealoma... and germinoma... .".

In 53 years' observations at the Mayo Clinic (DONAT et al. 1978) there were 10 germinomas and 10 pineal cell tumors in 34 patients. This seems to me to be one of the tumor groups where the World Health Organization ought to have allowed a double classification into germinomas *and* pinealomas according to the histological characteristics, and in fact this was changed only in the last moment.

Epidemiology (Age – Sex – Frequency – Site)

Age: It is difficult now, because of the difference in terminology and concept, to give precise details about germinomas or the two groups of pinealomas and germinomas (less than 2% of primary brain tumors: DONAT et al. 1978). The earlier data all combine the two groups. Of SANO's 48 cases of both types 33 patients were younger than 20 years and 15 patients were 20 years old or older; thus, there was a preference for the first two decades.

Sex: In all tumors of the pineal region there seems to be a pronounced male preponderance, already shown in BERBLINGER's series (1944) of patients under 17 years of age (92% were male and only 8% female). In SANO's series the total of 48 cases was made up of 41 male and 7 female patients.

Frequency: Reliable data on frequency must be considered with reference to the source. In CUSHING's (1932, 1935) series, for example, pinealoma was found in 0.7%, while in our collection of 9000 cases pinealomas accounted for 0.5%.

It is an old notion that in Oriental races these tumors of the pineal region are encountered in a percentage several times higher than that seen in westerners. For instance, UEKI (1963) reported 3.9% pineal tumors in 5794 brain tumors. ARAKI and MATSUMOTO (1969) gave the following figures: between 1958 and 1964 there were 87395 autopsies, revealing 1977 intracranial tumors in Japan. Of these, 1802 cases were histologically verified. Pineal tumors (136 cases) constituted 8% of the total of verified tumors. These 136 embraced 81 pinealomas in the pineal region, 16 ectopic pinealomas, and 39 teratomas in the pineal region; approximately 10% of the pinealomas were diagnosed as pineoblastomas. SANO (1985) found 4% pinealomas in the Japan Tumor Registry.

This was definitely many times higher than in the west; MATSUMOTO, while in Cologne, made a count of our collection with the following result: 3799 cases; of these, 0.5% pinealomas and 0.7% ectopic pinealomas and true genuine teratomas of various sites.

TAKEUCHI et al. (1978) found 132 germinomas and teratomas amongst 2609 tumors, i.e., 5% of the total series, 3.3% being histologically proven; 2.1% of these were germinomas.

In summary, in the western races around 0.5%–0.7% of a surgical brain tumor series will probably be accounted for by pineal tumors of the pinealoma or the germinoma type. In the eastern races 4%–4.5% of all intracranial neoplasms will be tumors in the pineal region.

Site: The most usual site of the two-cell-type tumors is the pineal region, and the next, the suprasellar localization; such tumors do also occur at other locations.

Of SANO's 48 cases, 28 were located in the pineal region, 11 in the suprasellar area, and 9 at other sites. Bifrontal tumors have been recorded (10 cases in Japan): KAWAMOTO et al. 1980.

The suprasellar "ectopic" two-cell pattern tumors pose the problem as to whether they are always *primary* genuine tumors of the suprasellar region, of whether and how often they are actually metastases, as in our own case (ZÜLCH 1956, Fig. 251; ZÜLCH 1963c; Fig. 82). In particular, we should like to draw attention to the case of KALM and MAGUN (1950) which in large celloidin sections show the primary in the pineal region, seeding throughout the ventricular system, and the localized large mass in the hypothalamic region that induced the clinical typical syndrome of the ectopic pinealoma. It is well known that metastases of two-cell-pattern tumors occur throughout the CNS, and we have depicted a case that was diagnosed only in the cauda equina. The pineal tumor was not detected until later, stimulated by the two-cell pattern histology (see HBT, Fig. 90d).

In our clinical case (ZÜLCH 1963c) it was also proven by PEG that there was a *primary* pineal tumor and a large (secondary) suprasellar mass, which responded well to radiation (survival time more than 5 years).

On the other hand, WARZOK and ARNOLD (1972) claim to have proven that in their cases the pineal gland was normal. DAYAN et al. (1966) refer to "multifocal pineal and suprasellar simultaneous" tumor growth. Other cases have been published by PEREY et al. (1955), RUBIN and KRAMER (1965), SIMSON et al. (1968), GHATAK et al. (1969), KAGEYAMA (1971), LEBLANC et al. (1976), and STEFANKO et al. (1979).

The primary and the seeding of the neoplastic process are exemplified in FAN and AGBATA's (1976) observation that beside the suprasellar tumor the connective tissue in the pineal gland was infiltrated (by "lymphocytic cells" corresponding to the small tumor cells and furthermore a few large epitheloid cells identical with the suprasellar large elements).

Although the embryology, anatomy, and pathology of the pineal gland (see Ariens KAPPERS 1965, 1976) have been exhaustively investigated, much has to be clarified before a convincing concept of the pathology and pathogenesis in the pineal region is achieved.

Gross Pathology

The mass of a germinoma compresses the adjacent anatomical structures, displacing the quadrigeminal plates downward (Fig. 144; GP, Figs. 243–246) and later pushing the posterior third of the corpus callosum and the deep cerebral veins upward. The thalami may be shifted to either side by the tumor. The

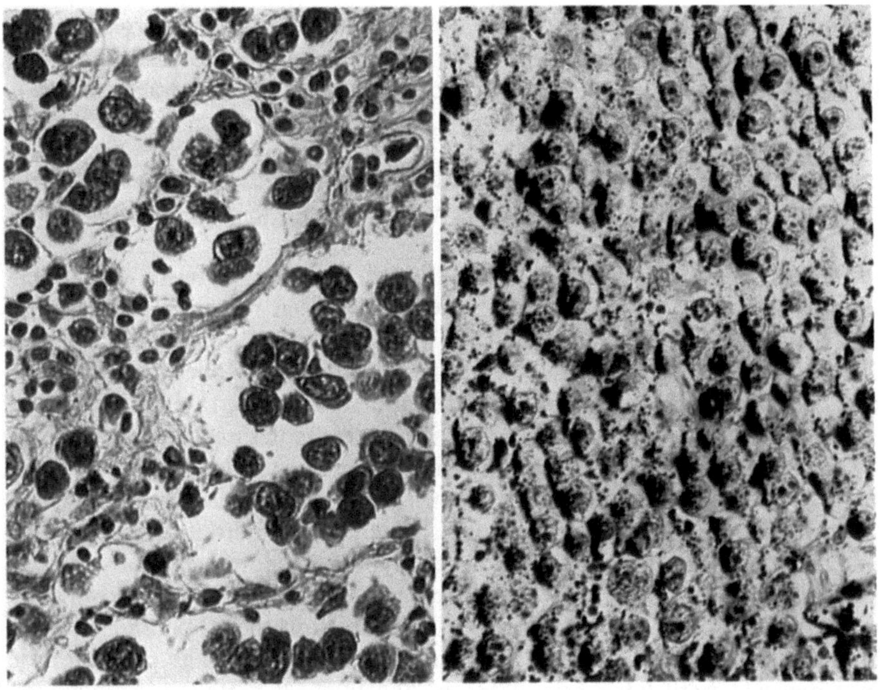

a b

Fig. 145. a The "two-cell" architecture of the germinoma can mimic the "two-cell pinealoma". H&E, ×312. **b** A striking feature is the intense staining with PAS. ×250

tumors infiltrate the surrounding area (HBT, Fig. 91a) and many have a marked tendency to calcify, as was already known to the classical neuroradiologists (half the cases seen at the Mayo Clinic in 53 years: DONAT et al. 1978).

Histologic Appearance

The basic two-cell pattern of these tumors (HBT, Figs. 89, 90) is the juxtaposition of large clear cells and small lymphoid elements (Fig. 145a). Large cells in the germinoma are thought to be larger than those in the pinealoma. Moreover, they have a tendency to form large dark nuclei and not infrequently even polynuclear (Fig. 146a, b) giant cells (HBT, Fig. 90c). In the marginal zone they may be infiltrating (HBT, Fig. 91a) and there may occasionally be epithelial tubules, from which the tumor cells apparently have developed by metaplasia (HBT, Fig. 91c).

We have emphasized above the negative results of impregnation with Di Girolami's method and the highly positive staining with PAS, showing large amounts of mucoproteins (Fig. 145b).

Electron Microscopy

Ultrastructural studies have been reported by WARZOK and ARNOLD (1972), TANI et al. (1974), HIRANO et al. (1975c), FAN and AGBATA (1976), and MARKESBERY et al. (1976). Germinomas are thought to have specialized intercellular junctions of three types.

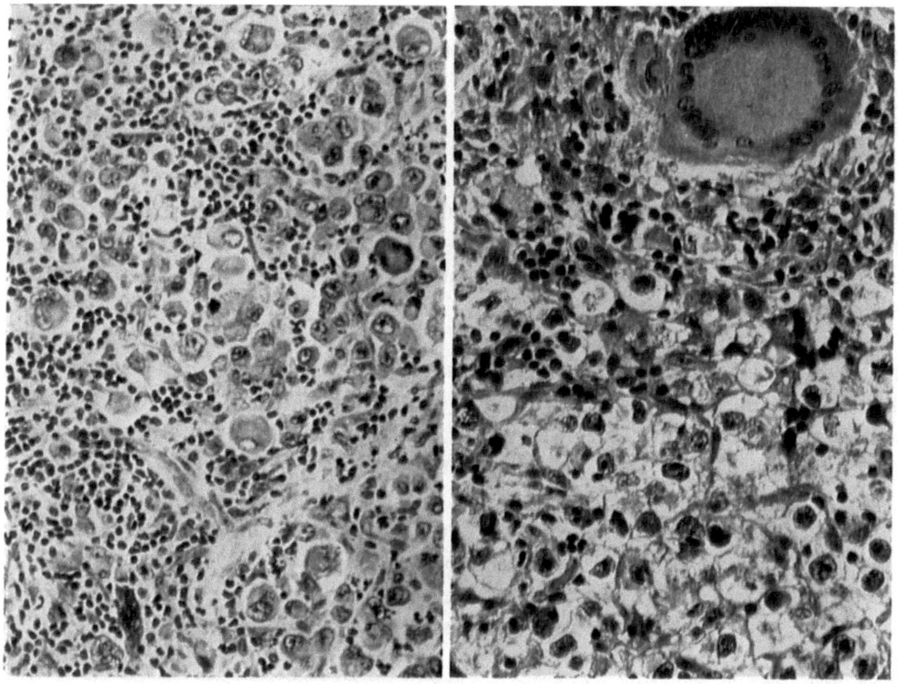

a b

Fig. 146a, b. The germinoma is composed of large spheroidal cells, including multinucleated giant cells and lymphoid cells, which can be a prominent feature. H&E, ×324 (**a**) and ×250 (**b**)

Differential Diagnosis

The characteristic differences between the pinealoma as defined by KRABBE (1923) and the germinoma as defined by FRIEDMAN (1947) have already been adequately treated.

Biologic Behavior (Grading), Metastasis, and Recurrence

The biologic behavior of pineal two-cell-pattern tumors, when successfully operated on and subsequently radiated, is promising; survival times of 5 and many more years are well known, particularly since HORRAX and WYATT's (1947) demonstration of the high radiosensitivity. Pinealoma, germinoma, and mature teratoma show a good prognosis according to SANO's (1983a) report, and should therefore be surgically attacked, the first two should also be irradiated after surgery.

The biologic behavior of the germinomas is expressed in the WHO classification by grades II and III. FUJITA et al. (1980) emphasize that following radiation 50%–60% of patients survive for more than 5 years (survival time 1–8 years).

Seeding via the CSF is not rare (WERNER 1939). Metastases to the body were first described in GOLDZIEHER's (1913) report of the seeding of a pineal tumor into the lungs, the lymph nodes, and the liver; this was followed by the cases of STOWELL et al. (1945), TOMPKINS et al. (1950), MOTOMICHI et al. (1980), and many others.

Recurrence is common, although following radiation an apparently disease-free interval of 5–10 years can be expected.

Operability: The first tumors in the pineal region were successfully operated on by OPPENHEIM and KRAUSE (1913a – probably a meningioma; see ZÜLCH 1981b), and later a pinealoma by FOERSTER (1928) and 2 mature teratomas by TÖNNIS (see WEBER 1939). In my report about the operability of the mesencephalic region I have listed the unsuccessful and the successful surgical attempts. In the series of SANO (1983a) "there was no operative mortality." The patients all received postoperative radiation. The 5-year survival rate (83.8%) and 10-year survival rate (78.9%) give an extremely good prognosis for patients undergoing surgery. Cases under 20 years of age showed better results than those of 20 years or over. The microsurgical approach makes tumor extirpation a theoretical possibility (NEUWELT et al. 1979); CSF shunting and radiotherapy are applied by ABAY et al. (1981) and SUNG et al. (1978).

Variants: KOBAYASHI et al. (1981) reported that 10% of all intracranial germinomas were located unilaterally in the basal ganglia and thalamus, in contrast to 70% in the pineal region and 20% ectopic tumors in the suprasellar region. The mean age of the patients in this study was 15.2 years and they were all male. We have seen a typical two-cell pattern tumor in the parietal lobe (described by KLEINSASSER and KLOSS 1958).

Clinical Course

A study of the various forms of the pineal tumors (FEDERMANN 1983) shows that the quadrigeminal syndrome prevailed in all sorts of space-occupying lesions in the pineal region (pinealomas, germinomas, teratomas etc.; see p. 291). Only the ventriculogram gave any indications of the different pathology (TÖNNIS, see WEBER 1939). The CT can now probably yield more information. SANO's (1983a, 1985) excellent results may suggest that surgery should be attempted more frequently. Diagnosis can be made by conventional neuroradiology including CT (TAKEUCHI et al. 1979).

One curious case is that of a patient who had a typical pineal teratoma totally removed, but developed a typical germinoma 15 years later (TSUCHIDA et al. 1976).

Further References: ASKANAZY (1921), BENEDEK (1936), BAGGENSTOSS and LOVE (1939).

20.2 Embryonal Carcinomas

Synonyms: Endodermal tumors, sinus tumors, yolk sac carcinomas

Introduction

Several tumors, particularly in the pineal region, have been identified with reference to similar species in general pathology and are therefore also mentioned in the WHO classification.

Historical Note and Definition

D. RUSSELL pointed out in 1944 that many of the so-called pinealomas were in fact atypical teratomas, and since then various variants have been described. FRIEDMAN and MOORE (1946) introduced the classification of embryonal and germ cell tumors, and DIXON and MOORE (1952) continued this attempt. TEILUM (1959, 1971) described several cases seemingly also proving the existence of endodermal sinuses within such or similar tumors (BESTLE 1968; BORIT 1969; JELLINGER et al. 1970b). TEILUM (1965) had also pointed out that tumors of this region showed structures like a selected overgrowth of yolk sac endoderm. Probably these rare neoplasms in the pineal region are derived from parenchymal cells of the gland itself, analogously to comparable lesions in the gonads (PIERCE and ABELL 1970).

Epidemiology (Age – Sex – Frequency – Site)

Age: The mean age at diagnosis is around 15 years; otherwise no age preference has been recorded.

Sex: The male:female ratio is around 20:6.

*Frequency:*The frequency is about 1 intracranial germ cell tumor to 200 intracranial tumors; in the series of ALBRECHTSEN et al. (1972) it amounted to 20 of 4000 tumors (9 germinomas, 5 teratomas, 2 endodermal sinus tumors, 4 mixed germ tumors). In the Osaka Neurosurgical Department it comprised 5.1% of 512 cases (ARITA et al. 1979); in the series of JELLINGER (1973) 0.48% of 3550 neoplasms belonged to this group.

Gross Pathology

These rare neoplasms are sometimes encapsulated, in which case they are totally removable (KHANTANAPHAR and BUNYARATVEJ 1974). Otherwise, they are not recognizable by any specific macroscopical features.

Histologic Appearance

Microscopically there is an analogy between the germinal tumors of the brain and those of the gonads (JELLINGER et al. 1970b). There are solid cell strands and gland-like structures, small cavities lined with flat cells, and a vacuolated network with wide meshes and microcysts. Necroses and hemorrhages occur (BORIT 1969; LEE et al. 1978; EBERTS and RANSBURG 1979). There are then acinar, tubular, cuboidal, papillary, and solid formations and gland-like structures. Sometimes a mixture of embryonal carcinoma and malignant teratoma in germinoma-like areas is observed (JELLINGER et al. 1970b); thus, they can occur in pure forms or as mixtures.

Differential Diagnosis

Analysis of the various structural formations described here should make it easy to recognize and distinguish the tumor in the pineal region.

Biologic Behavior (Grading), Metastasis, and Recurrence

The postoperative survival time is very short (1–2 years) because of the invasiveness and malignancy. The prognosis is therefore very poor (EBERTS and RANSBURG 1979). Surgery is often palliative, and the operative mortality high. More success is obtained with radiotherapy (up to 5.5 years of survival).

20.3 Choriocarcinomas

Synonym: Chorionepithelioma

Introduction

Choriocarcinomas are a separate entity in the subgroup of germ cell tumors in the WHO classification.

Historical Note and Definition

The first description of a tumor as chorionepithelioma came from ASKANAZY in 1906, but it turned out to be a two-cell-pattern pinealoma/germinoma. Many reports have appeared in the literature (e.g., STOWELL et al. 1945; GLASS and CULBERTSON 1946; BRUTON et al. 1961; NISHIYAMA et al. 1966; BORIT 1969; KELLY et al. 1971; JELLINGER 1973).

The microscopical features of some pineal tumors correspond to the pattern of choriocarcinomas. These are highly malignant tumors composed of elements identical with those of syncytiotrophoblast and cytotrophoblast. Most of them occur in patients below 20 years of age, the mean age being around 10 years (KELLY et al. 1971; HASEGAWA et al. 1974). One case has been reported in a newborn child. In 13 cases in the literature the mean age was 10.8 years, and all patients were under 19 years of age. HASEGAWA et al. (1974) reported 34 cases collected from the literature. GIUFFRE and DI LORENZO (1975) reported the development of a primary intrasellar germinomatous teratoma into a choriocarcinoma. Most of the cases seem to have been reported in a Japanese population. KAWAKAMI et al. (1980) emphasized that good results can be obtained by surgical removal followed by simultaneous chemotherapy and Co irradiation (ESTEBAN et al. 1979; NAKAGAWA et al. 1979; FUJII et al. 1981). – Metastases seem to be not uncommon (e.g., STOWELL et al. 1945; metastasis to the lung).

Further Reference: FRIEDMAN (1951).

20.4 Teratomas

Introduction

The teratomas exist as a well-defined subgroup of the *germ cell tumors* in the WHO classification.

Historical Note and Definition

The teratomas (VIRCHOW 1863/65) are tumors originating from several germ layers and – according to classic pathology – they can be subdivided into "teratomas" with three and "teratoid" tumors with two germ layers. The intracranial teratomas are typically composed of three germinal layers. The earlier category of teratoid tumors (see MÜLLER and WOHLFAHRT 1947) is not in common use any longer, because it seemed somewhat artificial. These tumors have been integrated into the teratoma group.

The teratomas of the pineal region have long been a subject of particular interest, since the correlation with the clinical syndrome of pubertas praecox was observed. MARBURG (1909) introduced the concept of an endocrinological function of this particular tumor. BERBLINGER (1925, 1944) observed clinical signs of pubertas praecox in 18 of 36 patients under 17 years with teratoma of the pineal region. Thus, in 50% – as also in the four cases, operated on by TÖNNIS (WEBER 1939) – this syndrome can be absent (classic cases listed in GREENHOUSE and NEUBUERGER's paper 1960; WILLIS 1971).

Epidemiology (Age – Sex – Frequency – Site)

Age: There is a preponderance in the first two decades, and within this period, for early infancy (TAKAKU et al. 1973: of 71 tumors in the first 2 months of life were 44 teratomas). The mean age in a Japanese study was 12.4 years (TAKEUCHI et al. 1975).

Sex: There is a marked male preponderance and teratomas of the pineal region almost always occur in the male sex (of 25 cases in the literature 1 patient was female; BERBLINGER 1925).

Frequency: At our count of 1956 the percentage of true three-layer teratomas was 0.3%. Other data were similar (CRITCHLEY 1925: 0.2%; ARSENI et al. 1969: 0.05% (!); MCCORMACK et al. 1978: 0.2–0.9%). According to SACHS and HORRAX (1949) teratomas are exceedingly rare and most common in childrens' hospitals (INGRAHAM and O.T. BAILEY 1946: 2% in subjects below 15 years).

Site: The teratomas in our series had a marked preponderance in the pineal region. In 71 cases (WEBER 1939) in the literature there were 32 teratomas of the pineal and 12 of the chiasma region; 11 in the spinal cord; 4 in the lateral ventricles; 2 in the orbit; and 10 at different sites (many of these being sacrococcygeal tumors). The distribution in the cases reported by TAKEUCHI et al. (1975) was similar: among 2419 intracranial tumors there were 21 pineal teratomas and 5 suprasellar teratomas, and all the others were located in the frontal area, the posterior fossa (STRANG et al. 1960), the lateral ventricles (GÜTHERT 1938; GAUPP 1942), or the fourth ventricle (MORELLI 1973). And lastly, of 99 intracranial teratomas tabulated by ACQUAVIVA et al. (1966) 49 were pineal, 14 were in the ventricles, 8 in the pituitary, 21 at other supratentorial sites, 4 in the posterior fossa (excluding fourth ventricle), and 5 at undefined sites. Of all teratomas seen in Nigerian children two-thirds were localized in the sacrococcygeal region (WILLIAMS et al. 1970).

This tumor has been found in combination with diastematomyelia (LAKE and PITTS 1969; ROSENBAUM et al. 1978). In the spinal region teratomas are extremely rare (SACHS and HORRAX 1949; HANSEBOUT and BERTRAND 1965; ROSENBAUM et al. 1978), as they are in the cauda equina/conus (BLACK and GERMAN 1950). An intramedullary localization was recorded by LIEBALDT (1963) in a child 1 year of age. Heredity may play a role in presacral teratomas (HUNT et al. 1977). Occurrence has been noted in a neonate (GREENHOUSE and NEUBUERGER 1960) and in two brothers (WAKAI et al. 1980).

Gross Pathology

The teratomas are well-defined masses ranging in size from that of a pinhead to that of a child's fist (or even 20 × 13.5 × 5 cm; 790 g: GREENHOUSE and NEUBUERGER 1960; 10 × 8 × 6 cm: HERRSCHAFT 1968). In isolated cases they can be very large and can displace the supratentorial brain (IMMISCH 1952; OBERMANN 1964; VRAA-JENSEN 1974). They are nodular (ZÜLCH 1956, Figs. 398, 399; GP, Figs. 268, 269) and encapsulated, and brownish red in color; not infrequently they have dark-colored cysts on the surface. The cyst fluid can be yellow and clear, but is more commonly dark brown or greenish. The tumors are usually hard, almost cartilage-like, and are occasionally calcified or crisscrossed by bony spicules.

Histologic Appearance

The microscopical appearance of the teratomas is well described in the textbooks of pathology. However, a more detailed account of the occurrence of nervous tissue in intracranial teratomas has been given by WILLIS (1971).

Tissue Culture – Electron Microscopy – Histochemistry

In cases of such tumors (see textbooks of general pathology) in the CNS there are no particular features that can be detected by these means.

Biologic Behavior (Grading), Metastasis, and Recurrence

The majority of teratomas grow extremely slowly and are benign (grade I). Small ones may be found incidentally. Patients with teratomas can live to an advanced age when the tumors do not block the CSF pathway (spinal teratomas, 21 years: FURTADO and MARQUES 1951). Malignant changes have been described by INGRAHAM and O.T. BAILEY (1946), and invasion and seeding into the meninges by MORI et al. (1974) and MICKLE and MCLENNAN (1975).

Differential Diagnosis

The observation of the typical elements of two or three germ blades makes differential diagnosis unnecessary.

Treatment

The operability of the teratomas is generally excellent, because of the formation of a capsule; sometimes, however, fixation by adjacent vessels make removal more difficult. TÖNNIS was probably the first to achieve successfully total removal of four teratomas of the pineal region, of whom three survived (WEBER 1939; see also KRABBE 1944).

Rupture of squamous epithelium-lined cysts containing fatty acids can produce an intense inflammatory reaction in the CSF system and subarachnoid space, as in the case of epidermoids (GAUPP 1942).

For reports on special cases see: lateral ventricle: GÜTHERT (1938); fourth ventricle: MORELLI (1973); posterior fossa: STRANG et al. (1960); teratoma with absence of falx and corpus callosum: FERRY et al. (1972).

21 Other Malformative Tumors and Tumor-Like Lesions

21.1 Craniopharyngiomas

Synonyms in the older literature: Tumors or cysts of the hypophyseal duct, cysts or tumors of Rathke's pouch, tumors of Rathke's cleft, cranopharyngeal pouch tumors, suprasellar cysts, pituitary stalk tumors, Erdheim's tumors, adamantinomas or ameloblastomas of the pituitary region

Introduction

This well-known tumor was described very early and is listed in the WHO classification system as *craniopharyngioma.*

Historical Note and Definition

Some of the older descriptions of "Markschwämme" or medullary carcinomas of the pituitary gland were most probably true craniopharyngiomas. However, we are indebted to ERDHEIM (1904) for the first correct interpretation and adequate description of these tumors. STRADA (1911) and CRITCHLEY and IRONSIDE (1926) listed the early cases. Among subsequent contributions the following especially are worth mentioning: MCLEAN (1930), FRAZIER and ALPERS (1931), WITTERMANN (1936), LOVE et al. (1939), MÜLLER and WOHLFAHRT (1950), MATSON (1964), SVIEN (1965), BANNA (1976).

Epidemiology (Age – Sex – Frequency – Site)

Age: The craniopharyngiomas can definitely be generally considered as tumors of childhood and adolescence, but they do also occur in adults (Fig. 9k). CUSHING (1932, 1935) himself saw two patients over 60 years of age; CAMPBELL and HUDSON (1960) had three patients over 60 years; KITANO et al. (1981), one of 3 years; and TABADDOR et al. (1974) reported one case of a neonatal craniopharyngioma. The peak incidence is between the ages of 10 and 25 (Fig. 9k). The oldest of our patients was 62, the youngest 5 years old. In childhood and adolescence craniopharyngiomas of the chiasmal region are one of the most common tumors. In FRAZIER and ALPERS' series (1931) 70% of the patients were younger than 20 years; however, in our early series (1956) only 43.18% fell in this age group.

Sex: There is a certain male proponderance with a ratio of around 3:2 (116 male and 69 female patients in our series of 9000 cases). In MÜLLER and WOHLFART's series (1950) it was only 5:4.

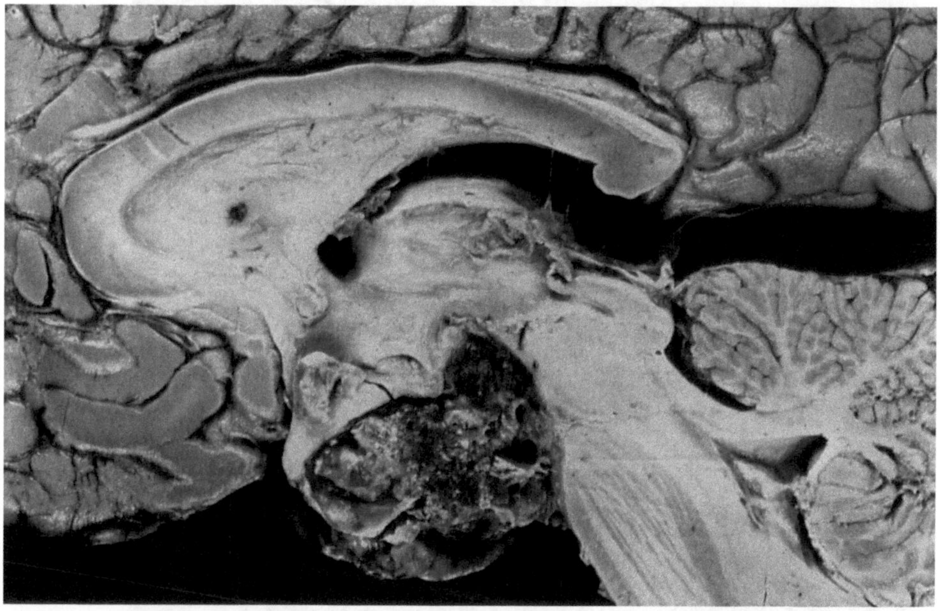

Fig. 147. Typical, partially cystic large craniopharyngioma, which has extended to the anterior border of the pons and the posterior portions of the 3rd ventricle

Frequency: The craniopharyngiomas accounted for 1.2% of all tumors in our series of 9000 cases and for 4.6% in the series of CUSHING (1932, 1935). In the tumors collected by FRAZIER and ALPERS (1931, 1934), of 244 lesions around the sella only 14 were craniopharyngiomas (11 of these were histologically verified). In the publications of McLEAN (1930, 1936a) they made up 30% of the "hypophyseal tumors." In the series of BENNET (1946) and of FRAZIER and ALPERS (1931) they accounted for 5.7% of the sellar and parasellar tumors. However, like the pineal tumors, their frequency is several times as high (SANO 1983a, 5.6%) in the Far East.

Site: Since craniopharyngiomas occur exclusively in the region of the sella, they are thought to originate from vestigial remnants of the craniopharyngeal duct (Rathke's pouch). The only ways they vary in site are in their relation to the diaphragma sellae (Figs. 147, 148) and in the direction of extension from this point. Thus, both *intra*sellar and *supra*sellar craniopharyngiomas (Fig. 148; GP, Figs. 258, 259) occur, and also combined growth in both spaces.

Of these, the intrasellar types are initially separated from the brain by the dura and arachnoid. As they grow, however, they push the diaphragma upward – generally breaking through it – growing in the direction of the third ventricle, where they excavate a bed for themselves from below (GP, Fig. 258). The suprasellar (Fig. 149) type starts in the arachnoid of the basal cisterns and pushes directly against the third ventricle; the ventricular floor then becomes paper-thin and tears, so that the tumor capsule abuts directly onto the ventricular wall.

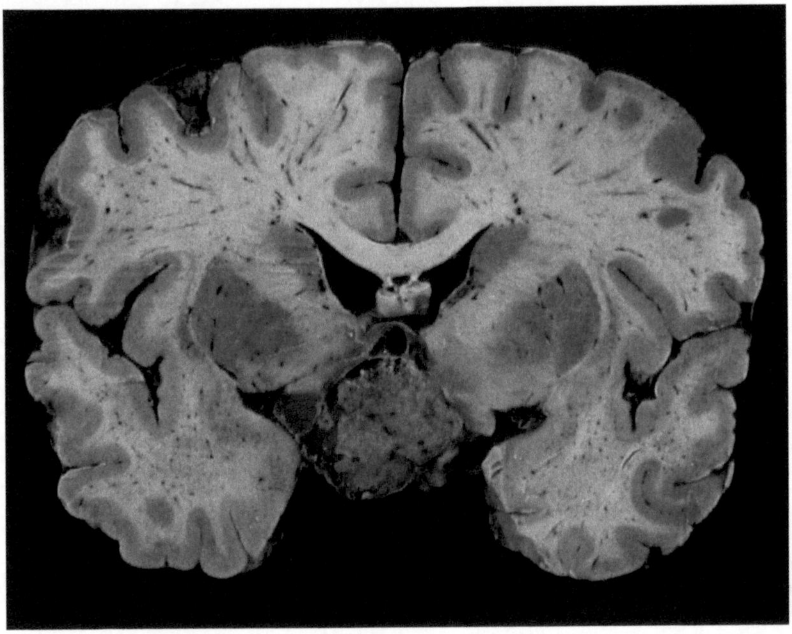

Fig. 148. Predominantly suprachiasmatic craniopharyngioma with only moderate degree of cyst formation. (ZÜLCH 1975a)

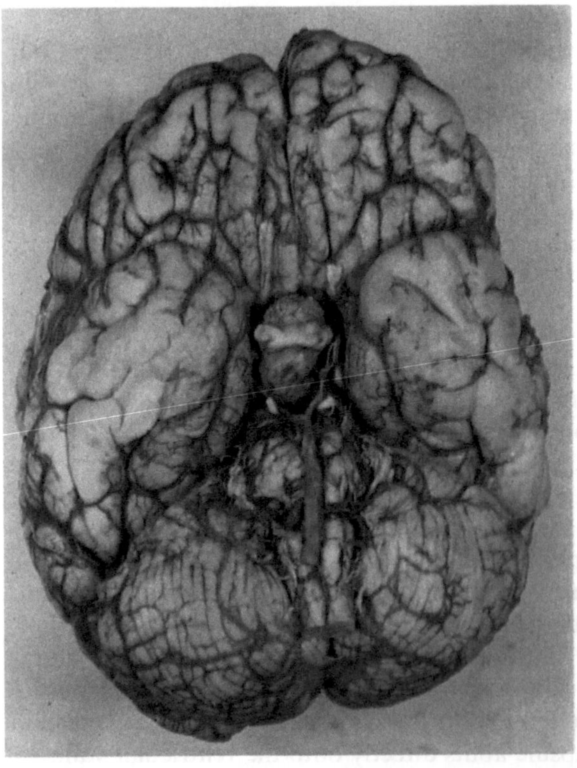

Fig. 149. Craniopharyngioma with origin in the parasellar and suprasellar regions. (ZÜLCH 1975a)

The relation of the tumor to the chiasm varies. Some tumors displace it forward and upward, stretching it into a thin band. Others develop above the chiasm from the first (Fig. 149), and force it downward. Still others lie primarily "in the lumen" of the third ventricle and can scarcely be seen on the base of the brain (GP, Figs. 265, 266; KUBOTA et al. 1980). They always stretch the surrounding arteries. All this is very important for interpretation of the angiogram and CT and subsequent surgical removal of these tumors.

They also occasionally grow toward the back of the head, i.e., in the direction of the thalamus and pons, and displace the third ventricle backward. They can expand to either side and occupy the region of the frontal or temporal lobes (GP, Figs. 261, 262, 263; KITANO et al. 1981); we have seen tumors the size of a men's fist at both these sites. In such cases the pituitary gland will be displaced downward, flattened out, and damaged by the intrasellar craniopharyngiomas, the floor of the sella being markedly eroded. However, the suprasellar craniopharyngiomas often leave the hypophysis and the bony sella undamaged (see schematic drawing of BUESS 1938), but extension through the base of the skull to involve the orbits, etc., is unusual (MAJLESSI et al. 1978). These various ways of growth can be explained embryologically by the varying primary site of the corresponding "rest" of the hypophysial duct. Occasionally, primary craniopharyngeal cysts are encountered that do not form a solid tumor (see p. 432, Rathke's cleft cysts).

Gross Pathology

Craniopharyngiomas are solid or cystic, well-encapsulated tumors, which grow purely by expansion. The size of most varies from a pea to a walnut; at times they reach the size of a tennis ball. They have a smooth encapsulated or finely nodular surface, and a grayish pink color (Fig. 148). The cut surface is spongy and porous and is permeated with various-sized cavities, depending on the degree of cystic degeneration (GP, Fig. 264). The bulk of the tumor is often made up of a single cyst (GP, Fig. 267). The cyst cavity is filled with a thick brownish yellow fluid (like motor oil with small glistening cholesterol crystals suspended in it; this is type specific for this tumor). The tumor has a tough consistency and is rather hard in parts because calcification occurs.

In the course of tumor growth a zone of reactive gliosis (HBT, Fig. 95c, d) may arise in the floor of the third ventricle, and Rosenthal fibers may then even be formed: this zone sometimes reaches the thickness of 0.5 cm and resembles a pilocytic astrocytoma, both macro- and microscopically. We interpret this as a cicatricial reaction to the fatty acids produced by the regressive processes and, particularly, to cholesterin, which is also capable of producing a marked inflammatory reaction (MAHONEY 1936).

Histologic Appearance

Where they have not degenerated the craniopharyngiomas consist – like the basal cell tumors – of broad communicating cords of stratified squamous epithelium in a system of epithelial bands and bridges, held together and nourished by the vascularized connective tissue stroma (HBT, Figs. 94, 95). The epithelial

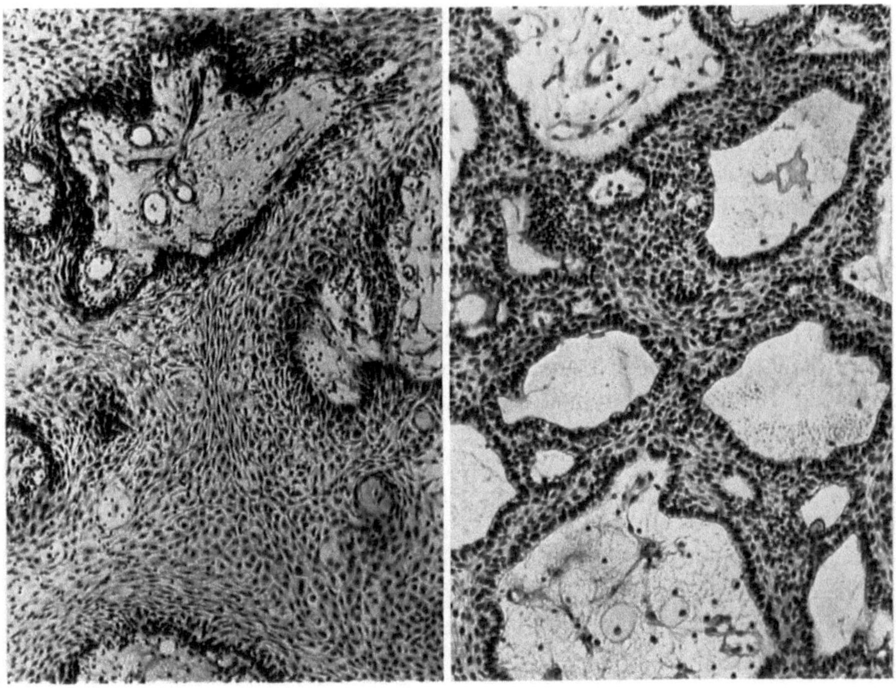

Fig. 150. a In epithelial bands the central transformation into "prickle cells" can be clearly discerned. The stroma is considerably increased and is undergoing mucoid degeneration. Individual capillaries are still clearly apparent. The stroma contains round cells and macrophages., Cresyl violet, ×84. **b** Within the epithelial bands large cysts occur. The marginal epithelium has become transformed into a columnar shape. H&E, ×125

zones are about 8–20 layers thick; and on their outside they are usually covered by high columnar epithelium (Fig. 150), while toward the inside they are less organized and form a progressively more spongy syncytium. This histological picture has been compared to the three strata of the Malpighian layer of the skin: the stratum cylindricum, stratum intermedium, and stratum spinosum. The presence of the latter stratum in the tumor, however, depends on the degree to which regressive changes have taken place. The architecture of the epithelial zones can be either more "adenomatous" or more "papillary" depending on regressive processes and the variation in the amount of stroma (Figs. 150). Regressive changes are numerous and consist in liquefaction of the cells, ranging in degree from the first stage, the spiny cell, all the way up to complete disintegration of the tissue. In addition, there is a type of degeneration in which the cells swell to the point where they lose all stainability *without showing* any tendency toward cornification and its particular staining properties or the early stages of *keratohyalin* formation (see Sect. 21.3). True cornified epithelial "keratin" pearls are not seen. Only a "*keratoid*" substance is deposited. Sometimes irritation phenomena are visible in the cells in the presence of pleomorphism of the epithelium; this must not be mistaken for cancerization.

The craniopharyngiomas grow very slowly and mitoses do not occur.

Electron Microscopy

The reader is referred to the sections dealing with other epithelial tumors and to the details published by HOSSMANN and WECHSLER (1971a), GENTH et al. (1974), and TOGA (1976).

Tissue Culture

In tissue culture the cell migration varies in speed (see also YOUNG et al. 1976).

Histochemistry

More recent observations refer to true keratin, but this is not compatible with the light-microscope observations. The deposition of calcium salts in these keratoid regions is a recognized characteristic of the craniopharyngiomas, allowing them to be visualized on x-ray. Moreover, ossification is sometimes encountered. The stroma also undergoes regressive changes; it swells, becomes edematous and relatively acellular, and finally undergoes cystic degeneration, so that cyst formation can be observed in both the ectodermal and the mesodermal portions.

Differential Diagnosis

It is necessary to differentiate (see the misinterpretation of von LEHOCZKY 1929) between epidermoids and those craniopharyngiomas that have been completely transformed into cysts, or "craniopharyngeal cysts" (p. 427). In the latter large cavities are formed, covered with a thin capsule of neoplastic tissue with small mural tumor nodules. Not only is the cyst content of craniopharyngiomas and epidermoids different – epidermoids contain concentric layers of swollen shed-off epithelial pearls (cholesteatomatous material) because of the regular deposition of layers of "epidermis," and particularly the true cornification of epidermoids (with keratohyalin granules; see p. 435). Craniopharyngiomas, on the other side, contain a brownish, oily fluid. This difference allows a distinction. Both secondarily cystic craniopharyngiomas and primary craniopharyngeal cysts (p. 432) have to be distinguished from ependymal cysts (p. 528) in the region of the foramen of Monro (p. 437). Only in the earlier literature was there any confusion between the choroid plexus papillomas or the hypophyseal adenomas of fetal type (p. 469) and the craniopharyngiomas.

Biologic Behavior (Grading), Metastasis, and Recurrence

Craniopharyngiomas are classed as grade I. Up to now, malignant degeneration of the craniopharyngioma has not been described. Metastasis is unknown.

The likelihood of postoperative recurrence depends on the kind and extent or surgery (cyst aspiration, incomplete/radical removal; see Table "Operative mortality", p. 171 in BINGAS and WOLTER 1968; KAHN et al. 1973) and whether radiation in the form of deep x-ray therapy is administered (SHAPIRO et al. 1979). In the case of recurrence following incomplete removal tumor growth is likely to be very slow. In the series of SHAPIRO et al. (1979), cyst aspiration with subsequent deep x-ray therapy was followed by recurrence in 50% of cases within a mean of 4.4 years, and in 23% of cases recurrence was observed even after so-called radical excision, within a mean of 2.2 years.

Radical excision, however, is recommended in all cases where it is possible; it is naturally more problematic in the aged and in the case of suprasellar masses.

Whether entirely cystic tumors have a better prognosis and are more amenable to radical excision or not has not yet been decided (see in contrast KATZ 1975, who saw more frequent recurrences). In summary, the prognosis is highly variable, depending on the method and extent of surgery, particularly since growth is sometimes so slow that an operation may not be indicated (BARTLETT 1971: 25 years without any operation).

Operative mortality is higher in the suprasellar type. Craniopharyngiomas are fairly radioresistant and do not have a pronounced response to chemotherapy. Aspiration of the cyst fluid or the production of a permanent opening in the cyst wall is adequate to improve the picture for a time. The final aim must always be total removal of the tumor or at least the restoration of the CSF circulation and shunting. However, the mortality is definitely lower than before; it was zero in a series of 40 patients reported by MATSON and CRIGLER (1969). An "aseptic" meningitic complication can occur if the cyst fluid drains into the CSF system.

Clinical Course

The slow growth of the craniopharyngiomas accounts for the long clinical course, which may be characterized by a hormonal and chiasmal syndrome. The diagnosis of these tumors can frequently may be made on plane x-ray because of the sellar lesion and the calcification of the tumor. It is important to remember that CSF serology is occasionally positive in craniopharyngiomas. Unfortunately, clinicians' indifference about endocrine disturbances – hypopituitarism – and visual defects may still be prevalent; this has sometimes meant that patients were not referred to hospital until they had increased intracranial pressure; at this stage the tumor is already enormous. Ophthalmic signs are extremely rare (FREEMAN et al. 1980).

Further References: BECKMANN and KUBIE (1929), PINTO and PINTO (1957), FOTAKIS (1961a), KRAYENBÜHL and PRADER (1962), ROUGERIE and FARDEAU (1962), ORTHNER and RETTINGER (1965), VAN DEN BERGH and BRUCHER (1970), CASHION and YOUNG (1971), GHATAK et al. (1971), ARSENI and MARETSIS (1972), BACKLUND (1972), COOPER and RANSOHOFF (1972), KUNICKI et al. (1972), BOLLATI et al. (1973), CHOUX et al. (1973), PATRICK et al. (1974), PERTUISET (1975), SATO et al. (1975).

21.2 Rathke's Cleft Cysts

Synonyms: Pituitary cysts, epithelial cysts of pituitary

Introduction

In the WHO classification these tumors are listed as a separate entity.

Historical Note and Definition

Rathke's cleft cysts are intrasellar cysts lined with remnants of Rathke's pouch, i.e., cuboidal (nonciliated, squamous?) or columnar epithelium, sometimes containing mucous Goblet cells (FAIRBURN and LARKIN 1964).

ERDHEIM (1904, p. 563) emphasized the occurrence of cystic remnants of the former hypophyseal anlage, i.e., the "Rathke's pouch," and preferred the name "Rathke's cysts."

The epithelium is identical with the lining of the small cysts frequently found between the pars anterior and the infundibular process of the pituitary gland (ZÜLCH 1956, Fig. 374c).

These cysts are occasionally very large; they may be surgically significant, in which case they have to be emptied. FRAZIER and ALPERS (1934) emphasized the distinction from common cysts in the pituitary adenomas or craniopharyngiomas or even the rare mucoceles from the sphenoidal sinus. This distinction is possible on the basis of the type of epithelium, which is partly cylindrical and ciliated, partly cuboid, and partly squamous (SMITH and BUCY 1953).

RUSSELL and RUBINSTEIN (1977) reported an intrasellar dumbbell cyst with a cuboidal and ciliated intrasellar and a squamous suprasellar part (see also DUFFY 1920; SMITH and BUCY 1953; EL-BANHAWY and AHMED 1962; FAGER and CARTER 1966). RINGEL and O.T. BAILEY (1972) have discussed the pathogenesis in detail. They collected 32 cases, 18 of which were surgically removed.

The differential diagnosis of intrasellar cysts is necessary because cystic sacs may occur which are remnants of an intrasellar hemorrhage and/or infarction of the pituitary gland (WEBER et al. 1970). HOLBACH and GULLOTTA (1977) compared these mono- or multiple-layer cysts with mucus-secreting cells to the foramen of Monro cysts.

Electron microscopy and *tissue culture* of these cysts have been described by YOSHIDA et al. (1977).

Further References: SHANKLIN (1949), ROWBOTHAM and CLARKE (1956), BERRY and SCHLEZINGER (1959).

21.3 Epidermoid and Dermoid Cysts

Synonyms in the older literature: Pearly tumors, tumeurs perlées, cholesteatomas with and without hair, sebaceous cysts

Introduction

The epidermoid and dermoid cysts feature as specific entities within the malformative tumors and tumor-like lesions in the WHO classification.

Historical Note and Definition

In the early literature descriptions of epidermoid and dermoid cysts are found because of the unusual and fatty content.

CRUVEILHIER, as early as 1829/35, reported on "pearly tumors," and Johannes MÜLLER in 1838 gave a very detailed account of "perlmutterglänzende Fettgeschwülste" ("fatty tumors shining like mother of pearl"). VIRCHOW in 1855 described pearly tumors in some detail. For the fundamental work dealing with embryological explanations of their origin we are indebted to von REMAK (1854) and to the elder BOSTROEM (1897). BAILEY (1920/1924), LOVE and KERNOHAN (1936), MAHONEY (1936), WETTLER (1948), LEPOIRE and PERTUISET (1957, 1958) followed with detailed reports.

The epidermoid and dermoid cysts are now sharply separated both from other squamous epithelium-containing tumors, e.g., the craniopharyngiomas, and from the "inflammatory cholesteatomas" of the middle ear. We therefore avoid the name cholesteatoma for this intracranial space-occupying malformative condition.

Epidermoid cysts in the sense of this chapter are space-occupying lesions containing cholesteatomatous material. They have an external, very tender capsule lined with keratin-producing squamous epithelium. Dermoid cysts also contain skin appendages.

Epidemiology (Age – Sex – Frequency – Site)

Age: The age curve of the epidermoid and dermoid cysts (at the time of operation) shows a definite peak around the age of 40 (MAHONEY 1936). In our own material it lies between 25 and 40 years (time of operation or autopsy), while in the curve representing the age of onset of the condition the peak comes far earlier, around the age of 15. They are therefore very slow-growing space-occupying lesions.

Sex: The sexes were equally represented in our series (83 male versus 83 female patients). A rather different distribution with 19 male and 12 female patients was encountered in the series of GUIDETTI and GAGLIARDI (1977). VERBIEST (1939), however, reported 6 male patients among 8 spinal cases.

Frequency: In the total count of epidermoid and dermoid cyst and teratomas we encountered 166 out of 9000 cases, i.e., 1.8%. In CUSHING's material (1932, 1935) the epidermoids *and* dermoids comprised 0.7%. FINDEISEN and TÖNNIS (1937) found 48 cases of *epidermoids* among 5185 intracranial tumors, i.e., 0.9%. Dermoids are certainly less frequent than epidermoids.

Site: Since the epidermoid and dermoid cysts develop in all probability from embryonic malformative rests, their predilection for certain sites is understandable. They occur most frequently in the lateral or midline positions. Epidermoid cysts are found in the arachnoidal spaces or in the diploe (BUCY 1935) and by preference at the following sites (MAHONEY 1936; RENGACHARY et al. 1978): cerebellopontine angle or parapontine; chiasmal region or parapituitary; longitudinal fissure and anterior corpus callosum; around the quadrigeminal plate and posterior corpus callosum; Sylvian fissure; third ventricle; fourth ventricle and midline cerebellum; diploe of the skull; spinal cord.

The most frequent localizations are the cerebellopontine angle (GP, Fig. 272), the supra- and parasellar regions, in the lateral and fourth ventricles, and the quadrigeminal region (GP, Fig. 271). Multiple epidermoid cysts apparently do not occur.

Gross Pathology

The *epidermoids* are readily recognized by their whitish shining mother-of-pearl capsule (GP, Fig. 270); they can be smooth, lobulated, or nodular with daughter nodules. The blood vessels run in the capsule. Section reveals shining masses of friable leafy material arranged in layers like onion skin. The inside is occasionally softened.

Sometimes they are firmly attached to the surrounding tissue, in some cases even the falx, because of the focal sterile meningitis and encephalitis (KRIEG 1936a; MAHONEY 1936; MAHONEY did some experimental work on this issue). It is important to recognize that epidermoid cysts can "melt" the adjacent parenchyma via irritation setting up an inflammatory process, so that an epidermoid cyst of the fourth ventricle, for example, may have a broad connection with the cerebellopontine angle through the lateral recess (BIRKMAYER and HASENJÄGER 1940). When located in the ventricles or the subarachnoid space these tumors are particularly likely to rupture and to extrude their contents into the CSF, causing meningeal reactions. Sometimes a subependymal proliferation of spongioblastic cells with Rosenthal fibers is encountered below the epidermoid cysts. MAHONEY (1936) interpreted this as an irritation phenomenon, while VUIA (1973) in contrast saw it as a sign of dysraphic origin. Our own experience supports Mahoney's interpretation.

The size of epidermoid cysts varies from that of a pinhead to that of an orange (see the unusually large epidermoid cyst in Fig. 6 of PINTO et al. 1957; see also BUCY 1935; LOVE and KERNOHAN 1936; GP, Figs. 270–273).

The *dermoid* cysts, on the other hand, are particularly apt to lie around the pituitary gland, the pons, or along embryonic closure lines. They are more common along the line of closure between the maxillae and the orbits (the embryonic naso-optic furrow) and may actually grow into one orbit (STENDER 1937). They are also encountered along the posterior fossa in the midline and in the sacral region.

Dermoid cysts have a firm pod or shell, and are generally filled with a greasy, soapy mass containing numerous short hairs (and even teeth) (GP, Fig. 274). The contents are formed by the continual proliferation of the new cells of the germinal layer, degeneration of these cells (deposition of keratohyalin granules), and finally cornification, as well as secretion of fatty material.

Histologic Appearance

Epidermoid cysts are characterized by a very monotonous histological picture, since they form cysts lined with keratin-producing squamous epithelium. In their small external capsule we see the three normal layers of the epidermis: the stratum germinativum, granulosum, and corneum, with a total of between two and five, or occasionally as many as ten, cell layers. Some epidermoid cysts are conspicuous by a papillary architecture of this capsular layer. Their content is brittle. Calcification of the epidermoid is very rare (Trabant and Mohr 1979; see HBT, Fig. 97a, b). *Dermoids,* on the other hand, differ from epidermoid cysts in that they contain the accessory structures of skin: the dermis with hair follicles, hairs, sebaceous glands, and (sometimes) sweat glands.

The inflammatory effect of the capsule contents upon the surrounding parenchymatous tissue is highly significant. This is particularly true of the epidermoid cysts, less so of the dermoids (HBT 97c, d). If epidermoid or dermoid cysts rupture and the contents enter the CSF spaces, or if contamination occurs at operation, a very intense aseptic inflammatory reaction of the meninges can arise (Krieg 1936a; Mahoney 1936; Verbiest 1939; recurrent: Leal and Miles 1978). Arachnoiditis and ependymitis, and even subsequent aqueduct stenosis may follow. The clinical symptoms are described below.

Differential Diagnosis

It is necessary to distinguish these tumor-like conditions from other squamous epithelium-containing tumors that produce cholesterin-bearing masses, such as the craniopharyngioma. This can be difficult if the neoplastic capsule itself is very thin. Attention should be paid to the epidermoid cysts' three-layered structure, and particularly to their true cornification with formation of keratohyalin granules, which does not take place in the craniopharyngioma or craniopharyngeal cysts.

Biologic Behavior (Grading), Malignancy, Metastasis, and Recurrence

The biologic behavior is characterized by slow growth; it corresponds therefore to grade I in the WHO classification, and if the cysts are totally removed a cure can be expected. Metastasis is not known. Recurrence always takes place if the capsule of such a cyst has not been completely removed. In some cases carcinomatous degeneration has been discovered in epidermoid cysts (Hug 1942; Davidson and Small 1960; Fox and South 1965: after 6 years; Landers and Danielski 1960; Gluszcz 1962; Nosaka et al. 1979; Garcia et al. 1981).

Origin: It is generally believed that these lesions originate from malformations during embryogenesis. There are, however, cases that are traumatically induced during therapeutic maneuvers (Gutin et al. 1980). This was observed particularly after World War II, when tuberculosis was still common in Europe. Lumbar punctures led to the introduction of microscopic pieces of epidermis into the spinal canal, with ensuing epidermoid cysts.

Clinical Course

We have emphasized the possibility of an aseptic meningitis with remissions in cases where the epidermoid capsule has torn and cholestomatous masses introduced into the spinal CSF chambers (Amendola et al. 1978). In contrast, rupture of an aneurysm into an epidermoid cyst is exceptional (Sakaki et al.

1981). Dermoid cysts can be unusually translucent, like lipomas (HANDA et al. 1979). Since the area surrounding these cysts often has a firm consistency due to the chronic sterile encephalitis and meningitis and since they are sometimes in unfavorable sites, operation still involves a considerable degree of risk (22.7% mortality in 21 cases, GRANT and AUSTIN 1950; see also GUIDETTI et al. 1959; GUIDETTI and GAGLIARDI 1977). BRÜCK (1952) has described some details of the clinical course: 16 epidermoids in 1017 operations.

Further References: BLECHER (1905), LEHOCZKY (1929), LEARMONTH and KERNOHAN (1930a), OLIVECRONA (1932, 1949), BAUDITZ (1933), DAVID et al. (1936b), KRIEG (1936b), VERBIEST (1939), HUG (1942), KRAYENBÜHL and SCHMID (1943), MARTIN and DAVIS (1943), RAND and REEVES (1943), SCHEINKER (1948), TYTUS and PENNYBACKER (1956), BAUCHHENSS and SCHÜRMANN (1962), MATHON and FILSAK (1962), KUNICKI and KALUZA (1963), FOX and SOUTH (1965), DECKER and GROSS (1967), V. GILDER and SCHWARTZ (1967), REEVES (1967), BISCHOF and NITTNER (1969), I.C. BAILEY (1970), KIRSCH and STEARS (1970), NEBLETT et al. (1970), TAN (1972), MILLER and EPSTEIN (1975), MATSUDA et al. (1976), MCDONNEL (1977), HAMEL et al. (1980).

21.4 Colloid Cysts

Synonyms: Paraphyseal, neuroepithelial, ependymal cysts

Introduction

In the WHO classification the cysts between the foramina of Monro are listed as an entity and distinguished from other forms (see p. 441).

Historical Note and Definition

The colloid cyst were first described by WALLMAN (1858) and named correctly by SJÖVALL (1910). By the investigations of MCLEAN (1936b) the position of these cysts towards plexus and tela chorioidea has been clarified. This can be confirmed by our own findings (ZÜLCH 1956, Fig. 240) which show the microcyst below the fornices. At the lower side the ependymal layer is doubled and consists (a) of the ependymal layer of the cyst, and (b) of the roof of the third ventricle.

Epidemiology (Age – Sex – Frequency)

Age: The majority of patients (YENERMEN et al. 1958) with such cysts are in the third and fourth decades (54 personal cases) or the third to fifth decades (200 cases in the literature). Of the 300 cases in the world literature only 6 patients were under 10, and 2 under 2 years of age (BUCHSBAUM and COLTON 1967). The youngest patients in our personal series were 2 and 3 years old, the oldest 72.

Sex: The sexes are about equally represented in the world literature.

Frequency: It is still impossible to define the frequency (BUCHSBAUM and COLTON 1967: 300 cases from the world literature).

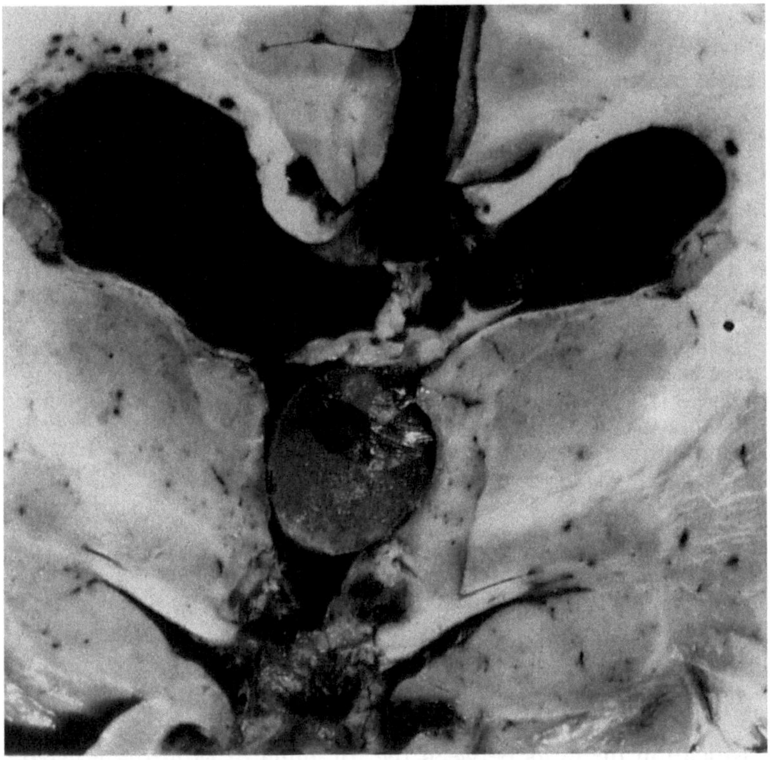

Fig. 151. Cherry-sized colloid cyst (ependymal cyst) of the foramina of Monro in situ. The lesion had been approached surgically by a transcallosal route. (ZÜLCH 1975a)

Gross Pathology

Macroscopically, in autopsy cases these colloid cysts of the foramen of Monro can be the size of a pea when encountered as incidental findings (GP, Fig. 74), or of a cherry (Fig. 151) when they are revealed by neurosurgery because they have occluded the foramina of Monro, producing obstructive hydrocephalus.

It is of historical interest that Harvey Cushing himself had a small colloid cyst (1 cm in diameter) in his third ventricle, so far as is known without clinical symptoms (FULTON 1946, p. 713).

The larger, i.e., cherry-sized, cysts are usually situated in the anterior third of the third ventricle between the two foramina of Monro, more rarely unilaterally.

HAYMAKER and YENERMEN (1955), on the basis of an extensive study of 60 cases, determined the diameters of the cysts as 1.0–3.5 cm. In the whole of their series only 7 were smaller and asymptomatic, and only 2 were positioned to one side causing unilateral hydrocephalus.

Histologic Appearance

A microscopical specimen has a few layers of connective tissue located on the outside, which are sometimes infiltrated by lymphocytes and plasma cells and sometimes even by macrophages containing hemosiderin. The innermost layer, however, either contains flatter cells reminiscent of ependyma or has a higher cylindrical epithelium with blepharoplasts. The center contains an amorphous material made up mainly of mucus.

Electron Microscopy

The first report of COXE and LUSE (1964) described the epithelium as separated from the connective tissue by a basement membrane. These authors also described cells with cilia and blepharoplasts containing mucus-positive material which gave a positive PAS reaction (see also HIRANO and GHATAK 1974).

Tissue Culture

SHUANGSHOTI and NETSKY (1966b) described three types of cells, a lighter cell which was ciliated, a second, denser one, which was not ciliated but was coated with electron-dense material; and a third type, which had already been described in the literature as having a secretory-cell-like structure.

Cells with microvilli were most frequent (LANDOLT-WEBER 1973), followed by the mucin-producing cells with club-shaped processes, and then by a cell type containing PAS-positive substances (granules), which had apparently accumulated these substances until the cells were expelled into the cyst.

Origin

In the literature several possibilities were discussed by HIRANO and GHATAK (1974), who conceived a neuroepithelial origin or an origin from the choroid plexus epithelium, or finally from the paraphysis (MACLEAN 1936b). Other authors compared the epithelium to the enterogenous cysts of the spinal canal.

Since such ependymal cysts were seen in combination with mucin producing ependymomas by SHUANGSHOTI et al. (1979) in the lateral and third ventricle, these authors also came to the opinion that they originated from the choroid plexus. A final possibility was discussed by LANDOLT-WEBER (1973), who noted that even the possibility of a diverticulum of the diencephalon had to be considered.

Clinical Course

The clinical diagnosis has been described in an excellent study by HAYMAKER and YENERMEN (1955) and YENERMEN et al. (1958), and also by KELLY (1951: 29 cases). Paroxysmal headache has occurred as the most characteristic symptom.

Biological Behavior (Grading), Metastasis, and Recurrence

The treatment of choice is certainly surgery, in spite of the poor prognosis (YENERMEN et al. 1958: of 27 patients undergoing surgery only 7 subsequently had a reasonable quality of life). Lately freehand puncture of the cyst has been favored (GUTIERREZ-LARA et al. 1975), or stereotaxic aspiration after a thorough CT study (BOSCH et al. 1978). However, in some cases sudden death resulting from blockage of the foramen of Monro with fatal obstructive hydrocephalus has been reported when the cystic sac has not been removed.

Further References: ZIMMERMAN and GERMAN (1933), HAMBÜCHEN (1952), LAUSBERG (1965), LITTLE and MACCARTY (1974).

21.5 Enterogenous Cysts

Synonyms: Neuroenteric, enterogenic, archenteric, foregut cyst

Introduction

The enterogenous cysts are listed as an entity in the WHO classification.

Historical Note and Definition

Apparently SCHLESINGER (1898), SCHMIDT (1904), KUBIE and FULTON (1928), and GUILLERY (1937) were among the first to describe these cysts, which are most commonly located near the spinal cord (NEUHAUSER et al. 1958; SCOVILLE et al. 1963; DORSEY and TABRISKY 1966; KAHN et al. 1971; MILLIS and HOLMES 1973; PIRAMOON and ABBASSIOUN 1974; ROSENBAUM et al. 1978), but occasionally also in the fourth ventricle (AFSHAR and SCHOLTZ 1981; PARKINSON and CHILDE 1952). These cysts consist of well-differentiated epitheliated cells with a basement membrane of fibrovascular tissue. They are generally also mucin producing. They are explained as anomalies on the basis of an embryological dysgenesis during the anlage stage (FABINYI and ADAMS 1979).

Epidemiology (Age – Sex – Frequency – Site)

This is a rare cause of spinal cord compression and the preferential age at manifestation is childhood or early adult life. The predilection sites are the thoracic and lower cervical regions.

Frequency: ELSBERG et al. (1934) reported 3 cases among 250 space-occupying spinal lesions.

Gross Pathology

These cysts are usually rostral to the spinal cord or more lateral, and are occasionally combined with malformations (MILLIS and HOLMES 1973) or even malformative neoplasias.

Further References: GIMENO et al. (1972), SYPERT et al. (1973), YAMASHITA et al. (1973), ODAKE et al. (1976), EVANS et al. (1979).

21.6 Other Cysts ("Ependymal Cysts")

There are other types of cysts of ependymal origin, which arise from separation of parts of the ventricular system. They form one or several small chambers, which may or may not stay in open communication with the CSF system. They are commonly found at the horns of the ventricles, have no growth tendency, and are therefore usually not of any surgical importance. However, they are covered with ventricular ependyma.

The cysts of the septum pellucidum are occasionally space occupying, and neurosurgical treatment is then emphasized (VASILIU et al. 1937; DE MORSIER 1962). They are not covered with ependyma, however, but arise apparently by a sort of softening of the glia within the septum pellucidum.

Ependymal sacs in the lateral recess have been described by ALEXANDER (1937). We have never seen one, despite witnessing autopsies of thousands of brains, though they can occur extremely rarely.

Ependymal Cysts with Growth Tendency

These are cystic cavitations described in many areas of the CNS and act as space-occupying lesions, e.g., the colloid cysts in the lateral ventricles. These may be part of the choroid plexus (BAKER and GOTTLIEB 1956; SHUANGSHOTI et al. 1975; SHIMA et al. 1976). They are also found in the fourth ventricle (SHARPE and DECK 1977).

Similar infratentorial cysts between inferior colliculum and vermis have been reported by CHALLA and MARKESBERY (1978), in the pons by MORTARA et al. (1974), and as large polycystic ependymal cavitations by FOERSTER and GAGEL (1933c).

Peculiar diencephalic cysts, probably also of a malformative character, have been described by FOERSTER (1939b), who called them "diverticulum paraphysarium". Furthermore, ependymal cysts have been described in the mesencephalic region by ourselves (ZÜLCH 1956, Fig. 239; GP, Fig. 75) (see also REMAGEN and MISSONI 1964). Finally, intradural but extramedullary ependymal cysts have been reported in the spinal cord, e.g., in the cervical region (MOORE and BOOK 1966). Such neuroepithelial cystic colloid containing sacs have also been found in close correlation with particular tumors, such as xanthogranulomas (SHUANGSHOTI et al. 1975).

Arachnoid cysts are discussed elsewhere (see Chap. 29).

21.7 Lipomas

Synonym: Fatty tumors

Introduction

The lipomas are categorized separately in the WHO classification as a type of malformative tumor.

Historical Note and Definition

Lipomas were first observed by neuroanatomists (MECKEL, J.F., 1781–1833: chiasma opticum) and pathologists (ROKITANSKY 1855/56; BOSTROEM 1897). BOSTROEM (1897) saw them particularly in aplasia of the corpus callosum. In his comprehensive report on epidermoids and lipomas he tried to derive the malformations from the particularities of the site. He classified the 28 cases of lipomas, collected in the literature, into two groups.

Eugen SCHERER (1935b) and KRAINER (1935) published excellent reports, the latter's distinguished particularly by his schematic drawings showing sites and extension of lipomas near the central nervous structures. Critical discussions of the cases in the world literature followed, by SPERLING and ALPERS (1936), EHNI and ADSON (1945), and VONDERAHE and NIEMER (1944: excellent photographs). Lipomas are malformative slow-growing tumors consisting of localized masses of adipose tissue, occurring usually in the meninges.

Epidemiology (Age – Sex – Frequency – Site)

Age: All age groups are affected, a certain preference for the second and fourth decades being apparent. A general feature seems to be that the space-occupying lipomas manifest themselves in earlier decades of life whereas the incidental findings at autopsy have no symptomatology.

Sex: Equal involvement of both sexes is manifest from the literature (DEMUS 1967, around 200 cases).

Frequency: Up to now no reliable data are available. Of our collection of 6000 cases lipomas together with the osteomas and chondromas accounted for 0.9%. They are thought to represent 1% of the spinal tumors (EHNI and LOVE 1945). GASTAUT et al. (1980), using CT, found 4 cases of corpus callosum lipomas in 13000 (0.03%) patients. THOMALSKE (personal communication to Gastaut) saw 1 lipoma in 11500 patients examined by CT.

However, these tumors do not seem to be actually so rare as suggested by the few cases reported in the literature (see above DEMUS 1967: 200 cases). For instance, 6 cases were reported within 3 years in one mental hospital.

Site: Lipomas occur predominantly in six areas:

1. Above the site of corpus callosum (Fig. 14, no. 44) in association with absence of all or part of the corpus callosum itself. They can have the circumscribed form of a bean or appear as a plaque a few millimeters thick.
2. At the infundibulum as a pea-sized lesion.
3. On the quadrigeminal plate, also as a pea-sized lesion, or between the mamillary bodies.
4. Attached to the choroid plexus of the lateral or third ventricles as a bean- or egg-sized tumor (GP, Fig. 276).
5. In the other cisterns – cerebellopontine angle – or over the convexity (rare).
6. Alongside the spinal cord where they are found (a) in the lower thoracic region extending over a few segments; (b) extending over the whole spinal

cord; or (c) in the region of the cauda equina. They usually lie dorsally over the posterior columns (see GIUFFRÈ 1966, 1976).

On average, lipomas probably affect the corpus callosum in around 50% of cases and the spinal cord in about 25%, as shown by DEMUS (1967) in a series of 200 cases.

Some spinal lipomas lie extradurally (BENDER et al. 1974), particularly in the sacral region (ALAVA et al. 1965); only rarely are they multiple. Often they show pimples on the skin, firmly and densely connected to the surface (BENDER et al. 1974). Most are intradurally located (WILSON et al. 1940; CARAM et al. 1957; GIUFFRÈ 1966). Some have been encountered in the medulla (BISCHOFF and W. MÜLLER 1966). A good description with tabulation of 35 cases has been published by BARRAQUER-FERRÈ et al. (1950), and one of 100 cases by BISCHOFF and W. MÜLLER (1966).

Specific descriptions have been given on cases affecting the corpus callosum (GAUPP and JANTZ 1942; LUTEN 1951; KETZ 1956; MANGANIELLO et al. 1966; WOLPERT et al. 1972; KRETSCHMER 1974a; GASTAUT et al. 1980). Other descriptions of lipomas at specific locations, such as mamillary bodies (FLAMENT and FLAMENT-DURAND 1964), quadrigeminal region (DAVISON 1944; HALMAGYI and EVANS 1978), cerebellopontine angle (FUKUI et al. 1977b), infundibulotuberal region and mamillary bodies (VONDERAHE and NIEMER 1944), cerebellum (SCHMID 1973), and lumbosacral region (LASSMAN and JAMES 1967), offer specialized knowledge about these particular cases. Multiple lipomas (lipomatosis) have been reported by BAKER and ADAMS (1938), and a wide extension by Eugen SCHERER (1936).

Gross Pathology

Lipomas are sharply circumscribed, but tightly fastened to the adjacent nervous structures along the blood vessels by penetrating strands of connective tissue. Some of them may be rich in vessels ("angiolipomas") and there may be an osseous nucleus with lipomatous tissue around the vessels (SCHEIDEGGER 1939).

Calcification in the overlying meninges is common (Fig. 152a) and sometimes, curiously, even only on half a side of the tumor. It may be mild (CRADDOCK and RIDDERWOLD 1972).

Histologic Appearance

The lipomas consist of typical fatty tissue, are sometimes angiomatous with abundant vessels, and they resemble lipomas in other localizations in the body.

They have to be distinguished from xanthomas, in which lipids are contained in very small droplets and have a different chemical composition.

Differential Diagnosis

Computed tomography reveals precisely the lipomatous nature of a space-occupying hypodense lesion by the number of Hounsfield units. Preoperative diagnosis is also possible on the basis of x-ray characteristics. In the corpus callosum they are easily recognized by their outward displacement of the lateral ventricles

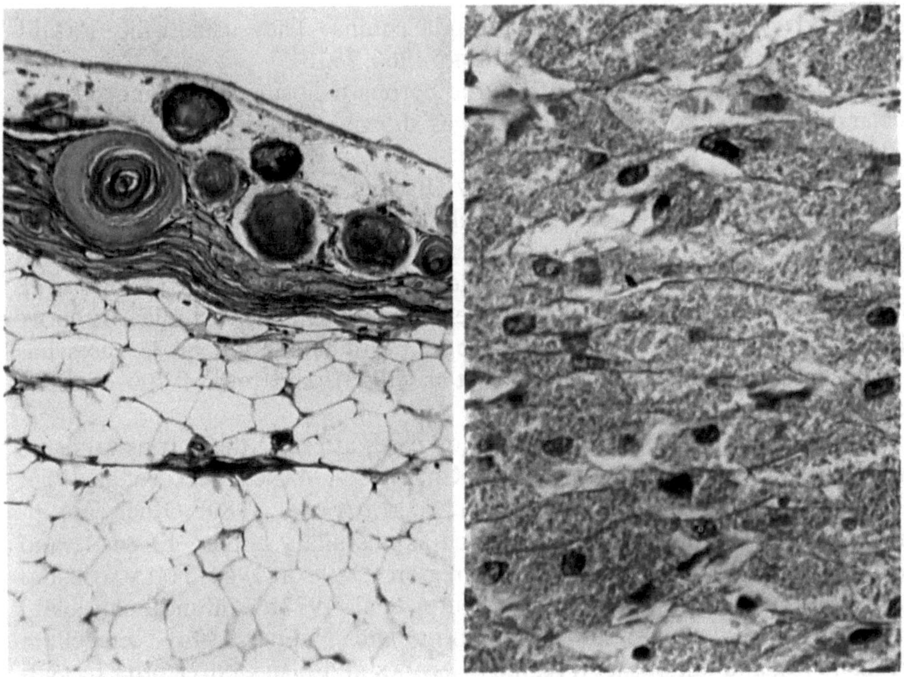

a b

Fig. 152. a Lipoma of the spinal cord. The overlying leptomeninges contain psammoma bodies. H&E ×104. **b** Granular cell myoblastoma (also known as choristoma or pituicytoma) consists of a mass of cells with eosinophilic granular cytoplasm. H&E, ×500

(BIANCHEDI and PELIZZA 1962) or by the usually mild calcification (see LINDGREN 1954, Fig. 46). According to GASTAUT et al. (1980) calcification was present in 68% of the cases in the literature.

Spinal lipomas must be distinguished from "lipomyelomeningoceles," in which the lipomatous part is a firm subcutaneous or intradural mass of lipomatous tissue from where strands lead directly to the conus medullaris along a fibrolipomatous band (WALSH and MARKESBERY 1980).

Biologic Behavior (Grading), Metastasis, and Recurrence

The lipomas are slow-growing, benign tumors. Excision is sometimes difficult because of the penetration of the adjacent nervous tissue by strands of connective tissue along the blood vessels. Metastases are unknown, but recurrences are not uncommon. Their grade in the WHO classification is I; but see p. 445: liposarcomas.

Clinical Course

Sometimes the CSF pathways are blocked by a lipoma and then surgery is necessary (KAZNER et al. 1980). In the clinical course epileptic fits (9 out of 11 patients; 86%: GASTAUT et al. 1980; ZETTNER and NETSKY 1960) can be the first sign of clinical manifestation.

Origin: Lipomas apparently originate from a closure defect caused by malformation during embryogenesis, thus resembling the epidermoid and dermoid cysts. However, KRAINER (1935) emphasized the maximum development in the cisterns, and the spinal cases occur at all levels (BISCHOFF and MÜLLER 1966, Fig. 3). BUDKA (1974) stressed the appearance together with medulloblastomas, colloid cysts, and epidermoid cysts, as well as with angiomatous malformations.

Further References: KASPER and COWAN (1929), TAKAHASHI et al. (1980), MATTERN et al. (1980), NABAWI et al. (1981).

Liposarcomas

Liposarcomas are rare tumors within the cranial cavity, usually extradurally localized (NAKAJIMA et al. 1976; SIMA et al. 1976). I cannot share the opinion of NOETZEL and HAUPTMANN (1964) that liposarcomas are identical with monstrocellular sarcomas.

Further References: FENDER (1933), KOTHANDARAM (1970).

21.8 Choristomas

Synonyms: Pituicytoma, granular cell "myoblastoma"; in the older literature: Sternberg-Priesel's choristoma, tumorettes, Abrikossoff myoblastic myomas, granular neuromas, granular cell tumors

Introduction

The choristomas are categorized in the WHO classification under the malformative tumors and tumor-like lesions. They are now considered as one entity with slight variations, although discussion may yet be continued.

Historical Note and Definition

The first description of such processes came apparently from BOYCE and BEADLESS (1893), and further reports about very small incidental findings in the pituitary gland from STERNBERG (1921) and PRIESEL (1922), who used the name *choristoma,* which was coined by ALBRECHT (1907a, b). They were found in 17% of an autopsy series (SHANKLIN 1947), and were also described as "tumorettes" [6.45% in the anterior lobe by LUSE and KERNOHAN (1955), and 5.7% by DORON et al. (1965)]. ULE et al. (1975) and ULE and WAIDELICH (1976) discussed the neurosecretory character of some of the cells. LISS and KAHN (1958) distinguished four different types of "pituicytes" yet did not believe that the various processes indicated by the different synonyms actually formed one entity.

However, a comparison of the pictures in the various publications shows that the granular cells of ULRICH et al. (1974), the glial tumors of the posterior pituitary lobe of TZONOS and MÜLLER (1967), and the granular cell myoblastomas of DORON et al. (1965) are all apparently identical with the granular cell tumors of MARKESBERY et al. (1973).

As will be emphasized in the section on differential diagnosis, most hamartomas of the pituitary region are not classifiable under this entity.

Epidemiology (Age – Sex – Frequency – Site)

The number of descriptions is too small for the data to yield information on preferential age and sex or on the actual frequency. ULE et al. (1975) believe that microscopic tumorettes (SHANKLIN 1947) can be found in about 17% of autopsies, but as choristomas without any mass character (see also "Historical Note and Definition"). The most usual site is the anterior lobe of the pituitary.

Gross Pathology

These choristomas range from the size of a pinhead to rare large forms that are space occupying (walnut sized) (LISS and KAHN 1958) and should be treated surgically (TZONOS and MÜLLER 1967).

Histologic Appearance

This mass is composed of cells with eosinophilic granular cytoplasm (Fig. 152b), which may be large and oval or epithelioid. The granules will be impregnated black by some reticulin (Laidlaw) or axon (Bodian) impregnations (HAMPERL and LATTES 1957).

Electron Microscopy

Ultrastructurally two cell types can be distinguished: (a) abundant cytoplasm filled with dense bodies, multivesicular bodies and vacuoles; and (b) a smaller cell type with only a few of the above-mentioned organelles. There can be inclusions resembling mitochondria and sometimes desmosome-like adhesions.

Differential Diagnosis

The choristomas with their different variants have to be distinguished from the hamartomas, which are either of a more neuronal character (p. 447) or may be lipomas or small ependymoma-like masses (p. 443). Histologically there is no possibility of confusion with the aforementioned cell and tissue types.

Biologic Behavior (Grading), Metastasis, and Recurrence

Space-occupying choristomas are treated surgically (SYMON et al. 1971), but little experience with information on survival times is so far available. All cases belong to grade I. Primary malignant granular cell tumors of the cerebral hemispherical white matter have been rarely observed (ULE et al. 1975).

Metastasis: Cerebral forms with metastasis have apparently not been described.

Origin: There are still various ideas about the origin, some authors postulating a neurogenic origin caused by a blastomatous change of Schwann cells, while others discuss a mesenchymal origin with undifferentiated mesenchymal cells and nonstriated muscle cells as a starting point.

Further References: ABRIKOSSOFF (1931), LAUCHE (1944), SCHWIDDE et al. (1951), LÜTHY and KLINGLER (1951), GLAZER et al. (1956), LISS (1958), WOLMAN (1959), BURSTON et al. (1962), FISHER and WECHSLER (1962), MOSCOVICH and AZAR (1967), POPOVITCH et al. (1970), STEIMLE et al. (1980).

21.9 Hypothalamic Neuronal Hamartomas

Introduction

The hamartomas of neuronal origin are listed in the WHO classification within the category of malformative tumors and tumor-like lesions.

Historical Note and Definition

Hamartomas were defined by ALBRECHT (1907a, b) as tumor-like masses arising from faulty embryonic development. They occur frequently in the hypothalamic region, when they harbor a vast number of large neuronal cells of the type of Cajal's infundibular nucleus. They are round masses 1 cm or more in diameter, are nodular, and arise between infundibulum and corpora mamillaria.

Interest in this group was actually raised (after the report of a case by LE MARQUAND and RUSSELL 1934/35) by a publication of DRIGGS and SPATZ (1939), which was followed by numerous other similar reports, e.g., those by WEINBERGER and GRANT (1941), J.E. MEYER (1948), RICHTER (1951), LANGE-COSACK (1951, 1952), and SCHMID et al. (1958).

However, it was at once apparent that *other hamartomas,* though rare, also occurred in this hypothalamic region, e.g., the "ependymoglioma" of HEUYER et al. (1931), the "glioma" of the posterior pituitary lobe of ROZYNEK (1942), the five cases of small lipomas of KRAINER (1935), and finally some cases reported by ANTONI (1950).

Two types should therefore be *distinguished:* the *neuronal* hamartoma of DRIGGS and SPATZ (1939), and the *hamartomas* of *different nature.* They project from the base of the brain and are attached to the tuber cinereum or mamillary bodies.

Whereas the original case of DRIGGS and SPATZ (1939) was characterized by pubertas praecox and gave rise to a long and interesting discussion on the point of origin (CAJAL's nucleus), other masses did not cause this symptom.

Epidemiology (Age – Sex – Frequency – Site)

According to SCHMIDT et al. in 1958 already 20 cases of pubertas praecox associated with neuronal hamartomas and in which the first symptoms already presented in the first or second year of life had been described in the literature. In one case the patient lived to the age of 62 years, after having presented with the first symptoms at 7 (WOLMAN and BALMFORTH 1963).

The frequency cannot be even roughly estimated; SCHMIDT et al. (1958), however, collected 27 cases of pubertas praecox with hamartomas (see above) from the literature, but not all of these could be classified with sufficient precision.

Site: These tumors are found in the tuber cinereum, between pituitary stalk and mamillary body.

Gross Pathology

The hypothalamic neuronal hamartomas consist of neuronal elements ending in nerve fiber bundles without any orderly structure. The neurons vary in size and form, but are all mature and have a normal appearance. SCHMIDT et al. (1958) found small closely packed neurons with roundish dark cytoplasm and excentric vesicular nuclei. Other cells were relatively large neurons in small groups or singly in the tissue.

Differential Diagnosis

We have emphasized above (p. 446) the various types of masses that arise near the hypophysis. In the hypothalamic region small heterotopias are not infrequently found. These hamartomas can be interpreted as hyperplastic forms of the inactive malformations that usually arise from the tuber cinereum or, more rarely from the mamillary body (i.e., that these tumor-like masses result from faulty embryonal development of the tissue normally present in the organ).

Biologic Behavior (Grading), Metastasis, and Recurrence

Biologically these tumors correspond to grade I. Metastases, recurrences, and anaplasia are unknown.

Clinical Course

Most of the patients so far reported have had an early puberty, some of them with epileptic fits, adipositas, and dwarfism. The symptoms usually start as soon as the first or second year of life.

Further References: HALLERVORDEN (1959), BEDWELL and LINDENBERG (1961), LICHTENSTEIN (1971, p. 1905).

21.10 Nasal Glial Heterotopias

Synonyms: Nasal glioma, "neurogenic", "gliomatous" tumor of nose

Introduction

The nasal glial heterotopia features in the WHO classification within the category of malformative tumors and tumor-like lesions.

Historical Note and Definition

Apparently BERGER (1890) was the first to describe nasal gliomas, but the first adequate description stems from M.B. SCHMIDT (1900) and was completed by BERBLINGER (1921), BLACK and SMITH (1950) collected 34 literature cases and gave a comprehensive list of references with tabulation.

SMITH et al. (1963) has published the most informative paper. The nasal heterotopias were localized intranasally (20 cases), extranasally (39 cases), or both (6 cases) in a series of 65 cases. They lie in the nasal lumen or on the dorsum of the nose and can be genuine heterotopias, i.e., not growing; or malformative tumors, i.e., of surgical importance (DEUTSCH 1965; HIRSCH et al. 1977).

Epidemiology (Age – Sex – Frequency – Site)

Age: Most of these heterotopias are visible at birth; however, they may not be of any clinical importance until one to two decades later.

Sex: In a list of cases there is a male preponderance (3:2).

Frequency: The frequency has not yet been defined, but the condition is fairly rare.

Site: The tumors are located intra- or extranasally or near the root of the nose and are usually subcutaneous. The overlying skin is reddish because of its vascularity.

Gross Pathology

There may be a firm paraseptal mass covered by normal mucosa or skin. The size may be that of a pea up to an apple. They can be asymptomatic and only a malformation, or have growth properties. Particles of glial tissue and collagenous stroma sometimes extend into the depths of the lesion connect with the intracranial contents (SMITH et al. 1963). The mass is elastic and occasionally cystic. There can be a defect of the frontal bone and bulging of cerebral tissue. The masses may lie inside the nasal lumen or outside at the dorsum of the nose.

Histologic Appearance

Histologically these tumors consist of nests of glia (mature astrocytes) in islands or encircled by wide irregular bands of a collagenous stroma resembling the architecture of marginal tissue in encephaloceles. There may occasionally be encased ganglion cells, there is no capsule; the masses are quite heavily vascularized and may grow by infiltration.

Electron Microscopy

SMITH et al. (1963) collected 93 literature cases. Electron microscopy reveals small mitochondria, few organelles, short dense tonofilaments, and thin plasma membranes.

Differential Diagnosis

Dermoid cysts, hemangiomatous growth (sinus pericranii) (KATZ and LEWIS 1971; MACGAVRAN 1970), meningiomas, esthesioneuroepitheliomas (BERGER et al. 1924), and extracerebral gliomas of surrounding tissue (OEHMICHEN 1971) have to be considered.

Biologic Behavior (Grading), Metastasis, Anaplasia, and Recurrence

Most of these masses are amenable to surgical treatment. HAGE (1958, 1960) reported on 39 cases; 11 recurred after operation.

Further References: DAVIS (1942), BRATTON and ROBINSON (1946), NEW and DEVINE (1947), DEL VILLAR (1956), AGARWAL et al. (1968), BIRNBAUM and OWSLEY (1968), HIRSCH et al. (1977).

22 Vascular Malformations

Synonyms: Angiomas, aneurysms, etc.

Introduction

In the WHO classification the vascular malformations are subdivided into the following entities:
1. Capillary teleangiectasia
2. Cavernous angioma
3. Arteriovenous malformation
4. Venous malformation
5. Sturge-Weber disease

To complete the description we add here:
6. Cryptic malformations (microangiomas)
7. Moya-Moya Disease

This classification is based mainly on the morphological structure of the entities, since adequate analysis by angiography has not yet been accomplished, except in the case of arteriovenous malformation (AVM).

Since the malformations, angiomas, and aneurysms are by definition not "brain tumors," one could question the inclusion of these entities in this volume, particularly since they are frequently non-space-occupying lesions. However, they are included because they can – and often do – produce a mass effect either through hemorrhage or by reactive changes of the adjacent tissue, and require surgery in most cases.

Historical Note and Definition

The classification goes back in its original concept to Virchow (1863/65) and has been defined in sufficient detail by Bergstrand, Olivecrona and Tönnis (1936). Only the entity of "arterial angiomas" has been omitted; up to now it has not been possible to verify these angiomas by arteriography. – A similar classification devised by Turner and Kernohan (1941) has not been used in the literature.

The following schematic classification also describes the preferential site of each type of malformation:

Type (Synonyms)	Meninges and bone	Brain and spinal cord
1. Capillary teleangiectasia (angioma racemosum, angioma capillare ectaticum)	–	Pons and quadrigeminal plate
2. Cavernous angioma	Skull and vertebral column	Cerebrum and brain stem, sellar and parasellar region, vertebral column
3. Arteriovenous malformations (angiomas, aneurysms)	Leptomeninges and convolutions in the distribution of the middle cerebral artery; rarer in distribution of anterior cerebral artery, very rare in that of the vertebral and middle meningeal arteries	
4. Venous malformation (angioma)	Dura, in vicinity of sagittal sinus; leptomeninges of Sylvian fissure, particularly of base	–
5. Sturge-Weber disease (angioma capillare et venosum calcificans, cerebrofacial or cerebrotrigeminal angiomatosis	Leptomeninges and sometimes the outer layers of the cortex; all lobes of the brain, but with a certain predilection for the parietooccipital region	
6. Cryptic malformations (microangiomas)		Thalamomesencephalic region, otherwise no preferential site

22.1 Capillary Teleangiectasia (Angioma Racemosum Capillare Ectaticum)

These angiomas form a tangled cluster of dilated capillaries of different sizes and lie most frequently in the midbrain and pons (NEUBUERGER and SILCOTT 1941; 18 cases of Courville). Such vascular malformations are usually discovered accidentally, because they are sometimes very small. However, they can be the source of recurrent and ultimately fatal hemorrhages. The overlying leptomeningeal vessels are unchanged. Many of them belong to the midline intracranial angiomas (PERRIA et al. 1971) and may be calcified (PENFIELD and WARD 1948). Some of them occur as microangiomas and cannot be classified before operation or autopsy (see p. 458; see also TEILMANN 1953).

22.2 Cavernous Angiomas

The rare cavernous angioma is composed of large vascular spaces with walls that simultaneously border the lumina of several vessels. There is thus no brain parenchyma between them.

"While in the skin the cavernous angioma is common and the racemose angioma rare, this relationship is exactly reversed in the central nervous system" (HAMPERL 1944). Thus, cavernous angiomas are not very common in the CNS.

They have been encountered, however, in all lobes of the cerebrum, in the diencephalon (MIZUTANI et al. 1981), in the brain stem, in the pineal region (VAQUERO et al. 1980), in the bones of the skull, and especially in the vertebral column (CORTEN 1921; BAILEY and BUCY 1929a; Dorothy RUSSELL 1931; ANTONI 1936a; BERGSTRAND et al. 1936).

In the angiogram they look like sinusoids (GIOMBINI and MORELLO 1978). Quite often the cavernous angiomas (AOKI et al. 1971) undergo calcification (some of the cases of TURNER and KERNOHAN 1941; HUBER and SORGO 1942; PENFIELD and WARD 1948; DI TULLIO and STERN 1979). Clinically epileptic seizures are particularly common in the presence of these calcified cavernomas. – There are also rare localizations, e.g., the sella (FINKEMEYER and KAUTZKY 1968; ORF 1970a; SANSONE et al. 1980).

Intramedullary cavernous angiomas have also been described (EVRARD et al. 1963; SCHRÖDER and BRUNNGRABER 1965 from our institute). VOIGT and YASARGIL (1976) reported on 164 literature cases, three-quarters of which were supratentorial and the rest infratentorial, 4% being were multiple. Of these tumors, 11% were calcified: every age group and each sex were equally represented; and 12.8% were successfully treated by operation (see also RAMINA et al. 1980). Exceptionally, a cavernous angioma in the posterior fossa of a newborn girl was described by CORTEN (1921). We have also observed multiple occurrence (see THIENEMANN 1975, case 9; and p. 459).

22.3 Arteriovenous Malformations

Synonyms: Arteriovenous aneurysmatic angioma, congenital arteriovenous angioma or aneurysm, cirsoid or serpentine angioma

Introduction

The group of vascular malformations includes arteriovenous malformation, describing it as "a mass of abnormally formed arteries and veins."

Historical Note and Definition

Apparently the arteriovenous malformation was theoretically already known to VIRCHOW (1863/65). It was not described until 1928, however (by DANDY 1928 and by CUSHING and BAILEY 1928b).

According to TÖNNIS (in BERGSTRAND et al. 1936; TÖNNIS 1948), the first precise clinical observation is thought to be that described by STEINHEIL (1895). The most detailed description of the entity is found in TÖNNIS' contribution to the monography of BERGSTRAND et al. (1936). Since then, RÖTTGEN (1937), SORGO (1938), LANGE-COSACK (1948), OLIVECRONA (1950), OLIVECRONA and LADENHEIM (1957) have all made important contributions to our knowledge. An interesting description was published by WYBURN-MASON (1943).

The exact morphological functional pattern of arteriovenous malformation was not clarified until angiography became available. Therefore, the first descriptions came from European neurosurgical departments in Sweden and Germany. The definition of this entity is that it consists of fairly correctly formed arteries and veins with entangled masses of undefined, partly sinusoid, partly capillary vessels between.

Epidemiology (Age – Sex – Frequency – Site)

Age: Bergstrand et al. (1936) believed that the peak manifestation was in the age group 11–30 years (see their p. 64, Table 5). Details will be found in the work of Lange-Cosack (1966, Fig. 45).

The frequency is different in our last series of 9000 cases, where they accounted for about 1.5% (malformations and aneurysms together: 3.8%).

The sites in which AVMs arise, in declining order of predilection, are the distribution of the middle cerebral artery, the anterior cerebral artery, with only a few cases occurring in the distribution area of the vertebrobasilar system and the external carotid artery. AVMs of the posterior cerebral artery are thought to be rarer (Sorgo 1949). The spinal AVM has been known since Rosenhagen (1933) and has been described by Schöpe (1941), Djindjian et al. (1970), and Pia (1973). Good documentation was found by Brion et al. (1952, Figs. 3, 4).

We have to emphasize here that most cases have been described as "varicosis" of the spinal cord and that only spinal angiography has clarified their mysterious nature (see R. Djindjian et al. 1970; M. Djindjian 1976).

Gross Pathology

The AVMs have a characteristic appearance: an area of the cortex, varying in size from a quarter to the whole of the palm of the hand, is covered by a network of tangled arteries, veins, and capillaries, often forming a plexus that is supplied with blood and drained by vessels ranging in thickness from that of a knitting needle to that of a pencil. The circumscribed AVM itself can be seen lying predominantly on the cortical surface, buried in the brain substance or even located within the lateral ventricles. The vessels are interconnected in part by "fistulous" connections of intermediate wall structure and by larger capillary-like vessels. The tangled cluster consists of a mass of blood vessels in which both thin and thick (aneurysmatically dilated) vessels are filled with bright red blood and form alternate loops around one another. However, the capillary system is usually not actually represented and therefore no oxygen is used for the brain tissue, which accounts for the bright red color even in the draining segments of the vasculature of the AVM and the subsequent atrophy of the adjacent brain tissue.

Not infrequently the angiomas have a wedge-shaped appearance of the frontal cuttings of the brain, where the point almost reaches the ventricular wall. There may be a small warty protuberance extending towards the ventricle (E. Fischer 1941, p. 235; Guillaume and Rogé 1949). In the spinal cord the AVMs are adapted, longer and narrower.

Histologic Appearance

Histologically we find vessel lumens of widely varying caliber and structure: some have a thick hyaline wall with no elastic layer; some have a normal architecture, including an elastic layer; and lastly there are sometimes cavities surrounded by a single layer of undifferentiated connective tissue; all lumina are packed with blood.

There are other vessels with good lamination of the wall in three layers or a wall formed by the median muscular layers. There is a last, less well-represented group of vessels consisting of lumina with one-layer endothelium (see SORGO 1938). Near the vascular lumina round cell infiltration and rusty-brown pigment (a remnant of earlier hemorrhages) are encountered.

The parenchyma around such an AVM is widely destroyed and replaced by foci of scavenger cells. The brain parenchyma is then softened and atrophic and scarred.

Large hemorrhages may occur and result in a not inconsiderable cystic cavity, which may communicate with the ventricle. Calcified blood vessels occasionally show up histologically as well as on x-rays.

Further References: Giant AVM: GUIDETTI and GAMBARCORTA (1971), LONG et al. (1974); dural AVM: VERBIEST (1951), KOSNIK et al. (1974); brain and spinal cord AVM: HASH et al. (1975); choroid plexus AVM: CARLETON and CAUTHEN (1975); see also RÖTTGEN (1937), OLIVECRONA and RIIVES (1948), OLIVECRONA (1950), POTTER (1955).

I discussed in Paris (1971 c) the correlations between the spinal (venous?) angiomas and the AVM with the so-called Foix-Alajouanine disease (subacute necrotizing myelitis). My concept was that it corresponded to a venous and capillary angiomatosis, which was located intra- and extradurally within the spinal canal.

Differential Diagnosis

Good differentiation is only possible if pertinent angiograms or autopsy observations are available. Descriptions in the older literature are usually not sufficient.

Clinical Course

The clinical symptoms were hemorrhage in 86% of cases; in 6%, headache; and in 8%, seizures. Surgical excision is the treatment of choice (SORGO 1949; NIEMEYER and AKERMAN 1953; TÖNNIS and SCHIEFER 1955; AMACHER et al. 1972: surgical mortality 2%; MORELLO and BORGHI 1973: 154 cases).

A more surgical procedure is embolization (see KUSSKE and KELLY 1974; R. DJINDJIAN et al. 1970, 1978).

Further Reference: LANGE-COSACK (1954).

Spinal Angiomas

Since arteriography of this part of the nervous system has only recently been perfected, subdivision of the angiomas is still incomplete.

A survey on 150 cases surgically operated on in Olivecrona's clinic has been given by FOERSTER et al. (1972), who on the basis of a 15-year follow-up recommended operation. PIA (1973) has reported on 93 spinal angiomas in 74 cases, with an emphasis on surgery. Later, in a complete monograph by

PIA et al. (1975; PIA and DJINDJIAN 1978) subdivision into extradural (vertebral, epidural) and intradural forms was attempted (see PIA and VOGELSANG 1965; LIETZ 1966).

Functional analysis on the basis of angiography is described in the excellent monographs by R. DJINDJIAN et al. (1970) and M. DJINDJIAN (1976).

Spinal angiomas generally seem to be rare, accounting for 4% of all cervical tumors (DRESSLER et al. 1968; W.L. BAILEY and SPERL 1969).

Further References: ANTONI (1936a), D. RUSSELL (1941), BUNTS (1949), VAN BOGAERT (1950), BISCHOF and SCHETTLER (1967), WALTER et al. (1967), ARONSON (1971), DECKER et al. (1978).

22.4 Venous Malformations (Angioma Venosum)

Synonyms: Plexiform angioma, Rankenangiom

Introduction

Venous angioma is listed as a subgroup in the WHO classification.

Historical Note and Definition

The early literature contains reports of malformations of a venous nature: VIRCHOW (1863/65) encountered "varicocele"-like masses of veins at the surface of the dura or leptomeninges. BAILEY and CUSHING (1928) observed a venous "wedge-shaped" angioma of the cerebrum. However, their differentiation from the arteriovenous type does not seem to be well documented. The same is true for two of the cases of BERGSTRAND (in BERGSTRAND et al. 1936), whereas DANDY (1928, Fig. 1) reported what seems to be a very typical case in a child of $2^1/_2$ years with a venous mass on both sides in the Sylvian fissures and a second characteristic case (his Fig. 2) which was more ball-like. TÖNNIS' case 1 (in BERGSTRAND et al. 1936) seems similar.

Therefore, precise classification of the cases in the literature is not simple, and we agree with TRUPP and SACHS (1948) that venous and arterial angiomas are difficult to distinguish; probably only a good angiogram makes it possible to diagnose this subgroup.

At best, cases that show a mass of abnormally formed veins which look like a varicocele (e.g., in the Sylvian fissure and over the spinal cord) can be included, but distinction from simple varices is still necessary. There may also be "cryptic" venous angiomas (WOLF et al. 1967; see "Microangiomas", p. 458).

Differential diagnosis from glioblastoma is sometimes only possible by angiography, where the venous malformation shows up in the last arterial phase (PREISSIG et al. 1976).

Further References: MONIZ (1942), HABERLAND (1950), SCOTTI et al. (1975), SARWAR and MCCORMICK (1978).

22.5 Sturge-Weber Disease

Synonyms: Cerebrofacial or cerebro-trigeminal angiomatosis, angioma capillare et venosum calcificans

Introduction

Sturge-Weber disease is listed as a well-described entity in the WHO classification.

Historical Note and Definition

Apparently the first description was published by STURGE (1879), and the first radiologic report by WEBER (1929). Further histological examinations were conducted by BERGSTRAND (BERGSTRAND et al. 1936), PETERS and TEBELIS (1937), GREEN (1945), and GREEN et al. (1950). An interesting clinical study was performed by KAUTZKY (1949), who emphasized that this was a systematic disease of some "head segments," involving brain, leptomeninges, and the corresponding skin in the trigeminal area simultaneously. However, a facial nevus alone is the most common manifestation, followed by the combination of facial and cerebral nevi. When fully developed, Sturge-Weber disease presents a true syndrome in the same manner as Lindau's disease: glaucoma, nevus flammeus of the face, and calcified angioma of the brain. Other vascular malformations can occur, so that Sturge-Weber disease can be classed as one of the systematic phakomatoses, hamartoblastomatoses, or neuroectodermal dysplasias (VAN BOGAERT 1935; KOCH 1940).

In South America particularly, the name is extended to Sturge-Weber-Dimitri-Krabbe disease.

Its association with other diseases has been discussed by WOHLWILL and YAKOVLEV (1957), ALEXANDER and NORMAN (1960), BARO (1964), BRUENS et al. (1968), and TÖNNIS and FRIEDMANN (1964). – Heredity may be dominant (KAMMER 1955). The most detailed study of this question has been made by KOCH (1973), who also made a survey of the literature up to 1973 (with 1081 references).

These angiomas are recognized by increased vascularity in the leptomeninges, caused by a sinuous network of venous and large vessels. The angiomatous malformation covers the cortex only with a fine calcification of the capillaries. However, there are rare cases without calcification.

Epidemiology (Age – Sex – Frequency – Site)

Predominantly the younger age group is affected. There is no sex preference and the frequency is not yet well defined: OLIVECRONA reported 5 personal cases, while BERGSTRAND collected 108 cases from the literature (BERGSTRAND et al. 1936). TÖNNIS and BORCK (1953) reported on 12 personal cases. In the meantime reports are more common, since the characteristic x-ray is better understood. No preferential site is known, although the parietal region is particularly involved. Apparently the angiomas do not occur at the median cortex of the two hemispheres or in the posterior fossa.

Gross Pathology

There is an increased vascularity of the leptomeninges owing to small worm-like venous vessels reaching down into the sulci and no thicker than pins, while a few larger vessels up to the thickness of a pencil overlie the angioma. The brain convolutions look "malformed" and the consistency of the brain is harder than normal (calcification); the leptomeninges look whitish gray.

Histologic Appearance

Brain parenchyma is atrophic, scarred and grossly calcified by an incrustation of the second and third layers and glial fibers are sometimes accumulated around the former capillaries. Scavenger cells are a prominent finding. Heterotopias are said also to be encountered (DI TULLIO and STERN 1979).

In differential diagnosis the dominant characteristic is the venous and capillary angioma of the leptomeninges. The same cortical calcification may occur overlying oligodendrogliomas, which is also where the double-lined garland-like ("crumb-line" or "railroad track") pattern occurs in the x-ray, and is explained by the particular projection of the calcified gyri (LINDGREN 1954, p. 36–39, Figs. 53a, b, 54).

Clinical Course

There is mental deterioration and focal seizures; nevus flammeus of the face is probably present in the majority of cases, and glaucoma occasionally.

The question as to whether this was a coordinated disturbance of leptomeninges and cortex was discussed by PETERS (1939), but he changed his earlier interpretation and accepted the concept of a secondary atrophic scarring process within the underlying cortex.

22.6 Cryptic Malformations (Microangiomas)

Synonyms: Cryptic angiomas, microangiomatous malformations

Introduction

This group is not included in the WHO classification, since it is morphologically not a uniform entity. It can be capillary in type (teleangiectasia, see p. 452), cavernous (see p. 452), or arteriovenous. Neurosurgically it has emerged in the last two decades as a uniform entity always causing the same problems. It will therefore be dealt here as a special subgroup.

Historical Note and Definition

These small angiomas less than 1 cm in diameter have been mentioned by many authors (D. RUSSELL 1954a; CRAWFORD and RUSSELL 1956; GERLACH and JENSEN 1960; COURVILLE 1963; GERLACH 1969). They have been called cryptic vascular malformations (MCCORMICK and NOFZINGER 1966) and microangiomatous malformations (McCONNELL and LEONARD 1967). However, GERLACH's term of "microangiomas" seem to be the most commonly used expression.

By definition these microangiomas are up to 1 cm in diameter and are seen in the angiogram or in the CT (TERAO et al. 1979). they are also often visible because of their calcification.

Epidemiology (Age – Sex – Frequency – Site)

Age: The cases recorded have been in patients between 21 and 81 years of age; however, there is a peak in the twenties.

Sex: No sex difference has been noted.

Frequency: Our series of 9000 tumors included 13 cases, which were compared by THIENEMANN (1975) with the 41 cases he collected from the literature. Our 13 cases were made up of 4 cases of teleangiectasia, 3 of cavernoma, 3 of arteriovenous malformations, and 1 "racemous" angioma, all in the supratentorial space.

Since these microangiomas have very fragile vascular walls, they tend to bleed. Alternating bleedings, particularly in the brain stem, can simulate the syndrome of multiple sclerosis (BRITT et al. 1981).

I was shown a similar case in 1953 in the University Clinic St. Louis as a possible case of multiple sclerosis; by chance, I suggested a bleeding angioma as the cause of the multiple recurrences of the tetraspastic syndrome. When the patient died a few days later autopsy revealed a capillary angioma below the tectum.

Multiple microangiomas have been reported by NOETZEL (1960), WOLF et al. (1967), and SCOTTI et al. (1975; angiography). We found around 35 microangiomas up to 0.5 cm in diameter distributed throughout the brain in one patient aged 63 years (see case 9, THIENEMANN 1975).

22.7 Moya-Moya Disease

This entity occurs almost exclusively in the Far East in the yellow races; in all probability it is a phenomenon of an unusual collateral circulation rather than a real malformation. The angiographic and histological observations suggest that it is caused by a proliferating stenosing arterial disease (possibly with some resemblance to Takayashu's disease, i.e., with a hyperallergic constitution) (see ZÜLCH 1981 a).

In Moya-Moya disease there is always a more peripheral or a proximal stenosis in the carotid artery with occlusion of the middle cerebral artery and often of the anterior cerebral artery as well.

A bundle of spiral, thickly twisted arterial channels extends from the siphon toward the basal ganglia, i.e., along the course of the medial and lateral striated vessels, and also along other perforating arteries supplying the basal ganglia.

In some cases (ZÜLCH et al. 1974b) a connection even with the cortical arteries, which perforate deep into the white matter and through the centrum semiovale, has been noted (for details of Moya-Moya syndrome see ZÜLCH 1981a).

We saw a case of secondary Moya-Moya syndrome in a white female patient aged 52, with stenosis of the carotid siphon and occlusion of the left middle cerebral artery distal to the striated arteries. These were patent. An angiogram 23 months later showed a typical Moya-Moya syndrome. Since there was no indication that the primary lesion was not atherosclerosis we referred to the condition as Moya-Moya *syndrome* rather than *disease* (ZÜLCH et al. 1974b). Whether the manifestation of a Moya-Moya syndrome presupposes a certain anlage of the vasculature remains to be clarified.

23 Tumors of the Anterior Pituitary

23.1 Pituitary Adenomas

Synonyms: Hypophyseal tumors, struma, epithelioma, carcinoma of the pituitary gland

Introduction

In no other group of intracranial tumors have the change in classification and the progress in identification of their nature been so striking as in the pituitary adenomas. In their excellent book on *The Pituitary Adenoma* POST et al. (1980) enumerate the following seven developments that have combined to bring about such radical progress:

1. Refinement of transphenoidal neurosurgery
2. Advances in radiological diagnosis of microadenomas (1 cm and smaller) by CT
3. Development of radioimmunoassay for prolactin detection
4. Isolation and synthesis of pituitary hormones
5. Medical treatment of endocrinological disturbances
6. Progress in finer morphological classification of pituitary tumors
7. Protein chemistry for pituitary disorders in man

These, they believe, "have virtually revolutionized our approach to pituitary adenoma."

Instead of a grouping according to the histology, which POST et al. (1980) call "anachronistic," the hormonal functions expressed in particular structures of the tumor cells are now the leading principle of an "ideal" examination. However, most pathologists are not yet able to perform such examinations in their routine work, because they need the combination of many different techniques, some highly sophisticated, including aniline staining, histochemical tests, radioimmunocytological studies, and EM. There is still a wide gap between the routine classification possible and the desired clinical (functional) grouping of these pituitary tumors.

The new WHO histological typing of CNS tumors has therefore not taken account of the aforementioned progress, but is based rather on the traditional entities. Yet, in the WHO Blue Books devoted to the histological typing of endocrine tumors (WILLIAMS et al. 1980) the modern histological classification of tumors of the "anterior pituitary" (adenohypophysis) is discussed.

Historical Note and Definition

It is surprising how little the older clinicians knew about the pituitary tumors (see NOTHNAGEL 1879), in spite of the frequently grotesque external disfigurement of those patients. The real study of this group of tumors did not begin until the discovery by Pierre MARIE (1886) of the connection between acromegaly and the eosinophilic pituitary adenomas. Comprehensive morphological studies followed, which opened up the way both for pituitary surgery and for morphological and functional research on the hypophysis (MARIE 1886; BABINSKI 1900; BENDA 1900, 1932b; FRÖHLICH 1901; ERDHEIM 1903, 1926; KRAUS 1914, 1926; SIMMONDS 1919; BIEDL 1922, 1930; P. BAILEY and DAVIDOFF 1925; FALTA 1928, 1940; P. BAILEY 1932b; BERBLINGER 1932, 1936; ROMEIS 1940; LABHART and ZACHMANN 1975).

In parallel, the surgical approach to this region was developed, which had been mastered by HORSLEY (1906), SCHLOFFER (1907, patient already operated 1906), F. KRAUSE (1908, already 1900 pistol bullet from chiasm removed), HIRSCH (1911, 1912, 1930, 1950). Harvey CUSHING (1912), as so many times, was the first to publish a comprehensive monograph on the diseases of the pituitary and their treatment (for details see WALKER 1951, p. 155ff.).

In the last 25 years the functional analysis of the pituitary hormones in the blood and urine and their correlation with the clinical syndromes (OBERDISSE and TÖNNIS 1953; FAHLBUSCH and VON WERDER 1978; POST et al. 1980) have formed the basis of all real progress.

We have to decide now which form of classification and description to use: since this book is meant for the clinician and the morphologist, both aspects have to be combined. It will start from the "anachronistic eosinophil, basophil, and chromophobe tinctorial designation" and proceed to "functional and practical classification."

In an attempt to find a compromise, we reproduce here a classification given in WHO Blue Book No. 23, Table 1 (WILLIAMS et al. 1980).

Structure and function in pituitary adenomas

H&E	PAS – orange G	Immunohistochemistry and electron microscopy	Clinical syndrome caused by the tumour[a]
Acidophil	Acidophil	Somatotroph cells[b] Lactotroph cells[b]	Acromegaly/gigantism Galactorrhoea-amenorrhoea
Chromophobe	Chromophobe	Agranular small cells	No known function
Basophil	Mucoid	ACTH-MSH cells[b]	Cushing's syndrome Melanodermia
		Thyrotroph cells[b] Gonadotroph cells[b]	Thyrotoxicosis ?
Oncocytic	Oncocytic	Oncocytic	No known function

[a] Excluding hypopituitarism, which may be caused by any type of pituitary tumour
[b] These cells may be well to poorly granulated

On the other hand, the grouping of HORVATH and KOVACZ (1976) seems to be adequate; they divide these tumors into adenomas with

1. HGH (human growth hormone activity)
2. PRL (prolactin) activity
3. HGH *and* PRL activity
4. ACTH (adrenocorticotrophic hormone) and MSH (melanostimulating hormone) activity and into those containing
5. Undifferentiated cells
6. Oncocytes
7. TSH (thyreostimulating hormone)
8. FSH (follicle-stimulating hormone)
9. LH (luteinizing hormone)

A correlation between these two principles will be found in the following grouping:

Adenomas secreting	Adenomas with cells of the traditional classification
HGH	Acidophilic
PRL	Acidophilic – often also chromophobe
Oncocytic	Acidophilic
ACTH	Basophilic
TSH	Basophilic
FSH	Chromophobe, occasionally acidophilic
LH	Chromophobe, occasionally acidophilic
Secretory-inactive	Chromophobe

However, it has to be emphasized here that for the neurosurgeon the pathomorphology of a tumor may not be the primary problem, although the surgery he has to perform may be directed by the endocrinological state. Therefore much of the old way of describing pituitary tumors has to be retained in this chapter. (For today's concepts see BERGLAND 1975; O.A. MÜLLER and VON WERDER 1977; SAEGER 1977).

Yet, RUSSELL and RUBINSTEIN (1977) may have been correct in emphasizing that "such a classification does not have any morphological equivalent with the three classic types of pituitary adenomas recognized by light microscopy."

Epidemiology (Age – Sex – Frequency – Site)

The space-occupying pituitary adenomas may account for around 8% of all intracranial tumors. In our personal series of 9000 cases they represented 6.6% and in the series of OLIVECRONA (1967), 8.6%, whereas in the series of CUSHING (1932) the disproportionately high percentage of these tumors was 17.8. ARENDT (1964b) had 9.1% and SCHELIN (1962) 10% of pituitary adenomas in their series.

Age: The rather blunt peak of the age curve lies around 35–45 years (Fig. 9 l), but with a generally earlier manifestation of clinical symptoms in the patients

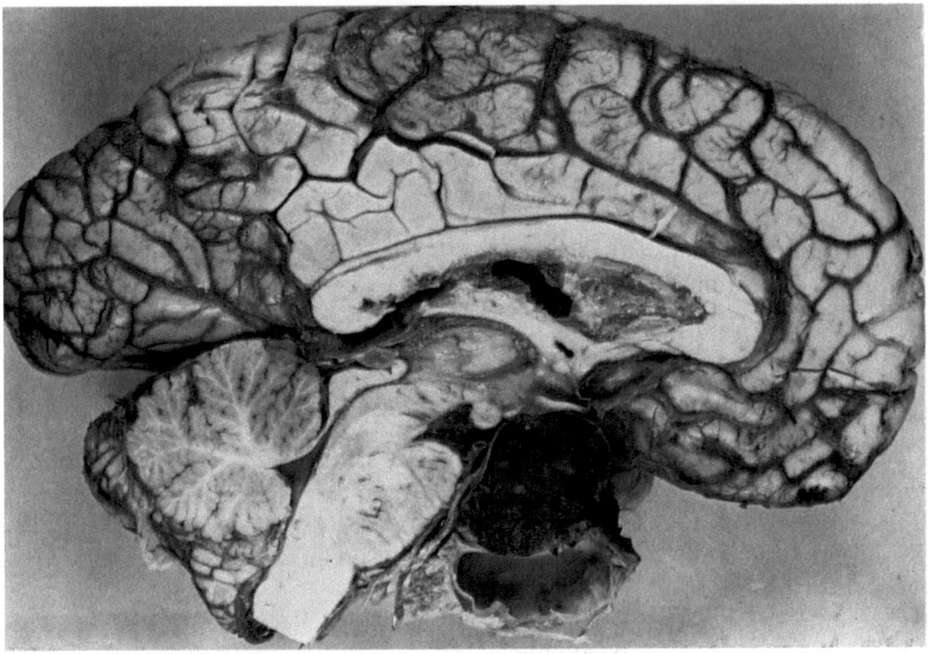

Fig. 153. Eosinophilic adenoma with diffuse intraparenchymatous hemorrhages which gave the tumor a brownish-black color at autopsy. (ZÜLCH 1975a)

with hormonally active adenomas than in those with hormonally inactive tumors. The latter have their peak later, around 55–60 years (W. MÜLLER 1969). Only rarely are patients under 16 years of age affected (KOOS and MILLER 1971). The age incidence of the three morphological traditional types is probably the same (see, however, W. MÜLLER 1969, above).

Sex: The ratio of the two sexes is assumed to be equal by JÄNISCH et al. (1976, Table 65), who collected 2140 cases from the literature, with a mean percentage of 49.7% male patients. However, the extreme figures for the male oscillated between 41.3% and 47.4% in the different series. In our own series the male patients always outnumbered the female patients by 15 to 13. Familial occurrence has been reported in a mother and daughter by LINQUETTE et al. (1967) and in two sisters by HIMURO et al. (1976).

Gross Pathology

By their intrasellar growth the pituitary adenomas produce an expansion of the pituitary fossa so that its dural and bony walls are forced sideways and downward towards the sphenoid sinus (Fig. 153), whereby the dura of the sella may be extremely thin; when they expand the borders of the sella the neoplasms are brought into contact with sensitive structures of the surrounding tissue, such as the optic fascicles and the chiasm. Later, the large chromophobe ad-

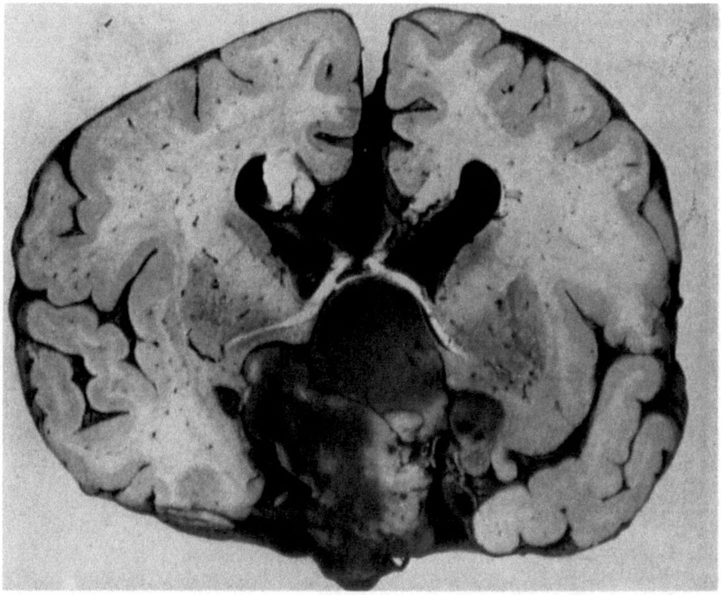

Fig. 154. Enormous chromophobe adenoma of the pituitary, which has extended mainly into the region of the 3rd ventricle and has also impinged on both temporal lobes by way of nodular growth. (ZÜLCH 1975a)

enomas (Fig. 154), in particular, may extend well beyond the sella (they were very large in 39% of cases in the series of KRAYENBÜHL 1961; GP, Figs. 247, 248, 251). They then compress the optic tracts or the caudal portion of the chiasm, depending on the anatomical variations in the form and position of these structures (GP, Figs. 249, 254). Apparently about two-thirds of pituitary adenomas have a suprasellar growth (GP, Figs. 253, 254, 256; HEIMBACH 1959). Erosion of the sella is almost inevitable in the larger tumors (GILBERTSON and GOOD 1956: 95 of 99 cases).

In still later stages of growth the chiasm may be displaced forward or, more commonly, pushed upward and stretched over the tumor, while the carotid arteries are usually displaced laterally. After rupturing the diaphragma sellae the tumor may grow toward the floor of the third ventricle and may even occupy its lumen (Fig. 154). The chiasm is displaced so far that it can be cut into by the overlying anterior communicating artery, while the constricting effect of the chiasm can produce an indentation or "waist" in the tumor itself. The larger adenomas may grow around both carotids or may extend forward into the frontal fossa (GP, Fig. 247) or laterally towards the temporal lobes (GP, Figs. 248); extension into direction of the paranasal sinuses is usually less pronounced (GP, Fig. 255). There are exceptional cases in which the suprasellar growth is so much more marked than the intrasellar component that the chiasm is compressed without any gross changes in the sella. It is very rare for it to extend into the diploe of the base of the skull (GP, Figs. 255, 256) from

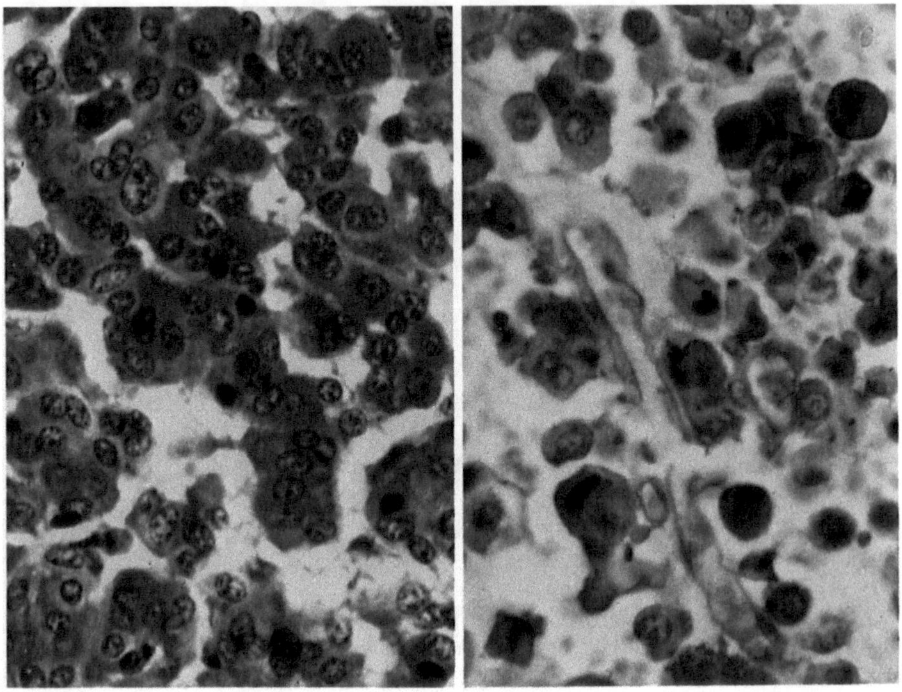

a b

Fig. 155. a Marked basophilia and true polymorphic epithelium of an adenoma of the hypophysis. H&E, ×350. **b** Moderately polymorphous epithelium in an eosinophilic adenoma of the hypophysis. H&E, ×500

which the tumor emerges by forming large nodules (GP, Fig. 253). The pituitary adenomas appear to be well encapsulated, and range in size from that of a plum to that of a child's fist. Because of frequent hemorrhages into the tumor, the eosinophilic adenomas often have a brownish color. The capsule of the tumor is quite tough, whereas its contents are commonly so soft that they can be removed with a surgical sucker. The capsules can be calcified, as can the tumor tissue itself (E. Lindgren 1954: 3.2% of 315 cases). The adenomas grow toward the brain purely by extension, and their capsule can be freely removed from the adjacent structures. They are characterized by a tendency to degeneration of the tumor tissue, which leads to the formation of smaller or larger degeneration cysts (GP, Fig. 251). This is well known in the chromophobe tumors; almost an entire tumor with a diameter of several centimeters can consist of a cyst.

The acidophilic adenomas generally produce marked clinical (endocrine) changes before they reach the chiasm. Large space-occupying tumors therefore usually belong morphologically to the chromophobe type, although they can now be diagnosed earlier if endocrinologically active. Basophilic tumors are rare and are rarely of any significant size or concern to the neurosurgeon from the mechanical standpoint. They can now be detected by the modern CT even while less than 1 cm in diameter, because of their early clinical manifestations.

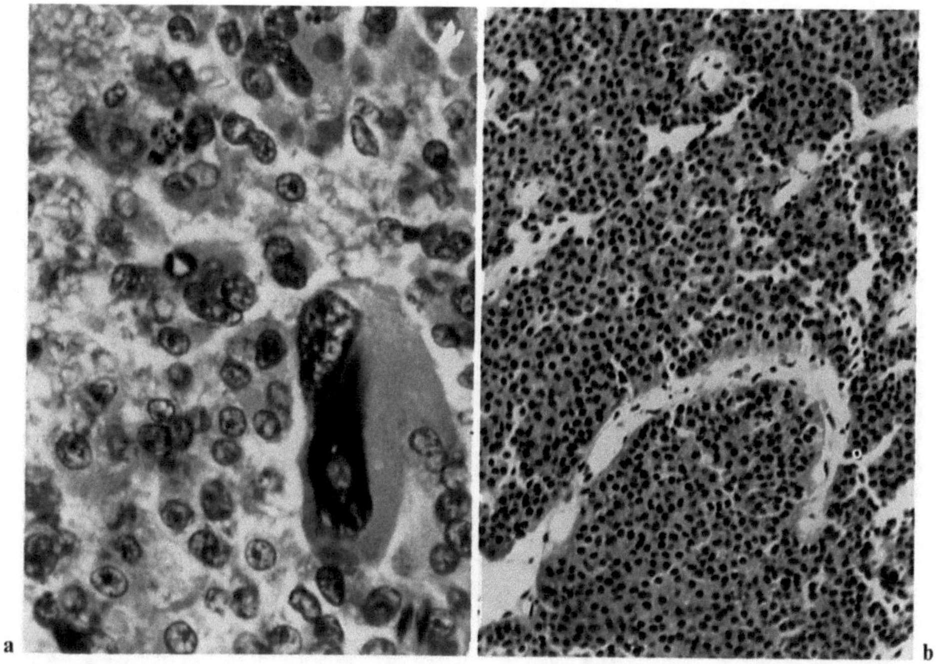

Fig. 156. a Polymorphous eosinophilic adenoma of the hypophysis. Note the giant cells with hyperchromatic nuclei and the mitotic figures. H&E, ×500. **b** Massively packed cells in a pituitary adenoma. H&E, ×136

A double tumor has been described: craniopharyngioma plus eosinophilic tumor (TZONOS and PFINGST 1964). These tumors also occur in combination with other malignant neoplasms (PINTO 1969). Isolated localization within the third ventricle without any sellar involvement is very rare (SHANKAR et al. 1976).

Histologic Appearance

We have emphasized above that routine histological examination is not sufficient if only H&E stains are applied. The PAS-orange G technique is necessary to recognize the mucoid (in H&E called basophil) elements. This is the minimum requirement. Radioimmunoassay and EM are desirable (WECHSLER and HOSSMANN 1965a; MOSCA and VASALLO 1970; FONCIN 1971; PELLETIER 1971; DONIACH 1972; RACADOT et al. 1975).

Acidophil (Eosinophilic) Adenomas

These are highly cellular, consisting of large neoplastic acidophilic cells (Fig. 155a) with a variable admixture of chromophobe cells. The elements usually lie in islands separated from each other by scant stroma (Fig. 155b). Not infrequently polynuclear giant cells occur (HBT, Fig. 92b), particularly if the tumor is markedly pleomorphous (Fig. 156a). They are usually seen when they are not yet so large, since the hormone activities are noted early. The cells

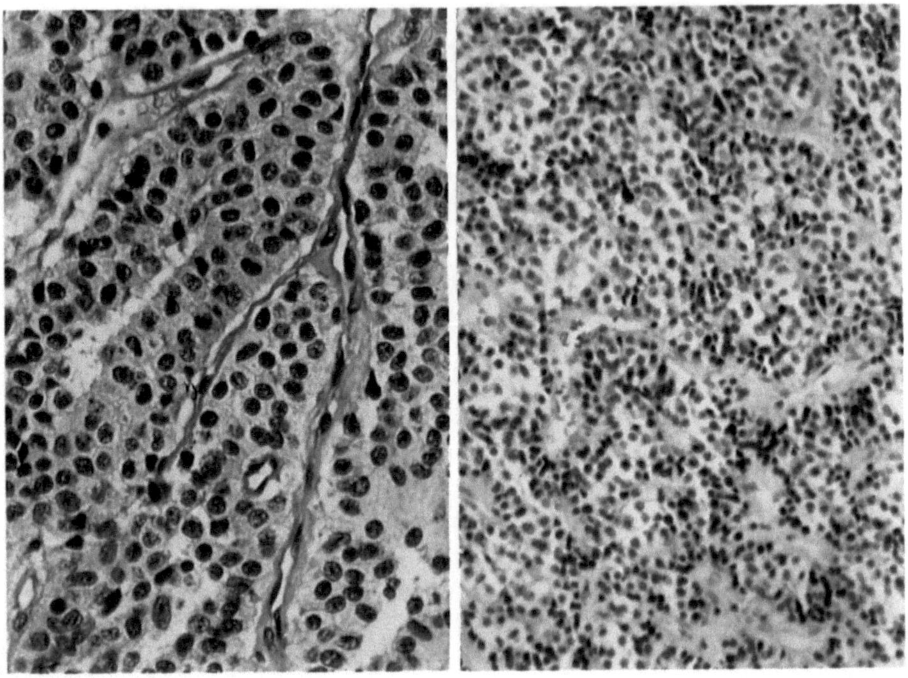

Fig. 157. a Typical chromophobe adenoma: The large cells with moderately chromatin-rich nuclei lie along the capillaries. H&E, ×262. **b** Chromophobe adenoma with mucoid degeneration. H&E, ×172

are stained with orange G and finely granulated. Their shape is polygonal (Fig. 156b) and the cytoplasm well delimited; the so-called alpha granules are distinctly stained with ethyl violet, iron-hematoxylin, or Gomori-chromhematoxylin stain. The nucleus is usually small, rich in chromatin and almost pyknotic. It often has an eccentric position.

Mucoid Cell ("Basophil") Adenomas

The term basophil is used when an H&E stain is applied. "Mucoid" can only be applied when PAS staining gives positive results. Although basophil and mucoid are not synonyms, most mucoid cells are also basophils (HBT, Fig. 92d).

These usually smaller tumors, often the size of a pinhead, consist of cells resembling the elements of the normal hypophysis. Their nuclei are roundish and pale, have little chromatin, and are sometimes overshadowed by the strongly stained cytoplasm. Besides these PAS-positive cells variable admixtures of chromophobe elements can be seen. They can now be clinically detected by modern CT techniques.

Microadenomas were found in early investigations by LÖWENSTEIN (1907) and COSTELLO (1936). They were encountered in around 25% of 1000 pituitary glands, but interestingly enough, never in juveniles.

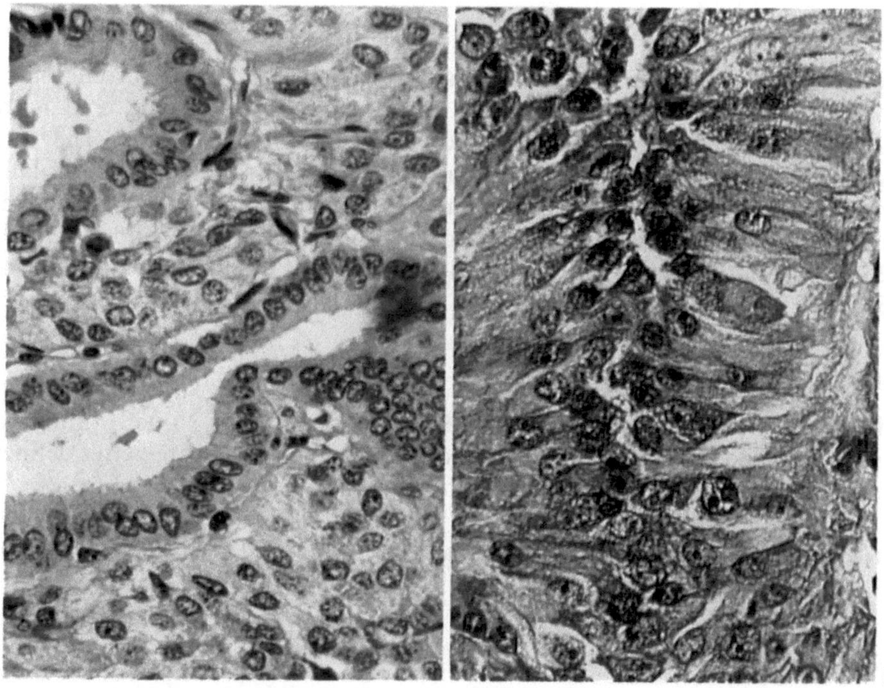

a b

Fig. 158. a Cuboidal epithelium-lined cysts in a chromophobe adenoma. They resemble the similar cysts occurring between the pars anterior and the infundibular process. H&E, ×272. **b** The epithelial cells of a chromophobe adenoma of the hypophysis appear aligned along blood vessels. H&E, ×336

Chromophobe Adenomas

These tumors consist only of chromophobe cells, and no neoplastic acidophil or mucoid cells at all can be demonstrated. The cells may have a cylindrical appearance, the scarce cytoplasm is sometimes not clearly limited, and the nucleus shows only a weak chromatin network. However, their architecture is indicative. They may be situated along the capillaries (HBT, Fig. 93a, b) in long bands (Fig. 157a) or more rarely as a papillary architecture, particularly in the case of regressive phenomena (Fig. 157b) when cells far distant from the capillary are liquefied. However, this process must not be mistaken for the genuine fetal type (see below), where arrangement in broad columns and an "epithelial" pattern prevail. – Epithelium lined cysts near the middle lobe of the pituitary may be encountered.

Fetal Type

These are pituitary adenomas with an almost papillary architecture (Fig. 158b), which can easily be confused with choroid plexus papillomas or papillary ependymomas, particularly after some dissociation of the tissue between the capillaries due to liquefaction which characterizes this architecture (see Kraus 1926; Zülch 1956, Fig. 388).

Transitional or Mixed Forms

There are some adenomas that fall histologically between the chromophobe and acidophil types and in which the architecture and cell type tend more to one or to the other. The granulation may be dense or scarce. They are now analyzed by endocrinological methods (see below), since they are usually hormonally active in nature. Their name of "transitional" or "mixed" forms in the literature was based on the cytological appearance (BAILEY and DAVIDOFF 1925; DOTT and BAILEY 1925; BAILEY 1932b; TÖNNIS et al. 1953; W. MÜLLER 1954; MÜLLER and TZONOS 1967).

Oncocytic Adenomas

This tumor is heavily stained with H&E (eosinophilic), less so with orange-G (acidophilic) and only poorly with trichrome techniques. They are better defined because of their typical closely packed mitochondria in EM.

Further References: HAMPERL (1962), LANDOLT and OSWALD (1973), MARTINS (1974, handbook article).

Growth and Regressive Changes

The growth of *all adenomas* is slow, and mitoses are rare. Regressive processes, however, are frequent. Hydropic swelling progressing to liquefaction and cyst formation, for instance, is very common in the chromophobe tumors, but also occurs in the eosinophilic type, and it can cause the architecture of a tumor to become completely blurred. Calcification is found histologically in a higher percentage of cases than radiologically (7.4%; W. MÜLLER and HOFFMANN 1967), yet computed tomography has changed this statement.

It is necessary, however, to distinguish the characteristic colloid cysts within the tumor tissue (Fig. 158a), some of which are ciliated (ZÜLCH 1956, Fig. 374c).

Biologic Behavior (Grading), Metastasis, and Recurrence

The growth of most of the pituitary adenomas is slow, and the clinical history is therefore long (average preoperative history 9.6 years: HOFELDT et al. 1973). However, the endocrine symptoms of the different adenoma types are now better known to practitioners, gynecologists, endocrinologists, and neurologists and therefore diagnosis is likely to be made earlier in the future.

Infarction and hemorrhages into the tumor can bring about an *apoplectiform* worsening of the symptoms and start up a clinical syndrome (BROUGHAM et al. 1950; LIST et al. 1952; RÖTTGEN and PETERS 1952; W. MÜLLER and PIA 1953: 7%).

It is almost impossible now to discuss the frequency of recurrences, because of the medical and combined surgical and radiological treatment. In former times recurrences were said to be more frequent in mixed adenomas than in the purely chromophobe types (see SAMII et al. 1975).

Histologically all pituitary adenomas correspond to grade I.

Attempts at New Classification on the Basis of Secretory Activity

Identification of a particular subtype of secreting tumor cannot be achieved by light microscopy alone. Histochemical tests, EM, and immunochemistry have to be used for the process of morphological classification.

HGH adenomas

These adenomas consist of acidophilic (eosinophilic) cells and are usually observed in acromegaly (general ratio: 14 out of 15 cases). They can be densely or sparsely granulated, according to the phase of granulation: regenerating/storage/secretory phase (KINNMAN 1978). The grade of acromegalism depends on the quantity of granulation. In the series of HORVATH and KOVACS (1976) the densely and sparsely granulated types were nearly equally represented. LEWIS and VAN NOORDEN (1974) reported 110 cases, only 23 of which were sparsely granulated. From p. 463 it is apparent that apart from the purely acidophilic also mixed adenomas occur, with HGH and PRL secretion (CORENBLUM et al. 1976). Whether in these cases both hormones are secreted by the same cell, as might be deduced from experiments in rats, remains open.

The group of HGH adenomas is thought to be the most common "functional" tumor of the pituitary. If, however, the chromophobe architecture prevails nuclei may appear more pleomorphic and real multinuclear cells may be seen as well as an eccentric arrangement of nuclei. Sometimes even globular fibrous bodies occur.

In a large series of acromegalics (YOUNG et al. 1965) it was demonstrated that only some of the adenomas were eosinophilic, and that of 44 adenomas all were of the "mixed chromophobe" type, with only a small proportion of acidophilic cells. RAY and HORWITH (1964), on radical exenteration of the sella found only 65% acidophilic tumors, but the material was somewhat heterogenous. SCHELIN (1962) in a series of patients undergoing transphenoidal surgery, recorded only 10% acidophilic tumors.

This discrepancy shows the difficulties inherent in a morphological classification.

Some Remarkable Clinical Syndromes. After bilateral adrenectomy rapidly growing mucoid adenomas of large size have been reported. Pituitary stalk compression is said to induce hypopituitarism with excessive prolactin production. The frequency of prolactin secretion adenomas seems to be increasing spectacularly (PEILLON et al. 1978). This may be due to improved diagnosis; understandably there is a female predominance of 4:1. It induces amenorrhea/galactorrhea in female patients; galacturia is rare in men, in whom impotence and loss of libido are the main symptoms.

PRL Adenomas

This group also belongs mainly to the eosinophilic type of adenomas of the traditional classification. However, since FORBES et al. (1954) called attention to the PRL-producing pituitary tumors with an amenorrhea/galactorrhea syndrome, it has been noted that many chromophobe adenomas are often secreting tumors (KOVACS et al. 1975: 8 chromophobe out of 44 with PRL granules). Later they were separated from the HGH adenomas (PEAKE et al. 1969). Modern techniques, particularly immunoperoxidase (ROBERT and HARDY 1975; HORVATH et al. 1977) allow their identification. They may account for around one-sixth of all chromophobe adenomas (KOVACS et al. 1976).

HGH and PRL Adenomas

HGH- and PRL-secreting cells may occur "mixed" in some tumors, but only rarely. This has been seen in a girl almost 5 years of age (GUYDA et al. 1973).

ACTH/MSH-Secreting Adenomas

This form of adenoma has been particularly frequently observed in patients with Nelson's syndrome after bilateral adrenalectomy indicated by a pre-existing Cushing syndrome (DEGENNES and TURPIN 1978). Such tumors occur either as a genuine neoplasia or only as a hyperplastic proliferation of the pituitary gland. Classically they can be basophilic, but can also occur as mixed chromophobe adenoma or even as an eosinophilic type (ERZIN et al. 1977).

Undifferentiated Chromophobe, Nonfunctional Pituitary Adenomas

These adenomas cannot be linked to any known normal pituitary cell type (see HORVATH and KOVACS 1976, LANDOLT et al. 1978). They comprise at least 20% of all adenomas in a modern hormonal classification. Most are said to be sparsely granulated (SAEGER et al. 1976). Small amounts of eosinophilic or basophilic granules may be demonstrated. Immunochemistry is important for confirmation of the diagnosis. There may be small amounts of normal hormones or an increased prolactin secretion but without galactorrhea, and there may be a male preponderance (1.7 male:1 female patients).

Because of these uncertainties the ratio in a modern hormonal classification varies very widely (MCCORMICK and HALMI 1971: 64% acidophil, 4% chromophobe; LANDOLT 1975: 36% acidophil, 57% chromophobe; see also Table II of MCCARTY et al. 1978).

Technical factors may be responsible for these wide differences; chromophobe adenomas do not stain distinctly with H&E or Mallory's stain. However, if they contain acidophilic cells they may be positive for Horlant's stain. On the other hand, they sometimes contain single granules and yet are clinically silent (see also LEWIS and VAN NOORDEN 1974). Adenomas of the secreting type that produce FSH or TSH are rare (DUELLO and HALMI 1977).

23.2 Pituitary Adenocarcinomas (Carcinoma of the Anterior Pituitary Cells)

Cytologically these tumors have a high mitotic activity but may be even less pleomorphous than other adenomas. Malignant (anaplastic) transition is more frequent in the chromophobe type than in other forms. Histologically the adenocarcinoma corresponds to grade III.

Histologically – if the adjacent tissue is present – they are recognized by the evidence of invasion and destructive growth or by metastasis (see CUSHING 1932; KRAYENBÜHL 1961 etc.). Some of them have infiltrated the dura, according to the literature.

Whether it is legitimate to use the term "carcinoma" in cases is debatable, when there are apparently no extracranial metastases (see below). Probably it would here be preferable to call these tumors "anaplastic" (or malignant) adenomas. This was also recommended by WILLIS (1960), who accepted only one case in the literature as a true carcinoma. I have published a critical discussion of the descriptions of these cases in the literature (ZÜLCH 1956): in the series of CUSHING (1935) there were 11 such adenocarcinomas among 338 cases; WINKELMAN et al. (1952) reported 11 cases from the literature, only 5 of which were called "probable"; EPSTEIN et al. (1964) called this type "an extreme rarity." NEWTON et al. (1962) accepted 4 out of 93 patients as compromised by such tumors.

Very rarely, cases of high malignancy are observed with extracranial metastases (SHELDON et al. 1954: liver; GRAF et al. 1962: lung and lymph nodes; BRAUN and TZONOS 1965).

Seeding within the CSF has been reported by RICOY et al. (1974: after operation) and MADONICK et al. (1963: without surgery). Highly invasive adenomas, on the other hand (GP, Figs. 253, 254, 255), do not seem to be too rare (ROBERT et al. 1973).

Perhaps malignancy could be characterized by three forms: (a) locally invasive type; (b) seeding within the CSF; and (c) with metastases in the body organs. The last form could then correctly be called adenocarcinoma (see GEROULANOS 1969: one case of his own with seeding into liver and bone; 13 cases in the literature with hematogenous seeding).

24 Local Extensions From Regional Tumors

24.1 Glomus Jugulare Tumors

Synonyms: Chemodectomas, nonchromaffin paragangliomas, carotid-body-type tumors

Introduction

Amongst the tumors that can extend into the CNS and present as a neurosurgical problem the WHO classification includes tumors of the glomus jugulare. These have gained in surgical importance in recent decades, particularly since ROSENWASSER (1945) called attention to this particular type of neoplasm.

Historical Note and Definition

Tumors of the carotid fork originating in the carotid body have long been familiar to ear, nose, and throat surgeons. However, only since more specific study of the carotid body (VON HALLER 1762) became possible, and particularly since the detection of tissue similar to that of the carotid and aortic bodies (W. KRAUSE 1878: "Glandula tympanica") and the research by GUILD (1941, 1953) has sufficient information been available to identify the "glomus jugulare" (glomus vagale) tumors. Tumors of the carotid body had been described at an early stage by BEVAN and MCCARTHY (1929), and the report was later extended by LUBBERS (1937). For further descriptions we are indebted to LATTES and WALTNER (1949), BICKERSTAFF and HOWELL (1953), and particularly to LE COMPTE (1951), who have published excellent pictures and informative texts. The excellent chapter of KLEINSASSER (1960) gives sound basic information.

Epidemiology (Age – Sex – Frequency – Site)

These are rare tumors occurring in middle age (41–70 years). There seems to be a female preponderance (KLEINSASSER 1960: 72.5%), but the frequency is unknown (KLEINSASSER had collected 160 cases up to 1960). The tumors are localized in the middle ear and they originate either from the glomus jugulare (GUILD 1941) or from the paraganglion tympanicum (W. KRAUSE 1878). They are locally invasive, usually starting at the hypotympanic recess; they destroy the petrous part of the temporal bone and sometimes present as heavily bleeding polyps of the ear. They invade the mastoid process or the tip of the pyramid, and can even grow down to the neck. They may extend to involve the brain near the jugular foramen, but can also infiltrate the cranial nerves, even to the existence of a Garcin syndrome. Infiltration of the brain has not been observed, although the dura can be invaded as well as the venous sinuses.

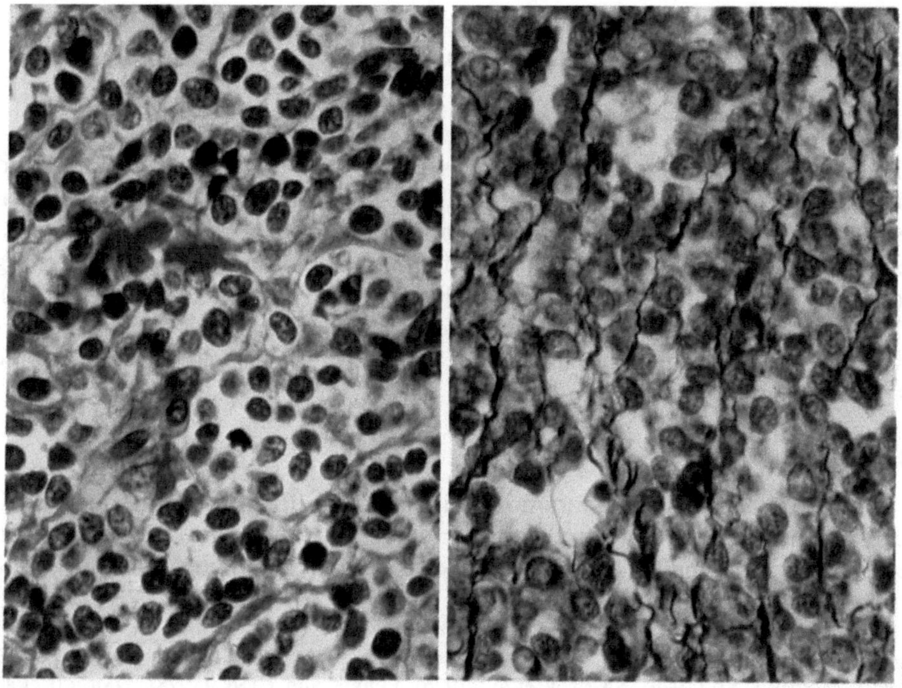

Fig. 159a, b. Typical carotid body/glomus tumor (chemodectoma). **a** H&E, ×500; **b** silver impregnation, ×372

Gross Pathology

These are highly vascularized tumors made up of a red soft tissue. The vasculature usually consists of small vessels, which may, however, adopt a cavernoma-like pattern. They are sometimes very large (ROUZAUD and LEBON 1965).

Histologic Appearance

The typical architecture is the intermingling of cell nests (Fig. 159a) or *Zell-Ballen,* surrounded by fibrous stroma rich in capillaries. The clusters of chief cells vary in nuclear size. They can be impregnated by special silver impregnation methods (HAMPERL and LATTES 1957), small granules suggestive of a glomus tumor. The cells are arranged in lobules (Fig. 159b), they sometimes mimic meningotheliomatous meningiomas.

Differential Diagnosis

These tumors may bulge beneath the tympanic membrane, and paracentesis can lead to severe hemorrhage. The intracranial extensions of the tumor are also highly vascular, and surgical removal can provoke massive hemorrhages. They must therefore be distinguished from other, similar tumors; preoperative angiography is a particularly reliable method.

However, modern methods of embolization have been successful in the hands of RUGGIERO et al. (1976), MERLAND et al. (1977), and VALDAZO et al. (1978).

Biologic Behavior (Grading), Metastasis, and Recurrence

The extreme vascularity of these tumors makes surgical removal difficult and causes operative problems (CAPPS et al. 1957). Early radiotherapy has been recommended, although the tumors seem to be fairly radioresistent. They often recur and metastasis is probably also common. Anaplastic development, among other conditions, has been described as lymph metastasis (ROSENWASSER 1968). The malignancy of these tumors is caused mainly by their invasive and destructive growth throughout the base of the skull (see above) and the high degree of vascularization (grade II and III).

Origin

It is generally agreed that the tumors originate from the jugular glomus, which corresponds biologically to the carotid glomus. Ultrastructural examination in recent decades seems to prove that the cells act as chemoreceptors (hence the name chemodectomas).

Further References: HUGHES and SMITT (1955), GRCEVIC (1956), WEIBÜLL (1961), PARKINSON (1969), MOODY et al. (1976), SPECTOR et al. (1976), GIBBIN and HENK (1978), NAIDICH et al. (1978).

24.2 Chordomas

Synonyms: Chordoblastomas, ecchondrosis physaliphora, chordocarcinomas/chordosarcomas

Introduction

In the WHO classification chordomas are listed among the "extensions" from the base of the skull.

Historical Note and Definition

The history starts with the discussions between VIRCHOW (1857, p. 58, Table VI, Figs. 16, 17), who had first described this type of tumor and called them "ecchondrosis physaliphora," and H. MÜLLER (1858), who correctly recognized the connection with notochordal rests. LUSCHKA (1856) and KLEBS (1864) took part in this discussion. However, RIBBERT's co-worker STEINER (RIBBERT and STEINER 1894) was the first to find the original tissue of these tumors, in 2% of 500 autopsies; with this the ultimate derivation from the chorda was obvious. COENEN (1925) gave the first classification, which in its general structure is still valid today, and distinguished the benign accidental findings from the clinically important space-occupying forms; a similar grouping was devised by LIVINGSTONE (1935). A comprehensive study has been published by DAHLIN and MACCARTY (1952). Details of the history have been given by FURLOW (1935).

In recent decades KLEINSASSER and FRIEDMANN (1958a) and KRAYENBÜHL and YASARGIL (1975a) have given excellent introductions and descriptions discussing all the variants and referring to the world literature (114 references).

The chordomas are rare tumors (around 0.2% of our series) and vary in size.

Epidemiology (Age – Sex – Frequency – Site)

Age: In older people these tumors are encountered as incidental findings in the clivus and scarcely act as space-occupying lesions (the so-called benign chordomas). They occur most often in the 21–40 age group but can occur at any age (KLEINSASSER and FRIEDMANN 1958a; KLEINSASSER 1960; KRAYENBÜHL and YASARGIL 1975a). Only the sacrococcygeal type of chordoma seems to occur earlier (FLETCHER et al. 1935).

Sex: In two large series (KRAYENBÜHL and YASARGIL 1975a; MACCARTY et al. 1975) no clear predominance of either of the sexes was seen, whereas DAHLIN and MACCARTY (1952) found a male predominance and furthermore an age range of 3–76 years, with a peak in the 6th decade and a mean age of 49 years (MACCARTY et al. 1961: 15 male and 3 female patients with sacrococcygeal chordomas). KLEINSASSER (1960) gave the following figures: 100 cases in the literature included 60 in male patients. This corresponds to the old rule that they were more common in the male than in the female sex at a ratio of 3:2.

Frequency: We have cited the average percentage in our series of 6000 as 0.2%. However, the increase, in the series of 9000 personal cases, to 0.8% stems from the great number of cases sent in for classification and is therefore unnatural. In STEWART and MORIN's (1926) series they accounted for 1.5%, while in CUSHING's series (1932, 1935: 2023 cases) only 2 chordomas had occurred (see BAILEY and BAGDASAR 1929). In HARVEY and DAWSON's (1941) series also, among 16000 tumors of all sorts 14 certain and 5 probable cases were found; PETIT-DUTAILLIS et al. (1952) reported an incidence of 0.1%, whereas in SCHISANO's series the incidence was 0.15% (SCHISANO and TOVI 1962).

Site: The old COENEN (1925) classification included the following groups by site: (a) the clivus; (b) the sella; (c) the nasopharyngeal system; (d) the dens epistrophi; and (e) extrachordal regions. FALCONER et al. (1968) only distinguished sellar, parasellar, and clival (intracranial) chordomas. HARVEY and DAWSON (1941) gave the following breakdown of their 240 cases: cranial 37%, vertebral 12%, sacrococcygeal 51%; while DAHLIN and MACCARTY (1952) reported: clivus 15 cases, cervical 9, thoracic 1, lumbar 2, sacrococcygeal 32. According to FLETCHER et al. (1935) two-thirds of the chordomas in their series were in the sacrococcygeal region. Of the others, eight were on the clivus, four cervical, two thoracic, and three lumbar.

The combination of intrasellar chordoma and suprasellar craniopharyngioma has been described (BELZA 1966).

With rare exceptions, chordomas are midline tumors occurring at the base of the skull at intrasellar, or subsellar sites or on the clivus, from where they expand, causing much bone destruction in the direction of the nasopharynx, the chiasm, or the foramen magnum (clivus chordomas). Spinal chordomas are found predominantly in the vicinity of the dens of the axis and in the sacrococcygeal region (see SUNDARESAN et al. 1979: 54 cases). Intracranial forms comprise 39% of all chordomas (SCHECHTER et al. 1974).

Gross Pathology

The chordomas are whitish pink in color, translucent and gelatinous, or (after hemorrhages) brownish red. Their consistency may be soft, mucous, or elastic. Their surface is finely nodular or occasionally they are even broken up into larger nodular segments. In size they vary from that of a millet seed, or cherry (noted only incidentally, RIBBERT and STEINER 1894) to that of a man's fist. Indeed, in the true pelvis they can attain the size of a child's head by growing with an anteroposterior orientation. Calcification is apparently more common than reports suggest (SCHECHTER et al. 1974). Some chordomas penetrate the skull and invade connective tissue and musculature.

Histologic Appearance

The tumor tissue is rather typical and corresponds to the basic pattern of notochordal tissue, i.e., it consists of vesicular cells with chromatin-rich nuclei, which in a way resemble plant cells. Collagen or less hyalinized connective tissue or osteoid regions sometimes extend through the tumor. The center of the growth often contains closely packed cells that are less vesicular than the others and have smaller eccentrically sited nuclei.

Generally it can be said that the more immature tumor cells are smaller and more like stellate elements, whereas the more mature cells are larger, contain a well-differentiated cytoplasm that will soon undergo mucous degeneration.

Regressive processes consist mainly of mucoid degeneration, while hemorrhages, calcification, and necrosis can occur.

Ultrastructure and Tissue Culture

SOFFER et al. (1970), GESSAGA et al. (1973), FU and PRITCHETT (1975), TRIPIER et al. (1975), and MIKRUZ et al. (1977) have described these processes.

Differential Diagnosis

All tumors occurring at the predilection sites of the chordomas have to be subjected to differential diagnosis. Calcification and invasion of bone make it difficult to distinguish the chordomas from the chondromas or chondrosarcomas. Some types of pituitary adenomas can be slightly similar.

Biologic Behavior, Metastasis, and Recurrence

Anaplasia has been defined by an elevated number of mitoses, hypercellularity, pleomorphism, and low vacuolization; it occurs according to KERNOHAN and

SAYRE (1952) and KRAYENBÜHL and YASARGIL (1975a) in 10% of chordomas. This problem has been also discussed by BOEMKE and JOEST (1936), POPPEN and KING (1952), and BRANDENBURG (1958). Invasiveness was considered an undoubted sign of malignancy by SCHISANO and TOVI (1962) and DAHLIN and HENDERSON (1962).

However, the problem of malignancy needs further clarification. To my mind the elevated cellularity and number of mitoses and the lack of differentiation of the cells, the occurrence of necrosis, and perhaps even the abundant vascularity may be characteristic signs, but invasiveness alone occurs too often to count as a sign of malignancy.

Metastasis has been described by HASS (1934), and MACCARTY et al. (1961, 1975, 2 of whose patients died from generalized seeding); according to STOUGH et al. (1971), and SASSIN (1974) it occurs in less than 10% of cases.

Clinical Course and Diagnosis

Complete erosion of the sacrococcygeal region (KAMRIN et al. 1964) may help in diagnosis by x-ray, whereas CT gives a better picture of destruction not visible on x-ray (SCHECHTER et al. 1974). Vascular chordomas are visualized by angiography (SMINCK et al. 1977).

Treatment

As long ago as 1929, BAILEY and BAGDASAR expressed the opinion that there was little hope that chordomas could be totally removed. However, sacrococcygeal forms have been completely excised (KAMRIN et al. 1964). FALCONER et al. (1968) achieved good improvement in five of nine cases. Recurrent surgery was discussed by POPPEN and KING (1952) and CANCILLA et al. (1964); a combination of surgery and radiation was used in the last decade (BECKER et al. 1975) in a child of 21 months, probably the youngest patient.

Survival Times

The typical survival times mentioned in the literature are 2–3 years for cranial, and 6–7 years for sacrococcygeal cases (JENNY 1941).

Further References: JELLIFFE and LARKIN (1911), HÄSSNER (1912), KADOTA et al. (1980). Handbook articles: ZÜLCH (1956, vast literature), KLEINSASSER (1960), STEEGMANN (1971), SASSIN (1974).

24.3 Chondromas

Synonyms: Enchondromas, enchondrosis

Introduction

The chondromas feature in the WHO classification as *local extensions from regional tumors.*

Historical Note and Definition

Apparently the first description came from Sir Astley COOPER (see BIRKENFELD 1930). Later, general pathologists described the various forms (JOH. VON MÜLLER 1838; VIRCHOW 1863/65, 1875; VON RECKLINGHAUSEN 1866; COHNHEIM 1867; OLLIER 1900; M.B. SCHMIDT 1900; and others). E. MÜLLER (1913) gave a review of the literature and JAFFÉ and LICHTENSTEIN (1942, 1948), a definition.

The chondromas are whitish pink tumors (ZÜLCH 1956, Fig. 358; GP, Fig. 275), hard and firm in consistency with a nodular surface. They adhere firmly to the dura or the bone, which they invade and may destroy.

Epidemiology (Age – Sex – Frequency – Site)

Age: According to KLEINSASSER's (1960) data there is a peak in the age group 11–50 years (see also KLINGLER 1951). Chondromas occur in babies (15 months: DUTTON 1978).

Sex: According to KLEINSASSER (1960) there is a female preponderance (3:2) in chondromas of the base of the skull, whereas in the other intracranial forms they occur equally in both sexes (KRAYENBÜHL and YASARGIL 1975a, b: in 68 patients).

Frequency: These are probably very rare tumors (9 cases in over 6000 brain tumors, KLEINSASSER and FRIEDMANN 1958b; 3 cases in 2023, CUSHING 1932/1935; 4 cases in 4135, LEITHOLF 1956, Olivecrona's series; in our own series in 1956: 0.3% in 4000 CNS tumors). VENZONI (1942) found only 30 cases in the literature.

Site: Chondromas can arise from the dura of the falx (VERBRUGGHEN and LEARMONTH 1932; OBRADOR ALCALDE and SOTO 1953) but occur most commonly in the dura at the base of the skull close to the foramen lacerum, e.g., at the synchondroses (KLEINSASSER 1960, Fig. 15). They can also be found in the choroid plexus of the lateral ventricles or occasionally in multiple sites on the spinal dura. They have been observed in the parasellar region, the cerebellopontine angle (ARONSON and OTIS 1962), and in "intrapontine" (ISHII et al. 1974) and supra- and retrosellar sites, in the sphenoid wing, and in the paranasal sinuses. According to KRAYENBÜHL and YASARGIL (1975a, b), the sinuses, the convexity of the skull, and the basal synchondroses (sphenopetrosal, petro-occipital, spheno-occipital) are most commonly involved. In rare cases they occur in the vertebral column (GROTE and HOFFMANN 1957; SLOWIK et al. 1968), in craniospinal sites (EVERKE 1966), or in the lateral ventricle (WAGNER 1847; FENYES et al. 1965), or they are simply recorded as being in the middle fossa (HIRSCHFELD 1851) on the posterior wall of the petrous bone extending into the posterior fossa (ISAMAT et al. 1968; good pictures reproduced in the work of GREEN and CHILDREY 1939).

Chondromas are mostly solitary, but two extradural tumors occurring simultaneously in the temporal and posterior fossa have been described (SCHULZE

1954). If they occur in multiple sites in the spinal dura they do not usually act as space-occupying lesions (VOLLAND 1938).

Gross Pathology

Usually these are nodular lobulated tumors, with an opalescent surface of a soft to elastic consistency and with regressive changes taking place by mucinous alteration; formation of small cysts, calcification, and ossification are seen as secondary changes. They are encapsulated by the dura and have no boundary on the side facing the bone, which they not infrequently destroy.

They can be very large (9 × 6 × 5 cm; FENYES et al. 1965): in rare cases they can even almost fill one hemisphere (DE BUSSCHER 1939); attain the size of a fist (BRÜTT 1931; VENZONI 1942; BORMANN 1951); or attain a weight of 128 g (SMITT 1929).

Histologic Appearance

Cranial chondromas are similar to those elsewhere in the body, but they are more irregular in pattern and grow predominantly by expansion. Chondromas form hyaline cartilage, which is trabeculated and lobulated. The nuclei are isomorphous, small, roundish, and dark. Double-nucleated cells are rare. The connective tissue trabeculae house the vessels. There is a granulation of the hyaline substance, and myxomatous change is common with a formation of microcysts; calcification occurs and is seen as a diffuse or powdery incrustation. Sometimes lamellae of bony tissue are formed.

Biologic Behavior (Grading), Metastasis, and Recurrence

Chondromas are commonly the most benign tumors of the base of the skull. Malignant forms do occur, which are characterized by abundant cells, and these invade brain, muscle, and skin (KLEINSASSER 1960; see also Sect. 23.4). Extracranial metastases have been described (EL-GINDI et al. 1974). Destruction of bone (together with calcification) is considered typical (HIMURO et al. 1977) and cannot count as a sign of malignancy. Recurrences are not likely when the whole dura is removed or not sooner than 5–10 years after excision; radical removal is sometimes difficult because of the infiltration of bone (KRAYENBÜHL and YASARGIL 1975b).

Clinical Course

Surgery is the treatment of choice since no improvement has been observed following radiotherapy (PIEPGRAS et al. 1972). The prognosis of surgery is "gloomy, but not hopeless" (FALCONER et al. 1968). Late operations have been reported (LOEW 1953, from the Tönnis clinic, and LEITHOLF 1956, from the department of Olivecrona). A 44-year survival has been described (R.W. HARDY et al. 1978).

Further Reference: Handbook article: KLEINSASSER (1960).

24.4 Chondrosarcomas – Mesenchymal Chondrosarcomas

Synonyms: Chondroplastic sarcomas, chondrofibro-chondromyxosarcomas

Introduction

Both primary chondrosarcomas and malignant (anaplastically transformed benign) chondromas occur (see p. 479). In the literature a distinction is made between the mesenchymal and the subdural skeletal types, which is said to be important since they have different prognoses (ALVIRA and MCLAURIN 1978). The primary mesenchymal chondrosarcomas (RASKIND and GRANT 1966) do not arise from the bones of the cranium. They are mentioned as an entity in the WHO classification.

Historical Note and Definition

Apparently one of the first authors to report malignant chondromas or chondrosarcomas was WEBER (1866), followed later by SCHWERDTFEGER (1911), GESCHICKTER and COPELAND (1936), and LIST (1943a). Chondrosarcomas are malignant tumors of cells that form a chondroid substance but never any osteoid matter.

Epidemiology (Age – Sex – Frequency – Site)

Patients are usually between 20 and 60 years of age when they develop chondrosarcomas; in most series the male sex is twice as frequently affected as the female. They occur at the same sites as chondromas.

Gross Pathology

These are whitish gelatinous or hard lobular tumors infiltrating the brain (WOLF and ECHLIN 1936), muscles, bone and skin.

Histologic Appearance

The tumors are characterized by high cellularity with undifferentiated cells not forming real cartilage; the pronounced mitotic activity and the highly invasive properties are well known. Formation of osteoid is never encountered.

Biologic Behavior (Grading), Metastasis, and Recurrence

The prognosis is apparently very poor, since radical removal is rarely possible. However, they may be asymptomatic (ALVIRA and MCLAURIN 1978).

Metastasis: There may be extracranial skeletal metastases (WAGA et al. 1972; EL-GINDI et al. 1974).

Recurrence: Even after a fairly radical operation recurrence is common.

24.5 Liposarcomas

Liposarcomas are apparently extremely rare or nonexistent in the cranial cavity but are listed among the orbital tumors. They consist of polymorphous sarcomatous tissue rich in cells infiltrated with foamy fat cells.

24.6 Olfactory Neuroblastomas (Esthesioneuroblastomas)

Synonyms: Esthesioneuromas/neurocytomas/neuroepitheliomas

Introduction

The olfactory neuroblastoma is a tumor entity included in the WHO classification under *other tumors,* forming *local extensions from regional tumors.*

Historical Note and Definition

The olfactory neuroblastomas were first described by BERGER et al. (1924) and BERGER and COUTARD (1926), and probably develop from the olfactory mucosa. They can be induced as an experimental tumor in rodents (MENNEL 1972).

These tumors are rare, presenting usually as masses in the nasal cavity; in about 20% of cases there are also neurological symptoms, such as progressive visual loss, caused by intracranial invasion.

Epidemiology (Age – Sex – Frequency – Site)

Age: These are apparently tumors of middle age: no sex predominance has yet been established.

Frequency: The exact incidence is not yet known, but FAIRBANKS-BARBOSA et al. (1971) found 4.5% olfactory neuroblastomas among 104 malignant tumors of the nasal region. In 1963 HUTTER et al. apparently found descriptions of 18 cases; in 1973, A.E. HAMILTON et al. found 128.

Gross Pathology

The olfactory neuroblastomas are neoplasms invading the paranasal sinuses, the nasopharynx, the palate, the orbit, the base of the cranium, and even the brain, and they are locally aggressive in all directions (KINOSHITA et al. 1975). Growth seems to be slow.

Histologic Appearance

The olfactory neuroblastomas consist of long cells arranged in blocks with a lobular pattern, or of lymphoid cells. There are apparently two types of differentiation; (a) cells are arranged in neuroblastic true rosettes (Fig. 160), i.e., with neuronal tubules and agyrophilic processes extending toward a central blood vessel, or (b) they have no particular architecture.

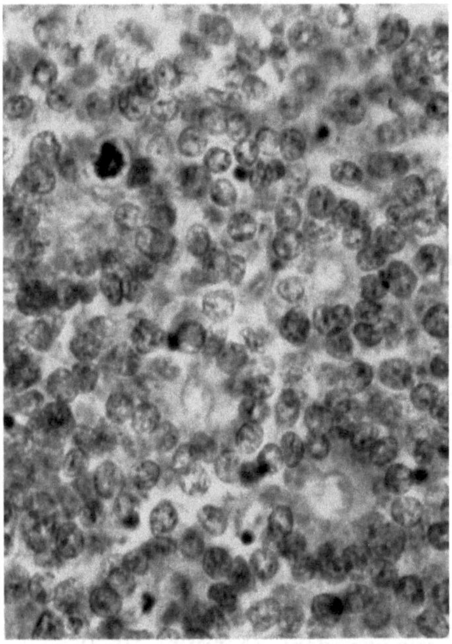

Fig. 160. True rosettes appear typically in retinoblastomas. Similar patterns are encountered in olfactory neuroblastomas. Cresyl violet, × 500

In the undifferentiated types the cytoplasm is scarce; in parts where they form rosettes there may be some resemblance to medulloepitheliomas. Argyrophilic processes may extend toward blood vessels.

In EM neurites with neurofilaments, neurotubules, synapses, and biogenic amine granules are sometimes observed, as is a poorly differentiated stroma (KAHN 1974; SCHOCHET et al. 1975; BERARD et al. 1976).

Differential Diagnosis

As MENNEL (1972) has emphasized, at least in experimental series there seem to be two types of tumor in this region: a genuine cancer of the nasal mucosa and a neuroepithelial neoplasm, i.e., the olfactory neuroblastoma.

Biologic Behavior (Grading), Metastasis, and Recurrence

This form of neuroblastoma is thought to be as malignant as the other types (grade IV), but survival times of 4 and 14 years have been recorded (JAKUMEIT 1971). Recurrences occur even if the tumors are thought to have been totally excised. Metastases are encountered in the CSF and visceral organs (A.E. HAMILTON et al. 1973: in 23 of 128 cases; SKOLNICK et al. 1966: in 11 cases in the cervical lymph nodes and in 11 instances in distant organs in a series of 97 patients).

Furthermore, intracranial extension with destruction of the cribriform plate and invasion of the frontal basis is possible, as are infections caused by invasion of the paranasal sinuses with consequent brain abscess.

Chemical treatment and radiotherapy are indicated even after local resection (ROBINSON and SOLITARE 1966). The clinical diagnosis can be in error when histories are particularly long (24 years: BERARD et al. 1976). Before the rare olfactory neuroblastoma is diagnosed, lymphosarcoma, anaplastic carcinoma, and similar tumors must be excluded (GERARD-MARCHAND and MICHEAU 1965).

Further References: FRÜHLING and WILD (1954), OBERT et al. (1960), DASTUR and LALITHA (1968), GOLDHAMMER et al. (1980).

24.7 Adenoid Cystic Carcinomas

Synonyms: Cylindromas, cylindromatous epitheliomas, adenoid cylindromatous carcinomas, adenocystic carcinomas

Introduction

These tumors are listed in the WHO classification as separate entity. Their position in the system of tumors has been discussed at length elsewhere (ZÜLCH 1956, p. 542).

Historical Note and Definition

The cylindromas were first recognized as surgical lesions by BILLROTH (1868), and their pathology was described by MARCHAND (1907), who himself described nine cases from the literature, five of which belonged to our group. He gave an exact description of these lesions from the morphological standpoint. For a precise description we are indebted to LEARMONTH and KERNOHAN (1930b), who described the tumor in a female patient aged 28 as a "neuroma originating from the capsule cells of the trigeminal ganglion." This case is recognizably an example of this tumor group.

Another case description ("muco-epitheliomas") came from JEFFERSON (1953). These cases were mentioned in the first edition of this book; my co-worker WALTER (1955) discussed our own experiences, which were also described elsewhere (ZÜLCH 1956), and a further extensive paper was later published by my group (see GONZALEZ and ZÜLCH 1964).

Epidemiology (Age – Sex – Frequency – Site)

Age: The age of our patients was between 40 and 65 years.

Sex: The group was made up of eight women and only one man.

Frequency: Data on the frequency of these tumors are vague. TITRUD and PEYTON (1940) recorded 5 "mixed tumors" (probably adenoid cystic carcinomas) among 159 nasopharyngeal space-occupying lesions.

Site: These rare epithelial tumors of "cylindromatous" architecture occur at the base of the cranium particularly in two sites, beginning as "nasopharyngeal"

tumors in the first instance. In these cases they force their way from the nasopharynx through the crista galli, displacing the fronto-orbital part of the frontal lobes upward like an olfactory groove meningioma (ZÜLCH 1956, Fig. 389; GP, Fig. 277). However, the adenoid carcinoma can be distinguished by the bone destruction that is always seen at the base of the tumor, and also by a corresponding change in the radiological appearance (plane x-ray) of the ethmoidal and sphenoid sinuses.

More commonly, however, they expand backward (ZÜLCH 1956, Fig. 390; GP, Fig. 278) in the direction of the Gasserian ganglion, which they usually invade, and also impinge the base of the temporal lobe. In this position they resemble the neurilemmomas in macroscopic appearance (see LEARMONTH and KERNOHAN 1930b), and regressive changes accompanied by the formation of small cysts are common. They can even expand so widely as to cause Garcin's syndrome (MASSEY and BRANNON 1980).

Gross Pathology

These tumors may be tangerine-sized, as in our autopsy cases (see above), or the size of a walnut when removed from the cerebellopontine angle. The site of the more anterior type is midline to the sella, usually eroding the ethmoidal anterior fossa.

Histologic Appearance

These are highly cellular epithelial tumors and form large epithelial islands, bands, and processes, which apparently liquefy centrally (Fig. 161), thereby forming the "cylinder." These regressive changes can progress to the point of a colloid-filled network similar to colloid goiter being formed (ZÜLCH 1956, Fig. 391a, b; GONZALEZ and ZÜLCH 1964, Fig. 6b). The possibility of actual secretion has to be considered. These tumors never infiltrate the brain.

Biologic Behavior (Grading), Metastasis, and Recurrence

Anaplastic alteration is not uncommon. We ourselves have noted a metastasis to the femur. They are classed as grade II or semibenign.

Origin

These tumors probably originate from the paranasal sinuses or the Eustachian tubes with their cylindrical epithelium.

Clinical Course

There is generally a history of several years, usually more than 4.

Operability: These neoplasms seem to be operable, particularly in the cerebellopontine angle as in our series and the case of LEARMONTH and KERNOHAN (1930b).

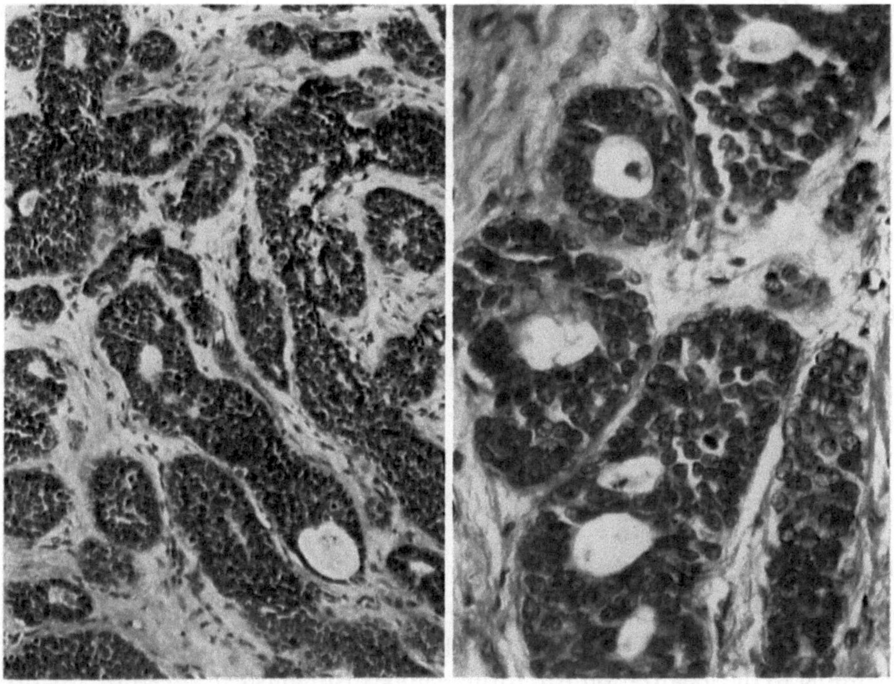

Fig. 161 a, b. Typical adenoid cystic carcinoma ("cylindroma"). The commencement of regressive changes can be recognized in the centre of the cellular islets. Later it leads to the cylindrical formations. H&E, ×125 (**a**) and ×272 (**b**)

Detailed descriptions have been given by ZÜLCH 1956, Handbuch der Neurochirurgie, Band III, p. 540ff.; KLEINSASSER 1960, Handbuch der Neurochirurgie, Band IV/1, p. 476ff.

Further Reference: SHINMURA et al. (1980).

24.8 Others

24.8.1 Osteomas

Synonyms: Fibro-osseous tumors, fibro-osteomas, osteofibromas

Introduction

The fibro-osseous tumors were well known to the classic scientists such as MALPIGHI (1628–1694) and MORGAGNI (1682–1771), and were closely studied by VIRCHOW (1863/1865) and BORST (1902a). They are of neurosurgical importance because of their appearance at the cranial vault, the synchondroses and the pneumatic chambers. These are mostly benign tumors (GESCHICKTER and COPELAND 1936; EWING 1939; HERZOG 1944; COPELAND 1950; HELLNER 1950; LICH-

TENSTEIN 1952; and others; see also the excellent and complete handbook chapter of O. KLEINSASSER 1960, with extensive references).

The osteomas appear as small tumors of the vault or in the frontal sinus (pneumatic chambers); they can grow also as large spongious tumors of the vault, and histologically as ossifying fibromas (osteoid fibromas).

Some forms, such as the "benign osteoblastoma" or "osteoid osteoma" are very rare in the cranium [personal observation in a 14-year-old girl, extradural site on lesser wing of sphenoid (unpublished)].

24.8.2 Osteosarcomas

Synonyms: Osteoplastic sarcomas, osteogenic sarcomas, osteofibrosarcomas, osteo-osteoid sarcomas

Introduction

These forms are only mentioned in the WHO classification of 1979.

Historical Note and Definition

VIRCHOW (1857, 1863–65) subdivided these tumors into malignant osteoid tumors, which consisted of the "osteoid chondromas," and "osteoid sarcomas." According to the localization two forms can be distinguished, (a) a rare "periosteal" form and (b) a common "central" form (for details see GESCHICKTER and COPELAND 1951; LICHTENSTEIN 1956; KLEINSASSER 1960).

Epidemiology (Age – Sex – Frequency – Site)

The osteosarcomas occur most commonly between the 10th and 25th years, and the male sex is affected twice as frequently as the female; the osteosarcomas are rare in the skull (20 cases up to 1960; KLEINSASSER 1960). CHRISTENSEN (1925) saw 8 such skull tumors amongst 441 osteogenic sarcomas.

Gross Pathology

These are invasive and infiltrating cranial tumors, which destroy the ground tissue; they have grayish and reddish areas and sometimes contain rests of bone.

Histologic Appearance

Microscopically they are highly cellular; they consist of fairly polymorphous elements, and have a tendency to form osteoid tissue, but chondroid parts are also encountered. More fibroblastic parts also occur (DAHLIN 1957). Necroses are sometimes formed, with secondary hemorrhages into the tissue.

Biologic Behavior (Grading), Metastasis, and Recurrences

Apparently the osteosarcomas are the most malignant bone tumors (DAHLIN 1957; 19% cure for 5 years, 15% for 10 years after surgery). GESCHICKTER

(1935b) reported metastases. Secondary brain metastases from osteosarcomas in the body have been observed (HARDING and COURVILLE 1934).

Further Reference: KLEINSASSER (1960, handbook chapter).

24.8.3 Nasopharyngeal Tumors

This is an ill defined group of partly benign, partly malignant tumors of the anterior base of the cranium, e.g., the benign juvenile fibroma-like tumors of the nose and pharynx and the so-called adenoid cystic carcinomas (cylindroma), which do not usually infiltrate the brain (see p. 485). The malignant tumors are of several kinds, e.g., carcinomas of keratinizing epithelium, lymphosarcomas, reticulosarcomas, and other "lymphomas"; probably the "lymphoepithelioma" (SCHMINCKE 1921) also belongs to the large group of lymphomas (WOLTMAN 1922; STOPPANI 1937; LOEPP 1939; TITRUD and PEYTON 1940). However, extradural parasellar meningiomas can also extend to the nasopharynx, and some pituitary adenomas extend sideways, undermining the cavernous sinus, in a similar way to the carcinomas that extend from the mucous membrane in the sphenoid sinus or from the nasopharynx (TAVERAS and WOOD 1964). In some cases, juvenile angiofibromas also extend from the nasopharynx, and may even destroy the foramen lacerum (THIBAUT 1963; SIEMSSEN et al. 1967).

The most common tumors of the nasopharyngeal region are transitional cell carcinoma and carcinoma with keratinizing epithelium; malignant papilloma and fibroepithelioma can also be highly invasive and destructive (BERENDES 1961). MARTIN and BLADY (1940) emphasized this region as the origin of most carcinomas of the base of the cranium, and WALTHER (1948) also found invasion of the skull base or the palate in 90% of nasopharyngeal tumors.

Most of these tumors have in common invasion from the nasopharynx toward the sphenoidal and ethmoidal zones and penetration of the foramen lacerum, which causes corresponding symptoms in the cranial nerves.

Other extensions are discussed in the sections on retinoblastoma, p. 301, rhabdomyosarcoma, p. 390, and primary malignant lymphoma, p. 394.

Further References: HANSEL (1932), DÖRING (1940), GODTFREDSEN (1940/41), NEW (1947), LEGLER (1949), RADCLIFFE (1951), ERICH (1955), LEMOYNE (1956), CANTRIL (1962).

25 Metastatic Tumors

Synonyms: Secondary brain tumors, *Tochtergeschwülste*

Introduction

Metastatic tumors feature in the WHO classification as a special group.

Historical Note and Definition

Classic pathology clearly recognized the process of metastasis, though some workers continued to assume a "coordinated neoplastic degeneration of the brain in the presence of general cancer disease of the body" (HASSE 1869, who also gave the first statistics on the condition). VIRCHOW (1863–1865) clearly recognized the process of seeding, but preferred the concept of the action of a cancerigenic agent (a "miasma") than the promotion of tissue parts or even cells, though he did not deny the latter process. The first well-documented reports were published by BUCHHOLZ (1898), GALLAVARDIN and VARAY (1903), GUTMANN (1904), KAUFMANN (1906), KRASTING (1906), and later ones by HASSIN and SINGER (1922), BRUNNER (1936), ZAAIJER (1938), MINKOWSKY (1941), WALTHER (1948), and GÄRTNER (1955b). For later detailed reports see: JÄNISCH, GÜTHERT and SCHREIBER (1976) and TAKAKURA, SANO, HOJO and HIRANO (1982).

The existence of a secondary spread to the brain from tumors elsewhere in the body has received a great deal of attention because of the increasing incidence of some of the primary tumors (bronchogenic carcinoma). In some cases brain metastases of body tumors are operated on knowingly, in others without recognition of their nature.

Metastasis is by definition the origin of a blastoma, which is morphologically identical with a primary tumor from which the secondary is separated. Metastases from primary brain tumors to the body are described on p. 183 and by JÄNISCH et al. (1976).

Epidemiology (Age – Sex – Frequency – Site)

Age: The age incidence for brain metastases corresponds to that for the primary tumor, but there are many exceptions from this rule. Seeding may have effects that are delayed by up to 20 years, as described in the literature (15 years after mammectomy: BAKER and WEYAND 1951; 16 years after pneumonectomy: DANIEL 1964; 15 years even after operation of solitary tumors: MCNEEL and LEAVENS 1968).

The age incidence depends on the type of tumor and it is therefore difficult to give figures. Our own age curves showed a peak around the age of 60 for men, and around 55 for women (Fig. 9m). Our youngest patient was 14 years old, the oldest 80 years. More detail has been given by JÄNISCH et al. (1966).

Sex: Apart from the different ages at manifestation of the sex-dependent tumors there does not seem to be any difference between the two sexes in the seeding of body tumors to the CNS. The apparent contemporaneous sex dependence of bronchogenic carcinoma, for instance, is also expressed by our figures; we had a 9:7.5 ratio of male to female in our global figures for metastatic tumors. ZAAIJER (1938) also reported a male predominance (27 males, 10 females). Other pertinent data are given by LILL (1952), and BRIHAYE (1963).

Frequency: The average frequency of brain metastases varies more widely than that of any other type of brain tumor for which statistics are available, and depends on the source of the clinical patients (e.g., 3%–5% in the present author's series). It can be up to 37% in a pathology institute. In the contrary metastases comprised 3.2% of the brain tumors in the series of CUSHING (1935); 4.7% of the cases of ELSBERG and GLOBUS (1929); and 5% (740 cases) in ZAAIJER's tabulation of SCHÖNBAUER's cases (1938) in the First Surgical Department in Vienna.

The figure is higher, however, in other series: over 10% in that of LILL (1952) and 12%–13% in others (ELKINGTON 1935). Yet, most figures oscillate around 4% in Tönnis' neurosurgical series (TOBIAS 1943) and 3.5% in Olivecrona's series of 4444 cases (STÖRTEBECKER 1954); WILLIS (1960) reported 4.6%; and GRANT and SAYERS (1951), 4%. On the other hand, in a tabulation prepared by HENSCHEN (1955, p. 649, literature cases) the proportion of metastases ranged from 37% to 40%! This shows better than anything else how the percentages depend on the institutions.

Another important proposal has been reported by POSNER (1977), viz. that in patients with systemic cancer there will be cerebral seeding in around 12%, the same percentage as has been given by CAIRNCROSS et al. (1979).

In more recent series examined at the pathology institutes of Erfurt and Halle (1954–1970: German Democratic Republic), 7.3% of the malignancies observed had a cerebral localization.

It is well known that the relative frequency of some tumors has been increasing in the last decades, e.g., that of bronchogenic carcinomas; HENSCHEN's figure of 1955 shows 27.4% metastases into the cerebrum, as against 50.9% in the 1205 metastases of JÄNISCH et al. in 1976 (66001 autopsies, 16584 malignancies). The increase in the figures of O. KOCH (1950) is also typical: for the years 1920–1923, 3.6% bronchogenic carcinomas; in 1948 as many as 35.5%. Similar figures have been published by HEPPNER (1952: tabulation), TREVISAN and DETTORII (1972), and EARLE (1954). This is also, finally, in keeping with the increase from 9.7% metastatic tumors in the series of KRASTING in 1906 to 25.1% in the global figures of JÄNISCH et al. in 1976 in pathology institutes.

There are some data, which is important to know, i.e., those for the relative frequency with which the different body organs are affected by the process of seeding. In the older statistics carcinomas of the lung, the breast, and the gastrointestinal system, etc. featured most prominently.

In neurosurgical series such as that of STÖRTEBECKER (1954, patients of Olivecrona), the various types of body cancer occurred in the following sequence of frequency: bronchogenic carcinomas, clear cell carcinomas of kidney, breast carcinomas, sarcomas, melanosarcomas. HENSCHEN (1955, Table 15, p. 650) had the identical order in 1542 metastases: bronchial carcinomas (27.4%), breast carcinomas (21.1%), kidney cancer (9.6%), gastrointestinal tumors (6.8%), melanomas (4.7%), sarcomas (3.9%). Similar figures were given by WALTHER (1948), GAMA (1949), LILL (1952), and GÄRTNER (1955b).

In one of the most recent neurosurgical series (BUSHE and KLENGEL 1972, cited in BUSHE 1972, Table 2) the following body cancer types were representative: among 202 cases there were 84 of lung cancer, 20 of breast cancer, 17 of renal cancer, 14 of gastrointestinal cancer, and 14 of melanomas.

Site: It used to be claimed that metastasis to the posterior fossa was more frequent than metastasis to the supratentorial space. This, however, has not been proven by data and it can be assumed that the ratio of supra- to infratentorial metastases probably corresponds to the ratio of space volume of the cerebrum to the cerebellum, viz. 8:1. Generally, localization of metastases will depend on the mechanism of seeding, that is to say it will be different in hematogenous (for details see JÄNISCH et al. 1976), lymphogenous (which is yet not proven), and CSF paths of propagation, as discussed by BLINZINGER and HENN (1966). Moreover, it can be imagined that parts with denser capillarization would have a higher percentage of metastases.

R.A. PFEIFFER, Leipzig (1951) has shown a particularly clear example of seeding into layer IV a/b in the optic areas of the occipital lobe. However, this mechanism cannot be accepted as a frequent event. Generally, dural involvement must be distinguished from subdural, leptomeningeal, and intraparenchymatous involvement (OI and GALICICH 1978; HOJO et al. 1978).

Early opinions that the left side is more frequently affected by the process of seeding (KRASTING 1906; SILVAN 1914; BRUNNER 1936; MCLEAN 1936a) have not been proven by later figures.

Whether a site of low resistance (traumatic contusion) can offer a preferential localization for seeding is still an open question (see ZÜLCH 1956, p. 580).

The following types of localization can be found in the CNS:

1. Brain and spinal cord
2. Pia and arachnoidea
3. Dura
4. Intradural parts of the cranial and spinal nerves

The metastases can also be subdivided into dural, subdural, leptomeningeal, intraparenchymatous involvement (OI and GALICICH 1978; HOJO et al. 1978). In the brain the most common localizations in declining order of frequency are (BRUNNER 1936): occipital, frontal, cerebellar, parietal, temporal. KRASTING (1906) was of the opinion that the cortex was more frequently involved than the white matter.

Special Localizations: There are a number of special reports on seeding in particular organ parts, such as the pineal body (OUYANG and ROZDILSKY 1966; HOL-

NESS and SANGALANG 1976) and intramedullary sites (rare: WALKER 1967; SMITH and TURNER 1968; EDELSON 1972; KAWAKAMI and MAIR 1973; HIROSE et al. 1980; own observation); in the literature we find frequencies of 1.6%–3.4% for metastases in series of spinal tumors. Yet, WEST (1979) emphasized a higher relative frequency, viz. 20%–30%.

Seeding into the pituitary gland (HÄGERSTRAND and SCHÖNEBECK 1969; SCHNEIDER et al. 1972; STINTZ 1974), into the choroid plexus (ASKANAZY 1914), and into the base of the skull (GREENBERG et al. 1981), has been described. Metastases into the cauda equina are rare according to PUTSCHAR (1930).

Other special localizations are reported by KINDT (1964) at the "borderlines" of the source arteries in the brain (HERRMANN 1961). We have seen here, as in the "Dreiländereck" between a temporal, parietal, and occipital lobe, predilection site for infarction but never for seeding (ZÜLCH 1981 a, 1985).

On the other hand we know of a very unusual site (GO KIAN GWAN 1961), namely on both sides of the septum pellucidum 3–5 mm thick (GP, Fig. 306; see also 1956, Fig. 429; HERZOG 1950).

Metastases can be either single or multiple [KRASTING 1906, in KAUFMANN's material: one-third of the metastatic carcinomas and over half the sarcomas were multiple; ZAAIJA 1938: of 37 cases 12 were multiple; STÖRTEBECKER (Olivecrona's series) 1954: one-third of the metastases were solitary]. It is therefore estimated that about one-third to one-half of the metastases are multiple.

This multiplicity can be enormous: the case of BUCHHOLZ (1898), with about 100 secondaries, is particularly well known. VORDERWINKLER (1951), in a large Nissl section through one hemisphere, showed numbers of metastases that could hardly be counted. HERRMANN (1961) has counted 6071 single metastases in the supratentorial cerebrum (see also PENZHOLZ 1968).

Seeding into primary brain tumors has even been reported as has seeding into a pituitary adenoma (VAN DER ZWAN et al. 1971; SCHÜRMEYER and BETTMANN 1956), an acoustic neurilemmoma (WALLACH and EDBERG 1959; WONG and BENNINGTON 1962; LE BLANC 1974), a meningioma (BERNSTEIN 1933; BEST 1963 a; PEISON and FEIGIN 1961; WILSON et al. 1967; KAWAKAMI and MAIR 1973; SAVOIARDO and LODRINI 1980), a cavernoma (HIRTZLER et al. 1975), an oligodendroglioma (STRANG 1965), and, finally, a glioma (POSNIKOFF and STRATFORD 1960). (For details see JÄNISCH et al. 1976, p. 403, Table 109).

Gross Pathology

The size of the secondaries ranges from that of a pinhead to that of a tennis ball (Fig. 162). They can be sharply delineated (GP, Figs. 300, 303) and in rare cases they have an attachment to the dura (GP, Fig. 301) and may therefore be initially misinterpreted as meningiomas on operation. Metastases can also be diffuse and cystic (GP, Fig. 302); they can be soft or hard (Fig. 162; GP, Figs. 307, 308). In some cases only, the delineation from the normal tissue is sharp (Fig. 162), so that the diagnosis can be made by the naked eye. On the other hand, in rare cases seeding is so diffuse that the diagnosis of an inflammatory process seems more likely at first sight. The metastases are often nodular and round, or rather wedge-shaped with the apex pointing towards

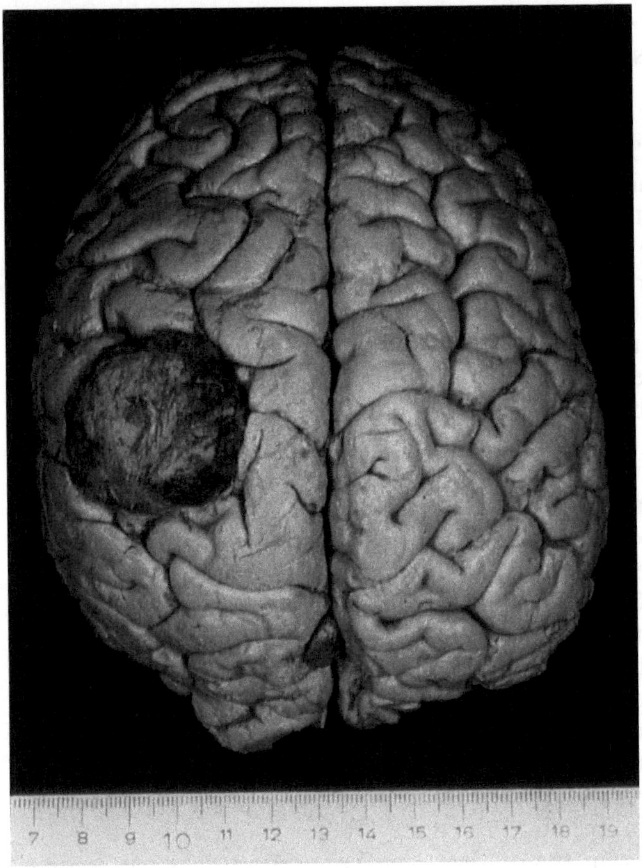

Fig. 162. Nodular, sharply demarcated, firm metastasis of a squamous cell carcinoma to the left parietal lobe. (ZÜLCH 1975a)

the ventricles. Metastasis to the leptomeninges (carcinomatosis of the meninges) results either in a diffuse whitish deposit, or in a formation of flat patches resembling sugar icing, particularly in the cisterns. Their cut surface is either finely tufted like asbestos (small cell necrotizing bronchial carcinoma), or smoother (squamous cell carcinoma). Liquefaction can lead to cysts (Fig. 163), predominantly in the bronchogenic carcinomas. Hemorrhages occur particularly in clear cell cancer of the kidneys, melanoblastomas, and chorionepitheliomas. The attachment to the surrounding tissue varies; either it is loose, in which case secondaries practically "fall out" of the brain tissue at autopsy, or the tumor is firmly fixed to the surrounding tissue, mostly the dura.

During the regressive processes, liquefaction (ARSENI et al. 1967) leads to an abscess-like appearance, and fatty degeneration is not uncommon.

Histologic Appearance

It seems superfluous to describe the histology of metastases, which depends on the primary, although it may be more dedifferentiated (see APITZ 1943), in which case it can be difficult to recognize the primary.

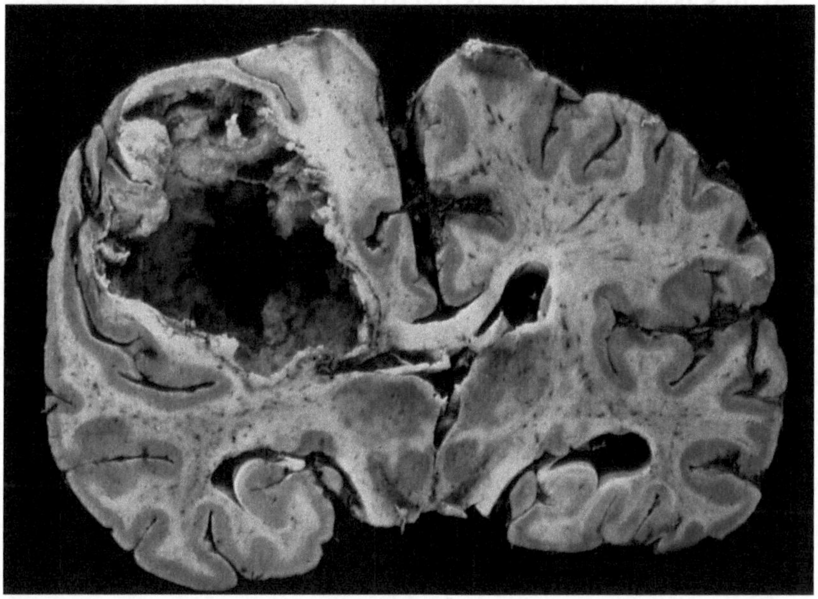

Fig. 163. Large cystic metastasis from a bronchial carcinoma (oat cell)

In one case of great legal importance we were able to recognize seeding of a small melanosarcoma on the skull to the brain by the occurrence of intranuclear "inclusions," which are a very typical characteristic of melanosarcomas. In this case there was a fist-sized leukometastasis to the brain (see APITZ 1937).

The production of brain edema and swelling must be emphasized; this can increase the volume of the "space-occupying lesion" in the case of a metastasis to many times the volume of the secondary. The yellow coloration of edema in the case of metastasis of a melanoma is a familiar feature (see Sect. 6.5). The various forms of propagation in secondaries are well known, as is the invasion of the cortex from the leptomeninges in cases of carcinomatosis following penetration of the pia by the vessels.

Examination by tissue culture, EM, and histochemistry has been described the various body tumors in the corresponding textbooks of general pathology.

Differential Diagnosis

There may sometimes be difficulties in recognizing the nature of an unknown tumor that is probably of secondary nature. We have mentioned above the occurrence of nuclear vacuoles (inclusions) in a case of melanoma (see APITZ 1937). The similarities between clear cell carcinoma (hypernephroma) and angioblastoma Lindau in its epithelial form should be emphasized (see p. 405).

Together with an experienced general pathologist, we ourselves once misdiagnosed a Lindau tumor as a secondary clear cell carcinoma, until the long survival and the negative result in diagnosis of a kidney tumor led us to the correct interpretation. The 15-year survival in a case of Olivecronas suggests to think that this may have been a similar situation.

At this point the reader is referred to our report (p. 493) of seeding of body tumors into primary brain tumors, which gives a very puzzling pattern particularly in the case of meningiomas.

Anaplastic oligodendrogliomas (see p. 255) can easily be misinterpreted, both macroscopically (reddish brown areas around a hemorrhage, black color of the edema in this case) and even microscopically, as metastases (melanomas, clear cell carcinomas, BURGER and VOGEL 1976). A melanoma sometimes simulates a subdural hematoma (PALMER and POULGRAIN 1978).

Surgical methods of differential diagnosis have been discussed by SCHIEFER et al. (1955a), and radiological methods, by TREVISAN and DETTORI (1972). Sometimes the removal of a metastatic tumor may precede the discovery of the primary tumor in the body by quite a long time. Clinically the long latency of seeding must always be borne in mind (e.g., 15 years after mastectomy; BAKER and WEYAND 1951). The question also arises as to whether a single cerebral metastasis should be extirpated even when the primary is not under control (BRENNER 1963: 4 years survival).

Results of Treatment (Surgery/Radiation)

The general rule is that solitary carcinomas should be attacked by surgery if the primary tumor is well controlled. This situation is not unusual in clear cell carcinomas of the kidney. Even in bronchial carcinomas the removal of a metastasis with pneumonectomy has led to survival for 16 years in one case (DANIEL 1964). Other long-term survivals have been reported by MCNEEL and LEAVENS (1968: 15 years). Even the removal of a recurrence of a solitary metastasis to the brain has been reported.

Yet, the figures generally given in the literature for survival of patients with metastases are very depressing: 2 months (BLATT and HØJGAARD 1963); 0–8 months (GRANT 1926); 3–12 months (LOKICH 1975). On the other hand we have optimistic reports such as that of SALERNO et al. (1978), who recorded that 13% of their lung cancer patients survived for more than 10 years; JACOBS et al. (1977) showed that 6% of patients with bronchogenic cancer had "silent" cerebral metastasis.

Table 101 of JÄNISCH et al. (1976) confirms the statements of both very short and long survivals; 22 (2.3%) of 947 patients had survived for between 6 and 15 years; HAAR and PATTERSON (1972) reported 10-year survival in 7 of 159 patients. Patients with solitary secondaries may have a longer average survival than 1 year (MAGILLIGAN et al. 1976).

The high operative mortality has been emphasized above (LILL 1952: 39%; GRANT 1956: 31%). Radiation alone may slow down growth and prolong survival (ZÜLCH 1969b, p. 93). More modern results have been recorded in larger series of patients treated with combined radiation and chemotherapy (LOKICH 1975).

Report on Special Types of Body Tumors

Bronchial Carcinoma

The proportion of bronchial carcinomas amongst the primaries of cerebral metastases has increased steadily (GUTTING 1940: 21.6%; GALLUZZI and PAYNE

1956: 25.7%; HOJO et al. 1978: 40%; JÄNISCH et al. 1966: 27.4% up to 1955, and 46.1% in subsequent years). The proportion has even been recorded as 65% (RICHARDS and MCKISSOCK 1968). Adenocarcinomas have been the most common (48%), and then squamous cell carcinomas with SALERNO et al. (1978); even adenomatosis of the lungs can seed (BINGAS and BÖHME 1964).

Renal Cancer (Clear Cell Carcinomas, Hypernephromas)

In older statistics these accounted for 16.38% (GUTTING 1940; HENSCHEN 1955, Table 15, p. 650: 9.6%); the proportion shrank to 8.4% in 1976 according to JÄNISCH et al.

Breast Cancer (Mammary Carcinomas)

Older series showed a 5% metastasis to the brain in patients with this body tumor (GUTTING 1940); however, this proportion later increased to 20% (JÄNISCH et al. 1966; HOJO et al. 1978), and even to 37% according to CHASON et al. (1963; see also YAP et al. 1978).

Gastrointestinal Cancer

Esophageal carcinomas are rare primaries for brain metastases (IRIE et al. 1978), though found more commonly by HERMAN and COURVILLE (1965); they accounted for 8% in the series of HOJO et al. (1978) but only for 1.8% in the series of JÄNISCH et al. (1976). This corresponds to the decreasing incidence of gastrointestinal tumors in the western world. The incidence is still very high in some provinces of mainland China.

One particular feature of gastric carcinoma has to be emphasized, viz.: the high proportion of cases of cerebral carcinomatosis, particularly with EBERTH's (1870) syndrome (53 cases of a gastric cancer primary in 143 cases of meningeal cancer; FISCHER-WILLIAMS et al. 1955; MAYER et al. 1978) in which it is involved. This is an old notion, although control of the primary may promote metastasis owing to the longer survival time.

A personal observation of Eberth's syndrome in cerebral carcinomatosis – which was later controlled for a long time by intrathecal chemotherapy – led to the discovery of a mucus-producing adenocarcinoma of the stomach.

Melanoma

Cerebral seeding has been reported in various percentages of patients with melanoma (AMER et al. 1978: 46% of 120 patients according to clinical examination and 75% at autopsy). Other figures have been supplied by HOJO et al. (1978: 50%); MCCANN et al. (1968: also 50%); PALMER and POULGRAIN (1978: similar 50%); GUPTA and BRASFIELD (1964: the highest figure with 90%). In the large autopsy material of JÄNISCH et al. (1976), 41% of the melanoma patients had cerebral involvement.

Further References: COURVILLE and SCHILLINGER (1939), MOERSCH et al. (1940).

Chorioepithelioma

A tabulation of the cases in the literature in 1975 (MEESE and GRUMME) contained 28 cases plus 2 personal observations. The percentage of cerebral seeding in choriocarcinoma in mainland China was 22.5% in 392 cases and 2.4% in 414 cases of malignant moles (HONGZHAO and BAOZHEN 1979). Intracranial hemorrhages were reported by KELLY et al. (1971) and VAUGHAN and HOWARD (1962), and emboli of chorioepithelioma simulating strokes by AGUILAR and RABINOVITCH (1964).

Thyroid Tumor

Seeding of thyroid tumors to the skull (HAMER and PIOTROWSKI 1973) and to the skull and vertebral column (PASSERINI and BERTAZZOLLI 1965) has been encountered, where surgery has been beneficial. Surprisingly, even struma colloides (ROHR 1958) and other benign tumors (ZAPATA and IGLESIAS 1964) seem to induce cerebral seeding. Spread from thyreogenic tumors along the spinal roots has been described by O. FOERSTER (1939a).

Others

Rarer types of body tumors also metastasize, e.g., adamantinoma of the mandible (I.C. BAILEY 1966), sweat gland carcinoma (MINCY and LEE 1966, only case), cylindroma (BIELEFELD 1955; see p. 485), thymoma (McDONALD et al. 1978), prostatic cancer (I. LEWIS 1967), hemangioendothelioma (NURICK and MAIR 1970), pleural mesothelioma (GRUMME and BINGAS 1973; JÄNISCH and ZIMMERMANN 1975), liposarcoma (LU and LEE 1961, with references), leiomyosarcoma (NIRMEL 1978), fibrosarcoma (ZUCKER et al. 1978), malignant lymphoma (in 25% as leptomeningeal seeding: OI and GALICICH 1978). the various forms of spread in leukemias have been discussed by SCHMITT (1970).

As a general comment we want to emphasize that we ourselves have seen predilections in particular cases of metastases, e.g., to the white matter more frequently than to the cortex. However, we have never managed to formulate any particular rule for the localization of the secondaries, or to note any difference between the two hemispheres.

Further References: WOJTEK (1949), FURLOW (1961), ARONSON et al. (1964), PIOTROWSKI et al. (1984).

26 Unclassified Tumors

Introduction

The series of CUSHING (1932, 1935) included 192 unclassified tumors, i.e., approximately 9.5% of the total. In our collection of 9000 tumors 3.2% were unclassified. We must expect, then, that 3%–8% of tumors in any series will not fall in any of the categories described above according to the system we have proposed. This may be attributable to the particular nature of some tumors, and these are the "unclassifiable" tumors in the strict sense of the word. However, it can also be due to inadequate technical requisites for study.

In some instances, owing to the nature of the surgery performed only a small amount of material could be retrieved from the aspiration flask, earlier, or be obtained now from stereotactic biopsy. The neoplastic nature of the specimen can be established in such cases, but a specific diagnosis of the tumor type cannot be made. This is particularly true of the pituitary tumors. CUSHING (1932, 1935) also included gliomas that were verified only clinically by demonstration of cyst fluid with the unclassified tumors, for example. Our cases were all histologically confirmed and *this seems necessary*.

It is often impossible to fit a particular specimen into the WHO classification system. CUSHING in 1935 mentioned a series of such tumors in which various diagnoses, such as sarcoma, ependymoma, spongioblastoma, and neuroblastoma, had been made. After a thorough study (see p. 191) we have designated such tumors "unclassified" and attempted to indicate their kinship or similarity to a known group by the addition of such designations as "ependymoma-like". In no case have we tried to *force* them into the classification, although we have given them a general biological characterization, such as malignant or benign, according to the recognized principles (see Sect. 2.1.1). As we have shown elsewhere (ZÜLCH 1950a, 1956, pp. 573–578, 1982a), some of these tumors may subsequently be assembled into a new group, along with other tumors, and be classified (see also FRIEDE et al. 1982).

New tumors are still encountered in our daily observations, which we have never previously seen; these have to remain unclassified, as I have recently discussed (ZÜLCH 1982a), until their nature has been clarified and a more frequent occurrence ascertained.

Yet, in concluding, we believe that one point cannot be sufficiently emphasized: *Never force a tumor into one of the classic groups*. For each of these the prognosis is well known and will spring to mind at once if the tumor is classed in one of them. A prognosis assumed on unjustifiable grounds can cause a great deal of trouble.

27 Parasitic Conditions

27.1 Cysticercosis

Historical Note and Definition

This most common parasite of man, occurring in the brain as small bean-sized cysts, is the larva of *Taenia soleum,* which is thought to have been known as long ago as in the Renaissance (MÜLLER 1558). Parasitism in man with spread to the CNS has been exhaustively described by HENNEBERG (1912, 1936), MATTOS-PIMENTA and BRANDT (1960), and more recently by TRELLES and TRELLES (1978).

Epidemiology (Age – Sex – Frequency – Site)

Cysticercosis does not single out any particular age groups. The occurrence of cysticercosis has varied from one century to another and from country to country and is generally decreasing steadily; it is still common in India, in Latin America, and in Eastern Europe (STEPIEN and CHOROBSKY 1949; STEPIEN 1962). VIRCHOW (1860) in Berlin found cysticerci in 2% of his autopsies; SIMMONDS (1907) in Hamburg in 0.025%; PINHEIRO and MELLO (1943) in South America in up to 1%; and FISCHER (1955) in only 1%. The frequency in 5469 patients in neurosurgical hospitals in South America was 1.3% (ARANA-INIGUEZ and ASENJO 1945); however, these patients accounted for 12.5% of their tumor series; in Mexico the corresponding figure was as much as 25%. The brain is thought to be affected in around 80% of cases of generalized cysticercosis.

The cysticerci settle diffusely throughout the brain, while outside the brain proper they infest the leptomeninges especially in the cisterns. It was stated early (HENNEBERG 1936) that cysticercosis is found particularly often in the aqueduct and in the fourth ventricle (giant cysticercus: CABRAL et al. 1974; HINZPETER and FLIEDNER 1975; POON et al. 1980).

Cysticerci sometimes attach themselves firmly to the neighboring tissue, in which they induce an inflammatory reaction (TSUKAMOTO et al. 1976 in the meninges). Sometimes they flow freely. There may be as many as 120–150 cysticerci in a single brain (personal observation 1956, Fig. 430; GP, Fig. 323). Spinal cases have been reported (MATTOS-PIMENTA and BRANDT 1960: in 10%; ROY et al. 1976), and even an "*intra*medullary" location has been encountered (GARZA-MERCADO 1976).

Gross Pathology

To the naked eye the cysticerci appear as floppy gray-red vesicles the size of lentils or peas, and filled with a clear or cloudy fluid. The watery contents contain either the larvae themselves or whitish crumbly masses. The cyst wall is later often calcified. It is reported to be visible on x-ray in 50% of cases (WAGNER and LANGE-COSACK 1936), 75% (DIXON and HARGREAVES 1944), or 30% (OBRADOR ALCALDE 1948).

In the racemose form, cysts – usually in the cisterns – lie one on top of the other, like a bunch of grapes (BICKERSTAFF et al. 1952; ZÜLCH 1956, Fig. 431; GP, Fig. 321; TRELLES et al. 1957). In our case (BEHREND et al. 1966, Fig. 2) these racemose cysticerci associated with a chronic meningitis induced a "stenosis" of one of the carotid arteries with an ensuing cerebral infarction.

Histologic Appearance

The picture is very uniform histologically: on suitable sections the outer membrane of the cyst and the larva within it can be seen. The cyst wall borders immediately upon the encapsulating inflammatory reaction of the brain or leptomeninges. This zone contains giant cells, epithelioid cells, further out, granulation tissue with fibroblasts, lymphocytes, and plasma cells, and lastly a capsule, consisting partly of glia and partly of connective tissue (ZÜLCH 1956, Fig. 432b). This capsule becomes calcified with time (JANSSEN 1955; see also above).

The condition can be recognized clinically if the cysticerci occur in the skin or eye, or if – when calcified – they are seen on x-ray. Because of their multiplicity, the cysticerci are difficult to attack operatively. Nevertheless, O. FOERSTER (1936) and many other authors (STEPIEN 1962; TSUKAMOTO et al. 1976) have successfully removed single vesicles from the Rolandic region (O. FOERSTER 1936, Fig. 71) or tumorous accumulations (or from the 4th ventricle) (ROCCA and MONTEAGUDO 1953; OBRADOR ALCALDE and LAMAS 1955; MATTOS-PIMENTA and BRANDT 1960: 35 personal cases; MADRAZO et al. 1979). Others have performed only decompression (TOLOSA 1954) in cases of increased intracranial pressure (LATOVITZKI et al. 1978). When cysticercus meningitis gives rise to hydrocephalus (DE FEO et al. 1975) atrioventricular shunts may be necessary (DIAZ et al. 1975).

Further References: ISAMAT DE LA RIVA (1957), INNES and SAUNDERS (1962), ARANA-INIGUEZ and LOPEZ-FERNANDEZ (1967), ŠLAIS (1968), RONGE et al. (1978).

27.2 Echinococcosis

Synonyms: "Hydatid cysts", *E. unilocularis* or *cysticus, E. multilocularis*

Introduction

Echinococcus cysts occur in the nervous system most commonly either intracranially (cerebral incidence is between 2% and 7.5% of the total cases) or in the spinal canal (1.94% of cases). The echinococcus or the hydatid cyst is a large uni- or multilocular parasite developing after tapeworm egg infestation.

It is well known and has long been described in Latin America, particularly in Argentina, Uruguay, Paraguay, and other countries raising cattle and sheep, and also in Algeria, Egypt, Palestine, Syria, Iran, Greece (GRIPONISSIOTIS 1957), and Turkey (KAYA et al. 1975: 17 cases among 500 brain tumors).

Epidemiology (Age – Sex – Frequency – Site)

The incidence of echinococci is definitely decreasing with the improvements in hygiene and veterinary services. Therefore, reliable frequencies cannot be reported (for Tehran ABBASSIOUN et al. 1978 reported 5 cases in 1500 CTs of patients with space-occupying lesions).

The age involvement data reveal that children are far more frequently compromised than adults (SCHROEDER and MEDOC 1951: 9 adults out of 42 observations: other statistics show a frequency 7 times higher in children). In Tunisia there was an incidence of 10 per 100000 population observed.

Gross Pathology

The unilocular cystic type and the multilocular form of echinococcus are different in appearance. The former are smooth-walled cysts (formerly 2% of all brain cysts?) the size of a cherry or a goose egg, with volumes up to 500–700 ml: ARANA-INIGUEZ and LOPEZ-FERNANDEZ 1967). They occur either singly or multiply with a daughter vesicle lying inside or outside, or floating free (POSSELT 1932; KAUFMANN 1922, Fig. 828, p. 1503). In the rarer multilocular form, however, the gelatinous vesicles are compressed and the membranes wrinkled. The skull may be eroded by underlying cortical vesicles and large areas of destruction occur, almost as holes (von LOESSL and von PAP 1941).

The echinococci in the vicinity of the vertebral column characteristically penetrate into the epidural space of the vertebral canal (DEVÉ 1928; our own case 1956, Fig. 433; GP, Fig. 322), as reported by ZEHNDER (1938a). In this event the vesicles extended over many segments in the form of long chains. Calcification is rare (OOSTHUIZEN and FAINSINGER 1949). Males are thought to be more frequently affected (3:2), and the age group affected seems to be particularly that up to 30 years (5–23 years: ÖZGEN et al. 1979).

Histologic Appearance

In a general way the histological description given for cysticercosis – as for other parasites of the same sort – applies here too: e.g., there is the parasite hyaline membrane, and the reactive zone with macrophages and granular corpuscles. Between the vesicles septa may proliferate and glial cells are often present.

Clinical Course

During ventricular puncture the vesicle may happen to be perforated, in which case specific diagnosis is possible on x-ray (ARANA-INIGUEZ et al. 1951a). The results of surgery are only fair, since cerebral echinococcosis is rarely primary and more commonly represents metastases from infestation elsewhere (see THIERRY et al. 1978, report on the East of France; SCHROEDER and MEDOC 1951). Former reports indicated that scarcely half the cases operated on have survived for any length of time. However, the results have improved meanwhile (ARANA-INIGUEZ et al. 1951b, 1952). A. SCHROEDER developed particular surgical techniques (see above). Vertebral cases can also be successfully treated by surgery (IVANISEVICH 1934, ZEHNDER 1938a). Diagnosis is now easier owing to the work of ABBASSIOUN et al. (1978), ÖZGEN et al. (1979), and HAMZA et al. 1982).

Further References: SALJMAN (1949), PINTO PUPO and MATTOS PIMENTA (1949), GOINARD and DESCUNS (1952), ARANA-INIGUEZ and SAN JULIAN (1955), INNES and SAUNDERS (1962), ARANA-INIGUEZ (1978), THOMSON (1978).

27.3 Others

Schistosomiasis (Bilharziosis)

Infection by *Schistosoma mansoni* takes place by permigration through the skin into the intestinal tract and from thereon by way of the blood stream. Thus, they gain access into the brain and spinal cord, where they produce granulomas up to the size of a pea or even of a hen's egg. The dura can adhere to these granulomas (CARMICHAEL and COWLEY 1952). The infection was common in South and East Africa, Egypt, Central America, also Brazil, and finally in Japan.

Macroscopically an abscess is formed. These "pseudotuberculomas" are surrounded by lymphatic and eosinophilic infiltrations (HUNT et al. 1948). Not infrequently the lesions caused by *Schistosoma mansoni* are localized within the spinal canal (PANNIER et al. 1977), provoking paraplegias. Apparently the most frequent cerebral abscess was caused by *Schistosoma japonicum* (see also SHIMIDZU 1935). Histologically chronic granulations with caseous necroses containing schistosoma eggs are apparent.

For the pathogenesis a venous localization is discussed, as is arterial embolism caused by the eggs. According to MATTOS-PIMENTA and BRANDT (1960), only 60 cases have been reported in the world literature.

Further References: BASSETT and LOEWENBERG (1949), COUTO and COSTA (1949), LICHTENSTEIN and SIMON (1951), GARCEZ DE SENA (1963), EL DIN MANSOUR and REESE (1964), BIRD (1978).

Paragonimiasis

This benign parasitic infection, occurring predominantly in the Far East, can lead to immigration along the vessels into the CNS (165 cases known in the mid-1950s); space-occupying lesions with cystic granulomas up to the size of a hen's egg have been described (KIM 1955). About 20 cases have been observed in the Southwest of Japan (WADA et al. 1975: 20 cases reported in 10 years in Kyushu). The lesions show small multiple calcifications and can be surgically removed (BUSCH and COOPER 1952; MATTOS-PIMENTA and BRANDT 1960; KIM and WALKER 1961; GALATIUS-JENSEN and UHM 1965; OH 1968; and WADA et al. 1975).

Further References: OH (1978).

Trichinosis

The very rare cases of granulomatous encephalitis caused by trichinella have a closer resemblance to encephalitides than to real space-occupying lesions of neurosurgical importance. In the western technological world they were extremely rare (see HASSIN and DIAMOND 1926; CHASANOW 1928; DANDY 1943).

Further References: ESCOBAR and NIETO (1972), KRAMER and AITA (1978).

Toxoplasmosis

Infection by *Toxoplasma gondii* occurs transplacentally and provokes severe encephalitis in the subependymal layers. The trend to formation of toxoplasma granulomas is less common than the formation of gross atrophic lesions caused by scarring of the subependymal white substances with subsequent atrophic hydrocephalus. Calcification of the compromised regions is constant. Our own cases have been described in detail by HECKER (1969). Good reference lists can be found in the publications of PINKERTON and WEINMAN (1940), FRENKEL (1949), CAIN (1953), WEISSE and KRÜCKE (1953), EICKE (1954), and COUVREUR and DESMONTS (1978).

Chagas' Disease

Similar pseudocysts to those seen in toxoplasmosis were also observed in Chagas' disease, which can cause inflammatory encephalopathy in children. This disease is not uncommon, particularly in Brazil (GARCEZ DE SENA 1963).

Further Reference: SPINA-FRANÇA and MATOSINHO FRANÇA (1978).

Amoebiasis

This was primarily a disease of the gastrointestinal tract, and as long ago as 1951 ORBISON et al. reported that they had collected 83 cases from the literature and added 5 new cases. Eleven cases located in the cerebrum have been reported (TAKARO and BOND 1958). As long ago as 1962 96 cases were already listed (LOMBARDO et al. 1964). Cerebral involvement was thought to occur in around 8% of 210 autopsy cases of amoebiasis. Cerebral cases can be successfully treated surgically (LENSHOEK et al. 1958). Histologically they present as necrosis and an inflammatory exudate varying in extent.

Further Reference: DUMA (1978).

28 Granulomas

The granulomas discussed here form either mass lesions or heavily scarred processes of the leptomeninges caused by the tubercle bacillus or the spirochaeta.

28.1 Tuberculomas

Historical Note and Definition

The tuberculomas of the brain and spinal cord previously constituted one of the most important and common space-occupying lesions encountered in neurological practice. They are now only rarely seen by neurosurgeons in the western world, though still very frequent in underdeveloped countries. In addition to the contributions of STARR (1886, 1893, 1894) and BRUNS (1904) and the comprehensive reports of VAN WAGENEN (1927) and VAN RASDOLSKY (1935) we will mention only the paper of DOTT and LEVIN (1939), who collected all the cases of cerebral tuberculomas seen within the British Society of Neurological Surgeons.

Historically interesting that the first space-occupying condition diagnosed solely by neurological means and operated upon successfully in 1882 – the case of Wernicke-Hahn (see ZÜLCH 1975b) – was a tuberculoma. Unfortunately the patient died a few weeks later of tuberculous meningitis.

Epidemiology (Age – Sex – Frequency – Site)

Age: Tuberculomas occur in all age groups but were formerly more common in childhood and adolescence whereas nowadays perhaps adults in the third and fourth decades are more frequently compromised in the western world (WHITENER 1978). The youngest patient in the literature is probably the one reported by the elder DEMME, quoted by BRUNS (1904), a child only 23 days old. Certainly these figures vary and depend on the way the material is collected, for there is hardly any other type of space-occupying lesion in which the figures vary as much as in tuberculomas: for instance there is a wide difference between Scandinavian and some South American countries.

Sex: Male subjects are thought to be affected twice as often as female ones (DESCUNS et al. 1954).

Frequency: In older statistics (PETERSON 1894, cited in RASDOLSKY 1935) tuberculomas accounted for 49.5% of 335 collected cases of brain "tumor." According to STARR (1886, 1893, 1894), there were 32.2% tuberculomas among 600 brain tumor patients, and in this group the incidence was as high as 50.8% in childhood and adolescence, but only 13.6% in patients over 20 years of age. Some decades later McLEAN (1935, 1936a) reported an incidence of 5–6 tuberculomas in 100 brain tumors for the year 1916, and only 1.4% for 1927; in 1941 OLIVECRONA noted only 1.7%. They are rare now in the United States of America, but may still be the most common space-occupying lesion in tropical countries (MATHAI and CHANDY 1967).

At the Charité, Berlin, only 3 cases occurred during a 5-year period (WENDT et al. 1969), a figure that corresponds to the observations of MAYERS et al. (USA, Bronx, 1978), who noted 12 cases in a 16-year period. In contrast, in Vallore (India) the incidence in children below 12 years of age was still 21.5%, and in DASTUR and DESAI's series (1965) these tumors accounted for 20% of all space-occupying lesions.

In our series tuberculomas comprised 0.5% and these figures correspond to those of CUSHING, who, however, did not advise surgery, so that they are understandably rare in his series of 2223 tumors.

Site: According to older reports tuberculomas are thought to occur 6 times more often infratentorially in children than supratentorially, while in adults the reverse was the case (MATHAI and CHANDY 1967, Figs. 8, 10–14); however, these figures vary, as in VAN WAGENEN's (1927) series only 3 of 17 were in the cerebellum. They are also encountered in the spinal canal intradurally (PARSONS and PALLIS 1965). They can involve the vertebral body (Pott's disease); less commonly they are found in the pedicle, the spine, and the transverse processes. The brain stem has remained a rare site (SUMRA et al. 1973).

Gross Pathology

Tuberculomas consist of a firm mass, nodular on the surface (ZÜLCH 1956, Fig. 434; GP, Fig. 325). They are grayish in color and usually well delineated. The center is usually necrotic with caseous material (ZÜLCH 1956, Fig. 435; GP, Fig. 324), which may liquefy so that at operation an abscess with fluid pus may be encountered. The size of a tuberculoma depends on the location of the infected region and its neurological importance (e.g., the time at which diagnosis can be made). It can grow as big as an apple (OTTOMO et al. 1976: 60 g). Not infrequently confluent tuberculomas are present. They are probably often multiple (24%–60% of cases reported earlier).

Histologic Appearance

Histologically the usual pattern of epitheloid cells, large polymorphous, polynuclear Langhans cells, some features of specific endarteritis, and marked cellular lympho/plasma cell inflammation in the marginal zones and the overlying meninges is encountered. Moreover, in some cases edema formation may be excessive, so that a real encephalopathy may be apparent. Transdural spread to the calvarium with specific osteomyelitis is rare (SINH et al. 1968). Tuberculomas are thought to begin their growth deep inside a sulcus and usually only circumscribed meningitis develops, although naturally diffuse spread can also occur.

Occasionally "growth rings" can be recognized on cut sections. Older tuberculomas can be recognized on the plane x-ray because of their calcification of some of the necrotic portions.

At operation, if there is neither an associated miliary meningeal tuberculosis nor a specific tuberculous meningitis, only the characteristic caseous consistency of the tumor's central necrotic core indicates tuberculoma. Diagnosis is easier, however, since CT is available.

Prognosis

Today, with antibiotic treatment, the prognosis of tuberculoma is better and not so hopeless as it was earlier: of VAN WAGENEN's (1927) cases only five were alive after 1 year. The combined statistics of DOTT and LEVIN (1939) already allowed a more optimistic impression (of 94 patients 16 died postoperatively; in 1956 SIBLEY and O'BRIEN: of 102 cases 23 died, 18 of these during surgery).

To date, total removal of cerebral tuberculomas is still the method of choice, even for miliary tuberculosis (LIEBERMAN et al. 1970). However, pre- and postoperative protection with antibiotics is absolutely indicated.

Further References: CAMERER (1940), CARRILLO (1940), OBRADOR ALCALDE and URQUIZA (1950), HOSSMANN and SCHÜTZ (1966), WILKINSON et al. (1971), REINA (1975), TYSON et al. (1978).

28.2 Gummas

Synonyms: Syphiloma, luetic granuloma

Of the various manifestations of lues, only the space-occupying lesions will be dealt with here, the so-called gummas. The description of luetic meningitis belongs rather in the textbooks of neuropathology and neurology. Gummas, just like tuberculomas, are steadily decreasing in frequency. There was still a 3.6% incidence of gummas in STARR's (1886, 1893, 1894) statistics, 0.5% in the series of CUSHING (1932, 1935), and the same percentage in GRANT and SAYERS' (1951) series. COURVILLE (1950) found 6 gummas (4 space-occupying) in a series of 15000 autopsies.

Apparently the incidence has now dwindled to 0.4%–0.5%. However, the same objections that were raised above about such statistics apply here too. The incidence given depends entirely on the region of the investigation.

According to earlier data, gummas had no special age preference, but nowadays infection is seen in the young and middle aged, and congenital syphilis is absolutely in the decline. In former times central, the hypothalamic and pituitary involvement were said to be frequent. The gumma of the calvarium that goes on to involve the brain is a genuine rarity, but multiple gummas are not infrequent.

Gross Pathology

A gumma can occasionally be identified by jelly-like infiltration of the leptomeninges, or chronic circumscribed meningitis. The leptomeninges may adhere to the dura. Symmetrical forms in both frontal lobes were described (PILLERI et al. 1974). Gummas are more difficult to separate from the brain than tuberculomas, since they are often fastened to the connective tissue of the vessels in their surroundings. They are softer and more elastic in consistency than tuberculomas, because of the preservation of connective tissue in their necrotic portions. They are rubbery (hence the name of "gumma"). Information about the histology and the differential diagnosis between tuberculous and luetic granulomas has been given in the classic neuropathology and pathology textbooks.

However, for diagnostic purposes three zones can be looked for (VON BAUMGARTEN 1881):

1. The "inner" nucleus of a necrosis with a firm network of reticular fibers between necrosis and scavenger cells.
2. Fusiform fibroblasts, intermingled with giant cells.
3. Marginal zones of chronic inflammation with lymphocytes, plasma cells, and giant cells.

The first surgical results were published by HORSLEY (1890) and MECEWEN (1893) followed later by DANDY (1938); the trend now is for conservative treatment.

I have briefly described a gumma in the cerebellopontine angle presenting as a mass lesion mimicking a neurilemmoma (ZÜLCH 1949a).

Further References: BECHTEREW (1904), COHN (1923), NONNE (1924), A. JAKOB (1927), JAHNEL (1929), BAGDASAR (1929), MARTIN (1929), D'AUNOY et al. (1930), SEZARY (1938), ALPERS (1939), ROGER and PAILLAS (1939), SHEPS and SIMON (1943), PAILLAS et al. (1950), BIANCHI and FRERA (1957), SALLES and PECKER (1961), OBLU et al. (1964), STORM-MATHISEN (1978).

28.3 Other Granulomas

Neurosarcoidosis

Synonym: Sarcoid granuloma, Besnier-Boeck-Schaumann disease

Historical Note and Definition

This disease of still unknown cause was described almost 90 years ago by BESNIER, who distinguished it from tuberculosis of the skin. Apart from BESNIER (1889), BOECK (1905) and SCHAUMANN (1917) made further important contributions to knowledge of this entity, which CRAVIOTO and FEIGIN (1959) already called a well-delineated disease. However, MATTHEWS (1965) gives a completely different ancestry.

KOLODNY et al. (1968) tried to sum up all entities well known up to now that could belong to this disease, e.g., granulomatous angiitis of CNS, allergic and hyperergic granulomatosis, and the Besnier-Boeck-Schaumann forms. In the discussion of differential diagnosis this will be referred to again.

Frequency: Sarcoidosis is called a rare disease (ASZKANAZY 1952), the CNS being affected in 2%–8% (HÖÖK 1954; SILVERSTEIN et al. 1965; WIEDERHOLT and SIEKERT 1965; SUCHENWIRTH 1963, 1968).

All age groups are probably affected, with a certain predilection for the 16- to 45-year group; in the cerebral forms probably slightly more male than female patients are affected (SCHUBERT et al. 1971).

Localization is mainly cerebral, with a predilection for the pituitary gland, the diencephalon, and the thalamus; however, the spinal cord is affected in only 7% of cases. Lesions of the cranial nerves are very frequent.

Gross Pathology

Sarcoidosis occurs either as an individual granuloma or as coalescent large masses without any signs of caseous degeneration. However, according to GERAUD et al. (1965) this is not uncommon and therefore differentiation from tuberculosis may be difficult. The granulomas may be scattered in the arachnoidal spaces where there is opaque discoloration. The process is pronounced in the basal cisterns and around the optic chiasm. The granulomas occur also in the ependymal lining of the ventricles and in the choroid plexuses (HERRING and URICH 1969). Most cases are recognized even macroscopically, by the nodular and granulomatous appearance of the lesions and by the adhesions of the arachnoid to the dura. The mass lesions present as single space-occupying processes and are amenable to surgery.

Histologic Appearance

Sarcoidosis granulomas are encountered as clusters of densely packed cells with a certain perivascular arrangement. They tend to have a condensation in the cerebral regions with a high vasculature, as in the hypothalamus (see WILCKE 1956). The chronic inflammatory process consists of fibrocytes, epitheloid cells, and giant cells, sometimes with a calcified Schaumann body (HOLBACH and GADDONI 1971). The dense reticular network may ultimately be collagenized. The inflammatory cells are mainly lymphocytes and plasma cells. The heavy involvement of the arachnoidal spaces is evident even to the naked eye. Since the picture is not so different from that of other granulomatous encephalitides the differential diagnosis is by no means sufficiently clarified.

Differential Diagnosis

The diagnosis is easy only in cases with a generalized or peripheral manifestation of the disease. In the neuroradiological picture CT-dense masses (77%), which are enhanced by contrast medium, and sometimes the occurrence of an obstructive hydrocephalus may suggest the correct diagnosis (BAHR et al. 1978; LUKIN et al. 1975, obstruction of the outlets of the fourth ventricle; KENDALL and TATLER 1978).

Although CT has contributed (HORI and NAGAI 1974) much to the diagnosis, it was still described as difficult by LAUSCHKE (1964) and SCHUBERT et al. (1971), particularly since other methods of neuroradiology, e.g., angiography, are not helpful (KENDALL and TATLER 1978). The main difficulty arises from the far from simple classification of the various granulomatous encephalitides. The correlations to giant cell arteriitis and allergic and hyperergic angiitis have been emphasized in this regard (ZOLLINGER 1941; KOLODNY et al. 1968). Granulomatosis of the lymphomatoid type in the brain may culminate in leukoencephalopathy (VERITY and WOLFSON 1976; KOKMEN et al. 1977). Such granulomatous angiitis may occur in herpes zoster and lymphosarcoma (ROSENBLUM and HADFIELD 1972). GAGEL's (1941) case has only recently been claimed to be histiocytosis X; SCHOEPES' (1939) type of "blastoma encephalitis" and the various Wilke's type cases (1950) of encephalitis have not yet been adequately classified.

It is particularly difficult to distinguish the various hypothalamic granulomas (VOIGT and DIETZ 1972) that may have a different pathology from sarcoidosis; for instance, they may frequently be classifiable as histiocytosis X (e.g., GAGEL's case 1941; see below).

Surgery of the well-circumscribed mass lesions is possible (LAUSCHKE 1964; HOLBACH and GADDONI 1971). The effects of corticoid treatment, however, are not yet well defined.

The uncertainty in this regard stems from the lack of information about the nature of this disease, which has been called a "hyperergic" or an "antigen antibody" reaction (JEFFERSON 1957), an "autoallergic disease" (KOLODNY et al. 1968), or even a "virus disease" (ROSENBLUM and HADFIELD 1972).

Further References: KNAPP (1942), BUCY and OVERHILL (1950), ZEMAN (1952), SKILLICORN and GARRITY (1955), MATTOS PIMENTA et al. (1956), GARCIN (1960), PLAIR and PERRY (1962), VUIA (1966), BOELLAARD (1971), MATTHEWS (1979).

Histiocytosis X

Introduction

Histiocytosis X is a relatively rare granulomatous (inflammatory?) lesion presenting in the form of one of the traditional nosological entities such as Abt-Letterer-Siwe disease, Hand-Schüller-Christian lipoid granuloma, or eosinophilic granuloma.

Historical Note and Definition

LICHTENSTEIN (1953) coined the term of histiocytosis X for the combination of eosinophilic granuloma of the bone, Abt-Letterer-Siwe disease, and Hand-Schüller-Christian lipoid granuloma as related manifestations of a single entity. Later the well-known case of GAGEL's (1941) "hypothalamic granuloma" was also included as a "form of an eosinophilic granuloma" (KEPES and KEPES 1969; KEPES 1979). An excellent survey of the historical development of the concepts of the three entities has been published by KEPES (1979).

Classification

One could classify the diseases according to the three entities (see above) and the localization as follows:

Site (Common): Cranial bones, cerebral and spinal parenchyma, particularly hypothalamus, and also pituitary gland, meninges; also combined forms.

Site (Special): Spinal cord (SALCMAN et al. 1974), cauda equina (HEWLETT and GANZ 1976), intraventricular (MÜLLER and ORTHNER 1965). Of particular clinical importance are the forms within the hypothalamic region (GAGEL 1941; BERNARD and AGUILAR 1969; TIBBS et al. 1978). GAGEL gave an extensive report of circumscribed destruction of the hypothalamus without involvement of the pituitary gland. He excluded tuberculosis and discussed the syphilitic nature. The morphological picture was characterized by epithelioid cells, lymphocytes, plasma cells, Langhans cells, and a feltwork of silver fibers with eosinophilic cells present (see also TZONOS and BRAUN 1965).

Histologic Appearance

The histology of all three entities is characterized by the presence of mono- and multinuclear histiocytes with lymphocytes and plasma cells, and of eosinophilic granulocytes. Lipid material in the cytoplasm is present to various degrees. There is a dense network of reticular fibers. As a rule of thumb it can be emphasized that the degree of eosinophilic representation corresponds to the malignancy of the entity concerned (KEPES 1979). This, however, hardly counts for the eosinophilic granuloma.

Since Abt-Letterer-Siwe and Hand-Schüller-Christian lesions are mainly of medical importance, only the third entity, the eosinophilic granuloma, will be described below in more detail.

Etiology

The etiology has not yet been clarified for any of the entities. They have been classified as "inflammatory (?)" lesions with fulminating forms, like Abt-Letterer-Siwe granuloma (MILLER et al. 1978).

Treatment

Except for the eosinophilic granuloma (see below), medical treatment is required.

Prognosis

Abt-Letterer-Siwe disease is usually fatal: in Hand-Schüller-Christian disease a cure may be possible even with medical treatment. Eosinophilic granuloma can be cured by combined surgical and radiological treatment.

Eosinophilic Granuloma

Because of its surgical and prognostic importance this entity will be described in more detail. Eosinophilic granuloma presents with bone defects 1–5 cm in diameter, usually in the cranial bones with a predilection for the parietal and frontal region, and is either unilocular or multilocular (BRANDT et al. 1976: 21 patients, of these 8 with multiple lesions; of 38 foci 15 were parietal, 8 frontal). The base of the skull is sometimes involved (MILLER et al. 1978: foramen rotundum; see also LICHTENSTEIN 1964; SCHULZE and SCHNEPPER 1967; HELWIG 1972). The foci have irregular, more or less sharply defined edges, and the lesion contains a grayish green or pinkish necrotic material under a local elastic painful swelling and a bulge of the calvarium. The externa of the cranial bones and the diploë may be destroyed, but the dura, periosteum, and brain are never invaded in these cases (BECK 1943; SOLDATOV et al. 1954; BRANDT et al. 1976).

There may be a predilection for the first 20 years of life; no sex predilection is prominent.

Histologic Appearance

Granulation tissue consisting of epithelioid cells, fibroblasts, reticular cells and histiocytes, giant cells, foam cells, and abundant infiltration with eosinophilic leukocytes characterizes the picture.

Differential Diagnosis

Other osteolytic processes, such as metastases, reticular sarcomas, tuberculomas, gummas, have to be excluded. In the particular cases of involvement of the cerebral tissue (see above) eosinophilia of blood and CSF (SIVALINGAM et al. 1977) are significant [although not present in GAGEL's (1941) case, in spite of the abundant eosinophilic leukocytosis within the granuloma].

Therapy

The therapy of choice seems to be combined surgery and radiation.

Prognosis

With such therapy the patients may be cured, but recurrences or multilocular manifestation and occasionally also transition of eosinophilic granuloma to other more malignant forms of histiocytosis X (LICHTENSTEIN 1964; SCHULZE and SCHNEPPER 1967; HELWIG 1972) have been reported.

The question arises, then, whether a consistent standpoint should be preserved in the definition when there are two points of growth: the more benign form, or eosinophilic granuloma, and the absolutely fulminating forms (MILLER et al. 1978), where particularly an inflammatory nature is suggested. One could also ask whether in future eosinophilic granuloma should be excluded, again because it is so amenable to surgery and radiotherapy, from the entity of histiocytosis X, which would still include Abt-Letterer-Siwe disease (prognosis fatal) and Hand-Schüller-Christian disease, the latter having the potential for either a benign or a malignant course.

Other Granulomas

There are also rare granulomas that must sometimes be differentiated from true tumors. These include multiple, often diffuse, lesions with chronic inflammatory infiltration, giant cells, and frequently eosinophilic elements, which in some cases form dense reticulin fiber networks. In the differential diagnosis, encephalomyelitides have to be considered, and some cases are even reminiscent of multiple sclerosis (H.J. SCHERER 1938) or diffuse sarcomatosis of the leptomeninges (see p. 386). These are probably specific granulomas (WILKE 1955) – possibly due to viruses – that may be related to Hodgkin's disease (SCHÖPE 1938, 1939). Furthermore, many cases of histiocytosis X have been described that are difficult to subclassify (GUARNASCHELLI et al. 1979; VAQUERO et al. 1979; KHAN et al. 1980; TAYLON and DUFF 1980).

28.4 Mycotic (Fungal) Infections

(see also FETTER et al. 1967; RIPPON 1978)

Actinomycosis

Synonym: Nocardiosis is occasionally classified as a subgroup of actinomycosis

Introduction

A well-known fungus infection is caused by the Wolf-Israel Actinomyces. The granulomas caused by *Nocardia asteroides* are now regarded by some authorities as a separate entity (FINKEMEYER et al. 1967; see also COTTIER 1980, p. 1994). Intracranial forms of actinomycosis are not so rare.

Historical Note and Definition

LANGENBECK (1845) seems to have been the first to describe actinomycosis in man, followed by PONFICK (1882) and EPPINGER (1890), who already noted abscess formation. In 1887 BOLLINGER is thought to have described the first actinomycotic granuloma within the third ventricle, followed by STERNBERG (1931) and finally HALLERVORDEN (1931), who even then gave the characteristic description of a translucent mass, clay colored and of soup-like consistency. The mass was thought to have a gelatinous center. Nocardiosis was formerly not distinguished from actinomycosis, since *Nocardia asteroides* and *brasiliensis* were said to belong to the "actinomycotic mycetomas."

Epidemiology (Age – Sex – Frequency – Site)

Actinomycosis is thought to affect persons in their twenties and thirties. The male sex is somewhat more often affected than the female.

The frequency varies with the region. FRIEDMANN and LEVY (1937) found 108 cases in the literature up to 1937. STEFANKO and GROCHMAL had already collected 138 cases of cerebral actinomycosis by 1962. In the series of FABIANI et al. (1975) of 3300 tumors in North Italy only 1 case of actinomycotic granuloma was diagnosed. MATTOS-PIMENTA and BRANDT (1960) estimate the frequency at 0.2%, which is similar to the figure given by TYSON et al. (1979).

Extracranial actinomycotic abscesses tend to disseminate to the brain (PRESANT et al. 1973: in 36%). The actinomycotic mass frequently grows extradurally (cranial nerves, vertebral column). Later it localizes as a meningoencephalitis with abscesses. These granulomatous masses or abscesses are then present throughout the brain and frequently multiple, they may also form subdural empyemas.

Gross Pathology

Most commonly, actinomycotic infection occurs as an *actinomycoma,* but there can be secondary ruptures into the ventricles (ELSAESSER 1950 in 60% of cases) (also in colloid cysts?). Well-circumscribed granulomas have been described. Two different forms of involvement can be differentiated: (a) diffuse invasion of the meninges; and (b) granuloma, often transforming to abscess.

Histological Appearance

A typical granulomatous process with the actinomyces drusa within the pus is diagnostically convincing (see MATTOS-PIMENTA and BRANDT 1960, Fig. 17).

Therapy

MUNSLOW (1954) and SCHNEIDER and RAND (1949), like BRANDT (1960), have reported successful recovery after surgery.

Further References: LEY et al. (1951), KRÜGER et al. (1954), TURNER (1954), KLOSS and THURNER (1955), CAUSEY (1978), CAUSEY and LEE (1978).

Nocardiosis

Synonym: occasionally classified as a subgroup of actinomycosis

Nocardiosis (asteroides) is now considered by some authorities to be a separate entity. It is thought to be particularly harmful to the human organism (STEVENS 1953). Nocardia infections commonly prefer the hematogenous route after entering the lung, while Actinomyces spreads by direct invasion. KRÜGER et al. (1954) reported 18 processes caused by Nocardia, and MUNSLOW (1954) one recovery after Nocardia abscess formation, which is the most common cerebral form of involvement. In a review of 147 cases of nocardiosis PRESANT et al. (1973) found a 36% incidence of cerebral abscesses. The mortality is still high despite sulfonamide administration (COOK and FARRAR 1978).

Further References: INNES and SAUNDERS (1962), FINKEMEYER et al. (1967).

Aspergillosis of the CNS

Introduction

Of the many hundreds of different types of aspergillus, only a few are pathogenic for man. The first case is thought to have been described by OPPE (1897).

Up to 1971 only 11 cases of solid aspergillotic granulomas had been described (LINARES et al. 1971), but by 1973 reports of 65 cases had been collected (VISUDHIPHAN et al. 1973), and 30 more up to 1978 (MOHANDAS et al. 1978). The typical patient is a middle-aged man, living in a rural district and showing signs of an expanding process.

Gross Pathology

The lesions caused by aspergillus can be

1. Granulomatous, nodular, forming micro- or macroabscesses, situated usually in the cerebrum and rarely in the spinal cord (DESHPANDE et al. 1975)
2. Aneurysms or thromboses of extra- or intracranial arteries (KAUFMAN et al. 1976), with either infarction or subarachnoid hemorrhage

The typical surgical lesions can be isolated (left parietal granuloma: VISUDHIPHAN et al. 1973; LINARES et al. 1971) or even multiple (bilobed frontal and left parietal: KAUFMAN et al. 1976). Occasionally the lesion is located within the ventricular system (fourth ventricle: CORREA et al. 1975). Not so infrequently local aspergillosis follows surgical treatment of a neoplasm (olfactory meningioma: GALASSI et al. 1978). In the literature some cases are reported in which the mass was located in the paranasal sinuses (intrasphenoidal) (LE CLECH et al. 1978; MOHANDAS et al. 1978).

Entrance of the aspergillus infection by the nose can lead either to diffuse involvement taking the form of meningitis at the base of the brain or to a brain abscess (EGER and KÜHRT 1954; MUKOYAMA et al. 1969).

Prognosis

According to BRANDT (1960), infections by aspergillus fumigatus all had a fatal outcome. GALASSI et al. (1978) reported that there are survivors but the prognosis is poor.

Further Reference: SARAVIA-GOMEZ (1978a).

North American Blastomycosis

CNS involvement was found in 8 of 25 autopsied cases (Veterans Administration Hospitals 1964) with North American blastomycosis. Altogether only 17 cases of blastomycotic meningitis have been reported (CARMODY and TAPPEN 1959). The only treatment, however, is nonspecific antibiotics (UTZ 1967).

Further References: North American blastomycosis (34 cases reviewed): HABTE-GABR and SMITH (1973), LEERS (1978); Paracoccidiomycosis (skull): KRIVOY O et al. (1978). For comparison South American blastomycosis (posterior fossa tumor): ARAUJO et al. (1978).

Candidiasis

Synonym: Moniliasis

In Kentucky – in an area where fungal infection is endemic – 1752 consecutive complete autopsies performed in 1964–1973 were reviewed, among which 14 patients (0.8%) had histologically confirmed fungal infections in the brain. The most prevalent fungus was *Candida albicans,* which was observed in 6 patients (PARKER et al. 1976). The use of antimicrobial agents, corticosteroids, and other immunosuppressive drugs has reinforced the action of *Candida albicans* in the human. Cerebral candida infection can occur as part of a generalized infection. Candida usually causes meningitis; granulomas may be caused by *Candida tropicalis* (KUMAR et al. 1979).

In typical cases the brain is affected by basal granulomatous meningoencephalitis; no gross lesions are seen but mininecroses or microabscesses are found scattered haphazardly.

UTZ (1967) found 27 cases in the literature, with a marked male predominance; most of the men had candida meningitis.

Further References: GREENFIELD and PRITCHARD (1937), MATTOS-PIMENTA and BRANDT (1960), TVETEN (1978).

Coccidiosis

Synonym: Coccidioidomycosis

The first case was described by WERNICKE (1892). The organism of *Coccidiodes immitis* was named by RIXFORD and GILCHRIST (1896). The granulomas may resemble tuberculomas; they are mostly smaller (ABBOTT and CUTLER 1936) and usually have a relation to the leptomeninges (see MÜLLER and SCHALTENBRAND 1948). Their frequency differs understandably: in 15000 autopsies in Los Angeles 7 cases of coccidiosis were found (ABBOTT and CUTLER 1936). These authors identified 23 cases in the world literature.

Further References: GOLDSTEIN and LAWRENCE (1978), SARAVIA-GOMEZ (1978b).

Cryptococcosis

Synonyms: Torulosis, Buschke's disease, European blastomycosis

Historical Note and Definition

The first original description of "torulosis" is thought to have been published by von HANSEMANN (1905), followed by LE COUNT and MYERS (1907; see LE COUNT 1909). (This condition must not be confused with North American blastomycosis; see p. 515).

Epidemiology (Age – Sex – Frequency – Site)

SELBY and LOPES (1973) found 37 cases in the literature and added 3 new ones. According to EVERETT et al. (1978), the number of reported cases was 600 in 1978. Male patients are involved twice as commonly as female ones, and apparently in 81% of all cases signs of CNS involvement have been seen (MATTOS-PIMENTA and BRANDT 1960).

Gross Pathology

There are apparently four different forms of involvement of the CNS by *Cryptococcus neoformans:*

1. The purely meningitic form, occurring predominantly in the basal leptomeninges.
2. The meningoencephalitic form, with invasion of the parenchyma along the perivascular spaces and a gelatinous appearance.
3. Formation of granulomas in cerebellum, spinal cord, and even within ventricles following chronic meningitis (DEMME and MUMME 1932; QUODBACH 1938; DANDY 1938; MANGANIELLO and NICHOLS 1955; VIJAYAN et al. 1971).
4. Granuloma formation in the choroid plexuses.

A very detailed and precise report on the various types of fungi, including the involvement of the nervous system, has been published by MATHEIS (1960), with excellent pictures of brain involvement, Figs. 1a, b, 3a, b, 4, 6, and fungi, black and white and in color. The macroscopical appearance of torulomas has also been well described. Cystic degeneration may occur. The work includes many references to the international literature.

Histologic Appearance

Identification of *Cryptococcus neoformans* is necessary for diagnosis, as are gelatinous destruction of tissue with replacement by mucus and sparse leukocytic infiltration.

The diagnosis is facilitated by CSF antigen levels and CT (TRESS and DAVIS 1979), which may also reveal multiple granulomas (EVERETT et al. 1978). Since earlier the prognosis was invariably fatal, surgery has seldom been performed. However, some authors (RISH and MEACHAM 1968; SELBY and LOPES 1973; EVERETT et al. 1978) have reported successful operations of cryptococcic granulomas. Therefore, the neurological surgeon must be aware of this disease. Antibiotic treatment is mentioned by UTZ (1967).

Scientists ask whether South or North American blastomycosis should be included into this entity (paracoccidioidomycosis, ARAUJO et al. 1978; North American blastomycosis, HABTE-GABR and SMITH 1973). Most authorities favor separate treatment of these conditions. Combination with lupus erythematodes has been discussed by COLLINS et al. (1971).

Further References: INNES and SAUNDERS (1962), WEENINK and BRUYN (1978).

Histoplasmosis

The rare infection by histoplasma – which is, however, common in Ohio and the Mississipi Valley (SCHOCHET et al. 1980) – occurred in 65 patients between 1952 and 1960 (COOPER and GOLDSTEIN 1963). The disease is not conspicuous in the CNS, because it does not cause circumscribed neurosurgical lesions (UTZ 1967).

Further References: LAWRENCE and GOLDSTEIN (1978)

Phycomycosis/Mucormycosis of the CNS

Infection with the saprophytic fungi of the class of Phycomycetes has already been reported in some 160 patients, 44 of whom had involvement of the paranasal sinuses, orbit, and CNS, to where it had usually spread by invasion of the intracranial blood vessels (WILSON et al. 1979). Only 8 have survived (PROCKOP and SILVA-HUTNER 1967). This disease is now found throughout the world and has been noted in the United States of America, England, and Canada. Surgery has been performed in individual cases of granuloma (RAO et al. 1978).

The infection is principally a complication of other, usually debilitating, diseases (lymphomas etc); however, diabetes mellitus is the most common (42% of the patients have been diabetics). Only 6 survivors of cerebral phycomycosis have been reported, and all these had residual neurological deficits (see REEVES et al. 1965).

An exceptionally rare entity is apparently *maduromycosis* of the brain (NATARAJAN et al. 1975), in which a brain abscess has been reported.

Further Reference: DHERMY (1978).

29 Arachnoiditis and Arachnoid Cysts

Synonyms: Leptomeningitis cystica, circumscribed meningitis, arachnopathia cystica proliferans, meningeal cysts

Introduction

Acute or subacute leptomeningeal infections (probably even some transmitted transplacentally) can be followed by a chronic reaction in the arachnoid leading to the formation of arachnoid cysts. Moreover, specific lesions may be induced by developmental errors. These all are not discussed in the WHO classification.

Historical Note and Definition

Early description were apparently given by QUAIN (1855: supratentorial cyst) and MAUNSELL (1889: posterior fossa). For the first pathogenetic explanation we are indebted to STROEBE (1904a, b), who in discussing the "hydrops meningeus" emphasized that probably local cystic collections of a watery fluid in the arachnoid are formed in places of former inflammatory reactions. Since adhesions and atresias of arachnoid spaces also follow these inflammatory lesions their barriers may occlude the communication of a localized area in the arachnoidal space to the CSF pathway. Similar changes had been emphasized by SCHLESINGER (1898), and the first surgical discussion of these lesions was published by PLACZEK and FEDOR KRAUSE (1907; see also PETTE 1936a, b).

The neurosurgical importance of either "cut off" and space-occupying ("cystic") lesions or "strangulating" lesions caused by scarring makes it necessary to discuss their morphology, etiology and pathogenesis.

Epidemiology (Age – Sex – Frequency – Site)

Further information about the age of the patients and the frequency of the condition can be found in the section on etiology and pathogenesis.

The *site* is fairly dependent on these factors as well as on the classification. A clear *age* preference has not yet been recognized except for the well-studied arachnoiditis of the chiasmal region, where a definite peak of frequency has been observed in the 3rd decade. KNUDTZON (1944) thought that the age curve peaked in the 2nd and 3rd decades and that male patients were compromised more often. The Dandy-Walker syndrome has been observed from the 1st year of life up to the 6th decade.

About the frequency of arachnoiditis data are not available (apart from reports from the Paris authors VINCENT et al. 1931; PETIT-DUTAILLIS 1933; PUECH and MAHOUDEAU 1935; DAVID et al. 1936a), who recorded 71 cases of arachnoiditis opto-chiasmatica among 155 space-occupying lesions of the sella region. Familial intradural cysts have been observed by AARABI et al. (1979).

Classification

The cystic formations within the cranial cavity have been classified by TÖRMÄ and HEISKANEN (1961; see also p. 137).

Of these, only the various types of arachnoidal (HANDA and BUCY 1956) and ependymal cysts (excluding the "colloidal" cysts of the foramen of Monro; see p. 437) will be considered here. They have been subdivided into *supratentorial* and *posterior fossa* cysts (DICK and GRUSKIN 1977) and also into "*primary*" and "*secondary*" forms (WEINMAN 1965). Detailed surgical descriptions published early by TÖNNIS (1937: his experience with 3 cerebellomedullary, 3 fossa sylvii, and 2 cisterna interhemispherica cysts) and by ZEHNDER (1938b). Broad morphological and pathogenetic descriptions will be found in the excellent monograph of D. RUSSELL (1949). ZÜLCH (1950b) discussed the neurosurgical importance.

The localization and the type of lesion direct the following description: the *arachnoid* cysts are almost exclusively located in the region of the large cisterns (GP, Figs. 326–332). According to their site and its relation to the brain they have been divided into "intra-axial" (Dandy-Walker syndrome) and "extra-axial" cysts (however, it seems doubtful whether this helps in description and understanding of the condition). We will therefore describe the various types according to site.

Arachnoid cysts occur near the

a) Cisterna magna: open forms
b) Cisterna magna: closed sac-like (chambered, cystic) forms
c) Cerebellopontine angle
d) Quadrigeminal region
e) Chiasm
f) Sylvian fissure
g) Sagittal (interhemispheric) cleft

a) The *open* forms of cyst formation within the cisterna magna are due to an arachnitic occlusion of the foramen of Magendie and of Luschka. Here only one caudal membrane embraces the arachnoidal sac consisting of the outer fibrous membrane of the cistern. However, this sac-like cyst acts like a corresponding tumor and can extend laterally to the cerebellopontine angle (GP, Fig. 330; see also GIBSON 1955).

b) Enormous *closed* cysts (Fig. 164) occur in the cisterna magna (ZÜLCH 1956, Fig. 441; ZÜLCH 1950b, Figs. 4–8; GP, Fig. 330); they form a closed sac up to the size of a chestnut or larger, and are characterized by closure of the foramina of Magendie and Luschka. They form the enlarged fourth ventricle, so to speak. The tonsils are pressed upward and to the side (Fig. 164) and can effectively obstruct the normal flow of CSF over the hemispheres. Furthermore, there is significant hydrocephalus affecting all four ventricles. The vermis may be displaced toward the oral cavity, but is never defective or absent (ROTH-

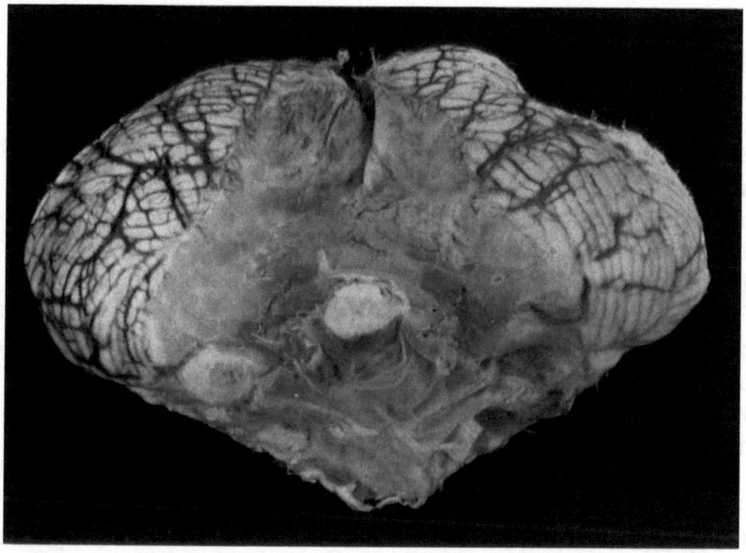

Fig. 164. Extensive formation of arachnoidal cysts in the cisterna magna and the adjacent basal cisterns. The foramen of Magendie was obstructed, resulting in a massive hydrocephalus. (ZÜLCH 1975a)

MANN 1939; TROWBRIDGE and FRENCH 1952a; GIBSON 1955; LAPRAS et al. 1963; McDONALD and COLGAN 1964). Our own photographs of surgical interventions have been reproduced by ZEHNDER (1938b, Figs. 2, 3).

c) In the *cerebellopontine angle* arachnoidal cysts have been reported in the literature to simulate acoustic neurilemmoma (NICHOLS and MANGANIELLO 1953; THIJSSEN et al. 1976) though on operation no tumor was found. It is apparent that the cases reported by TROWBRIDGE and FRENCH (1952a: "parafloccular") and SCHENK (1966: adjacent to recessus lateralis) belong to the same group. There is no communication to the fourth ventricle.

These cysts can be a part of a general process of cyst formation in the basal cisterns (GP, Fig. 326) resulting from meningeal irritation, as shown by our own picture (ZÜLCH 1956, Fig. 442; GP, Fig. 326). We have described (ZÜLCH 1956, Fig. 259) such cysts in the cerebellopontine angle in the presence of real acoustic neurilemmomas (Fig. 109).

d) Arachnoid cysts of the *quadrigeminal region* (GP, Fig. 332) form a closed sac, which lies over the midbrain and displaces the tectum, closes the aqueduct, and usually extends under the tentorium. It can also reach the size of a chestnut and acts as a tumor of the pineal region. Obstructive hydrocephalus of the first three ventricles is the consequence.

This has to be distinguished from a similar arachnoidal sac-like formation that in the case of occlusion of the aqueduct, for instance, can be formed by rupture of the medial wall of the brain mantle at the trigonum with bulging of the arachnoid to the point of formation of a real cystic sac. This presses from above and laterally on the quadrigeminal region (DE LANGE 1929; RIESSNER and ZÜLCH 1939, p. 17; PENNYBACKER and RUSSELL 1943). Moreover they have to be distinguished from genuine ependymal cysts of the quadrigeminal region (p. 528; see also HAMBY and GARDNER 1935; NOETZEL 1940; ALEXANDER 1953; LOURIE and BERNE 1961; ALVORD and MARCUSE 1962; LEWIS 1962; KRUYFF 1965; HAYASHI et al. 1980).

e) In the region of the *chiasm* cicatricial arachnoiditis is said to be of particular importance; it can culminate with the formation of small cysts. Amidst a ring of adhesions at this point the arachnoid cysts are usually not so well delimited and do not have such obvious predilection sites as in the other forms described. They form more a chambered system of closed formations (see ZÜLCH 1950b, Fig. 6; ZÜLCH 1956, Fig. 442; GP, Fig. 326). A network of small arachnoid cysts and cicatrices, some of them with fluid-containing compartments, compromises the chiasm and optic fascicles; the floor of the third ventricle is elevated. They frequently act as a real space-occupying lesions, with pressure mainly on the optic systems.

Extensive literature is cited by KNUDTZON (1944; see also RINGERTZ 1937; FOERSTER 1937; TÖNNIS 1937; TÖNNIS 1948, p. 756; SPOTA 1951; CARILLO et al. 1951), and a variant of arachnoid cyst may also have been present in the tabetic patients reported by DAVID et al. (1936). This form, well known in past decades as arachnitis opto-chiasmatica, has been particularly well studied and described by the French school, and especially by PETIT-DUTAILLIS (1933), PUECH and MAHOUDEAU (1935), DAVID et al. (1936a), and BOLLACK et al. (1937). These groups of authors emphasized the three forms of this cicatricial arachnoiditis: (i) a feltwork of fine fibrous strands; (ii) the formation of large cysts; (iii) a mainly atrophic form (see also FOERSTER 1937; DICKMANN et al. 1951; YUHL and RAND 1951; OBENCHAIN and BECKER 1972).

SPOTA (1951) called the clinical syndrome "Balado's syndrome" since apparently BALADO was the first to stress its occurrence.

An intrasellar arachnoid diverticulum has been described by CALKINS et al. (1968).

f) *Arachnoid cysts* in the *cistern* of the *Sylvian fissure* are particularly well known (ZÜLCH 1956, Figs. 436, 437; GP, Figs. 327, 328; WEINMAN 1965; SEUR and KOOMAN 1976). These are large, mainly "congenital" cysts (see below), usually the size of an apple (Fig. 165) and producing a corresponding displacement of the brain substance, the whole middle temporal lobe being pushed over the midline to the contralateral side. Moreover, a bulge of the temporal bone is apparent and has already been diagnosed on plane x-rays.

E. SCHERER's (1935a) case showed four such cystic accumulations (also in front of the pons and other spaces of the base). The pathogenesis of these cysts is probably twofold. The fact that the content of these cysts can also be of two kinds, waterclear CSF or milky CSF with cloudy yellowish detritus at the base, may also indicate the correctness of this distinction. Since in the latter case (personal observations in a man of 42 and a woman of 40; ZÜLCH 1950b, 1956) they show entirely different histological features, i.e., a high epithelium that apparently proliferates as in an epidermoid and sends the detritus into the cysts, genesis as an embryonic malformation in this form seems very likely (see p. 525). These cysts have been described by TÖNNIS (1948, Fig. 429) and ZEHNDER (1938b; see also BARRE et al. 1936; OKONEK 1938; MACGREGOR

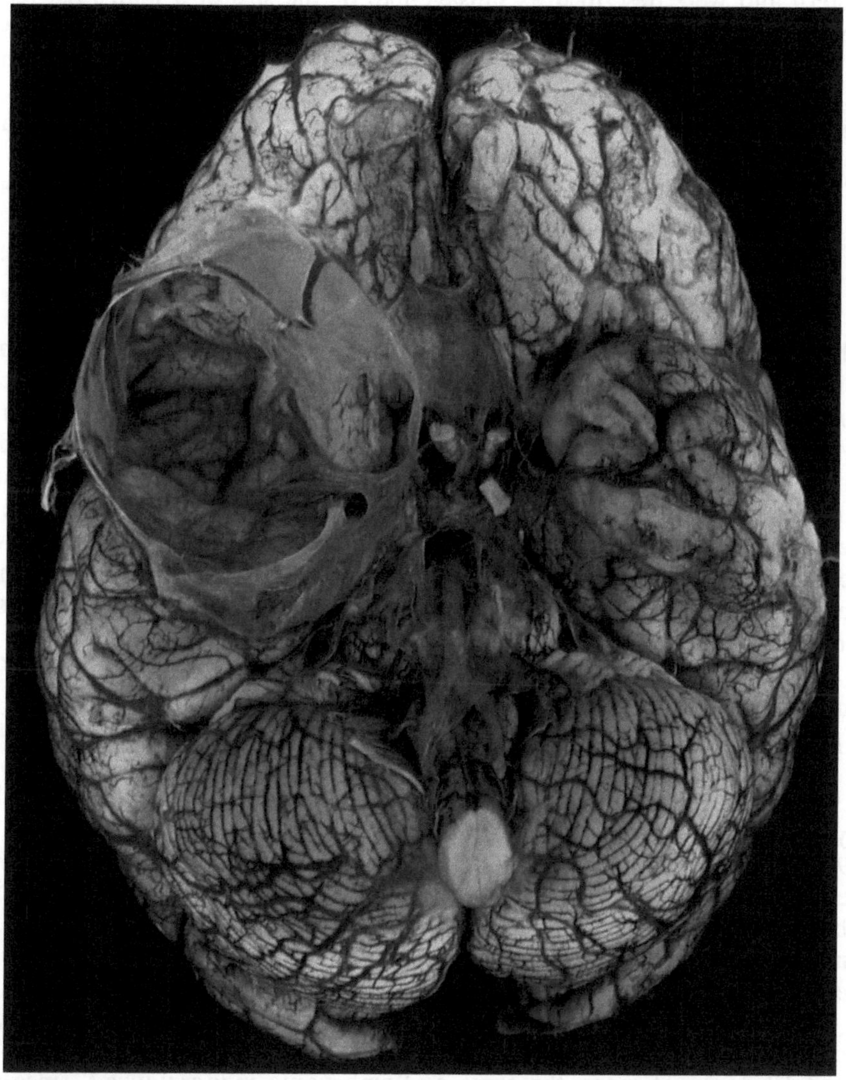

Fig. 165. Apple-sized, probably congenital, cyst of unknown etiology in the right Sylvian fissure (incidental finding)

et al. 1976). The other type of a cyst is an arachnoidal sac (see above). Differential diagnosis from porencephalic cysts is discussed elsewhere (GP, Fig. 327).

g) *Interhemispheric cisterns* of the median cleft are large cysts over the corpus callosum between the two hemispheres. They are not very common. They can press down on the corpus callosum so that it becomes atrophic or may be even absent (atretic?).

FOERSTER (1939b) described a "diverticulum" at this site which was not, however, of "ependymal" origin, as he reported, but of arachnoid origin. ZEHNDER's (1938b) cases were located in the anterior or middle third of the cistern and were described as sausage-like or the size of a man's fist (content 160 ml). A similar arachnoid cyst was described by VAN DEN HERREWEGEN (1954). The large arachnoid parietal cyst near the median cleft – but not in the cistern – does not seem to bear any relation to this type (see ZÜLCH 1956, Figs. 438, 439; GP, Figs. 333, 334). Again a large bulge of bone in the parietal region was noted in the case just cited, which was observed incidentally.

Arachnoid cysts in the cisterna ambiens have been described by NOETZEL (1940) and by GROLLMUS et al. (1976: "para-mesencephalic").

Dandy-Walker Syndrome

The Dandy-Walker syndrome appears as an anomaly of the cerebellum characterized by a balloon-like hydrocephalus of the fourth ventricle and an arachnoidal sac beneath and between the two cerebellar hemispheres; apart from the cystic dilatation of the fourth ventricle it is characterized by obstructive hydrocephalus of the other three ventricles, by a cleft formation between the two cerebellar hemispheres originating from a hypoplasia or complete absence of the cerebellar vermis, and by closure of the foramina of Magendie and Luschka, which according to the literature, however, can also be absent. These formations can be the size of a man's fist; the posterior fossa is enlarged; and the transverse sinus runs in an abnormal curve.

The syndrome was originally described by DANDY and BLACKFAN (1914) and then by TAGGART and WALKER (1942) and COLEMAN and TROLAND (1948: 3 personal cases, 3 of DANDY), and it was finally named by BENDA in 1954.

The pathogenetic mechanism has not yet been established. D'AGOSTINO et al. (1963a) believed it to be an embryonic malformation. This opinion was shared by many authors, who believed that the foramina failed to open (HALLER et al. 1971). In some cases peripheral malformations also suggested embryonic maldevelopment. However, PORTUGAL and BROCK (1964) assumed that early hydrocephalus caused the roof of the fourth ventricle to bulge, producing the cyst and preventing closure of the cerebellar vermis. So far about 150 cases have been reported in the literature (PALMA et al. 1979).

The discussion as to whether this is an embryonic or congenital or congenital postinfectious formation continues. However, it must be emphasized that "congenital" does not mean the same as "embryonic *malformative,*" since as we will point out later, EICKE (1943, 1959) has convincingly shown the "fetal type" of meningitis that has histological sequelae.

Certainly GARDNER et al. (1960) were correct in stating that final definition and distinction of the lesions in the posterior fossa (e.g., Arnold-Chiari syndrome and Dandy-Walker syndrome) had not yet been precisely achieved.

Gross Pathology

The arachnoid cysts appear as focal collections of fluid; they form a translucent sac, whitish in parts and varying in size from chestnut size up to that of a man's fist. They are filled with a clear CSF-like fluid. However, some of the larger cysts, usually located in the parasagittal cleft or the Sylvian fissure, contain a milky fluid with a whitish detritus sediment. The histology of these is also different.

These cysts produce a corresponding displacement of the brain substance and ventricles, and large cysts of the convexity can even cause a bulge of the bony calvarium (ZÜLCH 1956, Fig. 439; GP, Fig. 334), which is apparent on plane x-ray pictures. In some cases of arachnoiditis due to a general rise of intracranial pressure – obstructive hydrocephalus – the tonsillar pressure cone may develop and remain "kept down" in the future by adhesions even though the pressure syndrome has already faded away, which can lead to recurrent bouts of increased intracranial pressure (TÖNNIS 1948). If the arachnoid sacs are still communicating with the ventricular system they will be enlarged and bulging like part of the obstructive hydrocephalic ventricular system, because the pathway of the CSF to the site of absorption is blocked.

The fact that in a considerable number of cases the single cysts form only a part of a general cicatricial process in the basal cisterns of the brain suggests an external causative factor, such as a pre-existing (even congenital) irritation syndrome of the leptomeninges. From the descriptions it seems apparent that the arachnoid spaces were more frequently seen in a cicatricial state in former times (as described by the Paris school: VINCENT et al. 1931; CLAUDE 1933; BOLLACK et al. 1937).

Histologic Appearance

These different types of leptomeningeal irritations with cyst formation involve a thickening of the arachnoid with incipient fibrosis and increased homogeneity, sometimes with round cell infiltration and single gitter cell admixture. Depending on the stage of development there are either prominent signs of chronic inflammation, or cellular and fibrous proliferation, of the arachnoid mesothelium with fibrous scarring, but with very little infiltration of other kind of cells. Biopsies of so-called cured streptomycin-treated meningeal tuberculosis often revealed membranes still showing the specific histological pictures, even with polynuclear giant cells (see also SCHACHENMAYR and FRIEDE 1979).

In some of the large arachnoidal cysts, however, different structures are sometimes seen that point to a fetal origin. This is indicated even on examination by the naked eye, by the milky and cloudy contents of the cyst sac. The walls in such cases consist of a single layer of epithelium (ZÜLCH 1956, Fig. 445a, b), which occasionally forms psammoma bodies. It constantly produces new cell layers, which swell up, become amorphous, and are finally shed into the cyst as detritus in a manner similar to that seen in the epidermoid (ZÜLCH 1950b, Figs. 9, 10). This explains the milky appearance and the cloudiness of the cyst fluid (ZEHNDER 1938b).

Microscopically, either translucent membranes or thicker connective strands or even a feltwork of the arachnoid may be most prominent, with cyst formation in parts. Degenerative manifestations are particularly apparent in the optic nerve and chiasm when arachnoiditis is present.

Etiology and Pathogenesis

We pointed out the difference between "embryonic," "malformative," and "congenital" forms of cyst formation above (see also RENGACHARY and WATANABE 1981). Earlier, most of these cysts were thought to be sequelae of external factors such as acute, subacute, or chronic leptomeningeal infections, which were most frequent at that time in the first 2 or 3 years of life and were sometimes even transmitted transplacentally. The most important conditions formerly were meningococcal meningitis, hemophilus influenza, hemolytic streptococcus, and pneumococcus infections. Meningitides caused by *B. coli* and *Flexner's bacillus* (see D. RUSSELL 1949) were also seen.

The spread of an *infection* to the fetal brain during pregnancy has been well demonstrated by EICKE (1943, 1959), an observation of the utmost importance for our discussion. Arachnoiditis of syphilitic origin (particularly, probably, in the chiasmal region) was often assumed in former times. Even the so-called cured tuberculous meningitis, particularly around the cisterna ambiens, was not uncommon in the 1950s (ZÜLCH 1956, Fig. 444; GP, Fig. 331). Today, besides bacterial infections originating from the pneumatic chambers, viral CSF lesions are a more common cause.

Acute circumscribed meningeal irritation, probably arising again from infectious foci, is a second cause, in which local adhesions, less commonly cyst formations, near the sinuses and the other pneumatic chambers of the base of the skull irritate the adjacent meninges in the case of suppuration. More rarely, such localized meningeal irritations follow traumatic changes with subarachnoid hemorrhage (see below), particularly in the spinal canal.

Chronic adhesive forms can be formed adjacent to arachnoid cysts and can be the end-result of infection or acute meningeal irritation.

The *posttraumatic form* of arachnoidal irritation with scar and cyst formation has been described by TÖNNIS (1936), SCHALTENBRAND and TÖNNIS (1936/37), ROUQUES and DAVID (1949), ROUQUES et al. (1949: vertebral L2 fracture); NICHOLS and MANGANIELLO (1953: after fall followed by unconsciousness), THOMPSON (1946: 60 days after a jump from a parachute tower); and STENDER (1939) and DAVIDOFF et al. (1947: postoperative descriptions). *Spinal* postoperative arachnitis is of considerable surgical importance (see EPSTEIN et al. 1978). TIBERIN and GRUSZKIEWICZ (1961), LEWIS (1962), LITTLE et al. (1973) have also published reports.

Chemical irritation caused by the action of intrathecal positive oil contrast media has been described by MARCOVICH et al. (1941) and MORELLO and COOPER (1953). Their use is now avoided.

To give an impression of the relative frequency of the various etiologic factors we can list here those in the cases of LITTLE et al. (1973): unknown 8, infections 8, trauma 1, congenital 1, ectopic 1.

BURGER and VOGEL (1976) emphasized that actually the arachnoid cysts were not "true" cysts but only distended chambers of subarachnoid space, which are cut off and circumscribed by pial arachnoid adhesions. This is certainly correct. However, their concept that the lack of any communication with the ventricular system implies a developmental origin may be erroneous.

Operability

The surgical results reported on early by TÖNNIS (1937) and by KRAUS (1948) have improved meanwhile, since the wide spread introduction of CT diagnosis (ANDERSON et al. 1979). There are survival times even for Dandy-Walker syndrome of 6 months to 20 years (FISCHER 1973): of the 50% survivors in this series 30 had a normal or near-normal life. PALMA et al. (1979) reported on 4 patients with good and 1 with a fair result, and 3 in whom postoperative death occurred. The opening of a closed suprasellar cyst with a ventriculoscope has been described by MURALI and EPSTEIN (1979).

Further Reference: BHANDARI (1972).

30 Ependymitis – Ependymal Cysts

Introduction

Ependymitis and its sequelae are not described in the WHO classification. Some of its entities, however, are of neurosurgical importance and are therefore described below.

Concurrent ependymitis during the acute stage of meningitis is one of the manifestations of infection of the CSF spaces. The exudate lying on the ependyma or in the subependymal region can cause subsequent patchy or wart-like growth of acellular glial tissue (ependymitis granularis sive plastica; see DAHL and HARBITZ 1938). Cicatricial processes such as these can result in the occlusion of narrow points in the CSF circulation, as has been convincingly demonstrated by the pathology of aqueduct occlusion (Dorothy RUSSELL 1949; ZÜLCH 1956, Fig. 448; ZÜLCH and NACHTWEY 1958; GP, Figs. 363, 364).

This can lead, as in one personal case, to subsequent partial hydranencephalus (ZÜLCH 1954, Fig. 2; GP, Figs. 378, 379). Inflammatory blockage of the foramen of Monro has been described by ECTORS (1935) and ZÜLCH (1941c, Fig. 7) and can be revealed by CT.

Ependymitis consecutive to contrast injection into the ventricle was described formerly, and such injections are now avoided.

We have seen a block of the inferior one-third of the fourth ventricle in two cases (ZÜLCH 1950b, Fig. 1; 1956, Fig. 449; GP, Fig. 365). The adhesion arose as a result of a general inflammatory process with adhesions between the ventricular floor, the choroid plexus of the roof, and the meninges of the tonsils undersurfaces and the nodules, finally forming a cicatricial mass block in the foramina of Magendie and Luschka. Obstructive hydrocephalus of the first three ventricles and the upper portion of the fourth develops in these cases.

Ependymal cysts, on the other hand, seem to be mainly of embryonic origin as described in detail elsewhere (ZÜLCH 1956, p. 328).

We distinguish four forms of ependymal cysts:

1. Separations of ventricular parts, particularly at the end-formations (frontal, temporal, occipital horns), usually do not "grow."
2. Ependymal cysts have a tendency to increase in volume. We have described two walnut-sized cysts in the quadrigeminal region (ZÜLCH 1956, Fig. 239; MARX et al. 1968, Fig. 15d; GP, Figs. 75, 76). The case of HAMBY and GARDNER (1935) is more like the frequent arachnoidal cysts, particularly since neither cilia nor blepharoplasts have been described.
3. A rare formation of a cyst originating from the pineal region and protruding like a sac into the third ventricle, occluding the aqueduct, was observed together with ROER (1956, Figs. 2, 4).

Convincing examples of polycystic ependymal formations have been described by FOERSTER and GAGEL (1934b: eight cysts), HILL (1933), and HARDMAN and JEFFERSON (1938).

The case of TANDON et al. (1972), however, was one of the congenital "embryonic" forms of arachnoid cyst so commonly seen in the Sylvian Fissure (see p. 523; also ZÜLCH 1956, p. 610; PALMA 1975; PALMA et al. 1979).

4. The formation of ependymal bands and ependyma-lined grooves occurs frequently in the region of the aqueduct and these are described elsewhere (ZÜLCH 1956, Fig. 238; GP, Fig. 76).

The septum pellucidum cysts have no resemblance to the true ependymal cysts described above, but result from liquefaction of glial tissue within the organ part affected. They are usually "closed."

The so-called colloid cysts in the fourth ventricle, which were described by PARKINSON and CHILDE (1952), cannot be classified in this system (see Sect. 21.4).

Ependymal transverse bands (ZÜLCH and NACHTWEY 1958, Figs. 1, 3, 4) may occur in the aqueduct. At sites of previous postinflammatory stenosis of the aqueduct there is gliotic tissue intermingled with islands of ependymal canals and proliferations (see ZÜLCH and NACHTWEY 1958, Fig. 10).

Sometimes the medial wall of the trigonum is ruptured by the pressure of an obstructive hydrocephalus. Then the leptomeninx protrudes as a real sac into the quadrigeminal cistern (see ZÜLCH and NACHTWEY 1958, Fig. 16). It acts there as a space-occupying lesion.

31 "Pseudotumor Cerebri"

Synonym: Benign intracranial hypertension; BIH

NONNE's (1904) concept of pseudotumor cerebri, a syndrome seen in the classic period of neurology, is a purely clinical one. The term was meant to characterize a condition in which clinically the diagnosis of "tumor cerebri" was adequate but the outcome (cure or autopsy) could not confirm this diagnosis. In these circumstances it signifies a local or general increase in intracranial presssure that is not attributable to a tumor. It is related rather to a local or general increase of the volume of the brain resulting from something other than neoplasm. Its pathogenetic mechanism is not yet clear and not uniform, but it occurs after such processes as sinus thrombosis (KALBAG and WOOLF 1972), "otitic hydrocephalus" (ZÜLCH 1964; VENABBLE 1975), occupational or industrial intoxications, endocrinological or metabolic dysfunctions, particularly after prolonged steroid therapy or its withdrawal (WALKER and ADAMKIEWICZ 1964), occasionally after oral contraception or in association with obesity in women, or together with posttraumatic or posthemorrhagic cysts with a tendency to increase in size, or after arachnoiditis etc. This condition was broadly discussed in 1949 (see Congress of German Neurosurgeons, Göttingen, Zentralbl. Neurochir. 10, pp. 56–61, 1950).

KEHRER (1949) opposed Nonne's concept, enumerating 22 different and frequent causes of this pseudotumorous state. General reviews were given by CAESAR (1941), FOLEY (1955), and GREER 1960, 1974).

Further References: DAVIDOFF (1956), VAN BOGAERT (1959), N. MÜLLER (1961), GUIDETTI et al. (1968).

32 Tumors of the Spinal Cord, the Cauda Equina, and the Vertebral Column

Introduction

The WHO classification does not include a specific survey of space-occupying lesions by localization.

Historical Note and Definition

Apparently the first intradural, but *extramedullary,* tumor of the spinal cord was operated on successfully by Sir Victor HORSLEY after being diagnosed neurologically by GOWERS (see GOWERS and HORSLEY 1888).

Although brain surgery as such started at the same time, it was not until 1907 that the first *intramedullary* tumor was successfully removed by EISELSBERG (see EISELSBERG and RANZI 1913). The next reports of successful removal of intramedullary tumors were published by O. FOERSTER (1917, 1921); these reports were supplemented by descriptions of a series of spinal gliomas subjected to surgery (FOERSTER and GAGEL 1935; FOERSTER and BAILEY 1936; KERNOHAN 1941; WEBB et al. 1953). These publications included an excellent description of the histology of the intramedullary tumors. A list documenting the history of the pathology of spinal tumors has been published by SLOOFF et al. (1964), beginning with BRUNNER (1653–1727) and MORGAGNI (1682–1771).

Basically the same types of tumors are encountered in the spinal cord, cauda equina, and vertebral column as in the brain and the cranium (see BAILEY and BUCY 1930b; ZÜLCH 1980). However, there is a difference in relative frequency (NITTNER 1972). Due to the preponderance of the dural tissue and the coverings of the spinal roots, meningiomas and neurilemmomas are far more frequent near the spinal cord than near the brain. Even sarcomas and angiomatous tumors are more common in the vicinity of the spinal cord, due to the preponderance of such tissues of the epidural space and the vertebral bodies. The high number of lymphomas (reticular sarcomas) can be explained in the same way.

On the other hand, of the gliomatous tumors the ependymomas are far more frequent than astrocytomas, while oligodendrogliomas are very rare and glioblastomas almost never occur in these sites. The particular structure of the conus medullaris with its many ependymal cells explains the specific pathology of this region with the preponderance of myxopapillary ependymomas. Cystic degeneration is also far more common in the vertebral canal than in the cranium; it is – in my opinion wrongly in most cases – called "syringomyelia."

Classification

It seems necessary first to bring some order into the vast field of terminology for spinal tumors.

We can distinguish the following different localizations: (a) intramedullary and filum terminale; (b) extramedullary, intradural, and intraspinal sites; and (c) "spinal"[1] sites, i.e. neoplasms of the vertebral column.
Alternatively, a distinction can be made between primary tumors of (a) gliomatous and (b) nongliomatous nature; and finally the secondary tumors.

A last classification is based on the specific histology:

Primary lesions

Gliomas	*Nongliomatous tumors*
Astrocytomas, proper	Neurilemmomas
Astrocytomas, pilocytic	Meningiomas
Oligodendrogliomas	Tumors of the blood vessels
Ependymomas	Malformative tumors (epidermoid cysts, dermoid cysts, other cysts, lipomas, teratomas)
Glioblastomas	Vascular malformations (cavernous angioma, arteriovenous malformation, venous malformation)
Gangliocytomas, etc.	Sarcomas
	Lipomas
	Chordomas, chondromas, chondrosarcomas

Secondary lesions

Metastatic tumors
Parasites
Granulomas (fungus, etc.)

Epidemiology (Age – Sex – Frequency – Site)

Age: The age preferences are listed with the various histological groups. There is a vast amount of data about spinal cord tumors in *younger* age groups. Ross and O.T. Bailey (1953) recorded 13 patients aged below 16 years in a group of 63 tumors, i.e., around 20%. Anderson and Carson (1953) saw 21 cases under 16 years of age in a series of 164, i.e., 12.8% (see also Siwe 1956; Vigouroux et al. 1963; Ueda et al. 1975). A detailed description is given in the monograph by Rand and Rand (1960).

Bailey (1936b) discussing the paper of Sperling and Mayfield (see Anderson and Carson 1953) gave a ratio of 1:20 for spinal versus cranial tumors in the younger age group, i.e., below 15 years. Hamby (1935, 1944) also reported on a series of 114 cases below 15 years. Dodge et al. (1956) had 32.1% intramedullary versus 67.9% extramedullary tumors in infants and children in their series, and Rand and Rand (1960) and Rand (1963) had 64 childhood cases.

[1] "Spinal" tumors is the term commonly used in clinical practice for *all tumors* at and inside the vertebral column.

Sex: Any sex preponderance will be described in the notes on the histological groups.

Frequency: It is best to give a *general* survey on the frequencies of the histological groups and their preferential sites here.

Publications on large series of spinal tumors have been issued by the Mayo Clinic (KERNOHAN and SAYRE 1952; SLOOFF et al. 1964) and by the Neurosurgical Clinic in Cologne (1976). NITTNER (1972) had already reported on 4885 histologically classified spinal cord tumors of the literature. The table below shows the average proportions.

	KERNOHAN and SAYRE (1952)	NITTNER (1976)	NITTNER (1976) Childhood and youth
Neurilemmomas	29.9%	23.1%	9.3%
Meningiomas	25.9%	22.4%	4.4%
Gliomas	22.5%	13.3%	24.7%
Sarcomas etc.	11.2%	7.6%	15.3%
Extramedullary: hemangiomas, etc.	5.8%	6.2%	–

The cases of the Mayo Clinic (COHEN et al. 1964) were more finely classified:

Metastasis	121	Osteogenic sarcomas	8
Chordomas	72	Hemangiomas	8
Myelomas	55	Ependymomas	7
Chondrosarcomas	26	Fibrosarcomas	6
Giant cell tumors	16	Neurilemmomas	6
Osteochondromas	16	Angiosarcomas	3
Lymphomas	15	Chondromas	2
Giant osteoid osteomas	11	Undetermined sarcomas	11
Aneurysmal bone cysts	11		

This table shows the high preference of nongliomatous spinal tumors.

Distribution in various segments has been determined:

a) Cervical segments	19.0%
b) Thoracic segments	48.5%
c) Lumbosacral segments, cauda equina and filum terminale	31.5%
d) Several segments	1.0%

These percentages show the distribution of 979 intraspinal tumors seen at the Mayo Clinic (KERNOHAN and SAYRE 1952).

Multiple occurrences have been described by LINDAU (1926), GAMPER and STIEFLER (1929), LICHTENSTEIN (1941), NITTNER and SCHIEFER (1955), and NITTNER (1976, extensive report).

Gliomatous Tumors

Epidemiology (Age – Sex – Frequency – Site)

The general data on frequency of the gliomatous tumors are important.

Frequency: Early publications (SCHLESINGER 1898: 151 intraspinal tumors in 3500 autopsies, of these 20 intramedullary) gave a general idea of the frequency. A great deal of modern epidemiological data is available (e.g., KURLAND 1958; ALTER 1975).

The incidence of spinal tumors compared with that of primary brain tumors found by KURLAND (1958) was 2.5:7.7; that found by GUDMUNDSSON for Iceland (1970), 1.1:7.8; and later for the district of Rochester PERCY et al. (1972) found 1.3:12.5 for a 34-year period. The prevalence was 12.9 in Rochester, and 10.1 in Iceland. GOLDBERG and KURLAND (1962) estimated that spinal cord tumors account for 10% of all tumors of the nervous system.

However, the data for *gliomas* were different; for instance, the estimated proportion for the spinal forms was 2.57% of all gliomas of the nervous system, whereas actually they amounted to 7%. The spinal cord was, then, a preferential site for gliomas.

This preponderance was even more striking in the case of ependymomas, where 169 occurred in the spinal canal in a total of 452 ependymomas, i.e., 37.4% were encountered in the spinal canal and filum terminale. The actual number of astrocytomas, in contrast, was in fair agreement with the expected percentage. The tendency to develop in the brain substance is smaller for ependymomas than the tendency to develop in the spinal cord.

The annual incidence for spinal tumors was estimated at between 2.5 and 9 per 100000 population, and the corresponding figure for brain tumors at 7.7 by KURLAND (1958). The data for Israel and Iceland are very similar, as are those for ten fairly large cities in the United States of America, viz. 3.6 per 100000 for brain tumors and 1 per 100000 population for spinal cord tumors (DORN and CUTLER 1955). Similar ratios were shown in other figures of KURLAND (1958) and ALTER (1975). KURLAND (1958) reported on 8784 tumors, 85% of which were in the intracranial cavity and 15.1% in the spinal canal. Among the population of Rochester (30000 inhabitants) over a 10-year period there were 50 cases of intracranial neoplasm versus 12 intraspinal tumors. ALTER (1975) gave a percentage ratio of 0.9 spinal :2.5 intracranial for a population of 100000 (Israel).

Local environmental factors apparently play little if any part in determining the frequency of spinal cord tumors.

Difficulties, however, arise from the entries on death certificates (PERCY et al. 1972). Even with the more detailed distribution, problems can occur if gumma, metastasis, and vascular anomalies are excluded. A last point has to be emphasized: no distinct contrast in the distribution of the various types of spinal cord tumors among different populations has been confirmed, although initially the first impression had arisen that black populations might have a lower frequency, especially of meningiomas (CUSHING and EISENHARDT 1938). Contrasting reports in this respect probably depend on sociological and environmental factors (but see p. 148).

Pilocytic and Other Astrocytomas

Most of the astrocytomas in the spinal canal are pilocytic. The total number in the series of Slooff et al. (1964) was 86, among 1322 such tumors of the spinal canal. More than half of these were classified as grade I, and one-quarter as grade II. It is impossible, then, to define how many tumors of the pilocytic and how many of the other astrocytic varieties were observed, particularly since the authors mentioned that only 10% had Rosenthal fibers, a very characteristic phenomenon of the pilocytic type [for instance, a patient of O'Brien et al. (1968) had "café-au-lait spots," a forme fruste of von Recklinghausen's disease?]. Altogether, according to Burger and Vogel (1976), astrocytomas in the brain are 40 times more frequent than those in the spinal cord. Most of those in the spinal cord occur in the thoracic part.

Age: The average age of the patients in the series of Slooff et al. (1964) was around 35 years, with the highest percentage in the third decade. Of the 86 cases 48 were found in male and the rest in female patients. Location and extent of the tumors showed a preponderance of the thoracic area of the spinal column for astrocytomas (see above). Again, they very commonly appeared in the form of pencil-like gliomas with large cystic cavities (so-called syringomyelias?). Some of these apparently become "sclerotic" and are described as collagenous nodules (Gass et al. 1971). We reported these vascular, very collagenous parts in pilocytic astrocytomas in our first description of the so-called astrocytoma of the cerebellum or polar spongioblastoma (Zülch 1940a). With regard to the cyst formation, however, it has to be emphasized that in Kernohan and Sayre's series (1952) one-quarter of the astrocytomas only had these large cysts, whereas of seven ependymomas five had a large syrinx, as did two of three hemangioendotheliomas, though none of the oligodendrogliomas did.

Since two-thirds of the main groups of intramedullary tumors contained such cysts, the problem arises of deciding whether this is a primary or a secondary cavity formation (Lichtenstein and Zeitlin 1937; Shenkin and Alpers 1944; Lima Costa and Couto Cesar 1951; Ferry et al. 1969). The question as to whether astrocytomas or other intramedullary tumors may arise in the wall of a pre-existing syrinx has not been confirmed by large series of case studies (Levy and Elvidge 1956; Poser 1956) (see above our concept about syringomyelia and glial tumors).

Oligodendrogliomas

Oligodendrogliomas are not very common in the spinal cord, accounting for only "eight"[1] of 1322 tumors of the spinal canal (Slooff et al. 1964), 291 of which were gliomatous in nature. These thus formed only 2.3% of the total series of oligodendrogliomas. The average age was about the same as that for the astrocytomas, i.e., around 35 years. The sexes were almost equally represented, and the site again showed a preponderance of the thoracic region, as for the astrocytomas.

[1] There is a discrepancy in the number of oligodendrogliomas in the series, where the number of oligodendrogliomas is sometimes indicated "nine" (Kernohan and Sayre 1952).

Differential Diagnosis

We have emphasized above the difficulties of classification of the oligodendrogliomas in some cases, since KERNOHAN and SAYRE (1952) not infrequently observed "oligodendroglial" parts in ependymomas. We defined these as regressive changes and have observed them frequently. Moreover the pilocytic astrocytomas very commonly produce patterns during the process of liquefaction (see p. 51a, Fig. 51) that are difficult to distinguish at first sight from those in an oligodendroglioma (see also CHIGASAKI and PENNYBACKER 1968: 1 oligodendroglioma amongst 85 gliomas).

Ependymomas

The first systematic study of spinal ependymomas was performed by KERNOHAN and FLETCHER-KERNOHAN (1935), who at the same time described the papillary type of ependymoma, followed at once by the excellent clinicopathological report of FOERSTER and GAGEL (1936) on ependymomas of the filum terminale. This latter type is commonly of a myxopapillary nature caused by degeneration of the stroma, and there is also atrophy of parenchymal cells. Both lead to a blurring of the architecture, so that the original pattern is lost. If this degeneration pattern – which is specific for this particular type – is not present classification is difficult.

The ependymomas are the most common neuroepithelial tumors in the spinal cord (see FISCHER and TOMMASI 1976, filum terminale and conus). A ratio of 27 spinal cases to 47 intracranial was found in a total series of 2186 gliomas (BARONE and ELVIDGE 1970).

The average age of the patients is around 35–40 years. The male:female ratio is 6:4. The youngest patient in the Mayo Clinic series (see SLOOFF et al. 1964) was 6 years old, the oldest 82 years.

Gross Pathology

The gross pathology of these tumors is that of the typical *Stiftgliom,* i.e., pencil-like glioma, extending over large parts of the spinal cord (Fig. 39 in KERNOHAN and SAYRE 1952: between C-1 and L-4). Intramedullary ependymomas involving the whole of the spinal cord were described by HORRAX and HENDERSON as long ago as 1939. The formation of cysts (sometime mistaken as syringomyelias) is very common and will be discussed below.

Ependymomas of the cauda equina and filum terminale are massive tumors measuring up to 8 cm × 3 cm, and have been well described clinically and histologically by FOERSTER and GAGEL (1936), SCHATTENFROH (1962), and PIGANIOL et al. (1964). The predominance of ependymomas in the cauda equina was also emphasized by NORSTROM et al. (1961: 100 cases, 88 of which were ependymomas: 52 filum terminale, 17 conus, 31 both structures).

Multiple ependymomas were described by GAMPER and STIEFLER (1929), giant ependymomas with intrathecal extension (90 g, myxopapillary type), by VARA-THORBECK and SANZ-ESPONERA (1970). An extension from the pelvis into the abdomen was described by HEATH (1963). ADSON et al. (1939) saw 90 tumors in front of the sacrum, 7 of which were ependymomas; and ROSS (1948) another 55, of which 6 were ependymomas.

An extradural site (from ectopias) has not only been described for the ependymomas of the filum terminale and cauda equina but also for other ependymomas of the spinal cord (COOPER et al. 1950: 15 cases, 9 of which were ependymomas; ANDERSON 1966; WOLF et al. 1972).

Histologic Appearance

The frequent occurrence of ependymal canals and small true rosettes is emphasized by Figs. 41–44 of KERNOHAN and SAYRE (1952). It had been already well depicted and described in the original description of "neuroepitheliomas" of the spinal cord (ROSENTHAL 1898; SEIFARTH 1948). Neurons rarely occur (AYRES 1958); ours is one of the groups that has encountered this.

The formation of the so-called syringomyelia (57.6%, or 19 of 33 necropsies) was discussed by SLOOFF et al. (1964, p. 183). These authors also emphasized the occurrence of Rosenthal fibers. The syringomyelic cavity is always in direct topographical correlation to the tumor tissue. We have always thought that this cavity formation is caused by a particular trend to liquefaction within the ependymomas, as it is also seen just as often in the extraventricular ependymomas that occur in childhood and in youth (SCHATTENFROH 1962; see also p. 262).

In the EM secretory phenomena are seen at the mucopapillary type (MILLER and TORACK 1970).

Description of the metastases, e.g., by RUBINSTEIN and LOGAN (1970), into lung, pleura, and aortic lymph nodes from an ependymoma originating in the cauda or filum terminale is important (see also PATTERSON et al. 1961: patient with metastasis after 17 years' illness).

Subependymomas

In the series of SLOOFF et al. (1964) two tumors were classed as subependymomas ("extremely rare"). However, the definition is not very convincing, since we had already shown in 1956 that a very similar pattern can arise from a degenerative process in ependymomas when they are under pressure (see GIAMPALMO 1937). BOYKIN et al. (1954) also described such tumors (ZÜLCH 1956, Fig. 229a–d; HBT, Fig. 11a–d).

Mixed Gliomas

We have emphasized above how swelling of the cells can mimic the oligodendroglioma pattern; this process is very commonly seen in operation material that has remained for more than 2 hours on the operating table. We are inclined to explain most of the "mixed gliomas" of the ependymoma/oligodendroglioma type by this process; on the other hand, astrocytomas with the admixture of oligodendroglioma are not uncommon (see also ARENDT 1976; and Sect. 15.2.2).

Extramedullary Gliomas?

Many reports, beginning with that of KERNOHAN et al. (1931), have described extramedullary gliomas (which the authors consider might have arisen from heterotopias). COOPER et al. (1950) reviewed this problem of extramedullary gliomas, and claimed to have found a still larger group, for which again they assumed an origin in spinal heterotopias.

Glioblastomas

Cases of tumors in this group have been described by SLOOFF et al. (1964). They found 15 cases out of a total of 79 grade III astrocytomas, which according to the WHO nomenclature would be called anaplastic astrocytomas, and 5 grade IV astrocytomas, which corresponded to glioblastoma multiforme. BOUCQUEY (1967) described 3 cases of glioblastomas among 7 intramedullary tumors (although there may have been some errors in classification).

Neuronal Tumors

There are descriptions of spinal ganglion cell tumors and their precursors, although no such case is mentioned in KERNOHAN's series (see SLOOFF et al. 1964). Dumbbell ganglioneuromas in cervical spine have been described, however (STRANG and NORDENSTAM 1962); one ganglioneuroma and 9 neuroblastomas, probably originating in infancy, are listed in the paper of BALAKRISHNAN et al. (1974), and finally one description of a ganglioneuroblastoma has been given by LICHTENSTEIN and ZEITLIN (1937). Furthermore, lumbar dumbbell ganglioneuromas were described by NITTNER (1952). We encountered several tumors of this sort in our series. Neuronal tumors apparently originate at the ganglion, i.e., in the foramen intervertebrale, and also at the filum terminale (LERMAN et al. 1972).

Neurilemmomas

Synonyms: Neurinomas, schwannomas

Introduction

The spinal neurilemmomas are one of the common types of space-occupying lesions and are of particular neurosurgical interest.

Historical Note and Definition

Our present-day knowledge is based mainly on the two extensive series published from large neurosurgical units: the Mayo Clinic (see SLOOFF et al. 1964) and TÖNNIS' unit (see NITTNER 1976). In SLOOFF's series 29% of the neurilemmomas were intraspinal and attached to the nerve roots, whereas 31.8% were extradural, and 6.2% intra/extradural. NITTNER (1976) reported 1129 cases, i.e., 23.1% of a total of 4885 space-occupying spinal lesions collected from the literature. The relative percentage for the neurilemmomas, with 23.1%, was far higher than in our intracranial series, where of 9000 intracranial tumors only 614, i.e., 6.8%, neurilemmomas were encountered. A count of Tönnis' series was published by BACKUS (1965).

Most of the neurilemmomas of clinical importance are located along the posterior roots, more frequently before than after the foramen intervertebrale, where they may widen the outlet. Not too rarely they are structured as a dumbbell (hourglass) tumor. Here the larger part has usually developed outside the foramen intervertebrale and in localization they favor the thoracic cavity (T 3/4 → T 9–12).

TÖNNIS and NITTNER (1968) observed 14.2% dumbbell tumors among 513 patients with spinal cord neoplasms. The frequency of the dumbbell form among neurilemmomas has not yet been defined, however. The figures given so far vary between 25% and 50% (see NITTNER 1976). FIELDS, ZÜLCH et al. (1972) described a special group of neurilemmoma with a predilection site C 2/3.

Intramedullary Neurilemmomas

According to WOLTMAN et al. (1951) this type of neurilemmoma is certainly a very rare lesion (1 case among 74 neurilemmomas). However, such tumors do exist and have been described as fairly small intraspinal neurilemmomatous structures near the anterior roots (SCHÖPE 1951). However, these should be considered more as findings of an academic interest than of neurosurgical importance, because most frequently they are accumulations of Schwann cells sited strictly around the vessels, having a typical architecture but with a very small extension and not surgical lesions. A very typical figure is reproduced in the literature (SCOTT and BENTZ 1962, Fig. 2). MCCORMICK (1964) collected nine cases of intramedullary neurilemmoma from the literature, and recent reports have come from ISU et al. (1976). An intramedullary neurilemmoma was detected during a neurosurgical operation by RAMAMURTHI et al. (1958) when a midline incision of the spinal cord was made.

Epidemiology (Age – Sex – Frequency – Site)

Age: The majority of neurilemmomas occur in middle age, with the peak incidence between 25 and 40 years (SLOOFF et al. 1964: 43.5 years). In KURLAND's (1958) series the youngest patient was 11 months old and the oldest, 80 years.

Sex: NITTNER (1976) found an almost equal sex distribution with only a slight female preponderance (43:39), whereas the opposite was the case in the Mayo Clinic series (SLOOFF et al. 1964: 221 male:162 female patients = 4:3). KURLAND's (1958) series showed quite a striking male preponderance (221 versus 162) for neurilemmomas.

Frequency: The frequency cannot be determined exactly at present, but rough figures have been given above.

Site: The neurilemmomas are almost equally distributed over the spinal segments, with a particular group in vertebrae C1 and C2 (FIELDS, ZÜLCH et al. 1972). In the series of RASMUSSEN et al. (1940) neurilemmomas were not found at root C1, though as his Fig. 4 shows, there were 3 tumors in C2 (see also NITTNER 1976, Fig. 49a).

Neurilemmomas seem to have two slight preferences in the thoracic cord, namely between T 3/4 and T 9/12.

Gross Pathology

The spinal neurilemmomas can be small and pea-like in size (ZSCHAU 1929) or the size of a horse-bean when asymptomatic (GP, Fig. 176). They can also become larger, finger-shaped lesions, which in the caudal region have a length of 8–10 cm. Giant tumors of the cauda have been described (NATARAJAN et al. 1975: 6 cm × 2.5 cm × 1.5 cm). They are usually harder than the intracranial forms, with a smooth and glistering surface. Infiltration of the adjacent tissue (ORF 1970b) has been described, but this must be accepted with reservations; it must be an extremely rare event.

The neurilemmomas in the spinal canal are distributed over one or more segments, and are attached to the posterior roots or the cauda equina. In the dumbbell forms it must be borne in mind that they may be accompanied by a very large segmental artery, which may be inadvertently divided and lead to a subsequent neurological deficit. Spinal neurilemmomas quite often show mucoid degeneration and cyst formation, occasionally with various-sized hemorrhages into these cysts.

Histologic Appearance

The histology of the spinal neurilemmomas is very similar to that of their intracranial counterparts, but with a particular tendency (Fig. 113a) to form almost "ideal" palisades (see ZÜLCH 1956, Fig. 264a, b). The tendency to liquefaction and cyst formation has been emphasized above and led to the observation of KRAYENBÜHL and LÜTHY (1947), who described hemorrhage into cystic cavities in spinal neurilemmomas in children. This had given rise to an acute onset of symptoms and seems to be characteristic for this tumor type (one personal observation). Subarachnoidal hemorrhages have been also described in neurilemmomas of the cauda after physical exertion (review of 17 similar cases: PRIETO and CANTU 1967).

Multiple spinal neurilemmomas can sometimes be present (Fig. 111) without causing any symptom (GP, Fig. 176; SLOOFF et al. 1964, Fig. 73).

Anaplastic changes (malignant degeneration) can occur in the spinal neurilemmomas (see MENNEL and ZÜLCH 1971b), but this is very rare (see history of our case of intrasacral neurofibrosarcoma in a 49-year old patient with a 10-year clinical history).

Meningiomas

The meningioma in the spinal canal is one of the very frequent tumors (Mayo Clinic series: 979 spinal tumors, 25.9% meningiomas, whereas in our series of 9000 cases of ZNS neoplasms they represented only 16.6% within the spinal meningiomas.

Again our knowledge is mainly based on the two series of the Mayo Clinic and Tönnis' Clinic.

Epidemiology (Age – Sex – Frequency – Site)

Age: The average age of patients with spinal meningiomas was 49.9 years, the youngest patient being 3 and the oldest 88 years old in the Mayo Clinic series; there is a peak in the fifties.

Sex: There is a very marked female preponderance, which has been discussed at great length in the literature. In the series of HOSSMANN and ZÜLCH (1966) the sex ratio was 3.6:1. However, this ratio varied very widely if the selection criteria of the series were changed: for psammomatous meningiomas of all levels the ratio was 10:1, in the same class of tumors in the thoracic spine only it was as high as 20:1, the same ratio as formerly published in the series of LAPRESLE et al. (1952). In NITTNER's (1976) series there was also a very marked female preponderance (83.7% female versus 16.3% male patients, i.e., a ratio of 5:1).

Site: In the distribution in the vertebral column a certain preponderance of the thoracic region is encountered. Furthermore, HOSSMANN and ZÜLCH (1966) have emphasized that spinal cord tumors in women in their fifties are very likely to be psammomatous meningiomas in the thoracic region.

Gross Pathology

Spinal meningiomas are mostly globoid, and less commonly flattened. They rarely invade bone, in contrast to their cranial counterparts. With rare exceptions they are attached to the dura; they can be the size and shape of a plum or a bean and are unusual in having a very wide spread, e.g., as finger-like lesions over ten segments (Fig. 122; ODDSSON 1947; BURGER and VOGEL 1976). The largest meningiomas are found in the cervical and lumbosacral areas.

Histologic Appearance

Histologically most of the variants may occur, but there is a vast preponderance of the psammomatous type (see above), particularly in the thoracic spine and particularly in women. Anaplastic changes are exceptional. Multiple tumors occur (GP, Fig. 209). Calcification may be visible on plane x-ray (ORNOS 1939).

Extradural spinal meningiomas have been described (BORGHI 1973: 5 personal cases among 118 spinal meningiomas and 15 cases from the literature; BULL 1953: 6 cases). SINGH et al. (1968) calculated the incidence of extradural forms as 3.5% of the total number of spinal meningiomas.

ARENDT et al. (1962) emphasized the occurrence of diffuse spinal meningiomatosis with a large extension into the leptomeningeal space (RAND 1952; NITTNER and SCHIEFER 1955). The association of spinal meningiomas and metastases from elsewhere has been described in the literature (see p. 114).

Melanomas

Primary malignant spinal melanomas have been encountered (KING et al. 1952: 2 cases). They seem to occur very rarely and their origin is unresolved (leptomeningeal melanocytes?) (HIRANO and CARTON 1960; KIEL et al. 1961; CLIFFORD et al. 1968).

Vascular Tumors

"Vascular" tumors are "rare" (TURNER and KERNOHAN 1941: 10 cases). In KERNOHAN's series (SLOOFF et al. 1964) they made up 6.2% of the large sample of 1322 tumors; 12 (9.5%) of the vascular tumors were in intramedullary locations.

The divergence in the data originates from the poor definition of the term "vascular tumors." Therefore, the specific entities will be distinguished below.

Generally it was assumed that the male sex was predominantly affected (10 males to 3 females). The average age was around 36 years, with the youngest patient being 13 and the oldest, 51 years.

In cases of necropsy all vascular tumors had large cysts (were they hemangioblastomas?), i.e., so-called syringomyelias. In histology these were very similar to their intracranial counterparts (see also CUSHING and BAILEY 1928b).

Hemangioblastomas

The occurrence of hemangioblastomas in the spinal cord is thought to be "rare" (HUK and KLINGER 1973): apparently 1.5%–2.4% of all spinal cord tumors are such hemangioblastomas (BROWNE et al. 1976; UMBACH and KUNFT 1976). BROWNE et al. (1976) examined 85 cases with a median age of 30 years and an equal distribution between the two sexes. Other data, however, show a male predominance.

In a series of 40 patients with hemangioblastomas the tumors were located in the retina in 77.5%, cerebellum in 40%, spinal cord in 7.5%, and medulla oblongata in 5% of cases, and there was no supratentorial representation (BROWNE et al. 1976). In the same statistics multiple hemangioblastomas were not a rare item (see also RAWE et al. 1978).

Familial spinal hemangioblastomas (3 generations) were described by OTENASEK and SILVER (1961).

If the hemangioblastomas are intramedullary they can extend over many segments, or even the whole spinal cord – as in a personal observation – and their tendency to form large pencil-like cysts is as pronounced as that of the ependymomas and pilocytic astrocytomas (KERNOHAN and SAYRE 1952). There are older statistics on hemangioblastomas (ELSBERG 1941), which put their frequency at 1%–2% of the spinal cord tumors and suggested an epidural location in the majority of cases (see also BRONFMAN and ECTORS 1949).

The various locations were studied by BROWNE et al. (1976), who gave proportions of 3.6% for the extradural, 1.7% for the extra/intradural, and 3.3% for the intradural forms in the entire series of tumors (see also WYBURN-MASON 1943; GUIDETTI and FORTUNA 1967).

UMBACH (1962) and UMBACH and KUNFT (1976) emphasized that the hemangioblastomas can grow *within* the spinal cord but that some very soft tumors lie over the posterior columns as reddish/brownish masses, most commonly observed between the ages of 31 and 50 and with a male predominance of 60%–70%. The predilection site is thought to be the thoracic or thoracolumbar spinal cord.

Spinal Vascular Malformations and Malformative Tumors

Spinal vascular malformations account for around 6%–8% of space-occupying lesions in the spinal canal (YASARGIL 1976). Their classification corresponds to that of the other vascular lesions (see Chap. 22). MARINESCO and DRAGANESCO (1935) described the teleangiectasias of the spinal cord and suggested a connection with FOIX-ALAJOUANINE's angiomatosis. This was also discussed by ZÜLCH in 1971c.

BRION et al. (1952) collected 32 cases of such vascular malformations that led clinically to transverse myelitis (first described by FOIX and ALAJOUANINE in 1926).

Angiomas

The spine is the commonest site for *osseous* angiomas (10%–12% of autopsy cases, MAKRYCOSTAS 1927). Vascular tumors of the spine were found in 6.2% of 4858 tumors of the spinal canal (TÖNNIS and NITTNER 1957). UMBACH (1962) found 2.5% of such vascular lesions under 192 spinal tumors. The angiomas occur particularly in the thoracic lumbar spine, are usually solitary, and can compromise the laminae, the joints, or even the entire vertebra. Most commonly they belong to the variant of the cavernous angioma (see also BERGSTRAND et al. 1936).

The interest in the *spinal cord* vascular tumors has been stimulated particularly by the introduction of spinal angiography. In the series of PIA and R. DJINDJIAN (1978) and PIA (1979) the spinal angiomas were classified according to the *site* as extradural or vertebro-extradural or even intradural, and according to their *formation* as arteriovenous, capillary, or complex angiomas (see also R. DJINDJIAN et al. 1969).

Hemangiopericytomas

In the Mayo Clinic series five cases were reported as hemangiopericytomas (PITLYK et al. 1965). They were observed predominantly in extramedullary positions but with one intradural site (WISOFF et al. 1978). The definition of this group is still controversial and therefore the frequency data oscillate.

HARRIS et al. (1978) define the hemangiopericytoma as a vascular neoplasm consisting of capillaries outlined by an intact basement membrane that separates the endothelial cells of the capillaries from the spindle-shaped tumor cells in the extravascular area (see also STOUT and MURRAY 1942; STOUT 1949). This description is repeated here because of the divergence of the interpretations of the hemangiopericytomas (see p. 372).

Epidermoids, Dermoids, Teratomas

In the classifications of the Mayo Clinic these tumors together made up 1.4% of 1322 tumors of the spinal canal, half of them being in intramedullary positions (SLOOFF et al. 1964).

Epidermoids

The epidermoid cysts occurred in four patients, with an average age of 45 years, in the series. These cysts were described in some detail by MANNO et al. (1962), and represent about 0.2%–1% of all spinal canal tumors in large series. The aforementioned authors collected eight cases from the literature and added two of their own. MAHONEY (1936) described 142 epidermoids of the CNS; only seven were of spinal origin; see also the important contribution of VERBIEST (1939) on the spinal epidermoids.

It must be borne in mind that in the post war time of frequent tuberculous meningitis with very frequent lumbar punctures in many cases, epidermoids were encountered and ascribed to the penetrating mechanism of the needle point, by which a deep implantation of epidermis was thought to be made. GROTE and LUND (1957) discussed such postoperative or posttraumatic implantations in detail.

Dermoid Tumors

The dermoid tumors were also represented by four cases in the Mayo Clinic series, with an average age of 31.5 years. (See also I.C. BAILEY 1970: with 10 cases, 8 of which were lumbar.)

Teratomas

Teratomas are commonly operated on soon after birth because of enormous deformities of the caudal region. These tumors probably originate in the coccygeal or presacral parts of the vertebral column. They consist of solid and cystic areas (about lumbosacral teratomas see BUCY and HAYMOND 1932). The Mayo Clinic series included only two teratomas.

Histology

The histology of all these three tumor forms corresponds to that in other locations (see BURGER and VOGEL 1976).

Lipomas

Intraspinal lipomas are not common. The first series from the Mayo Clinic (EHNI and LOVE 1945) included four cases and 25 cases were added from the literature.

Epidemiology (Age – Sex – Site)

Age and Sex: There is apparently a certain male preponderance and the age distribution is equal between the 1st and 7th decades. GIUFFRÈ (1976) estimates the frequency at 2% (based on a published series of 154 cases).

Site: According to BISCHOF and MÜLLER (1966) lipomas in all age groups and at any level are mainly in dorsal positions, with an equal male:female ratio. They are abundant in the extradural space, but rare in intradural or intramedullary locations. The unfavorable characteristic of this tumor type is the attachment at the inner side of the pial membrane with an indentation into the substance of the spinal cord or the roots of the cauda equina. In these circumstances the tumor cells follow the mesodermal septa, a process that leads to a very close connection between the tumor and the underlying nervous tissue and hampers surgery.

Histologic Appearance

Histologically the lipoma in the spinal canal is a very typical tumor of its kind: it is yellowish in color and stands out clearly from the adjacent tissue. Lipomas are frequently lobulated and have a fine whitish fibrous capsule. They may be penetrated by non-adipose tissues such as blood vessels, smooth muscle, or osteoid. They may adhere firmly to the spinal cord. Predominant growth follows the midline. In around 14% of cases they are multiple (GIUFFRÈ 1976). There is never any evidence of malignancy.

Chordomas

The cervical chordoma is most common (ADSON et al. 1935; DAHLIN and MCCARTY 1952), less commonly chordomas are encountered in the thoracic region. ALLEN and KERR (1968) described nine cases, eight of which affected the clivus and one C-5.

In the total series of 155 patients 49% of chordomas were in the sacrococcygeal region, 36% in the spheno-occipital region, and the remaining 15% in the various parts of the vertebral column (BEAUGIÉ et al. 1969). These authors found one presacral chordoma among 40000 autopsy cases. WHITTAKER and PEMBERTON (1938) emphasized the site of such tumors in the ventral sacrum and MAYO et al. (1953) described 161 such presacral tumors.

Gross Pathology

To the naked eye chordomas appear whitish and gelatinous with some reddish streaking. They consist of a soft, semitranslucent tissue (BURGER and VOGEL 1976). A content of calcium is not infrequent. They can erode the vertebral bones without infiltration and can extend over several vertebrae. As they grow they pass through the bone and destroy the disk. Chordomas infiltrate along the line of least resistance but never grow into brain and viscera. Distant metastasis may occur in 10% of all chordomas.

Chondromas

Chondromas (NAG and FALCONER 1966) are benign bone tumors composed of mature hyalin cartilage, and can occur in any part of the vertebral column (JAFFE 1958) and even be multiple. They occur equally in both sexes and preferentially in the age group 30–40 years.

Osteochondromas

Osteochondromas are rare in the spine (MITSUMORI et al. 1975). In SUNDARESAN's et al. (1979) series of 54 patients, the lesion was in the sacrococcygeal region in 36. There were almost twice as many male as female patients and 5-year survival was noted in two-thirds of the patients with osteochondromas in the sacrococcygeal region. With regard to the localization, on collecting 600 cases of the literature the authors found 50% located in the sacrum, 35% in the clivus region, and 15% in other parts of the vertebral column. In TÖRMÄ's (1957, 1975) series the osteochondromas were the largest group of benign tumors arising from precartilaginous connective tissue in the skeleton, but it was rare for them to occur only in the vertebral column, where the predilection site was the dorsal spine.

Benign chondroblastic tumors were very rare, and chondromyxomas sporadic (see also DAHLIN's series in 1957: 2276; in 1967: 3987 bone tumors).

PAILLAS et al. (1963) reported on 70 tumors of the vertebral column, 6 of which were benign; they included 5 personal observations (DAHLIN 1957: 4 cases in the vertebral column among 96 chondromas).

Osteoblastic Tumors

The osteoblastic tumors are relatively uncommon in the spine (ELSBERG 1925; PUUSEP 1933; ANTONI 1936a). ANTONI (1936a) examined 6840 necropsies and found 12 cases of benign osteogenic tumors. TÖRMÄ (1957) collected a series of 1119 tumors of the spine from five large Scandinavian clinics, only 12 of which were benign osteogenic neoplasms. They are classified in the WHO classification by SCHAJOWICZ et al. (1972: osteomas, osteosarcomas, chondrosarcomas, chondromyxoid fibromas; etc.).

Osteomas can occur at any age and the female sex is more frequently affected than the male; any part of the vertebra can be compromised. The preferred site for osteoid osteomas is the arch of the vertebra, but at this site they affect males more commonly than females. The preferential age is 10–25 years (see JAFFE 1956, 1958).

Osteoblastomas have a distinct predilection for the vertebral column; male subjects are more commonly compromised; and the preferential age group is up to 30 years. Osteoblastomas are usually calcified, forming osteoid substance, and quite a larger number of multinucleated giant cells are observed.

The *osteosarcomas* compromise single vertebrae, with a preference for the upper lumbar spine. They consist of grayish tumor masses infiltrating also the paravertebral muscles. The preferential age is from early adulthood onward.

Sarcomas

The report on the Mayo Clinic series did not cite any publications dealing with primary sarcomas of the spinal cord or the filum terminale (SLOOFF et al. 1964). However, the Mayo Clinic researchers themselves had encountered a fibrosarcoma of the filum terminale. Nonetheless, very many reticulosarcomas (see lymphomas, p. 394ff.) have been described in the epidural space (see p. 547).

However, there were 157 such sarcomas amongst the 1322 spinal tumors in the series of the Mayo Clinic, 7 of which were at intramedullary sites.

The reticular sarcomas (including Ewing's sarcomas) accounted in the series of PAILLAS et al. (1976) for 34.5% of the primary malignant tumors of the spine. They formed 23% of the entire series of 335 spinal tumors with an average patient age of 11–45 years.

Malignant Lymphomas

The new classification of the malignant lymphomas (LENNERT 1978; see p. 394) contains many entities already well known to the clinician and morphologist under different names, e.g., the reticulosarcomas etc. Hodgkin's disease is more prominent in frequency than lymphocytic or histiocytic lymphomas (BURGER and VOGEL 1976). We have emphasized their occurrence in the thoracic section of the spine above. They can occur in younger age groups (KLEIN 1961; BUCY 1962), and were extensively described by BINGAS and ZÜLCH (1964).

The vertebral myelomas may lead to a collapse of the bony structure or to rib fractures. The series of the Mayo Clinic included 145 cases (ONOFRIO and SVIEN 1976). They can be either solitary or multiple, occurring usually in patients over 40 years and with predilection sites in the middle and lower thoracic spine.

Multiple myelomas (plasmocytomas) very commonly involve the vertebral column and are associated with infiltration of the epidural space. The preferential age group for these tumors is 41–70 years.

Classification – Summary of the Intravertebral Tumors

A detailed classification of the primary tumors of the spine was given by PAILLAS et al. (1976). They distinguished (a) skeletal tissue tumors such as chondromas, osteochondromas, osteomas etc.; (b) reticular tissue tumors such as reticulosarcomas, reticuloxanthomas, plasmocytomas, myelomas; (c) blood vessel tumors (connective tissue angiomas, aneurysms, cysts, giant cell tumors (CARDAUNS and FRIEDMANN 1961), or bone marrow tumors, lipomas, fibromas etc.); and (d) tumors of the embryonal rests such as chordomas and teratomas. They also list pseudotumors such as granulomas of the type histiocytoma X (Gaucher's disease, etc.).

However, the reader will note that this classification is not in keeping with the terminology described above, where several intravertebral tumors have already been described.

The same is true of the classification of GOLDHAHN and GOLDHAHN (1976), who reviewed the spinal epidural tumors: they listed lipomas and angiolipomas, which do not penetrate the dura; spinal angiomas, which are round, well demarcated, grow in the body of the vertebra and more rarely in the arches (only 10%–12%; cavernomas?); eosinophilic granulomas; malignant teratomas (see also CHRETIEN et al. 1970); malignant lymphomas; lymphogranulomatosis, malignant osteogenic tumors, etc.

And finally, TÖRMÄ's (1957) report on 1119 tumors of the spine (12 benign) is certainly also the result of an intensive study, but again he used a different terminology system. He emphasized the benign osteogenic tumors. He distinguished the benign and malignant forms of bone- and cartilage-forming tumors, adding the giant cell tumors, the bone marrow tumors, the vascular tumors and other connective tissue tumors. Furthermore, he considered "other" forms, such as chordomas, adamantinomas, neurilemmomas, neurofibromas, and finally unclassified tumors. TÖRMÄ (1964, cited in NITTNER 1976, p. 192), however, classified 540 cases according to the following groups: 1. Teratoma (see McDONALD 1973); 2. Neuroblastoma; 3. Lipoma; 4. Dermoid cyst; 5. Sarcoma; 6. Others.

These confusing classifications are reproduced here to emphasize that a critical review was needed and that a new classification must be adopted, which we have tried to define above according to the recommendations of the World Health Organization and some authorities writing in relevant handbooks.

Cystic Lesions of the Meninges and Nerve Roots

There may be several kinds of cystic lesions within the spinal canal, e.g., the meningeal epidural cysts, which are an extension of the arachnoidal space into the epidural space (dorsally); and the epidermoid cysts that are not infrequently situated dorsal to the spinal cord, ventral ependymal cysts, and finally enterogenous cysts extending from the ventral abdominal cavities through the vertebral body towards the ventral surface of the spinal cord. Perineural cysts form an extension of the leptomeninges around a nerve root and are of importance for disk operations.

Spinal Intradural Cysts

MOSSO and VERITY (1975) mentioned that ependymal cysts are very rare. They found only four cases in the literature. MORELLO and LOMBARDI (1964) had a case (their Fig. 4) with ependymal lining. This was in a 32-year-old patient with a history going back 14 years.

Spinal Extradural Cysts

Extradural cysts occur particularly in youth, as shown by KRUMBHOLZ et al. (1966). KRONBORG (1967) observed that these cysts occurred preferably in the thoracic region and that 42% communicated between the extradural and the subdural spaces. These cysts can be the consequence of infections or trauma, or can even be congenital.

There are certainly also secondary (partly iatrogenic) postoperative or post-traumatic spinal meningeal outpouchings, for instance after disk operations (see Fig. 3 in RINALDI and PEACH 1969). The number of descriptions of such cases has increased so much that CLOWARD in 1968 had already collected 92, and BODOSI in 1970, 97 cases in the literature.

Spinal arachnitis is dealt with on p. 519 (first description, SCHLESINGER 1898). The spinal extradural cysts have been examined with more interest only in the last decade. WILKINS and ODOM (1976) found 160 cases in the literature.

Some were observed as multiple congenital extradural space-occupying lesions (NUGENT et al. 1959) along the nerve roots and sheaths. They were filled with a clear and colorless fluid and were covered by flattened layers of cells resembling arachnoidal cells.

An intrasacral site of a cyst below a meningocele is illustrated in a figure of BAKER and WEBB (1952).

There is a particular form of epidural "*enterogenous cysts*" whose pathogenesis is still unclear. They are covered with an endothelium of cylindrical, sometimes mucus-producing cells and may be of dumbbell shape, with a small cyst located intradurally and a larger one in the epidural space, extending from the ventral abdominal cavity through the vertebral body towards the ventral surface (PALMA and DI LORENZO 1970; BURGER and VOGEL 1976).

Primary Aneurysmal Bone Cysts

These cystic degenerations of the bone are rare (1.5% of all bone tumors). The vertebrae may collapse, subluxations can occur, and an approachment of the spinal canal follow (see also DAHLIN et al. 1955; TILLMAN et al. 1968; MACCARTY and DAHLIN 1976; DI LORENZO et al. 1979). They consist of smaller or larger channels arounded by delicate or thick walls of blood-filled spaces, benign giant cells etc.

Multiple Tumors

Multiple tumors occur within the vertebral canal as described by NITTNER and SCHIEFER (1955: 3 meningiomas), by GAMPER and STIEFLER (1929: multiple ependymoblastomas), and LICHTENSTEIN (1941: multiple intramedullary tumors of the spinal cord – ependymomas – associated with neurinomas and meningiomas). Most multiple tumors are meningiomas, although there are no other features of von Recklinghausen's disease in these cases (LIST 1943b; RAND 1952; NITTNER and SCHIEFER 1955). They are mostly benign (NITTNER 1976). Multiple myelomas (plasmocytomas) not infrequently involve the vertebral column, including the infiltration of the epidural space (age group 41–70 years).

Metastases of Primary Spinal Tumors

Intracranial seeding of primary spinal cord tumors is apparently extremely rare (TASHIRO et al. 1976: 9 literature cases). Metastases to multiple visceral organs (liver, lung, pleura etc.) were described by PATTERSON et al. (1961), in one instance in a patient who had been ill for 17 years.

Metastatic Tumors

KRETSCHMER (1979) emphasized that over 5% of cancer patients may have spinal symptoms. He reported on 105 patients operated on in 10 years because of spinal metastases: 10% had bronchocarcinomas (COHEN et al. 1964: 14%); 9.5% breast carcinomas (COHEN et al. 1964: 10%); 9.5% clear cell carcinomas

(COHEN et al. 1964: 12%); 5.7% melanomas (COHEN et al. 1964: 1%); and 4.8% prostatic cancer (COHEN et al. 1964: 22%). KRETSCHMER (1979) also listed 9.5% plasmocytomas and 7.6% Hodgkin's tumors.

COHEN et al. (1964) added three more groups: lower bowel carcinomas, 10%; uterine carcinomas 6%; and bladder carcinomas 3%. In this series the metastases of thyroid tumors, seminomas, etc. were rare. The work gives an extensive reference list.

MOFFI and STEFANKO (1979, unpublished data) described *intramedullary* metastases with an incidence of 5%; we have observed such tumors not infrequently in our own material. Metastatic intramedullary neoplasms have a much lower incidence in the spinal cord, and correspond to the relative volume of the organ (see STRANG 1962; EDELSON et al. 1972). In their report on intramedullary spinal cord metastases JELLINGER et al. (1979) listed lung and breast tumors together with melanomas as the most common primaries; the lymphomas were the second commonest tumors metastasizing into the spinal cord.

CHADE (1968, 1976) reported on metastatic tumors and found that the carcinomas were not so often represented in the lumbar and cervical spine as in the thoracic segment. The comprehensive report of CHADE (1976) on the Zurich series gave the following sequence of primaries metastasizing to the spinal cord: bronchial carcinomas first, followed by carcinoma of the kidneys, the breast, the thyroid, the prostate, the intestine, and the uterus, and "others."

The sequence for frequency of primaries of spinal *epidural* metastases recorded by AULD and BUERMAN (1966) in 50 cases was: lung carcinoma; prostate carcinoma; kidney carcinoma; breast carcinoma; lymphomas; and others (see also JELLINGER et al. 1979). Granulomas and parasites as metastases were described by LUYENDIJK and LINDEMANN (1975, see p. 502). FIREMARK (1978) reported on spinal and AKIGUCHI et al. (1979), on intramedullary cysticercosis.

Rare Clinical Signs in Spinal Cord Lesions

The occurrence of *papilledema* was described some years ago by NITTNER (1956) and RAYNOR (1969), in spinal vascular malformations among other conditions, and by ULBRICHT (1966) in epidural meningiomas. Papilledema was also seen by SATO et al. (1977), and by ISHIKAWA et al. (1974). Increased intracranial pressure was also encountered by GLASAUER (1964) in thoracic and lumbar tumors, as well as by NITTNER (1956). He added 20 cases from the literature (see also MITTAL et al. 1970).

The pathogenesis of this phenomenon is not quite clear. Was it caused by the high protein content of the spinal fluid? Or by the site of the tumor? Generally speaking, raised intracranial pressure occurs only in 1%–3% of all cases of intraspinal tumors.

Clinically the craniospinal tumors have to be excluded from this discussion (BOGORODINSKII and SUVOROV 1961; KRENKEL and FRIEDMANN 1967: apparent frequency 9.4% of 341 spinal cases). Those observed were meningiomas, neurilemmomas, chordomas, angioblastomas, sarcomas, ependymomas, pilocytic astrocytomas, and "other gliomas" at this particular location. COOPER et al. (1952) mentioned 15 neoplasms with a relative paucity of symptoms (9 astrocytomas, 1 ependymoma, 1 oligodendroglioma, 4 Lindau's hemangioblastomas). The occurrence of subarachnoid hemorrhage in rare cases of spinal tumors is discussed elsewhere (p. 354; neurilemmomas); it is also encountered in extramedullary upper thoracic astrocytoma (RUNNELS and HANBERY 1974).

It may be mentioned here that sometimes even giant tumors of the medulla oblongata may remain almost asymptomatic (see BRUGGER 1954; GP, Fig. 158).

The clinical prognosis will not be discussed here. For most spinal tumor groups it is well defined and broadly described in Vol. 19 of the Handbook of Clinical Neurology. Special follow-up studies were conducted by CHIGASAKI and PENNYBACKER (1968) on the basis of 677 intraspinal tumors, 118 of which were intramedullary.

33 The Orbit: Space-Occupying Lesions

Amongst the main lesions of the orbit the space-occupying processes of the eye and optic fascicle are most important.

The retrobulbar pilocytic astrocytoma of the optic fascicle (see p. 231) has a characteristic form, namely a blowing-up of the fascicle (ZÜLCH and NOVER 1960), which is diffusely infiltrated by the tumor so that the arachnoidal sheath itself is grossly enlarged by direct invasion. The same type of pilocytic astrocytoma can also grow more in the retina itself or exclusively in that location, or it can have an hourglass or dumbbell form.

There is only a slight similarity between this and the second form of tumor of the optic fascicle, i.e., the meningioma of the optical sheath. It is said to be not so spindle-like in shape as the astrocytoma, but more nodular.

For comparison see the excellent schematics (Figs. 20 and 21) of LUNDBERG (1935), which are redrawn after GOLOVINE (1918).

In the meningioma the tumor growth is only subdural and takes place in the arachnoidal sheath *around* the fascicle, whereas the nerve itself is not invaded but only strangulated.

According to LUNDBERG (1935) the ratio of gliomas to meningiomas is about 5:2, and the remaining one-eight is made up of "other" space-occupying lesions.

The others include the angioblastic tumors, which are particularly typical and common in the form of the cavernous angioma, a well-encapsulated lesion, or – exceedingly rare – of the hemangioblastoma.

Of the entirely *retinal* tumors we have already mentioned the retinoblastoma (p. 301) and the retinal melanoma (p. 391).

Extraocular but infraorbital lesions are the carcinomas of the lacrimal gland and the retrobulbar lymphomas, and all possible secondaries into the orbit. Meningioma from outside the sphenoid wing can involve the orbital cavity, as well as meningiomas within the orbital roof occur.

Finally, Basedow-Graves disease and other swellings of rheumatic/allergic nature of the eye muscles must be borne in mind (for general review see UNSÖLD 1982).

References

Aarabi B, Long DM (1979) Dynamics of cerebral edema. The role of an intact vascular bed in the production and propagation of vasogenic brain edema. J Neurosurg 51:779–784

Aarabi B, Pasternak G, Hurko O, Long DM (1979) Familial intradural arachnoid cysts. J Neurosurg 50:826–829

Abay EO II, Laws ER, Grado GL, Bruckman JE, Forbes GS, Gomez MR, Scott M (1981) Pineal tumors in children and adolescents. Treatment by CSF shunting and radiotherapy. J Neurosurg 55:889–895

Abbassioun K, Rahmat H, Ameli NO, Tafazoli M (1978) Computerized tomography in hydatid cyst of the brain. Neurosurgery 49:408–411

Abbott KH, Cutler OI (1936) Chronic coccidioidal meningitis. Review of literature and report of seven cases. Arch Pathol 21:320–330

Abbott KH, Glass B (1955) Intracranial extracerebral (leptomeningeal) glioma. Excerpta Med (Amst) Sect VIII: 786

Abbott KH, Kernohan JW (1943) Primary sarcomas of the brain. Review of the literature and report of twelve cases. Arch Neurol Psychiatry 50:43–66

Abbott M, Killeffer FA, Crandall PH (1968) Melanotic meningioma. Case report. J Neurosurg 29:283–286

Abrikossoff AI (1931) Weitere Untersuchungen über Myoblastenmyome. Virchows Arch [A] 280:723–740

Abtahi H (1975) Multiple meningiomas. Adv Neurosurg 2:48–50

Achucarro N (1912) Sobre los nucleos de las celulas gigantes de un glioma. Trab Lab Biol 10:262–272

Acquaviva R, Charbit E, Benkiran-Malbos D, Lebascle J (1966) Les tératomes intracrâniens (Revue de la littérature à propos d'une observation). J Méd Maroc 2:272–314

Adams JE (1953) Familial hemangioblastoma of the cerebellum. Pedigree of two families. J Neurosurg 10:421–422

Adams JH (1970) The various forms of microgliomatosis. In: Proceedings of the International Congress of Neuropathology, Paris, 1970. Masson, Paris, pp 437–438

Adams JH (1975) The classification of microgliomatosis with particular reference to diffuse microgliomatosis. Acta Neuropathol [Suppl] (Berl) VI:119–123

Adams JH, Jackson JM (1966) Intracerebral tumors of reticular tissue: the problem of microgliomatosis and reticulo-endothelial sarcomas of the brain. J Pathol Bact 91:369–381

Adelman LS, Aronson SM (1972) Intramedullary nerve fiber and Schwann cell proliferation within the spinal cord (schwannosis). Neurology (Minneap) 22:726–731

Adeloye A, Odeku EL (1969) Metastatic neoplasms of the brain in Nigeria. Br J Cancer 23:340–348

Adler (1898) Über das Auftreten von Hirngeschwülsten nach Kopfverletzungen. Arch Unfallheilkd 2:189–225

Adson AW, Kernohan JW, WoltmanWH (1935) Cranial and cervical chordomas. Arch Neurol Psychiatry 33:247–261

Adson AW, Moersch FP, Kernohan JW (1939) Neurogenic tumors arising from the sacrum. Arch Neurol Psychiatry 41:535–555

Aebi M, Kraus-Ruppert R (1978) Oligodendroglioma with a twenty-two year history. J Neurol 219:139–144

Afra D, Turóczy L, Deák G (1981) Ependymomas extending into both lateral ventricles: CT-diagnosis and operability. Report of 2 cases. Zentralbl Neurochir 42:255–262

Afshar F, Scholtz CL (1981) Enterogenous cyst of the fourth ventricle. J Neurosurg 54:836–838

Agarwal S, Gandagule VN, Chouhan SS (1968) Neurogenic tumours of the nose. Indian J Cancer 5:127–131
Agduhr E (1922) Über ein zentrales Sinnesorgan bei den Vertebraten. Z Anat Entwickl Gesch 66:223–360
Aguilar MJ, Rabinovitch R (1964) Metastatic chorionepithelioma simulating multiple strokes. Neurology (Minneap) 14:933–937
Aita JA (1968a) Genetic aspects of tumors of the nervous system: I. Nebr Med J 53:121–124
Aita JA (1968b) Genetic aspects of tumors of the nervous system: II. Nebr Med J 53:302–304
Akiguchi I, Fujiwara T, Matsuyama H, Muranaka H, Kameyama M (1979) Intramedullary spinal cysticercosis. Neurology (Minneap) 29:1531–1534
Alava AG, Ortiz Gonzalez JM, Castroviejo IP (1965) Lipomas extradurales sacros. Arch Neurobiol (Madr) 28:481–490
Albert DM, Dalton AJ, Rabson AS (1970) Microtubules in retinoblastoma. Am J Ophthalmol 69:296–299
Albert F (1982) Spontaneous haemorrhage in intracranial tumours. A clinical report of 50 cases. Acta Neurochir (Wien) 62:143–144
Albrecht E (1907a) Die Grundprobleme der Geschwulstlehre. Frankfurt Z Pathol 1:221–247
Albrecht E (1907b) Randbemerkungen zur Geschwulstlehre. Frankfurt Z Pathol 1:347
Albrechtsen R, Klee IG, Möller JE (1972) Primary intracranial germ cell tumours including five cases of endodermal sinus tumors. Acta Pathol Microbiol Scand [Suppl 233] 80:32–38
Alexander E Jr (1953) Benign subtentorial supracollicular cyst as a cause of obstructive hydrocephalus. J Neurosurg 10:317–323
Alexander GL, Norman RM (1960) The Sturge-Weber syndrome. Wright, Bristol
Alexander L (1937) Tumors and cysts of the cerebellopontine angle and their relation to the lateral recesses of the fourth ventricle. Williams and Wilkins, Baltimore, pp 266–314 (Association for Research in Nervous and Mental Disease: Tumors of the nervous system, vol 16)
Alexander L (1939) A note on the differential diagnosis of experimentally produced brain tumors and their relation to brain tumors in man. Am J Cancer 37:395–399
Alexander WS (1948) Multiple primary intracranial tumors. J Neuropathol Exp Neurol 7:81–88
Allen JC, Epstein F (1982) Medulloblastoma and other primary malignant neuroectodermal tumors of the CNS. J Neurosurg 57:446–451
Allen KL, Kerr WA (1968) Chordomas of the clivus and cervical spine. S Afr Med J 42:1165–1174
Allen RA, Latta H, Straatsma BR (1962) Retinoblastoma. A study of two cases by electron microscopy. Invest Ophthalmol 1:728–744
Alpers BJ (1931) Origin and development of giant cells in gliomas. Arch Neurol 25:281–298
Alpers BJ (1939) Gumma of the brain. Am J Syphil 23:233–240
Alpers BJ, Grant FC (1931) The ganglioneuromas of the central nervous system. Arch Neurol 26:501–523
Alpers BJ, Rowe SN (1937) The astrocytomas. Am J Cancer 30:1–18
Alpers BJ, Grant FC, Yaskin J (1932) Primary fibroblastoma of the brain. Arch Neurol Psychiatry 27:270–281
Alter M (1975) Statistical aspects of spinal cord tumors. In: Vinken PJ, Bruyn GW (eds) Tumours of the spine and spinal cord. North-Holland, Amsterdam/American Elsevier, Oxford (Handbook of clinical neurology, vol 19, part 1, pp 1–22)
Altmann H-W (1961) Ein Beitrag zur Pathologie des cellulären Zentralapparates. Nach Beobachtungen an einem Hirntumor. Virchows Arch [A] 334:132–159
Alvira MM, McLaurin RL (1978) Asymptomatic subdural chondrosarcoma. J Neurosurg 48:825–828
Alvord EC Jr, Marcuse PM (1962) Intracranial cerebellar meningo-encephalocele (posterior fossa cyst) causing hydrocephalus by compression of the incisura tentorii. J Neuropathol Exp Neurol 21:50–69
Alzheimer A (1910) Beiträge zur Kenntnis der pathologischen Neuroglia und ihrer Beziehungen zu den Abbauvorgängen im Nervengewebe. Histol Histopathol Arb Großhirnrinde 3:401–562

Amacher AL, Allcock JM, Drake CG (1972) Cerebral angiomas: the sequelae of surgical treatment. J Neurosurg 37:571–575

Ambler M, Pogacar S, Sidman R (1969) Lhermitte-Duclos disease (granule cell hypertrophy of the cerebellum). Pathological analysis of the first familiar cases. J Neuropathol Exp Neurol 28:622–647

Ameli NO, Haddadian A, Kamalian N (1979) Incidence of intracranial tumours in Iran. Neurosurg Rev 2:67–71

Amendola MA, Garfinkle WB, Ostrum BJ, Katz MR, Katz RI (1978) Preoperative diagnosis of a ruptured intracranial dermoid cyst by computerized tomography. J Neurosurg 48:1035–1037

Amer MH, Al-Sarraf M, Baker LH, Vaitkevicius VK (1978) Malignant melanoma and central nervous system metastases. Incidence, diagnosis, treatment and survival. Cancer 42:660–668

Amstad E (1937) Beitrag zur Klinik und Histopathologie des Gangliocytoms der Medulla oblongata. Schweiz Arch Neurol Psychiatr 39:5–25

Anderson FM, Carson MJ (1953) Spinal cord tumors in children: A review of the subject and presentation of twenty-one cases. J Pediatr 43:190–207

Anderson FM, Segall HD, Caton WL (1979) Use of computerized tomography scanning in supratentorial arachnoid cysts. J Neurosurg 50:333–338

Anderson JW (1879) Tumors of the dura mater. Convulsions. Removing of tumor by trephining. Recovery. Glasgow Med J 12:210

Anderson MS (1966) Myxopapillary ependymomas presenting in the soft tissue over the sacrococcygeal region. Cancer 19:585–590

Anderson Hospital (1974) Nomenclature of neoplastic disease. Department of Pathology, University of Texas System Cancer Center, Houston, Texas

Andrioli GC, Scanarini M (1979) Intrinsic haematopoietic activity of cerebellar hemangioblastomas. Ultrastructural study of three cases. Neurochirurgia (Stuttg) 22:24–28

Annegers JF, Schoenberg BS, Okazaki H, Kurland LT (1981) Epidemiologic study of primary intracranial neoplasms. Arch Neurol 38:217–219

Ansbacher L, Low N, Beck D, Boarini D, Jacoby C, Cancilla PA (1981) Neoplastic angioendotheliosis: a clinicopathological entity with multifocal presentation. J Neurosurg 54:412–415

Anton G (1904) Gehirnoedem und Compression. In: Flatau E, Jacobsohn L, Minor L (eds) Handbuch der pathologischen Anatomie des Nervensystems, vol I. Karger, Berlin, pp 396–467

Antoni N (1920) Über Rückenmarkstumoren und Neurofibrome. Bergmann, München

Antoni N (1936a) Tumoren der Wirbelsäule einschließlich des epiduralen Spinalraumes. In: Bumke O, Foerster O (eds) Erkrankungen der Wirbelsäule, des Schädels mit Nebenhöhlen, und der Hüllen. Springer, Berlin (Handbuch der Neurologie, vol X, pp 51–109)

Antoni N (1936b) Tumoren des Rückenmarks, seiner Wurzeln und Häute. In: Bumke O, Foerster O (eds) Raumbeengende Prozesse. Springer, Berlin (Handbuch der Neurologie, vol XIV, pp 1–131)

Antoni N (1950) Gliomas of the neurohypophysis and hypophysial stalk. J Neurosurg 7:521–531

Aoki H, Ogashiwa M, Wakutani K, Ito E (1971) Cavernous hemangioma of the cerebral hemisphere, a case report (In Japanese). No To Shinkei 23:931–932

Aoyagi T, Kyuno K (1912) Über die endothelialen Zellzapfen in der Dura mater cerebri und ihre Lokalisation in derselben nebst ihrer Beziehung zur Geschwulstbildung in der Dura mater. Neurologia (Tokyo) 11:1–11

Apitz K (1937) Über Pigmentbildung in den Zellkernen melanotischer Geschwülste. Virchows Arch [A] 300:89–112

Apitz K (1943) Die Geschwülste und Gewebsmißbildungen der Nierenrinde. Virchows Arch [A] 311:285–305

Arai H, Yamazaki K, Yamazaki Y, Ueki K (1976) A statistical study of brain tumors (In Japanese). No To Shinkei 28:779–791

Araki C (1937) Meningioma in the pineal region. A report of two cases removed by operation (In Japanese). Nippon Geka Hokan 14:1181–1192

Araki C, Matsumoto S (1969) Statistical reevaluation of pinealoma and related tumors in Japan. J Neurosurg 30:146–149

Arana-Iñiguez R (1978) Echinococcus. In: Vinken PJ, Bruyn GW (eds) Infections of the nervous system. North-Holland, Amsterdam (Handbook of clinical neurology, vol 35, part III, pp 175–208)

Arana-Iñiguez R, Asenjo A (1945) Ventriculographic diagnosis of cysticercosis of the posterior fossa. J Neurosurg 2:181–190

Arana-Iñiguez R, López-Fernández JR (1967) Parasitosis of the nervous system with special reference to echinococcosis. Clin Neurosurg 14:123–144

Arana-Iñiguez R, San Julian J (1955) Hydatid cysts of the brain. J Neurosurg 12:323–335

Arana-Iñiguez R, Gorlero Armas A, San Julian J (1951a) Angiografia en el quiste hidático cerebral. IVth South American Congress of Neurosurgery, Porto Alegre, 6–12 May 1951

Arana-Iñiguez R, Rodriguez-Barrios R, San Julian J (1951b) Nueva técnica para la extirpación del quiste hydatico nota precia. Prensa Méd Argent 38:891–897

Arana-Iñiguez R, Rodriguez Barrios R, San Julian J (1952) Surgical treatment of hydatid cysts of the brain. Trans Am Neurol Assoc 77:210–211

Araoz C, Moore JJ, Sun C, Angel C (1979) Melanotic neuroectodermal tumor of the middle fossa. Ultrastructural and biochemical study. J Neuropathol Exp Neurol 38:303

Araujo JC, Werneck L, Cravo MA (1978) South American blastomycosis presenting as a posterior fossa tumor. Case report. J Neurosurg 49:425–428

Archangelsky VV, Golubew VJ, Kasumova SJ, Kotelnikow VM, Kondakowa LJ (1972) Study of cell populations, kinetics and cytogenetics of human macroglial tumors (Proceedings of the 4th European Congress of Neurosurgery, Prague). Avicenum, Prague

Arendt A (1964a) Die gewebliche Entdifferenzierung der Gliome. Oncologia (Basel) 17:16–30

Arendt A (1964b) Histologisch-diagnostischer Atlas der Geschwülste des Zentralnervensystems und seiner Anhangsgebilde. Fischer, Jena

Arendt A (1965) An attempt to grade the factor of malignancy in cases of cerebral tumour. J Neurol Sci 2:442–445

Arendt A (1976) Spinal gliomas. In: Vinken PJ, Bruyn GW (eds) Tumors of the spine and and spinal cord. North-Holland, Amsterdam/American Elsevier, Oxford (Handbook of clinical neurology, vol 20, part II, pp 323–351)

Arendt A, Möller B (1973) Hirngeschwülste im Kindesalter. Arch Geschwulstforsch 41:164–176

Arendt A, Senitz D (1972) Histologische Kriterien zur biologischen Wertigkeit beim Ependymom. Arch Geschwulstforsch 40:44–50

Arendt A, Fischer W, Schneider HJ (1962) Diffuse spinale Meningeomatose. Neurochirurgia (Stuttg) 5:161–170

Arita N, Ushio Y, Hayakawa T, Watanabe M, Maeda Y, Kanai N, Mogami H (1979) Primary intracranial germ cell tumor (In Japanese). No Shinkei Geka 7:465–474

Arjona V, Aneiros J, Linares J, Aguilar D, Diaz-Flores L (1978) Sarcomatoid transformation of the vascular walls in giant cell glioblastoma. Morf Norm B 1:319–334

Arlant PA, Grunnet ML, Heilbrun MP (1977) Primary malignant melanoma of the pineal region. Surg Neurol 7:121–123

Arlt HG (1936) Multiple Meningeome des Gehirns und diffuse Meningiomatosis des Rückenmarks. Z Gesamte Neurol Psychiatr 156:713–734

Armstrong RM, Hanson CW (1969) Familial gliomas. Neurology (Minneap) 19:1061–1063

Arnold A, Bailey P, Laughlin JS (1954) Effects of betatron radiations on brain of primates. Neurology (Minneap) 4:165–178

Arnold H, Zimmerman HM (1943) Experimental brain tumors: III. Tumors produced with dibenzanthracene. Cancer Res 3:682–685

Arnold H, Grubel G, Franke H, Grosch I, Marsmann G (1978) Results of medulloblastoma treatment under the influence of modern therapy. Adv Neurosurg 5:253–256

Arnvig J, Christensen E (1939) Primary benignant intracranial melanoma. Acta Chir Scand 82:217–226

Aron BS (1971) Medulloblastoma in children. Am J Dis Child 121:314–317

Aronson HA, Otis RD (1962) Intracranial chondroma involving the cerebellopontine angle. Report of a case. J Neurosurg 19:529–531

Aronson SM (1971) Vascular malformations. In: Minckler J (ed) Pathology of the nervous system, vol II. McGraw-Hill, New York, pp 1884–1897
Aronson SM, Garcia IH, Aronson BE (1964) Metastatic neoplasms of the brain: their frequency in relation to age. Cancer 17:558–563
Arseni C, Maretsis M (1972) Craniopharyngioma. Neurochirurgia (Stuttg) 15:25–32
Arseni C, Simionescu M, Carp N, Guran C (1967) The abscess-like form of brain metastases. Acta Neurochir (Wien) 17:113–125
Arseni C, Mestes E, Georgian M (1968) La cyto-oncologie de la pinéale. Ann Anat Pathol 13:119–136
Arseni C, Danaila L, Nicola N, Georgian M, Istrati C (1969) Intracranial teratomas. Acta Neurochir (Wien) 20:37–51
Arseni C, Constantinescu A, Danaila I, Carp I (1975) Multiple cerebral tumors of varying histological origin. Neurol Psychiatr (Bucur) 13:111–116
Asbury AK, Ojemann RG, Nielsen SL, Sweet WH (1972) Neuropathologic study of fourteen cases of malignant brain tumor treated by boron-10 slow neutron capture radiation. J Neuropathol Exp Neurol 31:278–303
Ascherl GF Jr, Hilal SK, Brisman R (1981) Computed tomography of disseminated meningeal and ependymal malignant neoplasms. Neurology (NY) 31:567–574
Askanazy M (1906) Teratom and Chorionepitheliom der Zirbel. Verh Dtsch Ges Pathol 10:58–76
Askanazy M (1914) Zur Physiologie und Pathologie der Plexus chorioidei. Verh Dtsch Ges Pathol 17:85–103
Askanazy M (1921) Die Zirbel und ihre Tumoren in ihrem funktionellen Einfluß. Frankfurt Z Pathol 24:58–77
Aszkanazy CL (1952) Sarcoidosis of the central nervous system. J Neuropathol Exp Neurol 11:392–400
Auer RN, Rice GPA, Hinton GG, Amacher AL, Gilbert JJ (1981) Cerebellar astrocytoma with benign histology and malignant clinical course. J Neurosurg 54:128–132
Auer RN, Budny J, Drake CG, Ball MJ (1982) Frontal lobe perivascular schwannoma. J Neurosurg 56:154–157
Auld AW, Buerman A (1966) Metastatic spinal epidural tumors. Arch Neurol 15:100–108
Aulich A, Wende S, Meese W, Meinig G, Reulen HJ (1976) Follow-up studies in cerebral tumors using CT. In: Lanksch W, Kazner E (eds) Cranial computerized tomography. Springer, Berlin Heidelberg New York, pp 135–142
Auster LS (1961) The role of trauma in oncogenesis. A juridical consideration. JAMA 175:946–950
Ayres WW (1958) Ependymoma of the cauda equina: A report of the clinico-pathologic aspects and follow-up studies of 18 cases. Milit Med 122:10–35
Azzarelli B, Richards DE, Anton AH, Roessmann U (1977) Central neuroblastoma. Electron microscopic observations and catecholamine determinations. J Neuropathol Exp Neurol 36:384–397
Baba M, Iseki H, Kumagai Y, Sugiyama H, Nawada H (1980) Acoustic neurinoma with massive hemorrhage within the tumor tissue. A case report (In Japanese). No Shinkei Geka 8:193–198
Babinski J (1900) Tumeur de corps pituitaire sans acromégalie et avec arrêt de développement des organes génitaux. Rev Neurol (Paris) 8:531–535
Bachmann K-D (1979) Neuroblastoma sympathicum. Dtsch Ärzteblatt 6:339–344
Backlund E-O (1972) Studies on craniopharyngiomas: I. Treatment: past and present. Acta Chir Scand 138:743–747
Backus ML (1965) Untersuchungen zur Statistik der Biologie und Pathologie intrakranieller und spinaler raumfordernder Prozesse. Medical dissertation, University of Cologne
Badt B (1937) Mikroskopische Schnelldiagnose bei hirnchirurgischen Eingriffen. Zentralbl Neurochir 2:123–140
Baethmann A (1978) Pathophysiological and pathochemical aspects of cerebral edema. Neurosurg Rev 1:85–100
Bagdasar D (1929) Le traitement chirurgical des gommes cérébrales. (Leur incidence par rapport aux tumeurs). Rev Neurol (Paris) 36:1–30

Baggenstoss AH, Love JG (1939) Pinealomas. Arch Neurol 41:1187–1206

Bahr AL, Krumholz A, Kristi D, Hodges FJ (1978) Neuroradiological manifestations of intracranial sarcoidosis. Radiology 127:713–717

Bailey IC (1966) Intracranial spread of adamantinoma. Case report. J Neurosurg 25:455–457

Bailey IC (1970) Dermoid tumors of the spinal cord. J Neurosurg 33:676–681

Bailey OT (1936) Relation of glioma of the leptomeninges to neuroglial nests: Report of a case of astrocytoma of the leptomeninges. Arch Pathol 21:584–600

Bailey OT (1940) Histology of meningioma. Arch Pathol 30:42–69

Bailey OT, Ford R (1942) Sclerosing hemangiomas of the central nervous system: Progressive tissue changes in hemangioblastomas of the brain and in so-called angioblastic meningiomas. Am J Pathol 18:1–27

Bailey P (1920) Cruveilhier's tumeurs perlées. Surg Gynceol Obstet 31:390–401

Bailey P (1924) Further observations on pearly tumors. Arch Surg 8:524–534

Bailey P (1927) Further remarks concerning tumors of the glioma group. Bull Johns Hopkins Hosp 40:354–389

Bailey P (1929) Intracranial sarcomatous tumors of leptomeningeal origin. Arch Surg 18:1359–1402

Bailey P (1930) Further notes on cerebellar medulloblastomas. The effects of roentgen radiation. Am J Pathol 6:125–135

Bailey P (1932a) Cellular types in primary tumors of the brain. In: Penfield W (ed) Cytology and cellular pathology of the nervous system. Hoeber, New York, pp 905–951

Bailey P (1932b) Tumors of the hypophysis cerebri. In: Penfield W (ed) Cytology and cellular pathology of the nervous system. Hoeber, New York, pp 1133–1144

Bailey P (1933) Intracranial tumors. Baillière, Tindall and Cox, London

Bailey P (1936a) Die Hirngeschwülste, 1st edn. Enke, Stuttgart

Bailey P (1936b) Tumors of the nervous system in infancy and childhood. In: Brennemann's loose leaf pediatrics, vol 4, chap 21. Prior, Hagerstown, p 28

Bailey P (1951) Die Hirngeschwülste, 2nd edn. Enke, Stuttgart

Bailey P, Bagdasar D (1929) Intracranial chordoblastoma. Am J Pathol 5:439–450

Bailey P, Bucy PC (1929a) Cavernous hemangioma of the vertebrae. JAMA 92:1748–1751

Bailey P, Bucy PC (1929b) Oligodendrogliomas of the brain. J Pathol 32:735–751

Bailey P, Bucy PC (1930a) Astroblastomas of the brain. Acta Psychiatr Neurol Scand 5:439–461

Bailey P, Bucy PC (1930b) Tumors of the spinal canal. Surg Clin North Am 10:233–257

Bailey P, Bucy PC (1931) The origin and nature of meningeal tumors. Cancer Res 15:15–54

Bailey P, Cushing H (1925) Medulloblastoma cerebelli: a common type of midcerebellar glioma of childhood. Arch Neurol 14:192–223

Bailey P, Cushing H (1926) A classification of the tumors of the glioma group on a histogenetic basis with a correlation study of prognosis. Lippincott, Philadelphia

Bailey P, Cushing H (1928) Blood vessel tumors of the brain. Thomas, Springfield

Bailey P, Cushing H (1930) Die Gewebsverschiedenheit der Gliome und ihre Bedeutung für die Prognose. Fischer, Jena

Bailey P, Davidoff LM (1925) Concerning the microscopic structure of the hypophysis cerebri in acromegaly. Am J Pathol 1:185–207

Bailey P, Eisenhardt L (1932) Spongioblastomas of the brain. J Comp Neurol 56:391–430

Bailey P, Hiller F (1924) The interstitial tissues of the nervous system. J Nerv Ment Dis 59:337–361

Bailey P, Sánchez M (1946) Neurinoma de nervio vago derecho en forma de reloj de arena. Arch Neurol Mexico 8:125–133

Bailey P, Cushing H, Eisenhardt L (1928) Angioblastic meningiomas. Arch Pathol 6:953–990

Bailey P, Buchanan DN, Bucy PC (1948) Intracranial tumors of infancy and childhood, 2nd edn. (1st edn 1939) University Chicago Press, Chicago

Bailey Pearce, Jelliffe SE (1911) Tumors of the pineal body. Arch Intern Med 8:851–880

Bailey WL, Sperl MP (1969) Angiomas of the cervical spinal cord. J Neurosurg 30:560–568

Bakay L, Cares HL (1972) Olfactory meningiomas. Report on a series of twenty-five cases. Acta Neurochir (Wien) 26:1–12

Baker AB, Adams JM (1937) Primary fibroblastoma of the brain. Am J Pathol 13:129–137

Baker AB, Adams JM (1938) Lipomatosis of the CNS. Cancer Res 34:214–219
Baker GS, Bailey AA (1952) Neurofibroma of the trigeminal nerve root in the posterior fossa. Proc Staff Meet Mayo Clin 27:118–120
Baker GS, Gottlieb CM (1956) Cyst of the choroid plexus of the lateral ventricle causing disabling headache and unconsciousness. Proc Staff Meet Mayo Clin 31:95–97
Baker GS, Webb JH (1952) Intrasacral meningocele causing backache and sacral nerve pain. Report of case. Proc Staff Meet Mayo Clin 27:231–234
Baker GS, Weyand RE (1951) Metastatic tumor of the brain fifteen years after resection of primary tumor of the breast. Proc Staff Meet Mayo Clin 26:250–252
Balakrishnan V, Rice MS, Simpson DA (1974) Spinal neuroblastomas. Diagnosis, treatment and prognosis. J Neurosurg 40:631–638
Balaparameswara Rao S, Dinakar I, Sreenivasa Rao K (1971) Giant intracranial epidural meningioma. J Neurosurg 35:748–750
Balhuizen JC, Bots GTAM, Schaberg A, Bosman FT (1978) Value of cerebrospinal fluid cytology for the diagnosis of malignancies in the central nervous system. J Neurosurg 48:747–753
Ballinger WE Jr, Schimpff RD (1979) An experimental model for cerebral metastasis preliminary light and ultrastructural studies. J Neuropathol Exp Neurol 38:19–34
Balsys R, Norton GA (1980) Intracranial meningioma presenting as a mass in the neck. Neuroradiology 19:89–91
Banerjee AK, Blackwood W (1971) A subfrontal tumour with the features of plasmocytoma and meningioma. Acta Neuropathol (Berl) 18:84–88
Bangert L, Orthner H (1959) Über diffuse Gliose. Zentralbl Allg Pathol 101:48–68
Banna M (1976) Review article: Craniopharyngioma, based on 160 cases. Br J Radiol 49:206–223
Barboni E (1940) Contributo allo studio dei gliomi dell'encefalo nel bovino. Tumori 26:361–393
Barbosa-Coutinho L, Mennel HD, Zülch KJ (1974) Die Morphologie der Tumoren der Nasenhöhle und des Bulbus olfactorius bei Ratten. Acta Neurochir (Wien) 31:73–88
Bargmann W (1943) Die Epiphysis cerebri. In: Möllendorf W (ed) Blutgefäß- und Lymphgefäßapparat, intersekretorische Drüsen. Springer, Berlin (Handbuch der mikroskopischen Anatomie des Menschen, vol VI/4, pp 309–502)
Barker DJP, Weller RO, Garfield JS (1976) Epidemiology of primary tumours of the brain and spinal cord: a regional survey in Southern England. J Neurol Neurosurg Psychiatry 39:290–296
Barnard RO (1968) The development of malignancy in oligodendrogliomas. J Pathol Bacteriol 96:113–123
Barnard RO (1974) Tumour biopsy in brain tumour. In: Vinken PJ, Bruyn GW (eds) Tumors of the brain and skull. North-Holland, Amsterdam/American Elsevier, New York (Handbook of clinical neurology, vol 16, part I, pp 708–726
Barnard RO, Scott T (1975) Pattern of proliferation in cerebral lymphoreticular tumours. Acta Neuropathol (Berl) 6:125–130
Baro F (1964) Angiomatose méningée non calcifiante, état granulaire de l'écorce, sclérose diffuse axiale et cutis marmorata congenita. Acta Neurol Belg 64:1042–1063
Barone BM, Elvidge AR (1970) Ependymomas. A clinical survey. J Neurosurg 33:428–438
Barraquer-Ferré L, Tolosa E, Barraquer-Bordas L, Duran F (1950) Intradural lipoma of the spinal cord. Acta Psychiatr Neurol Scand 25:7–17
Barré JA, Leriche R, Gilard (1936) Arachnoïdite primitive. Crises douloureuses. Section de quatre racines sensitives. Guérison immédiate et durable. Rev Neurol (Paris) 65:339–343
Barrer SJ, Simeone FA, Han SS (1980) An unusual presentation of an oligodendroglioma. J Neurosurg 53:560–561
Barrows HS, Harter DH (1962) Tentorial meningiomas. J Neurol Neurosurg Psychiatry 25:40–44
Bartlett IR (1971) Craniopharyngiomas: a summary of 85 cases. J Neurol Neurosurg Psychiatry 34:37–41
Basauri L, Asenjo A (1967) Trigeminal neurinomas. Acta Neurochir (Wien) 17:1–6
Bassett RC, Lowenberg K (1949) Cerebral schistosomiasis. J Neuropathol Exp Neurol 8:220–225

Bastian FO (1971) Papova-like virus particles in a human brain tumor. Lab Invest 25:169–175

Batson R, Shapiro J, Christie A, Riley HD Jr (1955) Acute nonlipid disseminated reticuloendotheliosis. Am J Dis Child 90:323–343

Battista AF, Bloom W, Loffman M, Feigin I (1961) Autotransplantation of anaplastic astrocytoma into the subcutaneous tissue of man. Neurology (Minneap) 11:977–981

Batzdorf U (1966) Chemotherapy of glioblastoma multiforme: an appraisal. Bull Los Angeles Neurol Soc 31:164–176

Batzdorf U, Malamud U (1963) The problem of multicentric gliomas. J Neurosurg 20:122–136

Batzdorf U, Pokress SM (1968) Architectural features of ependymomas in tissue culture. J Neuropathol Exp Neurol 27:333–347

Bauchhenss G, Schürmann K (1962) Die intracraniellen Epidermoide. Zentralbl Neurochir 22:129–161

Bauditz A (1933) Über Dermoide und Epidermoide des Gehirns. Z Gesamte Neurol Psychiatr 144:135–147

Bauer KH (1928) Mutationstheorie der Geschwulstentstehung. Springer, Berlin

Bauer KH (1949) Das Krebsproblem. Springer, Berlin Göttingen Heidelberg

Baumgarten PC von (1881) Über gummöse Syphilis des Gehirns und des Rückenmarks, namentlich der Hirngefäße und über das Verhältnis zu den tuberkulösen Affektionen. Arch Pathol Anat (Berl) 86:179–221

Beal MF, Kleinman GM, Ojemann RG, Hochberg FH (1981) Gangliocytoma of third ventricle: Hyperphagia, somnolence and dementia. Neurology (NY) 31:1224–1228

Beatty RA (1972) Malignant melanoma of the choroid plexus epithelium. J Neurosurg 36:344–347

Beaugié JM, Mann CV, Butler EG (1969) Sacrococcygeal chordoma. Br J Surg 56:586–588

Bebin J, Tytus JS (1955) Ossification in gliomas. J Neurosurg 12:577–583

Bebin J, Tytus JS (1956) Gliomatosis cerebri. Neurology (Minneap) 6:815–822

Bechterew W von (1904) Die Syphilis des Centralnervensystems. In: Flatau E, Jacobsohn L, Minor L (eds) Handbuch der pathologischen Anatomie des Nervensystems, vol I. Karger, Berlin, pp 580–635

Beck C (1943) Über das gutartige Knochenmarkretikulom mit Eosinophilie. Virchows Arch [A] 311:569–592

Beck DJK, Russell DS (1942) Oligodendrogliomatosis of the cerebrospinal pathway. Brain 65:352–372

Becker D, Norman D, Wilson CB (1979) Computerized tomography and pathological correlation in cystic meningiomas. J Neurosurg 50:103–105

Becker DP, Benyo R, Roessmann U (1967) Glial origin of monstrocellular tumor. Case report of prolonged survival. J Neurosurg 26:72–77

Becker LE, Yates AJ, Hoffman HJ, Norman MG (1975) Intracranial chordoma in infancy. J Neurosurg 42:349–352

Beckmann JW, Kubie LS (1929) Tumor of the hypophyseal stalk. Brain 52:127–170

Beckmann O (1930) Gliom and Trauma. Medical dissertation, University of Kiel

Beckwith JB, Perrin EV (1963) In situ neuroblastomas: a contribution to the natural history of neural crest tumors. Am J Pathol 43:1089–1104

Bedwell SF, Lindenberg R (1961) A hypothalamic hamartoma with dendritic proliferation and other neuronal changes associated with "blastomatoid" reaction of astrocytes. J Neuropathol Exp Neurol 20:219–236

Behrend CM (1957) Fedor Krause und die Anfänge der Neurochirurgie in Deutschland. Dtsch Med Wochenschr 82:519–520

Behrend RC (1962) Diagnostik von Meningiomen der dritten Stirnhirnwindung. Dtsch Med Wochenschr 38:1899–1906

Behrend RC (1974) Epidemiology of brain tumors. In: Vinken PJ, Bruyn GW (eds) Tumors of the brain and skull. North-Holland, Amsterdam/American Elsevier, New York (Handbook of clinical neurology, vol 16, part I, pp 56–88)

Behrend RC, Zülch KJ, Kleihues P, Kalm H, Schultze-Bergmann G, Wack H-O (1966) La clinique des sténoses carotidiennes et la portée du traitement médical. Rev Neurol (Paris) 115:673–694

Behrendt W, Schultrich S (1963) Das maligne Neurinom. Z Krebsforsch 65:524–528

Beller AJ, Feinsod M, Sahar A (1972) The possible relationship between small dose irradiation to the scalp and intracranial meningiomas. Neurochirurgia (Stuttg) 15:135–143

Belza J (1966) Double midline intracranial tumors of vestigial origin: contiguous intrasellar chordoma and suprasellar craniopharyngioma. J Neurosurg 25:199–204

Benda C (1900) Beiträge zur normalen und pathologischen Histologie der menschlichen Hypophysis cerebri. Klin Wochenschr 37:1205–1210

Benda C (1932a) Zirbeldrüse. In: Handbuch der inneren Sekretion, vol I. Kabitzsch, Leipzig

Benda C (1932b) Hypophysis cerebri. In: Handbuch der inneren Sekretion, vol I. Kabitzsch, Leipzig

Benda CE (1954) The Dandy-Walker syndrome or the so-called atresia of the foramen Magendie. J Neuropathol Exp Neurol 13:14–29

Benda P (1968) Protéine S-100 et tumeurs cérébrales humaines. Rev Neurol (Paris) 118:368–372

Bender JL, Van Landingham JH, Manno NJ (1974) Epidural lipoma producing spinal cord compression. J Neurosurg 41:100–103

Bender W, Panse FR (1932) Familiäres Gliom (zur Genetik der Gliome). Monatsschr Psychiatr Neurol 83:253–285

Benedek L (1936) Über die autochthonen Dysembryome (Pinealome) des Gehirns. Z Gesamte Neurol Psychiatr 156:677–693

Benedek L, Juba A (1941a) Die Gewebsstruktur der Gliome mit besonderer Berücksichtigung der Einteilungsmöglichkeit. Arch Psychiatr Nervenkr 113:233–283

Benedek L, Juba A (1941b) Über das Mikrogliom. Dtsch Z Nervenheilkd 152:159–169

Benedek L, Juba A (1943) Über den histologischen Aufbau und die systematischen Beziehungen der Ependymome. Dtsch Z Nervenheilkd 155:69–90

Beneke R (1926) Trauma und Gliom. Verh Dtsch Ges Pathol 21:441–450

Beneke R (1932) Klinische und anatomische Beiträge zur traumatischen Ätiologie der Geschwülste des Zentralnervensystems und seiner Häute. Ergeb Allg Pathol 26:893–1027

Bennet AM, Godlee RJ (1885) Case of cerebral tumor. The surgical treatment. Br Med J I:988–989

Bennett WA (1946) Primary intracranial neoplasms in military age group world war II. Milit Surg 99:594–652

Bennington JL, Jones RE (1962) Primary sarcoma of the cerebellum (cerebellar sarcoma) with extracranial metastases. Case reports. J Neurosurg 19:685–690

Bérard M, Tripier MF, Choux R, Gambarelli D, Grisoli F, Toga M (1976) Esthésioneurocytome olfactif. Acta Neuropathol (Berl) 35:139–150

Berblinger W (1921) Gliom von seltener Lokalisation. Zentralbl Allg Pathol 31:201

Berblinger W (1922) Zur Frage der Zirbelfunktion. Virchows Arch [A] 237:144–153

Berblinger W (1925) Zur Kenntnis der Zirbelgeschwülste. Z Gesamte Neurol Psychiatr 95:741–761

Berblinger W (1926) Die Glandula pinealis. In: Lubarsch O, Henke F, Rössle R (eds) Handbuch der speziellen pathologischen Anatomie und Histologie, vol 8. Springer, Berlin, pp 681–759

Berblinger W (1928) Kurze Bemerkung zu der Arbeit von A. Schuback über die Angiomatosis des ZNS (Lindausche Krankheit). Z Gesamte Neurol Psychiatr 112:315–316

Berblinger W (1930) Physiologie und Pathologie der Zirbel. Erg Inn Med Kinderheilkd 14:245–312

Berblinger W (1932) Pathologie und pathologische Morphologie der Hypophyse. In: Handbuch der inneren Sekretion, vol 1. Kabitzsch, Leipzig

Berblinger W (1936) Die Adenome der Hypophyse. Nervenarzt 9:329–340

Berblinger W (1944) Zur Kenntnis der Pinealocytome nebst Bemerkungen über die cerebrogene Frühreife. Schweiz Z Pathol 7:107–128

Berendes I (1961) Das maligne Papillom der Nasennebenhöhlen. HNO 9:265–269

Berg NO, Lindgren M (1958) Time-dose relationship and morphology of delayed radiation lesions of the brain in rabbits. Acta Radiol [Suppl] (Stockh) 167

Berg BO, Ablin AR, Wang W, Skoglund R (1974) Encephalopathy associated with occult neuroblastoma. J Neurosurg 41:567–572

Bergdahl L, Boquist L, Liliequist D, Thulin C-A, Tovi D (1972) Primary malignant melanoma of the central nervous system. A report of 10 cases. Acta Neurochir (Wien) 26:139–149

Berger EC, Elvidge MD (1963) Medulloblastomas and cerebellar sarcomas. A clinical survey. J Neurosurg 20:139–144
Berger L, Coutard H (1926) L'estésioneurocytome olfactif. Bull Assoc Fr Cancer 15:404–414
Berger L, Luc R, Richard J (1924) L'esthésioneuroépithéliome olfactif. Bull Assoc Fr Cancer 13:410–421
Berger P (1890) Considerations sur l'origine, le mode de développement et le traitement de certaines encéphalocéles. Rev Chir (Paris) 10:269
Berghorn WJ (1982) Untersuchungen zur biologischen Wertigkeit des klassischen und des desmoplastischen Medulloblastoms. Medical dissertation, University of Düsseldorf
Bergland RM (1975) Pathological considerations in pituitary tumours. Prog Neurol Surg 6:62–94
Bergmann E von (1866–1873) Verletzungen und chirurgische Krankheiten des Kopfes. In: Pitha, Billroth T (eds) Handbuch der allgemeinen und speziellen Chirurgie, vol 3. Enke, Stuttgart, pp 1–314
Bergmann E von (1890) Surgical treatment of diseases of the brain. In: Woods medical and surgical monographs, vol 6. Wood, New York, pp 765–968
Bergmann E von (1895) Über einige Fortschritte in der Hirnchirurgie. Verh Dtsch Ges Chir 24:1–17
Bergstrand A, Höök O, Lidvall H (1963) Vertebral haemangiomas compressing the spinal cord. Acta Neurol Scand 39:59–66
Bergstrand H (1932a) On gliomas of the cerebral hemispheres. Acta Pathol Microbiol Scand 11:100–113
Bergstrand H (1932b) Über das sogenannte Astrozytom des Kleinhirns. Virchows Arch [A] 287:538–552
Bergstrand H (1933) Über das Gliom in den Großhirnhemispheren. Virchows Arch [A] 287:797–822
Bergstrand H (1937) Weiteres über sogenannte Kleinhirnastrozytome. Virchows Arch [A] 299:725–739
Bergstrand H, Olivecrona H (1935) Angioblastic meningiomas. Am J Cancer 24:522–530
Bergstrand H, Olivecrona H, Tönnis W (1936) Gefäßmißbildungen und Gefäßgeschwülste des Gehirns. Thieme, Leipzig
Berkheiser SW (1956) Oligodendrogliomas in the young-age group. J Neurosurg 13:170–175
Bernard JD, Aguilar MJ (1969) Localized hypothalamic histiocytosis X. Report of a case. Arch Neurol 20:368–372
Bernat JL (1976) Glioblastoma multiforme and the meningeal syndrome. Neurology (Minneap) 26:1071–1074
Bernell WR, Kepes JJ, Seitz EP (1972) Late malignant recurrence of childhood cerebellar astrocytoma. Report of two cases. J Neurosurg 37:470–474
Bernhard W (1961) Elektronenmikroskopischer Beitrag zum Studium der Kanzerisierung und des malignen Zustandes der Zelle. Verh Dtsch Ges Pathol 45:8–37
Bernhardt M (1881) Beiträge zur Symptomatologie und Diagnostik der Hirngeschwülste. Hirschwald, Berlin
Bernhuber K (1935) Die Angioblastome des Kleinhirns. Medical dissertation, University of Würzburg
Bernstein SA (1933) Über Carcinommetastasen in einem Duraendotheliom. Zentralbl Allg Pathol 58:163–166
Berry RG, Schlezinger NS (1959) Rathke-cleft cysts. Arch Neurol 1:648–658
Bertha H (1939) Beitrag zur Morphologie der Gefäßverteilung bei Hirntumoren. Z Gesamte Neurol Psychiatr 167:563–604
Bertha H (1940) Morphologische Studien der Gefäße bei einem sogenannten „apoplektischen Gliom". Z Gesamte Neurol Psychiatr 169:617–636
Bertha H (1942) Die Spiegelschrift der linken Hand. Z Gesamte Neurol Psychiatr 175:68–96
Bertha H (1955) Zur Gefäßmorphologie bei Hirntumoren. Acta Neurochir [Suppl] (Wien) III:181–189
Bertha H, Sorgo W (1940) Über einen operativ geheilten Fall eines Plexuspapilloms. Chirurg 12:714–718
Besnier E (1889) Lupus pernio de la face. Ann Dermatol Syph 10:333

Besold G (1986) Über 2 Fälle von Gehirntumor (Hämangiosarkom oder sog. Peritheliom) in der Gegend des dritten Ventrikels bei zwei Geschwistern. Dtsch Z Nervenheilkd 8:49–74

Best PV (1963a) Metastatic carcinoma in a meningioma. Report of a case. J Neurosurg 20:892–894

Best PV (1963b) Intracranial oligodendrogliomatosis. J Neurol Neurosurg Psychiatry 26:249–256

Best PV (1973) A medulloblastoma-like tumor with melanin formation. J Pathol 110:109–111

Best PV (1974) Posterior fossa medulloepithelioma. Report of a case. J Neurol Sci 22:511–518

Bestle J (1968) Extragonadal endodermal sinus tumours originating in the region of the pineal gland. Acta Pathol Microbiol Scand 74:214–222

Bestle J (1969) Oligodendroglioma with unusual meningeal spread. Acta Neuropathol (Berl) 12:94–97

Betty MJ (1964) Quality of survival in treated patients with supratentorial gliomata. J Neurol Neurosurg Psychiatry 27:556–561

Bevan AD, McCarthy ER (1929) Tumors of the carotid body. Surg Gynecol Obstet 49:764–779

Bhandari YS (1972) Noncommunicating supratentorial subarachnoid cysts. J Neurol Neurosurg Psychiatry 35:763–770

Bhangui GR, Roy S, Tandon PN (1977) Multiple primary tumors of the brain including a medulloblastoma in the cerebellum. Cancer 39:293–297

Bhrany D, Murphy MG, Horenstein S, Silbert SH (1974) Diffuse periventricular and meningeal glioma. Acta Neuropathol (Berl) 30:243–249

Bianchedi S, Pelizza A (1962) Il lipoma del corpo calloso. Minerva Pediatr 14:1015–1020

Bianchi M, Frera C (1957) A case of brain gumma. J Neurol Neurosurg Psychiatry 20:133–135

Bickerstaff ER, Howell JS (1953) Neurological importance of tumors of the glomus jugulare. Brain 76:576–593

Bickerstaff ER, Cloake PCP, Hughes B, Smith WT (1952) The racemose form of cerebral cysticercosis. Brain 75:1–18

Bickerstaff ER, Conolly RC, Woolf AL (1967) Cerebellar medulloblastoma occurring in brothers. Acta Neuropathol (Berl) 8:104–107

Bicknell JM (1967) Chromosome studies of human brain tumors. Neurology (Minneap) 17:485–490

Bicknell JM, Carlow TJ, Kornfeld M, Stovring J, Turner P (1978) Familial cavernous angiomas. Arch Neurol 35:746–749

Biedl A (1922) Physiologie und Pathologie der Hypophyse. Verh Dtsch Ges Inn Med 34:1–81

Biedl A (1930) Die Hypophyse. In: Bethe A, Von Bergmann G, Embden G, Ellinger A (eds) Handbuch der normalen und pathologischen Physiologie, vol 16, part 1

Biedler JL, Roffler-Tarlov S, Schachner M, Freedmann LS (1978) Multiple Neurotransmitter synthesis by human neuroblastoma cell lines and clones. Cancer Res 38:3751–3758

Bielfeld K (1955) Über ein metastasierendes Zylindrom. Zentralbl Allg Pathol 93:353–357

Bielschowsky M (1914) Über tuberöse Sclerose und ihre Beziehung zur Recklinghausenschen Krankheit. Z Gesamte Neurol Psychiatr 26:133–155

Bielschowsky M (1915) Zur Kenntnis der Beziehungen zwischen tuberöser Sclerose und Gliomatose. J Psychol Neurol 21:101

Bielschowsky M (1924) Zur Histopathologie und Pathogenese der tuberösen Sclerose. Neue Beiträge. J Psychol Neurol 30:167–200

Bielschowsky M (1925) Das multiple Ganglioneurom des Gehirns und seine Entstehung. J Psychol Neurol 32:1–20

Bielschowsky M (1932) Neuroblastic tumors of the sympathetic nervous system. In: Penfield W (ed) Cytology of the nervous system. Hoeber, New York, pp 1085–1094

Bielschwosky M, Gallus J (1913) Über tuberöse Sclerose. J Psychol Neurol 20 (1):1–88

Bielschowsky M, Henneberg R (1922) Zur Histologie und Histogenese der zentralen Neurofibromatose. Libro en Honor de D.S. Ramon y Cajal, vol 1. Madrid, pp 505–536

Bielschowsky M, Henneberg R (1928) Über Bau und Histogenese der zentralen Ganglioneurome. Monatsschr Psychiatr Neurol 68:21–51

Bielschowsky M, Rose M (1927) Zur Kenntnis der zentralen Veränderungen bei Recklinghausenscher Krankheit. J Psychol Neurol 35:42–63

Bielschowsky M, Simon A (1930) Über diffuse Hamartome (Ganglioneurome) des Kleinhirns und ihre Genese. J Psychol Neurol 41:50–75
Bielschowsky M, Unger E (1906) Zur Kenntnis der primären Epithelgeschwülste der Adergeflechte des Gehirns. Arch Klin Chir 81:61–82
Bielschowsky M, Unger E (1920) Syringomyelie mit Teratom und extramedullärer Blastombildung. J Psychol Neurol 25:173
Biemond A (1974) Cerebellar tumors. In: Vinken PJ, Bruyn GW (eds) Tumors of the brain and skull. North Holland, Amsterdam/American Elsevier, New York (Handbook of clinical neurology, vol 17, part II, pp 707–718)
Bierring F, Egeberg J, Jensen OA (1967) A contribution to the ultrastructural study of retinoblastomas. Acta Ophthalmol (Copenh) 45:424–428
Bigner DD (1978) Role of viruses in the causation of neural neoplasia. In: Laerum OD, Bigner DD, Rajewsky MF (eds) Biology of brain tumors. UICC, Genf (UICC technical report, vol 30, No 5, pp 85–111)
Bigner DD, Pegram CN (1976) Virus-induced experimental brain tumors and putative associations of viruses with human brain tumors: a review. Adv Neurol 15:57–83
Bigner DD, Swenberg JA (1977) Virally induced CNS tumors. In: Bigner DD, Swenberg JA (eds) Jänisch and Schreiber's experimental tumors of the central nervous system. 1st English edn. Upjohn, Kalamazoo, pp 91–93
Billroth T (1868) Allgemeine chirurgische Pathologie und Therapie. Berlin 1868
Bingas B (1964a) On the primary sarcomas of the brain. Acta Neurochir [Suppl] (Wien) X:186–189
Bingas B (1964b) Das monstrozelluläre Sarkom des Gehirns. Arch Psychiatr Nervenkr 205:223–236
Bingas B (1964c) Das Retikulumzellsarkom des Gehirns. Zentralbl Neurochir 24:143–148
Bingas B (1965) Das Fibrosarkom der Dura. Neurochirurgia (Stuttg) 8:20–25
Bingas B (1966) Enzymhistochemische Befunde an intracraniellen Tumoren. Naturwissenschaften 53:87
Bingas B (1970) Klassifikation und Prognose semibenigner Gliome. Fortschr Med 88:625–626
Bingas B (1972) Klinische, histologische und fermenthistochemische Befunde an semibenignen Gliomen. Acta Neuropathol (Berl) 20:43–54
Bingas B, Böhme D (1964) Ein Fall von Hirnmetastasen bei knotiger Lungenadenomatose. Zentralbl Neurochir 25:125–129
Bingas B, Brunngraber CV (1964) Das gleichzeitige Vorkommen von Meningeom und Glioblastom. Zentralbl Neurochir 24:271–275
Bingas B, Grumme T (1971) Die Bedeutung hydrolytischer Fermente für die Klinik der Meningiome. Zentralbl Neurochir 32:261–271
Bingas B, Schulze A (1964) Das Problem der malignen Entartung des Astrocytoms nach Operation und Bestrahlung. Arch Psychiatr Nervenkr 205:600–609
Bingas B, Wolter M (1968) Das Kraniopharyngiom. Fortschr Neurol Psychiatr 36:117–195
Bingas B, Zülch KJ (1964) Epidurale Sarkome des Spinalkanals. Acta Neurochir (Wien) 12:11–30
Bingas B, Zülch KJ (1966) Zur Klinik und Morphologie des sogenannten „adventitiellen Sarkoms". Acta Neurochir (Wien) 15:11–27
Biran S, Herishianu Y (1972) Brain involvement in Hodgkin's disease. Report of a case. Eur Neurol 8:352–358
Bird AV (1978) Schistosomiasis of the central nervous system. In: Vinken PJ, Bruyn GW (eds) Infections of the nervous system. North-Holland, Amsterdam New York Oxford (Handbook of clinical neurology, vol 35, part III, pp 231–241)
Birkenfeld W (1930) Zur Erblichkeit der multiplen kartilaginären Exostosen (Exostosen bei eineiigen Zwillingen). Dtsch Z Chir 226:397–403
Birkmayer W, Hasenjäger T (1940) Ventilverschluß des vierten Ventrikels durch ein Epidermoid. Zentralbl Neurochir 5:177–184
Birnbaum LM, Owsley JQ (1968) Frontonasal tumors of neurogenic origin. Plast Reconstr Surg 41:462–470
Bischof W, Müller W 1966) Beitrag zur Biologie der intramedullären Lipome. Dtsch Z Nervenheilkd 189:1–10

Bischof W, Nittner K (1969) Epidermoide und Dermoide des Spinalkanals. Zentralbl Neurochir 30:101–118
Bischof W, Schettler G (1967) Zur Klinik und Therapie der arteriovenösen Angiome und Varicosen des Rückenmarks. Dtsch Z Nervenheilkd 192:46–68
Bischoff A (1961) Erfahrungen mit der Tumorzelldiagnostik im Liquor cerebrospinalis. Acta Neurochir (Wien) 9:510–524
Bito S, Sakaki S, Gohma T, Kozumi T, Matsuoka K (1974) Incisural tumor. Two cases of dumbbell type tumor in the incisural region (In Japanese). No Shinkei Geka 2:771–777
Bittorf A von (1904) Beiträge zur pathologischen Anatomie der Gehirn- und Rückenmarksgeschwülste. Beitr Pathol Anat 35:169
Bizzozero G, Bozzolo C (1874) Studi sui tumori primitivi della dura madre. Riv Clin Bologna 4:223–267
Black BK, Kernohan JW (1950) Primary diffuse tumors of the meninges (so-called meningeal meningiomatosis). Cancer 3:805–819
Black BK, Smith DE (1950) Nasal glioma. Two cases with recurrence. Arch Neurol Psychiatry 64:614–630
Black SPW, German WJ (1950) Four congenital tumors found at operation within the vertebral canal. With observations on their incidence. J Neurosurg 7:49–61
Blagoweschtschenskaja NS (1952) Die Arachnoidendotheliome der hinteren Schädelgrube und Funktionsstörungen des Nervus acusticus. (In Russian) Vopr nevrokhir 4:15
Bland J (1936) Tissue culture of gliomata. J Anat 71:149
Bland J, Russell D (1938) Histological types of meningioma. J Pathol 47:291–309
Blatt B, Højgaard K (1963) Cancer metastaticus cerebri. Acta Neurol Scand 39:356–368
Blecher D (1905) Über Cholesteatome (Epidermoide) der Schädelknochen. Dtsch Z Chir 70:352–362
Bleher EA, Poretti PG, Veraguth PC (1982) Radiotherapy of medulloblastoma: Radiation technique, results, and complications. In: Voth D, Gutjahr P, Langmaid C (eds) Tumours of the central nervous system in infancy and childhood. Springer, Berlin Heidelberg New York, pp 344–348
Blinzinger K, Henn R (1966) Carcinose der Hirnkammern infolge Geschwulstzellaussaat auf dem inneren Liquorweg. Acta Neuropathol (Berl) 6:14–24
Bloom HJG, Wallace ENK, Henk JM (1969) The treatment and prognosis of medulloblastoma in children. A study of 82 verified cases. Am J Roentgenol 105:43–62
Blümcke S (1965) Elektronenoptische Untersuchungen an Schwannschen Zellen während der Wallerschen Degeneration peripherer Nerven. Verh Dtsch Ges Pathol 49:346–349
Blümcke S, Niedorf HR (1966) Electron microscope studies of Schwann cells during the Wallesian degeneration with special reference to the cytoplasmic filaments. Acta Neuropathol (Berl) 6:46–60
Blumenfeld CM, Gardner WJ (1945) Disseminated oligodendroglioma. Arch Neurol Psychiatry 54:274–276
Bochnik HJ (1953) Nekrosekalk und kalzifierende Organisation im Gehirn. Dtsch Z Nervenheilkd 169:358–382
Bodechtel G (1934) Ein Neuroepitheliom (Neuroblastom) unter dem klinischen Bild eines Meningioms der Olfactoriusrinne. Arch Psychiatr 101:617–622
Bodosi M (1970) Die angeborene spinale extradurale Zyste. Acta Neurochir (Wien) 23:275–283
Bodsch W, Hürter T, Hossmann K-A (1982) Immunochemical method for quantitative evaluation of vasogenic brain edema following cold injury of rat brain. Brain Res 249:111–121
Boeck C (1905) Fortgesetzte Untersuchungen über das multiple benigne Sarkoid. Arch Dermatol Syph 71:301
Böhmig KH (1918) Gehirntumor bei zwei Geschwistern. Arch Psychiatr 59:527–533
Boellaard JW (1964) Ein Medulloblastom mit quergestreiften Muskelfasern. Arch Psychiatr Nervenkr 206:228–236
Boellaard JW (1971) Über einen Fall von Granulomenzephalitis mit ungewöhnlicher Lokalisation. Arch Psychiatr Nervenrk 214:17–32
Boemke F, Joest W (1936) Chordome im Bereich des Schädels. Virchows Arch [A] 297:351–367
Boesel CP, Suhan JP (1979) A pigmented choroid plexus carcinoma: Histochemical and ultrastructural studies. J Neuropathol Exp Neurol 38:177–186

Boesel CP, Suhan JP, Sayers MP (1978) Melanotic medulloblastoma. Report of a case with ultrastructural findings. J Neuropathol Exp Neurol 37:531–543

Bofin PJ, Ebels E (1963) A case of medullomyoblastoma. Acta Neuropathol (Berl) 2:309–311

Boggan JE, Rosenblum ML, Wilson CB (1979) Neurilemmoma of the fourth cranial nerve. Case report. J Neurosurg 50:519–521

Bogorodinskii DK, Suvorov GP (1961) On clinical aspects of craniovertebral tumors. (In Russian) Zh Nevropatol Psikhiatr 61:497–500

Bohm E, Strang R (1961) Choroid plexus papillomas. J Neurosurg 18:493–500

Boivin P, Bousser J, Brion S, Guiot G (1965) Polyglobulie et hémangiome du cervelet. Rapport de deux cas avec mise en évidence d'une substance érythropoiétique dans la tumeur et le plasma. Presse Med 73:2799–2803

Bojsen-Møller M (1977) Primary cerebral melanomas. Report of six cases and a review of the literature. Acta Pathol Microbiol Scand [A] 85:447–454

Bojsen-Møller M, Spaun E (1978) Peripheral nerve tumour composed of neurilemmoma and haemangioma elements. Acta Neurochir (Wien) 40:299–305

Boll F (1874) Die Histologie und Histogenese der nervösen Zentralorgane. Arch Psychiatr 4:1–138

Bollack J, David M, Puech P (1937) Les arachnoidites optochiasmatiques. Masson, Paris

Bollati A, Giunta F, Lenzi A, Masini G (1973) Third ventricle intrinsic craniopharyngioma. J Neurosurg Sci 17:316–317

Bollinger VO (1887) Über primäre Aktinomykose des Gehirns beim Menschen. MMW 34:789–792

Bond WH, Richards D, Tumer E (1965) Experiences with radioactive gold in the treatment of craniopharyngioma. J Neurol Neurosurg Psychiatry 28:30–38

Bonebrake RA, Siqueira EB (1964) The familial occurrence of solitary hemangioblastoma of the cerebellum. Neurology (Minneap) 14:733–743

Bonikos DS, Bensch KG, Kempson RL (1976) The contribution of electron microscopy to the differential diagnosis of tumors. Beitr Pathol 158:417–444

Bonis G (1961) Über das Vorkommen von Kerneinschlüssen in Meningiomen. Dtsch Z Nervenheilkd 183:194–198

Bonnal J, Sedan R, Pellet W, Fabre J, Laviéille J, Paillas J (1966) Le pronostic opératoire des tumeurs bénignes intracrâniennes. Neurochirurgie 12:361–372

Bookallil AJ (1975) Tumours of the pineal region. A review of 49 cases. Abstracts 5th Congress European Association of Neurosurgical Societies, Oxford, pp 79–81

Borchers (1910) Tumoren des Plexus chorioideus des Gehirns. Medical dissertation, University of Leipzig

Borck WF (1950) Geschlechtsverteilung bei Hirngeschwülsten. Medical dissertation, University of Hamburg

Borck WF, Zülch KJ (1951) Über die Erkrankungshäufigkeit der Geschlechter an Hirngeschwülsten. Zentralbl Neurochir 11:333–350

Borden S, Weber AL, Toch R, Wang CC (1973) Pineal germinoma. A long term survival. Am J Dis Child 126:214–216

Borghi G (1973) Extradural spinal meningiomas. Acta Neurochir (Wien) 29:195–202

Borit A (1969) Embryonal carcinoma of the pineal region. J Pathol 97:165–168

Borit A, Richardson EP (1982) The biological and clinical behaviour of pilocytic astrocytomas of the optic pathways. Brain 105:161–187

Borit A, Blackwood W, Mair WGP (1980) The separation of pineocytoma from pineoblastoma. Cancer 45:1408–1418

Bormann H (1951) Artdiagnose der seltenen Schädelbasisgeschwülste. Zentralbl Neurochir 11:33–45

Borovich B, Mayer M, Gellei B, Peyser E, Yahel M (1976) Multifocal glioma of the brain. J Neurosurg 45:229–232

Borst M (1902a) Die Lehre von den Geschwülsten. Bergmann, Wiesbaden

Borst M (1902b) Ein Sakraltumor von eigenartigem Bau. Beitr Pathol Anat 31:419

Borst M (1924) Allgemeine Pathologie der malignen Geschwülste. In: Zweiffel P, Payr E (eds) Die Klinik der bösartigen Geschwülste. Hirzel, Leipzig, pp 1–180

Bosch DA, Rähn T, Backlund EO (1978) Treatment of colloid cysts of the third ventricle by stereotactic aspiration. Surg Neurol 9:15–18
Bostroem E (1897) Über die pialen Epidermoide, Dermoide und Lipome etc. Zentralbl Allg Pathol 8:1–98
Bots GTAM, Went LN, Schaberg A (1964) Results of a sedimentation technique for cytology of cerebrospinal fluid. Acta Cytol (Baltimore) 8:234–241
Bots GTAM, Went LN, Schaberg A (1968a) Sedimentation technique for cerebrospinal fluid. In: Koss LG (ed) Diagnostic cytology and its histological bases, 2nd edn. Lippincott, Philadelphia, pp 622–623
Bots GTAM, Kroes R, Feron VJ (1968b) Spontaneous tumours of the brain in rats. A report of three cases. Vet Pathol 5:290–296
Bouchard J (1966) Radiation therapy of tumors and disease of nervous system. Lea and Febiger, Philadelphia
Bouchard J, Peirce CB (1960) Radiation therapy in the management of neoplasma of the central nervous system, with special note in regard to children. Twenty years' experience. Am J Roentgenol 84:610–628
Boucquey JP (1967) Les tumeurs non kystiques intramédullaires cervicales. Acta Neurol Psychiatr Belg 67:527–538
Boudouresques G, Boudouresques J, Grisoli F, Hassoun J, Delpuech F, Vincentelli F, Khalil R (1980) Neuroblastoma cérébral de l'adulte. Aspects cliniques et scanographiques. Rev Neurol (Paris) 136:879–881
Bourneville DM (1880) Sclérose tubéreuse des circonvolutions cérébrales: idiotie et épilepsie hémiplégique. Arch Neurol (Paris) 1:81–91
Bouteille M, Houdart R, Delarue G (1965) Arguments ultrastructuraux en faveur de unicité histogénétique des astrocytomes, glioblastomes polymorphes et oligodendrogliomes. Rev Neurol (Paris) 112:69–71
Boveri T (1914) Zur Frage der Entstehung maligner Tumoren. Fischer, Jena
Boyce R, Beadless CF (1893) A further contribution to the study of the pathology of the hypophysis cerebri. J Pathol 1:359–383
Boykin FC, Cowen D, Jannucci CAJ, Wolf A (1954) Subependymal glomerate astrocytomas. J Neuropathol Exp Neurol 13:30–49
Bracken MM (1957) Von Recklinghausen's disease with medullary ependymoma, acoustic neurilemmoma etc. Cancer Seminar 2:64–69
Bradford FK (1948) Hemangioblastoma of the posterior fossa (Lindau's disease). Report of two cases with familial history. J Neurosurg 5:196
Brain Tumor Registry in Japan (1978) (In Japanese). Shinkei Kenkyo No Shinpo 22:5–14
Bramann V (1893) Über Extirpation von Hirntumoren. Arch Klin Chir 45:365–400
Bramwell B (1894) On intracranial surgery. Edinburgh Med J 39:1007–1090
Brand MM, Maker HS, Lehrer GM, Schein HM (1971) Metabolic characteristic cells. J Neuropathol Exp Neurol 30:121–122
Brandenburg W (1958) Maligne Chordome der Schädelbasis (Clivus- und sogenanntes hypophysäres Chordom). Zentralbl Allg Pathol 98:512–521
Brandt M, Langhans P, Clemens M, Heger RA (1976) Das esosinophile Granulom des Schädels. Klinikarzt 5:981–984
Brandt P (1960) Aspergillose. In: Mattos-Pimenta A, Brandt P (eds) Die tierischen Parasiten und Pilzinfektionen im zentralen Nervensystem. Springer, Berlin Göttingen Heidelberg (Handbuch der Neurochirurgie, vol IV/l, pp 713–714)
Brasseur R (1961) Etude clinique, anatomopathologique et „in vitro" d' un hémangioblastome cérébral. Acta Neurol Psychiatr Belg 61:1102–1107
Brasseur R, Andre-Balisaux G, Gonsette R (1964) La culture „in vitro" de tumeurs de la lignée astrocytaire. Résultats personnels et considérations ontogéniques. Acta Neurol Psychiatr Belg 64:590–606
Bratton AB, Robinson SHG (1946) Gliomata of the nose and oral cavity. J Pathol Bacteriol 58:643–648
Braun W, Tzonos T (1965) Über ein ungewöhnlich rasch wachsendes Hypophysencarcinom mit intracerebralen Metastasen. Acta Neurochir (Wien) 12:615–624

Braun W, Tzonos T (1968) Zur Frage der extracraniellen Metastasierung von Gliomen durch Implantation. Acta Neurochir (Wien) 19:149–162

Braunstein H, Martin F (1952) Congenital papilloma of choroid plexus. A report of a case, with observations on pathogenesis of associated hydrocephalus. Arch Neurol 68:475–480

Brem S (1976) The role of vascular proliferation in the growth of brain tumors. Proceedings of the Congress of Neurological Surgeons, 1975, Atlanta. pp 440–453

Brenner H (1963) Hirnmetastasenoperationen bei bestehendem Primärtumor. Wien Klin Wochenschr 75:723–725

Brihaye J (1963) Les tumeurs métastatiques du système nerveux central. A propos de 239 observations. Acta Chir Belg 62:43–59

Brion S, Netsky MG, Zimmerman HM (1952) Vascular malformations of the spinal cord. Arch Neurol Psychiatry 68:339–345

Brisman R, Housepian EM, Chang C, Dufty P, Balis E (1976) Adjuvant nitrosourea therapy for glioblastomas. Arch Neurol 33:745–750

Britt RH, Connor WS, Enzmann DR (1981) Occult arteriovenous malformation on the brainstem simulating multiple sclerosis. Neurology (NY) 31:901–903

Broders AC (1920) Squamous-cell epithelioma of the lip. A study of 537 cases. JAMA 74:656–664

Broders AC (1926) Carcinoma: Grading and practical application. Arch Pathol 2:376–381

Brodie BB, Gilette JR, La Du BN (1958) Enzymatic metabolism of drugs and other foreign compounds. Annu Rev Biochem 27:427–454

Brody JI, Rodriguez F (1961) Cerebellar hemangioblastoma and polycythemia (erythrocythemia). Am J Med Sci 242:579–584

Bronfman S, Ectors L (1949) Hémangioblastome épidural. Acta Neurol Psychiatr Belg 49:433–440

Bronfman S, Reumont M (1947) La sarcomatose méningée primitive. (Etude clinique et histopathologique). Acta Neurol Psychiatr Belg 47:3–31

Bronson SM (1953) Sympathoblastoma in adults with special emphasis on its differential diagnosis. Medical dissertation, University of Basel

Brougham M, Heusner AP, Adams RD (1950) Acute degenerative changes in adenomas of the pituitary body – with special reference to pituitary apoplexy. J Neurosurg 7:421–439

Brouwer B, Van den Hoeve J, Mahoney W (1937) A fourth type of phakomatosis: Sturge-Weber syndrome. Verh Kon Akad Wet Amsterdam [II] 36:1–33

Brown M (1975) Tuberous sclerosis with malignant astrocytoma. Med J Aust 1:811–814

Brown RC, Gunderson L, Plenk HP (1977) Medulloblastoma, a review of the LDS Hospital experience. Cancer 40:56–60

Browne TR, Adams RD, Roberson GH (1976) Hemangioblastoma of the spinal cord. Review and report of five cases. Arch Neurol 33:435–441

Brucher JM (1962) Le sarcome monstrocellulaire du cerveau. Etude anatomoclinique de sept cas. Acta Neurol Psychiatr Belg 62:193–200

Brucher JM (1964) The classification and diagnosis of intracranial sarcomas. Acta Neurochir (Suppl) (Wien) 10:190–200

Brucher JM, Van den Bergh R (1959) Un cas de gangliocytome du cervelet. Acta Neurol Psychiatr Belg 3:367–374

Brucher JM, Soffer D, Wechsler W (1970) Feinstruktur eines polymorphen Hypophysenadenoms. Pathol Eur 5:442–453

Brucher JM, Hizawa K, Wechsler W (1971) Fibrome et fibrosarcome intracérébraux, étude histologique et ultrastructurale. Pathol Eur 6:227–249

Brück WE (1952) Einige Besonderheiten des klinischen Verlaufs der Cholesteatome der seitlichen Zisterne der Pons Varoli. Vopr Nevrokhir 4:23

Bruens JH, Guazzi GC, Martin JJ (1968) Infantile form of meningeal angiomatosis with Sudanophilic leucodystrophy associated with complex abiotrophies. Study of a second family. J Neurol Sci 7:417–425

Brütt H (1931) Intracranielles Chondrom als Hirntumor. Dtsch Z Chir 231:497–503

Brugger G (1954) Über einen fast symptomlos verlaufenden riesigen Tumor der Medulla oblongata. Zentralbl Neurochir 14:301–304

Brugger G (1955a) Ventrikeltumoren bei tuberöser Sklerose. Zentralbl Allg Pathol 93:421–422

Brugger G (1955b) Über ein riesiges Meningeom mit intra- und extrakraniellem Wachstum. Zentralbl Neurochir 15:223–225

Brunner H (1936) Über die Häufigkeit von Gehirnmetastasen bösartiger Geschwülste besonders des primären Lungentumors und ihre Bedeutung für die Klinik. Z Gesamte Neurol Psychiatr 154:793–798

Bruns L (1897) Die Geschwülste des Nervensystems. Karger, Berlin

Bruns L (1904) Hirngeschwülste und Hirnparasiten. In: Flatau E, Jacobson L, Minor L (eds) Handbuch der pathologischen Anatomie des Nervensystems, vol I, Karger, Berlin, pp 515–578

Bruns L (1908) Die Geschwülste des Nervensystems. Karger, Berlin

Bruns V von (1854) Die chirurgischen Krankheiten und Verletzungen des Gehirns und seiner Umhüllungen. In: von Bruns V (ed) Handbuch der praktischen Chirurgie für Ärzte und Wundärzte. vol I/14. Laupp, Tübingen, p 1096

Bruton OC, Martz DC, Gerard ES (1961) Precocious puberty due to secreting chorionepithelioma of the brain. J Pediatr 59:719–725

Brutschin P, Culver GJ (1973) Extracranial metastases from medulloblastomas. Neuroradiology 107:359–362

Brzustowicz RJ, Kernohan JW (1952) Cell rests in the region of the fourth ventricle: I. Their site and incidence according to age and sex. Arch Neurol Psychiatry 67:585–591

Buchholz A (1898) Kasuistischer Beitrag zur Kenntnis der Karzinome des Zentralnervensystems. Monatsschr Psychiatr 4:183

Buchmann E, Zülch KJ (1959) Zur Frage der postoperativen Überlebensdauer und der Fernmetastasierung beim Medulloblastom des Kleinhirns. Acta Neurochir (Wien) 7:263–273

Buchsbaum HW, Colton RP (1967) Anterior third ventricular cysts in infancy. J Neurosurg 26:264–266

Buck K (1909) Die Bedeutung des Traumas für die Entstehung von Hirngeschwülsten. Zentralbl Nervenheilkd 32:193–208

Buckley RC (1929) Tissue culture studies of the glioblastoma multiforme. Am J Pathol 5:467–472

Buckley RC, Eisenhardt L (1929) Study of a meningioma in supravital preparations, tissue culture and paraffin sections. Am J Pathol 5:659–664

Bucy PC (1935) Intradiploic epidermoid (cholesteatoma) of the skull. Arch Surg 31:190–199

Bucy PC (1942) Tumors of the central nervous system. Tice's system of medicine. Prior, Hagerstown

Bucy PC (1946) Intrinsic tumors of the cerebellum and brain stem. In: Bancroft FW, Pilcher C (eds) Surgical treatment of nervous system. Lippincott, Philadelphia

Bucy PC (1947) Tumors of the brain in childhood. Round table discussion on tumors, benign and malignant. J Pediatr 30:716–738

Bucy PC (1962) Some primary (malignant?) tumors of the spine. In: Proceedings congress of neurological surgeons, Chicago, 1960. Clin Neurosurg 8:32–63

Bucy PC, Gustafson WA (1939) Structure, nature and classification of the cerebellar astrocytomas. Am J Cancer 35:327–353

Bucy PC, Haymond HE (1932) Lumbosacral teratoma associated with spina bifida occulta. Report of a case with review of the literature. Am J Pathol 8:339–345

Bucy PC, Jerva MJ (1962) Primary epidural spinal lymphosarcoma. J Neurosurg 19:142–158

Bucy PC, Muncie WS (1929) Neuroepithelioma of the cerebellum. Am J Pathol 5:157–170

Bucy PC, Overhill HR (1950) Intradural spinal granulomas. J Neurosurg 7:1–12

Budka H (1974) Intracranial lipomatous hamartomas (intracranial „lipomas“). A study of 13 cases including combinations with medulloblastoma, colloid and epidermoid cysts, angiomatosis and other malformations. Acta Neuropathol (Berl) 28:205–222

Budka H (1975) Partially resected and irradiated cerebellar astrocytoma of childhood; malignant evolution after 28 years. Acta Neurochir (Wien) 32:139–146

Budka H, Pilz P, Guseo A (1975) Primary leptomeningeal sarcomatosis. Clinicopathological report of six cases. J Neurol 211:77–93

Budka H, Podreka I, Reisner T, Zeiler K (1980) Diagnostic and pathomorphological aspects of glioma multiplicity. Neurosurg Rev 3:233–241

Bücheler J, Kleihues P (1977) Excision of O^6-methylguanine from DNA of various mouse tissues following a single injection of *N*-methyl-*N*-nitrosourea. Chem Biol Interact 16:325–333
Bürki E (1944) Über den primären Sehnerventumor und seine Beziehungen zur Recklinghausenschen Neurofibromatose. Bibl Ophthalmol 30:1–64
Buess H (1938) Chiasmadurchtrennung: Gefäßruptur aus basalem Aneurysma bei intrasellärer Hypophysengangcyste. Beitr Pathol Anat 101:335
Buffoni L (1955) Un caso di neuroblastoma simpatico congenito ad evoluzione eccezionalmente favorevole. Minerva Pediatr 7:3–20
Bull JWD (1953) Spinal meningiomas and neurofibromas. Acta Radiol (Stockh) 40:283–300
Bunts AT (1949) Malformations vasculaires du cerveau. Rev Neurol (Paris) 81:442–452
Burger PC, Vogel FS (1976) Surgical pathology of the nervous system and its coverings. Wiley, New York
Burkitt DP, Wright DH (1970) Burkitt's lymphoma. Livingstone, Edinburgh
Burstein SD, Kernohan JW, Uihlein A (1963) Neoplasms of the reticuloendothelial system of the brain. Cancer 16:289–305
Burston J, John R, Spencer H (1962) „Myoblastoma" of the neurohypophysis. J Pathol Bacteriol 83:455–461
Busch E, Christensen E (1937) Das Oligodendrocytom der Sehnervenkreuzung. Zentralbl Neurochir 2:315–320
Busch E, Christensen E (1947a) The three types of glioblastoma. J Neurosurg 4:200–220
Busch E, Christensen E (1947b) Tumors of peripheral nerves with special reference to neurogenous sarcomas. Acta Psychiatr Neurol Scand [Suppl] 46:72–93
Busch E, Cooper M (1952) Paragonimiasis, a case with metastasis to the brain. Surgical removal. Acta Med Scand [Suppl 266] 142:343–348
Bushe K-A (1958) Beitrag zur Frage der Meningeomentstehung durch Trauma. Hefte Unfallheilkd 56:164–168
Bushe K-A (1972) Intrakranielle Metastasen. Bedeutung und therapeutisches Konzept. Langenbecks Arch Chir 332:369–375
Bushe K-A, Glees P (1968) Chirurgie des Gehirns und Rückenmarks im Kindes- und Jugendalter. Hippokrates, Stuttgart
Cabral G, Pianetti G, Carneiro FA, Lauar EH (1974) Riesenzystizerkus des 4. Ventrikels. Zentralbl Neurochir 35:61–65
Cacudi G, Cazzato G (1960) Su di un caso di melanoblastoma primitivo delle leptomeningi. G Psichiatr Neuropathol 88:799–809
Caesar KC (1941) Über Erkrankungen, die unter dem Bilde einer Hirngeschwulst verlaufen, mit besonderer Berücksichtigung des sog. Pseudotumor cerebri. Arch Psychiatr Nervenkr 113:655–676
Cain H (1953) Encephalitis und Toxoplasmose. Frankfurt Z Pathol 64:171–184
Cairncross JG, Chernik NL, Kim J-H, Posner JB (1979) Sterilization of cerebral metastases by radiation therapy. Neurology (Minneap) 29:1195–1202
Cairns H (1929) A study of intracranial surgery. Privy Council of the Medical Research Council. MRC, pp 1–83 Special reports series no. 125
Cairns H (1936) The ultimate results of operations for intracranial tumours. Yale J Biol Med 8:421–492
Cairns H, Adelaide MB (1936) Late results in the operative treatment of intracranial tumours. Lancet I:1223–1228 and 1291–1294
Cairns H, Russell DS (1931) Intracranial and spinal metastases in gliomas of the brain. Brain 54:377–421
Calkins RA, Pribram HFW, Joynt RI (1968) Intrasellar arachnoid diverticulum. Neurology (Minneap) 18:1037–1040
Calogero JA, Moossy J (1972) Extradural spinal meningiomas. Report of four cases. J Neurosurg 37:442–447
Calvo W (1952) Influencia de los traumatismos en le génesis de los tumores encéfalomedulares. Rev Esp Otoneurooftalmol Neurocir 62:3–6
Calvo W (1954) Tumores encefalomedulares. Estudio morfológico y biológico Arch Esp Morfol (Suppl) 5

Calvo W (1964) Observations on the metallic impregnations of brain tumours. In: Zülch KJ, Woolf AL (eds) Classification of brain tumors. Acta Neurochir (Suppl) 10:85–93
Calvo W, Barcia JL (1952) La malignidad y frecuencia de los tumores del sistema nervioso en relación con el sexo y la edad de los pacientes. Med Españ 28:280–290
Camerer JW (1940) Hirntuberkulome im Kindesalter. Monatsschr Kinderheilkd 83:163–178
Campbell JB, Hudson FM (1960) Craniobuccal origin, signs, and treatment of craniopharyngiomas. Surg Gynecol Obstet 111:183–191
Cancilla PA, Zimmerman HM (1965) The fine structure of a cerebellar hemangioblastoma. J Neuropathol Exp Neurol 24:621–628
Cancilla PA, Morecki R, Hurwitt ES (1964) Fine structure of a recurrent chordoma. Arch Neurol 11:289–295
Canti RG, Bland JOW, Russell DS (1935) Tissue culture of gliomata. Assoc Res Nerv Dis Proc 16:1–24
Cantril ST, Parker RG, Lund PK (1962) Malignant tumors of the maxillary sinus. Acta Radiol (Stockh) 58:105–128
Capps FCW, Kemp Harper RA, Williams IG (1957) Tumours of the glomus jugulare. J Fac Radiol (Lond) 8:312–338
Caram PC, Scarcella G, y Carton CA (1957) Intradural lipomas of the spinal cord with particular emphasis on the intramedullary lipomas. J Neurosurg 14:28–42
Cardauns H (1957) Über ein malignes Plexuspapillom. Zentralbl Neurochir 17:349–353
Cardauns H, Friedmann G, Nittner K (1961) Bericht über 4 Riesenzelltumoren der Wirbelsäule. Zentralbl Neurochir 21:3–14
Carleton CC, Cauthen JC (1975) Vascular („arteriovenous") malformations of the choroid plexus. Arch Pathol 99:286–288
Carmichael F (1928) Cerebral gliomata. J Pathol 31:493–510
Carmichael FA Jr, Cowley HS (1952) Schistosomiasis of the brain. J Neurosurg 9:620–634
Carmody DC, Tappen W (1959) Blastomycosis meningitis: report of a case successfully treated with amphotericin. B. Ann Intern Med 51:780–791
Carrillo R (1940) Metastatic tuberculoma of cauda equina. Prensa Med Argent 27:1547
Carrillo R, Oribe M (1939) Neuroblastomas leptomeningea. Dos observationes anátomo clinicas. Arch Argent Neurol 20:172–207
Carrillo R, Prado J, Matera RF, et al. (1951) Patologia de la aracnoiditis optoquiasmatica. Arch Neurochir 8:23–63
Carrillo R, Ricoy JR, Herrero-Vallejo J, Bravo G (1975) Fibrous xanthomas of the brain. Report of two cases. Clin Neurol Neurosurg 78:34–40
Carter P, Beggs J, Waggener JD (1972) Ultrastructure of three choroid plexus papillomas. Cancer 30:1130–1136
Casentini L, Rigobello L, Gerosa M, Pardatscher K, Andrioli GC (1979) Choroid plexus carcinoma. Case report. Zentralbl Neurochir 40:239–244
Cashion EL, Young JM (1971) Intraventricular craniopharyngioma. Report of two cases. J Neurosurg 34:84–87
Castaigne P, Escourolle R, Poirier J (1966a) L'ultrastructure des méningiomes. Étude de 4 cas en microscopie électronique. Rev Neurol (Paris) 114:249–261
Castaigne P, Cambier J, Escourolle R, Masson M (1966b) Réticulose cérébrale circonscrite à double localisation hypothalamique et protubérantielle. Presse Med 76:1213–1216
Castaigne P, David M, Pertuiset B, Escourolle R, Poirier J (1968) L'ultrastructure des hémangioblastomes du système nerveux central. Rev Neurol (Paris) 118:25–26
Castaigne P, Rondot P, Escourolle R, Ribadeau Dumas J-L, Cathala F, Hauw J-J (1974) Leucoencéphalopathie multifocale progressive et „gliomes" multiples. Rev Neurol (Paris) 130:379–392
Castellano F, Ruggiero G (1953) Meningiomas of the posterior fossa. Acta Radiol [Suppl] (Stockh) 104
Castellano F, Guidetti B, Olivecrona H (1952) Pterional meningiomas „en plaque". J Neurosurg 9:188–196
Causey WA (1978) Actinomycosis. In: Vinken PJ, Bruyn GW (eds) Infections of the nervous system. North-Holland, Amsterdam (Handbook of Clinical Neurology, vol 35, part III, pp 383–394

Causey WA, Lee R (1978) Nocardiosis. In: Vinken PJ, Bruyn GW (eds) Infections of the nervous system. North-Holland, Amsterdam (Handbook of clinical neurology, vol 35, part III, pp 517–530
Cervós-Navarro J (1967) Zur Feinstruktur endotheliomatöser Meningeome des Menschen. Acta Neuropathol (Berl) 8:141–148
Cervós-Navarro J (1971) Elektronenmikroskopie der Hämangioblastome des ZNS und der angioblastischen Meningiome. Acta Neuropathol (Berl) 19:184–207
Cervós-Navarro J, Gullotta F (1961) Contributo della microscopia elettronica alla conoscenza del glioblastoma. Arch Ital Anat Istol Pathol 35:365–378
Cervós-Navarro J, Matakas F (1968) Elektronenmikroskopischer Beitrag zur Histogenese der Neurinome. Verh Dtsch Ges Pathol 52:391–395
Cervós-Navarro J, Matakas F (1970) La contribution de la microscopie électronique à l'origine tissulaire des medulloblastomes. Neurochirurgie 16:551–557
Cervós-Navarro J, Menozzi V (1959) Das Verhalten des Mensenchyms bei Hirntumoren. Seishin Shinkeigaku Zasshi 61:371–392
Cervós-Navarro J, Pehlivan N (1981) Ultrastructure of oligodendrogliomas. Acta Neuropathol [Suppl] (Berl) 7:91–93
Cervós-Navarro J, Vasquez J (1966) Elektronenmikroskopische Untersuchungen über das Vorkommen von Cilien in Meningeomen. Virchows Arch [A] 341:280–290
Cervós-Navarro J, Vasquez J (1969) An electron microscopic study of meningiomas. Acta Neuropathol (Berl) 13:301–323
Cervós-Navarro J, Matakas F, Lazaro M-C (1968) Das Bauprinzip der Neurinome. Ein Beitrag zur Histogenese der Nerventumoren. Virchows Arch [A] 345:276–291
Cervós-Navarro J, Ferszt R, Brackertz M (1981) The ultrastructure of oligodendrogliomas. Neurosurg Rev 4:17–31
Chade HO (1968) Metastasen der Wirbelsäule und des Rückenmarks. Schweiz Arch Neurol Neurochir Psychiatr 102:257–287
Chade HO (1976) Metastatic tumours of the spine and spinal cord. In: Vinken PJ, Bruyn GW (eds) Tumors of the spine and spinal cord. North Holland, Amsterdam/American Elsevier, New York (Handbook of clinical neurology, vol 20, pp 415–433)
Challa VR, Markesbery WR (1978) Infratentorial neuroepithelial cyst (colloid cyst). J Neurosurg 49:457–459
Changaris DG, Powers JM, Perot PL, Hungerford GD, Neal GB (1981) Subependymoma presenting as subarachnoid hemorrhage. J Neurosurg 55:643–645
Chasanow M (1928) Meningitis bei Trichinose. Dtsch Z Nervenheilkd 103:197–205
Chason IL, Walker FB, Landers IW (1963) Metastatic carcinoma in the central nervous system and dorsal root ganglia. Cancer 16:781–787
Chatty EM, Earle KM (1971) Medulloblastoma. A report of 201 cases with emphasis on the relationship of histologic variants to survival. Cancer 28:977–983
Chaudhari AB, Ladapo F, Duncan JTK (1978) Fibrosarcoma of the scalp. J Neurosurg 49:893–897
Cherington M, Schneck SA (1966) Clivus meningiomas. Neurology (Minneap) 16:86–92
Chigasaki H, Pennybacker JB (1968) A long follow-up study of 128 cases of intramedullary spinal cord tumours. Neurol Med Chir (Tokyo) 10:25–66
Chiovenda M (1933) I gliomi dell'encefalo. Arch Ital Anat Istol Pathol 4:261–692
Cho E-S, Connolly E, Porro RS (1974) Primary reticulum cell sarcoma of the brain in a renal transplantation recipient. J Neurosurg 41:235–239
Choi NW, Schuman LM, Gullen WH (1970a) Epidemiology of primary central nervous system neoplasms: I. Mortality from primary central nervous system neoplasms in Minnesota. Am J Epidemiol 91:238–259
Choi NW, Schuman LM, Gullen WH (1970b) Epidemiology of primary central nervous system neoplasms: II. Case-control study. Am J Epidemiol 91:467–485
Choux R, Hassoun J, Berard M, Pellissier JM, Choux M, Toga M (1973) Ultrastructure d'un craniopharyngiome étude in vivo et in vitro. Arch Anat Pathol 21:179–188
Choux R, Hassoun J, Gambarelli D, Sedan R, Toga M (1975) Etude ultrastructurale d'un „méningiome humide" de Masson. Bull Cancer (Paris) 62:125–136
Chretien PB, Milam JI, Foote FW, Miller TR (1970) Embryonal adenocarcinomas (a type

of malignant teratoma) of the sacrococcygeal region. Clinical and pathological aspects of 21 cases. Cancer 26:522–535
Christensen E (1937) Über Ganglienzellgeschwülste im Gehirn. Virchows Arch [A] 300:567–581
Christensen E, Lara DE (1953) Intracranial sarcomas. J Neuropathol Exp Neurol 12:41–56
Christensen E, Højgaard K, Winkel Smith CC (1961) Congenital malignant mesenchymal tumours in a two-month-old child. Acta Pathol Microbiol Scand 53:237–242
Christensen FC (1925) Bone tumors. Analysis of one thousand cases with special reference to location, age, and sex. Ann Surg 81:1074–1092
Christian HJ (1961) So-called gangliocytoma of the cerebellum. J Neurosurg 18:125–128
Ciesielski-Treska J, Stefanovic V, Mandel P (1975) Activité acétylcholinestérasique des cellules de neuroblastome et des cellules gliales en coculture. CR Acad Sci [D] (Paris) 281:1261–1264
Clara M (1959) Das Nervensystem des Menschen, 3rd edn. Barth, Leipzig
Clarenbach P, Kleihues P, Metzel E, Dichgans J (1979) Simultaneous clinical manifestation of subependymoma of the fourth ventricle in identical twins. Case report. J Neurosurg 50:655–659
Clark JV (1970) Familial occurrence of cavernous angiomata of the brain. J Neurol Neurosurg Psychiatr 33:871–876
Claude H (1933) L'arachnoido-piemérite séreuse cérébrale. Rev Neurol (Paris) 40:824–850
Claveria LE, Kendall BE, du Boulay GA (1977) Computerized axial tomography in supratentorial gliomas and metastases. In: du Boulay GH, Moseby JF (eds) Computed tomography in clinical praxis. Springer, Berlin Heidelberg New York, pp 85–93
Clifford JH, McClintock HG, Lubchenco AE (1968) Primary spinal cord malignant melanoma, case report. J Neurosurg 29:410–413
Cloward RB (1968) Congenital spinal extradural cysts. Case report with review of literature. Ann Surg 168:851–864
Coakham HB, Lakshmi MS (1975) Tumour-associated surface antigen(s) in human astrocytoma. Oncology 31:233–243
Coenen H (1925) Das Chordom. Bruns' Beitr Klin Chir 133:1–77
Cohen A, Modan B (1968) Some epidemiologic aspects of neoplastic diseases in Israel immigrant population: 3. Brain tumors. Cancer 22:1323–1328
Cohen DM, Dahlin DC, MacCarty CS (1964) Apparently solitary tumours of the vertebral column. Mayo Clin Proc 39:509–528
Cohen ME, Duffner PK (1983) Brain tumors in childhood: principles of diagnosis and treatment. Raven Press New York (International review of child neurology series)
Cohen MS, Kushner MJ, Dell S (1981) Frontal lobe astrocytoma following radiotherapy for medulloblastoma. Neurology (NY) 31:616–619
Cohen SL, Aronson SM (1968) Secondary brain stem hemorrhages. Arch Neurol 19:257–263
Cohn A, Zimmerman HM (1955) Growth behaviour of chemically induced mouse brain tumours in the chick embryo. Excerpta Med (Amst) Sect VIII 8:818
Cohn E (1923) Gummen der Hypophyse. Virchows Arch [A] 240:452–468
Cohnheim J (1867) Ein Fall von multiplen Exostosen. Virchows Arch [A] 38:561–565
Cohnheim J (1882) Vorlesungen über allgemeine Pathologie, 2nd edn. vol I. Hirschwald, Berlin
Coleman CC, Troland CE (1948) Congenital atresia of foramina of Luschka and Magendie. J Neurosurg 5:84–88
Collins DN, Oppenheim IA, Edwards MR (1971) Cryptococcosis associated with systemic lupus erythematosus. Arch Pathol 91:78–88
Connor CL, Cushing H (1927) Diffuse tumors of the leptomeninges. Arch Pathol 3:374–392
Cook FV, Farrar WE (1978) Treatment of nocardia asteroides infection with trimethoprim-sulfametaxazole. South Med J 71:512–515
Cook T, Holt S, Yates PO (1962) Diffuse hypertrophy of the cerebellum. J Neurol Neurosurg Psychiatry 25:218–221
Cooper EH, Bedford AI, Kenny TE (1975) Cell death in normal and malignant tissues. Adv Cancer Res 21:59–120
Cooper ERA (1935) The relation of oligocytes and astrocytes in cerebral tumours. J Pathol 44:259–266

Cooper IS, MckCraig W, Kernohan JW (1950) Tumours of the spinal cord: Primary extramedullary gliomas. Coll Papers Mayo Clin 42:493–495
Cooper IS, Kernohan JW, MckCraig W (1952) Tumors of the medulla oblongata. Arch Neurol Psychiatry 67:269–282
Cooper JR (1971) Brain tumors in hereditary multiple system hamartomatosis (tuberous sclerosis). J Neurosurg 34:194–202
Cooper PR, Ransohoff J (1972) Craniopharyngioma originating in the sphenoid bone. Case report. J Neurosurg 36:102–106
Cooper RA, Goldstein E (1963) Histoplasmosis of the central nervous system. AM J Med 35:45–57
Copeland MM (1950) Benign tumors of bone. Surg Gynecol Obstet 90:697–712
Corenblum B, Sirek AMT, Horvath E, Kovacs K, Ezrin C (1976) Human mixed somatotrophic and lactotrophic pituitary adenomas. J Clin Endocrinol Metab 42:857–863
Cornell SH, Hibri NS, Menezes AH, Graf CJ (1979) The complementary nature of computed tomography and angiography in the diagnosis of cerebellar hemangioblastoma. Neuroradiology 17:201–205
Corradini W, Browder J (1948) Angioblastic neoplasms of the brain. J Neuropathol Exp Neurol 7:299–308
Correa AJE, Brinckhaus R, Kesler S, Martinez E (1975) Aspergillosis of the fourth ventricle. J Neurosurg 43:236–238
Corten MH (1921) Über ein Haemangioma sarcomatodes des Gehirns bei einem Neugeborenen. Frankfurt Z Pathol 24:693–705
Costello RT (1936) Subclinical adenoma of the pituitary gland. Am J Pathol 12:205–215
Costero I (1962) Pathology of glial neoplasm. In: Fields WS, Sharkey PC (eds) The biology and treatment of intracranial tumors. Thomas, Springfield, pp 178–211
Costero I, Pomerat CM (1955a) Cellular prototypes of central gliomata. In: Proceedings Second International Congress of Neuropathology, London 1955, Part I. Excerpta Medica Foundation, Amsterdam, pp 273–277
Costero I, Pomerat CM (1955b) Normal and neoplastic brain in time-lapse cinematography. In: Proceedings of the Second International Congress of Neuropathology, London 1955, part II. Excerpta Medica Foundation, Amsterdam, pp 629–634
Costero I, Pomerat CM (1955c) Standard cellular morphology in vitro as compared with explanted normal brain cells. Excerpta Med (Amst) Sect VIII 8:821
Costero I, Pomerat CM, Jackson IJ, Barroso-Moguel R, Chévez A (1955a) Tumors of human nervous system in tissue culture; cultivation and cytology of meningioma cells. JNCI 15:1319–1339
Costero I, Pomerat CM, Barroso-Moguel R, Chévez A (1955b) Tumors of human nervous system in tissue culture; analysis of fibroblastic activity in meningiomas. JNCI 15:1341–1365
Costero I, Barroso-Moguel R, Chévez A (1979) Biologia de los gliomas. Instituto Nacional de Neurologia y Neurocirurgia, Mexico
Cottier H (1980) Pathogenese. Springer, Berlin Heidelberg New York
Couch JR, Weiss SA (1974) Gliomatosis cerebri. Report of four cases and review of the literature. Neurology (Minneap) 24:504–511
Coulon RA, Till K (1977) Intracranial ependymomas in children. Childs Brain 3:154–168
Courville CB (1930) Ganglioglioma. Tumor of the central nervous system; review of the literature and report of two cases. Arch Neurol Psychiatry 24:439–491
Courville CB (1931) Gangliogliomas. A further report with special reference to those occurring in the temporal lobe. Arch Neurol Psychiatry 25:309–326
Courville CB (1936) Multiple primary tumors of the brain. Review of the literature and report of twenty-one cases. Am J Cancer 26:703–731
Courville CB (1950) Pathology of the central nervous system, 3rd edn. Pacific Press, Mountain View California
Courville CB (1956) Trauma and intracranial tumor. J Forensic Med 3:16–26
Courville CB (1958) Gangliocytoma myelinicum diffusum of the cerebellar cortex. Bull Los Angeles Neurol Soc 23:72–80

Courville CB (1963) Small arteriovenous malformation of the temporal isthmus. Some observations on its architecture. Bull Los Angeles Neurol Soc 28:27–30

Courville CB, Abbott H (1940) The angioblastic group of meningiomas. Bull Los Angeles Neurol Soc 5:47–72

Courville CB, Abbott H (1941) On the classification of meningiomas. Bull Los Angeles Neurol Soc 6:21–31

Courville CB, Abbott H (1942) The histogenesis of meningiomas. J Neuropathol Exp Neurol 1:337–343

Courville CB, Abbott H (1955) Malignant changes in cerebral ganglioglioma. Report of two cases. Excerpta Med (Amst) Sec VIII 8:786

Courville CB, Schillinger RJ (1939) Metastatic melanoblastomas of the brain. Bull Los Angeles Neurol Soc 4:8–22

Coutinho LMB, Zülch KJ (1974) Reticulossarcomas epidurais intraespinais. Estudo de 34 casos. Arq Neuropsiquiatr 32:263–274

Couto D, Costa N (1949) Esquistossomose da medula. J Bras Neurol 1:189–241

Couvreur J, Desmonts G (1978) Toxoplasmosis. In: Vinken PJ, Bruyn GW (eds) Infections of the nervous system. North-Holland, Amsterdam (Handbook of clinical neurology, vol 35, part III, pp 115–141)

Cox LB (1933) The cytology of the glioma group; with special reference to the inclusion of cells derived from invaded tissue. Am J Pathol 9:839–898

Cox LB, Cranage ML (1937) Studies on the tissue culture of intracranial tumors. J Pathol Bacteriol 45:477–499

Cox WS, Luse SA (1964) Colloid cyst of third ventricle. J Neuropathol Exp Neurol 23:431–445

Craddock WE, Riddervold HO (1972) Unilateral calcification in a lipoma of the corpus callosum. J Can Assoc Radiol 23:192–194

Cramer F, Kinsey MW (1952) The cerebellar hemangioblastomas. Arch Neurol Psychiatry 67:237–252

Cravioto H (1969) The ultrastructure of acoustic nerve tumors. Acta Neuropathol (Berl) 12:116–140

Cravioto H, Dart D (1973) The ultrastructure of „pinealoma“ (seminoma-like tumor of the pineal region). J Neuropathol Exp Neurol 32:552–565

Cravioto H, Feigin J (1959) Noninfectious granulomatous angiitis with a predilection for the nervous system. Neurology (Minneap) 9:599–609

Cravioto H, Lockwood R (1969) The behaviour of acoustic neuroma in vitro. Acta Neuropathol (Berl) 12:141–157

Cravioto H, Palekar L, Weiss E, Bennett K (1972) Experimental neurinoma in tissue culture. Acta Neuropathol (Berl) 21:154–164

Crawford JV, Russell DS (1956) Cryptic arteriovenous and venous hamartomas of the brain. J Neurol Neurosurg Psychiatry 19:1–11

Creagan ET, Fraumeni JF (1972) Brief communication: Deaths from brain tumors in Eastern Kentucky, 1950–69. JNCI 51:1717

Crisp DE, Thompson JA (1981) Primary malignant melanomatosis of the meninges. Clinical course and computed tomographic findings in a young child. Arch Neurol 38:528–529

Critchley MD (1925) Brain tumors in children. Br J Child Dis 22:251–264

Critchley MD, Ironside RN (1926) The pituitary adamantinomas. Brain 49:437–481

Crompton MR, Gautier-Smith PC (1970) The prediction of recurrence in meningiomas. J Neurol Neurosurg Psychiatry 33:80–87

Crouse SK, Berg BO (1972) Intracranial meningiomas in childhood and adolescence. Neurology (Minneap) 22:135–141

Crue BL, Todd EM, Lockwood RW (1967) Medulloblastoma: II. Therapy with triethylene melamine and cobalt 60 irradiation. Bull Los Angeles Neurol Soc 30:161–168

Cruveilhier JC (1829/35) Anatomie pathologique du corps humain. Baillière, Paris

Cumberlin RL, Luk KH, Wara WM, Sheline GE, Wilson CB (1979) Medulloblastoma. Treatment results and effect on normal tissues. Cancer 43:1014–1020

Cuneo HM, Rand CW (1952) Brain tumors of childhood. Thomas, Springfield

Cushing H (1908) Technical methods of performing certain cranial operations. Surg Gynecol Obstet 6:227–246

Cushing H (1912) The pituitary body and its disorders, clinical states produced by disorders to the hypophysis cerebri. Lippincott, Philadelphia
Cushing H (1917) Tumors of the nervous acusticus and the syndrome of the cerebello-pontine angle. Saunders, Philadelphia
Cushing H (1925) Studies in intracranial physiology and surgery. Oxford University Press, London
Cushing H (1927) The intracranial tumors of preadolescence. Am J Dis Child 33:551–584
Cushing H (1930) Experiences with the cerebellar medulloblastomas. Acta Pathol Microbiol Scand 7:1–86
Cushing H (1931) Experiences with the cerebellar astrocytomas. Surg Gynecol Obstet 52:129–204
Cushing H (1932) Intracranial tumors. Thomas, Springfield
Cushing H (1935) Intrakranielle Tumoren. Springer, Berlin
Cushing H, Bailey P (1928a) Hemangiomas of cerebellum and retina. Arch Ophthalmol 57:447–463
Cushing H, Bailey P (1928b) Tumors arising from the blood vessels of the brain; angiomatous malformations and hemangioblastomas. Thomas, Springfield
Cushing H, Eisenhardt L (1938) Meningiomas, their classification, regional behaviour, life history and surgical end results. Thomas, Springfield
D'Agostino AN, Kernohan JW, Brown JR (1963a) The Dandy-Walker syndrome. J Neuropathol Exp Neurol 22:450–470
D'Agostino AN, Sowle EH, Miller RH (1963b) Primary malignant neoplasms of nerves (malignant neurilemmomas) in patients without manifestations of multiple neurofibromatosis (von Recklinghausen's disease). Cancer 16:1003–1114
Dahl B, Harbitz F (1938) Om stenose i aquaeductus sylvii fra anatomisk synspunkt. Norsk Mag Laegevidensk 99:961–974
Dahlin DC (1957) Bone tumors. General aspects and an analysis of 2276 cases. Thomas, Springfield
Dahlin DC (1967) Bone tumors. General aspects and data on 3987 cases, 2nd edn. Thomas, Springfield
Dahlin DC, Henderson ED (1962) Mesenchymal chondrosarcoma. Cancer 15:410–417
Dahlin DC, MacCarty CS (1952) Chordoma. A study of 59 cases. Cancer 5:1170–1178
Dahlin DC, Besse BE, Pugh DG, Ghormley RK (1955) Aneurysmal bone cysts. Radiology 64:56–65
Dahme E, Schiefer B (1960) Intracranielle Geschwülste bei Tieren. Zentralbl Veterinärmed 7:341–363
Dalforno S, Gigliardi MR (1968) Maturazione di metastasi di neuroblastoma con trasformatione in ganglioneuroma. Cancro 21:669–675
Dammer M (1930) Unfall und Hirngeschwulst. Med Klin 26:1280–1283
Dandy WE (1928) Venous abnormalities and angiomas of the brain. Arch Surg 17:715–793
Dandy WE (1938) Hirnchirurgie. Barth, Leipzig
Dandy WE (1943) Infections of brain, meninges and skull. In: Lewis' practice of surgery, vol 14. Prior, Hagerstown
Dandy WE, Blackfan KD (1914) Internal hydrocephalus: An experimental, clinical, and pathological study. Am J Dis Child 8:406–482
Daniel PM (1964) The management of metastases in the central nervous system. Proc R Soc Med 57:1151–1154
Danziger J, Bloch S, Podlas H (1975) Schwannomas of the central nervous system. AJR 125:692–701
Dargeon HW (1947) Round table discussion on tumours, benign and malignant. J Pediatr 30:716–738
Dastur DK, Lalitha VS (1968) Pathological analysis of intracranial space-occupying lesions in 1000 cases including children: II. Incidence, types and unusual cases of glioma. J Neurol Sci 8:143–170
Dastur DK, Sinh G, Pandya SK (1967) Melanotic tumor in the acoustic nerve. Case report. J Neurosurg 27:166–170
Dastur DK, Lalitha VS, Prabhakar V (1968) Pathological analysis of intracranial space-occu-

pying lesions in 1000 cases including children: Age, sex and pattern; and the tuberculomas. J Neurol Sci 6:575–592
Dastur HM, Desai AD (1965) A comparative study of brain tuberculomas and gliomas based upon 107 case records of each. Brain 88:375–396
Daum S, Le Beau J (1963) Hémangioblastome du cervelet opéré au même âge chez la mère et le fils (maladie de Von Hippel-Lindau) Rev Neurol (Paris) 108:50–54
Daum S, Billet R, Janau J, Comoy J (1967) Ganglioneurome diffus du cortex cérébelleux (maladie de Lhermitte et Duclos) opéré avec succès. Neurochirurgie 13:665–671
D'Aunoy R, Friedrichs A, Zoeller A (1930) Gumma of the brain. Am J Syph 14:175–187
David M, Berdet H, Guillaumat L, Askenazy H (1936a) Arachnoidite syphilitique de la grande cîterne. Rev Neurol (Paris) 66:759–767
David M, Lacroix A, Thieffry S, Brun M (1936b) Cholestéatome suprasellaire. Rev Neurol (Paris) 2:1–12
David M, Hecaen H, Bonis A (1956) Tumeurs du système nerveux central et maladie de Recklinghausen. Sem Hop Paris 32:5
David M, Garcin R, Sachs M, Metzger J (1966) Maladie de von Hippel-Lindau à localisations multiples. Cérébelleuses et médullaires, révélées avant l'intervention par l'angiographie vertébrale avec soustraction, incidence hérédofamiliale hautement probable. Neurochirurgia (Stuttg) 9:121–132
Davidoff LM (1940) A thirteen year follow-up study of a series of cases of verified tumors of the brain. Arch Neurol Psychiatry 44:1246–1261
Davidoff LM (1956) Pseudotumor cerebri. Neurology (Minneap) 6:605–615
Davidoff LM, Gass H, Grossman J (1947) Postoperative spinal adhesive arachnoiditis and recurrent spinal cord tumors. J Neurosurg 4:451–464
Davidson S, Small IM (1960) Malignant change in an intracranial epidermoid. J Neurol Neurosurg Psychiatry 23:176–178
Davis EW (1942) Gliomatous tumors in the nasal region. J Neuropathol Exp Neurol 1:312–319
Davis FA (1940) Primary tumors of the optic nerve. (A phenomenon of the Recklinghausen's disease) Arch Ophthalmol 23:735–821, 957–1022
Davis L, Martin J, Goldstein SL, Ashkenazy M (1949) A study of 211 patients with verified glioblastoma multiforme. J Neurosurg 6:33–44
Davis L, Martin J, Padberg F, Anderson RK (1950) A study of 182 patients with verified astrocytoma, astroblastoma and oligodendroglioma of the brain. J Neurosurg 7:299–312
Davis LE (1924) A physiopathologic study of the choroid plexus with a report of a case of villous hypertrophy. J Med Res 44:521–534
Davis LE, Cushing H (1925) Papillomas of the choroid plexus. With a report of six cases. Arch Neurol Psychiatry 13:681–710
Davis RL, Fox GE (1970) Acinar choroid plexus adenoma. Case report. J Neurosurg 33:587–590
Davison C (1944) Lipoma in quadrigeminal plate with hydrocephalus. J Neuropathol Exp Neurol 3:427–428
Davison C, Brock S, Dyke CG (1936) Retinal and central nervous hemangioblastomatosis with visceral changes (von Hippel-Lindau's disease). Bull Neurol Inst NY 5:72–93
Dayan AD, Marshall A, Miller A, Pick FJ, Rankin NE (1966) Atypical teratomas of the pineal and hypothalamus. J Pathol Bacteriol 92:1–28
Dean MRF, Newton KA, Swann GF (1967) Percutaneous intraarterial chemotherapy in the treatment of intracranial neoplasms. A review of 36 cases. Br J Radiol 40:828–833
De Armond SJ, Eng LF, Rubinstein LJ (1980) The application of glial fibrillary acidic (GFA) protein immunohistochemistry in neurooncology. A progress report. Pathol Res Pract 168:374–394
De Blasi A (1930) Un melanosarcoma primitivo del midollo spinale. Oliveri, Genova
Debnam IW, Staple TW (1973) Osseous metastases from cerebellar medulloblastoma. Radiology 107:363–365
De Busscher J (1939) Deux chondromes intracrâniens. J Belge Neurol Psychiatr 2:81–102
De Busscher J, Scherer HJ (1942) Les gliomes de l'encéphale. L'edition Universelle, Bruxelles
Deck JHN (1969) Cerebral medulloepithelioma with maturation into ependymal cells and ganglion cells. J Neuropathol Exp Neurol 28:442–454

Decker RE, Gross SW (1967) Intraspinal dermoid tumor presenting as chemical meningitis. J Neurosurg 27:60–62
Decker RE, San Augustin W, Epstein JA (1978) Spinal epidural venous angioma causing foraminal enlargement and erosion of vertebral body. J Neurosurg 49:605–606
Deery EM (1932) Some features of glioblastoma multiforme. Bull Neurol Inst NY 2:157–193
Deery EM (1934) Histologic features of glioblastoma multiforme. Arch Neurol Psychiatry 31:212–215
De Feo D, Foltz EL, Hamilton AE (1975) Double compartment hydrocephalus in a patient with cysticercosis meningitis. Surg Neurol 4:247–251
De Gennes IL, Turpin G (1978) Adénomes corticotropes avec mélanodermie. Nouv Presse Med 7:1185–1189
De Girolami U (1977) Pathology of tumors of the pineal region. In: Schmidek HH (ed) Pineal tumors. Masson, Paris, pp 1–19
De Girolami U, Schmidek H (1973) Clinicopathological study of 53 tumors of the pineal region. J Neurosurg 39:455–462
De Girolami U, Zvaigzne O (1973) Modification of the Achucarro-Hortega pineal stain for paraffin-embedded formalin-fixed tissue. Stain Technol 48:48–50
Deiters O (1865) Untersuchungen über Gehirn und Rückenmark des Menschen und der Säugetiere. Vieweg, Braunschweig
De Lange C (1929) Klinische und pathologisch-anatomische Mitteilungen über Hydrocephalus chronicus congenitus und acquisitus. Z Gesamte Neurol Psychiatr 120:433–500
Delleman JW, De Jong JGY, Bleeker GM (1978) Meningiomas in 5 members of a family over 2 generations, in one member simultaneously with acoustic neurinomas. Neurology (Minneap) 28:567–570
Demme H, Mumme C (1932) Blastomykose des Zentralnervensystems. Dtsch Z Nervenheilkd 127:1–26
De Morsier G (1962) Les kystes épendymaires colloides du septum lucidum et des ventricules latéraux. Schweiz Arch Neurol Neurochir Psychiatr 90:34–56
Demus H (1967) Neue Gesichtspunkte zur Entstehung der pialen Lipome. Arch Psychiatr Nervenkr 209:426–442
Den Hartog JC, Guazi GC, Nunes Vicente A (1960) Reticulo-endothéliose cérébrale primitive (dite encéphalite granulomateuse) et granulome infundibulo-tubérien. Rev Neurol (Paris) 102:20–43
Den Harto Jager WA (1969) Cytopathology of the cerebrospinal fluid examined with the sedimentation technique after Sayk. J Neurol Sci 9:155–177
Denny-Brown D (1938) Adenoma sebaceum, without epilepsy, in a woman: epilepsy without adenoma sebaceum in her son. Proc R Soc Med 31:717–718
Dereymaeker A, Brucher JM, De Somer P, Brasseur R (1958) La culture des tumeurs cérébrales humaines. Premièrs resultats personnels. Acta Neurol Psychiatr Belg 58:772–777
Descuns P, Garrée H, Phéline C (1954) Tuberculomas of the brain and cerebellum. J Neurosurg 11:243–250
Deshpande DH, Desai AP, Dastur HM (1975) Aspergillosis of the central nervous system. Neurology (Bombay) 23:167–175
Deutsch HJ (1965) Intranasal glioma. Ann Otol Rhinol Laryngol 74:637–644
Devadiga KV, Abraham J, Chandy J (1969) Primary choroid plexus papilloma of the cerebellopontine angle. J Neurosurg 30:286–288
Dévé F (1928) L'échinococcose vertébrale. Son processus pathogénique et ses lésions. Ann Anat Pathol 5:841–859
Devesa SS (1975) The incidence of retinoblastoma. Am J Ophthalmol 80:263–265
Dexter D, Howell DA (1965) Medulloblastomas and arachnoidal sarcomas. Brain 88:367–374
Dhermy P (1978) Phycomycosis (mucormycosis). In: Vinken PJ, Bruyn GW (eds) Infections of the nervous system. North-Holland, Amsterdam (Handbook of clinical neurology, vol 35, part III, pp 541–555)
Diaz G, Schoihet S, Poblete R (1975) Neurocisticercosis, evaluacion del tratamiento mediante derivativa ventriculo-atrial. Neurocirugia (Santiago) 33:160–166
Diba J, Frowein RA, Stammler A (1979) Gangliocytoma: operability and follow-up. Neurosurg Rev 2:47–53

Dickmann GH, Cramer FK, Kaplan AD (1951) Opto-chiasmatic arachnoiditis. J Neurosurg 8:355–359
Dietrich A (1941) Krebs und Kriegsverletzung. Z Krebsforsch 52:91–103
Dietrich A (1950) Krebs im Gefolge des Krieges. Hirzel, Stuttgart
Dietrich F (1952) Pathologisch-anatomische Auswertung von sechzehn Fällen von Neuroblastoma sympathicum (Sympathogoniom), davon zwei bei Neugeborenen. Medical dissertation, University of Zurich
Diezel P (1949) Gliom nach Trauma. Frankfurter Z Pathol 60:316–326
Diezel PB (1954) Die Geschwülste der Hirnhäute. Ein Beitrag zur formalen Genese der Meningeome. Virchows Arch [A] 325:441–454
Diezel PB, Rottmann E (1958) Histochemische Untersuchungen an „Rosenthalschen Fasern" in Ependymgranulationen und im Spongioblastom. Dtsch Z Nervenheilkd 177:222–234
Di Lorenzo N, Palma L, Nicole S (1977) Lymphocytic infiltration in long-survival glioblastomas: possible host's resistence. Acta Neurochir (Wien) 39:27–33
Di Lorenzo N, Nolletti A, Palma L (1978) Late cerebral radionecrosis. Surg Neurol 10:281–290
Di Lorenzo N, Savino S, Nicole S, Mercuri S (1979) Aneurysmal bone cysts of the spine. Report of 7 cases treated by surgery only. Neurosurg Rev 2:25–30
Di Tullio MV, Stern WE (1979) Hemangioma calcificans. J Neurosurg 50:110–114
Dixon FJ, Moore RA (1952) Tumors of the male sex organs. Armed Forces Institute of Pathology, Washington
Dixon HBF, Hargreaves WH (1944) Cysticercosis, its radiology. Q J Med 13:107–121
Djindjian M (1976) Les malformations artério-veineuses de la moëlle épinière et leur traitement. Thesis, University of Paris
Djindjian R, Houdart R, Hurth M (1969) Les angiomes de la moëlle épinière. Sandoz, Paris
Djindjian R, Houdart R, Hurth M (1970) L'angiographie de la moëlle épinière. Masson, Paris
Djindjian R, Picard L, Manelfe C, Merland JJ, Théron J (1978) Développement de la neuroradiologie thérapeutique. Neuroradiology 16:381–384
Dobberstein J (1955) Die Geschwülste der Vögel. Verh Dtsch Ges Pathol 39:320–323
Dodge HW, Keith HM, Campagna MJ (1956) Intraspinal tumors in infants and childhood. J Int Coll Surg 26:199–215
Döring G (1940) Über das Retothelsarkom des Nasenrachenraums mit neurologischen Komplikationen. Z Gesamte Neurol Psychiatr 168:432–447
Doernbach J (1949) Über cystische und zellige Geschwülste der Hirnventrikel. Virchows Arch [A] 316:51–75
Dohrmann GJ, Collias JC (1975) Choroid plexus carcinoma. J Neurosurg 43:225–232
Dohrmann GJ, Dunsmore RH (1975) Glioblastoma multiforme of the cerebellum. Surg Neurol 3:219–223
Dohrmann GJ, Farwell JR (1976) Ependymal neoplasms in children. Trans Am Neurol Ass 101:125–129
Dohrmann GJ, Farwell JR, Flannery JT (1976a) Glioblastoma multiforme in children. J Neurosurg 44:442–448
Dohrmann GJ, Farwell JR, Flannery JT (1976b) Ependymomas and ependymoblastomas in children. J Neurosurg 45:273–283
Dohrmann GJ, Farwell JR, Flannery JT (1978) Oligodendrogliomas in children. Surg Neurol 10:21–25
Doljanski L, Roulet F (1933) Studien über die Entstehung der Bindegewebsfibrille. Virchows Arch [A] 291:260
Dolman CL, Sweeney VP, Magil A (1979) Neoplastic angioendotheliosis. The case of the missed primary? Arch Neurol 36:5–7
Dom R, Brucher JM (1969) Hamartoblastome (gangliocytome diffus) unilatéral de l'écorce cérébrale associé à une dégénérescence soudanophile de la substance blanche du côté opposé. Rev Neurol (Paris) 120:307–318
Donat JF, Okazaki H, Gomez MR, Reagan TJ, Baker HL Jr, Laws ER Jr (1978) Pineal tumors. A 53-year experience. Arch Neurol 35:736–740
Donat R (1944) Pseudoverkalkung des Gehirns bei tumorähnlicher chronisch-encephalitischer Gliaproliferation. Virchows Arch [A] 312:726

Donegani G, Grattarola FR, Wildi E (1972) Tuberous sclerosis, Bourneville disease. In: Vinken PJ, Bruyn GW (eds) The phakomatoses. North Holland, Amsterdam (Handbook of clinical neurology, vol 14, pp 340–389)
Doniach Y (1972) Cytology of pituitary adenomas. J R Coll Physicians Lond 6:299–308
Donnell MS, Meyer GA, Donegan WL (1979) Estrogen-receptor protein in intracranial meningiomas. J Neurosurg 50:499–502
Donohue WL, Jaffe FA, Rewcastle NB (1967) Radiation-induced neurofibromata. Cancer 20:589–595
Dorn HF, Cutler SJ (1955) Morbidity from cancer in the United States. Government Printing Office, Washington (Public Health monograph no. 29)
Doron Y, Behar A, Beller AJ (1965) Granular-cell „myoblastoma" of the neurohypophysis. J Neurosurg 22:95–99
Dorsey JF, Tabrisky J (1966) Intraspinal and mediastinal foregut cyst compressing the spinal cord. Report of a case. J Neurosurg 24:562–567
Dosik GM, Rodriguez V, Benjamin RS, Bodey GP (1978) Neuroblastoma in the adult. Effective combination chemotherapy. Cancer 41:56–63
Dos-Santos R (1950) Arteriography in bone tumors. J Bone Joint Surg [Br] 32:17–29
Dott NM, Bailey P (1925) Hypophysial adenomata. Br J Surg 13:314–366
Dott NM, Levin E (1939) Intracranial tuberculoma. Edinburgh Med J 46:36–41
Dressler F, Schliack H, Wende S (1968) Halsmarkangiom mit rezidivierenden Insulten. Dtsch Med Wochenschr 93:1852–1855
Dretler J (1938) Über eine diffuse, ausgereifte – durch abortive tuberöse Sklerose komplizierte – Hirngeschwulst. Dtsch Z Nervenheilkd 148:84–106
Drew JH, Grant FC (1948) Benign cyst of the brain. J Neurosurg 5:107–123
Driggs M, Spatz H (1939) Pubertas praecox bei einer hyperplastischen Mißbildung des Tuber cinereum. Virchows Arch [A] 305:567–592
Druckrey H (1975) Chemical carcinogenesis on *N*-nitroso derivates. GANN Monogr Cancer Res 17:107–132
Druckrey H, Ivankovic S, Preussmann R (1965) Selektive Erzeugung maligner Tumoren im Gehirn und Rückenmark von Ratten durch *N*-Methyl-Nitrosoharnstoff. Z Krebsforsch 66:389–408
Druckrey H, Ivankovic S, Preussmann R (1966) Teratogenic and carcinogenic effects in the offspring after single injection of ethylnitrosourea to pregnant rats. Nature 210:1378–1379
Druckrey H, Preussmann R, Ivankovic S, Schmähl D (1967) Organotrope carcinogene Wirkungen bei 65 verschiedenen *N*-Nitroso-Verbindungen an BD-Ratten. Z Krebsforsch 69:103–201
Druckrey H, Schagen B, Ivankovic S (1970) Erzeugung neurogener Malignome durch einmalige Gabe von Äthylnitrosoharnstoff (ÄNH) an neugeborene und junge BD-IX-Ratten. Z Krebsforsch 74:141–161
Druckrey H, Ivankovic S, Preussmann R, Zülch KJ, Mennel HD (1972) Selective induction of malignant tumors of the nervous system by resorptive carcinogens. In: Kirsch WM, Grosso-Paoletti E, Paoletti P (eds) The experimental biology of brain tumors. Thomas, Springfield, pp 85–147
Duckett S, Wilson RR (1964) Fetal spongioblastoma. J Neuropathol Exp Neurol 23:560–564
Duckett S, Poirier J, Galle P (1978) Electron microprobe study of calcifications in human brain tumors. Acta Neuropathol (Berl) 44:145–146
Duello TM, Halmi NS (1977) Pituitary adenoma producing thyrotropin and prolactin. Virchows Arch [A] 376:255–265
Duffell D, Farber L, Chou S, Hartmann JF, Nelson E (1963) Electron microscopic observations on astrocytomas. Am J Pathol 43:539–554
Duffner PK, Klein DM, Cohen ME (1978) Calcification in brainstem gliomas. Neurology (Minneap) 28:832–834
Duffy PE (1983) Astrocytes: normal, relative, and neoplastic. Raven, New York
Duffy WC (1920) Hypophyseal duct tumors. A report of three cases and a fourth case of cyst of Rathke's pouch. Ann Surg 72:537–555, 725–757
Duinkerke SJ, Slooff JL, Gabreëls FJM, Renier WO, Thijssen HOM, Biesta JH (1981) Melano-

tic rhabdomyomedulloblastoma or teratoid tumour of the cerebellar vermis. Clin Neurol Neurosurg 83:29–33
Duma RJ (1978) Amoebic infections of the nervous system. In: Vinken PJ, Bruyn GW (eds) Infections of the nervous system. North-Holland, Amsterdam (Handbook of clinical neurology, vol 35, part III, pp 25–66)
Dunn J Jr, Kernohan JW (1957) Gliomatosis cerebri. Arch Pathol 64:82–91
Dunsmore RH, Roberts M (1974) Trauma as a cause of brain tumor. A medicolegal dilemma. Conn Med 38:521–523
Durante F (1887) Contribution to intracranial surgery. Lancet II:654–655
Duret H (1905) Les tumeurs de l'encéphale. Alcan, Paris
Durity FA, Dolman CL, Moyes PD (1968) Ganglioneuroblastoma of the cerebellum. J Neurosurg 28:270–273
Dutton J (1978) Intracranial solitary chondroma. J Neurosurg 49:460–463
Dyck P, Gruskin P (1977) Supratentorial cysts in adults. Arch Neurol 34:276–279
Earle KM (1954) Metastatic and primary intracranial tumors of the adult male. J Neuropathol Exp Neurol 13:448–454
Earle KM, Rentschler EH, Snodgras SR (1957) Primary intracranial neoplasms. J Neuropathol Exp Neurol 14:321–331
Earnest F, Kernohan JW, MckCraig W (1950) Oligodendrogliomas. Arch Neurol Psychiatry 63:964–976
Ebels EJ, Go KG (1974) A presumably unique intracranial tumour (elastoma). Clin Neurol Neurosurg 77:20–25
Eberth CJ (1870) Über Entwicklung des Epithelioms der Pia und der Lunge. Virchows Arch [A] 49:51–62
Eberts TJ, Ransburg RC (1979) Primary intracranial endodermal sinus tumor. Case report. J Neurosurg 50:246–252
Ebhardt G, Cervós-Navarro J (1981) Feinstructure of cells in astrocytomas of various grades of malignancy. Acta Neuropathol [Suppl] (Berl) VII:88–90
Ebhardt G, Heiss WD (1984) Tumors in the central nervous system in the presence of malignant extracranial neoplasms. Adv Neurosurg 12:62–67
Ebhardt G, Müller W, Thun F, Wilcke O, Fischer R (1983) Spontaneous hemorrhages in intracerebral brain tumors and leukemia. Adv Neurosurg 11:157–164
Echlin F (1934) Cranial osteomas and hyperostoses produced by meningeal fibroblastoma. A clinical pathologic study. Arch Surg 28:357–403
Echols DH (1938) Spongioblastoma polare. Arch Neurol Psychiatry 39:494–512
Echols DH (1941) Multiple meningioma. Removal of ten intracranial tumors from a patient. Arch Neurol Psychiatry 46:440–443
Ectors L (1935) La ventriculographie dans les cas d'imperméabilité du trou de Monro. Rev Neurol (Paris) 63:149–157
Ectors L (1945) Les méningiomes de la 3e frontale. Desoer, Liège/Masson, Paris
Ectors L, Achslogh J (1959) Le syndrome pyramidal homolatéral précoce et les méningiomes de la IIIe frontale. Neurochirurgie 5:388–400
Edelson RN, Deck MDF, Posner JB (1972) Intramedullary spinal cord metastases. Neurology (Minneap) 22:1222–1231
Eger W, Kührt P (1954) Über akute Pilzencephalitis (Aspergillose) beim Menschen und im Tierexperiment. Dtsch Z Nervenheilkd 171:370–387
Ehni G, Adson AW (1945) Lipoma of the brain. Report of cases. Arch Neurol Psychiatry 53:299–304
Ehni G, Love JG (1945) Intraspinal lipomas: Report of cases. Review of the literature, and clinical and pathologic study. Arch Neurol Psychiatry 53:1–28
Eicke WJ (1943) Zur Frage der fetalen Encephalitis, Meningitis und ihrer Folgeerscheinungen. Arch Psychiatr Nervenkr 116:568–592
Eicke WJ (1952) Bindegewebige Substitution eines Oligodendroglioms nach Röntgenbestrahlung. Dtsch Z Nervenheilkd 169:273–288
Eicke WJ (1954) Toxoplasmose-Encephalitis. Nervenarzt 25:387–388
Eicke WJ (1959) Les maladies inflammatoires de l'encéphale chez le fetus. In: Heuyer MMG, Feld M, Gruner J (eds) Malformations congénitales du cerveau. Masson, Paris, pp 81–92

Eiselsberg AF, Ranzi E (1913) Über die chirurgische Behandlung der Hirn- und Rückenmarkstumoren. Arch Klin Chir 102:309–468
Eisenberg HM, McComb JG, Lorenzo AV (1974) Cerebrospinal fluid overproduction and hydrocephalus associated with choroid plexus papilloma. J Neurosurg 40:381–385
Eisenhardt L (1935) Long postoperative survivals in cases of intracranial tumor. Assoc Res Nerv Ment Dis Proc 16:390–416
Eisenhardt L, Cushing H (1930) Diagnosis of the intracranial tumors by supravital technique. Am J Pathol 6:541–552
El-Banhawy A, Ahmed KEK (1962) Classification of intracranial cysts. J Egypt Med Assoc 45:649–661
El-Banhawy A, Walter W (1962) Meningiomas with acute onset. Acta Neurochir (Wien) 10:194–206
El-Banhawy A, Sheldon PWE, Pennybacker J (1963) On missing meningiomas. J Neurol Neurosurg Psychiatry 26:462–467
El Din Mansour S, Reese HH (1964) Neuromuscular schistosomiasis (clinicopathological and experimental studies). University of Wisconsin, Madison
El-Gindi S, Salama M, El-Henawy M, Farac S (1973) Metastases of glioblastoma multiforme to cervical lymph nodes. J Neurosurg 38:631–634
El-Gindi S, Abd-El-Hafeez M, Salama M (1974) Extracranial skeletal metastases from an intracranial meningeal chondrosarcoma. Case report. J Neurosurg 40:651–653
Elkington JSC (1935) Metastatic tumors of brain. Proc R Soc Med 28:1080–1096
Elsaesser KH (1950) Über die Aktinomykose und ihre Lokalisation im Zentralnervensystem. Dtsch Z Nervenheilkd 164:123–142
Elsberg CA (1925) Some aspects of the diagnosis and surgical treatment of tumors of the spinal cord with a study of the end result in a series of 119 operations. Ann Surg 81:1057–1073
Elsberg CA (1941) Surgical diseases of the spinal cord, membranes and nerve roots: Symptoms, diagnosis and treatment. Hoeber, New York
Elsberg CA, Globus JH (1929) Tumors of the brain with acute onset and rapidly progressive course. „Acute brain tumor". Arch Neurol Psychiatry 21:1044–1078
Elsberg CA, Hare CC (1932) The blood supply of the gliomas. Bull Neurol Inst NY 2:210–246
Elsberg CA, Dyke DG, Brewer ED (1934) The symptoms and diagnosis of extradural cysts. Bull Neurol Inst NY 3:395–417
Elschnig (1913) Nystagmus retractorius, ein cerebrales Herdsymptom. Med Klin 9:8
Elvidge AR (1968) Long-term survival in the astrocytoma series. J Neurosurg 28:399–404
Elvidge AR, Martinez-Coll A (1956) Long-term follow-up of 106 cases of astrocytoma, 1928–1939. J Neurosurg 13:230–243
Emanuel C (1900) Ein Fall von Gliom der Pars ciliaris retinae. Virchows Arch [A] 161:338–364
Eng LF, Rubinstein LJ (1978) Contribution of immunohistochemistry to diagnostic problems of human cerebral tumors. J Histochem Cytochem 26:513–522
Eng LF, Gerstl B, Vanderhaeghen JJ (1970) A study of proteins in old multiple sclerosis plaques. Trans Am Soc Neurochem 1:42
Engel H (1951) Ein Beitrag zu den Syndromen der Stirnhirngeschwülste (Oligodendrogliom). Medical dissertation, University of Hamburg
Engelhardt P, Lang W (1977) Primary melanocytoblastoma of the leptomeninges. J Neurol 215:73–79
Eppinger H (1890) Über eine neue, pathogene Cladothrix und eine durch sie hervorgerufene Pseudotuberculosis (cladothrichica). Beitr Pathol Anat 9:287–328
Epstein JA, Epstein BS, Molho L, Zimmerman HM (1964) Carcinoma of the pituitary gland with metastases to the spinal cord and roots of the cauda equina. J Neurosurg 21:846–853
Epstein JA, Epstein BS, Lavine LS, Rosenthal AD, Decker RE, Carras R (1978) Obliterative arachnoiditis complicating lumbar spinal stenosis. J Neurosurg 48:252–258
Erbslöh F (1956) Zur Pathologie der diffusen Pigmentgeschwülste im Meningealraum. Arch Geschwulstforsch 9:103–143
Erdheim J (1903) Zur normalen und pathologischen Histologie der Glandula thyreoidea, parathyreoidea and hypophysis. Beitr Pathol Anat 33:158–236

Erdheim J (1904) Über Hypophysenganggeschwülste und Hirncholesteatome. SB Akad Wiss Wien, Math-Natl Kl 113:537–726
Erdheim J (1926) Pathologie der Hypophysengeschwülste. Ergeb Allg Pathol 21:482–561
Erich JB (1955) Juvenile fibromas of the nasopharynx. Arch Otolaryngol 62:277–281
Ermel AE (1974) Histogenesis of angiomatous areas in meningiomas. An electron microscope study. Pathol Eur 9:217–231
Ermel AE, Brucher JM (1974) Arguments ultrastructuraux en faveur de l'appartenance du médulloblastome à la lignée neuronale. Acta Neurol Belg 74:208–220
Escalona-Zapata J (1966) Über die Einordnung des sogenannten malignen Astrozytoms. Acta Neurochir (Wien) 14:126–140
Escalona-Zapata J (1972) Neuroblastische Tumoren der Großhirnhemisphäre. Zentralbl Neurochir 33:35–44
Escalona-Zapata J (1981) Uncommon oligodendrogliomas. Acta Neuropathol [Suppl] (Berl) 7:94–96
Escalona-Zapata J, Baez O (1963) Contribuciòn al encuadramiento nosológico de llamado granuloma óseo eosinófilo. Acta Oncol (Madr) 2:2–27
Escalona-Zapata J, Diez-Nan MD (1981) The astrocytic nature of glioblastoma demonstrated by tissue culture. Acta Neuropathol (Berl) 53:155–160
Escobar A, Nieto D (1972) Parasitic diseases (trichinosis). In: Minckler J (ed) Pathology of the nervous system, vol III. McGraw Hill, New York, pp 2518–2519
Escourolle R, Poirier J (1967) L'ultrastructure du médulloblastome cérébelleux. Ann Anat Pathol (Paris) 12:121–136
Essbach H (1943) Die Meningeome. Vom Standpunkt der organoiden Geschwulstbetrachtung. Ergeb Allg Pathol 36:185–490
Esslen E (1950) Ein Beitrag zu den Syndromen der Stirnhirngeschwülste (Gliome ohne Oligodendrogliome). Medical dissertation, University of Hamburg
Esteban HM, Villanueva JP, Bueno G, Puentes F (1979) Primary intraventricular choriocarcinoma. Surg Neurol 11:21–23
Ethelberg S, Jensen VA (1952) Obscurations and further time-related paroxysmal disorders in intracranial tumours. Syndrome of initial herniation of parts of brain through the tentorial incisure. Arch Neurol Psychiatry 68:130–149
Evans DC, Netsky MG, Allen VE, Kasantikul V (1979) Empty sella secondary to suprasellar colloid cyst of foregut (respiratory) origin. J Neurosurg 51:114–117
Evans N (1926) Mitotic figures in malignant tumors as affected by time before fixation of tissues. Arch Pathol 1:894–898
Everett BA, Klusske JA, Rush JL, Pribram HW (1978) Cryptococcal infection of the central nervous system. Surg Neurol 9:157–163
Everke H (;966) Ein Myxochondrom-Chondromyxoid-Fibrom der Schädelbasis mit Ausdehnung in den Canalis spinalis. Acta Neurochir (Wien) 15:150–158
Evrard E, Reznik M, Divry P, Molders V (1963) Angiome caverneux intramédullaire du renflement cervical et pseudosclérose latérale amyotrophique. Acta Neurol Psychiatr Belg 63:527–544
Ewing J (1928) Neoplastic diseases: A treatise on tumors, 3rd edn. Saunders, Philadelphia
Ewing J (1935) Modern attitude toward traumatic cancer. Arch Pathol 19:690–728
Ewing J (1939) A review of the classification of bone tumors. Surg Gynecol Obstet 68:971–976
Eyre-Brook AL, Hewer TF (1962) Spontaneous disappearance of neuroblastoma with maturation to ganglioneuroma. J Bone Joint Surg (Br) 44-B:886–890
Eyster EF, Nielsen SL, Sheline GE, Wilson CB (1974) Cerebral radiation necrosis simulating a brain tumor. Case report. J Neurosurg 39:267–271
Ezrin C, Horvath E, Kovacs K (1977) The pituitary gland. Presented at the 1977 endocrine pathology course. Harvard Medical School, Boston
Fabiani A, Peres B, Torta R, Trebini F (1975) Cerebral actinomycotic granuloma. Zentralbl Neurochir 36:195–198
Fabiani A, Favero M, Trebini F (1980) On the primary meningeal tumors with special concern to the hemangiopericytoma pathology and biology. Zentralbl Neurochir 41:273–286
Fabing H (1934) Tuberous sclerosis with epilepsy (epiloia) in identical twins. Brain 57:227–238

Fabinyi GCA, Adams JE (1979) High cervical spinal cord compression by an enterogenous cyst. Case report. J Neurosurg 51:556–559
Fager CA, Carter H (1966) Intrasellar epithelial cysts. J Neurosurg 24:77–81
Fahlbusch R, von Werder K (1978) Treatment of pituitary adenomas. Thieme, Stuttgart
Fairbanks-Barbosa J, Luisi A, Rapoport A, Araujo J (1971) Estesioneuroblastoma. Bol Oncol (Sao Paulo) 61:27–34
Fairburn B, Larkin IM (1964) A cyst of Rathke's cleft. J Neurosurg 21:223–225
Fairburn B, Ulrich H (1971) Malignant gliomas occurring in identical twins. J Neurol Neurosurg Psychiatry 34:718–722
Falconer MA, Bailey IC, Duchen LW (1968) Surgical treatment of chordoma and chondroma of the skull base. J Neurosurg 29:261–275
Falta W (1928) Die Erkrankungen der Blutdrüsen. Springer, Wien-Berlin
Falta W (1940) Diabetes und Hypophyse. Verh Dtsch Ges Inn Med 52:424–436
Fan KJ, Agbata A (1976) Intracranial germinomas. J Natl Med Assoc 68:309–311
Fan KJ, Kovi J, Earle KM (1977) The ethnic distribution of primary central nervous system tumors: AFIP 1958 to 1970. J Neuropathol Exp Neurol 36:41–49
Fankhauser R, Luginbühl H (1968a) Tumoren des Zentralnervensystems. In: Dobberstein J, Pallaske G, Stünzi H (eds) E. Joest's Handbuch der speziellen pathologischen Anatomie der Haustiere, 3rd edn, vol 3 Parey, Berlin, pp 366–423
Fankhauser R, Luginbühl H (1968b) Pathologische Anatomie des zentralen und peripheren Nervensystems der Haustiere. Parey, Berlin
Fankhauser R, Luginbühl H, McGrath JT (1974) Tumors of the nervous system. Bull WHO 50:53–69
Farwell J, Flannery JT (1984) Cancer in relatives of children with central-nervous-system neoplasms. N Engl J Med 311:749–753
Farwell JR, Dohrmann GJ, Flannery JT (1978) Intracranial neoplasms in infants. Arch Neurol 35:533–537
Faust DS, Tatem HR, Brady LW, Olsen AK, Osterholm JL, Kazem I, Mancall EL (1970) Radiation therapy in the management of medulloblastomas. Neurology (Minneap) 20:519–522
Federmann M (1983) Die klinische Symptomatik der Tumoren der Pinealisregion. Medical dissertation, University of Cologne
Feigin I (1971) The nerve sheath tumor, solitary and in von Recklinghausen's disease: A unitary mesenchymal concept. Acta Neuropathol (Berl) 17:188–200
Feigin I (1975) The occurrence and characteristics of non-myelinated neuromas within central nervous tissue. J Neuropathol Exp Neurol 34:478–491
Feigin IH, Gross SW (1955) Sarcoma arising in glioblastoma of the brain. Am J Pathol 31:633–653
Feigin IH, Allen LB, Lipkin L, Gross SW (1958) The endothelial hyperplasia of the cerebral blood vessels with brain tumors and its sarcomatous transformation. Cancer 11:264–277
Fein SB, Newill VA (1954) Cerebral Hodgkin's disease. Case report of Hodgkin's granuloma with cerebral invasion. Am J Med 17:291–294
Feiring EH, Davidoff LM (1947) Two tumors, meningioma and glioblastoma multiforme, in one patient. J Neurosurg 4:282–289
Feiring EH, Foer WH (1968) Meningioma following radium therapy. Case report. J Neurosurg 29:192–194
Felix Y, González A, Ambrosius K (1976) Medulomioblastoma. Bol Med Hosp Infant Mex 33:1033–1039
Fender FA (1933) Liposarcoma. Report of a case with intracranial metastases. Am J Pathol 9:909–914
Fenstermacher JD, Patlak CS (1976) The movements of water and solutes in the brain of mammals. In: Pappius HM, Feindel W (eds) Dynamics of brain edema. Springer, Berlin Heidelberg New York, pp 86–94
Fényes G, Kepes J (1956) Über das gemeinsame Vorkommen von Meningeomen und Geschwülsten anderen Typs im Gehirn. Zentralbl Neurochir 16:251–260
Fényes G, Slowik F (1972) Über extracraniell metastasierende Meningiome. Zentralbl Neurochir 33:131–135

Fényes G, Slowik F, Deák G (1965) Über ein operiertes intracranielles Chondrom. Zentralbl Neurochir 26:22–28
Fernandez-Moran H (1948) Examination of the brain tumor tissue with the electron microscope. Arkh Zoologi 40A:1–15
Ferner H (1940) Untersuchungen über die „zelligen Knötchen" (Epithelgranulation) und die Kalkkugeln in den Hirnhäuten des Menschen. Z Mikrosk Anat Forsch 48:592–605
Ferrer Y, Ysamat F, Acebes J (1979) A Golgi and electron microscopic study of a dysplastic gangliocytoma of the cerebellum. Acta Neuropathol (Berl) 47:163–165
Ferry DJ, Hardman JM, Early KM (1969) Syringomyelia and intramedullary neoplasms. Med Ann DC 38:363–365
Ferry DJ, Mylander MCK, Hardman I (1972) Radiographic identification and surgical removal of a teratoid tumor of the roof of the third ventricle. J Neurosurg 36:231–234
Fetter BF, Klintworth GK, Hendry WS (1967) Mycoses of the central nervous system. Williams and Wilkins, Baltimore
Fewer D, Wilson CB, Boldrey EB, Enot KJ, Powell MR (1972) The chemotherapy of brain tumors. Clinical experience with carmustine (BCNU) and vincristine. JAMA 222:549–552
Fields WS, Zülch KJ, Maslenikov V (1972) High cervical neurinoma. Special neurologic and radiologic features. Zentralbl Neurochir 33:89–102
Fincher EF, Coon GP (1929) Ependymomas. Arch Neurol Psychiatry 22:19–44
Findeisen L, Tönnis W (1937) Über intracranielle Epidermoide. Zentralbl Neurochir 2:301–315
Finkemeyer H (1961) Das Glioblastom in den verschiedenen Hirnregionen. Beihefte Zentralbl Neurochir, Barth, Leipzig
Finkemeyer H, Behrend RC (1956) Hirntrauma und Gliomentstehung. Zentralbl Neurochir 16:318–324
Finkemeyer H, Kautzky R (1968) Das Kavernom des Sinus cavernosus. Zentralbl Neurochir 29:23–30
Finkemeyer H, Pfingst E (1966) Das Meningeom des Orbitadaches. Zentralbl Neurochir 27:81–94
Finkemeyer H, Tzonos T (1965) Die klinische Diagnostik der diffusen Gliomatose. Acta Neurochir (Wien) 13:86–112
Finkemeyer H, Krämer W, Pfingst E, Tzonos T (1965) Malignität und Rezidiv bei den hirneigenen Tumoren. Zentralbl Neurochir 25:281–299
Finkemeyer H, Tzonos T, Stanisic M (1967) Ein Nokardia-Granulom des Ganglion Gasseri. Zentralbl Neurochir 28:137–146
Finkemeyer H, Pfingst E, Zülch KJ (1975) The astrocytomas of the cerebral hemispheres. In: Vinken PJ, Bruyn GW (eds) Tumors of the brain and skull. North-Holland, Amsterdam/American Elsevier, New York (Handbook of clinical neurology, vol 18, part III, pp 1–47)
Finzi O (1929) Mieloma con prevalenza delle cellule eosinofile, circonscritto all'oso frontal in un giovanne de 15 ani. Minerva Med 91:239
Firemark HM (1978) Spinal Cysticercosis. Arch Neurol 35:250–251
Fischer AW, Hohlfelder H (1930) Lokales Amyloid im Gehirn. Eine Spätfolge von Röntgenbestrahlungen. Dtsch Z Chir 227:475–483
Fischer B (1918) Das Wesen und die Benennung der Gliome (Neuroblastome). Zentralbl Allg Pathol 29:545–553
Fischer EG (1973) Dandy-Walker syndrome: an evaluation of surgical treatment. J Neurosurg 39:615–621
Fischer G, Tommasi M (1976) Spinal ependymomas. In: Vinken PJ, Bruyn GW (eds) Tumors of the spine and spinal cord. North Holland, Amsterdam/American Elsevier, New York (Handbook of clinical neurology, vol 20, part II, pp 353–387)
Fischer W (1955) Die parasitären Erkrankungen des Zentralnervensystems und seiner Hüllen. In: Lubarsch O, Henke F, Rössle R (eds) Handbuch der speziellen pathologischen Anatomie und Histologie, vol XIII/3. Springer, Berlin-Göttingen-Heidelberg, pp 372–412
Fischer[-Brügge] E (1941) Gefäßbedingte Schädigungen bei offenen Hirnverletzungen. Zentralbl Neurochir 6:232–274
Fischer-Brügge E (1949) Das „Klivuskanten-Syndrom". Eine durch die Klivuskante hervorgerufene Druckfurche des N. oculomotorius. Zentralbl Chir 74:403

Fischer-Brügge E (1950) Anatomische Ursachen funktionaler Kreislaufstörungen des Gehirns und am N. oculomotorius. Bruns Beitr Klin Chir 181:323–336

Fischer-Brügge E (1951) Das Klivuskantensyndrom. Acta Neurochir (Wien) 2:36–68

Fischer-Wasels B (1927) Regenerationsgeschwülste. Verh Dtsch Ges Pathol 22:69

Fischer-Wasels B (1932) Die traumatische Entstehung der Gliome und Piatumoren nach R. Beneke. Monatsschr Unfallheilkd 39:489–527

Fischer-Williams M, Bosanquet FF, Daniel PM (1955) Carcinomatosis of the meninges. A report of three cases. Brain 78:42–58

Fisher ER, Wechsler H (1962) Granular cell myoblastoma – a misnomer. Electron microscopic and histochemical evidence concerning its Schwann cell derivation and nature (granular cell schwannoma). Cancer 15:936–954

Flament J, Flament-Durand J (1964) Etude anatomo clinique d'un cas de lipome de la région des tubercules mamillaires. Acta Neurol Psychiatr Belg 64:607–616

Flaschka G, Popper H (1981) Die primäre Melanoblastose der Leptomeninx. Nervenarzt 52:350–355

Flenker H (1972) Zur Frage des Kausalzusammenhanges zwischen Schädelhirnverletzungen und Hirntumoren. Lebensversicherungsmedizin 24:115–117

Fletcher EM, Woltman HW, Adson AW (1935) Sacrococcygeal chordomas. Arch Neurol Psychiatr 33:283–299

Flexner S (1891) A peculiar glioma (neuroepithelioma?) of the retina. Johns Hopkins Hosp Bull 2:115

Flossdorf R, Reinhardt V, Gerhard L (1981) Morphological studies in malignant tumors of the peripheral nervous system (neurofibrosarcoma, malignant schwannoma, Schwann cell sarcoma). Acta Neuropathol [Suppl] (Berl) 7:129–133

Flyger G (1956) Epilepsy following radical removal of parasagittal and convexity meningiomas. Acta Psychiatr Scand 31:245–251

Foerster DMC, Steiner L, Håkanson S (1972) Arteriovenous malformations of the brain. J Neurosurg 37:562–570

Foerster O (1917) Fall von intramedullärem Tumor, erfolgreich operiert. Berl Klin Wochenschr 58:338

Foerster O (1921) Zur Diagnostik und Therapie der Rückenmarkstumoren. (10. Jahresversammlung der Gesellschaft deutscher Nervenärzte, Leipzig 1920). Dtsch Z Nervenheilkd 70:64–74

Foerster O (1928) Ein Fall von Vierhügeltumor durch Operation entfernt. Arch Psychiatr Nervenkr 84:515–516

Foerster O (1934) Die Diagnostik und Behandlung der Geschwülste des Großhirns. Klin Wochenschr 13:1737–1742

Foerster O (1936) Motorische Felder und Bahnen. In: Bumke O, Foerster O (eds) Großhirn. Vegetatives Nervensystem. Körperbau und Konstitution. Springer, Berlin (Handbuch der Neurologie, vol 6, pp 1–357)

Foerster O (1937) „Chiasmal syndrome". Discussion of Society of British Neurological Surgeons and Berliner Medizinische Gesellschaft. Zentralbl Neurochir 2:364–365

Foerster O (1939a) Thyreogene intrarachideale Geschwülste. Zentralbl Neurochir 4:198–214

Foerster O (1939b) Ein Fall von Agenesie des Corpus callosum verbunden mit einem Diverticulum paraphysarium des Ventriculus tertius. Z Gesamte Neurol Psychiatr 164:380–391

Foerster O, Bailey P (1936) A contribution to the study of gliomas of the spinal cord with special reference to their operability. In: Jubilee Volume for Davidenkov. State Institute for Publication of Biological and Medical Literature, Leningrad

Foerster O, Gagel O (1931) Ein Fall von sogenanntem Gliom des Nervus opticus – Spongioblastoma multiforme ganglioides. Z Gesamte Neurol Psychiatr 136:335–366

Foerster O, Gagel O (1932a) Ein Fall von Gangliocytoma der Oblongata. Z Gesamte Neurol Psychiatr 141:797–823

Foerster O, Gagel O (1932b) Ein Fall von Gangliogliom der Rautengrube. Z Gesamte Neurol Psychiatr 142:507–518

Foerster O, Gagel O (1932c) Ein Fall von Recklinghausenscher Krankheit mit fünf nebeneinander bestehenden verschiedenartigen Tumorbildungen. Z Gesamte Neurol Psychiatr 138:339–360

Foerster O, Gagel O (1933a) Ein Fall von Gangliogliom des Bodens des dritten Ventrikels. Z Gesamte Neurol Psychiatr 145:29–37
Foerster O, Gagel O (1933b) Ein Fall von Gangliocytoma dysplasticum des Kleinhirns. Z Gesamte Neurol Psychiatr 146:792–803
Foerster O, Gagel O (1933c) Ein Fall von Ependymzyste des 3. Ventrikels. Ein Beitrag zur Frage der Beziehungen psychischer Störungen zum Hirnstamm. Z Gesamte Neurol Psychiatr 149:312–344
Foerster O, Gagel O (1934a) Zentrale diffuse Schwannose bei Recklinghausenscher Krankheit. Z Gesamte Neurol Psychiatr 151:1–16
Foerster O, Gagel O (1934b) Ein Fall von Ependymoma polycysticum des Kleinhirns. Z Gesamte Neurol Psychiatr 150:515–527
Foerster O, Gagel O (1935) Klinik und Pathohistologie der intramedullären Rückenmarkstumoren. Dtsch Z Nervenheilkd 136:239–240
Foerster O, Gagel O (1936) Das Ependymom des Filum terminale. Zentralbl Neurochir 1:5–18
Foerster O, Gagel O (1939) Das umschriebene Arachnoidalsarkom des Kleinhirns. Z Gesamte Neurol Psychiatr 164:565–580
Foerster O, McLean AJ, Gagel O (1933a) Ein Fall von Ganglioneuroma amyelinicum des Hirnstammes. Z Gesamte Neurol Psychiatr 143:635–650
Foerster O, McLean AJ, Gagel O (1933b) Ein Fall von Gangliogliom der Regio hypothalamica. Z Gesamte Neurol Psychiatr 145:17–28
Foerster O, McLean AJ, Gagel O (1933c) Ein Fall von Ganglienzellgeschwulst des Hirnstammes (N. caudatus). Z Gesamte Neurol Psychiatr 147:713–745
Foix C, Alajouanine T (1926) La myélite nécrotique subaigue. Rev Neurol (Paris) 2:1–42
Fokes EC, Earle KM (1969) Ependymomas: clinical and pathological aspects. J Neurosurg 30:585–594
Foley J (1955) Benign forms of intracranial hypertension – „toxic" and „otitic" hydrocephalus. Brain 78:1–41
Folkman J (1976) The vascularization of tumors. Sci Am 234:58–73
Foncin JF (1971) Morphologie ultrastructurale de l'hypophyse humaine. Neurochirurgie 17 [Suppl 1]:10–24
Font RL, Croxatto JO (1980) Intracellular inclusions in meningothelial meningioma. J Neuropathol Exp Neurol 39:575–583
Foot NC (1949) The histology of tumours of the peripheral nerves. Adv Surg 2:385–415
Foot NC, Cohen S (1933) Report of a case of retothelial sarcoma (reticulosarcoma) of the cerebral hemispheres. Am J Pathol 9:123–132
Forbes AP, Henneman PH, Griswold GC, Albright F (1954) Syndrome characterized by galactorrhea, amenorrhea and low urinary FSH: Comparison with acromegaly and normal lactation. J Clin Endocrinol Metab 14:265–271
Fornari M, Savoiardo M, Morello G, Solero CL (1981) Meningiomas of the lateral ventricles. Neuroradiological and surgical considerations in 18 cases. J Neurosurg 54:64–74
Fotakis NS (1961a) Über die formale Genese von Keratinformationen in Kraniopharyngiomen (Erdheim-Tumor). Dtsch Z Nervenheilkd 181:581–592
Fotakis NS (1961b) Zur Histochemie der Rosenthalschen Fasern. Dtsch Z Nervenheilkd 182:445–454
Fowler FD, Matson DD (1957) Gliomas of the optic pathways in childhood. J Neurosurg 14:515–528
Fowler M (1968) Embryonic ependymoma arising in a cerebral hemisphere. Cancer 21:1150–1156
Fowler M, Simpson DA (1962) Malignant melanin-forming tumour of the cerebellum. J Pathol Bacteriol 84:307–311
Fox H, South A (1965) Squamous cell carcinoma developing in an intracranial epidermoid cyst (cholesteatoma). J Neurol Neurosurg Psychiatry 28:276–281
Fox H, Emery JL, Goodboy RA, Yates PO (1964) Neurocutaneous melanosis. Arch Dis Child 39:508–516
Fraenkel J, Hunt JR (1903) Tumors of the ponto-medullo-cerebellar space. Acoustic neuromata. (Central neurofibromatosis). Med Rec NY 64:1001–1008

François J, Hanssens M, Lagasse A (1965) The ultrastructure of retinoblastomata. Ophthalmologica 149:53–67

Frankel SA, German WJ (1958) Glioblastoma multiforme; review of 219 cases with regard to natural history, pathology, diagnostic methods and treatment. J Neurosurg 15:489–503

Frauchiger E (1968) Hirngeschwülste bei Tieren im Vergleich zum Menschen. Selecta 12:870–874

Frauchiger E, Fankhauser R (1949) Die Nervenkrankheiten unserer Hunde. Huber, Bern

Frauchiger E, Fankhauser R (1957) Vergleichende Neuropathologie der Menschen und Tiere. Springer, Berlin Göttingen Heidelberg

Frazier CH, Alpers BJ (1931) Adamantinoma of the craniopharyngeal duct. Arch Neurol Psychiatr 26:905–965

Frazier CH, Alpers BJ (1933) Meningeal fibroblastomas of the cerebrum. Arch Neurol Psychiatry 29:935–989

Frazier CH, Alpers BJ (1934) Tumors of Rathke's cleft (hitherto called tumors of Rathke's pouch). Arch Neurol Psychiatry 32:973–984

Freedman H, Forster FM (1948) Bone formation and destruction in hyperostoses associated with meningiomas. J Neuropathol Exp Neurol 7:69–80

Freeman D, Zimmerman HM (1944) Experimental brain tumors: V. Behavior in intraocular transplants. Cancer Res 4:273–278

Freeman JW, Cox TA, Batnitzky S, Morantz RA, Lansky LA (1980) Craniopharyngioma simulating bilateral internal ophthalmoplegia. Arch Neurol 37:176–177

Freeman L, Feigin D (1963) Oligodendroglioma with 35 years of survival. J Neurosurg 20:363–365

French JD (1947) Plasmocytoma of the hypothalamus. Clinical-pathological report of a case. J Neuropathol Exp Neurol 6:265–270

Frenkel JK (1949) Pathogenesis, diagnosis and treatment of human toxoplasmosis. JAMA 140:369–377

Fresh CB, Takei Y, O'Brien MS (1976) Cerebellar glioblastoma in childhood. J Neurosurg 45:705–708

Freudenberg K (1955) Neuere Untersuchungen über die Krebssterblichkeit. Ärztl Mitt 2:38–42

Friede RL (1966) Topographic brain chemistry. Academic Press, New York

Friede RL, Pollak A (1978) The cytogenetic basis for classifying ependymomas. J Neuropathol Exp Neurol 37:103–118

Friede RL, Janzer RC, Roessmann U (1982) Infantile small cell gliomas. Acta Neuropathol (Berl) 57:103–110

Friedman NB (1947) Germinoma of the pineal. Its identity with germinoma ("seminoma") of the testis. Cancer Res 7:363–368

Friedman NB (1951) The comparative morphogenesis of the extragenital and gonadal teratoid tumors. Cancer 4:265–276

Friedman NB, Moore RA (1946) Tumors of the testis. Report on 922 cases. Milit Surg 99:573–593

Friedmann ED, Levy HH (1937) Actinomycosis of the central nervous system. Report of a case and a review of literature. Int Clin 2:36–61

Friedmann ED, Plaut A (1935) Tumor of the pineal gland (pinealocytoma) with meningeal and neural metastases. Arch Neurol Psychiatry 33:1324–1341

Fröhlich (1901) Ein Fall von Tumor der Hypophysis cerebri ohne Acromegalie. Wien Klin Rundsch 15:883

Froelich JS, Lapham LW (1965) Tissue culture studies of gliomas: 1. Intranuclear inclusions in glial cells. Am J Pathol 47:147–158

Froman C, Lipschitz R (1970) Demography of tumors of the central nervous system among the Bantu (African) population of the Transvaal, South Africa. J Neurosurg 32:660–664

Frowein RA (1949) Trauma und Hirngeschwulst. Medical dissertation, University of Düsseldorf

Frühling L, Wild C (1954) Olfactory esthesioneuroepitheliomas of Louis Berger. Arch Otolaryngol 60:37–48

Fu YS, Pritchett PS (1975) Tissue culture study of a sacrococcygeal chordoma with further ultrastructural study. Acta Neuropathol (Berl) 32:225–233

Fu YS, Chen ATL, Kay S, Young HF (1974) Is subependymoma (subependymal glomerate astrocytoma) an astrocytoma or ependymoma? A comparative ultrastructural and tissue culture study. Cancer 34:1992–2008

Fujii T, Itakura T, Hayashi S, Komai N, Nakamine H, Saito K (1981) Primary pineal choriocarcinoma with hemorrhage monitored by computerized tomography. Case report. J Neurosurg 55:484–487

Fujita K, Obora Y, Fujiwara K, Tamaki N, Matsumoto S, Matsukura S (1980) Suprasellar germinoma and primary suprasellar choriocarcinoma. Report of ten cases (In Japanese). No Shinkei Geka 8:819–826

Fujiwara S, Hachisuga S, Numaguchi Y (1980) Intracranial hypoglossal neurinoma: Report of a case. Neuroradiology 20:87–90

Fukaya T, Yoshida I, Banno T, Kageyama N, Ito M (1976) Intracranial collision tumor (In Japanese). No Shinkei Geka 4:585–591

Fukui M, Kitamura K, Ohgami S, Takaki T, Kinoshita K, Watanabe K, Mihara K (1977a) Radiosensitivity of meningioma-analysis of five cases of highly vascular meningioma treated by preoperative irradiation. Acta Neurochir (Wien) 36:47–60

Fukui M, Tanaka A, Kitamura K, Okudera T (1977b) Lipoma of the cerebellopontine angle. J Neurosurg 46:544–547

Fukumitsu T (1964) Giant-celled glioblastoma. Nature of so-called giant-celled glioblastomas; an electron microscopic study (In Japanese). Nippon Geka Hokan 33:350–360

Fukuo (1914) Über die Teratome der Glandula pinealis. Medical dissertation, University München

Fukuyama Y, Arima M, Nagahata M, Kubota T (1957) Cerebral tumors in childhood. Statistics of autopsy cases of past 73 years. Folia Psychiatr Neurol Jpn [Suppl] 4:57–58

Fulton JF (1946) Harvey Cushing. A biography. Blackwell Scientific, Oxford

Furlow L (1935) Intracranial chordoma. Report of a case. Arch Neurol Psychiatry 34:839–343

Furlow LT (1961) Metastatic tumors of the brain. Proceedings of the Congress of Neurological Surgeons, Miami Beach 1959, vol 7. Williams and Wilkins, Baltimore

Furtado D, Marques V (1951) Spinal teratoma. J Neuropathol Exp Neurol 10:384–393

Furukawa T, Shinizu T, Toyokura Y (1973) Facial hemihypertrophy and cerebellar hemangioblastoma. Neurology (Minneap) 23:1324–1328

Gabryel P (1962) Morphologische Veränderungen im Hirngewebe beim experimentellen Ödem. Phasenkontrast- und elektronenmikroskopische Untersuchungen. In: Jacob H (ed) IV. Internationaler Kongress für Neuropathologie, München 1961, vol 3. Thieme, Stuttgart, pp 173–176

Gänshirt H, Schiefer W (1954) Zur Kreislaufpathologie des arteriovenösen Hirnangioms und des multiformen Glioblastoms. Dtsch Z Nervenheilkd 172:58–80

Gärtner J (1955a) Statistische Untersuchungen an 654 intrakraniellen raumfordernden Prozessen. Ein Beitrag zur Biologie der Hirngeschwülste. Zentralbl Neurochir 15:333–351

Gärtner J (1955b) Über intracranielle Geschwulstmetastasen. Zentralbl Allg Pathol 93:171–183

Gagel O (1936) Neurofibromatose (Recklinghausensche Krankheit). In: Bumke O, Foerster O (eds) Angeborene früh erworbene heredofamiliäre Erkrankungen. Springer, Berlin (Handbuch der Neurologie, vol 16, pp 289–318)

Gagel O (1938) Über Hirngeschwülste. Z Gesamte Neurol Psychiatr 161:69–113

Gagel O (1941) Eine Granulationsgeschwulst im Gebiete des Hypothalamus. Z Gesamte Neurol Psychiatr 172:710–722

Gagel O (1942) Tuberöse Sklerose. Klinische Fortbildung. Neue Deutsche Klinik, 8. Ergänzungsband. Urban and Schwarzenberg, Berlin

Gagel O, Kreissel H (1948) Die Geschwülste des Nervensystems. In: Schaltenbrand G (ed) Neurologie, part II: Nervenkrankheiten. Dietrich'sche Verlagsbuchhandlung W Klemm, Wiesbaden (Naturforschung und Medizin in Deutschland 1939–1946 [special edition of the Fiat Review of German Science for sale in Germany] vol 81, pp 49–71)

Gainer JV, Chou SM, Chadduck WM (1975) Familial cerebral sarcomas. Arch Neurol 32:665–668

Galanski M, Benz G (1978) Nativdiagnostische Befunde am Schädel bei der Neurofibromatose von Recklinghausen. ROFO 129:757–761

Galassi E, Pozzati E, Poppi M, Vinci A (1978) Cerebral aspergillosis following intracranial surgery. J Neurosurg 49:308–311
Galatius-Jensen F, Uhm IK (1965) Radiological aspects of cerebral paragonimiasis. Br J Radiol 38:494–502
Gallavardin L, Varay F (1903) Etude sur le cancer secondaire du cerveau, du cervelet et de la moëlle. Rev Med (Paris) 23:441–449
Galluzzi S, Payne PM (1956) Brain metastases from primary bronchial carcinoma: a statistical study of 741 necropsies. Br J Cancer 10:408–414
Gama C (1949) Tumormetastasen im Encephalon und Metastasen verursachende Tumoren des Nervensystems. Neurobiologia (Recife) 12:1–33
Gamper E (1929) Zur Kenntnis der zentralen Veränderungen beim Morbus Recklinghausen. J Psychol Neurol 39:39–84
Gamper E, Stiefler G (1929) Über Rückenmarkstumoren mit dem klinischen Bilde einer rasch tödlich verlaufenden spinalen Erkrankung. Dtsch Z Nervenheilkd 111:239–258
Gandolfi A, Brizzi RE, Tedeschi F, Paini P, Bassi P (1981) Symptomatic subependymoma of the fourth ventricle. J Neurosurg 55:841–844
Garcez de Sena P (1963) Aspectos anátomo clinico dos parasitoses do sistema nervoso. Neurobiologia (Recife) 26:115–139
Garcia CA, McGarry PA, Rodriguez F (1981) Primary intracranial squamous cell carcinoma of the right cerebellopontine angle. J Neurosurg 54:824–828
Garcia JH, Lemmi H (1970) Ultrastructure of oligodendroglioma of the spinal cord. Am J Clin Pathol 54:757–765
Garcia-Bengochea F, Collins GH (1969) Monstrocellular sarcoma of the brain: 6-year postoperative survival. Case report. J Neurosurg 31:686–689
Garcin R (1960) Les atteintes neurologiques et musculaires dans la maladie de Besnier-Boeck-Schaumann. Psychiatr Neurol Neurochir (Amst) 63:285–297
Gardner WJ, Frazier CH (1930) Bilateral acoustic neurofibromas: a clinical study and field survey of a family of five generations with bilateral deafness in thirty-eight members. Arch Neurol 23:266–302
Gardner WJ, Turner OA (1940) Acoustic neurofibromas. Further clinical and pathologic data on hereditary deafness and Recklinghausen's disease. Arch Neurol 44:76–99
Gardner WJ, McCormack LJ, Dohn DF (1960) Embryonal atresia of the fourth ventricle. The cause of "arachnoid cyst" of the cerebello-pontine angle. J Neurosurg 17:226–237
Garrido DO, Kepes JJ (1978) Histologic variants of meningiomas: Interrelations between subgroups (Abstract). J Neuropathol Exp Neurol 37:616
Garza-Mercado R (1976) Intramedullary cysticercosis. Surg Neurol 5:331–332
Gass H, Van Wagenen WP (1950) Meningioma and oligodendroglioma adjacent in the brain. Case report. J Neurosurg 7:440–443
Gass H, Goodman PA, Miller J, Chason JL (1971) Intramedullary sclerosing astrocytoma of the spinal cord. Case report. J Neurosurg 34:693–696
Gastaut H, Regis H, Gastaut JL, Yermenos E, Low MD (1980) Lipomas of the corpus callosum and epilepsy. Neurology (NY) 30:132–138
Gaupp R (1942) Ein Teratom des Gehirnseitenventrikels bei gleichzeitig bestehendem Verschluß des IV. Ventrikels und mit ungewöhnlichem Liquorbefund. Nervenarzt 15:363–373
Gaupp R, Jantz H (1942) Zur Kasuistik der Balkenlipome. Nervenarzt 15:58–68
Gawish HHA (1976) Primary Burkitt's lymphoma of the frontal bone. Case report. J Neurosurg 45:712–715
Gazso L, SLowik F (1975) Primary lymphomas of the central nervous system; in vitro culture observations. Acta Neuropathol [Suppl] (Berl) 6:103–106
Geigy: Angeborene Geschwülste des Auges. Das „Glioma retinae". Folia Ophthalmologica. Geigy, Basel
Geile G, Mogharei M (1965) Ein Angioblastom des linken Schläfenlappens. Zentralbl Neurochir 26:317–322
Geissinger JD, Bucy PC (1971) Astrocytoma of the cerebellum in children. Arch Neurol 24:125–135

Genth J, Gullotta F, Serra JP (1974) Elektronenoptische und enzymhistochemische Vergleichsuntersuchungen an Kraniopharyngiomen und ihren Gewebekulturen. Acta Neuropathol (Berl) 28:331–341
Gerard-Marchand R, Micheau C (1965) Microscopical diagnosis of olfactory esthesioneuromas: general review and report of five cases. JNCI 35:75–82
Géraurd I, Rascol A, Jorda P, Caizergues P, Karkous E (1965) La sarcoidose cérébrale. Rev Neurol (Paris) 112:85–98
Gerhardt C (1882) Das Gliom. Festschrift on the tricentenary of the University of Würzburg, II
Gerlach J (1969) Intracerebral hemorrhage caused by microangiomas. Prog Neurol Surg 3:363–396
Gerlach J, Jensen H-P (1960) Mikroangiome des Gehirns. Langenbecks Arch Klin Chir 293:481–493
German WJ (1961a) The gliomas: A follow-up study. Clin Neurosurg 7:1–20
German WJ (1961b) Acoustic neurinomas: a follow-up study. Clin Neurosurg 7:21–39
Geroulanos S (1969) Chromophobes Hypophysencarcinom mit Leber- und Knochenmetastase. Schweiz Med Wochenschr 99:1817–1824
Gerstner L, Wöber G, Jellinger K (1977) The diagnostic accuracy of imprint cytology for neurosurgical biopsies. In: Wüllenweber R, Brock M, Hamer J, Klinger M, Spoerri O (eds) Lumbar disc adult hydrocephalus. Springer, Berlin Heidelberg New York
Geschickter CF (1935a) Tumors of the peripheral nerves. Am J Cancer 25:377–410
Geschickter CF (1935b) Bone tumors. Am J Roentgenol 34:1–29
Geschickter CF, Copeland MM (1936) Tumors of bone. Am J Cancer 26:489–562
Geschickter CF, Copeland MM (1951) Parosteal osteoma of bone: A new entity. Ann Surg 133:790–807
Gessaga E (1968) Über einen Fall eines malignen Meningeomes mit extracraniellen Metastasen. Sist Nerv 4:258–270
Gessaga EC (1980) Lhermitte-Duclos disease (diffuse hypertrophy of the cerebellum). Report of two cases. Neurosurg Rev 3:151–158
Gessaga EC, Anzil AP (1975) Rod-shaped filamentous inclusions and other ultrastructural features in a cerebellar astrocytoma. Acta Neuropathol (Berl) 33:119–127
Gessaga EC, Mair WGP, Grant DN (1973) Ultrastructure of a sacrococcygeal chordoma. Acta Neuropathol (Berl) 25:27–35
Geyer H, Pedersen O (1939) Zur Erblichkeit der Neubildungen des ZNS und seiner Hüllen. Z Gesamte Neurol Psychiatr 165:284–294
Ghatak NR, McWhorter JM (1976) Ultrastructural evidence for CSF production by a choroid plexus papilloma. J Neurosurg 45:409–415
Ghatak NR, Hirano A, Zimmerman HM (1969) Intrasellar germinomas. J Neurosurg 31:670–675
Ghatak NR, Hirano A, Zimmerman HM (1971) Ultrastructure of a craniopharyngioma. Cancer 27:1465–1475
Giampalmo A (1937) Zur Frage der extraventrikulären Ependymome. Zentralbl Neurochir 2:283–290
Gibbin KP, Henk JM (1978) Glomus jugulare tumours in South Wales. A twenty-year review. Clin Radiol 29:607–609
Gibson AAM, Hendrick EB, Conen PE (1966) Intracerebral schwannoma. Report of a case. J Neurosurg 24:552–557
Gibson JB (1955) Congenital hydrocephalus due to atresia of the foramen of Magendie. J Neuropathol Exp Neurol 14:244–262
Gibson JB, Burrows D, Weir WP (1957) Primary melanoma of the meninges. J Pathol Bacteriol 74:419–438
Gilbert C, Gillman J (1958) Spontaneous neoplasms in the albino rat. S Afr J Med Sci 23:257–272
Gilbertson EL, Good CA (1956) Roentgenographic signs of tumors of the brain. Am J Roentgenol 76:226–247
Gimeno A, Lopez F, Figuera D, Rodrigo L (1972) Neuroentheric cyst. Neuroradiology 3:167–172

Giombini S, Morello G (1978) Cavernous angiomas of the brain. Acta Neurochir (Wien) 40:61–82

Girard PF, Trillet M, Confavreux C, Chazot G (1977) Méningiomatose multiple et familiale, un syndrome voisin de la neurofibromatose de Recklinghausen. Rev Neurol (Paris) 133:359–362

Giuffrè R (1966) Intradural spinal lipomas. Review of the literature (99 cases) and report of an additional case. Acta Neurochir (Wien) 124:69–95

Giuffrè R (1976) Spinal lipomas. In: Vinken PJ, Bruyn GW (eds) Tumors of the spine and spinal cord. North-Holland, Amsterdam/American Elsevier, New York (Handbook of clinical neurology, vol 20, part II, pp 389–414)

Giuffrè R (1984) Successful radical removal of an intracranial meningioma in 1835 by Professor Pecchioli of Sienna. J Neurosurg 60:47–51

Giuffrè R, Di Lorenzo N (1975) Evolution of a primary intrasellar germinomatous teratoma into a choriocarcinoma. Case report. J Neurosurg 42:602–604

Gjerris F, Klinken L (1978) Long-term prognosis in children with benign cerebellar astrocytoma. J Neurosurg 49:179–184

Gjerris F, Klinken JG, Klinken L (1976) Malignancy grade and long-term survival in brain tumors of infancy and childhood. Acta Neurol Scand 53:61–71

Glanzmann Ch, Jutz P, Horst W (1976) Ergebnisse der Strahlentherapie bei Hirnmetastasen (118 Fälle). Strahlentherapie 152:352–357

Glasauer FE (1964) Thoracic and lumbar intraspinal tumours associated with increased intracranial pressure. J Neurol Neurosurg Psychiatry 27:451–458

Glasauer FE, Yuan RHP (1963) Intracranial tumors with extracranial metastases. Case report and review of the literature. J Neurosurg 20:474–493

Glasberg MR, Kirkpatrick JB, Neuwelt EA (1979) Pineal parenchymal cell tumors: a light microscopic and ultrastructural study. J Neuropathol Exp Neurol 38:314

Glass LR, Culbertson CG(1946) Teratoma of pineal gland with choriocarcinoma and rhabdomyosarcoma. Arch Pathol 41:552–555

Glazer N, Hauser H, Slade H (1956) Granular cell tumor of the neurohypophysis. Am J Roentgenol 76:324–326

Gleeson RK, Butzer JF, Grin OD (1978) Acoustic neurinoma presenting as subarachnoid hemorrhage. J Neurosurg 49:602–604

Globus JH (1931) Die Umwandlung gutartiger Gliome in bösartige Spongioblastome. Ein Beitrag zur Frage der gliogenen Geschwülste des Nervensystems. Z Gesamte Neurol Psychiatr 134:325–360

Globus JH (1937) Meningiomas. Arch Neurol 38:667–712

Globus JH (1942) Infundibuloma. A newly recognized tumor of neurohypophysial derivation with a note on the saccus vasculosus. J Neuropathol Exp Neurol 1:59–80

Globus JH, Cares RM (1953) Neuroepithelioma. J Neuropathol Exp Neurol 12:311–348

Globus JH, Kuhlenbeck H (1944) The subependymal cell plate (matrix) and its relationship to brain tumors of the ependymal type. J Neuropathol Exp Neurol 3:1–35

Globus JH, Silbert S (1931) Pinealomas. Arch Neurol 25:937–985

Globus JH, Strauss I (1925) Spongioblastoma multiforme. Arch Neurol Psychiatry 14:139–151

Globus JH, Strauss I, Selinsky H (1932) Das Neurospongioblastom. Z Gesamte Neurol Psychiatr 140:1–29

Glowacki J (1963) Multiple cerebral tumors accompanying Recklinghausen's disease. Folia Med Cracov 5:99–130

Glowacki J, Selosse P (1965) Sur les sarcomes intracérébraux à cellules monstrueuses. Neurochirurgia 8:45–59

Gluszcz A (1962) A cancer arising in a dermoid of the brain. J Neuropathol Exp Neurol 21:383–387

Gluszcz A (1970) Morphogenesis and evolution of intracerebral monstrocellular tumours („sarcoma monstrocellulare"). Neuropathol Pol 8:5–22

Gluszcz A (1972) Grouping of supratentorial gliomas according to their dominant biomorphological features. Acta Neuropathol (Berl) 22:110–126

Gluszcz A, Giernat L, Habryka K, Alwasiak J, Lach B, Papierz W (1971) Rosenthal fibers, birefringent gliofibrillary changes and intracellular homogenous conglomerates in tissue culture of gliomas. Acta Neuropathol (Berl) 17:54–67

Godtfredsen E (1940/1941) Neurologische Symptome bei malignen Rhinopharynx-Tumoren. Acta Psychiatr Neurol Scand 15/16:47–67

Goebel HH, Cravioto H (1972) Ultrastructure of human and experimental ependymomas. J Neuropathol Exp Neurol 31:54–71

Gössinger SM (1983) Primäres malignes Melanom der Meningen. Fortschr Neurol Psychiatr 51:158–163

Go Kian Gwan (1961) Über eine eigenartige Lokalisation von Metastasen am Septum pellucidum. Zentralbl Neurochir 22:102–110

Goinard P, Descuns P (1952) Les kystes hydatiques du nevraxe. Rev Neurol (Paris) 86:369–415

Gol A (1961) The relatively benign astrocytomas of the cerebrum J Neurosurg 18:501–506

Gol A (1962) Cerebral astrocytomas in childhood. A clinical study. J Neurosurg 19:577–582

Gold E (1924) Ependymom am Boden der Rautengrube und cerebrale Luftembolie mit protrahiertem Verlauf. Arb Neurol Inst Univ Wien 25:223–226

Goldberg ID, Kurland LT (1962) Mortality in 33 countries from diseases of the nervous system. World Neurol 3:444–465

Goldhahn WE, Goldhahn G (1976) Neoplasms of the spinal epidural space, with special reference to lymphogranulomatosis. In: Vinken PJ, Bruyn GW (eds) Tumors of the spine and spinal cord. North-Holland, Amsterdam/American Elsevier, New York (Handbook of clinical neurology, vol 20, part II, pp 103–136)

Goldhammer Y, Sadeh M, Tadmor R, Leventon G (1980) Intracranial esthesioneuroblastoma associated with unilateral visual loss. J Neurosurg 53:836–840

Goldmann (1911) Studien zur Biologie der bösartigen Neubildungen. Bruns Beitr Klin Chir 72:1–90

Goldstein E, Lawrence RM (1978) Coccidioidomycosis of the central nervous system. In: Vinken PJ, Bruyn GW (eds) Infections of the nervous system. North-Holland, Amsterdam (Handbook of clinical neurology, vol 35, part III, pp 443–457)

Goldzieher M (1913) Über eine Zirbeldrüsengeschwulst. Virchows Arch [A] 213:353–365

Golgi C (1869) Sulla struttura e sviluppo degli psammomi, Morgagni 11:874–886

Golgi C (1884) Über die Gliome des Gehirns (Untersuchungen über den feineren Bau des Nervensystems). Fischer, Jena

Golovine SS (1918) Tumeurs intradurales bénignes du nerf optique et leur traitement chirurgical. Arch Ophthalmol 36

Gonatas NK, Besen M (1963) An electron microscopic study of three human psammomatous meningiomas. J Neuropathol Exp Neurol 22:263–273

Gonzalez C, Zülch KJ (1964) Über die zylindromatösen Epitheliome der Schädelbasis („Zylindrome") Zentralbl Neurochir 25:111–125

Goodbody RA, Gamlen TR (1974) Cerebellar Haemangioblastoma and genito-urinary tumours. J Neurol Neurosurg Psychiatry 37:606–609

Goodman J, Kleinholz E, Peck FC Jr (1964) Lindau's disease in the Hudson Valley. J Neurosurg 21:97–103

Goran A, Ciminello VJ, Fisher RG (1965) Hemorrhage into meningiomas. Arch Neurol 13:65–69

Gordon A, Maloney AFJ (1965) A case of metastasizing meningioma. J Neurol Neurosurg Psychiatry 28:159–162

Goridis C, Schachner M (1978) Immunological cell surface markers. In: Laerum OD, Bigner DD, Rejewsky MF (eds) Biology of brain Tumors. UICC, Geneva (UICC Technical report series, vol 30, rep. no. 5 pp 158–171)

Gowers WR (1888) A manual of diseases of the nervous system. Blackiston, Philadelphia

Gowers WR, Horsley VA (1888) A case of tumour of the spinal cord; removal; recovery. Trans Med Chir Soc (Edinb) 71:379–430

Grace JT Jr, Perese DM, Metzgar RS, Sasabe T, Holdridge B (1961) Tumor autograft responses in patients with glioblastoma multiforme. J Neurosurg 18:159–167

Graf CI, Blinderman EE, Terplan KL (1962) Pituitary carcinoma in a child with distant metastases. J Neurosurg 19:254–259

Grampa G, Baroldi G (1958) Sui gliomi con metastasi extracraniche. Oncology 11:1–15
Grant FC (1926) Intracranial malignant metastases; their frequency and value of surgery in their treatment. Ann Surg 84:635–646
Grant FC (1956) A study of the results of surgical treatment in 2326 consecutive patients with brain tumor. J Neurosurg 13:479–488
Grant FC, Austin GM (1950) Epidermoids: clinical evaluation and surgical results. J Neurosurg 7:190–198
Grant FC, Sayers MP (1951) Notes of a series of brain tumors. J Neurosurg 8, 510–514
Grcevic N (1956) Tumours of the glomus jugulare. Zentralbl Neurochir 16:260–267
Grcevic N, Yates PO (1957) Rosenthal fibres in tumours of the cerebral nervous system. J Pathol Bact 73:467–472
Green JR (1945) Encephalo-trigeminal angiomatosis. J Neuropathol Exp Neurol 4:27–42
Green JR, Foster J, Berens DL (1950) Encephalotrigeminal angiomatosis (Sturge-Weber syndrome). Am J Roentgenol 64:391–398
Green MJ, Childrey JH (1939) Intracranial chondroma. A case report. J Nerv Ment Dis 89:650–652
Greenberg HS, Deck MDF, Vikram B, Chu FCH, Posner JB (1981) Metastasis to the base of the skull: Clinical findings in 43 patients. Neurology (NY) 31:530–537
Greendyke RM (1965) Primary fibrosarcoma of brain with ossification. Report of a case. Arch Pathol 80:225–227
Greene HSN (1951a) The transplantation of tumors to the brains of heterologous species. Cancer Res 11:529–534
Greene HSN (1951b) A conception of tumour autonomy based on transplantation studies. A review. Cancer Res 11:899–903
Greene HSN, Harvey E (1968) The development of sarcomas from transplants of the hyperplastic stromal endothelium of glioblastoma multiforme. Am J Pathol 53:483–499
Greenfield JG (1934) Two cases of medulloepithelioma (Bailey and Cushing) with special reference to the relative malignancy of this type of tumor. J Pathol 38:11–16
Greenfield JG (1939) The histology of cerebral oedema associated with intracranial tumors (with special reference to changes in the nerve fibres of the centrum ovale). Brain 62:129–152
Greenfield JG, Pritchard B (1937) Cerebral infection with schistosoma japonicum. Brain 60:361–372
Greenfield JG, Robertson EG (1933) Cystic oligodendrogliomas of the cerebral hemispheres and ventricular oligodendrogliomas. Brain 56:247–264
Greenhouse AH, Neubuerger KT (1960) Intracranial teratomata of the newborn. Arch Neurol 3:718–724
Greenwood J Jr, McGuire TH (1957) Multiple primary neoplasms of the central nervous system. Report of a case. J Neurosurg 14:462–465
Greer M (1974) Benign intracranial hypertension. Pseudotumor cerebri. In: Vinken PJ, Bruyn GW (eds) Tumours of the brain and skull. North-Holland, Amsterdam/American Elsevier, New York (Handbook of clinical neurology, vol 16, part I, pp 150–166)
Griepentrog F (1952) Ein Beitrag zur diffusen meningealen Sarkomatose. Arch Psychiatr Nervenkrankh 188:549–555
Griepentrog F, Pauly H (1957) Intra- und extracranielle, frühmanifeste Medulloblastome bei erbgleichen Zwillingen. Zentralbl Neurochir 17:129–140
Grinker RR (1932) Tumors of the retina. In: Penfield's cytology and cellular pathology of the nervous system, chap XII. Hoeber, New York
Grinyo A (1968) Staining of oligodendroglia with silver ammino tungstate in unembedded and embedded material. Stain Technol 43:19–25
Griponissiotis B (1957) Hydatid cyst of the brain and its treatment. Neurology (Minneap) 7:789–792
Groeneveld A, Schaltenbrand G (1927) Ein Fall von Duraendotheliom über der Großhirnhemisphäre mit einer bemerkenswerten Komplikation: Läsion des gekreuzten Pes pedunculi durch Druck auf den Rand des Tentoriums. Dtsch Z Nervenheilkd 97:32–50
Grollmus JM, Wilson CB, Newton TH (1976) Paramesencephalic arachnoid cysts. Neurology (Minneap) 26:128–134

Gropp A (1955) Über ein metastasierendes „Gliom“. Z Krebsforsch 60:590–596
Grosz K, Plaschkes SJ (1960) The occurrence of cerebral tumors in a brother and sister. Isr Med J 19:302–305
Grote W, Hoffmann W (1957) Über Chondrome der Wirbelsäule. Zentralbl Neurochir 17:342–349
Grote W, Lund OE (1957) Bemerkungen zur Pathogenese eines ungewöhnlichen intraspinalen Epidermoids. Dtsch Z Nervenheilkd 176:48–54
Grove AS, Di Chiro G, Rabotti GF (1967) Experimental brain tumors with a report of those induced in dogs by Rous-sarcoma virus. J Neurosurg 26:465–477
Gruber GB (1935) Über raumbeengende Neubildungen im Schädel: 1. Fortschr Röntgenstr 52:319–329
Grün K (1936) Die Geschwülste des ZNS und seiner Hüllen bei unseren Haustieren. Dissertation, Faculty of Veterinary Medicine, University of Berlin
Grumme T, Bingas B (1969) Beitrag zur Prognose der Kleinhirn-Sarkome. Acta Neurochir (Wien) 21:23–30
Grumme T, Bingas B (1973) Die intracranielle Metastasierung des diffusen Pleuramesothelioms. Zentralbl Neurochir 34:41–48
Gruner JE (1960) Les lésions élémentaires de la neurofibromatose de Recklinghausen. Etude au microscope électronique. Rev Neurol (Paris) 102:525–529
Gruszkiewicz J, Doron Y, Gellei B, Peyser E (1972) Brain tumors during the first year of life. Zentralbl Neurochir 33:183–188
Guarnaschelli JJ, Wehry SM, Serratoni FT, Dzenitis AJ (1979) Atypical fibrous histiocytoma of the thoracic spine. Case report. J Neurosurg 51:415–416
Gudeman SK, Sullivan HG, Rosner MJ, Becker DP (1979) Surgical removal of bilateral papillomas of the choroid plexus of the lateral ventricles with resolution of hydrocephalus. J Neurosurg 50:677–681
Gudmundsson KR (1970) A survey of tumours of the central nervous system in Iceland during the 10-year period 1954–1963. Acta Neurol Scand 46:538–552
Guérin J, Bioulac B, Caillé JM, Pouyanne H (1974) Les hémangioblastomes multiples. Neurochirurgie 20:565–582
Güthert H (1938) Ein Teratoid im linken Seitenventrikel des Gehirns. Zentralbl Allg Pathol 70:295–300
Guidetti B, Fortuna A (1967) Surgical treatment of intramedullary hemangioblastoma of the spinal cord. J Neurosurg 27:530–540
Guidetti B, Gagliardi FM (1977) Epidermoid and dermoid cysts. J Neurosurg 47:12–18
Guidetti B, Gambacorta D (1971) Intracranial vascular malformation of unusual size. Complete surgical removal with excellent result. Acta Neurochir (Wien) 25:115–121
Guidetti B, Moscatelli G (1958) Considerazioni sui rapporti fra trauma e tumori cranici. Lav Neuropsichiatr 22:1–21
Guidetti B, Spallone A (1981) The surgical treatment of choroid plexus papillomas. Neurosurg Rev 4:129–137
Guidetti B, Corradi M, Riccio A (1959) Le cisti epidermoidi del cranio e del nevrasse. Lav Neuropsichiatr 24:3–111
Guidetti B, Giuffrè R, Gambacorta D (1968) Follow-up study of 100 cases of pseudotumor cerebri. Acta Neurochir (Wien) 18:259–267
Guild SR (1941) A hitherto unrecognized structure, the glomus jugulare in man. Anat Rec 79 [Suppl 2]:28
Guild SR (1953) The glomus jugulare, a nonchromaffin paraganglion in man. Ann Otol Rhinol Laryngol 62:1047–1071
Guillaume J, Rogé R (1949) Hémorragies méningées répétées par angiomes paraventriculaires. Deux cas opérés. Rev Neurol 81:600–602
Guillery H (1937) Eine in die Wirbelsäule eingewachsene mediastinale Zyste (Vorderarmzyste). Zentralbl Allg Pathol 69:49–53
Guiot G, Derome P (1966) A propos des méningiomes en plaque du ptérion. Le traitement chirurgical des méningiomes osseux hyperostosants. Ann Chir 20:1109–1127
Guleke A (1946) Gehäuftes Auftreten mehrfacher Krebsgeschwülste. Dtsch Gesundheitswes, 200

Gullotta F (1964) Zur in vitro-Diagnostik gliös-mesenchymaler Mischgeschwülste. Dtsch Z Nervenheilkd 186:323–335

Gullotta F (1966) Il medulloblastoma: un sarcoma embrionale a localizzazione specifica. Riv Patol Clin Sper 7:145–160

Gullotta F (1967a) Das sogenannte Medulloblastom. Springer, Berlin Heidelberg New York (Monographien aus dem Gesamtgebiete der Neurologie und Psychiatrie, Heft 118)

Gullotta F (1967b) Vergleichende Untersuchungen zur Morphologie und Genese der sogenannten Medulloblastome. Acta Neuropathol (Berl) 8:76–83

Gullotta F (1971) Die Kleinhirngeschwülste des Kindesalters (eine vergleichende elektronenoptische und Gewebekulturuntersuchung). Ver Dtsch Ges Pathol 55:315

Gullotta F (1973) The ultrastructure of neoplastic astroglia with special consideration of spongioblasts and Rosenthal fibers. In: Kuhlendahl H, Hensell V (eds) Modern aspects of neurosurgery. Excerpta Medica, Amsterdam (Proceedings of the German Society for Neurosurgery, Düsseldorf 1971, vol 3, pp 127–131)

Gullotta F, Bettag W (1967) Zur Frage der längeren Überlebenszeit bei Glioblastomen. Acta Neurochir (Wien) 16:122–128

Gullotta F, Entzian W (1975) Klinische und morphologische Betrachtungen über das „Medulloepitheliom". Neurochirurgia (Stuttg) 18:193–199

Gullotta F, Fliedner E (1972) Spongioblastomas, astrocytomas and Rosenthal fibers. Ultrastructural, tissue culture, and enzyme histochemical investigations. Acta Neuropathol (Berl) 22:68–78

Gullotta F, Kersting G (1972) The ultrastructure of medulloblastoma in tissue culture. Virchows Arch [A] 356:111–118

Gullotta F, Kersting G (1973) Ultrastruttura e comportamento in vitro dei sarcomi cerebrali. Acta Neurol (Napoli) 28:231–234

Gullotta F, Kreutzberg G (1963) Das Gliom des Opticus. Acta Neuropathol (Berl) 2:413–424

Gullotta F, Lanza C (1965) Malformazione retinica neoplastiforme (contributo alle genesi formale delle „rosette"). Riv Patol Clin Sper 6:477–488

Gullotta F, Melo AS de (1979) Das Karzinom des Plexus chorioideus. Klinische, lichtmikroskopische und elektronenoptische Untersuchungen. Neurochirurgia (Stuttg) 22:1–9

Gullotta F, Wüllenweber R (1968) Zur Frage der malignen Entartung bei Meningeom und Meningeom-Rezidiv. Acta Neurochir (Wien) 18:15–27

Gullotta F, Cervós Navarro J, Puig Serra J (1970) Istologia, ultrastruttura e comportamento in vitro di un ganglioglioma cerebrale. Acta Neurol (Napoli) 25:188–196

Gullotta F, Fliedner E, Wüllenweber R, Orf G (1973) Tissue culture, electron microscopic and enzyme histochemical investigations on a sympathetic ganglioneuroblastoma. Acta Neuropathol (Berl) 24:107–116

Gunther M, Penrose LS (1935) Genetics of epiloia. J Genet 31:413–430

Gupta TD, Brasfield R (1964) Metastatic melanoma. A clinicopathologic study. Cancer 17:1323–1339

Gusek W (1962) Submikroskopische Untersuchungen als Beitrag zur Struktur und Onkologie der Meningiome. Beitr Pathol Anat 127:274–326

Gutierrez-Lara F, Patino R, Hakim S (1975) Treatment of tumors of the third ventricle: a new and simple technique. Surg Neurol 3:323–325

Gutin PH, Boehm J, Bank WO, Edwards MS, Rosegay H (1980) Cerebral convexity epidermoid tumor subsequent to multiple percutaneous subdural aspirations. J Neurosurg 54:574–577

Gutjahr P, Voth D (1978) Successful treatment of childhood medulloblastoma – and what thereafter? In: Frowein RA, Wilcke O, Karimi-Nejad A, Brock M, Klinger M (eds) Tumors of the cerebellar region. Adv Neurosurg 5:257–258

Gutmann C (1904) Zur Kenntnis der metastatischen Geschwülste im Gehirn. Fortschr Med 22:141–145

Gutting J (1940) Hirnmetastase und Primärtumor. Dissertation, Faculty of Medicine, University of Düsseldorf

Guyda H, Robert F, Colle E, Hardy J (1973) Histology, ultrastructural, and hormonal characterisation of a pituitary tumor secreting both NGH and prolactin. J Clin Endocrinol Metab 36:531–547

Haar F, Patterson RH (1972) Surgery for metastatic intracranial neoplasm. Cancer 30:1241–1245

Haberich H, Zülch KJ (1959) Über die „Fernmetastasen" der Hirngeschwülste (unter besonderer Berücksichtigung der mesodermalen Tumoren). Zentralbl Neurochir 19:213–219

Haberland K (1950) Über ein spinales Angioma racemosum venosum. Arch Psychiatr Nervenkr 184:417–425

Habte-Gabr E, Smith IM (1973) North American blastomycosis in Iowa. Review of 34 cases. J Chronic Dis 26:585–594

Hadfield MG, Silverberg SG (1972) Light and electron microscopy of giant-cell glioblastoma. Cancer 30:989–996

Hägerstrand I (1961) Vascular changes in cerebral metastases. Acta Pathol Microbiol Scand 51:63–71

Hägerstrand I, Schönebeck J (1969) Metastasis to the pituitary gland. Acta Pathol Microbiol Scand 75:64–70

Haene A de, Hoffmann G, Hozay J (1953) Sur les gliomes du tronc cerebral I. Etude d'un gangliocytome du pont pénétrant dans la région hypothalamique. Acta Neurol Psychiatr Belg 53:355–365

Hässner O (1912) Über Chordome unter gleichzeitiger Mitteilung eines Falles von seltener Größe. Virchows Arch [A] 210:385–406

Haferkamp O, Risopatrón LS (1955) Eigentümliche Melanose der Leptomeningen. Zentralbl Allg Pathol 94:274–277

Hage J (1958) Zwei Fälle von Nasengliom. Fortschr Kiefer Gesichtschir 4:103–109

Hage J (1960) Surgical approach to the external and internal nose: a supplementary report on two cases of nasal glioma. Br J Plast Surg 12:327–339

Hager H (1964) Die feinere Cytologie und Cytopathologie des Nervensystems. Fischer, Stuttgart (Veröffentlichungen aus der morphologischen Pathologie, Heft 67)

Haglid KG, Stavrou D (1973) Water-soluble and pentanol-extractable proteins in human brain normal tissues and human brain tumours with special reference to S-100 protein. J Neurochem 20:1523–1532

Haglid KG, Carlsson C-A, Stavrou D (1973) An immunological study of human brain tumors concerning the brain specific protein S-100 and 14.3.2. Acta Neuropathol (Berl) 24:187–196

Hahn JF, Sperber EG, Netsky MG (1976) Melanotic neuroectodermal tumors of the brain and skull. J Neuropathol Exp Neurol 35:508–519

Haldeman KO (1927) Pineal gland tumors. Arch Neurol Psychiatry 18:724–754

Haller A von (1762) Elementa physiologiae corporis humani, vol 4. Grasset, Lausanne

Haller JS, Wolpert SM, Rabe EF, Hills JR (1971) Cystic lesions of the posterior fossa in infants: A comparison of the clinical, radiological and pathological findings in Dandy-Walker syndrome and extra-axial cysts. Neurology (Minneap) 21:494–506

Hallervorden J (1931) Ein Aktinomykom im 3. Ventrikel. Arch Psychiatr 95:527–536

Hallervorden J (1936) Erbliche Hirntumoren. Nervenarzt 9:1–8

Hallervorden J (1938) Aussprache: Hirngeschwülste. Z Gesamte Neurol Psychiatr 161:217

Hallervorden J (1948) Oligodendrogliom nach Hirntrauma. Nervenarzt 19:163–167

Hallervorden J (1952) Bemerkungen zur zentralen Neurofibromatose und tuberösen Sklerose. Dtsch Z Nervenheilkd 169:308–321

Hallervorden J (1959) Über die Hamartome (Ganglioneurome) des Kleinhirns. Dtsch Z Nervenheilkd 179:531–563

Hallervorden J, Krücke W (1956) Die tuberöse Hirnsklerose. In: Scholz W (ed) Nervensystem, part IV: Erkrankungen des zentralen Nervensystems. Springer, Berlin Göttingen Heidelberg (Handbuch der speziellen pathologischen Anatomie und Histologie, vol 13/IV, pp 602–663)

Halmagyi GM, Evans WA (1978) Lipoma of the quadrigeminal plate causing progressive obstructive hydrocephalus. J Neurosurg 49:453–456

Halmagyi GM, Bignold LP, Allsop JL (1979) Recurrent subependymal giant-cell astrocytoma in the absence of tuberous sclerosis. J Neurosurg 50:106–109

Hamada H, Kadota K, Vetsuhara K, Asakura T, Igakura T (1977) Extracalvarial meningioma (In Japanese). No Shinkei Geka 5:633–639

Hambüchen D (1952) Plexuscysten im 3. Ventrikel, ihre Herkunft und ihre Lokalisation. Beitr Pathol Anat 112:453–469

Hamby WB (1935) Tumors in the spinal canal in childhood. J Nerv Ment Dis 81:24–42

Hamby WB (1944) Tumors of the spinal canal in childhood: analysis of the literature of a subsequent decade (1933–1942); report of a case of meningitis due to an intramedullary epidermoid communicating with a dermal sinus. J Neuropathol Exp Neurol 3:397–412

Hamby WB, Gardner WJ (1935) An ependymal cyst in the quadrigeminal region. Report of a case. Arch Neurol Psychiatry 33:391–398

Hamel E, Frowein RA, Karimi-Nejad A (1980) Intracranial intradural epidermoids and dermoids. Neurosurg Rev 3:215–219

Hamer J, Piotrowski W (1973) Schädeldachtumor beim metastasierenden Schilddrüsenadenom. Zentralbl Neurochir 34:139–145

Hamilton AE, Rubinstein LJ, Poole GJ (1973) Primary intracranial esthesioneuroblastoma (olfactory neuroblastoma). J Neurosurg 38:548–556

Hamilton AM, Garner A, Tripathi RC, Sanders MD (1973) Malignant optic nerve glioma. Report of a case with electron microscope study. Br J Ophthalmol 57:253–264

Hammock MK, Milhorat TH, Breckbill DL (1976) Primary choroid plexus papilloma of the cerebellopontine angle presenting a brain stem tumor in a child. Childs Brain 2:132–142

Hamperl H (1944) Pathologisch-histologisches Praktikum. Springer, Berlin

Hamperl H (1952) Über die Gutartigkeit und Bösartigkeit von Geschwülsten. Verh Dtsch Ges Pathol 35:29–54

Hamperl H (1962) Benign and malignant oncocytoma. Cancer 15:1019–1027

Hamperl H, Lattes R (1957) A study of the argyrophilia of nonchromaffin paragangliomas and granular-cell myoblastomas. Cancer 10:408–413

Hamza R, Touibi S, Jamoussi M, Bardi-Bellagha I, Chtioui R (1982) Intracranial and orbital hydatid cysts. Neuroradiology 22:211–214

Handa H, Bucy PC (1956) Benign cysts of the brain simulating brain tumor. J Neurosurg 13:489–499

Handa J, Handa H, Nakano Y, Mukai T (1979) Radiolucent intracranial dermoid cyst. Report of an unusual case. Neuroradiology 17:211–214

Hanefeld P (1967) Histochemische Untersuchungen zur Verteilung und Aktivität hydrolytischer Enzyme im Gliomen. Dtsch Z Nervenheilkd 192:165–173

Hansebout RR, Bertrand G (1965) Intraspinal teratoma simulating protruded intervertebral disc. J Neurosurg 22:374–379

Hansel FK (1932) Malignant tumours of the nasopharynx with involvement of the nervous system. Ann Otol Rhinol Laryngol 41:74–93

Hansemann D von (1898) Studien über die Spezifität, den Altruismus und die Anaplasie der Zellen. Hirschwald, Berlin

Hansemann D von (1905) Über eine bisher nicht beobachtete Gehirnerkrankung durch Hefen. Verh Dtsch Ges Pathol 9:21–24

Hansemann D von (1920) Das Problem der Krebsmalignität. Z Krebsforsch 17:172–191

Hara M, Takeuchi K (1975) Study of long survival term in pontine tumors (In Japanese). No To Shinkei 27:1187–1191

Hara M, Takeuchi K (1977) A temporal study of survival of patients with pontine gliomas. J Neurol 216:189–196

Harbitz HF (1935) A case of multiple meningiomas combined with diffuse meningiomatosis. Acta Pathol Microbiol Scand [A] 12:24–37

Harder WA (1965) Zur pathologischen Anatomie und Pathogenese des Röntgenspätschadens des Zentralnervensystems. Untersuchungen am Kaninchenhirn. Med. Dissertation, Universität Köln

Harding WG, Courville CB (1934) Bone formation in metastasis of osteogenic sarcoma. Report of case with metastases to the brain. Am J Cancer 21:787–794

Hardman J (1940) The angioarchitecture of the gliomata. Brain 63:91–118

Hardman J, Jefferson G (1938) Cerebellopontine angle signs produced by ependymomata (cyst, tumor). Zentralbl Neurochir 3:137–145

Hardy DG, Hope-Stone HF, McKenzie CG, Scholtz CL (1978) Recurrence of medulloblastoma after homogenous field radiotherapy. Report of three cases. J Neurosurg 49:434–440

Hardy RW Jr, Benjamin SP, Gardner WJ (1978) Prolonged survival following excision of dural chondroma. Case report. J Neurosurg 48:125–127

Hare CC, Wolf A (1934) Intramedullary tumors of the brain stem. Arch Neurol Psychiatry 32:1230–1252
Harper CG, Stewart-Wynne EG (1978) Malignant optic gliomas in adults. Arch Neurol 35:731–735
Harris DJ, Fornasier VL, Livingston KE (1978) Hemangiopericytoma of the spinal canal. Report of three cases. J Neurosurg 49:914–920
Harris W, Cairns H (1932) Diagnosis and treatment of pineal tumours. Lancet I:3–9
Harrison F (1904) Neuere Versuche und Beobachtungen über die Entwicklung der peripheren Nerven. Sitz Ber der Niederrhein Ges f Naturheilkd zu Bonn
Hart MN, Petito CK, Earle KM (1974) Mixed gliomas. Cancer 33:134–140
Harvald B, Hauge M (1956) On the heredity of glioblastoma. J Natl Cancer Inst 17:289–396
Harvey WF, Dawon EK (1941) Chordoma. Edinburgh Med J 48:713–730
Hasegawa H, Ushio I, Hori M, et al (1974) Primary intracranial choriocarcinoma in the pineal region. Med J Osaka Univ 25:63–71
Hasenjäger T (1938) Über die Ausbreitung ventrikelnaher Gliosarkome. Z Gesamte Neurol Psychiatr 161:153–159
Hasenjäger T (1939a) Über seitenventrikelnahe Gliome als eine besondere Gruppe unter den Großhirngeschwülsten. Arch Psychiatr 110:570–604
Hasenjäger T (1939b) Über die Ependymitis blastomatosa bei seitenventrikelnahen Gliomen. Arch Psychiatr 110:605–632
Hash CJ, Grossman CB, Shenkin HA (1975) Concurrent intracranial and spinal cord arteriovenous malformations. J Neurosurg 43:104–107
Hass GM (1934) Chordomas of the cranium and cervical portion of the spine. Arch Neurol Psychiatry 32:300–327
Hass WK (1966) Soluble tissue antigens in human brain tumor and cerebral fluid. Arch Neurol 14:443–447
Hasse KE (1869) Darstellung der Krankheiten des Nervenapparates vom pathologisch-anatomischen Standpunkte. In: Hasse KE (ed) Krankheiten des Nervensystems. Enke, Erlangen (Handbuch der speziellen Pathologie und Therapie, 2nd edn, vol IV/1, pp 379–651)
Hasselbach H (1931) Ependymäres Gliom des 4. Ventrikels (Zusammenhang zwischen Schädeltrauma und Hirntumor). Beitr Pathol Anat 86:120–134
Hassin GB, Diamond IB (1926) Trichinosis encephalitis: a pathologic study. Arch Neurol Psychiatry 15:34–47
Hassin GB, Singer HD (1922) Histopathology of cerebral carcinoma. Arch Neurol Psychiatry 8:155–171
Hassoun J, Tripier MF, Pellisier JF, Bernard M, Choux R, Toga M (1973) Étude ultrastructurale d'un gliome "pseudo-sarcomateux" du cervelet. Arch Anat Pathol 21:73–79
Hassoun J, Hirano A, Zimmerman HM (1975) Fine structure of intercellular junctions and blood vessels in medulloblastomas. Acta Neuropathol (Berl) 33:67–78
Hassoun J, Gambarelli D, Pellisier JF, Henin D, Toga M (1981) Germinomas of the brain. Light and electron microscopic study. A report of seven cases. Acta Neuropathol [Suppl] (Berl) 7:105–108
Hatam A, Bergström M, Möller A, Olivecrona H (1978) Early contrast enhancement of acoustic neuroma. Neuroradiology 17:31–33
Hatanaka H, Sano K (1973) A revised Boron-neutron capture therapy for malignant brain tumours: 1. Experience on terminally ill patients after Co-60 radiotherapy. Z Neurol 204:309–332
Hauge M, Harvald B (1957) Genetics in intracranial tumours. Acta Genet Stat Med (Basel) 7:573–591
Hayashi T, Kuratomi A, Fukuda H, In S, Kuramoto S (1980) Arachnoid cyst of the quadrigeminal cistern. A case report and its clinical analysis based on the published cases (In Japanese). No To Shinkei 32:87–95
Hayes HM, Priester WA, Pendergrass TW (1975) Occurrence of nervous-tissue tumors in cattle, horses, cats and dogs. Int J Cancer 15:39–47
Haymaker W, Yenermen MH (1955) Pathological features of colloid cysts of the third ventricle. A consideration of 60 cases. Excerpta Med [Sect VIII] 8:788

Haymaker W, Rubinstein LJ, Miquel J (1972) Brain tumors in irradiated monkeys. Acta Neuropathol (Berl) 20:267–277

Heath NH (1963) Presacral ependymoma. Case report and review of the literature. Am J Clin Pathol 39:161–166

Hecker J (1969) Ausbreitung und Stadien der cerebralen Toxoplasmose. Dissertation, Faculty of Medicine, University of Cologne

Hedeman LS, Lewinsky BS, Lochridge GK, Trevor R (1978) Primary malignant schwannoma of the Gasserian ganglion. J Neurosurg 48:279–283

Hegedus B (1962) Recherches histochimiques sur la surcharge graisseuse du neurinome. In: Jacob H (ed) Histochemie und Biochemie/Histochemistry and biochemistry. Proceedings of the Fourth International Congress of Neuropathology, vol I. Thieme, Stuttgart, pp 58–60

Heienbrock W, Roters M, Linden WA (1978) Objective characterization of proliferation and malignancy in human brain tumors. In: Frowein RA, Wilcke O, Karimi-Nejad A, Brock M, Klinger M (eds) Head injuries. Tumors of the cerebellar region. Adv Neurosurg 5:285–287

Heimbach SB (1959) Follow-up study on 105 cases of verified chromophobe and acidophile pituitary adenomata after treatment by transfrontal operation and X-ray irradiation. Acta Neurochir (Wien) 7:101–155

Heine J (1931) Über die Vielgestaltigkeit und Kriechbewegungen der Sarkomzellen. Virchows Arch [A] 280:122

Heinlein H, Falkenberg K (1939) Beitrag zur Kasuistik der Ganglioneurome des Kleinhirns. Z Gesamte Neurol Psychiatr 166:128–135

Heiskanen O, Raitta C, Torsti R (1978) The management and prognosis of gliomas of the optic pathways in children. Acta Neurochir (Wien) 43:193–199

Heiss W-D, Turnheim M, Mamoli B (1978) Combination chemotherapy of malignant glioma. Effect of postoperative treatment with CCNU, vincristine, amethopterin and procarbazine. Eur J Cancer Clin Oncol 14:1191–1202

Held H (1909) Die Entwicklung des Nervengewebes bei den Wirbeltieren. Barth, Leipzig

Hellner H (1950) Die Knochengeschwülste. Springer, Berlin

Helwig H (1972) Das eosinophile Knochengranulom. Helv Chir Acta 39:479–501

Henderson WR (1939) The pituitary adenomata. A follow-up study of the surgical results in 338 cases (Dr. Harvey Cushing's series). Br J Surg 26:809–921

Henneberg R (1912) Die tierischen Parasiten des Zentralnervensystems. In: Lewandowsky M (ed) Spezielle Neurologie II. Springer, Berlin (Handbuch der Neurologie, vol 3, pp 643–713)

Henneberg R (1936) Die tierischen Parasiten des Zentralnervensystems. In: Antonini N, Henneberg R, McLean AJ (eds) Raumbeengende Prozesse. Springer, Berlin (Handbuch der Neurologie, vol 14, pp 286–322)

Henriquez AS, Robertson MD, Marshall WJ (1973) Primary neuroblastoma of the CNS with spontaneous intracranial metastases. J Neurosurg 38:226–231

Henry JM, Heffner RR, Earle KM (1978) Gangliogliomas of CNS. A clinicopathological study of 50 cases. J Neuropathol Exp Neurol 37:626

Henschen F (1910) Über Geschwülste der hinteren Schädelgrube, insbesondere des Kleinhirnbrückenwinkels. Fischer, Jena

Henschen F (1934) Referat über Gliome. Zentralbl Allg Pathol 60:8–39, 67–77

Henschen F (1955) Tumoren des ZNS und seiner Hüllen. In: Scholz W (ed) Nervensystem. Springer, Berlin (Handbuch der speziellen pathologischen Anatomie und Histologie, vol XIII/3, pp 413–1040)

Heppner F (1952) Die Erkennung und Behandlung von neoplastischen Hirnmetastasen. Zentralbl Neurochir 12:129–145

Heppner F (1954) Über Meningeome des 3. Ventrikels. Acta Neurochir (Wien) 4:55–67

Heppner F (1955) Meningiomas of the third ventricle in children. Review of the literature and report of two cases with uneventful recovery after surgery. Acta Psychiatr Neurol Scand 30:471–481

Herbst AL, Ulfelder H, Poskanzer DC (1971) Adenocarcinoma of the vagina. Association of maternal stilbestrol therapy with tumor appearance in young women. N Engl J Med 284:881–878

Herbst M (1982) Radiation therapy in the treatment of the astrocytomas and midline tumours of childhood. In: Voth D, Gutjahr P, Langmaid C (eds) Tumours of the central nervous system in infancy and childhood. Springer, Berlin Heidelberg New York, pp 325–332

Herman DL, Courville CB (1965) Pathogenesis of meningeal carcinomatosis. Report of case secondary to carcinoma of cecum via perineural extension, with a review of 146 cases. Bull Los Angeles Neurol Soc 30:107–118

Herman MM, Rubinstein LJ (1978) Divergent glial and neuronal differentiation in a human medulloblastoma maintained in an organ culture system. J Neuropathol Exp Neurol 37:627

Herndon RM, Rubinstein LJ, Freeman JM, Mathieson G (1970) Light and electron microscopic observations on Rosenthal fibers in Alexander's disease and in multiple sclerosis. J Neuropathol Exp Neurol 29:524–551

Herrick MK, Rubinstein LJ (1978) The true pinealomas. A clinicopathological review of 27 cases. J Neuropathol Exp Neurol 37:627

Herrick MK, Rubinstein LJ (1979) The cytological differentiating potential of pineal parenchymal neoplasms (true pinealomas). Brain 102:289–320

Herring AB, Urich H (1969) Sarcoidosis of the CNS. J Neurol Sci 9:405–422

Herrmann E (1963) Das Plasmocytom der Schädelbasis. Beitrag zu seiner Neurologie und Radiologie. Arch Psychiatr Nervenkr 204:262–270

Herrmann H (1961) Beitrag zur Frage der bevorzugten Lokalisation cerebraler Geschwulstmetastasen. Dissertation, Faculty of Medicine, University of Munich

Herrschaft H (1968) Die Teratome des Zentralnervensystems. Dtsch Z Nervenheilkd 194:344–365

Herschman HR (1978) Characteristics of cell culture lines derived from chemically induced neural tumors. In: Laerum OD, Bigner DD, Rajewsky MF (eds) Biology of brain tumors. UICC, Geneva (UICC technical report series, vol 30, report no. 5, pp 172–183)

Hertig AT, Gore H (1961) Tumors of the female sex organs: 3. Tumors of the ovary and fallopian tube. Armed Forces Institute of Pathology, Washington

Herxheimer G (1913) Über Tumoren des Nebennierenrindenmarks, insbesondere das neuroblastoma sympathicum. Beitr Pathol 57:112

Herzog G (1944) Spezielle Pathologie des Skelets und seiner Teile: Die primären Knochengeschwülste. Springer, Berlin (Henke/Lubarsch: Handbuch der speziellen pathologischen Anatomie und Histologie, vol IX/5)

Herzog W (1950) Über ein primäres Melanosarkom der Leptomeninx mit Ausbreitung auf dem Liquorwege. Zentralbl Allg Pathol 86:5–16

Hess IR (1978) Frequency of surface microprojections and coated vesicles with increased malignancy in human astrocytic neoplasms. Acta Neuropathol (Berl) 44:151–153

Hesselvik M, Tygstrup I (1965) Metastasizing cerebral ependymoma. Acta Neuropathol (Berl) 4:416–420

Heuyer G, Lhermitte J, De Martel T, Vogt C (1931) Un cas de macrogénitosomie précoce liée à un épendymogliome de la région mamillo-tubérale. Rev Neurol (Paris) 38:194–210

Hewlett RH, Ganz JC (1976) Histiocytosis X of the cauda equina. Neurology (Minneap) 26:472–476

Heyck H (1954) Glioblastom nach Leukotomie. Monatsschr Psychiatr Neurol 128:180–188

Higginson I (1968) Distribution of different patterns of cancer. Isr J Med Sci 4:457

Hildebrandt K (1906) Zur Kenntnis der gliomatösen Neubildungen des Gehirns mit besonderer Berücksichtigung der ependymären Gliome. Dissertation, Faculty of Medicine, University of Berlin

Hilding DA, House WF (1965) "Acoustic neuroma": Comparison of traumatic and neoplastic. J Ultrastruct Res 12:611–623

Hill L (1933) Congenital ependymal cyst of the 4th ventricle. J Nerv Ment Dis 77:358

Himuro H, Kobayashi E, Kono H, Jinbo M, Kitamura K (1976) Familial occurrence of pituitary adenoma (In Japanese). No Shinkei Geka 4:371–377

Himuro H, Suzuki H, Takeyama E, Jinbo M, Kitamura K (1977) A case of intracranial osteochondroma (In Japanese). No Shinkei Geka 5:1079–1083

Hinzpeter T, Fliedner E (1975) Solitärer Cysticercus cellulosae racemosus im 4. Ventrikel. Zentralbl Neurochir 36:117–120

Hirano A (1975) A comparison of the fine structure of malignant lymphoma and other neoplasms in the brain. Acta Neuropathol [Suppl] (Berl) 6:141–145
Hirano A (1978) Some contributions of electron microscopy to the diagnosis of brain tumors. Acta Neuropathol (Berl) 43:119–128
Hirano A (1983) Praktischer Leitfaden der Neuropathologie. Springer, Berlin Heidelberg New York
Hirano A, Carton CA (1960) Primary malignant melanoma of the spinal cord. J Neurosurg 17:935–944
Hirano A, Ghatak NR (1974) The fine structure of colloid cysts of the third ventricle. J Neuropathol Exp Neurol 33:333–341
Hirano A, Ghatak NR, Zimmerman HM (1973) The fine structure of ependymoblastoma. J Neuropathol Exp Neurol 32:144–152
Hirano A, Matsui T, Zimmerman HM (1975a) Electron microscopic observations of ependyma (In Japanese). No Shinkei Geka 3:237–244
Hirano A, Matsui T, Zimmerman HM (1975b) The fine structure of ependymoma. No Shinkei Geka 3:557–563
Hirano A, Llena JF, Chung HD (1975c) Same new observations in an intracranial germinoma. Acta Neuropathol (Berl) 32:103–113
Hirano A, Llena JF, Chung HD (1975d) Fine structure of a cerebellar "fibroma". Acta Neuropathol (Berl) 32:175–186
Hirose G, Shimazaki K, Takado M, Kosoegawa H, Ohya N, Mukawa A (1980) Intramedullary spinal cord metastasis associated with pencilshaped softening of the spinal cord. Case report. J Neurosurg 52:718–721
Hirsch A (1886) Die Organkrankheiten. In: Handbuch der historisch-geographischen Pathologie. Enke, Stuttgart
Hirsch EF, Elliot AR (1925) Ependymomas of the lateral and fourth ventricles of the brain. Am J Pathol 1:627–634
Hirsch LF, Stool SE, Langfitt TW, Schut L (1977) Nasal glioma. J Neurosurg 46:85–91
Hirsch O (1911) Über die endonasale Operationsmethode bei Hypophysentumoren mit Bericht über 12 operierte Fälle. Berl Klin Wochenschr 48:1933–1935
Hirsch O (1912) Die operative Behandlung von Hyphosistumoren nach endonasalen Methoden. Arch Laryngol Rhinol 26:529–686
Hirsch O (1930) Über Hypophysentumoren und deren Behandlung. Klin Monatsbl Augenheilkd 85:609–640
Hirsch O (1950) 40 Jahre transphenoidale Operation von Hypophysentumoren. Wien Klin Wochenschr 62:35–37, 640–644
Hirschfeld L (1851) Sur une tumeur cartilagineuse de la base du crâne (enchondrome) C R Soc Biol 3:94–96
Hirst LW, Miller NR, Allen GS (1979) Sphenoidal pneumosinus dilatans with bilateral optic nerve meningiomas. J Neurosurg 51:402–407
Hirtzler R, Pavelić Z, Kubović M, Šalić M (1975) Metastasen des Lungenkarzinoms in benignen Tumoren. Zentralbl Allg Pathol 119:272–275
His W (1904) Die Entwicklung des menschlichen Gehirns. Hirsel, Leipzig
Hitchock E, Sato F (1964) Treatment of malignant gliomata. J Neurosurg 21:497–505
Hitselberger WE, Kernohan JW, Uihlein A (1961) Giant cell fibrosarcoma of the brain. Cancer 14:841–852
Hizawa K, Wechsler W (1966) Zur Feinstruktur des Fibrosarkoms der Dura. Beitr Pathol Anat 134:449–463
Ho K-L (1981) Schwannoma of the trochlear nerve. J Neurosurg 55:132–135
Hoch A (1951) Geschwülste des Kindesalters. Zürcher Beobachtungen an Hand von 223 kindlichen und jugendlichen Tumorfällen. Oncologia 4:94–108
Höök O (1954) Sarcoidosis with involvement of the nervous system. Arch Neurol Psychiatry 71:554–575
Hoessly GF, Olivecrona H (1955) Report on 280 cases of verified parasagittal meningioma. J Neurosurg 12:614–626
Hofeldt FD, Levin SR, Schneider V, Becker U, Forsham P (1973) Clinical features of acromegaly and response to cryohypophysectomy. Rocky Mt Med J 70:21–24

Hoff JT, Bronson SR(1968) Cerebral hemangioblastoma occurring in a patient with von Hippel-Lindau disease. Case report. J Neurosurg 28:365–368
Hoffmann H (1919) Gehirntumoren bei 2 Geschwistern. Ein Beitrag zur Vererbung der Geschwülste. Z Gesamte Neurol Psychiatr 51:113–123
Hoffmann KJ, Hendrick EB, Humphreys RP (1976) Metastasis via ventriculoperitoneal shunt in patients with medulloblastoma. J Neurosurg 44:562–566
Hojo S, Llena J, Hirano A, Zimmerman HM (1978) Metastatic tumors in the central nervous system. 8th International Congress of Neuropathology Washington 1978. J Neuropathol Exp Neurol 37:628
Holanda FJCS, Holanda GMP (1980) Tuberous sclerosis. Neurosurgical indication in intraventricular tumors. Neurosurg Rev 3:139–150
Holbach K-H, Gaddoni G (1971) Die Sarkoidose des ZNS als neurochirurgisches Krankheitsbild. Acta Neurochir (Wien) 24:121–133
Holbach K-H, Gullotta F (1977) Zur Formalgenese intrasellärer und intraventrikulärer Zysten. Neurochirurgia (Stuttg) 20:186–188
Holimon JL, Rosenblum WI (1971) "Gangliorhabdomyosarcoma", a tumor of ectomesenchyme. Case report. J Neurosurg 34:417–422
Hollin SA, Drapkin AJ, Wancier J, Huang YP (1978) Mobile schwannoma of the cauda equina. J Neurosurg 48:135–137
Holness RO, Sangalang VE (1976) Myelomatous metastasis to the pineal body. Surg Neurol 5:97–98
Holt JF, Wright EM (1948) The radiologic features of neurofibromatosis. Radiology 51:647–664
Holtås S, Cronqvist S (1981) Cranial computed tomography of patients with malignant melanoma. Neuroradiology 22:123–127
Hongzhao S, Baozhen W (1979) Brain metastasis in choriocarcinoma and malignant mole. Analysis of 98 cases. Chin Med J [Engl] 92:164–174
Hooper R (1976) Intracranial tumours in childhood. Med J Aust 1:624–627
Hoover R, Fraumeni JF (1973) Risk of cancer in renal-transplant recipients. Lancet II:55–57
Hope DT, Symon L (1978) Metastasis of carcinoma to meningioma. Acta Neurochir (Wien) 40:307–313
Hope-Stone HF (1970) Results of treatment of medulloblastomas. J Neurosurg 32:83–87
Hoppe HJ (1952) Diskordantes Auftreten von Hirntumoren bei erbgleichen Zwillingen. Zentralbl Neurochir 12:34–36
Hori A (1973) Über intraspinale Schwannosen der Zona terminalis (Lissauer). (Formes frustes der Neurofibromatose Recklinghausen oder „reaktiv"?). Acta Neuropathol (Berl) 25:89–94
Hori K, Nagai I (1974) Brain scintiphotogramm in sarcoidosis of central nervous system. A case report (In Japanese). No Shinkei Geka 2:169–173
Hormes R (1974) Zur formalen Genese kristalliner Strukturen in Oligodendrogliomen. Acta Neuropathol (Berl) 27:369–375
Horrax G (1947) The role of pinealomas in the causation of diabetes insipidus. Ann Surg 126:725–739
Horrax G (1949) The diagnosis and treatment of pineal tumors. Radiology 52:186–192
Horrax G (1950) Treatment of tumors of the pineal body. Experience in a series of twenty-two cases. Arch Neurol Psychiatry 64:227–242
Horrax G, Bailey P (1925) Tumors of the pineal body. Arch Neurol Psychiatry 13:423–467
Horrax G, Bailey P (1928) Pineal pathology, further studies. Arch Neurol Psychiatry 19:394–413
Horrax G, Henderson DG (1939) Encapsulated intramedullary tumor involving the whole spinal cord from medulla to conus: complete enucleation with recovery. Surg Gynecol Obstet 68:814–819
Horrax G, Wu WQ (1951) Postoperative survival of patients with intracranial oligodendroglioma with special reference to radical tumor removal. A study of 26 patients. J Neurosurg 8:473–479
Horrax G, Wyatt JP (1947) Ectopic pinealomas in the chiasmal region. J Neurosurg 4:309–326
Horsley V (1886) Brain surgery. Br Med J II:670–675

Horsley V (1887) Remarks on ten consecutive cases of operations upon the brain and cranial cavity to illustrate the details and safety of the method employed. Br Med J I:863

Horsley V (1890) Remarks on the surgery of the central nervous system. Br Med J II:1286–1292

Horsley V (1906) On the technique of operations on the central nervous system. Br Med J II:411–423

Horten BC, Rubinstein LJ (1976) Primary cerebral neuroblastoma. A clinicopathological study of 35 cases. Brain 99:735–756

Horten BC, Ulrich H, Rubinstein LJ, Montagne SR (1977) The angioblastic meningioma: a reappraisal of a nosological problem. J Neurol Sci 31:387–410

Horvat B, Pena C, Fisher ER (1969) Primary reticulum cell sarcoma (microglioma) of brain. An electron microscopy study. Arch Pathol 87:609–616

Horvath E, Kovacs K (1976) Ultrastructural classification of pituitary adenomas. Can J Neurol Sci 3:9–21

Horvath E, Kovacs K, Singer W, Ezrin C, Kerenyi NA (1977) Acidophil stem cell adenoma of the human pituitary. Arch Pathol Lab Med 101:594–599

Hoshino T, Barker M, Wilson CB, Boldrey EB, Fewer D (1972) Cell kinetics of human gliomas. J Neurosurg 37:15–26

Hoshino T, Wilson CB, Rosenblum ML, Barker M (1975) Chemotherapeutic implications of growth fraction and cell cycle time in glioblastomas. J Neurosurg 43:127–135

Hosibuchi Y (1970) Virus-like particles in human schwannoma. Proceedings of the VIth International Congress of Neuropathology. Masson, Paris, p 998

Hossmann K-A (1964) Paper presented at the annual meeting of the German Society of Neurosurgery, Hamburg 1964 (unpublished)

Hossmann K-A (1966) Möglichkeiten der Elektronenmikroskopie in der Diagnostik menschlicher Hirntumoren. In: Lüthy F, Bischoff A (eds) Proceedings of the 5th International Congress of Neuropathology, Zürich 1965. Excerpta Medica Foundation, Amsterdam, pp 901–903

Hossmann K-A (1980) Pathophysiology of brain edema, recent observations on cytotoxic (ischemic) and vasogenic (peritumorous) brain edema. Seara Med Neuroc (Sao Paulo) 9:141–150

Hossmann K-A (1982) Pathophysiology of vasogenic and cytotoxic brain edema. In: Hartmann A, Brock M (eds) Treatment of cerebral edema. Springer, Berlin Heidelberg New York, pp 1–10

Hossmann K-A, Blöink M (1981) Blood flow and regulation of blood flow in experimental peritumoral edema. Stroke 12:211–217

Hossmann K-A, Schütz H (1966) Tuberkulome im Bereich eines alten Hirnschußkanales. Acta Neurochir (Wien) 14:254–263

Hossmann K-A, Schuier FJ (1979a) Pathophysiology of stroke edema. In: Zülch KJ, Kaufmann W, Hossmann K-A, Hossmann V (eds) Brain and heart infarct II. Springer, Berlin Heidelberg New York, pp 119–129

Hossmann K-A, Schuier FJ (1979b) Metabolic (cytotoxic) type of brain edema following middle cerebral artery occlusion in cats. In: Price TR, Nelson E (eds) Cerebrovascular diseases. Raven, New York

Hossmann K-A, Wechsler W (1965) Zur Feinstruktur menschlicher Spongioblastome. Dtsch Z Nervenheilk 187:327–351

Hossmann K-A, Wechsler W (1971a) Elektronenmikroskopie kindlicher Hirngeschwülste. In: Kraus H, Sunder-Plassmann M (eds) Pädiatrische Neurochirurgie. Report of the 1st European Congress, Vienna, 1967. Vienna Medical Academy, Vienna

Hossmann K-A, Wechsler W (1971b) Ultrastructural cytopathology of human cerebral gliomas. Oncology 25:455–480

Hossmann K-A, Zülch KJ (1966) Die spinalen psammomatösen Meningeome der Frau. Neurochirurgia (Stuttg) 9:106–113

Hossmann K-A, Schröder M, Wechsler W (1965) Das morphologische Substrat der Bluthirnschranke unter physiologischen und pathologischen Bedingungen. Verh Dtsch Ges Pathol 49:350–356

Hossmann K-A, Wechsler W, Wilmes F (1979) Experimental peritumorous edema. Acta Neuropathol (Berl) 45:195–203

Howarth IC, Bunts AT (1950) Intracranial meningioma following trauma. Report of case. Cleve Clin Q 17:14–18
Hoyt WF, Baghdassarian SA (1969) Optic glioma of childhood. Natural history and rationale for conservative management. Br J Ophthalmol 53:793–798
Hoyt WF, Meshel LG, Lessell S, Schatz NJ, Suckling RD (1973) Malignant optic glioma of adulthood. Brain 96:121–132
Hsy YK (1940) Primary intracranial sarcomas. Arch Neurol Psychiatry 43:901–924
Hu KH, Friede AL (1967) Cholesterol content of xanthogranulomas of the choroid plexus. J Neuropathol Exp Neurol 26:507–510
Huber K, Sorgo W (1942) Über zwei verkalkte Hirntumoren. Z Gesamte Neurol Psychiatr 174:80–88
Hueck W (1937) Morphologische Pathologie. Thieme, Leipzig
Hürter T, Bröcker W, Hossmann K-A (1981) Evaluation of vasogenic edema in experimental brain tumors by cathodoluminescence and fluorescence microscopy. Histochemistry 72:249–254
Huffmann G, Hienz HA, Petry R, Stammler A (1967) Primäre meningeale Blastomatose unter dem klinischen Bild einer chronischen Meningitis. Fortschr Neurol Psychiatr 35:139–147
Hug O (1942) Krebsbildung in einem pialen Epidermoid. Virchows Arch (Pathol Anat) 308:679–689
Hughes EB, Smitt WT (1955) An unusual tumor histologically resembling a chemodectoma removed surgically from the pineal region. Excerpta Med (Sect VIII) 8:790
Huk W, Klinger M (1973) The diagnosis of cervical spinal angioblastomas. Neuroradiology 5:174–177
Hung CC, Chang WY, Yao YT (1972) Post-traumatic intracranial meningioma. Taiwan J Hsueh Hui Tsa Chih (J Formosan Med Assoc) 71:214–219
Hunt PT, Davidson KC, Ashcraft KW, Holder TM (1977) Radiography of hereditary presacral teratoma. Radiology 122:187–191
Hunt WE, Abramson W, Weaver TA (1948) Cerebral schistosomiasis. Report of a case simulating cerebral neoplasm. JAMA 136:686–690
Husain MM, Sun CN, White HJ (1979) Neoplastic angioendotheliosis. 55th Annual Meeting of American Association of Neuropathologists. J Neuropathol Exp Neurol 38:322
Hutter RVP, Lewis JS, Foote FW Jr, Tollefsen R (1963) Esthesioneuroblastoma: A clinical and pathological study. Am J Surg 106:748–753
Iacono RP, Apuzzo MLJ, Davis RL, Tsai FY (1981) Multiple meningiomas following radiation therapy for medulloblastoma. Case report. J Neurosurg 55:282–286
Ibelgaufts H (1982) Are human DNA tumour viruses involved in the pathogenesis of human neurogenic tumours? Neurosurg Rev 5:3–24
Ibelgaufts H, Doerfler W, Scheidtmann KH, Wechsler W (1980) Adenovirus type 12-induced rat tumour cells of neuroepithelial origin: Persistence and expression of the viral genome. J Virol 33:423–437
Ibelgaufts H, Jones KW, Maitland N, Shaw JF (1982) Adenovirus-related RNA acid sequences in human neurogenic tumours. Acta Neuropathol (Berl) 56:113–117
ICD-O (1975) World Health Organization – International classification of diseases for oncology. WHO, Geneva
Ignelzi RJ, Bucy PC (1967) Intracranial hypoglossal neurofibroma. Case report. J Neurosurg 26:352–356
Iizuka J (1969) Rückfälle bei Lindautumoren. Beobachtungen von 57 Fällen von Hämangioblastom des Kleinhirns. Acta Neurochir (Wien) 20:281–298
Ikuta F, Kumanishi T (1973) Experimental virus-induced brain tumors. Prog Neuropathol 2:253–334
Ikuta F, Zimmerman HM (1965) Virus particles in reactive cells induced by intracerebral implantation of Dibenzanthracene. J Neuropathol Exp Neurol 24:225–243
Ilsen HW, Petrovici IN, Mennel HD, Zülch KJ, Szymaś J (1982) Die Wirkung kombinierter Chemotherapie (Adriamycin/VM 26/CCNU) bei hirneigenen Tumoren des Erwachsenenalters und im Tierexperiment. Fortschr Neurol Psychiatr 50:73–90
Immisch V (1952) Ein intrakraniales Teratom bei einer weiblichen Totgeburt. Zentralbl Allg Pathol 89:163–166

Ingraham FD, Bailey OT (1946) Cystic teratomas and teratoid tumors of central nervous system in infancy and childhood. J Neurosurg 3:511–532
Ingraham FD, Matson DD (1954) Neurosurgery of infancy and childhood. Thomas, Springfield
Innes JR, Saunders LZ (1962) Comparative neuropathology. Academic Press, New York
Irie K, Austin E, Morgenstern L (1978) Solitary meningocerebral metastasis from squamous cell carcinoma of the esophagus. A case report. Cancer 42:2461–2465
Isamat de la Riva F (1957) Cysticercosis cerebral, 1st edn. Vergara, Barcelona
Isamat F, Miranda AM, Ripoll M (1968) Parajugular foramen chondroma. J Neurosurg 28:490–494
Isamat F, Bartumeus F, Miranda AM, Prat J, Pons LC (1975) Neurinomas of the facial nerve. J Neurosurg 43:608–613
Isfort A, Sunder-Plassmann P (1965) Klinik und Diagnostik der Lindautumoren. Dtsch Z Nervenheilkd 187:548–565
Ishida Y (1973) Lymphoreticular tissue tumours of the nervous system with special regard to the problem of microgliomatosis. Recent Adv RES Res 13:77–95
Ishida Y (1975) Fine structure of primary reticulum cell sarcoma of the brain. Acta Neuropathol [Suppl] (Berl) 6:147–153
Ishida Y, Kawai S, Sato K, Niibe H (1964a) Electron microscopy of medulloblastoma. Gumma J Med Sci 13:71–78
Ishida Y, Kawai S, Sato S, Takayanagi T, Kawafuchi J-I (1964b) Electron microscopy of meningothelial meningioma. Gumma J Med Sci 13:181–197
Ishida Y, Nakazato Y, Nagaya T, Suzuki K (1978) Medulloblastoma-like tumor of the cerebellum with melanin formation. J Neuropathol Exp Neurol 37:634
Ishii R, Sato S, Ueki K, Oyake Y (1974) Myxoosteochondroma in the pons. J Neurosurg 41:240–243
Ishii R, Tsuchida T, Honda H, Ueki K, Oyake Y (1976) Radiation therapy and surgical management of pineal tumors. Follow-up study of 96 patients (In Japanese). No Shinkei Geka 4:263–270
Ishikawa S, Kajikawa H, Tomihara K, Watanabe K, Nosaka K, Shima T (1974) Intraspinal tumor associated with increased intracranial pressure and papilledema (In Japanese). No Shinkei Geka 2:409–413
Ishiyama R, Sakai H, Okasaki N, Shinozawa S, Nakamura N (1975) Intracranial neurinoma of the jugular foramen. A case report (In Japanese). No Shinkei Geka 3:1015–1021
Ishwar S, Taniguchi RM, Vogel FS (1971) Multiple supratentorial hemangioblastomas. Case study and ultrastructural characteristics. J Neurosurg 35:396–405
Isu T, Tashiro K, Mitsumori K, Sato M, Tsura M, Kashiwaba T (1976) A case of intramedullary spinal schwannoma (In Japanese). No Shinkei Geka 4:897–901
Ito J, Kadekaru T, Hayano M, Kurita I, Okada K, Yoshida Y (1981) Meningioma in the tela choroidea of the third ventricle: CT and angiographic correlations. Neuroradiology 21:207–211
Ito T (1958) Pathology of brain tumors. Acta Pathol Jpn 8:415–600
Ivanisevich O (1934) Hidatidosis ósea. Amorrortu, Buenos Aires
Ivankovic S, Druckrey H (1968) Transplacentare Erzeugung maligner Tumoren des Nervensystems. Z Krebsforsch 71:320–360
Ivankovic S, Preussmann R (1970) Transplazentare Erzeugung maligner Tumoren. Naturwissenschaften 57:460
Ivankovic S, Druckrey H, Preussmann R (1966) Erzeugung neurogener Tumoren bei den Nachkommen nach einmaliger Injektion von Äthylnitrosoharnstoff an schwangeren Ratten. Naturwissenschaften 53:410
Iwanaga H, Kamada K, Nakata Y, Iida N, Harada T, Tsukamoto M, Honda M (1980) Cystic meningioma. A case report (In Japanese). No Shinkei Geka 8:867–873
Izawa M, Manaka S, Nawata H (1976) Occipital tumor simulating pericranial sinus (In Japanese). No Shinkei Geka 4:479–487
Jackson JH (1906) Case of tumour of the middle lobe of the cerebellum – cerebellar paralysis with rigidity (cerebellar attitude) – occasional tetanus-like seizures. Brain 29:425–445
Jacob H (1934) Diffuse melanotische Geschwulstbildungen der weichen Hirnhäute Dtsch Z Nervenheilkd 133:167–187

Jacobs L, Kinkel WR, Vincent RG (1977) "Silent" brain metastases from lung carcinoma determined by computerized tomography (CT scanning). XIth World Congress of Neurology, Amsterdam, 11–16 September 1977
Jänisch W, Schreiber D (1967) Experimentelle Hirngeschwülste bei Kaninchen nach Injektion von Methylnitrosoharnstoff. Naturwissenschaften 54:171–172
Jänisch W, Schreiber D (1969) Experimentelle Geschwülste des Zentralnervensystems. Fischer, Jena
Jänisch W, Schreiber D (1974) Experimental brain tumours. In: Vinken PJ, Bruyn GW (eds) Tumors of the brain and skull. North Holland, Amsterdam/American Elsevier, New York (Handbook of clinical neurology, vol 17, part II, pp 1–41)
Jänisch W, Zimmermann K (1975) Häufigkeit von Metastasen im Zentralnervensystem bei Pleuramesotheliomen und Lungencarcinomen. Zentralbl Neurochir 36:37–39
Jänisch W, Unger H, Petermann A (1966) Über die Häufigkeit und Herkunft von Metastasen im Zentralnervensystem. Dtsch Z Nervenheilkd 189:79–86
Jänisch W, Schreiber D, Scholtze P, Gerlach H (1973) Über Beziehungen zwischen reticulohistiocytärer Enzephalitis und neoplastischen Retikulosen. Schweiz Arch Neurol Neurochir Psychiatr 112:263–270
Jänisch W, Güthert H, Schreiber D (1976) Pathologie der Tumoren des Zentralnervensystems. Fischer, Jena
Jänisch W, Schreiber D, Gerlach H (1980) Tumoren des Zentralnervensystems bei Feten und Säuglingen. Fischer, Jena
Jaffe HL (1956) Benign osteoblastoma. Bull Hosp Joint Dis 17:141–151
Jaffe HL (1958) Tumors and tumorous conditions of bones and joints. Lea and Febiger, Philadelphia
Jaffe HL, Lichtenstein L (1942) Benign chondroblastoma of bone: A reinterpretation of the so-called calcifying or chondromatous giant cell tumor. Am J Pathol 18:969–991
Jaffe HL, Lichtenstein L (1948) Chondromyxoid fibroma of bone. A distinctive benign tumor likely to be mistaken especially for chondrosarcoma. Arch Pathol 45:541–551
Jahnel F (1929) Allgemeine Pathologie und pathologische Anatomie der Syphilis des Nervensystems. In: Jadassohn J (ed) Handbuch der Haut- und Geschlechtskrankheiten, vol 17. Springer, Berlin, p 1
Jakob A (1927) Normale und pathologische Anatomie und Histologie des Großhirns. Deuticke, Leipzig (Handbuch der Psychiatrie, vol I, p 336)
Jakumeit HD (1971) Neuroblastoma of the olfactory nerve. Acta Neurochir (Wien) 25:99–108
James TGI, Pagel W (1951) Oligodendroglioma with extracranial metastases. Br J Surg 39:56–65
Janssen P (1955) Sur un cas de cysticercose cérébrale chez le noir. Acta Neurol Psychiatr Belg 55:86–93
Janssen P, Piraux A (1955) Tumeurs cérébrales chez le noir. Acta Neurol Psychiatr Belg 55:94–110
Jastrowitz M (1870) Studien über die Encephalitis und Myelitis des ersten Kindesalters. Arch Psychiatr Nervenkr 2:389–414
Jastrowitz M (1872) Studien über die Encephalitis und Myelitis des ersten Kindesalters. Arch Psychiatr Nervenkr 3:192–213
Jefferson G (1953) The Bowman lecture concerning injuries, aneurysms and tumors involving the cavernous sinus. Trans Ophthalmol Soc UK 73:117–152
Jefferson M (1957) Sarcoidosis of the NS. Brain 80:540–556
Jeffreys RV (1974) Supratentorial haemangioblastoma. Acta Neurochir (Wien) 31:55–65
Jelliffe SE, Larkin JH (1911) Über ein malignes Chordom mit Symptomen von seiten des Gehirns und Rückenmarks. Z Gesamte Neurol Psychiatr 5:590–604
Jellinger K (1972) Cerebral medulloepithelioma. Acta Neuropathol (Berl) 22:95–101
Jellinger K (1973) Primary intracranial germ cell tumors. Acta Neuropathol (Berl) 25:291–306
Jellinger K, Machacek E (1982) Rare intracranial tumours in infancy and childhood. In: Voth D, Gutjahr P, Langmaid C (eds) Tumours of the central nervous system in infancy and childhood. Springer, Berlin Heidelberg New York, pp 44–52
Jellinger K, Radaszkiewicz T (1976) Involvement of the CNS in malignant lymphomas. Virchows Arch [A] 370:345–362

Jellinger K, Slowik F (1975) Histological subtypes and prognostic problems in meningiomas. J Neurol 208:279–298

Jellinger K, Minauf M, Salzer-Kuntschik M (1969) Oligodendroglioma with extraneural metastases. J Neurol Neurosurg Psychiatry 32:249–253

Jellinger K, Minauf M, Brenner H (1970a) Primäres intrakranielles Neuroblastom. In: Bushe K-A (ed) Fortschritte auf dem Gebiet der Neurochirurgie. Hippokrates, Stuttgart, pp 276–282

Jellinger K, Minauf M, Kraus H, Sunder-Plassmann M (1970b) Embryonales Carcinom der Epiphysengegend. Acta Neuropathol (Berl) 15:176–182

Jellinger K, Radaszkiewicz T, Slowik F (1975) Primary malignant lymphomas of the central nervous system in man. Acta Neuropathol [Suppl] (Berl) 6:95–102

Jellinger K, Kothbauer P, Sunder-Plassmann E, Weiss R (1979) Intramedullary spinal cord metastases. J Neurol 220:31–41

Jellinger K, Gullotta F, Mossakowski M (1981) Experimental and clinical neuropathology. Springer, Berlin Heidelberg New York Vienna (Acta neuropathologica, suppl VII)

Jelsma R, Bucy PC (1967) The treatment of glioblastoma multiforme of the brain. J Neurosurg 27:388–400

Jelsma R, Bucy PC (1969) Glioblastoma multiforme. Its treatment and some factors affecting survival. Arch Neurol 20:161–171

Jenkin RDT, Simpson WJK, Keen CW (1978) Pineal and suprasellar germinomas. Results of radiation treatment. J Neurosurg 48:99–107

Jenny F (1941) Beitrag zur Klinik der Chordome. Schweiz Med Wochenschr 71:1061–1085

Jensen RD, Miller RW (1971) Retinoblastoma. Epidemiologic characteristics. N Engl J Med 285:307–311

Jentzer A, Fatzer H (1937) Ein Fall von Ganglioneurofibromatose des Mesenteriums und Darms mit maligner Umwandlung. Schweiz Med Wochenschr 67:569

Jéquier-Doge M (1941) A propos de la classification des tumeurs cérébrales. Schweiz Arch Neurol Neurochir Psychiatry 48:40–70

Jervis GA (1954) Spongioneuroblastoma and tuberous sclerosis. J Neuropathol Exp Neurol 13:105–116

Jestico JO, Lantos PL (1976) Malignant meningioma with liver metastases and hypoglycaemia. A case report. Acta Neuropathol (Berl) 35:357–361

Johannsson IH, Rekate HL, Roessmann U (1981) Gangliogliomas: pathological and clinical correlations. J Neurosurg 54:58–63

Jooma R, Kendall BE (1982) Intracranial tumours in the first year of life. Neuroradiology 23:267–274

Jordan (1901) Über die Entstehung von Tumoren, Tuberkulose und anderen Organerkrankungen nach Einwirkung stumpfer Gewalt (unter Ausschluß von Frakturen, Luxationen, Hernien und traumatischen Neurosen). Münch Med Wochenschr 44:1741–1746

Josephy H (1924) Ein Fall von Porobulbie mit solitärem zentralem Neurinom. Z Gesamte Neurol Psychiatr 93:62–82

Joughin JL (1928) Coincident tumor of the brain in twins. Arch Neurol Psychiatry 19:948–950

Juhàsz P (1942) Über ein diffuses Kleinhirnoligodendrogliom und das Oligodendrogliom der hinteren Schädelgrube. Z Gesamte Neurol Psychiatr 174:701–714

Jung R (1935) Über die Angiome Lindau's als eine charakteristische Gruppe unter den Kleinhirntumoren". Arch Psychiatr 103:580–626

Jungherr E, Wolf A (1939) Gliomas in animals. A report of two astrocytomas in the common fowl. Am J Cancer 37:493–509

Junqueira LCU, Montes GS, Kaupert D, Shigihara KM, Bolonhani TM, Krisztán RM (1981) Morphological and histochemical studies on the collagen in neurinomas, neurofibromas, and fibromas. J Neuropathol Exp Neurol 40:123–133

Kadota K, Sasahira M, Hamada H, Awa H, Matsuda K, Asakura T (1980) A case of intracranial chordoma with a special reference to the findings in computed tomography (In Japanese). No Shinkei Geka 8:173–180

Kagan H (1958) Anorexia and severe inanition associated with a tumour involving the hypothalamus. Arch Dis Child 33:257–260

Kageyama N (1971) Ectopic pinealoma in the region of optic chiasm. J Neurosurg 35:755–759

Kageyama N, Belsky R (1961) Ectopic pinealoma in the chiasma region. Neurology (Minneap) 11:318–327

Kahl R-J (1973) Ein Neurinom des Nervus infraorbitalis. J Neurol 204:155–158

Kahlden C von (1895) Über multiple wahre Neurome des Rückenmarks. Beitr Pathol Anat 17:587–601

Kahle W (1957) Zum Problem der diffusen Glioblastose. Dtsch Z Nervenheilkd 176:469–499

Kahn AP, Hirsch JF, DaLage C, Lyon G, Saporta L, Evrard P (1971) Les kystes entériques intrarachidiens. A propos de trois observations. Neurochirurgie 17:33–44

Kahn EA, Basset RC, Schneider RC, Crosby EC (1955) Correlative neurosurgery. Thomas, Springfield

Kahn EA, Gosch HH, Seeger JF, Hicks SP (1973) Forty-five years experience with the craniopharyngiomas. Surg Neurol 1:5–12

Kahn LB (1974) Esthesioneuroblastoma: a light and electron microscopic study. Hum Pathol 5:364–371

Kajikawa H, Harada K, Hirayama M, Okada T (1973) Primary tissue culture of brain tumor using glass fiber. Hiroshima J Med Sci 22:57–63

Kalbag RM, Woolf AL (1972) Thrombosis and thombophlebitis of cerebral veins and dural sinuses. In: Vinken PJ, Bruyn GW (eds) Vascular disease of the nervous system. North Holland, Amsterdam/American Elsevier, New York (Handbook of clinical neurology, vol 12, part II, pp 422–446

Kalbfleisch HH (1946) Spätveränderungen im menschlichen Gehirn nach intensiver Röntgenbestrahlung des Kopfes. Strahlentherapie 76:584–586

Kalbfleisch HH, Grebe H (1937) Über das Einwachsen der Schädelmeningeome in das umgebende Gewebe, namentlich in das Gehirn. Arch Klin Chir 188:118–137

Kalm H (1950) Ein malignes Tentorium-Meningeom mit Metastasierung in die Oblongata und in die subarachnoidalen Liquorräume. Dtsch Z Nervenheilkd 163:131–140

Kalm H (1959) Phasenkontrastbeobachtungen an Hirngeschwülsten. Dtsch Z Nervenheilkd 179:267–284

Kalm H, Magun R (1950) Beitrag zur Klinik und pathologischen Anatomie der Pinealome. Dtsch Z Nervenheilkd 164:453–468

Kalumpaheti R, Thumnoon K, Thanaphum U (1978) The pineal tumors in Thailand. J Neuropathol Exp Neurol 37:639

Kalvelage B (1976) Über den Einfluß einer Störung des hormonellen Gleichgewichts durch das synthetische Östrogen Diäthylstilbestrol auf die Erzeugung von Tumoren des Nervensystems durch neurotrope Resorptivcarcinogenese bei Ratten. Dissertation, Faculty of Medicine, University of Cologne

Kamisasa A, Kuwabara T, Inaba Y (1973) Intracranial ossifying fibroma. Report of an unusual case and its pathological study (In Japanese). No Shinkei Geka 1:519–525

Kammer G (1955) Beitrag zur Erbbiologie und Klinik der Sturge-Weberschen Erkrankung. Z Menschl Vererb Konstit Lehre 33:203–220

Kamrin RP, Potanos JN, Pool JL (1964) An evaluation of the diagnosis and treatment of chordoma. J Neurol Neurosurg Psychiatry 27:157–165

Kapp JP, Paulson GW, Odom GL (1967) Brain tumors with tuberous sclerosis. J Neurosurg 26:191–202

Kappers J Ariëns (1965) Survey of the innervation of the epiphysis cerebri and the accessory pineal organs of vertebrates. Prog Brain Res 10:87–153

Kappers J Ariëns (1976) The mammalian pineal gland, a survey. Acta Neurochir (Wien) 34:109–149

Karasick JL, Mullan SF (1974) A survey of metastatic meningiomas. J Neurosurg 39:206–212

Karch SB, Urich H (1972) Medulloepithelioma: definition of an entity. J Neuropathol Exp Neurol 31:27–53

Kasantikul V, Netsky MG (1979) Combined neurilemmoma and angioma. J Neurosurg 50:81–87

Kasantikul V, Netsky MG, Glasscock ME, Hays JW (1980) Acoustic neurilemmoma. Clinicoanatomical study of 103 patients. J Neurosurg 52:28–35

Kasper JA, Cowan A (1929) Extradural lipoma of the spinal canal. Arch Pathol 8:800–802

Katsura S, Suzuki J, Wada T (1959) A statistical study of brain tumors in the neurosurgical clinics in Japan. J Neurosurg 16:570–580
Katz A, Lewis JS (1971) Nasal gliomas. Arch Otolaryngol 94:351–355
Katz EL (1975) Late results of radical excision of craniopharyngiomas in children. J Neurosurg 42:86–90
Katzenstein R (1932) Über innere Recklinghausensche Erkrankung: Endotheliom, Neurinom, Gliome, Gliose, Hydromyelie. Virchows Arch [A] 286:42–61
Kaufman DM, Thal LJ, Farmer PM (1976) Central nervous system aspergillosis in two young adults. Neurology (Minneap) 26:484–488
Kaufmann E (1902) Diskussion zu Saxer. Zieglers Beitr Pathol Anat 32:
Kaufmann E (1906) Beitrag zur Statistik und Casuistik metastatischer Tumoren, besonders der Carcinommetastasen im Zentralnervensystem. Korrespondenz Bl Schweiz Arzte 36:255–261
Kaufmann E (1922) Lehrbuch der speziellen pathologischen Anatomie für Studierende und Ärzte, 7th and 8th edn. De Gruyter, Berlin
Kautzky R (1939) Zur Kenntnis der diffusen Glioblastose. Dtsch Z Nervenheilkd 148:143–158
Kautzky R (1948) Das gefäßreiche parietale Glioblastom. Dtsch Z Nervenheilkd 159:57–74
Katzky R (1949) Die Bedeutung der Hirnhaut-Innervation und ihrer Entwicklung für die Pathogenese der Sturge-Weber'schen Krankheit. Dtsch Z Nervenheilkd 161:506–525
Kautzky R (1951) Die Schnelldiagnose intrakranialer Erkrankungen mit Hilfe des supravital gefärbten Quetschpräparates. Virch Arch (Pathol Anat) 320:495–550
Kautzky R, Vierdt N (1953) Ein Angioblastom des Großhirns. Zentralbl Neurochir 13:158–163
Kautzky R, Zülch KJ (1955) Neurologisch-neurochirurgische Röntgendiagnostik Springer, Berlin Göttingen Heidelberg
Kautzky R, Zülch KJ, Wende S, Tänzer A (1976) Neuroradiologie auf neuropathologischer Grundlage. Springer, Berlin Heidelberg New York
Katzky R, Zülch KJ, Wende S, Tänzer A (1982) Neuroradiology. A neuropathological approach. Springer, Berlin Heidelberg New York
Kawaguchi S, Ito K, Onuma T, Yoshimura N (1975) Autopsy case of pinealoma with extranervous system metastasis (In Japanese). No To Shinkei 27:421–427
Kawakami Y, Mair WGP (1973) Haematomyelia due to secondary renal carcinoma. Acta Neuropathol (Berl) 26:85–92
Kawakami Y, Yamada O, Tabuchi K, Ohmoto T, Nishimoto A (1980) Primary intracranial choriocarcinoma. J Neurosurg 53:369–374
Kawamoto K, Tani S, Kawamura Y, Matsumura H, Someda K (1980) A case of large germinoma in bilateral frontal region (In Japanese). No Shinkei Geka 8:577–582
Kawamura J, Kamijyo Y (1975) A specific organelle in the vascular endothelial cells of cerebellar neoplasms (In Japanese). No Shinkei Geka 3:565–570
Kawamura J, Garcia JH, Kamijyo Y (1973) Cerebellar hemangioblastoma: histogenesis of stroma cells. Cancer 31:1528–1540
Kawano N, Yada K, Ogawa Y, Sasaki K (1977) Spontaneous transdural extension of malignant astrocytoma. J Neurosurg 47:766–770
Kaya U, Ozden B, Türker K (1975) Intracranial hydatid cysts. Study of 17 cases. J Neurosurg 42:580–584
Kazner E, Stochdorph O, Wende S, Grumme T (1980) Intracranial lipoma. Diagnostic and therapeutic consideration. J Neurosurg 52:234–245
Kazner E, Wende S, Grumme T, Lanksch W, Stochdorph O (1981) Computertomographie intrakranieller Tumoren aus klinischer Sicht. Springer, Berlin Heidelberg New York
Keegan HR, Mullan S (1962) Pigmented meningiomas, an unusual variant. Report of a case with review of the literature. J Neurosurg 19:696–698
Kehrer FA (1949) Zur Frage des „Pseudotumor cerebri". Dtsch Z Nervenheilkd 160:1–9
Keith MM, McCraig W, Kernohan JW (1949) Brain tumors in children. Pediatrics 3:839–844
Keller H (1933) Sogenannte „hyperplastische Capillarangiome" (Lindau) und Großhirncyste, zugleich ein Beitrag zur Tumor-Cystenfrage. Virchows Arch [A] 289:151–181
Kelly M (1951) Colloid cysts of the third ventricle. Analysis of 29 cases. Brain 74:23–65
Kelly DL, Kushner J, McLean WT (1971) Neonatal intracranial choriocarcinoma. Case report. J Neurosurg 35:465–471

Kempson RL, McGavran MH (1964) Atypical fibroxanthomas of the skin. Cancer 17:1463–1471

Kendall B, Shah S (1972) Investigation of meningiomas of cerebellar convexities. Neuroradiology 4:162–170

Kendall BE, Tatler GLV (1978) Radiological findings in neurosarcoidosis. Br J Radiol 51:81–92

Kennerdell JS, Jannetta P, Johnson BL (1974) A steroid-sensitive solitary intracranial plasmocytoma. Arch Ophthalmol 92:392–398

Kent SP, Pickering JE (1958) Neoplasms in monkey (*Macaca mulatta*): spontaneous and irradiation induced. Cancer 11:138–147

Kepes J (1961 a) Observations on the formation of psammoma bodies and pseudopsammoma bodies in meningiomas. J Neuropathol Exp Neurol 20:255–262

Kepes J (1961 b) Electron microscopic studies of meningiomas. Am J Pathol 39:499–510

Kepes JJ (1970) "Xanthomatous" changes in a papilloma of the choroid plexus. Acta Neuropathol (Berl) 16:367–369

Kepes JJ (1971) Differentialdiagnostic problems of brain tumors. In: Minckler J (ed) Pathology of the nervous system, vol 2. McGraw-Hill, New York, pp 2219–2237

Kepes JJ (1979a) Xanthomatous lesions of the CNS: Definition, classification, and some recent observations. Prog Neuropathol 4:179–213

Kepes JJ (1979b) Histiocytosis X. In: Vinken PJ, Bruyn GW (eds) Neurological manifestation of systemic disease. North-Holland, Amsterdam (Handbook of clinical neurology, vol 38, part I, pp 93–117)

Kepes JJ, Kepes M (1969) Predominantly cerebral forms of histiocytosis-X. A reappraisal of "Gagel's hypothalamic granuloma", "granuloma infiltrans of the hypothalamus" and "Ayala's disease" with a report of four cases. Acta Neuropathol (Berl) 14:77–98

Kepes JJ, Kepes M (1975) Lymphoreticular proliferative disorders of the CNS and other organs: analogies and differences. Acta Neuropathol [Suppl] (Berl) 6:75–79

Kepes JJ, Rubinstein LJ (1981) Malignant gliomas with heavily lipidized (foamy) tumor cells. A report of three cases with immunoperoxidase study. Cancer 47:2451–2459

Kepes JJ, MacGee EE, Vergara G, Sil R (1971) Malignant meningioma with extensive pulmonary metastases. A case report. J Kans Med Soc 72:312–316

Kepes JJ, Kepes M, Slowik F (1973) Fibrous xanthomas and xanthosarcomas of the meninges and the brain. Acta Neuropathol (Berl) 23:187–199

Kepes JJ, Rubinstein LJ, Eng LF (1978) Meningocerebral xanthoastrocytoma. In: Abstracts of the 8th International Congress of Neuropathology, Washington, 24–29 September

Kepes JJ, Rengachary SS, Lee SH (1979a) Astrocytes in hemangioblastomas of the central nervous system and their relationship to stromal cells. Acta Neuropathol (Berl) 47:99–104

Kepes JJ, Rubinstein LJ, Eng LF (1979b) Pleomorphic xanthoastrocytoma: A distinctive meningocerebral glioma of young subjects with relatively favorable prognosis. A study of 12 cases. Cancer 44:1839–1852

Kepes JJ, Lewis RC, Vergara GG (1980) Cerebellar astrocytoma invading the musculature and soft tissues of the neck. J Neurosurg 52:414–418

Kepes JJ, Rubinstein LJ, Chiang H (1984) The role of astrocytes in the formation of cartilage in gliomas. An immunohistochemical study of four cases. Am J Pathol 117:471–483

Kernohan JW (1930) Cortical anomalies, ventricular heterotopies and occlusion of aqueduct of sylvius. Arch Neurol Psychiatry 23:460–480

Kernohan JW (1932) Primary tumors of the spinal cord and intradural filum terminale. In: Penfield W (ed) Cytology and cellular pathology of the nervous system, vol 3. Hoeber, New York, pp 993–1025

Kernohan JW (1941) Tumors of the spinal cord. Arch Pathol 32:843–882

Kernohan JW (1971) Oligodendrogliomas. In: Minckler J (ed) Pathology of the nervous system, vol 2. McGraw-Hill, New York, pp 1993–2007

Kernohan JW, Fletcher-Kernohan EM (1935) Ependymomas. A study of 109 cases. Proc Assoc Res Nerv Ment Dis (Baltimore) 16:182–209

Kernohan JW, Parker HL (1932) A case of Recklinghausen's disease with observation on the associated formations of tumors. J Nerv Ment Dis 76:313–330

Kernohan JW, Sayre GP (1952) Tumors of the central nervous system. Armed Forces Institute of Pathology, Washington
Kernohan JW, Uihlein A (1962) Sarcomas of the brain. Thomas, Springfield
Kernohan JW, Woltman HW (1929) Incisura of the crus due to contralateral brain tumor. Arch Neurol Psychiatry 21:274–287
Kernohan JW, Woltman HW, Adson AW (1931) Intramedullary tumors of the spinal cord: A review of fifty-one cases, with an attempt at histologic classification. Arch Neurol Psychiatry 25:679–699
Kernohan JW, Learmonth JR, Doyle JB (1932) Neuroblastomas and gangliocytomas of the central nervous system. Brain 55:278–310
Kernohan JW, Mabon RF, Svien HJ, Adson AW (1949) A simplified classification of the gliomas. Symposium on a new simplified concept of gliomas. Proc Staff Meet Mayo Clin 24:71–75
Kerschner F (1928) Erfahrungen bei der operativen Behandlung von Hirntumoren. Bruns Beitr Klin Chir 144:458–487, 519–555
Kershman J (1938) The medulloblast and the medulloblastomas. Arch Neurol Psychiatry 40:937–967
Kershman J (1939) Genesis of microglia in the human brain. Arch Neurol Psychiatry 41:24–50
Kersting G (1961) Die Gewebszüchtung menschlicher Hirngeschwülste. Springer, Berlin Göttingen Heidelberg
Kersting G (1964) Tissue culture and the classification of brain tumors. In: Zülch KJ, Woolf AL (eds) Classification of brain tumours. Acta Neurochir [Suppl X] (Wien):68–72
Kersting G (1967) Die Gewebszüchtung der Medulloblastome. Acta Neuropathol (Berl) 8:100–103
Kersting G (1968) Tissue culture of human gliomas. Prog Neurol Surg 2:165–202
Kersting G (1973) Tissue culture of recurrent gliomas. In: Kuhlendahl H, Hensell V (eds) Modern aspects of neurosurgery. Proceedings of the German Society for Neurosurgery 1971, vol 3. Excerpta Medica, Amsterdam, pp 122–124
Kersting G, Finkemeyer H (1958) Das Wachstum menschlichen Neurinomgewebes in vitro. Zentralbl Neurochir 18:2–11
Ketz E (1956) Zur Klinik und Therapie der sogenannten Balkenlipome. Zentralbl Neurochir 16:80–84
Khan A, Fulco JD, Shende A, Rosenthal A, Marc JA (1980) Focal histiocytosis X of the parietal lobe. Case report. J Neurosurg 52:431–433
Khantanaphar S, Bunyaratvej S (1974) Embryonal carcinoma in the cerebellum. Case report. J Neurosurg 40:657–662
Khominsky BS (1958) Pathological morphology and classification of meningiomas (arachnoid endotheliomas). Arkh Patol 20:3–20
Khominsky BS (1969) Grades of malignancy of tumours of neuroectodermal origin. Neoplasma 16:651–666
Khominsky BS, Brodskaya IA (1973) Histochemistry of nucleic acids and proteins in cells of neuroectodermal tumours of different grades of malignancy. Neoplasma 20:281–296
Khominsky BS, Schamaev M-J (1971) Über die Vaskularisation der neuroektodermalen Geschwülste von verschiedenen Malignitätsgraden. Arch Geschwulstforsch 37:136–151
Kida H, Kojiro M, Yonekura A, Yamamoto M (1978) Malignant choroid plexus papilloma, an autopsy case report (In Japanese). No To Shinkei 30:99–105
Kido G, Takeuchi T, Tsukiyama T, Nakamura S, Tsubokawa T, Hemni A (1984) Tumor of the pineal region in three brothers (In Japanese). No Shinkei Geka 12:975–980
Kiel EW, Starr LB, Hansen JL (1961) Primary melanoma of the spinal cord. J Neurosurg 18:616–629
Kienecker EW, Piscol K, Artmann H, Schaaban M (1975) Diagnostical and clinical appearance of the sphenoidal ridge meningioma en plaque. Adv Neurosurg 2:68–71
Kiessling M, Anagnostopoulos J, Lombeck G, Kleihues P (1982) Diagnostic potential of stereotactic biopsy of brain tumors. A report of 400 cases. In: Voth D, Gutjahr P, Langmaid C (eds) Tumors of the central nervous system in infancy and childhood. Springer, Berlin Heidelberg New York, pp 247–256
Kim SK (1955) Cerebral paragonimiasis. J Neurosurg 12:89–94

Kim SK, Walker AE (1961) Cerebral paragonimiasis. Acta Psychiatr Neurol Scand 36 [Suppl 153]
Kim Y-B (1958) Histologische Untersuchungen zur Frage der Spongioblastome. Dissertation, Faculty of Medicine, University of Cologne
Kimura O (1921) Über die größeren Zellen in verschiedenen Gliomen (nebst Beiträgen zum Neuroglioma gigantocellulare, Neuroepitheliom und zur Lehre der tuberösen Hirnsclerose). Mitt Allg Pathol (Sendai) 1:321–374
Kindt GW (1964) The pattern of location of cerebral metastatic tumours. J Neurosurg 21:54–57
King AB, Chambers IW, Garey I (1952) Primary malignant melanoma of the spinal cord. Arch Neurol 68:226–275
King JS (1976) Trochlear nerve sheath tumor. J Neurosurg 44:245–247
Kinnman J (1978) Morphology of adenomas in acromegaly. In: Fahlbusch R, von Werder K (eds) Treatment of pituitary adenomas. Thieme, Stuttgart, pp 130–154
Kino F (1935) Zur Morphologie der Hirngliome und ihre Beziehung zum klinischen Verhalten. Z Gesamte Neurol Psychiatr 153:680–718
Kinomoto H, Iwasaki Y, Nakagawa Y et al. (1982) Extracranial metastases from intracranial meningioma. A report of 2 cases and review of literature (In Japanese). No To Shinkei 10:325–326
Kinoshita K, Marubayashi T, Tocuda H, Matsukado Y (1975) Primary intracranial olfactory esthesioneuroepithelioma (In Japanese). No To Shinkei 27:39–47
Kirchhoff D (1975) "Micromeningiomas" of cavum Meckeli. Adv Neurosurg 2:79–83
Kirsch WM, Stears JC (1970) Radiographic identification and surgical excision of an epidermoid tumor of the pineal gland. J Neurosurg 33:708–713
Kirsch WM, Grossi-Paoletti E, Paoletti P (1972) The experimental biology of brain tumors. Thomas, Springfield
Kirsch WM, Van Buskirk JJ, Schulz DW, Tabuchi K (1976) The biologic basis of malignant brain tumor therapy. Adv Neurol 15:301–313
Kishikawa T, Numaguchi Y, Fukui M, Komaki S, Ikeda J, Kitamura K, Matsuura K (1981) Primary intracranial sarcomas: Radiological diagnosis with emphasis on arteriography. Neuroradiology 21:25–31
Kissel P, Lepoire J, Dollander A, Duprez A, Montant J (1966) Auto-historadiographie in vivo de trois tumeurs cérébrales humaines par la thymidine H^3 et le P^{32}. Neurochirurgie 12:411–419
Kitano I, Yoneda K, Yamakawa Y, Fukui M, Kinoshita K (1981) Huge cystic craniopharyngioma with unusual extensions. Neuroradiology 22:39–42
Kitaoka K, Tashiro K, Abe H, Tsuru M (1980) A clinical survey of cerebellar astrocytoma – Comparison between childhood and adult cases (In Japanese). No Shinkei Geka 8:55–64
Kjellin K, Müller R, Åström KE (1960) The occurrence of brain tumors in several members of a family. J Neuropathol Exp Neurol 19:528–537
Klar E, Becker J, Scheer KE (1954) Eine kombinierte chirurgisch-radiologische Behandlung bei Glioblastoma multiforme mit radioaktivem Kobalt Co^{60}. Langenbecks Arch Klin Chir 280:55–65
Klatzo I (1967) Presidential address: Neuropathological aspects of brain edema. J Neuropathol Exp Neurol 26:1–14
Klatzo I, McMillan GC (1952) A new technic for the rapid diagnosis of brain tumors using chlorazol black E. Lab Invest 1:24–29
Klatzo I, Wisniewski H, Steinwall O, Streicher E (1967) Dynamics of cold injury edema. In: Klatzo I, Seitelberger F (eds) Brain edema. Springer, New York, pp 554–563
Klatzo I, Chui E, Fujiwara K, Spatz M (1980) Resolution of vasogenic brain edema. Adv Neurol 28:359–373
Klaus E, Nekula J, Minariková E, Fárková H (1978) Neurofibromatosis von Recklinghausen mit intrakranialer Stenose der A. carotis interna bei orbito-sphenoidaler Knochendysplasie. ROEFO 129:250–252
Klebs E (1864) Ein Fall von Ecchondrosis spheno-occipitalis amylacea. Virchows Arch [A] 31:396
Klebs E (1877) Die Geschwülste des nervösen Zentralapparates. Vjschr Prakt Heilkd (Prag) 34:133

Klebs E (1889) Die allgemeine Pathologie. Jena
Kleihues P (1965) Gibt es im Gehirn echte Kompositionstumoren? Z Krebsforsch 67:262–271
Kleihues P (1972) Alkylating agents and their effect on the adult mammalian brain. In: Cavanagh JB (ed) The brain in unclassified mental retardation. Churchill Livingstone, Edinburgh, pp 117–132
Kleihues P, Bücheler J (1977) Long-term persistance of O^6-methylguanine in rat brain DNA. Nature 269:625–626
Kleihues P (1978) Chemical carcinogenesis in the nervous system. In: Laerum OD, Bigner DD, Rajewsky MF (eds) Biology of brain tumors. UICC, Geneva (UICC Technical report series, vol 30, report no. 5, pp 113–128)
Kleihues P, Cooper HK (1976) Repair excision of alkylated bases from DNA in vivo. Oncology 33:86–88
Kleihues P, Magee PN (1973) Alkylation of rat brain nucleic acids by *N*-methyl-*N*-nitrosourea and methyl methanesulfonate. J Neurochem 20:595–606
Kleihues P, Margison GP (1974) Carcinogenicity of *N*-methyl-*N*-nitrosourea: possible role of repair excision of O^6-methylguanine from DNA. J Natl Cancer Inst 53:1839–1841
Kleihues P, Margison GP (1976) Exhaustion and recovery of repair excision of O^6-methylguanine from rat liver DNA. Nature 259:153–155
Kleihues P, Wechsler W, Zülch KJ (1966) Elektronenmikroskopische Befunde aus den perifokalen Ödemzonen des Katzengehirns nach lokaler Diphtherie-Intoxikation. Naturwissenschaften 53:202
Kleihues P, Zülch KJ, Matsumoto S, Radke U (1970) Morphology of malignant gliomas induced in rabbits by systemic application of *N*-methyl-*N*-nitrosourea. Z Neurol 198:65–78
Kleihues P, Lantos PL, Magee PN (1976) Chemical carcinogenesis in the nervous system. Int Rev Exp Pathol 15:153–232
Klein MR (1961) Les tumeurs de la moëlle chez l'enfant. Acta Neurochir (Wien) 9:69–86
Kleinman GM, Schoene WC, Walshe TM, Richardson EP Jr (1978) Malignant transformation in benign cerebellar astrocytoma. J Neurosurg 49:111–118
Kleinman GM, Liszczak T, Tarlov E, Richardson EP Jr (1979) Microcystic variant of meningioma. J Neuropathol Exp Neurol 38:326
Kleinsasser O (1960) Pathologie der Geschwülste des Hirnschädels. In: Olivecrona H, Tönnis W (eds) Klinik und Behandlung der raumbeengenden intrakraniellen Prozesse. Springer, Berlin Göttingen Heidelberg (Handbuch der Neurochirurgie, vol IV/1, pp 367–537)
Kleinsasser O, Friedmann G (1958a) Die Chordome der Schädelbasis. Ein Beitrag zur Klinik, Pathologie und Differentialdiagnose am Röntgenbild. Dtsch Z Nervenheilkd 177:263–285
Kleinsasser O, Friedmann G (1958b) Die Knorpelgeschwülste der Schädelbasis. Dtsch Z Nervenheilkd 177:378–404
Kleinsasser O, Kloss K (1958) Zur Frage der ektopischen Pinealome. Acta Neurochir (Wien) 6:20–29
Kleinsasser O, Monteleone M (1957) Das bösartige Neuroblastom des Sympathicus (Klinik, Pathologie und Differentialdiagnose seiner Knochenmetastasen gegen das sogenannte Ewing-Sarkom). Forsch Forscher Tiroler Med Ärzteschule Insbruck 3:127–151
Kleinsasser O, Scharfetter G (1957) Zeruminaldrüsenadenom mit Einbruch in Dura und Kleinhirn. Zentralbl Neurochir 17:4–12
Kline KT, Damjanov I, Katz SM, Schmidek H (1979) Pineoblastoma: an electron microscopic study. Cancer 45:2119–2130
Klingler M (1951) Über Knorpelgeschwülste der Schädelbasis mit intracranieller Ausdehnung. Acta Neurochir (Wien) 1:337–380
Klose HH (1961) Deutung des Zusammenhangs zwischen elastischen Fasern, Gefäßen und Psammomkörperbildung in Meningiomen. Acta Neurochir (Wien) 9:359–366
Kloss K (1952) Hirntumoren höherer Altersstufen. Acta Neurochir (Wien) 2:217–232
Kloss K, Thurner J (1955) Aktinomykotische Hirnabszesse. Klin Med (Wien) 10:489–502
Klüver H, Weil A (1948) Carcinomas of the tongue in monkeys and pathologic changes in the central nervous system. J Neuropathol Exp Neurol 7:144–153
Klug N (1978) Management and prognosis of medulloblastomas. Review series of 80 cases. In: Frowein RA, Wilcke O, Karimi-Nejad A, Brock M, Klinger M (eds) Tumors of the cerebellar region. Adv Neurosurg 5:245–252

Knapp P (1942) Besnier-Boeck'sches Sarcoid. Schweiz Med Wochenschr 72:827

Knoblauch (1843) De neuromate et gangliis accessoriis. Dissertation, Faculty of Medicine, University of Frankfurt

Knudson AG Jr, Amromin GD (1966) Neuroblastoma and ganglioneuroma in a child with multiple neurofibromatosis. Implications for the mutational origin of neuroblastoma. Cancer 19:1032–1037

Knudtzon K (1944) Arachnoiditis in primis cisternae chiasmatis. Acta Psychiatr Neurol Scand 19:201–231

Kobayashi S, Okazaki H, MacCarty CS (1971) Intraventricular meningiomas. Mayo Clin Proc 46:735–741

Kobayashi T, Kageyama N, Kida Y, Yoshida J, Shibuya N, Okamura K (1981) Unilateral germinomas involving the basal ganglia and thalamus. J Neurosurg 55:55–62

Koch G (1940) Beitrag zur Erblichkeit der Sturge-Weber'schen Krankheit. Z Gesamte Neurol Psychiatr 168:614–623

Koch G (1954) Beitrag zur Erblichkeit der Hirngeschwülste (vorläufige Mitteilung). Acta Genet Med Gemellol (Roma) 3:170–191

Koch G (1957) Ergebnisse aus der Nachuntersuchung der Berliner Zwillingsserie nach 20–25 Jahren (vorläufige Ergebnisse). Acta Genet Med Gemellol (Roma) 7:47–52

Koch G (1960a) Neuere Betrachtungen über die Erblichkeit der Sturge-Weberschen und von Hippel-Lindauschen Krankheit: I. Med Welt 38:1955–1961

Koch G (1960b) Neuere Betrachtungen über die Erblichkeit der Sturge-Weberschen und von Hippel-Lindauschen Krankheit: II. Med Welt 40:2104–2108

Koch G (1964) The genetics of cerebral tumours. In: Zülch KJ, Woolf AL (eds) Classification of brain tumours. Acta Neurochir [Suppl X] (Wien):24–29

Koch G (1972a) Humangenetisch-klinische Befunde bei Zwillingen. Ergebnisse aus der Nachuntersuchung der Zwillingsserie des ehemaligen Kaiser-Wilhelm-Institutes für Anthropologie, menschliche Erblehre und Eugenik (Eugen-Fischer-Institut) in Berlin-Dahlem nach 20–25 Jahren. Hoge, Erlangen

Koch G (1972b) Genetic aspects of the phacomatoses. In: Vinken PJ, Bruyn GW (eds) The phakomatoses. North-Holland, Amsterdam/American Elsevier, New York (Handbook of clinical neurology, vol 14, pp 488–561)

Koch G (1973) Die Sturge-Weber'sche Krankheit. Palm and Enke, Erlangen (Bibl Genet Med 2)

Koch G (1980) Sobre el problema del "cancer familiar". Folia Hum 18:577–581

Koch G (1981) Results of the 40-year longitudinal study of a series of twins of Berlin (450 monozygotic and dizygotic twins). Prog Clin Biol Res [C] 69:201–209

Koch G, Middendorf E (1960) Vorkommen von Glioblastoma multiforme bei 3 Schwestern im Alter von 50–54 Jahren. Med Welt 48:2541–2544

Koch O (1950) Der Lungenkrebs. Z Tuberk 94:23–43

Köhlmeier W (1943) Über multizentrisch entstandene Oligodendrogliome. Z Gesamte Neurol Psychiatr 175:385–402

Koella W (1947) Das Angioblastom. Schweiz Arch Neurol Psychiatr 59:208–238

Kölliker A von (1859) Handbuch der Gewebelehre des Menschen. Engelmann, Leipzig

Koeppe P, Oeser H (1982) Prognose der Krebsmortalität in der Bundesrepublik Deutschland 1976–2070. Lebensversicherungsmedizin 3:50–60

Koeppen AH, Cassidy RJ (1981) Oligodendroglioma of the medulla oblongata in a neonate. Arch Neurol 38:520–523

Környey S (1934) Eine sich entlang den Gefäßwandungen ausbreitende Hirngeschwulst (adventitielles Sarkom), zugleich Bemerkungen zu der Frage der Peritheliome des Gehirns. Z Gesamte Neurol Psychiatr 149:50–67

Környey S (1937) Über die diagnostische Bedeutung röntgenologisch darstellbarer Kalkherde in den Großhirnhemisphären von Erwachsenen nebst Bemerkungen zur Klinik und Pathologie des Oligodendroglioms. Zentralbl Neurochir 2:224–242

Koestner A (1975) Primary lymphoreticuloses of the nervous system in animals. Acta Neuropathol [Suppl] (Berl) 6:85–89

Koestner A, Zeman W (1962) Primary reticuloses of the central nervous system in dogs. Am J Vet Res 23:381–393

Koide O, Watanabe Y, Sato K (1980) A pathological survey of intracranial germinoma and pinealoma in Japan. Cancer 45:2119–2130

Koizumi J, Shiraishi H, Minei S, Nose T, Maki Y, Matsumoto Y (1973) Fine structural changes in the human cerebral cortex adjacent to meningioma. Folia Psychiatr Neurol Jpn 27:42–50

Kokmen E, Billman IK Jr, Abele MR (1977) Lymphomatoid granulomatosis clinically confined to the CNS. Arch Neurol 34:782–784

Kollmannsberger A, Kazner E, Prechtel K, Stochdorph O (1975) Zur Frage der extrakraniellen Metastasierung meningealer Tumoren. Malignes Meningeom mit regionalen Lymphknotenmetastasen. Zentralbl Neurochir 36:27–36

Kolodny EH, Rebeiz JJ, Caviness VS Jr, Richardson EP (1968) Granulomatous angiitis of the central nervous system. Arch Neurol 19:510–524

Komatsu S, Sato T, Katakura R, Sakurai Y, Wada T, Namiki T (1980) Pulmonary metastasis from cerebellar medulloblastoma (In Japanese). No Shinkei Geka 8:187–191

Koos W, Laubichler W (1967) Über die spinalen Geschwülste bei Kindern. Wien Z Nervenheilkd 24:247–263

Koos WT, Miller MH (1971) Intracranial tumors of infants and children. Thieme, Stuttgart

Koos WT, Jellinger K, Sunder-Plassmann M (1971) Intracerebral fibroma in an 11-month-old infant. Case report. J Neurosurg 35:77–81

Kosnik EJ, Hunt WE, Miller CA (1974) Dural arteriovenous malformations. J Neurosurg 40:322–329

Kostka VI, Drahozal H 1973) Méně obvykly připad sarkomatózy tvrdé pleny vytvářejici obraz subdurálniho hygromu (An unusual case of dural sarcomatosis simulating subdural hygroma). Cesk Neurol Neurochir 36:43–46

Kothandaram P (1970) Dural liposarcoma associated with subdural hematoma. Case report. J Neurosurg 33:85–87

Kovacs K, Horvath E, Corenblum B, Sirek AMT, Penz G, Ezrin C (1975) Pituitary chromophobe adenomas consisting of prolactin cells. Virchows Arch [A] 366:113–123

Kovacs K, Corenblum B, Sirek AMT, Penz G, Ezrin C (1976) Localization of prolactin in chromophobe pituitary adenomas: Study of human necropsy material by immunoperoxydase technique. J Clin Pathol 29:250–258

Krabbe KH (1916) Histologische und embryologische Untersuchungen über die Zirbeldrüse des Menschen. Anat Hefte 54:187–319

Krabbe KH (1923) The pineal gland, especially in relation to the problem of its supposed significance in sexual development. Endocrinology 7:374–414

Krabbe KH (1944) Un cas de tératome dans la glande pinéale guéri par intervention opératoire. Acta Psychiatr Neurol Scand 19:233–245

Krainer L (1935) Die Hirn- und Rückenmarkslipome. Virchows Arch [A] 295:107–142

Kramer MD, Aita JF (1978) Trichinosis. In: Vinken PJ, Bruyn GW (eds) Infections of the nervous system. North-Holland, Amsterdam (Handbook of clinical neurology, vol 35, part III, pp 267–290)

Kramer S, McKissock W, Concannon JP (1961) Craniopharyngiomas. Treatment by combined surgery and radiation therapy. J Neurosurg 18:217–226

Krasting K (1906) Beitrag zur Statistik und Kasuistik metastatischer Tumoren, besonders der Carcinommetastasen im Zentralnervensystem (auf Grund von 12730 Sektionen der Pathologisch-Anatomischen Anstalt Basel). Z Krebsforsch 4:315–379

Kraus EJ (1914) Die Beziehungen der Zellen des Vorderlappens der menschlichen Hypophyse zueinander etc. Beitr Pathol Anat 58:159

Kraus EJ (1926) Die Hypophyse. In: Uehlinger E (ed) Drüsen mit innerer Sekretion. Springer, Berlin (Handbuch der speziellen Anatomie und Histologie, vol 8, pp 810–950)

Kraus H (1948) Die Arachnitis chronica cerebralis und spinalis und ihre operative Behandlung. Langebecks Arch Chir 261:31–67

Krause F (1892) Resection des Trigeminus innerhalb der Schädelhöhle. Verh Dtsch Ges Chir 21:199–210

Krause F (1908) Chirurgie des Gehirns und Rückenmarks, vol I. Urban and Schwarzenberg, Berlin

Krause F (1909–1912) Surgery of the brain and spinal cord on personal experiences (3 vols). Rebman, New York

Krause F (1911) Chirurgie des Gehirns und Rückenmarks, vol II. Urban and Schwarzenberg, Berlin

Krause G (1950) Über die Häufigkeit der einzelnen Hirngeschwulstarten am verschiedenen Sitz. Dissertation, Faculty of Medicine, University of Hamburg

Krause G, Zülch KJ (1951) Über die Häufigkeit der Hirntumorarten in den verschiedenen Regionen. Zentralbl Neurochir 11:222–231

Krause W (1878) Die Glandula tympanica des Menschen. Zentralbl Med Wiss 16:736–739

Krayenbühl H (1936) Primary tumours of the root of the fifth cranial nerve: their distinction from tumours of the Gasserian ganglion. Brain 59:337–352

Krayenbühl H (1961) Hypophysenadenome und Kraniopharyngeome. Excerpta Medica, Amsterdam, D12–D14 (International congress series no. 36)

Krayenbühl H, Lüthy F (1947) Das spinale Neurinom und sympathische Ganglioneurom im Kindesalter. Schweiz Z Pathol 10:51–65

Krayenbühl H, Prader A (1962) Traitement endocrinien des troubles de la croissance chez des malades opérés d'un craniopharyngiome. Neurochirurgie 8:223–233

Krayenbühl H, Schmid AE (1943) Zur Lokalisation intrakranieller orbitaler Dermoide. Ophthalmologica 106:251–270

Krayenbühl H, Yasargil G (1958) Das Kleinhirnhämangiom. Schweiz Med Wochenschr 88:99–104

Krayenbühl H, Yasargil MG (1975a) Cranial chordomas. Prog Neurol Surg 6:380–434

Krayenbühl H, Yasargil MG (1975b) Chondromas. Prog Neurol Surg 6:435–463

Krebs E, Rappoport F, David M (1932) Méningiome de la gaine du trijumeau. Ablation. Guérison. Discussion du diagnostic et des indications opératoires dans les cas d'atteinte organique de la cinquième paire. Rev Neurol (Paris) 39:700–713

Kredel FE (1928) Tissue culture of intracranial tumors with note on the meningiomas. Am J Pathol 4:337–340

Kredel FE (1929) Intracranial tumors in tissue culture. Arch Surg 18:2008–2018

Krementz ET, Greene HSN (1953) Heterologous transplantation of human neural tumors. Cancer 6:100–110

Krenkel W, Friedmann G (1967) Diagnose und Therapie der kraniospinalen Tumoren. Fortschr Neurol Psychiatr 35:237–262

Kretschmer H (1974a) Callosal tumors. In: Vinken PJ, Bruyn GW (eds) Tumours of the brain and skull, part II. North-Holland, Amsterdam/American Elsevier, New York (Handbook of clinical neurology, vol 17, pp 490–554)

Kretschmer H (1974b) Die extrakranielle Metastasierung intrakranieller Geschwülste. Zentralbl Neurochir 35:81–112

Kretschmer H (1979) Spinal metastases as the cause of acute and subacute transverse spinal cord paralysis. Neurosurg Rev 2:65–72

Kreutzberg G, Langer E, Minauf M (1965) Beitrag zur Enzymhistochemie und Gewebekultur des Ganglioneuroms. Acta Neuropathol (Berl) 4:392–401

Kreutzberg GW, Minauf M, Gullotta F (1966) Enzyme histochemistry of human brain tumors and their tissue culture with special reference to the oxidoreductases in the glioblastoma multiforme. Histochemistry 6:8–16

Kricheff II, Becker M, Schneck SA, Taveras JM (1964) Intracranial ependymomas. Am J Roentgenol 91:167–175

Krieg W (1936a) Aseptische Meningitis nach Operation von Cholesteatomen des Gehirns. Zentralbl Neurochir 1:79–86

Krieg W (1936b) 164 Fälle von Cholesteatomen des Gehirns. Zentralbl Chir [no. 51] 3047

Kristensson K, Molin B, Sourander P (1967) Delayed radiation lesions of the human spinal cord. Report of five cases. Acta Neuropathol (Berl) 9:34–44

Krivoy O S, Belfort EA, Mondolfi A, Walzer I, Essenfeld E, Landaeta T (1978) Paracoccidioidomycosis of the skull. Case report. J Neurosurg 49:429–433

Kronborg O (1967) Extradural spinal cysts. A literature survey and a case of multiple extradural cysts. Dan Med Bull 14:46–48

Krücke W (1942) Zur Histopathologie der neuralen Muskelatrophie, der hypertrophischen Neuritis und Neurofibromatose. Arch Psychiatr 115:180–236

Krüger DW (1961) Über einen Fall multipler intracranieller Geschwülste mesodermaler Herkunft. Zentralbl Neurochir 21:62–66

Krüger EG, Morsa L, Kenney M, Price PA (1954) Nocardiosis of the central nervous system. J Neurosurg 11:226–233

Krumbein C (1925) Über die Band- oder Palisadenstellung der Kerne, eine Wuchsform des feinfibirillären mesenchymalen Gewebes. Zugleich eine Ableitung der Neurinome (Verocay) vom feinfibrillären Bindegewebe (Fibroma termifibrillare). Virchows Arch [A] 255:309–331

Krumbholz S, Hankowitz M, Schyra B (1966) Differentialdiagnose extraduraler Zysten im Spinalkanal. Zentralbl Neurochir 27:118–125

Kruyff E (1965) Paracollicular plate cysts. Am J Roentgenol 95:899–916

Krynauw RA, Jackson C (1948) Presence of parasitic agent in various intracranial tumors of man. Nature 162:147–148

Kubie LS, Fulton JF (1928) A clinical and pathological study of two teratomous cysts of the spinal cord, containing mucus and ciliated cells. Surg Gynecol Obstet 47:297–311

Kubo O, Okino T, Kamijo Y, Hamada H, Himuro H, Kitamura K (1974) Electron microscopic observations of two cases of monstrocellular sarcoma of the brain in vivo and in vitro (In Japanese). No Shinkei Geka 2:469–475

Kubo O, Kamijo Y, Himuro H, Kitamura K, Okino T (1976) Studies on neurinoma and neurofibroma in tissue culture (In Japanese). No Shinkei Geka 4:1149–1154

Kubota T, Fujii H, Ikeda K, Ito H, Yamamoto S, Nakanishi I (1980) A case of intraventricular craniopharyngioma with subarachnoid hemorrhage (In Japanese). No Shinkei Geka 8:495–501

Kufs H (1932) Klinik, Histopathologie und Vererbungspathologie der v. Hippel-Lindauschen Erkrankung. Z Gesamte Neurol Psychiatr 138:414–427

Kuhlendahl H, Stochdorph O, Hübner G (1975) Zur nosologischen Stellung und histologischen Herleitung des sogenannten Kleinhirnastrozytoms. Acta Neurochir (Wien) 32:235–245

Kumanishi T, Ikuta F, Yamamoto T (1970) Aldolase isozyme patterns of representative tumors in the human nervous system. Acta Neuropathol (Berl) 16:200–225

Kumanishi T, Koga M, Ogawa H, Nakamura N, Ikuta F, Oyake Y, Ueki K (1975) Malignant lymphoma in the central nervous system (In Japanese). No To Shinkei 27:21–34

Kumar S, Kaza RC, Tandon A, Nayar M (1979) Subdural spinal fungal granuloma due to candida tropicalis. J Neurosurg 50:395–396

Kummer RV, Volk B, Dorndorf W (1977) Extraneural metastasierendes Oligodendrogliom. Arch Psychiatr Nervenkr 223:287–293

Kunft H-D, Piotrowski W (1964) Über gleichzeitiges Vorkommen primärer intracranieller Gewächse verschiedener Keimblätter. Zentralbl Neurochir 24:189–198

Kung PC, Lee JC, Bakay L (1969) Vascular invasion by glioma cells in man. J Neurosurg 31:339–345

Kunicki A, Kaluza J (1963) Clinical and anatomical description of 10 cases of intracranial epidermoid. Acta Med Pol 4:143–157

Kunicki A, Lechowski S, Madroszkiewicz E, Szwagrzyk E (1972) Rathke's pouch tumors of childhood in the material of the department of neurosurgery, Medical Academy in Cracow. Pol Med J 9:986–990

Kurland LT (1958) The frequency of intracranial and intraspinal neoplasms in the resident population of Rochester, Minnesota. J Neurosurg 15:627–641

Kurland LT (1972) Geography of neuronal tumors. In: Minckler J (ed) Pathology of the nervous system, vol 3. Mac Graw-Hill, New York, pp 2803–2808

Kurland LT, Kurtzke JF (1972) Geographic neuropathology. In: Minckler J (ed) Pathology of the nervous system, vol 3. Mac Graw-Hill, New York pp 2771–2803

Kurland LT, Myrianthopoulos NC, Lessell S (1962) Epidemiologic and genetic considerations of intracranial neoplasms. In: Fields WS, Sharkey PC (eds) The biology and treatment of intracranial tumors. Thomas, Springfield, pp 5–48

Kurland LT, Kurtzke JF, Goldberg ID (1973) Epidemiology of neurologic and sense organ disorders. Harvard University Press, Cambridge

Kurtzke JF (1969) Geographic pathology of brain tumor. I. Distribution of deaths from primary tumors. Acta Neurol Scand 45:540–555

Kurumado K, Mori W (1976) Virus-like particles in human pinealoma. Acta Neuropathol (Berl) 35:273–276
Kusske JA, Kelly WA (1974) Embolization and reduction of the „steal" syndrome in cerebral arteriovenous malformations. J Neurosurg 40:313–321
Kwan ST, Alpers BJ (1931) The oligodendrogliomas. Arch Neurol Psychiatry 26:279–321
Labhart A, Zachmann M (1975) Clinical physiology of pituitary tumors. Prog Neurol Surg 6:1–61
Lach B, Weinrauder H (1978) Glia-specific antigen in the intracranial tumors. Immunofluorescence study. Acta Neuropathol (Berl) 41:9–15
Laerum OD, Bigner DD, Rajewsky MF (1978) Biology of brain tumors. A series of workshops on the biology of human cancer, report no 5. Unio Internationalis Contra Cancrum, Geneva (Technical report series vol 30)
Lagos JC, Gomez MR (1967) Tuberous sclerosis: Reappraisal of a clinical entity. Mayo Clin Proc 42:26
Laha RK, Huestis WS (1975) Unilateral acoustic neuroma and cerebellopontine angle lesions in children. Surg Neurol 4:371–374
Lake PA, Pitts FW (1969) Atypical myelomeningocele with associated anomalies. J Neurosurg 31:234–237
Lalitha VS, Rubinstein LJ (1979) Reactive glioma in intracranial sarcoma. A form of mixed sarcoma and glioma (sarcoglioma). Cancer 43:246–257
Lana-Peixoto MA, Lagos J, Silbert SW (1977) Primary pigmented carcinoma of the choroid plexus. J Neurosurg 47:442–450
Landau W (1910) Das diffuse Gliom. Frankfurt Z Pathol 5:469–514
Landau W (1911) Über Rückbildungsvorgänge in Gliomen. Frankfurt Z Pathol 7:351
Landers JW, Danielski JJ (1960) Malignant intracranial epidermoid cyst. Arch Pathol 70:419–423
Landolt AM (1975) Ultrastructure of human sella tumours. Acta Neurochir [Suppl] (Wien) 22:1–67
Landolt AM, Oswald WW (1973) Histology and ultrastructure of an oncocytic adenoma of the human pituitary. Cancer 31:1099–1105
Landolt AM, Rothenbühler V, Kistler GS (1978) Morphology of the chromophobe adenoma. In: Fahlbusch R, Werder KO (eds) Treatment of pituitary adenomas. Thieme, Stuttgart, pp 154–171
Landolt-Weber UM (1973) Ultrastruktur einer Kolloidcyste des dritten Ventrikels. Acta Neuropathol (Berl) 26:59–70
Lange-Cosack H (1948) Gefäßmißbildungen des Gehirns und seiner Häute. In: Kirschner M, Nordmann O (eds) Die Chirurgie, vol III. Urban and Schwarzenberg, Vienna, pp 613–660
Lange-Cosack H (1951) Verschiedene Gruppen der hypothalamischen Pubertas praecox. (1st communication.) Dtsch Z Nervenheilkd 166:499–545
Lange-Cosack H (1952) Verschiedene Gruppen der hypothalamischen Pubertas praecox. 2. Mitteilung. Dtsch Z Nervenheilkd 168:237–266
Lange-Cosack H (1954) Psychische Störungen beim arterio-venösen Rankenangiom des Gehirns. Dtsch Z Nervenheilkd 171:416–442
Lange-Cosack H (1966) Anatomie und Klinik der Gefäßmißbildungen des Gehirns und seiner Häute. In: Krenkel W, Olivecrona H, Tönnis W (eds) Klinik und Behandlung der raumbeengenden intrakraniellen Prozesse: II. Springer, Berlin Göttingen Heidelberg (Handbuch der Neurochirurgie, vol IV/2, pp 1–145)
Langenbeck B von (1845) cited in Mohr W (1952)
Langheim W, Kernohan JK, Uihlein A (1962) Arachnoidal sarcoma of the cerebellum. Cancer 15:705–716
Lanksch W, Kazner E (1976) Cranial computerized tomography. Springer, Berlin Heidelberg New York
Lapham LW (1959) Subdivision of glioblastoma multiforme on a cytologic and cytochemical basis. J Neuropathol Exp Neurol 18:244–262
Lapras C, Wertheimer J, Thierry A (1963) A propos d'un nouveau cas de kyste arachnoidien de las fosse cérébrale postérieure. Neurochirurgie 9:229–234

Lapresle J, Netsky MG, Zimmerman HM (1952) The pathology of meningiomas. A study of 212 cases. Am J Pathol 28:757–791
Laqueur GL (1964) Carcinogenic effects of cycad meal and cycasin, methylazoxymethanol glycoside in rats and effects of cycasin in germfree rats. Fed Proc 23:1386–1387
Laqueur GL, Mickelsen O, Whiting MG, Kurland LT (1963) Carcinogenic properties of nuts from *Cycas circinalis* L. indigenous to Guam. J Natl Cancer Inst 31:919–951
Lassman LP, Arjona VE (1967) Pontine gliomas in childhood. Lancet 1:913–915
Lassman LP, James CCM (1967) Lumbosacral lipomas: critical survey of 26 cases submitted to laminectomy. J Neurol Neurosurg Psychiatry 30:174–181
Latovitzki N, Abrams G, Clark C, Mayeux R, Ascherl G, Sciarra D (1978) Cerebral cysticercosis. Neurology (Minneap) 28:838–842
Lattes R, Waltner IG (1949) Non chromaffin paraganglioma of the middle ear (carotid-body-like tumor; glomus jugulare tumor). Cancer 2:447–468
Lauche A (1925) Über rhythmische Strukturen in menschlichen Geweben. Virchows Arch [A] 257:751
Lauche A (1944) Sind die sogenannten „Myoblastenmyome" Speicherzellgeschwülste? Virchows Arch [A] 312:335–345
Laurence KM (1974) The biology of choroid plexus papilloma and carcinoma of the lateral ventricle. In: Vinken PJ, Bruyn GW (eds) Tumors of the brain and skull, part II. North-Holland, Amsterdam/American Elsevier, New York (Handbook of clinical neurology, vol 17, pp 555–595)
Lausberg G (1965) Kolloid-Zysten der Seitenventrikel. Zentralbl Neurochir 26:42–50
Lauschke H (1964) Zur Differentialdiagnose intracranieller granulomatöser Geschwülste (Hirntumor bei Morbus Besnier-Boeck-Schaumann). Acta Neurochir (Wien) 11:429–438
Lawrence RM, Goldstein E (1978) Histoplasmosis. In: Vinken PJ, Bruyn GW (eds) Infections of the nervous system, part III. North-Holland, Amsterdam (Handbook of clinical neurology, vol 35, pp 503–515)
Laymon CW, Becker FT (1949) Massive metastasizing meningioma involving the scalp. Arch Dermatol 59:626–635
Leal O, Miles J (1978) Epidermoid cyst in the brain stem. J Neurosurg 48:811–813
Learmonth JR (1927) On leptomeningiomas (endotheliomas) of the spinal cord. Br J Surg 14:397–471
Learmonth JR, Camp JD (1933) Multiple tumor implants in the ventricles revealed by ventriculography. Report of a case. Am J Roentgenol 29:393–394
Learmonth JR, Kernohan JW (1930a) Three cases of epidermoid cyst of the brain. Proc Staff Meet Mayo Clin 5:853–865
Learmonth JR, Kernohan JW (1930b) Tumour of the gasserian ganglion: sheath neuroma. Brain 53:1–6
Leavitt FH (1928) Cerebellar tumors occurring in identical twins. Arch Neurol Psychiatry 19:617–622
Lebert H (1851) Über Krebs und die mit Krebs verwechselten Geschwülste im Gehirn und seinen Hüllen. Virchows Arch [A] 3:463–469
LeBlanc C (1868) Papilloma myxomathodes. Beitrag zur pathologischen Anatomie der Gehirntumoren. Dissertation Faculty of Medicine, University of Bonn
Leblanc G, Francoeur J, Copty M, Contreras C, Gagne F (1976) Intracranial dysgerminomas. Can J Neurol Sci 3:199–203
LeBlanc RA (1974) Metastasis of bronchogenic carcinoma to acoustic neurinoma. Case report. J Neurosurg 41:614–617
Le Clech G, Vallee B, Scarabin JM, Bourdiniere J, Ardonin M, Urvoy M (1978) Aspergillose pseudo-tumorale du sinus sphenoidal. Rev Otoneuroopthalmol 50:421–428
Le Compte PM (1951) Tumors of the carotid body and related structures (chemoreceptor system). Atlas of tumor pathology, sect IV, fasc 16. Armed Forces Institute of Pathology, Washington
Le Count ER (1909) Blastomycotic lesions of the brain. J Nerv Ment Dis 36:144–149
Le Count ER, Myers J (1907) Systemic blastomycosis (final report of the case described by Eisendrath and Ormsby in 1905 in JAMA). J Infect Dis 4:187–200
Lee BCP, Gawler J (1978) Tuberous sclerosis. Radiology 127:403–407

Lee JC, Glasauer FE (1968) Ganglioglioma: light and electron microscopic study. Neurochirurgia (Stuttg) 11:160–170
Lee KF, Suh JH, Lee YE, Berry RG (1979) Meningioma of the paranasal sinuses. Neuroradiology 17:165–171
Lee SH, Sundaresan N, Jereb B, Galicich JM (1978) Endodermal sinus tumor of the pineal region. Neurosurgery 3:407–412
Leech RW, Christofferson LA, Gilbertson RG (1977) Dysplastic gangliocytoma (Lhermitte-Duclos disease) of the cerebellum. J Neurosurg 47:609–612
Leers W-D (1978) North American blastomycosis. In: Vinken PJ, Bruyn GW (eds) Infections of the nervous system. North-Holland, Amsterdam (Handbook of clinical neurology, vol 35, part III, pp 401–411)
Lefèvre J, Klein MR, Lepintre J, Fauré C (1956) Etude radiologique des tumeurs médullaires chez l'enfant. Acta Radiol (Stockh) 46:48–54
Legier J, Wells H Jr (1967) Primary cerebellar rhabdomyosarcoma. Case report. J Neurosurg 26:436–438
Legler U (1949) Unsere Erfahrungen mit malignen Epipharynxtumoren. Z Laryng Rhinol 28:383–389
Legré J, Sedan R, Lavielle J, Clément JP, Paillas JE (1968) Maladie de von Hippel-Lindau. Ablation des angioreticulomes cérébelleux et gúerison. Etude neuro-radiologique avec exploration angiographique sélective des localisations viscérales. Neurochirurgie 14:583–597
Lehoczky T von (1929) Über die Anatomie und Klinik der Epidermoidzysten des Gehirns. Z Gesamte Neurol Psychiatr 122:756–799
Lehrer GM (1962) The quantitative histochemistry of human glial tumors. In: Fields WS, Sharkey PC (eds) The biology and treatment of intracranial tumors. Thomas, Springfield, pp 140–153
Lehrer GM, Maker HS (1971) Energy metabolism of glial tumors. J Neurosurg 34:452–453
Lehrer GM, Maker HS, Scheinberg LC (1967) The quantitative enzyme histochemistry of an experimental glioma. J Neuropathol Exp Neurol 26:142
Leibel SA, Sheline GE, Wara WM, Boldrey EB, Nielsen SL (1975) The role of radiation therapy in the treatment of astrocytoma. Cancer 35:1551–1557
Leibowitz U, Yablonski M, Alter M (1971) Epidemiology of tumors of the nervous system in Israel. Isr J Med Sci 7:1491–1499
Leitholf O (1956) Tumoren der Schädelknochen. Acta Neurochir (Wien) 4:287–319
Leksell L (1951) The stereotaxic method and radiosurgery of the brain. Acta Chir Scand 102:316–319
Le Marquand HS, Russell DS (1934/35) A case of pubertas praecox (macrogenitosomia praecox) in a boy associated with a tumour in the floor of the third ventricle. R Berkshire Hosp Rep 3:31–32
Lemke R (1950) Über Hirncysten. Dtsch Z Nervenheilkd 162:70–89
Lemoyne J (1956) Les examens oto-rhino-laryngologiques en neurologie. Masson, Paris
Lenče P (1937) Über seltene primäre Lokalisationen melanotischer Tumoren. Ergeb Allg Pathol 32:48–90
Lenhossek M von (1895) Der feinere Bau des Nervensystems im Lichte neuester Forschungen, 2nd edn. Fischer's Medicinische Buchhandlung H. Kornfeld, Berlin
Lennert K (1975) Morphology and classification of malignant lymphomas and so-called reticuloses. Acta Neuropathol (Berl) 6:1–16
Lennert K (1978) Malignant lymphomas other than Hodgkin's disease. Springer, Berlin Heidelberg New York
Lenshoek CH, Baumann C, Wielenga DK (1958) Brain abscess due to entamoeba histolytica. Case report with successful excision. Arch Chir Neerl 10:34–40
Lepoire J, Pertuiset B (1957) Les kystes épidermoides cranio-encéphaliques. Masson, Paris
Lepoire J, Pertuiset B (1958) Die Epidermoidcysten an Schädel und Hirn. Neurochirurgia (Stuttg) 1:1–26
Lerman RL, Kaplan ES, Daman L (1972) Ganglioneuroma – paraganglioma of the intradural filum terminale. J Neurosurg 36:652–658
Leszinsky WM (1907) Report of a case of intracranial tumor resulting from traumatism. JAMA 49:1361–1363

Leu HJ, Rüttner JR (1973) Angioretikulome des Zentralnervensystems. Acta Neurochir (Wien) 29:73–82
Leventhal HR (1959) Electron microscopy of brain tumors. Clin Neurosurg 7:56–62
Levin PM (1936) Multiple hereditary hemangioblastomas of the nervous system. Arch Neurol Psychiatry 36:384–391
Levin P, Gross SW, Malis LI, Kirshenbaum AH, Hollin SA (1964) Multiple intracranial meningiomas. Surgery 119:1085–1090
Levin VA, Wilson CB, Davis R, Wara WM, Pischer TL, Irwin L (1979) A phase III comparison of BCNU, hydroxyurea, and radiation therapy to BCNU and radiation therapy for treatment of primary malignant gliomas. J Neurosurg 51:526–532
Levinthal R, Bentson JR (1976) Detection of small trigeminal neurinomas. J Neurosurg 45:568–575
Leviton A, Fulchiero A, Gilles FH, Winston K (1978) Survival status of children with cerebellar gliomas. J Neurosurg 48:29–33
Levy LF, Elvidge AR (1956) Astrocytoma of the brain and spinal cord; a review of 176 cases, 1940–1949. J Neurosurg 13:413–443
Lewis AJ (1962) Infantile hydrocephalus caused by arachnoid cyst. J Neurosurg 19:431–434
Lewis AJ (1968) Melanoma with a coincidental acoustic neurinoma. J Neurosurg 29:280–282
Lewis AJ (1973) Medulloblastoma with striated muscle fibers. Case report. J Neurosurg 38:642–646
Lewis I (1967) Cerebellar metastasis from prostatic carcinoma. A case report. Neurology (Minneap) 17:698–702
Lewis MB, Nunes LB, Powell DE, Shnider BI (1973) Extra-axial spread of medulloblastoma. Cancer 31:1287–1297
Lewis P (1967) Carcinoma of the choroid plexus. Brain 90:177–186
Lewis PD, Van Noorden S (1974) Nonfunctioning pituitary tumors. Arch Pathol 97:178–182
Ley A, Walker AE (1936) Statistical review of 230 consecutive cases of intracranial tumor. Folia Neuropathol Eston 15/16:52–67
Ley A, Jacas R, Oliveras C (1951) Torula granuloma of the cervical spinal cord. J Neurosurg 8:327–335
Ley A, Campillo D, Oliveras C (1961) Extracranial metastasis of glioblastoma multiforme. J Neurosurg 18:313–330
Lhermitte J, Duclos P (1920) Sur un ganglioneurome diffus du cortex du cervelet. Bull Assoc Franç Cancer 9:99–106
Liber F (1937) The nature of Rosenthal fibers. J Nerv Ment Dis 85:286–304
Lichtenstein BW (1941) Multiple primary tumours of the spinal cord. Arch Neurol Psychiatry 46:59–71
Lichtenstein BW (1971) Hamartomas and phacomatoses. In: Minckler J (ed) Pathology of the nervous system, vol 2. McGraw-Hill, New York, pp 1897–1906
Lichtenstein BW, Simon A (1951) Cerebral schistosomiasis producing epilepsy in a veteran of the Pacific. J Neuropathol Clin Neurol 1:81–87
Lichtenstein BW, Zeitlin H (1937) Ganglioglioneuroma of spinal cord. Associated with pseudosyringomyelia: Histologic study. Arch Neurol Psychiatry 37:1356–1370
Lichtenstein L (1952) Bone tumors. Mosby, St. Louis
Lichtenstein L (1953) Histiocytosis X. Integration of eosinophilic granuloma of bone, "Letterer-Siwe disease" and "Schüller-Christian disease" are related manifestations of a single nosologic entity. Arch Pathol 56:89–103
Lichtenstein L (1956) Benign osteoblastoma. Cancer 9:1044–1052
Lichtenstein L (1964) Histiocytosis X (eosinophilic granuloma of bone, Letterer-Siwe disease and Schüller-Christian disease). J Bone Joint Surg 76:76–90
Lichtenstein L, Jaffe H (1940) Eosinophilic granuloma of the bone. Am J Pathol 16:595
Liebaldt G (1957) Trauma and Meningeomentstehung. Zentralbl Allg Pathol 96:260–263
Liebaldt G (1963) Zur Genese und Deutung intramedullärer Teratome. Dtsch Z Nervenheilkd 185:557–564
Lieberman A, Dart L, Bennett R (1970) Intracerebral tuberculoma. Case report. J Neurosurg 33:331–333

Lietz S (1966) Die Bedeutung des Wirbelhämangioms für Klinik und Praxis, mit einer Kasuistik von fünf Fällen. Fortschr Neurol Psychiatr 34:176–197
Liliequist B (1956) The anatomy of the subarachnoid cisterns. Acta Radiol (Stockh) 46:61–71
Liliequist B, Thulin C-A, Tovi D, Wiberg A, Öhman J (1972) Neurinoma of the labyrinthine portion of the facial nerve. Case report. J Neurosurg 37:105–109
Lill H (1952) Über metastatische Hirntumoren. Klinische Erfahrungen an einem Material von 97 Fällen. Wien Med Wochenschr 102:277–278
Lima Costa A, Couto Cesar H (1951) Siringomielia e tumor medular. J Brasil Neurol 3:1–50
Limas C, Tio FO (1972) Meningeal melanocytome (melanotic meningioma) Its melanocytic origin as revealed by electron microscopy. Cancer 30:1286–1294
Linares G, McGarry PA, Baker RD (1971) Solid solitary aspergillotic granuloma of the brain. Neurology (Minneap) 21:177–184
Lindau A (1926) Studien über Kleinhirncysten. Bau, Pathogenese und Beziehungen zur Angiomatosis retinae. Acta Pathol Microbiol Scand [Suppl] 1
Lindgren E (1954) Röntgenologie einschließlich Kontrastmethoden. In: Olivecrona H, Tönnis W (eds) Röntgenologie. Springer, Berlin Göttingen Heidelberg (Handbuch der Neurochirurgie, vol II, pp 1–296)
Lindgren M (1953) Radiotherapie des gliomes. Acta Radiol (Stockh) 40:325–334
Lindgren M (1958) On tolerance of brain tissue and sensitivity of brain tumors to radiation. Acta Radiol [Suppl] (Stockh) 170
Lindlar F (1970) Zur Biochemie der Hirngeschwülste. In: Kraus H, Sunder-Plassmann M (eds) Pädiatrische Neurochirurgie. Verlag der Wiener Medizinischen Akademie, pp 105–109
Lindlar F, Bingas B (1965) Die Lipide von Hirntumoren. Dtsch Z Nervenheilkd 187:737–748
Link K, Schleussing H (1950) Statistische Erhebung an 248 intracraniellen Geschwülsten. Arch Psychiatr Nervenkr 184:646–652
Linquette M, Herlant M, Laine E, Forsati P, Dupont-Lecompte MJ (1967) Adénome à prolactine chez une jeune fille dont la mère était proteuse d'un adénome hypophysaire avec aménorrhée-galactorrhée. Ann Endocrinol (Paris) 28:773–780
Lins E (1974) Das Medulloblastom des Erwachsenen. Acta Neurochir (Wien) 31:67–72
Lipčina LP (1952) Histochemische Untersuchungen des Glykogengehaltes in Arachnoidendotheliomen. (in Russian) Vopr Nevrochir 16:30–35
Liss L (1958) Pituitcytoma, a tumor of the hypothalamus. Arch Neurol Psychiatry 80:567–576
Liss L (1961) Oligodendrogliomas. J Neuropathol Exp Neurol 20:582–592
Liss L (1962) Morphology of nervous system tumors in vitro. In: Jacob H (ed) Electronmicroscopy of the central and peripheral nervous system. Proceedings of the IVth International Congress of Neuropathology, Munich 1961. Thieme, Stuttgart, pp 247–254
Liss L (1972) The use of tissue cultures in the study of brain tumors. Prog Exp Tumor Res 17:93–110
Liss L, Kahn EA (1958) Pituicytoma. Tumor of the sella turcica. J Neurosurg 15:481–488
List CF (1936) Epileptiform attacks in cases of glioma of the cerebral hemispheres. Relation to the location and histologic type of glioma. Arch Neurol Psychiatry 35:323–350
List CF (1943a) Osteochondromas arising from the base of the skull. Surg Gynecol Obstet 76:480–492
List CF (1943b) Multiple meningiomas: removal of four tumors from the region of the foramen magnum and upper cervical region of the cord. Arch Neurol Psychiatry 50:335
List CF, Dowman CE, Bagchi BK, Bebin J (1958) Hamartome des hinteren Hypothalamus und Gangliogliome als Ursache einer Pubertas praecox. Neurology (Minneap) 8:164–174
List CF, Williams JR, Balyeat GW (1952) Vascular lesions in pituitary adenomas. J Neurosurg 9:177–187
Little JR, MacCarty CS (1974) Colloid cysts of the third ventricle. J Neurosurg 40:230–235
Little JR, Gomez MR, MacCarty (1973) Infratentorial arachnoid cysts. J Neurosurg 39:380–386
Liu CT, Selbach G (1953) Primary sarcoma of the leptomeninges. Report of 3 cases. J Neuropathol Exp Neurol 12:186–193
Liu MH, Boggs J, Kidd J(1976) Ependymomas of childhood: I. Histological survey and clinicopathological correlation. Childs Brain 2:92–110
Livingstone G (1935) Chordoma of base of skull. Proc R Soc Med 28:1427–1429

Liwnicz BH (1979) Bilateral trigeminal neurofibrosarcoma. Case report. J Neurosurg 50:253–256
Ljungdahl I, Strang RR, Tovi D (1965) Intracerebral Hodgkin's granuloma. Report of a case and review of the literature. Neurochirurgia (Stuttg) 8:113–118
Llena JF, Chung HD, Hirano A, Feiring EH, Zimmerman HM (1975) Intracerebellar „fibroma". J Neurosurg 43:98–101
Löhlein W, Tönnis W (1949) Die operative Behandlung der das Foramen opticum überschreitenden Sehnervengeschwülste. Albrecht Von Graefes Arch Ophthalmol 149:318–354
Löhr H-H, Vieten H (1967) Die Strahlenbehandlung raumbeengender intrakranieller Prozesse. In: Olivecrona H, Tönnis W (eds) Klinik und Behandlung der raumbeengenden intrakraniellen Prozesse. Springer, Berlin Heidelberg New York (Handbuch der Neurochirurgie, vol IV/4, pp 421–566)
Löhr W, Jacobi W (1933) Die kombinierte Encephalo-Arteriographie. Arch Klin Chir 173:399–420
Løken AC (1952) Histological grouping of brain tumors in a 10 years material. Acta Pathol Microbiol Scand [Suppl] 93:135–148
Loepp W (1939) Die Pathologie der Schädelbasis im Röntgenbild. Fortschr Roentgenstr 59:451–474
Loessl J von, Pap Z von (1941) Über eine ungewöhnlich große primäre Echinococcuscyste im Gehirn. Nervenarzt 14:214–222
Loew F (1953) Operative Behandlungsmaßnahmen der Tumoren der Schädelbasis. Langenbecks Arch Chir 273:716–720
Loew F, Plogsties HR (1964) Kasuistischer Beitrag zur Frage der exogenen Meningeomentstehung. Acta Neurochir (Wien) 11:229–235
Loew F, Tönnis W (1954) Klinik und Behandlung der Neurinome des Nervus trigeminus. Zentralbl Neurochir 14:32–41
Löwenberg K, Waggoner RW (1939) Gross pathology of the oligodendrogliomas. Arch Neurol Psychiatry 42:842–861
Löwenstein C (1907) Die Entwicklung der Hypophysenadenome. Virchows Arch [A] 188:44–65
Löwenthal A (1950) Hémangioblastome cérébelleux, hémangioblastome méningé à métaplasie osseuse, hypertrophie des plexus choroides à surcharge calcaire amorphe, chez le même sujet. Acta Neurol Psychiatr Belg 50:185–198
Lokich JJ (1975) The management of cerebral metastases. JAMA 234:748–751
Lolova I, Bojinov S, Ivanova A, Christov V (1972) Cerebral medulloepithelioma. J Neurol Sci 15:173–182
Lombardo L, Alonso P, Arroyo LS, Brandt H, Mateos JH (1964) Cerebral amebiasis. J Neurosurg 21:704–709
Long DM, Seljeskog EL, Chon SN, French LA (1974) Giant arteriovenous malformations of infancy and childhood. J Neurosurg 40:304–312
Lopes de Faria J (1957) Rhabdomyosarcoma of cerebellum. Arch Pathol 63:234–238
Lopez DA, Silvers DN, Helwig EB (1974) Cutaneous meningiomas – a clinicopathologic study. Cancer 34:728–744
Lorenz R (1940) Differentialdiagnose der arteriographisch darstellbaren intrakraniellen Geschwülste. Glioblastom, Meningeom, Sarkom. Zentralbl Neurochir 4:30–60
Lorenz R (1949) Erfahrungen auf dem Gebiet der Röntgenbestrahlung von Hirntumoren. Zentralbl Neurochir 9:209–215
Loretz W (1870) Ein Fall von gangliösem Neurom (Gangliom). Virchows Arch [A] 49:435
Lo Schiavo F, Amici G (1971) Il neuroblastoma del simpatico. Considerazioni sui fenomeno dell regressione spontanea. Rass Int Clin Ter 51:420–430
Lotmar F (1935) Zur Kenntnis der Lindau'schen Krankheit. Schweiz Arch Neurol Psychiatr 36:257–270
Lotmar O (1918) Beiträge zur Histologie des Glioms. Histol Arb Gehirnrinde (Jena) 6:433
Louis A (1774) Mémoire sur les tumeurs fongueuses de la dure-mère. Mém Acad Roy Chir (Paris) 5:1–59
Lourie H, Berne AS (1961) Radiological and clinical features of an arachnoid cyst of the quadrigeminal cistern. J Neurol Neurosurg Psychiatry 24:374–378

Love JG, Kernohan JW (1936) Dermoids and epidermoidal tumors of the CNS. JAMA 107:1876–1882
Love JG, Shelden CH, Kernohan JW (1939) Tumors of the hypophysial duct (Rathke's cysts). Arch Surg 39:28–56
Lu AT, Lee CO (1961) Liposarcoma of chest wall with metastasis to the cerebrum. Review of literature and report of case. Bull Los Angeles Neurol Soc 26:217–224
Lu AT, Kypridakis G, Abbott KH, Vogel PJ (1963) Intramedullary neurofibromas of the cervical cord. Report of two cases. Bull Los Angeles Neurol Soc 28:31–36
Lubbers J (1937) Gezwel van het os petrosum met gecombineerde hersenzenuwverlamming (Syndrom foramen jugulare Burger) en gelijktijdig gezwel van glomus caroticum aan de andere zijde. Ned Tijdschr Geneeskd 81:2566–2567
Lubs HA, Salmon JH (1965) The chromosomal component of human solid tumors. J Neurosurg 22:160–168
Ludwin SK, Rubinstein LJ, Russell DS (1975) Papillary meningioma: a malignant variant of meningioma. Cancer 36:1363–1373
Lüthy F, Irsigler FJ (1952) Beitrag zur Klinik und Histologie der Ependymome der Cauda equina. Acta Neurochir (Wien) 2:354–368
Lüthy F, Klingler M (1951) Der Tumorettentumor des Hypophysenhinterlappens. Schweiz Z Allg Pathol Bact 14:721–729
Luginbühl H (1962a) Zur vergleichenden Pathologie der Tumoren des Nervensystems. Schweiz Arch Tierheilkd 104:305–322
Luginbühl H (1962b) Geschwülste des Zentralnervensystems bei Tieren. In: Frauchiger E, Seitelberger F (eds) Symposion über vergleichende Neuropathologie. Acta Neuropathol [Suppl] (Berl) 1:9–18
Luginbühl H (1963) Comparative aspects of tumors of the nervous system. Ann NY Acad Sci 108:702–721
Luginbühl H (1964a) A comparative study of neoplasms of the central nervous system in animals. In: Zülch KJ, Woolf AL (eds) Classification of brain tumors. Acta Neurochir [Suppl] (Wien) 10:30–42
Luginbühl H (1964b) Oligodendrogliomas in animals. In: Zülch KJ, Woolf AL (eds) Classification of brain tumors. Acta Neurochir [Suppl] (Wien) 10:173–184
Luginbühl H, Fankhauser R, McGrath JT (1968) Spontaneous neoplasms of the nervous system in animals. Prog Neurol Surg 2:85–164
Lukin RR, Chambers AA, Soleimanpour M (1975) Outlet obstruction of the fourth ventricle in sarcoidosis. Neuroradiology 10:65–68
Lumsden CE (1951) Aspects of neurite outgrowth in tissue culture. Anat Rec 110:145–179
Lumsden CE (1955a) Observations on the morphogenesis and growth rate of astrocytic gliomas in tissue culture. Excerpta Med (Amst) Sect VIII:792
Lumsden CE (1955b) Differentiation and de-differentiation in cultures of tumours of the astrocytoma-glioblastoma group. In: Proceedings of the Second International Congress of Neuropathology, London 1955. Excerpta Medica Foundation, Amsterdam, pp 279–285
Lumsden CE (1971) The study by tissue culture of tumours of the nervous system. In: Russell DS, Rubinstein LJ (eds) Pathology of tumors of the nervous system, 3rd edn. Arnold, London, pp 334–420
Lumsden CE (1974) Tissue culture of brain tumours. In: Vinken PJ, Bruyn GW (eds) Tumours of the brain and skull. North-Holland, Amsterdam/American Elsevier, New York (Handbook of clinical neurology, vol 17, part I, pp 42–103)
Lund M (1952) Epilepsy in association with intracranial tumor. Acta Psychiatr Scand [Suppl] 81
Lundberg A (1935) Über die primären Tumoren der Sehnerven und der Sehnervenkreuzung. Dissertation, Faculty of Medicine, University of Orburg
Lundberg A (1937) Le gliome primitif du nerf optique et du chiasma des nerfs optiques. Arch Ophthalmol (Paris) 1:97–107
Luschka H (1856) Die Altersveränderungen der Zwischenwirbelknorpel. Virchows Arch [A] 9:311–328
Luse SA (1958) Ultrastructure of reactive and neoplastic astrocytes. Lab Invest 7:401–417

Luse SA (1960) Electron microscopic studies of brain tumors. Neurology (Minneap) 10:881–905

Luse SA (1961a) An electron microscopic study of normal optic nerve and of an optic nerve glioma. J Neurosurg 18:466–478

Luse SA (1961b) Ultrastructural characteristics of normal and neoplastic cells. Prog Exp Tumor Res 2:6–35

Luse SA (1962) Electron microscopy of brain tumors. In: Fields WS, Sharkey PC (eds) The biology and treatment of intracranial tumors. Thomas, Springfield, pp 74–102

Luse SA, Kernohan JW (1955) Granular cell tumors of the stalk and posterior lobe of the pituitary gland. Cancer 8:616–622

Luten J (1951) Lipomas of corpus callosum. Ned Tijdschr Geneeskd 95:1416–1421

Luyendijk W (1954) Multiple meningiomas and meningiomatosis. Acta Neurochir (Wien) 3:263–274

Luyendijk W, Lindemann J (1975) Schistosomiasis (bilharziasis) Mansoni of the spinal cord simulating an intramedullary tumor. Surg Neurol 4:457–460

Luyendijk W, Staal A (1964) Über ein Großhirnependymom bei einem Säugling von zwei Monaten. Zentralbl Neurochir 24:100–103

Luzzato A (1942) Osservazioni sulla angioarchitectonica dei tumori cerebrali. Riv Patol Nerv Ment 59:293–375

Lynch HT, Krush AJ, Thomas RJ, Lynch J (1976) Cancer family syndrome. In: Lynch HT (ed) Cancer genetics. Thomas, Springfield, pp 355–388

Lynn JA, Panopio IT, Martin JH, Shaw ML, Race GJ (1968) Ultrastructural evidence for astroglial histiogenesis of the monstrocellular astrocytoma (so-called monstrocellular sarcoma of brain). Cancer 22:356–366

Lyser KM (1975) Human nervous system tumors. Observations by high voltage electron microscopy. Acta Neuropathol (Berl) 32:313–324

Mabon RT, Svien HJ, Gates EM, Kernohan JW (1950) Medullo-epithelioma. A critical reevaluation. J Neuropathol Exp Neurol 9:193–197

MacCarty CS, Dahlin DC (1976) Aneurysmal bone cysts of the neural axis. In: Vinken PJ, Bruyn GW (ed) Tumors of the spine and spinal cord. North Holland, Amsterdam/American Elsevier, Oxford (Handbook of clinical neurology, vol 20, part II, pp 1–7)

MacCarty CS, Waugh JM, Coventry MB, O'Sullivan DC (1961) Sacrococcygeal chordomas. Surg Gynecol Obstet 113:551–554

MacCarty CS, Dahlin DC, Heffelfinger MJ (1975) Chordomas of the neural axis. In: Vinken PJ, Bruyn GW (eds) Tumors of the spine and spinal cord. North Holland, Amsterdam/American Elsevier, Oxford (Handbook of clinical neurology, vol 19, part I, pp 287–292)

Macewen W (1881) Tumors of the dura mater (operated 1879). Lancet II:581–582

Macewen W (1885) Cases illustrative of cerebral surgery. Lancet I:881–883; 934–936

Macewen W (1888) An address on the surgery of the brain and spinal cord. Br Med J I:302

Macewen W (1893) Discussion of paper by V. Horsley: Treatment of cerebral tumors. Br Med J II:1367–1368

MacGregor BJL, Gawler J, South JR (1976) Intracranial epithelial cysts. Report of two cases. J Neurosurg 44:109–115

Mackay B, Luma MA, Butler JJ (1976) Adult neuroblastoma, electron microscopic observations in nine cases. Cancer 37:1334–1351

Madonick MJ, Rubinstein LJ, Rona Dacso M, Ribner H (1963) Chromophobe adenoma of pituitary gland with subarachnoid metastases. Neurology (Minneap) 13:836–840

Madrazo I, Sanchez Cabrera JM, Maldonado Leon JA (1979) Pipette suction for atraumatic extraction of intraventricular cysticercosis cysts. J Neurosurg 50:531–532

Maffei WE (1937) Tumores do sistema nervoso. Rev Neurol Psiquiatr (S. Paulo) 3:65–105

Magee PN, Barnes JM (1956) The production of malignant primary hepatic tumors in the rat by feeding dimethylnitrosamine. Br J Cancer 10:114–122

Magee PN, Pegg AE, Swann PF (1975) Molecular mechanisms of chemical carcinogenesis. In: Grundmann E (ed) Geschwülste/Tumors II. Virale and chemische Carcinogenese. Springer, Berlin Heidelberg New York (Handbuch der allgemeinen Pathologie, vol VI, part 6, pp 329–419)

Magilligan DJ Jr, Rogeis JS, Knighton RS, Davila JC (1976) Pulmonary neoplasm with solitary cerebral metastasis. Results of combined excision. J Thorac Cardiovasc Surg 72:690–698
Magnus R, De Kleijn A (1912) Die Abhängigkeit des Tonus des Extremitätenmuskels von der Kopfstellung. Pflügers Arch 145:455
Magrath IT, Mugerwa J, Bailey I, Olweny C, Kiryabuire Y (1974) Intracerebral Burkitt's lymphoma: pathology, clinical features and treatment. Q J Med 43:489–508
Mahaim C (1953) Les tumeurs pinéales et leurs formes malignes avec métastases spinales. Schweiz Arch Neurol Psychiatr 71:1–37
Mahaley MS, Brooks WH, Roszman TL, Bigner DD, Dudka L, Richardson S (1977a) Immunobiology of primary intracranial tumors. J Neurosurg 46:467–476
Mahaley MS, Gentry RE, Bigner DD (1977b) Immunobiology of primary intracranial tumors: 2. The evaluation of chemotherapy and immunotherapy. Protocols using the avian sarcoma virus glioma model. J Neurosurg 47:35–43
Mahoney W (1936) Die Epidermoide des Zentralnervensystems. Z Gesamte Neurol Psychiatr 155:416–471
Mair WGP, Erdohazi M (1978) Ultrastructure of the medulloblastoma. J Neuropathol Exp Neurol 37:652
Majerszky-Santha K (1943) Craniospinale Meningeome. Arch Psychiatr Nervenkr 116:648–657
Majlessi H, Shariat AS, Katirai A (1978) Nasopharyngeal craniopharyngioma. J Neurosurg 49:119–120
Makrycostas K (1927) Über das Wirbelangiom, -lipom und -osteom. Virchows Arch [A] 265:259–303
Mallory FB (1902) Three gliomata of ependymal origin: Two in the fourth ventricle, one subcutaneous over the coccyx. J Med Res 8:1–13
Mallory FB (1904/1905) A contribution to the classification of tumors. J Med Res 13:113
Mallory FB (1914) Principles of pathologic histology. Saunders, Philadelphia
Mallory T (1920) The type cell of the so-called dural endothelioma. J Med Res 41:349–365
Manasse (1896) Zur Histologie und Histogenese der primären Nierengeschwülste. Virchows Arch [A] 143:278, 145:113
Mancuso TF (1963) Tumors of the central nervous system. Industrial considerations. Acta Un Int Cancer 19:488–489
Mandybur TI (1974) Melanotic nerve sheath tumors. J Neurosurg 41:187–192
Manganiello LOJ, Nichols P (1955) Intraventricular Torula granuloma. J Neurosurg 12:306–310
Manganiello LOJ, Daniel EF, Hair LQ (1966) Lipoma of the corpus callosum. J Neurosurg 24:892–894
Mani RL, Hedgcock MW, Mass SI, Gilmor RL, Enzmann DR, Eisenberg RL (1978) Radiographic diagnosis of meningioma of the lateral ventricle. Review of 22 cases. J Neurosurg 49:249–255
Mann I, Yates PC, Ainslie JP (1953) Unusual case of double primary orbital tumor. Br J Ophthalmol 37:758–762
Manno NJ, Uihlein A, Kernohan JW (1962) Intraspinal epidermoids. J Neurosurg 19:754–765
Mannweiler K, Palacios O (1961) Ultrastrukturelle Untersuchungen an menschlichen Hirntumoren und deren Gewebskulturen. Untersuchungen an Oligodendrogliomen. Beitr Pathol Anat 125:325–356
Mansfield JB (1977) Primary fibrosarcoma of the skull. Case report. J Neurosurg 47:785–787
Mansuy L, Allègre G, Courjon J, Tommasi M, Thierry A (1967) Analyse d'une série opératoire de 49 oligodendrogliomes. Avec 3 localisations infra-tentorielles. Neurochirurgie 13:679–700
Mansuy L, Thierry A, Tommasi M (1975) Oligodendrogliomas. In: Vinken PJ, Bruyn GW (eds) Tumours of the brain and skull. North-Holland, Amsterdam/American Elsevier, Oxford (Handbook of clinical neurology, vol 18, part III, pp 81–104)
Manuelidis EE (1965) Long-term lines of tissue cultures of intracranial tumors. J Neurosurg 22:368–373
Manuelidis EE (1971) Glioma in trauma. In: Minckler J (ed) Pathology of the nervous system, vol II. McGraw-Hill, New York, pp 2237–2240

Manuelidis EE, Solitare GB (1971) Glioblastoma multiforme. In: Minckler J (ed) Pathology of the nervous system, vol II. McGraw-Hill, New York, pp 2026–2071
Manzini C, Serra P (1952) I gliomi multipli dell'encephalo. Acta Neurochir (Wien) 2:249–273
Marburg O (1909) Normale und pathologische Histologie der Zirbeldrüse. Arb Neurol Inst Univ Wien 17:217
Marburg O (1913) Die Klinik der Zirbeldrüsenerkrankungen. Ergeb Inn Med Kinderheilk 10:146
Marburg O (1921) Zur Kenntnis der neuroepithelialen Geschwülste. Blastoma ependymale. Arb Neurol Inst Univ Wien 23:192–221
Marburg O (1931) Zur Kenntnis der sog. Medulloblastome (Sphäroblastoma polymorph). Dtsch Z Nervenheilkd 117/119:289–308
Marburg O (1934) Unfall und Hirngeschwulst. Springer. Wien
Marburg O (1935) Über Reizgeschwülste und meningeale Tumoren. Virchows Arch [A] 294:759–773
Marchand F (1907) Beitrag zur Kenntnis der Geschwülste des Ganglion Gasseri. In: Festschrift für G.E. von Rindfleisch. Engelmann, Leipzig, pp 265–290
Marchesani O (1930) Untersuchungen über die Glia: II. Mitteilung (das Glioma retinae). Arch Augenheilkd 103:484–510
Marcos F (1954) Über ein hochgradig polymorphes Meningeom mit langsamem Wachstum. Angiomatöses Meningeom mit 15-jähriger Vorgeschichte. Zentralbl Neurochir 14:304–307
Marcovich AW, Jessico CM, Walker AE (1941) Immediate and late effects of intrathecal injection of iodised poppy seed oil. Arch Neurol Psychiatry 45:570
Marie P (1886) Sur deux cas d'acromégalie: hypertrophie singulière non-congénitale des extrémités supérieuses, inférieures, et céphaliques. Rev Méd 6:297
Marinesco G, Draganesco S (1935) Formations télangiectasiques méningées avec processus angiomateux intramédullaires. Rev Neurol (Paris) 63:809–827
Marinesco G, Goldstein M (1933) Sur une forme anatomique, non encore décrite, de médulloblastome: médullo-myoblastome. Ann Anat Pathol (Paris) 10:513–525
Mark J, Granberg I (1970) The chromosomal aberration of double-minutes in three gliomas. Acta Neuropathol (Berl) 16:194–204
Markesbery WR, Duffy PE, Cowen D (1973) Granular cell tumors of the central nervous system. J Neuropathol Exp Neurol 32:92–109
Markesbery WR, Brooks WH, Milsow L, Mortara RH (1976) Ultrastructural study of the pineal germinoma in vivo and in vitro. Cancer 37:327–337
Markiewicz T (1935) Über Spätschädigungen des menschlichen Gehirns durch Röntgenstrahlen. Z Gesamte Neurol Psychiatr 152:548–568
Markwalder TM, Markwalder RV, Markwalder HM (1979) Meningioma of the anterior part of the third ventricle. J Neurosurg 50:233–235
Marquardt B (1941) Über ein umschriebenes Arachnoidalsarkom des Kleinhirns. Z Gesamte Neurol Psychiatr 171:117–127
Marsden HB (1974) Cerebral rhabdomyosarcoma. Arch Dis Child 49:498
Martin F, Lemmen LJ (1952) Calcification in intracranial neoplasms. Am J Pathol 28:1107–1131
Martin HE, Blady JV (1940) Cancer of nasopharynx. Arch Otolaryngol 32:692–727
Martin J, Davis L (1943) Intracranial dermoid and epidermoid tumors. Arch Neurol Psychiatry 49:56–70
Martin JP (1931) Two cases of oligodendroglioma: with remarks on the general clinical features of such cases. Brain 54:330–349
Martin P (1929) Tumors of the brain and syphilis. Arch Surg 18:1531–1541
Martin P, Cushing H (1923) Primary gliomas of the chiasm and optic nerves. Arch Ophthalmol 52:209–241
Martinez R, Vaquero J, Cabezudo J, Areitio E, Bravo G (1981) Neurinomas of the jugular foramen in children. J Neurosurg 54:693–695
Martins AN (1974) Pituitary tumors and intrasellar cysts. In: Vinken PJ, Bruyn GW (eds) Tumors of the brain and skull. North-Holland, Amsterdam/American Elsevier, New York (Handbook of clinical neurology, vol 17, part II, pp 375–439)

Martuza RL, Kornblith PL, Liszczak TM (1977) Characteristics of human optic gliomas in tissue culture. J Neurosurg 46:78–84
Marty R, Minckler DS (1973) Radiation myelitis simulating tumor. Arch Neurol 29:352–354
Marx P, Kleihues P, Zülch KJ (1968) Normale und pathologische Anatomie des Mittelhirns. Radiologe 8:335–347
Maseritz IH (1942) Neurogenic sarcoma. J Bone Joint Surg 24:586–594
Mason GA, Hart-Mercer J, Millar EJ, Strang LB, Wynne NA (1957) Adrenaline-secreting neuroblastoma in an infant. Lancet II:322–325
Massey EW, Brannon WL (1980) Cylindroma causing Garcin's syndrome. Arch Neurol 37:786
Masson CB, Dreyfuss R (1925) Neurogliocytome embryonaire du vermis. Rev Neurol (Paris) 2:227
Masson MT (1934) Gliomes cérébraux et traumatismes craniens. Thesis University of Paris
Masson P (1970) Human tumors. Wayne State University Press, Detroit
Matakas F, Cervós-Navarro J (1970) The ultrastructure of medulloblastomas. Acta Neuropathol (Berl) 16:271–284
Mathai KV, Chandy J (1967) Tuberculous infections of the nervous system. Clin Neurosurg 14:145–177
Mathé G, Rappaport H, O'Conor GT, Torloni H (1976) Histological and cytological typing of neoplastic diseases of haematopoietic and lymphoid tissues. International histological classification of tumors 14. World Health Organization, Geneva
Matheis H (1960) Die Cryptococcose (Torulose) des Nervensystems. Dtsch Z Nervenheilkd 180:595–639
Mathon K, Filsak E (1962) Das supraselläre Epidermoid. Bemerkungen zu der neurologischen, ophthalmologischen und röntgenologischen Symptomatologie. Ophthalmologica 144:231–243
Matson DD (1964) Craniopharyngioma. Clin Neurosurg l10:116–129
Matson DD, Crigler JF Jr (1969) Management of craniopharyngioma in childhood. J Neurosurg 30:377–390
Matson DD, Crofton FDL (1960) Papilloma of the choroid plexus in childhood. J Neurosurg 17:1002–1027
Matsuda I, Kikuchi H, Furuse S, et al (1976) Dermoid tumor in left cerebellum. A case report. No Shinkei Geka 4:597–604
Matsukado Y, MacCarty CS, Kernohan JW (1961) The growth of glioblastoma multiforme (astrocytomas, grades 3 and 4) in neurosurgical practice. J Neurosurg 18:636–644
Matsukado Y, Yokota A, Marubayashi T (1975) Rhabdomyosarcoma of the brain. Case report. J Neurosurg 43:215–221
Matsuoka Y, Hossmann K-A (1981) Corticosteroid therapy of experimental tumour oedema. Neurosurg Rev 4:185–190
Matsutani M (1976) Ultrastructural study of pinealoma in view of its histogenesis (In Japanese). No To Shinkei 28:41–56
Matsutani M, Nagai M, Takakura K, Sano K (1975) Ultrastructural study of pinealoma in view of its histogenesis. In: Proceedings of the VII International Congress of Neuropathology, Budapest, September 1974. Excerpta Medica, Amsterdam/Akadémiai Kiado, Budapest, pp 413–416
Mattern WC, Blattner RE, Werth J, Shuman R, Bloch S, Leibrock LG (1980) Eight nerve lipoma. J Neurosurg 53:397–400
Matthews WB (1965) Sarcoidosis of the nervous system. J Neurol Neurosurg Psychiatry 28:23–29
Matthews WB (1979) Neurosarcoidosis. In: Vinken PJ, Bruyn GW (eds) Neurological manifestation of systemic diseases. North-Holland, Amsterdam (Handbook of clinical neurology, vol 38, part I, pp 521–542
Mattos-Pimenta A, Brandt P (1960) Die tierischen Parasiten und Pilzinfektionen im zentralen Nervensystem. In: Olivecrona H, Tönnis W (eds) Klinik und Behandlung der raumbeengenden intrakraniellen Prozesse. Springer, Berlin Göttingen Heidelberg (Handbuch der Neurochirurgie, vol 4/1, pp 673–727)
Mattos-Pimenta A, Maffei WE (1950) Neuroepithelioma cerebral. J Bras Neurol 2:21–29

Mattos-Pimenta A, Bastos de Olivera F, Maffei WE (1956) Die Boecksche Krankheit. Bericht über einen neurochirurgischen Fall. Acta Neurochir (Wien) 4:261–276
Maunoury R, Vedrenne C, Constans JP (1975) Infiltrations lymphocytaires dans les gliomes humains. Neurochirurgie 21:213–222
Maunsell HW (1889) Subtentorial hydatid tumor removed by trephining: recovery. N Zeal Med J 2:151–156
Mawas MJ, Autrevaux Y de (1930) Gliome du nerf optique. Bull Soc Ophthalmol Fr 43
Mayer RJ, Berkowitz RS, Griffiths CT (1978) Central nervous system involvement by ovarian carcinoma. A complication of prolonged survival with metastatic disease. Cancer 41:776–783
Mayers MM, Kaufman DM, Miller MH (1978) Recent cases of intracranial tuberculomas. Neurology (Minneap) 28:256–260
Mayo CM, Barron KD (1966) Concurrent glioma and primary intracranial sarcoma. Neurology (Minneap) 16:662–672
Mayo CW, Baker GS, Smith LR (1953) Presacral tumors: differential diagnosis and report of case. Proc Staff Meet Mayo Clin 28:616–622
McCann W, Weir BKA, Elvidge AR (1968) Long-term survival after removal of metastatic malignant melanoma of the brain. Report of two cases. J Neurosurg 28:483–487
McCarty KS, Bredesen DE, Vogel FS (1978) Neoplasms of the anterior pituitary. Neurosurgery 3:96–104
McConnell TH, Leonard JS (1967) Microangiomatous malformations with intraventricular hemorrhage. Neurology (Minneap) 17:618–620
McCormack TJ, Plassche WM, Lin S-R (1978) Ruptured teratoid tumor in the pineal region. J Comput Assist Tomogr 2:499–501
McCormick WF (1964) Intramedullary spinal cord schwannoma. A unique case. Arch Pathol 77:378–382
McCormick WF, Halmi NS (1971) Absence of chromophobe adenomas from a large series of pituitary tumor. Arch Pathol 92:231–238
McCormick WF, Nofzinger JD (1966) „Cryptic“ vascular malformations of the central nervous system. Neurosurgery 24:865–875
McCormick WF, Gerber HW, Mergner WJ (1967) Prolonged survival with extensive astrocytoma. J Neurosurg 27:449–455
McDonald JV, Colgan J (1964) Arachnoidal cysts of posterior fossa. Neurology (Minneap) 14:643–646
McDonald J, Parker JC, Brown S, Page LK, Wolfe DL (1978) Cerebral metastasis from a malignant thymoma. Surg Neurol 9:58–60
McDonald P (1973) Malignant sacrococcygeal teratoma. A report of 4 cases. Am J Roentgenol 118:444–449
McDonnell DE (1977) Pineal epidermoid cyst. Surg Neurol 7:387–391
McDonnell DE, Pollock P (1978) Cerebral cystic hemangioblastoma. Surg Neurol 10:195–199
McGavran MH (1970) Neurogenous nasal neoplasms. Ann Otol 79:547–550
McGrath JT (1962) Intracranial pathology of the dog. Acta Neuropathol [Suppl] (Berl) 1:3–4
MckCraig W (1937) Intracranial tumors of sisters, occurring at approximately the same age and presenting similar syndromes. Proc Staff Meet Mayo Clin 12:798–800
MckCraig W, Horrax G (1949) The occurrence of hemangioblastomas (two cerebellar and one spinal) in three members of a family. J Neurosurg 6:518–529
MckCraig W, Wagener HP, Kernohan JW (1941) Lindau-von Hippel disease. A report of four cases. Arch Neurol Psychiatry 46:36–54
McLean AJ (1930) Die Craniopharyngealtaschentumoren. Z Gesamte Neurol Psychiatr 126:639–682
McLean AJ (1934) Cytoid bodies. Arch Ophthalmol 12:391–403
McLean AJ (1935) Tuberkel des Gehirns. Z Gesamte Neurol Psychiatr 154:18
McLean AJ (1936a) Intracranial tumors. In: Bumke O, Foerster O (eds) Raumbeengende Prozesse. Springer, Berlin (Handbuch der Neurologie, vol 14, pp 131–168)
McLean AJ (1936b) Paraphysial cysts. Arch Neurol 36:485–512
McNeel DP, Leavens ME (1968) Long-term survival with recurrent metastatic intracranial melanoma. Case report. J Neurosurg 29:91–93

Mechtijeva ND (1954) Klinisch-histologische Analyse der Tumoren der Fossa cranii occipitalis. (in Russian) Vopr Nevrokhir 18:44–48
Medley BE, McLeod RA, Houser OW (1976) Tuberous sclerosis. Semin Roentgenol 11:35–54
Meduna LJ von (1930) Tuberöse Sklerose und Gliom. Z Gesamte Neurol Psychiatr 129:679–712
Meese W, Grumme T (1975) Hirnmetastasen des Chorionepithelioma malignum. Zentralbl Neurochir 36:93–99
Meller K (1963) Modifikation der Silberimprägnation zur Darstellung der Zellen des Oligodendroglioms im Paraffinmaterial. Acta Neuropathol (Berl) 2:497–500
Mena H, Garcia JH (1978) Primary brain sarcomas, light and electron microscopic features. Cancer 42:1298–1307
Mendiratta SS, Rosenblum JA, Strobos RJ (1967) Congenital meningioma. Neurology (Minneap) 17:914–918
Mennel HD (1966) Selektive Erzeugung von Carcinomen und Esthesioneuroepitheliomen in der Nasenhöhle von Ratten durh *N*-Nitrosopiperidin und *N,N'*-Dinitrosopiperazin bei subcutaner Injektion. Dissertation, Faculty of Medicine, University of Freiburg
Mennel HD (1972) Gewebekulturuntersuchungen an experimentell erzeugten, transplantierten malignen Neurinomen. J Neurol 201:269–278
Mennel HD (1974) Experimental tumors of the nervous system. Recent results. Cancer Res 44:158–169
Mennel HD (1977) Experimental tumors of the nervous system. In: Grundman E (ed) Special topics in carcinogenesis. Springer, Berlin Heidelberg New York, pp 158–169 (Recent results in cancer research, vol 44)
Mennel HD (1978) Transplantation of tumors of the nervous system, induced by resorptive carcinogens: I. Histological investigations of intracerebrally transplanted tumors of the central nervous system. Neurosurg Rev 1:123–131
Mennel HD (1980) Short-term tissue culture observations of experimental primary and transplanted nervous system tumors. J Neuropathol Exp Neurol 60:639–660
Mennel HD, Bücheler J (1974a) Experimental ependymomas: in vivo and in vitro morphology. Z Krebsforsch 82:65–74
Mennel HD, Bücheler J (1974b) Experimentally induced malignant neurinomas as transplantable tumors. Morphology and in vitro behaviour. Acta Neuropathol (Berl) 27:153–161
Mennel HD, Groneck P (1977) Quantitative aspects of transplantation of experimentally induced tumors of the nervous system. Acta Neuropathol (Berl) 40:145–150
Mennel HD, Szymas J (1978) Chemotherapy of brain tumors – Experimental results. In: Frowein RA, Wilcke O, Karimi-Nejad A, Brock M, Klinger M (eds) Head injuries, tumors of the cerebellar region. Springer, Berlin Heidelberg New York, pp 289–291
Mennel HD, Zülch KJ (1971a) The significance of recent experiments on the production of tumours of the nervous system. In: Proceedings of the German Society for Neurosurgery: Modern aspects of neurosurgery, vols 1–2. Excerpta Medica Foundation, Amsterdam, pp 381–387
Mennel HD, Zülch KJ (1971b) Die Morphologie maligner Tumoren des peripheren Nerven. Zentralbl Neurochir 32:11–24
Mennel HD, Zülch KJ (1972a) Formale Pathogenese experimenteller Hirntumoren. Acta Neuropathol (Berl) 21:140–153
Mennel HD, Zülch KJ (1972b) Zur Morphologie transplazentar erzeugter neurogener Tumoren beim Goldhamster. Acta Neuropathol (Berl) 21:194–203
Mennel HD, Zülch KJ (1976) Tumours of the central and peripheral nervous system. In: Turusov VS (ed) Pathology of tumours in laboratory animals: Tumours of the rat. World Health Organization, Lyon (IARC scientific publications, no 6, vol I, part II, pp 295–312)
Mennel HD, Sato K, Zülch KJ (1971) Traumatische Regeneration und Resorptivkarzinogene am Zentralnervensystem. Acta Neurochir (Wien) 25:197–206
Mennel HD, Wechsler W, Zülch KJ (1974) Morphologie und Morphogenese der durch Diäthylnitrosamin erzeugten Nasenhöhlentumoren beim Goldhamster. Beitr Pathol 151:134–156
Mennel HD, Bücheler J, Zülch KJ (1975) In vitro and in vivo morphology of experimental neuroepithelial tumors. VIIth International Congress of Neuropathology, Budapest 1974. Excerpta Medica Foundation, Amsterdam, pp 421–424

Mennel HD, Petrovici JN, Heiss WD, Zülch KJ (1982) Comparative studies of chemotherapeutic effectiveness upon brain neoplasia in men and experimental animals. In: Hildebrand J, Gangji D (eds) Treatment of neoplastic lesions of the nervous system. Pergamon Press, Oxford

Mennenga M (1936) Zur Klinik und Pathologie der Lindau'schen Erkrankung. Bruns Beitr Klin Chir 164:633–639

Mercuri S, Russo A, Palma L (1981) Hemispheric supratentorial astrocytomas in children. Long-term results in 29 cases. J Neurosurg 55:170–173

Meredith JM, Belter LF (1959) Malignant meningioma. Case report of a parasagittal meningioma of the right cerebral hemisphere with multiple extracranial metastases to the vertebrae, sacrum, ribs, clavicle, lungs, liver, left kidney, mediastinum and pancreas. South Med J 52:1035–1040

Merland JJ, Tempier P, Rancurel G, Bories J, Buge A (1977) Tentative de traitement par embolisation d'une volumineuse tumeur glomique tympano-jugulaire et rétropharyngée. Rev Neurol (Paris) 133:621–626

Merriam GR Jr (1950) Retinoblastoma; analysis of 17 autopsies. Arch Ophthalmol 44:71–108

Merzbacher L, Uyeda (1910) Gliastudien. Das reaktive Gliom und die reaktive Gliose. Z Gesamte Neurol Psychiatr 1:285–317

Metzel E (1963) Über die familiär gehäuften Gliome. Arch Psychiatr Nervenkr 204:537–555

Metzel E (1964) Betrachtungen zur Genetik der familiären Gliome. Acta Genet Med Gemellol (Roma) 13:124–131

Meyer A (1920) Herniation of the brain. Arch Neurol Psychiatry 4:387–400

Meyer HH (1937) Über Besonderheiten corticaler Gliome und ihre Abgrenzbarkeit gegen Tumoren der Meningen. Virchows Arch [A] 300:296–318

Meyer HH, Scheller H (1937) Über ein Fibromyxom des Gehirns. Virchows Arch [A] 300:473–486

Meyer JE (1948) Pubertas praecox bei einer hyperplastischen Mißbildung des Hypothalamus. Ein Beitrag zur Frage des Sexualzentrums und der Neurosekretion im Zwischenhirn. Arch Psychiatr Nervenkr 179:378–415

Meyer R (1979/1920) Beitrag zur Verständigung über die Namensgebung in der Geschwulstlehre. Zentralbl Allg Pathol 30:291–296

Meyermann R, Kletter G (1976) Comparative evaluation of various histological techniques for the rapid diagnosis of brain tumours. Acta Neurochir (Wien) 35:171–180

Meyer-Schwickerath G (1947) Über Gliomrosetten und ähnliche Gebilde. Albrecht von Graefes Arch Ophthalmol 148:139–151

Mickle JP, McLennan JE (1975) Malignant teratoma arising within a lipomeningocele. J Neurosurg 43:761–763

Mikruz G, Mydla F, Gütter W (1977) Chordoma: Ultrastructural, biochemical and cytophotometric findings. Beitr Pathol 161:150–165

Miller AA, Ramsden F (1963) Primary reticulosis of the central nervous system. „Microgliomatosis". Acta Neurochir (Wien) 11:439–478

Miller AA, Ramsden F (1966) A cerebral neuroblastoma with unusual fibrous tissue reaction. J Neuropathol Exp Neurol 25:328–340

Miller CA, Torack RM (1970) Secretory ependymoma of the filum terminale. Acta Neuropathol (Berl) 15:240–250

Miller CA, Lloyd TV, Johnson JC, Hunt WE (1978) Eosinophilic granuloma of the base of the skull. J Neurosurg 49:464–466

Miller NR, Epstein MH (1975) Giant intracranial dermoid cyst: Case report and review of the literature on intracranial dermoids and epidermoids. Can J Neurol Sci 2:127–134

Millis RR, Holmes AE (1973) Enterogenous cyst of the spinal cord with associated intestinal reduplication, vertebral anomalies, and a dorsal dermal sinus. Case report. J Neurosurg 38:73–77

Miltz H, Thal H-U (1978) Catamnestic examinations of patients with cerebellar tumors. Adv Neurosurg 5:266–268

Min K-W, Gyorkey F, Haplert B (1975) Primary rhabdomyosarcoma of the cerebrum. Cancer 35:1405–1411

Minauf M, Summer K (1972) Primäre Melanoblastose der Leptomeningen. Wien Z Nervenheilkd 30:150–157

Minauf M, Jellinger K, Grunnert V (1970) Zur Häufigkeit und Morphologie supratentorieller Ependymome im Erwachsenenalter. Acta Neurochir (Wien) 22:181–193

Mincy JE, Lee LC (1966) Intracranial metastasis of sweat gland carcinoma. J Neurosurg 25:564–566

Minkowski M (1941) Über metastatische Hirngeschwülste. Schweiz Arch Neurol Psychiatr 46:41–157

Minkowski M (1969) Über jahrzehntelanges Überleben mit erstaunlicher beruflicher Rehabilitation in einem Fall von nicht-operiertem Kleinhirnbrückenwinkeltumor. Schweiz Arch Neurol Neurchir Psychiatr 103:93–106

Misugi K, Liss L (1970) Medulloblastoma with cross-striated muscle. A fine structural study. Cancer 25:1279–1285

Misugi K, Liss L, Bradel EJ (1967) Electron microscopic study of an ectopic pinealoma. Acta Neuropathol (Berl) 9:346–356

Mitsumori K, Otsuka K, Iwasaki J, Yada K (1975) Osteochondroma of the high cervical spine – a case report – (In Japanese). No Shinkei Geka 3:867–871

Mittal MM, Gupta NC, Sharma ML (1970) Spinal epidural meningioma associated with increased intracranial pressure. Neurology (Minneap) 20:819–820

Mittelbach M (1935) Über Gliome mit Metastasen. Beitr Pathol Anat 95:538–572

Mitts MG, Walker AE (1964) Autotransplantation of gliomas. J Neuropathol Exp Neurol 23:324–333

Miyake E (1979) Establishment of a human oligodendroglial cell line. Acta Neuropathol (Berl) 46:51–55

Mizutani T, Goldberg HI, Kerson LA, Murtagh F (1981) Cavernous hemangioma in the diencephalon. Arch Neurol 38:379–382

Modan B, Mart H, Baidatz D, Steinitz R, Levin SG (1974) Radiation-induced head and neck tumours. Lancet II:277–279

Modesti LM, Binet EF, Collins GH (1976) Meningiomas causing spontaneous intracranial hematomas. J Neurosurg 45:437–441

Möller A, Hatam A, Olivecrona H (1978) The differential diagnosis of pontine angle meningioma and acoustic neuroma with computed tomography. Neuroradiology 17:21–23

Möller HU (1929) Familial angiomatosis retinae et cerebelli (Lindau's disease). Acta Ophthalmol (Copenh) 7:244–260

Möller HU (1944) Ophthalmic symptoms and heredity in cerebellar angioreticuloma. Acta Psychiatr Neurol Scand 19:275–292

Moersch FP, Love JG, Kernohan JW (1940) Melanoma of the central nervous system. Report of 34 cases. JAMA 115:2148–2155

Moersch FP, MckCraig W, Kernohan JW (1941) Tumors of the brain in aged persons. Arch Neurol Psychiatr 45:235–245

Moghimi M (1965) Giant-cell fibrosarcoma of brain. Case report. J Neurosurg 22:81–85

Mohandas S, Ahuja GK, Sood VP, Virmani V (1978) Aspergillosis of the central nervous system. J Neurol Sci 38:229–233

Mohr W (1952) Die Mykosen: Die Aktinomykose und verwandte Fadenpilzerkrankungen. In: von Bergmann G, Frey W, Schwiegk H (eds) Infektionskrankheiten. Springer, Berlin Göttingen Heidelberg (Handbuch der Inneren Medizin, vol I/I, pp 903–927)

Monakow C von (1924) Gliom und Schädeltrauma. Schweiz Arch Neurol Psychiatr 14:289–300

Money RA, Halliday GC (1965) Neurinomas of the facial nerve. J Neurosurg 23:539–541

Moniz E (1940) Die cerebrale Angiographie und Plebographie. Springer, Berlin (Monographien aus dem Gesamtgebiet der Neurologie und Psychiatrie, Heft 70, Ergänzungsserie zum Handbuch der Neurologie II)

Moniz E (1942) Angioma venoso do corpo estriado. Sindroma parquinsónico lateralizado. Communicação feita à Academia das Ciéncias na Sessão de 19 de Febereiro de 1942. Impr Méd (Lisboa) 4, Ano VIII

Monro P, Smith JF (1968) The distinction between central neurofibromatosis and tuberous sclerosis. Acta Neuropathol (Berl) 11:87–91

Moody DM, Ghatak NR, Kelly DL Jr (1976) Extensive calcification in a tumor of the glomus jugulare. Neuroradiology 12:131–135
Moore BW, McGregor D (1965) Chromatografic and electrophoretic fraction of soluble proteins of brain and liver. J Biol Chem 240:1647–1653
Moore BW, Perez VJ (1966) Specific acidic proteins of the nervous system. In: Carlson FP (ed) Physiological and biochemical aspects of nervous integration. Prentice Hall, New Jersey, pp 343–359
Moore MT (1954) Diffuse cerebrospinal gliomatosis masked by syphilis. J Neuropathol Exp Neurol 13:129–143
Moore MT, Book MH (1966) Congenital cervical ependymal cyst. J Neurosurg 24:558–561
Moore MT, Eisinger G (1963) Extra primary seeding of glioblastoma multiforme in the subarachnoid space and ependyma. Neurology (Minneap) 13:855–865
Moossy J, Wilson CB (1967) Solitary intracranial plasmocytoma. Arch Neurol 16:212–216
Morantz RA, Shain W (1978) Trauma and brain tumor: An experimental study. J Neuropathol Exp Neurol 37:662
Morantz RA, Feigin J, Ransohoff J (1976) Clinical and pathological study of 24 cases of gliosarcoma. J Neurosurg 45:398–408
Morantz RA, Shain W, Cravioto H (1978) Immune surveillance and tumors of the nervous system. J Neurosurg 49:84–92
Morantz RA, Kepes JJ, Batnitzky S, Masterson BJ (1979) Extraspinal ependymomas. J Neurosurg 51:383–391
Morelli RJ (1966) Intracranial neurilemmoma of the hypoglossal nerve. Neurology (Minneap) 16:709–713
Morelli RJ (1973) Teratoma of the fourth ventricle. J Neurosurg 38:355–357
Morello A, Cooper IS (1953) Cerebral lipoidolgranuloma. Neurology (Minneap) 3:886–889
Morello G, Bianchi M (1963) Cerebral hemangioblastomas. Review of literature and report of two personal cases. J Neurosurg 20:254–264
Morello G, Borghi GP (1973) Cerebral angiomas. Acta Neurochir (Wien) 28:135–155
Morello G, Lombardi G (1964) Choroido-ependymal cyst of the spinal roots. Case report. J Neurosurg 21:1103–1107
Morello G, Migliavacca F (1964) Primary choroid papillomas in the cerebello-pontine angle. J Neurol Neurosurg Psychiatry 27:445–450 (1964)
Morgan KT, Frith CH, Swenberg JA, McGrath JT, Zülch KJ, Crowder DM (1984) A morphologic classification of brain tumors found in several strains of mice. JNCI 72:151–160
Mori K, Iwayama K, Fujita Y (1974) Malignant suprasellar teratoma in a girl with elevated serum gonadotropin (In Japanese). No Shinkei Geka 2:243–248
Mori T, Takaku A, Mineura K, Hori S, Suzuki J (1977) Follow-up study of fourth ventricle tumors in childhood. Neurol Surg 5:965–972
Mørk SJ, Berg-Jensen M, Hangen A (1979) Cerebellar ganglioglioma. J Neurosurg 51:562–564
Morris AA (1947) The use of the smear technique in the rapid histological diagnosis of tumors of the central nervous system. J Neurosurg 4:497
Mortara RH, Markesberg WR, Brooks WH (1974) Pontine cyst presenting as trigeminal pain. Case report. J Neurosurg 41:636–639
Mosca L, Vasallo G (1970) Morfologia dei tumori ipofisari nell'uomo. Atti Soc Ital Endocrinol 13:339–401
Moscovic EA, Azar HA (1967) Multiple granular cell tumors („myoblastomas"). Cancer 20:2032–2047
Moser KD, Araoz CA, Smith PL (1972) Immunosuppressive therapy and reticulum cell sarcomas of the brain. A report of 2 cases. Panminerva Med 14:436–438
Mosso JA, Verity MA (1975) Ependymal cyst of the spinal cord. Case report. J Neurosurg 43:757–760
Motomochi M, Makita Y, Nabeshima S, Aojama I, Ichijima K, Yamabe H, Kobashi Y (1980) A case of intracranial germinoma with multiple remote metastases (In Japanese). No Shinkei Geka 8:563–570
Mühlichen H-H (1974) Unterschiedliche relative Häufigkeit normaler Mitosephasen und verschiedener charakteristischer Mitosestörungen an Schnittpräparaten von Oligodendro-

gliomen, Ependymomen und Sarkomen. Dissertation, Faculty of Medicine, University of Cologne
Müller D, Orthner H (1965) Intracerebrale Lipoidgranulomatose. Bericht über 2 Fälle. Dtsch Z Nervenheilkd 187:608–636
Müller E (1903) Zur Ätiologie und Pathologie der Geschwülste des Stirnhirns. Dtsch Z Nervenheilkd 23:378–416
Müller E (1913) Über hereditäre multiple cartilaginäre Exostosen und Enchondrosen. Beitr Pathol Natl 57:232–281
Müller E, Schaltenbrand G (1948) Coccidioidose der Meningen. Nervenarzt 19:327–333
Müller H (1858) Über das Vorkommen von Resten der Chorda dorsalis bei Menschen nach der Geburt und über ihr Verhältnis zu den Gallertgeschwülsten am Clivus. Z Rat Med 2:202–229
Müller H-R (1939) Unfall und Hirngeschwulst. Zentralbl Chir 66:1164–1165
Müller J von (1838) Über den feineren Bau und die Formen der krankhaften Geschwülste. Reimer, Berlin
Müller J, Mealey J Jr (1971) The use of time culture in differentiation between angioblastic meningioma and hemangiopericytoma. J Neurosurg 34:341–348
Müller N (1961) Über den sogenannten Pseudotumor cerebri. Med Welt 48:2508–2513
Müller OA, von Werder K (1977) Diagnostik bei Hypophysentumoren. Med Klin 72:1563–1577
Müller R, Wohlfart G (1947) Intracranial teratomas and teratoid tumors. Acta Psychiatr Neurol Scand 22:69–95
Müller R, Wohlfart G (1950) Craniopharyngiomas. Acta Med Scand 138:121–138
Müller W (1933) Änderung des Gewebscharakters nicht radikal operierter Gliome. Z Gesamte Neurol Psychiatr 148:469–477
Müller W (1940) Ungewöhnlicher Fall eines Ependymoma cerebri. Zentralbl Neurochir 5:199–206
Müller W (1954) Zur Frage der hypophysären Tumoren vom Mischtyp. Acta Neuroveg (Wien) 8:451–465
Müller W (1961) Zur Frage der Verkalkung bei der Sturge-Weberschen Krankheit. Zentralbl Neurochir 21:67–74
Müller W (1962a) Über das Pigment im Neurinom. Dtsch Z Nervenheilkd 183:331–339
Müller W (1962b) Beitrag zur Angioarchitektur der Meningeome. Dtsch Z Nervenheilkd 183:467–483
Müller W (1964) Remarks on the histochemistry of brain tumors. In: Zülch KJ, Woolf AL (eds) Classification of brain tumours. Acta Neurochir (Suppl) (Wien) 10:80–84
Müller W (1965) Untersuchungen über die Lipoide im Neurinom. Verh Dtsch Ges Pathol 49:338–341
Müller W (1967) Histochemische Untersuchungen an menschlichen Medulloblastomen. Acta Neuropathol (Berl) 8:96–99
Müller W (1969) Pathologie der Hypophysentumoren. In: Kracht J (ed) Oestrogene Hypophysentumoren. Paper presented at the 15th Symposium of the Deutsche Gesellschaft für Endokrinologie. Springer, Berlin Heidelberg New York, pp 206–222
Müller W (1973) Über das Vorkommen von Glioblastomen im kaudalen Hirnstamm. Acta Neurochir (Wien) 28:65–80
Müller W, Hoffmann H (1967) Über Verkalkungen in Hypophysenadenomen. Zentralbl Neurochir 28:287–290
Müller W, Nasu H (1960) Fermenthistochemische Untersuchungen an Neurinomen. Frankfurt Z Pathol 70:417–422
Müller W, Ojak W (1960) Über das Vorkommen von Mitochondrien in Hirntumoren. Dtsch Z Nervenheilkd 180:668–694
Müller W, Pia HW (1953) Zur Klinik und Ätiologie der Massenblutungen in Hypophysenadenomen. Dtsch Z Nervenheilkd 170:326–336
Müller W, Schaefer HE (1974) Beitrag zur morphologischen Onkotypie des Medulloblastoms. Acta Neuropathol (Berl) 30:51–61
Müller W, Schröder R (1968) Zur Diagnostik der Gliome. Neurochirurgia (Stuttg) 11:30–36

Müller W, Tzonos T (1967) Beitrag zur Klinik und Morphologie der Hypophysenadenome. Dtsch Z Nervenheilkd 191:97–124

Müller W, Slowik F, Schröder R (1978) Studies on the biology of medulloblastomas. Adv Neurosurg 5:232–235

Müller W, Klein PJ, Vierbuchen MJ, Uhlenbruck G (1980) Lectin binding sites in the choroid plexus and choroid plexus papillomas. Neurosurg Rev 3:57–65

Mugnaini E, Forstrønen PF (1967) Ultrastructural studies on the cerebellar histiogenesis. I. Differentiation of granule cells and development of glomeruli in the chick embryo. Z Zellforsch 77:115–143

Mukoyama M, Gimple K, Poser CM (1969) Aspergillosis of the central nervous system. Report of a brain abscess due to *A. funigatus* and review of the literature. Neurology (Minneap) 19:967–974

Mulcahy GM, Harlan WL (1976) Occurrences of central nervous system tumors, with special reference to relative genetic factors. In: Lynch HT (ed) Cancer genetics. Thomas, Springfield, pp 263–300

Mullan JF (1975) Introductory remarks. In: Hekmatpanah J (ed) Gliomas. Springer, Berlin Heidelberg New York, pp 3–5 (Recent results in cancer research, vol 51)

Mundinger F (1966) The treatment of brain tumors with radioisotopes. Prog Neurol Surg 1:202–257

Mundinger F, Metzel E (1968) Erfahrungen mit der lokalen Strahlenbehandlung inoperabler Zwischenhirn- und Basalganglientumoren mit der stereotaktischen Permanent-Implantation von Iridium-192. Arch Psychiatr Nervenkr 212:70–90

Munslow RA (1954) Actinomycotic (nocardia asteroides) brain abscess with recovery. J Neurosurg 11:399–402

Munslow RA, Hill AH (1955) Multiple occurrences of gliomas in a family J Neurosurg 12:646–656

Murali R, Epstein F (1979) Diagnosis and treatment of suprasellar arachnoid cyst. Report of three cases. J Neurosurg 50:515–518

Murphy ES, Lipscomb WR, Bouslog JS (1952) Neurogenic sarcoma treated by surgery and radiotherapy. J Neurosurg 9:214–218

Murray MR (1942) Comparative data on tissue cultures of acoustic neurilemmomas and meningiomas. J Neuropathol Exp Neurol 1:123–124

Murray MR, Stout AP (1947) Distinctive characteristics of the sympathicoblastoma cultivated in vitro. Am J Pathol 23:429–441

Murray MR, Stout AP (1948) A sympathetic ganglioneuroma cultivated in vitro. Cancer 1:242–247

Muthmann A, Sauerbeck E (1903) Über eine Gliageschwulst des 4. Ventrikels. Neuroepithelioma gliomatosum. Beitr Pathol Anat 34:445 (1903)

Myerson PG (1942) Multiple tumors of the brain of diverse origin. J Neuropathol Exp Neurol 1:406–415

Myles ST, Murphy SB (1973) Gliomas of the optic nerve and chiasm. Can J Ophthalmol 8:508–514

Nabawi P, Dobben GD, Mafee M, Espinosa GA (1981) Diagnosis of lipoma of the corpus callosum by CT in five cases. Neuroradiology 21:159–162

Nachlas MM, Tsou K-C, De Souza E, Cheng C-S, Seligman AM (1957) Cytochemical demonstration of succinic dehydrogenase by the use of a new *p*-nitrosophenyl substituted ditetrazole. J Histochem Cytochem 5:420–436

Naeslund J (1926) A study of neuro-epithelioma gliomatosum Upsala Läk-Fören Förh 31:193–222

Naffziger HC, Boldrey EB (1948) Cancer of the nervous system (brain, spinal cord, and peripheral nerves). JAMA 136:96–103

Nag TK, Falconer MA (1966) Enchondroma of the vertebral body: Report of a case causing bilateral sciatica. Br J Surg 53:1067–1071

Nagashima C, Nakashio K, Fujino T (1963) Meningioma and astrocytoma adjacent in the brain. J Neurosurg 20:995–999

Nager GT (1964) Meningiomas involving the temporal bone. Clinical and pathological aspects. With a foreword by Earl Walker. Thomas, Springfield

Nahser HC, Grote W, Löhr E, Gerhard L (1981) Multiple meningiomas. Clinical and computed tomographic observations. Neuroradiology 21:259–263

Naidich TP, Pudlowski RM, Leeds NE, Deck MDF (1978) Hypoglossal palsy: computed tomography demonstration of denervation hemiatrophy of the tongue associated with glomus jugulare tumor. J Comput Assist Tomogr 2:630–632

Nakagawa Y, Tashiro K, Isu T, Tsuru M (1979) Occlusion of cerebral artery due to metastasis of chorioepithelioma. Case report. J Neurosurg 51:247–250

Nakajima K, Ito Z, Fukasawa H (1976) Intracranial extradural liposarcoma in the posterior fossa. A case report. Neurol Surg 4:297–298

Nakamura S, Miyagami M, Morigasu N (1973) Electron microscopic study of ATP use activity in human brain tumors. J Neurosurg 38:420–427

Nakazato Y, Ishida Y, Kawabuchi J (1978) Ganglioneuroblastic differentiation in a pineocytoma. J Neuropathol Exp Neurol 37:665

Napolitano L, Kyle R, Fisher ER (1964) Ultrastructure of meningiomas and the derivation and nature of their cellular components. Cancer 17:233–241

Nass R, Whelan MA (1981) Gangliogliomas. Neuroradiology 22:67–71

Nassar SI, Mount LA (1968) Papillomas of the choroid plexus. J Neurosurg 29:73–77

Nasu H (1964) Fermenthistochemische Untersuchungen an Meningiomen. Acta Neuropathol (Berl) 3:627–637

Nasu H, Müller W (1964) Enzymhistochemische Untersuchungen an Gliomen. Dtsch Z Nervenheilkd 186:67–86

Natarajan M, Rajagopal T, Srinivasan K (1975) A giant schwannoma of cauda equina. Surg Neurol 4:367–368

Natarajan M, Balakrishnan D, Muthu AK, Arumugham K (1975) Maduromycosis of the brain. Case report. J Neurosurg 42:229–231

Navas JJ, Battifora H (1978) Choroid plexus papilloma: Light and electron microscopic study of three cases. Acta Neuropathol (Berl) 44:235–239

Neblett CR, Caram PC, Morris R (1970) Lateral congenital dermal sinus tract associated with an intradiploic dermoid tumor. J Neurosurg 33:103–105

Neidhardt MK (1982) Medulloblastoma treatment protocol of the [German] Society of Pediatric Oncology. Acta Neurochir (Wien) 62:128–129

Neller K, Brunngraber CV, Wechsler W (1969) Klinik, Pathologie und Differentialdiagnose der Großhirnangioblastome. Acta Neurochir (Wien) 21:227–252

Netsky MG (1964) Experimental induction and transplantation of brain tumors in animals. Acta Neurchir [Suppl] (Wien) 10:46–56

Netsky MG, August B, Fowler W (1950) The longevity of patients with glioblastoma multiforme. J Neurosurg 7:261–269

Netsky MG, Shapiro J, Hoffman M, Corsentino B, Freid JR, Zimmerman HM (1956) The effect of single doses of roentgen radiation on experimentally induced gliomas: with a critical review of the effects of roentgen radiation on gliomas in man. Am J Roentgenol 76:351–366

Neubuerger K (1925) Über das Auftreten von Gliomen nach Kriegsschußverletzungen. MMW 13:508–510

Neubuerger KT, Davis CL (1943) Cerebral tumor in a dog resembling human medulloblastoma. Cancer Res 3:243–247

Neubuerger KT, Greene LW (1946) Circumscribed arachnoidal sarcoma of cerebellum. J Neuropathol Exp Neurol 5:233–239

Neubuerger KT, Silcott WL (1941) Angioma simplex of the pons. J Nerv Ment Dis 94:586–592

Neuhauser EBD, Harris GBC Berrett A (1958) Roentgenographic features of neuroenteric cysts. Am J Roentgenol 79:235–240

Neuwelt EA, Glasberg M, Frenkel E, Clark WK (1979) Malignant pineal region tumors. J Neurosurg 51:597–607

Nevin S (1938) Gliomatosis cerebri. Brain 61:170–191

New GB (1947) Neurogenic tumors of nose and throat. Am Otol Rhinol Laryngol 56:228–229

New GB, Devine KD (1947) Neurogenic tumors of the nose and throat. Arch Otolaryngol 46:163–179

Newbill HP, Anderson GC (1944) Racial and sexual incidence of primary intracranial tumors: statistical study of 133 cases verified by autopsy. Arch Neurol 51:564–567

Newton TH, Burhenne HJ, Palubinskas AJ (1962) Primary carcinoma of the pituitary. Am J Roentgenol 87:110–120

Nichols P Jr, Manganiello LOJ (1953) Traumatic arachnoidal cyst simulating acoustic neurinoma. J Neurosurg 10:538–539

Nichols P, Wagner JA (1952) Primary intracranial sarcoma. Report of nine cases with suggested classification. J Neuropathol Exp Neurol 11:215–234

Nicola M, Stochdorph O, Thal HV, Miltz H (1976) Ein myxopapilläres Ependymom des Os sacrum. Zentralbl Neurochir 37:147–151

Nielsen SL, Wilson CB (1975) Ultrastructure of a "pineocytoma". J Neuropathol Exp Neurol 34:148–158

Niemeyer P, Akerman A (1953) Diagnostico e tratamento cirurgico dos aneurismas arterio-venosos do cerebro. Med Cirurg Farm 204:111–147

Nigogosyan G, De la Pava S, Pickren JW (1962) Brain tumor with extracranial metastases. Arch Neurol 6:300–306

Nirmel KN, Aleksie S, Sidhu G, Emancipator S, Ransohoff J, Budzilovich GN (1978) Leiomyosarcoma metastatic to the brain. Surg Neurol 10:147–151

Nisce LZ, Hilaris BS, Chu FCH (1971) A review of experience with radiation of brain metastasis. JAR 111:329–333

Nishii B (1929) Zur Kenntnis der diffusen Sarcomatose des Nervensystems. Arb Neurol Inst Univ Wien 31:116–129

Nishiura I, Takeuchi J, Handa H, Kang SS (1980) Intracranial malignant lymphoma (In Japanese). No Shinkei Geka 8:839–844

Nishiyama RH, Batsakis IG, Weaver DK, Simrall IH (1966) Germinal neoplasms of the central nervous system. Arch Surg 93:342–347

Nittner K (1952) Klinische Fehlbeurteilung eines lumbalen Sanduhrganglioneuroms. Zentralbl Neurochir 12:167–174

Nittner K (1956) Die raumbeschränkenden spinalen Prozesse im Kindes- und Jugendalter. Zentralbl Neurochir 16:348–352

Nittner K (1972) Raumbeengende Prozesse im Spinalkanal (einschließlich Angiome und Parasiten). In: Olivecrona H, Tönnis W (eds) Wirbelsäule und Rückenmark. Springer, Berlin Heidelberg New York (Handbuch der Neurochirurgie, vol 7, part II, pp 1–606)

Nittner K (1976) Spinal meningiomas, neurinomas and neurofibromas and hourglass tumours. In: Vinken PJ, Bruyn GW (eds) Tumours of the spine and spinal cord. North Holland, Amsterdam/American Elsevier, Oxford (Handbook of clinical neurology, vol 20, part II, pp 177–322)

Nittner K, Schiefer W (1955) Multiple Meningeome im Spinalkanal. Zentrabl Neurochir 15:99–103

Nizzoli V, Brizzi R (1964) Traumi cranici e meningiomi. Sist Nerv 16:178–191

Noël J, Méthot Y (1970) La radiothérapie du medulloblastome. Dix ans d'expérience. Union Med Can 99:1848–1851

Noetzel H (1940) Arachnoidalcysten in der Cisterna ambiens. Zentralbl Neurochir 4:281–294

Noetzel H (1951) Über Meningeome und ihre unterschiedlichen Auswirkungen am Gehirn. Beitr Pathol Anat 111:391–406

Noetzel H (1952) Angiome im Gehirn bei einem Fall von tuberöser Sklerose. Dtsch Z Nervenheilkd 168:401–405

Noetzel H (1953) Trauma und Gliom. Vortrag vor der Arbeitsgemeinschaft für Hirntraumafragen in Mainz

Noetzel H (1959) Gliome bei zwei Geschwisterpaaren. Zentralbl Neurochir 19:169–173

Noetzel H (1960) Multiple Angiome im Gehirn bei generalisierter Angiomatosis. Beitr Pathol Anat 123:251–258

Noetzel H, Hauptmann A (1964) Zur Frage der Identität des sogenannten monstrocellulären Hirnsarkoms und des Liposarkoms. Frankfurt Z Pathol 73:535–539

Nötzli M, Malamud M (1962) Postirradiation fibrosarcoma of the brain. Cancer 15:617–622

Nonne M (1904) Über Fälle von Symptomenkomplex „Tumor cerebri" mit Ausgang in Heilung

(Pseudotumor cerebri). Über letal verlaufene Fälle von „Pseudotumor cerebri" mit Sektionsbefund. Dtsch Z Nervenheilkd 27:162–216
Nonne M (1924) Syphilis und Nervensystem, 5th edn. Karger, Berlin
Norlén G (1950) Papillomas of the choroid plexus. Acta Chir Scand 99:273–279
Norstrom CW, Kernohan JW, Love JG (1961) One hundred primary caudal tumors. JAMA 178:1071–1077
Nosaka Y, Nagao S, Tabuchi K, Nishimoto A (1979) Primary intracranial epidermoid carcinoma. J Neurosurg 50:830–833
Nothnagel H (1879) Glandula pituitaria. In: Nothnagel H (ed) Topische Diagnostik der Gehirnkrankheiten. Hirschwald, Berlin, p 538
Nugent GR, Odom GL, Woodhall B (1959) Spinal extradural cysts. Neurology (Minneap) 9:397–406
Numaguchi Y, Kishikawa T, Ikeda J, Tsukamoto Y, Fukui M, Kitamura K, Matsuura K (1980) Angiographic diagnosis of acoustic neurinomas and meningiomas in the cerebellopontine angle – a reappraisal. Neuroradiology 19:73–80
Nurick S, Mair WGP (1970) Brain metastases from haemangioendothelioma of the spleen. Report of a case. Acta Neuropathol (Berl) 14:345–349
Nyström SH (1965) A study on supratentorial meningiomas. With special reference to gross and fine structure. Acta Pathol Microbiol Scand [Suppl] 176:1–90
Obenchain TG, Becker DP (1972) Head bobbing associated with a cyst of the third ventricle. Case report. J Neurosurg 37:457–459
Oberdisse K, Tönnis W (1953) Pathophysiologie, Klinik und Behandlung der Hypophysenadenome. Ergeb Inn Med Kinderheilkd 4:976–1057
Oberling C (1922) Les tumeurs des méninges. Bull Assoc Fr Cancer 11:365–384
Oberling C (1943) A propos des glioses méningées (gliose méningoencéphalique) des centres nerveux et du nerf optique. Rev Can Biol 2:120
Obermann B (1964) Intracranial teratoma replacing brain. Arch Neurol 11:423–426
Obert GJ, Devine KD, McDonald JR (1960) Olfactory neuroblastomas. Cancer 13:205–215
Oblu N, Stanciu A, Dobrescu G (1964) La gomme syphilitique cérébrale. Neurochirurgie 10:361–369
Obrador Alcalde S (1948) Clinical aspects of cerebral cysticercosis. Arch Neurol 59:457–468
Obrador Alcalde S, Lamas E (1955) Cisticerco solitario del cuarto ventriculo. Rev Clin Esp 59:42–64
Obrador Alcalde S, Escalona I (1963) Gliomas encefalicos en la enfermedad de Recklinghausen. Rev Esp Oncol 10:259–278
Obrador Alcalde S, Sanz Ibanez YJ (1955) Tumores intracraneales. Monogr Inst Nac Oncol, Madrid
Obrador Alcalde S, Soto F (1953) Condroma frontal de la hoz del cerebro. Rev Clin Esp 14:257–260
Obrador Alcalde S, Urquiza P (1950) The value of streptomycin in the surgical treatment of intracranial tuberculoma. J Neurol Neurosurg Psychiatry 13:66–70
O'Brien CP, Lehrer HZ, Harkin JC (1968) Extensive oligodendrogliomas of the spinal cord with associated bone changes. Neurology (Minneap) 18:887–890
O'Connor JS, Laws ER (1963) Histochemical survey of brain tumor enzymes. Arch Neurol 9:641–651
O'Connor JS, Laws ER (1969) Changes in histochemical staining of brain tumor blood vessels associated with increasing malignancy. Acta neuropathol (Berl) 14:161–173
Oda Y (1974) Studies on cellular immunity of brain tumors: glial carcinofetal antigens and serum blocking factors in gliomas (In Japanese). Nippon Geka Hokan 43:111–123
Odake G, Yamaki T, Naruse S (1976) Neurenteric cyst with meningomyelocele. J Neurosurg 45:352–356
Oddsson B (1947) Spinal meningioma. Thesis. Munksgaard, Copenhagen
Oehlecker F (1952) Eine ungewöhnlich große Geschwulst des Schädeldaches (Meningeom, Hyperostose). Zentralbl Chir 77:1433–1443
Oehmichen M (1971) Extracerebrale Gliome im Gesichtsbereich. Acta Neuropathol (Berl) 17:321–330
Oehmichen M (1976) Cerebrospinal fluid cytology. Thieme, Stuttgart

Oertelt R (1970) Klinisch-genetische Analyse des von Hippel-Lindau-Syndroms, ausgehend von den Angioblastomen des Kleinhirns (Lindau-Tumoren). Dissertation, Faculty of Medicine, University of Heidelberg

Oeser H (1982) Krebsangst schüren. Ist das ärztlich? Med Tribune 10:41–42

Oeser H, Zülch KJ (1974) Spinale Strahlenspätnekrose mit Querschnitt-Syndrom: eine Fehlbegutachtung? Strahlentherapie 148:303–312

Oestreich R, Slawyk (1899) Riesenwuchs und Zirbeldrüsengeschwulst. Virchows Arch [A] 157:475

Özgen T, Erbengi A, Bertan V, Sağlam S, Gürçay Ö, Pirnar T (1979) The use of computerized tomography in the diagnosis of cerebral hydatid cysts. J Neurosurg 50:339–342

Ogasawara N (1966) Zur Histochemie der Rosenthalschen Fasern. Wien Z Nervenheilkd 23:185–196

Ogawa K, Hamaya K, Fujii Y, Matsuura K, Endo T (1969) Tumor induction by adenovirus type 12 and its target cells in the central nervous system (In Japanese). Gan 60:383–392

Ogle C (1898) Melanotic sarcoma of the pineal body. Br Med J:1745

Oh SJ (1968) Roentgen findings in cerebral paragonimiasis. Radiology 90:292–299

Oh SJ (1978) Paragonimiasis in the central nervous system. In: Vinken PJ, Bruyn GW (eds) Infections of the nervous system. North-Holland, Amsterdam (Handbook of clinical neurology, vol 35, part III, pp 243–266)

Ohmori M (1965) Electron microscopic studies on the tumor induced by adenovirus type 12. Acta Med Okayama 19:199–208

Oi S, Galicich JH (1978) Intracranial metastasis of malignant tumors – The classification of parenchymal type, leptomeningeal type and diffuse type and its clinical significance: 1. Clinical manifestations (In Japanese). No Shinkei Geka 6:29–37

Oi S, Raimondi AJ (1980) Brain tumors in infants and children – factors affecting prognosis: 1. Ependymoma (In Japanese). No Shinkei Geka 8:1049–1055

Oka K, Kitamura K, Fukui M, Nishio S, Nakagaki H (1982) Clinical aspects of hemangioblastoma (In Japanese). No Shinkei Geka 10:909–921

Okawara S-H (1973) Solid cerebellar hemangioblastoma. J Neurosurg 39:514–518

Okonek G (1938) Extracerebrale Arachnoidalcyste der linken Großhirnhemisphäre. Zentralbl Neurochir 2:112–118

Olischer RM, Schröter P (1963) Zur Diagnostik der primären Melanoblastomatose des Zentralnervensystems. Nervenarzt 34:266–270

Olivecrona H (1919) Zwei Ganglioneurome des Großhirns. Virchows Arch [A] 226:1–17

Olivecrona H (1927) Die chirurgische Behandlung der Hirntumoren. Eine klinische Studie. Springer, Berlin

Olivecrona H (1932) On suprasellar cholesteatomas. Brain 55:122–134

Olivecrona H (1934) Die parasagittalen Meningeome. Thieme, Leipzig

Olivecrona H (1941) Chirurgische Behandlung der Geschwülste. In: Krause F (ed) Die spezielle Chirurgie der Gehirnkrankheiten, vol III. Enke, Stuttgart, pp 193–374

Olivecrona H (1947) The parasagittal meningiomas. J Neurosurg 4:327–341

Olivecrona H (1949) Cholesteatomas of the cerebello-pontine angle. Acta Psychiatr Scand 24:639–643

Olivecrona H (1950) Die arteriovenösen Aneurysmen des Gehirns. Dtsch Med Wochenschr 75:1169–1173

Olivecrona H (1952) The cerebellar angioreticulomas. J Neurosurg 9:317–330

Olivecrona H (1967) The surgical treatment of intracranial tumors. In: Olivecrona H, Tönnis W (eds) Klinik und Behandlung der raumbeengenden intrakraniellen Prozesse. Springer, Berlin Heidelberg New York (Handbuch der Neurochirurgie, vol IV, part 4, pp 1–301)

Olivecrona H, Ladenheim J (1957) Congenital arteriovenous aneurysms of the carotid and vertebral arterial systems. Springer, Berlin Göttingen Heidelberg

Olivecrona H, Riives J (1948) Arteriovenous aneurysms of the brain. Arch Neurol Psychiatry 59:567–602

Oliveras de la Riva C (1955) Sarcomas primitivos encefalicos. In: Obrador Alcalde S, Sanz Ibanez YJ (eds) Tumores intracraneales. Monogr Inst. Nac Oncol, Madrid, pp 149–161

Ollier M (1900) Sur une nouvelle affection: La dyschondroplasie. Rev Chir (Paris) 21:396–398

Olvera Rabiela JE, Poucell SL, González Fonseca R (1974) El meduloblastoma desmoplásico. Revision de algunos conceptos a propósito de 10 casos en sujetos adultos. Patologia (Mex) 12:99–111

Onofrio BM, Svien HJ (1976) Solitary and multiple vertebral myelomas. In: Vinken PJ, Bruyn GW (eds) Tumors of the spine and spinal cord. North-Holland, Amsterdam/American Elsevier, Oxford (Handbook of clinical neurology, vol 20, part II, pp 9–18)

Onofrio BM, Kernohan JW, Uihlein A (1962) Primary meningeal sarcomatosis. A review of the literature and report of 12 cases. Cancer 15:1197–1208

Oosthuizen SF, Fainsinger MH (1949) Hydatid disease. Radiology 53:248–254

Opalski A (1934) Studien zur allgemeinen Histopathologie der Ventrikelwände. Z Gesamte Neurol Psychiatr 150:42–74

Oppe W (1897) Zur Kenntnis der Schimmelmykosen beim Menschen. Zentralbl Allg Pathol 8:301–306

Oppenheim H (1907) Beiträge zur Diagnostik und Therapie der Geschwülste im Bereich des zentralen Nervensystems. Karger, Berlin

Oppenheim H, Krause F (1913a) Operative Erfolge bei Geschwülsten der Sehhügel und Vierhügelgegend. Berl Klin Wochenschr 50:2316–2322

Oppenheim H, Krause F (1913b) Partielle Entfernung des Wurms wegen Geschwulstbildung unter breiter Eröffnung des vierten Ventrikels. Berl Klin Wochenschr 50:333

Orbison JA, Reeves N, Leedham CL, Blumberg JM (1951) Amebic brain abscess. Medicine (Baltimore) 30:247–282

Orf G (1970a) „Angioretikulom" der Sella turcica. Acta Neurochir (Wien) 23:63–78

Orf G (1970b) Zur Klinik und Morphologie eines infiltrativen Spinalneurinoms. Arch Psychiatr Nervenkr 213:396–407

Orf G (1972) Neurochirurgische Manifestationsformen sympathischer Neuroblastome. Arch Psychiatr Nervenkr 215:293–314

Ornos M (1939) Positives Röntgenschattenbild eines extramedullären (psammösen) Meningeoms. Schweiz Arch Neurol Psychiatr 44:309–312

Orthner H, Rettinger E (1965) Ein intraventrikuläres Kraniopharyngeom, zugleich ein Beitrag zum hypothalamisch ausgelösten Korsakow-Syndrom. Vergleichende Übersicht über die hypothalamisch auslösbaren Störungen der Merkfähigkeit und des Trieblebens bei Mensch und Tier. Fortschr Neurol Psychiatr 33:299–331

Ortmann R (1961) Chemoarchitektonik des Gehirns. Dtsch Med Wochenschr 86:2062–2068

Ortmann R (1964) Über die chemische Spezifität von Neuronensystemen. Prog Brain Res 6:4–25

Orzechowski K von, Kuligowski ZW (1933) Ein Fall von Neuroblastoma verum des Stirnlappens. Z Gesamte Neurol Psychiatr 147:696–712

Osborne RL, Freis ED, Levin AG (1944) Eosinophilic granuloma of bone presenting neurologic signs and symptoms. Arch Neurol 51:452–456

Ostertag B (1936a) Die Einzelformen der Verbildungen (einschließlich Syringomyelie). In: Scholz W (ed) Nervensystem. Springer, Berlin (Handbuch der speziellen Pathologie, Anatomie und Histologie, vol XIII, part 4, pp 363–601)

Ostertag B (1936b) Einteilung und Charakteristik der Hirngewächse. Fischer, Jena

Ostertag B (1941) Pathologie der raumfordernden Prozesse des Schädelbinnenraumes. In: Krause F (ed) Spezielle Chirurgie der Gehirnkrankheiten, vol III. Enke, Stuttgart, pp 375–624

Ostertag B (1952) Die Onkotopik der Hirngewächse. J Nerv Ment Dis 116:726–738

Ostertag B, Buschmann H (1941) Wieweit kann Wehrdienstbeschädigung bei Geschwülsten angenommen werden. Med Klin 15:351–353

Osugi T, Matsui T, Hirano A (1977) Fine structure of endothelial cells in meningioma. Excerpta Medica, Amsterdam, pp 101–102 (International congress series, vol 427)

Otani G, Ehrlich JC (1940) Solitary granuloma of bone simulating primary neoplasm. Am J Pathol 16:479

Otenasek FJ, Silver ML (1961) Spinal hemangioma (hemangioblastoma) in Lindau's disease. Report of six cases in a single family. J Neurosurg 18:295–300

Ottomo M, Mita R, Tamura H, Suzuki S (1976) Successfully operated case of posterior fossa tuberculoma in childhood (In Japanese). No Shinkei Geka 4:707–713

Ouyang R, Rozdilsky B (1966) Metastasis of carcinoma to pineal body. Arch Neurol 15:399–403
Oxenhandler DC, Sayers MP (1978) The dilemma of childhood optic gliomas. J Neurosurg 48:34–41
Paarmann HF (1952) Das Retinagliom und seine Metastasen. Zugleich ein Beitrag zur Frage der Knochenmetastasen. Virchows Arch [A] 322:49–65
Pack GT, Ariel IM (1958) Trauma inducing sarcomas. In: Pack GT (ed) Tumors of soft somatic tissues. A clinical treatise. Hoeber-Harper, New York
Paillas JE, Combalbert A (1964) Evolution comparée des gliomes du cerveau: A propos d'une statistique opératoire de 333 cas observés avec les mêmes méthodes durant une même décennie. Rev Neurol (Paris) 111:43–60
Paillas J, Roger J, Bonnal J, Tamalet J (1950) Epilepsie partielle contenue de Kojewnikoff dans un cas de syphilome. Rev Neurol (Paris) 83:302–304
Paillas JE, Serratrice G, Legré J (1963) Les tumeurs primitives du rachis. Masson, Paris
Paillas JE, Alliez B, Pellet W (1976) Primary and secondary tumours of the spine. In: Vinken PJ, Bruyn GW (eds) Tumors of the spine and spinal cord. North-Holland, Amsterdam/ American Elsevier, Oxford (Handbook of clinical neurology, vol 20, part II, pp 19–54)
Paillas JE, Prince MA, Hassoun J, Pellet W, Peragut JC (1979) L'apport de la chimiothérapie au traitement conventionnel des gliomes malins du cerveau. Rev Neurol (Paris) 135:251–262
Pakula H, Mennel HD, Zülch KJ (1978) Gross vascularization of experimentally induced transplanted tumors of the central and peripheral nervous system. Acta Neuropathol (Berl) 43:185–190
Pal AK, Chopra SK, Samanta HK (1979) Primary melanoma of the leptomeninges. Indian J Pathol Microbiol 17:187–189
Palacios E, Azar-Kia B (1975) Malignant metastasizing angioblastic meningiomas. J Neurosurg 42:185–188
Palma L (1975) Supratentorial neuroepithelial cysts. Report of two cases. J Neurosurg 42:353–357
Palma L, DiLorenzo N (1976) Spinal endodermal cysts without associated vertebral or other congenital abnormalities. Acta Neurochir (Wien) 33:283–300
Palma L, DiLorenzo N, Guidetti B (1978) Lymphocytic infiltrates in primary glioblastomas and recidivous gliomas. J Neurosurg 49:854–861
Palma L, DiLorenzo N, Nicole S (1979) Developmental CSF cysts of the posterior fossa. Neurosurg Rev 2:159–169
Palmer FJ, Poulgrain AP (1978) Metastatic melanoma simulating subdural hematoma. Case report. J Neurol 49:301–302
Palmer JJ (1972) Haemangioblastomas. A review of 81 cases. Acta Neurochir (Wien) 27:125–148
Pannier S, Got C, Bourgeois-Gavardin M, Lacert P, Piera JB, Grossiord A (1977) Paraplégie et Bilharziose. Rev Neurol (Paris) 133:165–173
Papadakis N, Millan J, Grady DF, Segerberg LH (1971) Medulloblastoma of the neonatal period and early infancy. Report of two cases. J Neurosurg 34:88–91
Papo I, Salvolini U (1974) Meningiomas of the free margin of the tentorium developing in the pineal region. Neuroradiology 7:237–243
Pappenheim E, Bhattacharji SK (1962) Primary melanoma of the central nervous system: clinical-pathological report of a case with survey and discussion of the literature. Arch Neurol 7:101–113
Pappenheimer AM (1910) Über Geschwülste des Corpus pineale. Virchows Arch [A] 200:122
Parker EF, Kernohan JW (1931) The relation of injury and glioma of the brain. JAMA 97:535–539
Parker JC jr, McCloskey JJ, Solanki KV, Goodman NL (1976) Candidosis: the most common postmortem cerebral mycosis in an endemic fungal area. Surg Neurol 6:123–128
Parkinson D (1969) Intracranial phaeochromocytomas (active glomus jugulare). Case report. J Neurosurg 31:94–100
Parkinson D, Childe AE (1952) Colloid cyst of the fourth ventricle. Report of a case of two colloid cysts of the fourth ventricle. J Neurosurg 9:404–409

Parkinson D, Hall CW (1962) Oligodendrogliomas simultaneous appearance in frontal lobes of siblings. J Neursurg 19:424–426

Parr JC (1948) Tuberous sclerosis with cerebral neoplasm; report of case benefited by surgery. NZ Med J 47:550–559

Parsons M, Pallis CA (1965) Intradural spinal tuberculomas. Neurology (Minneap) 15:1018–1022

Pasquier B, Couderc P, Pasquier D, Hong PM, Pellat J (1975) Primary rhabdomyosarcoma of the central nervous system. Acta Neuropathol (Berl) 33:333–342

Pasquier B, Couderc P, Pasquier D, Panh HM, Arnould JP (1978) Primary malignant melanoma of the cerebellum. Cancer 41:344–351

Pasquier B, Pasquier D, N'Golet A, Panh MH, Couderc P (1979) Le potentiel métastatique des tumeurs primitives du système nerveux central. Rev Neurol (Paris) 135:263–278

Passerini A, Bertazzoli A (1965) Cranial and vertebral metastases from thyroid tumors and from "benign metastasising goitres". Acta Neurol Scand 41:419–430

Patrick BS, Smith RR, Bailey TO (1974) Aseptic meningitis due to spontaneous rupture of craniopharyngioma cyst. Case report. J Neurosurg 41:387–390

Patterson RH, Campbell WG, Parsons H (1961) Ependymoma of the cauda equina with multiple visceral metastases. Report of a case. J Neurosurg 18:145–150

Paul F (1926) Beitrag zur Histopathologie der Ganglioneurome des Zentralnervensystems. Beitr Pathol Anat 75:221–228

Peake GT, McKeel DW, Jarett L, Daughaday WH (1969) Ultrastructural, histologic and hormonal characterization of a prolactin-rich human pituitary tumor. J Clin Endocrinol Metab 29:1383–1393

Pearl GS, Mirra SS, Miles ML (1979) Medulloblastomas and related CNS neoplasms: An ultrastructural study. J Neuropathol Exp Neurol 38:334

Pedersen H, Gjerris F, Klinken L (1981) Computed tomography of benign supratentorial astrocytomas of infancy and childhood. Neuroradiology 21:87–91

Pedersen O, Geyer H (1938) Diskordantes Auftreten von Hirntumoren bei erbgleichen Zwillingen. Zentralbl Neurochir 3:53–63

Peers JH (1936) The occurrence of tumors of the CNS in routine autopsies. Am J Pathol 12:911

Peers JH (1940) The response of the central nervous system to the application of carcinogenic hydrocarbons. II. Methylcholanthrene. Am J Pathol 16:799–816

Peet MM cited in Kahn EA, Basset RC, Schneider RC, Crosby EC (1929) Correlated neurosurgery. Thomas, Springfield

Peillon F, Racadot J, Moussy D, Vila-Porcile E, Olivier L, Racadot O (1978) Prolactin-secreting adenomas. A correlative study of morphological and clinical data. In: Fahlbusch R, Werder K von (eds) Treatment of pituitary adenomas. Thieme, Stuttgart, pp 114–122

Peirce CB (1964) The efficacy of radiation therapy in the treatment of tumors of the brain and brain stem. Proceedings of the Congress on Neurologic Surgery, Houston 1962. Clin Neurosurg 10:195–211

Peison WB, Feigin I (1961) Suprasellar meningioma containing metastatic carcinoma. Report of case. J Neurosurg 18:688–689

Pelgrom von Motz I, Bots GTAM, Endtz LJ (1977) Astrocytoma in three sisters. Neurology (Minneap) 27:1038–1041

Pelletier G (1971) Classification et physiopathologie des tumeurs hypophysaires. Union Med Can 100:1779–1783

Peña CE, Felter R (1973) Ultrastructure of a composite glioma-sarcoma of the brain. Acta Neuropathol (Berl) 23:90–94

Pendl G (1975) Meningiomas in childhood. Adv Neurosurg 2:121–124

Penfield W (1927) Principles of the pathology of neurosurgery. In: Nelson's loose leaf surgery, New York, pp 303–347

Penfield W (1931) The classification of gliomas and neuroglia cell types. Arch Neurol Psychiatr 26:745–753

Penfield W (1932a) Cytology and cellular pathology of the nervous system. Hoeber, New York

Penfield W (1932b) Tumors of the sheaths of the nervous system. In: Penfield W (ed) Cytology and cellular pathology of the nervous system. Hoeber, New York, pp 955–990

Penfield W, Ward A (1948) Calcifying epileptogenic lesions (hemangioma calcificans). J Neuropathol Exp Neurol 7:111
Penfield W, Young AW (1930) The nature of v. Recklinghausen's disease and the tumors associated with it. Arch Neurol 23:320–344
Penfield W, Erickson TC, Tarlov I (1940) Relation of intracranial tumors and symptomatic epilepsy. Arch Neurol Psychiatr 44:300–315
Pennybacker J (1954) Recurrence in cerebellar haemangiomas. Zentralbl Neurochir 14:63–73
Pennybacker J, Meadows S (1938) Normal ventriculograms in tumours of the cerebral hemispheres. Lancet I:186–190
Pennybacker J, Russell DS (1943) Spontaneous ventricular rupture in hydrocephalus, with subtentorial cyst formation. J Neurol Neurosurg Psychiatry 6:38–45
Pennybacker J, Russell DS (1948) Necrosis of the brain due to radiation therapy. J Neurol Neurosurg Psychiatry 11:183–198
Penzholz H (1968) Die metastatischen Erkrankungen des Zentralnervensystems bei bösartigen Tumoren. Springer, Wien
Percy AK, Elveback LR, Okazaki H, Kurland LT (1972) Neoplasms of the CNS: epidemiological considerations. Neurology (Minneap) 22:40–48
Perey J, Chevrey ML, Beltau A, Richier ME (1955) Tumeur de la region hypophysaire à structure de séminome. Rev Neurol (Paris) 92:76–80
Perlmutter I, Horrax G, Poppen JL (1950) Cystic hemangioblastomas of the cerebellum: End results in 25 verified cases. Surg Gynecol Obstet 91:89–99
Perot P, Weir B, Rasmussen T (1966) Tuberous sclerosis. Surgical therapy for seizures. Arch Neurol 15:498–506
Perria L, Sacchi U (1950) Incidenza del fattore età e dello stroma tumorale sul decorso del glioblastoma. Sist Nerv 2:176–186
Perria L, Viale GL (1966) A chemical approach to the problem of cellular malignancy in tumours of the nervous system. Acta Neurochir (Wien) 15:33–39
Perria L, Viale G, Andreussi L, Ibba F, Viale E (1964) Istocitochimica dei tumori endocranici. Neuropsichiatria 20:420–538
Perria L, Viale GL, Rosa M (1971) Remarks on the pathology and surgery of midline intracranial angiomas. Neurochirurgia (Stuttg) 14:71–78
Perrin EV (1958) Extracranial metastases from intracranial gliomata. Am J Clin Pathol 30:244–251
Perthes P (1919) Glückliche Entfernung eines Tumors des Plexus chorioideus aus dem Seitenventrikel des Cerebrum. MMW 66:677–678
Pertuiset B (1975) Craniopharyngiomas. In: Vinken PJ, Bruyn GW (eds) Tumors of the brain and skull. North-Holland, Amsterdam/American Elsevier Oxford (Handbook of clinical neurology, vol 18, part III, pp 531–572)
Pertuiset B, Virot A, Metzger J (1976) Diagnosis of pinealoblastomas by positive response to cobalt-therapy. Acta Neurochir (Wien) 34:151–152
Peters G (1939) Zur Pathogenese der Sturge-Weberschen Krankheit. Z Gesamte Neurol Psychiatr 164:365–379
Peters G (1951) Beitrag zur Pathologie und Klinik der Meningiome. Dtsch Z Nervenheilkd 167:83–101
Peters G (1952) Hirntrauma und Gliom. Fortschr Neurol Psychiatr 20:403–422
Peters G, Tebelis F (1937) Beitrag zur Klinik, Anatomie und Pathogenese der Sturge-Weberschen Krankheit. Z Gesamte Neurol Psychiatr 157:782–794
Petit-Dutaillis D (1933) Traitement chirurgical des méningites séreuses. Rev Neurol (Paris) 40:919–938
Petit-Dutaillis D, Bertrand I (1932) Fibroblastome profond, intracérébral de l'hémisphère gauche, sans connexions méningées décelables. Ablation de la tumeur. Guérison operatoire. Rev Neurol (Paris) 2:96–100
Petit-Dutaillis D, Messimy R, Benhain (1952) A propos du diagnostic des chordomes sphéno-occipitaux. Rev Otoneuroophthalmol 24:202–206
Petrovici JN, Ilsen H-W (1978) Chemotherapy of brain tumors. In: Frowein RA, Wilcke O, Karimi-Nejad A, Brock M, Klinger M (eds) Head injuries, tumors of the cerebellar region. Springer, Berlin Heidelberg New York, pp 292–296

Pette H (1936a) Die verschiedenen Formen der Meningitis serosa. Zentralbl Neurochir 1:86–98

Pette H (1936b) Pachymeningitis und Leptomeningitis. In: Bumke O, Foerster O (eds) Erkrankungen der Wirbelsäule, des Schädels mit Nebenhöhlen und der Hüllen. Springer, Berlin (Handbuch der Neurologie, vol 10, pp 268–412)

Pfeifer RA (1951) Die Darstellungen von Lymphströmungen im inneren Milieu des Gehirns. Geest and Portig, Leipzig

Pfeiffer SE, Wechsler W (1972) Biochemically differentiated neoplastic clone of schwann cells. Proc Natl Acad Sci USA 69:2885–2889

Pfleger L, Tappeiner J (1959) Zur Kenntnis der systemisierten Endotheliomatose der cutanen Blutgefäße (Reticuloendotheliose?). Hautarzt 10:359–363

Pfreundschuh M, Shiku H, Takahashi T, Ueda R, Ransohoff J, Oettgen HF, Old LJ (1978) Serological analysis of cell surface antigens of malignant human brain tumors. Proc Natl Acad Sci USA 75:5122–5126

Phillips TL, Sheline GE, Boldrey E (1964) Therapeutic considerations in tumors affecting the central nervous system. Ependymomas. Radiology 83:98–105

Pia HW (1953) Prognose der Schläfenlappengeschwülste. Dtsch Z Nervenheilkd 171:137–147

Pia HW (1957) Die Schädigung des Hirnstammes bei den raumfordernden Prozessen des Gehirns. Acta Neurochir [Suppl] (Wien) 4

Pia HW (1973) Diagnosis and treatment of spinal angiomas. Acta Neurochir (Wien) 28:1–12

Pia HW (1977) Die Hirngliome. Dtsch Ärzteblatt 18:1189–1192

Pia HW (1979) Treatment of intramedullary angiomas. Adv Neurosurg 7:64–75

Pia HW, Djindjian R (1978) Spinal angiomas. Advances in diagnosis and therapy. Springer, Berlin Heidelberg New York

Pia HW, Vogelsang H (1965) Diagnose und Therapie spinaler Angiome. Dtsch Z Nervenheilkd 187:74–96

Pia HW, Gleave JRW, Grote E, Zierski J (1975) Cerebral angiomas. Springer, Berlin Heidelberg New York

Pick L, Bielschowsky M (1911) Über das System der Neurome und Beobachtungen an einem Ganglioneurom des Gehirns nebst Untersuchung über die Genese der Nervenfasern in „Neurinomen". Z Gesamte Neurol Psychiatr 6:391–437

Pickel VM, Reis DJ, Marangos PJ, Zomzely-Neurath CE (1975) Immunocytochemical localization of nervous system specific protein (NSP-R) in rat brain. Brain Res 105:184–188

Piepgras U, Hirth R, Städtler F, Kammerer V (1972) Chondroblastoma of the temporal bone, an unusual cause of increasing intracranial pressure. Neuroradiology 4:25–29

Pierce GB Jr (1966) Ultrastructure of human testicular tumors. Cancer 19:1963–1983

Pierce GB, Abell MR (1970) Embryonal carcinoma of the testis. Pathol Annu 5:27–60

Piganiol G, Billé J, Bérard U, Paillas JE (1964) Tumeurs géantes de la queue de cheval. Neurochirurgie 10:211–229

Pilleri G, Lechi A, Carreras M (1974) Symmetric syphilitic gummas of the frontal lobes. Arch Psychiatr Nervenkr 219:207–221

Pineda A (1964a) Multicentric gliomas. Report of a patient with a thalamic astrocytoma associated with a rare primary neurohypophyseal tumor. J Neurosurg 21:805–811

Pineda A (1964b) Submicroscopic structure of acoustic tumors. Neurology (Minneap) 14:171–184

Pineda A (1965) The "lemmocyte" in peripheral nerve tumors. J Neurosurg 22:594–601

Pinheiro J, Mello AR (1943) Consideracões sôbre a cisticercose encefalica. Arq Serv Nac Doenç (Rio):773

Pinkerton H, Weinman D (1940) Toxoplasma infection in man. Arch Pathol 30:374–392

Pinto F (1958) Meningeoma do cavum de meckel. Rev Bras Cirurg 35:100–102

Pinto F (1969) Zusammentreffen eosinophiler Hypophysenadenome mit nicht nervalen bösartigen Körpergeschwülsten. Zentralbl Neurochir 30:303–308

Pinto F, Pinto A (1957) Craniofaringeomas. Rev Bras Cirurg 34:226–230

Pinto F, Pinto A (1959) Beitrag zur chirurgischen Behandlung der Retinoblastome. Zentralbl Neurochir 19:13–20

Pinto F, Pinto A, Vaz JLM, Viera da Silva AS (1957) Colesteatomas. Rev Bras Cirurg 34:622–625

Pinto Pupo P, Mattos Pimenta A (1949) Cisticercose do IV ventriculo: consideracões anatomoclinicas e sobre a terapeutica cirurgica. Arq Neuropsiquiatr 7:274–291

Piotrowski W, Brock M, Klinger M (1984) CNS metastases. Neurosurgery in the aged. Springer, Berlin Heidelberg New York Tokyo

Piramoon AM, Abbassioun K (1974) Mediastinal enterogenic cyst with spinal cord compression. J Pediatr Surg 9:543–545

Piscol K, Hoffmann G (1961) Das primäre Melanoblastom des Zentralnervensystems (unter Berücksichtigung neurochirurgischer Probleme). Neurochirurgia (Stuttg) 4:1–26

Pitkethly DT, Hardman JM, Kempe LG, Earle KM (1970) Angioblastic meningiomas. Clinicopathologic study of 81 cases. J Neurosurg 32:539–544

Pitlyk PJ, Dockery MB, Miller RH (1965) Hemangiopericytoma of the spinal cord. Report of three cases. Neurology (Minneap) 15:649–653

Placzek S, Krause F (1907) Zur Kenntnis der umschriebenen Arachnitis adhaesiva cerebralis. Berl Klin Wochenschr 24:911–918

Plair CM, Perry S (1962) Hypothalamic-pituitary sarcoidosis. A clinical and pathological entity; report of a case. Arch Pathol 74:527–535

Plath von (1884) Hyperplasie der Plexus chorioidei laterales bei Hydrocephalus internus congenitus. Jb Kinderheilkd 21:419

Plewes JL, Jacobson I (1971) Familial frontonasal dermoid cysts. Report of four cases. J Neurosurg 34:683–686

Poche R, Hoffmann U (1968) Über die allgemeine Krebshäufigkeit und die Altersverteilung einzelner Organkrebse in Düsseldorf von 1908–1964. Ergeb Allg Pathol Pathol Anat 50:26–62

Poirier J, Escourolle R (1967) Ultrastructure des neurinomes de l'acoustique. Z Mikrosk Anat Forsch 76:509–529

Poirier J, Escourolle R (1970) Definition ultrastructurale des neurinomes de l'acoustique. Neurochirurgie (Suppl 1) 16:7–12

Poirier J, Escourolle R, Castaigne P (1968) Les neurofibromes de la maladie de Recklinghausen. Etude ultrastructurale et place nosologique par rapport aux neurinomes. Acta Neuropathol (Berl) 10:279–295

Polak M (1966) Blastomas del sistema nervioso central y periferico. Patologia y ordenación histogenética. Lopez Libreros Editores, Buenos Aires.

Polak M (1967) On the true nature of the so-called medulloblastoma. Acta Neuropathol (Berl) 8:84–95

Pollice L, Marzullo F (1970) Il medulloblastoma desmoplastico. Tumori 56:93–101

Polmeteer FE, Kernohan JW (1947) Meningeal gliomatosis. Arch Neurol Psychiatry 57:593–616

Pomerat CM, Goldblatt D (1961) Observations on glioblastoma multiforme transferred from Guinea pig eye to cell culture. Clin Neurosurg 7:123–137

Ponfick E (1882) Die Actinomykose des Menschen, eine neue Infektionskrankheit auf vergleichend pathologischer und experimenteller Grundlage geschildert. Berlin

Pool JL (1968) Gliomas in the region of the brain stem. J Neurosurg 29:164–167

Pool JL, Kamrin RP (1966) The treatment of intracranial gliomas by surgery and radiation. Prog Neurol Surg 1:258–299

Poon TP, Hirano A, Zimmerman HM (1971) Electron microscopic atlas of brain tumors. Grune and Stratton, New York

Poon TP, Arida EJ, Tyschenko WP (1980) Cerebral cysticercosis with aqueductal obstruction. Case report. J Neurosurg 53:252–255

Popoff NA, Ellsworth RM (1971) The fine structure of retinoblastoma. In vivo and in vitro observations. Lab Invest 25:389–402

Popoff NA, Malinin TI, Rosomoff HL (1974) Fine structure of intracranial hemangiopericytoma and angiomatous meningioma. Cancer 34:1187–1197

Popovitch ER, Sutton CH, Becker NH, Zimmerman HM (1970) Fine structure and histochemical studies of choristomas of the neurohypophysis. J Neuropathol Exp Neurol 39:155–156

Poppen JL, Marino R (1968) Pinealomas and tumors of the posterior portion of the third ventricle. J Neurosurg 28:357–368

Portugal JR, Brock M (1964) On the pathogenesis of the Dandy-Walker-Brodal syndrome. Zentralbl Neurochir 23:80–97
Poser CM (1956) The relationship between syringomyelia and neoplasm. Thomas, Springfield
Posner JB (1977) Management of central nervous system metastases. Semin Oncol 4:81–91
Posner JB, Shapiro WR (1975) Brain tumor. Current status of treatment and its complications. Arch Neurol 32:781–784
Posnikoff J, Stratford J (1960) Carcinoma metastasis to malignant glioma. Case report. Arch Neurol 3:559–563
Posselt A (1932) Die vielkammerige Blasenwurmgeschwulst außerhalb der Leber (extrahepatitischer Alveolarechinokokkus). Erg Allg Pathol 26:423–611
Post KD, Jackson JMD, Reichlin S (1980) The pituitary adenoma. Plenum, New York
Potter JM (1955) Angiomatous malformations of the brain: Their nature and prognosis. Ann R Coll Surg Engl 16:227–243
Pouillart P, Schwarzenberg L, Amiel JL, et al. (1975) Combinaisons chimiothérapiques de drogues se potentialisant: III. Applications aux tumeurs du système nerveux central. Nouv Presse Med 4:721–724
Pouillart P, Mathé G, Poisson M, et al. (1976) Essai de traitement des glioblastomes de l'adulte et des métastases cérébrales par l'association d'adriamycine, de VM 26 et de CCNU. Nouv Presse Med 5:1571–1575
Pouillart P, Mathé G, Thy TH, et al (1977) Treatment of malignant gliomas in adults using combination of adriamycin, VM 26 and CCNU. Results of a type-II trial. Eur J Cancer 13:419–424
Pou-Serradell A, Llovet-Tapies J, Galito E, Pascual J (1978) Neurinome intracrânien du nerf spinal. Rev Neurol (Paris) 134:803–805
Prakash B, Roy S, Tandon PN (1980) Schwannoma of the brain stem. J Neurosurg 53:121–123
Preissig RS, Preissig SH, Goree JA (1976) Angiographic demonstration of a cerebral venous angioma. J Neurosurg 44:628–631
Presant CA, Wiernik Ph, Serpick AA (1973) Factors affecting survival in nocardiosis. Am Rev Respir Dis 108:1444–1448
Priesel A (1922) Über Gewebsmißbildungen in der Neurohypophyse und am Infundibulum des Menschen. Virchows Arch [A] 238:423–440
Prieto A, Cantu RC (1967) Spinal subarachnoid hemorrhage associated with neurofibroma of the cauda equina. J Neurosurg 27:63–69
Pritchett PS, King TJ (1978) Dysplastic gangliocytoma of the cerebellum – an ultrastructural study. Acta Neuropathol (Berl) 42:1–5
Probert JC, Lederman M, Bagshaw MA (1973) Medulloblastoma – Treatment and prognosis. Calif Med 118:14–17
Probst A (1971) Kombination eines Cushing Syndroms, Hypophysenadenoms und suprasellären Meningeoms. Zentralbl Neurochir 32:75–82
Probst A, Ulrich J, Zdrojewski B, Hirt H-R (1979) Cerebellar ganglioglioma in a child. J Neuropathol Exp Neurol 38:57–71
Prockop LD, Silva-Hutner M (1967) Cephalic mucormycosis (Phycomycosis). A case with survival. Arch Neurol 17:379–386
Proctor NSF (1955) Intracranial tumors and cysts in the South African Bantu. Excerpta Med (Amst), Sect VIII:788
Pross E, Hill K, Schmitt-Köppler A (1972) Zur Klinik und Histogenese der neurogenen Tumoren des oberen Gastrointestinaltraktes. Dtsch Med Wochenschr 97:899–902
Puech P, Mahoudeau D (1935) Les arachnoidites opto-chiasmatiques. Leur diagnostic et les indications thérapeutiques. Gaz Med France 3:1–24
Putschar W (1930) Zur Pathologie und Symptomatologie der Carcinommetastasen des Zentralnervensystems. Z Gesamte Neurol Psychiatr 126:129–148
Putschar W (1935) Über Angiomatosis des Zentralnervensystems und der Netzhaut („v. Hippel-Lindausches Syndrom“) mit besonderer Berücksichtigung der Pankreasveränderungen. MMW II:1084–1088
Puusepp L (1933) Chirurgische Neuropathologie, vol 2: Das Rückenmark. Krüger, Tartu (Dorpat)
Quain R (1855) Large cyst from the cavity of the arachnoid. Trans Pathol Soc Lond 6:8–10

Quest DO, Brisman R, Antunes JL, Housepian EM (1978) Period of risk for recurrence in medulloblastoma. J Neurosurg 48:159–163
Quick D, Cutler M (1927) Neurogenic sarcoma. A clinical and pathological study. Ann Surg 86:810–829
Quodbach K (1938) Ein Beitrag zur Pathologie der Blastomykosen des Zentral-Nerven-Systems. Zentralbl Allg Pathol 69:227–231
Raaf JE, Kernohan JW (1944) Relation of abnormal collections of cells in posterior medullary velum of cerebellum to origin of medulloblastomas. Arch Neurol Psychiatry 52:163–169
Rabotti GF (1972) Experimental intracranial tumors of viral etiology. In: Kirsch WM, Paoletti D, Grossi-Paoletti E (eds) The experimental biology of brain tumors. Thomas, Springfield, pp 148–180
Racadot I, Vila-Porcile E, Olivier L, Peillon F (1975) Electron microscopy of pituitary tumors. Prog Neurol Surg 6:95–141
Radcliffe A (1951) Ethmoidal fibro-angioma. J Laryngol Otol 65:768–787
Radolsky I van (1935) Tuberkulome des Gehirns. Z Gesamte Neurol Psychiatr 154:18–31
Raimondi AJ (1966) Ultrastructure and the biology of human brain tumors. Prog Neurol Surg 1:1–63
Raimondi AJ, Beckman F (1967) Perineural fibroblastomas: Their fine structure and biology. Acta Neuropathol (Berl) 8:1–23
Raimondi AJ, Mullan S, Evans JP (1962) Human brain tumors. An electron microscopic study. J Neurosurg 19:731–753
Ramamurthi B, Anguli VC, Iyer CGS (1958) A case of intramedullary neurinoma. J Neurol Neurosurg Psychiatr 21:92–94
Ramani PS (1974) Chondromyxoid fibroma: a rare cause of spinal cord compression. Case report. J Neurosurg 40:107–109
Ramina R, Ingunza W, Vonofakos D (1980) Cystic cerebral cavernous angioma with dense calcification. J Neurosurg 52:259–262
Ramon y Cajal S (1908) Nouvelles observations sur l'évolution des neuroblastes. Anat Anz 11:255
Ramon y Cajal S (1952) Histologie du système nerveux de l'homme et des vertébrés. Consejo superior de investigaciones sientificas, vol 1. Instituto Ramon y Cajal, Madrid
Ramsey HJ (1966) Fine structure of hemangiopericytoma and hemangioendothelioma. Cancer 19:2005–2018
Ramsey HJ, Kernohan JW (1964) Circumscribed sarcoma of the cerebellum. J Neuropathol Exp Neurol 23:706–718
Ramsey HL (1965) Ultrastructure of a pineal tumor. Cancer 18:1014–1025
Ramsey RG, Brand WN (1973) Radiotherapy of glioblastoma multiforme. J Neurosurg 39:197–202
Rand CW (1963) Surgical experiences with spinal cord tumors. A survey over a 40-year period. Bull Los Angeles Neurol Soc 28:260–268
Rand CW, Reeves DL (1943) Dermoid and epidermoid tumors (cholesteatomas) of the central nervous system. Report of twenty-three cases. Arch Surg 46:350–376
Rand RW (1952) Multiple spinal cord meningiomas. J Neurosurg 9:310–314
Rand RW, Rand CW (1960) Intraspinal tumors of childhood. Thomas, Springfield
Ranke O (1911) Histologisches zur Gliomfrage. Z Gesamte Neurol Psychiatr 5:690–701
Rao VRK, Pillai SM, Mathews G, Radhakrishnan VV (1978) Cerebral mucormycosis. A case report. Neuroradiology 15:291–293
Rapoport Y, Ruben JR (1974) Malignant ependymoma involving the temporal bone with remote metastasis. Can J Otolaryngol 3:611–617
Rapp (1924) Über die Häufigkeit der Hirntumoren unter dem Sektionsmaterial des pathologischen Instituts Tübingen. Med. Dissertation, Universität Tübingen
Rappaport H (1966) Tumors of the hematopoietic system. Atlas of tumor pathology, sect 3, fasc 8. Armed Forces Institute of Pathology, Washington
Rappaport H (1974) Nouveaux concepts dans la classification des hémopathies malignes. Bull Cancer (Paris) 61:11–12
Raskind R, Beigel F (1964) Brain tumors in early infancy – probably congenital in origin. J Pediatr 65:727–732

Raskind R, Grant S (1966) Primary mesenchymal chondrosarcoma of the cerebrum. Report of a case. J Neurosurg 24:676–678
Rasmussen TB, Kernohan JW, Adson AW (1940) Pathologic classification, with surgical consideration of intraspinal tumors. Ann Surg 111:513–530
Rauch HJ (1944) Zur Entstehung der Ependymome. Z Gesamte Neurol Psychiatr 177:226–237
Raventos A, Gross SW, Pendergrass EP (1960) Sarcoma following radiation injury of skull. Am J Roentgenol 83:145–148
Rawe SE, Van Gilden JC, Rothman SLG (1978) Radiographic diagnostic evaluation and surgical treatment of multiple cerebellar, brain stem, and spinal cord hemangioblastomas. Surg Neurol 9:337–342
Rawlinson DG, Herman MM, Rubinstein LJ (1973) The fine structure of a myxopapillary ependymoma of the filum terminale. Acta Neuropathol (Berl) 25:1–13
Ray BS, Horwith M (1964) Surgical treatment of acromegaly. Clin Neurosurg 10:31–59
Raynor RB (1969) Papilledema associated with tumors of the spinal cord. Neurology (Minneap) 19:700–704
Reagan TJ, Bisel HF, Childs DS, Layton DD, Rhoton AL, Taylor WF (1976) Controlled study of CCNU and radiation therapy in malignant astrocytoma. J Neurosurg 44:186–190
Recklinghausen F von (1863) Ein Herz von einem Neugeborenen, welches mehrere theils nach aussen, theils nach den Höhlen prominierende Tumoren (Myome) trug. Verh Ges Geburtsh 15
Recklinghausen F von (1866) Ein Fall von multiplen Exostosen. Virchows Arch [A] 35:203–207
Recklinghausen F von (1882) Über die multiplen Fibrome der Haut und ihre Beziehungen zu den multiplen Neuromen. In: Virchow R (ed) Festschrift zur Feier des 25-jährigen Bestehens des pathologischen Institutes zu Berlin. Hirschwald, Berlin
Reeves DL (1967) Epidermoid (mixed) tumors of the central nervous system. J Neurosurg 26:21–24
Reeves DL, Dickson DR, Benjamin EL (1965) Phycomycosis (mucormycosis) of the central nervous system. J Neurosurg 23:82–84
Regato IA del (1958) Cancer in children. Cancer seminar, vol 2/III. Penrose Cancer Hospital, Colorado Springs
Reichardt M (1905) Zur Entstehung des Hirndrucks. Dtsch Z Nervenheilkd 28:306
Reichardt M (1957) Das Hirnödem. In: Scholz W (ed) Nervensystem. Springer, Berlin Göttingen Heidelberg (Handbuch der speziellen pathologischen Anatomie, vol 13, I/B, pp 1229–1283)
Reina A (1975) Tuberculous epidural granuloma simulating a herniated lumbar disc. Surg Neurol 4:335–338
Reinhardt G (1928) Trauma – Fremdkörper – Hirngeschwulst. MMW 75:399–401
Remagen W, Missoni L (1964) Außergewöhnlich große Ependymcyste im Mittelhirn. Dtsch Z Nervenheilkd 186:238–245
Remak R von (1854) Beitrag zur Entwicklungsgeschichte der krebshaften Geschwülste. Dtsch Klin 6:170–174
Rengachary SS, Watanabe I (1981) Ultrastructure and pathogenesis of intracranial arachnoid cysts. J Neuropathol Exp Neurol 40:61–83
Rengachary SS, Kishore PRS, Watanabe I (1978) Intradiploic epidermoid cyst of the occipital bone with torcular obstruction. J Neurosurg 48:475–478
Resnikoff S, Cardenas y C. J (1964) Meningioma at the foramen magnum. Case reports. J Neurosurg 21:301–302
Rettelbach E, Schutzbach (1942) Über Sehnerventumoren, ihre Beziehungen zur Neurofibromatosis Recklinghausen und ihr klinisches Krankheitsbild. Albrecht Von Graefes Arch Ophthalmol 145:179–241
Reulen HJ, Graham R, Spatz M, Klatzo I (1977) Role of pressure gradients and bulk flow in dynamics of vasogenic brain edema. J Neurosurg 46:24–35
Reulen HJ, Tsayumu M, Tack A, Fenske AR, Prioleau GR (1978) Clearance of edema fluid into CSF. A mechanism for resolution of vasogenic brain edema. J Neurosurg 48:754–764
Reymond A (1953) Méningites tumorales. Oncologia (Basel) 6:85–91
Reymond A, Ringertz N (1950) L'oligodendrogliome. Schweiz Arch Neurol Psychiatr 65:221–254

Rhodes RH, Davis RL, Kassel SH, Clague BH (1978) Primary cerebral neuroblastoma. A light and electron microscopic study. Acta Neuropathol (Berl) 41:119–124
Ribbert H (1904) Geschwulstlehre. Cohen, Bonn
Ribbert H (1910a) Über das Endotheliom der Dura. Virchows Arch [A] 200:141–151
Ribbert H (1910b) Neuroepithel in Gliomen. Zentralbl Allgem Pathol 21:145–148
Ribbert H (1918) Über das Spongioblastom und das Gliom. Virchows Arch [A] 225:195–213
Ribbert H, Steiner H (1894) Über die Ecchondrosis physalifora sphenooccipitalis, nach Untersuchungen von Hermann Steiner. Zentralbl Allg Pathol 5:457–461
Rich JR (1969) A survey of cerebrospinal fluid cytology. Bull Los Angeles Neurol Soc 34:115–131
Richards P, McKissock W (1968) Intracranial metastasis. Br Med J I:15–18
Richmond IL, Wilson CB (1978) Pituitary adenomas in childhood and adolescence. J Neurosurg 49:163–168
Richmond JJ (1953) Radiotherapy of intracranial tumours in children. J Fac Radiol (Lond) 4:180–189
Richter RB (1951) True hamartoma of the hypothalamus associated with pubertas praecox. J Neuropathol Exp Neurol 10:368–383
Ricoy I, Carillo R, Garcia J, Bravo G (1974) Dissemination of pituitary adenomas. Acta Neurochir (Wien) 31:123–130
Ridley A, Cavanagh JB (1971) Lymphocytic infiltration in gliomas: evidence of possible host resistance. Brain 94:117–124
Riessner D, Zülch KJ (1939) Über die Formveränderungen des Hirns (Massenverschiebungen, Zisternenverquellungen) bei raumbeengenden Prozessen. Dtsch Z Chir 253:1–61
Riggs HE, Clary WU (1957) A case of intramedullary sheath cell tumor of the spinal cord: consideration of vascular nerves as a source of origin. J Neuropathol Exp Neurol 16:332–336
Rinaldi I, Peach WF (1969) Postoperative lumbar meningocele. Report of two cases. J Neurosurg 30:504–507
Ringel SP, Bailey OT (1972) Rathke's cleft cyst. J Neurol Neurosurg Psychiatry 35:693–697
Ringertz N (1937) Histologische Untersuchungen bei Arachnitis. Zentralbl Neurochir 2:356–357
Ringertz N (1950) Grading of gliomas. Acta Pathol Microbiol Scand 27:51–64
Ringertz N (1955) On the question of different histologic types of medulloblastoma. Proceedings of the Second International Congress of Neuropathology, London 1955, part I. Excerpta Medica Foundation, Amsterdam, pp 249–250
Ringertz N (1971) Cancer incidence in Finnland, Iceland, Norway, and Sweden. Munksgaard, Copenhagen (Acta Pathol Microbiol Scand, [A] Suppl 224)
Ringertz N, Nordenstam H (1951) Cerebellar astrocytoma. J Neuropathol Exp Neurol 10:343–367
Ringertz N, Reymond A (1949) Ependymomas and choroid plexus papillomas. J Neuropathol Exp Neurol 8:355–380
Ringertz N, Tola JH (1950) Medulloblastoma. J Neuropathol Exp Neurol 9:354–372
Ringertz N, Nordenstam H, Flyger G (1954) Tumors of the pineal region. J Neuropathol Exp Neurol 13:540–561
Ringertz N, Törnberg B, Sjöstrom A, Swenson D (1962) Cancer incidence in Sweden 1959. National Board of Health, Cancer Registry, Stockholm
Ringertz N, Ericsson J, Mattsson B (1971) Cancer incidence in Sweden 1959–1965. National Board of Health and Welfare, Cancer Registry, Stockholm
Rinke HW (1933) Zur Kenntnis der Ependymome. Z Gesamte Neurol Psychiatr 148:736–752
Rio Hortega P del (1932) Estructura y systematisacion de los gliomas y paragliomas. Arch Esp Oncol 2:411–678
Rio Hortega P del (1944) Contribución al conocimiento citológico de los tumores del nervio y quiasma ópticos. Arch Histol (B. Aires) 2:307–358
Rio Hortega P del (1945) Nomenclatura y clasificacion de los tumores del sistema nervioso. Lopez and Etchefoyen, Buenos Aires [Arch Histol (B. Aires) 3:5–63]
Rio Hortega P del (1962) The microscopic anatomy of tumors of the central and peripheral nervous system. Thomas, Springfield

Rippon JW (1978) Mycosis (pathogenesis and epidemiology). In: Vinken PJ, Bruyn GW (eds) Infections of the nervous system. North-Holland, Amsterdam (Handbook of clinical neurology, vol 35, part III, pp 371–381)
Rish BL, Meacham WF (1968) Intracerebral cystic toruloma. J Neurosurg 28:603–604
Rivera E, Chason JL (1966) Cerebral hemangioblastoma. J Neurosurg 25:452–454
Riverson EA, Zülch KJ (1979) Pineal parenchymal tumours and germinomas (the problem of the so-called pinealomas). Neurosurg Rev 1:3–11
Riverson EA, Brunngraber CV, Zülch KJ (1973) Beitrag zur Frage der ektopischen Pinealome. Zentralbl Neurochir 34:31–40
Riverson EA, Kleihues P, Schultze B, Wechsler W (1966) Experimentelles Hirnödem nach epiduraler Kompression. Verh Dtsch Ges Pathol 50:441–446
Rixford E, Gilchrist TC (1896) Two cases of protozoan coccidioidal infection of the skin and other organs. Johns Hopkins Hosp Rep 1: 209–268
Robert CM, Feigenbaum IA, Stern WE (1973) Ocular palsy occurring with pituitary tumors. J Neurosurg 38:17–19
Robert F, Hardy J (1975) Prolactin-secreting adenomas. Arch Pathol 99:625–633
Roberts M, German WJ (1966) A long-term study of patients with oligodendrogliomas. Follow-up of 50 cases. Including Dr. H. Cushing's series. J Neurosurg 24:697–700
Roberts M, German WJ (1969) Oligodendroglioma: a 40-year survival. J Neurosurg 31:355–357
Robertson HE (1915a) Ein Fall von Ganglioneuroma am Boden des dritten Ventrikels mit Einbeziehung des Chiasma opticum. Virchows Arch 220:80
Robertson HE (1915b) Das Ganglioneuroblastom, ein besonderer Typus im System der Neurome. Virchows Arch [A] 220:147
Robertson DM (1964) Electron microscopic studies of nuclear inclusions in meningiomas. Am J Pathol 45:835–847
Robertson DM, Hetherington RF (1964) A case of ganglioneuroma arising in the pituitary fossa. J Neurol Neurosurg Psychiatry 27:268–272
Robertson DM, MacLean JD (1965) Nuclear inclusions in malignant gliomas. Arch Neurol 13:287–296
Robertson DM, Vogel FS (1962) Concentric lamination of glial processes in oligodendrogliomas. J Cell Biol 15:313–334
Robertson DM, Hendry WS, Vogel FS (1964) Central ganglioneuroma: a case study using electron microscopy. J Neuropathol Exp Neurol 23:692–705
Robinson F, Solitaire GB (1966) Olfactory neuroblastoma. J Neurosurg 25:133–139
Rocca E, Monteagudo E (1953) Tratamiento quirúrgico en la neurocisticercosis racemosa. Bol Acad Péruan Cir 6:34–38
Rochat GF (1931) Großhirnangiom bei der Lindauschen (v. Hippelschen) Erkrankung. Klin Monatsbl Augenheilkd 86:23–27
Rodriguez HA, Berthrong M (1966) Multiple primary intracranial tumors in von Recklinghausen's neurofibromatosis. Arch Neurol 14:467–475
Roemer F (1896) Ein Fall von Endotheliom der Dura mater. Jber Hambg Staats Krk Anst 4:41
Roer H (1956) Plötzlicher Tod durch Zirbelcyste bei einem Kind mit Pubertas praecox. Zentralbl Neurochir 16:229–336
Rössle R (1911) Zwei Fälle von Gliomen auf traumatischer Basis. MMW 58:2530
Rössle R (1939) Das Retothelsarkom der Lymphdrüsen. Seine Formen und Verwandtschaften. Beitr Pathol Anat 103:385–415
Rössle R (1950) Stufen der Malignität. S-Ber Dtsch Akad Wiss, Kl Math Nat Nr 5
Roessmann U, Weiss MH (1972) Giganto-cellular glioblastoma of the lumbosacral spinal cord. Acta Neuropathol (Berl) 20:264–266
Röttgen P (1937) Weitere Erfahrungen an kongenitalen arterio-venösen Aneurysmen. Zentralbl Neurochir 2:18–33
Röttgen P, Peters G (1952) Über „Massenblutungen“ in Hypophysenadenomen. Zentralbl Neurochir 12:65–73
Roger H, Paillas JE (1939) Syphilis et tumeurs cérébrales. Marseille Méd 76:831–837
Rohr H (1958) Hirn- und Rückenmarksläsionen durch metastasierende Kolloidstrumen. Acta Neurochir (Wien) 6:93–114

Rokitansky C von (1855/56) Lehrbuch der pathologischen Anatomie, vol I–II. Braunmüller, Wien
Roman B (1913) Zur Kenntnis des Neuroepithelioma gliomatosum. Virchows Arch [A] 211:126
Romansky SG, Crocker DM, Shaw KNF (1978) Ultrastructural studies of neuroblastoma. Evaluation of cytodifferentiation and correlation of morphology and biochemical and survival data. Cancer 42:2392–2399
Romeis B (1940) Innersekretorische Drüsen: II. Hypophyse. In: Möllendorff W von (ed) Blutgefäss- und Lymphgefässapparat, innersekretorische Drüsen. Springer, Berlin (Handbuch der mikroskopischen Anatomie des Menschen, vol VI/3, pp 1–625)
Romeis B (1968) Mikroskopische Technik, 16th edn. Oldenbourg, Munich
Ronge J, Aidoo GA, Krüger G (1978) Zystizerkose des Gehirns. Fortschr Neurol Psychiatr 46:269–286
Rosenbaum TJ, Soule EH, Onofrio BM (1978) Teratomatous cyst of the spinal canal. J Neurosurg 49:292–297
Rosenberg Ga, Herz DA, Leeds N, Strully K (1975) Meckel's cave meningiomas with subarachnoid hemorrhage. Surg Neurol 3:333–336
Rosenblum WI, Hadfield MG (1972) Granulomatous angiitis of the nervous system in cases of herpes zoster and lymphosarcoma. Neurology (Minneap) 22:348–354
Rosenhagen H (1933) Zur Klinik des Angioma racemosum arterio-venosum der Rückenmarkshäute. Z Gesamte Neurol Psychiatr 147:216–229
Rosenthal W (1898) Über eine eigentümliche mit Syringomyelie complicierte Geschwulst des Rückenmarks. Beitr Pathol Anat 23:111–143
Rosenwasser H (1945) Carotid body-like tumor involving the middle ear and mastoid bone. Arch Otolaryngol 41:64–67
Rosenwasser H (1968) Glomus jugulare tumors: I. Historical background. Arch Otolaryngol 88:29–66
Ross AT, Bailey OT (1953) Tumors arising within the spinal canal in children. Neurology (Minneap) 3:922–930
Ross AT, Dickerson WW (1943) Tuberous sclerosis. Arch Neurol Psychiatry 50:233–257
Ross ST (1948) Sacral and presacral tumors. Am J Surg 76:687–693
Roth IG, Elvidge AR (1960) Glioblastoma multiforme: A clinical survey. J Neurosurg 17:736–750
Rothman SM, Nelson JS, De Vivo DC, Coxe WS (1979) Congenital astrocytoma presenting with intracerebral hematoma. Case report. J Neurosurg 51:237–239
Rothmann A (1939) Eine ungewöhnlich große Arachnoidalcyste. Zentralbl Allg Pathol 73:5
Rougerie I, Fardeau M (1962) Les cranio-pharyngeomes. Masson, Paris
Roulet FC (1930) Das primäre Retothelsarkom der Lymphknoten. Virchows Arch [A] 277:15–47
Roulet FC (1932) Weitere Beiträge zur Kenntnis des Retothelsarkoms der Lymphknoten. Virchows Arch [A] 286:702–732
Roulet FC (1953) Die ausgesprochenen blastomatösen Retikulosen. Verh Dtsch Ges Pathol 37:105–127
Rouquès L, David M (1949) Le role des arachnoidites segmentaires dans les séquelles nerveuses des traumatismes fermés du rachis. Rev Neurol (Paris) 81:185–202
Roquès L, Patel J, Sors C (1949) A propos des arachnoidites segmentaires consécutives aux fractures fermées du rachis lombaire: présentation de pièce. Rev Neurol (Paris) 81:615–616
Roussy G, Cornil L (1928) A propos de la classification des tumeurs des méninges. Rev Neurol (Paris) 49:122
Roussy G, Oberling C (1930) Les tumeurs angiomateuses des centres nerveux. Press Med 11:1–32
Roussy G, Oberling C (1931) Atlas du cancer. Alan, Paris
Roussy G, Oberling C (1932) Histologic classification of tumors of the central nervous system. Arch Neurol Psychiatr 27:1281–1289
Roussy G, Lhermitte J, Cornil L (1924) Essai de classification des tumeurs cérébrales. Ann Anat Pathol (Paris) 1:333–378
Roussy G, Oberling C, Raileanu C (1931) Les neurospongiomes. Presse Med 12:977–981

Rouzaud M, Lebon P (1965) Volumineuse tumeur du glomus jugulaire à évolution particulièrement rapide. Rev Otoneuroophtalmol 37:284–288

Rowbotham GF (1939) The hyperostoses in relation with the meningiomas. Br J Surg 26:593–623

Rowbotham GF, Clarke PRR (1956) Colloid cyst of the pituitary gland causing chiasmal compression. Br J Surg 44:107–108

Roy RN, Bhattacharya MB, Chatterjee BP, Pal NC (1976) Spinal cysticercosis. Surg Neurol 6:129–131

Rozynek M (1942) Ein Gliom des Hypophysenhinterlappens. Virchows Arch [A] 308:776–782

Ruberti R, Carteri A (1961) Neurinomas del forame lacero posteriore. G Psichiatr Neuropathol 4:1–30

Rubin P, Kramer S (1965) Ectopic pinealomas – a radiocurable neuroendocrinologic entity. Radiology 85:512–523

Rubin R, Sutton CH, Zimmerman HM (1968) Experimental ependymoblastoma. J Neuropathol Exp Neurol 27:421–438

Rubin R, Ames RP, Sutton CH, Zimmerman HM (1969) Virus-like particles in murine ependymoblastoma. J Neuropathol Exp Neurol 28:371–387

Rubinstein LJ (1956) The development of contiguous sarcomatous and gliomatous tissue in intracranial tumors. J Pathol 71:441–459

Rubinstein LJ (1959) Extracranial metastases in cerebellar medulloblastoma. J Pathol 78:187–195

Rubinstein LJ (1964) Discussion on polar spongioblastomas. Acta Neurochir [Suppl] (Wien) 10:126–132

Rubinstein LJ (1967) Development of extracranial metastases from a malignant astrocytoma in the absence of previous craniotomy. J Neurosurg 26:542–547

Rubinstein LJ (1970) The definition of the ependymoblastoma. Arch Pathol 90:35–45

Rubinstein LJ (1971) Sarcomas of the nervous system. In: Minckler J (ed) Pathology of the nervous system, vol 2. McGraw-Hill, New York, pp 2144–2164

Rubinstein LJ (1972) Tumors of the central nervous system. Armed Forces Institute of Pathology, Washington (Atlas of tumor pathology, second series, fasc 6)

Rubinstein LJ (1976) Current concepts in neurooncology. Adv Neurol 15:1–25

Rubinstein LJ, Brucher JM (1981) Focal ependymal differentiation in choroid plexus papillomas. An immunoperoxidase study. Acta Neuropathol (Berl) 53:29–33

Rubinstein LJ, Herman MM (1972) A light- and electron microscopic study of a temporal-lobe ganglioglioma. J Neurol Sci 16:27–48

Rubinstein LJ, Herman MM (1975) Studies on the differentiation of human and experimental gliomas in organ culture systems. In: Hekmatpanah J (ed) Gliomas. Springer, Berlin Heidelberg New York (Recent results in cancer research vol 51, pp 35–51)

Rubinstein LJ, Logan WJ (1970) Extraneural metastases in ependymoma of the cauda equina. J Neurol Neurosurg Psychiatry 33:763–770

Rubinstein LJ, Northfield DWC (1964) The medulloblastoma and the so-called „arachnoidal cerebellar sarcoma". A critical re-examination of a nosological problem. Brain 87:379–410

Rubinstein LJ, Herman MM, Foley VL (1973) In vitro characteristics of human glioblastomas maintained in organ culture systems. Am J Pathol 71:61–75

Rubinstein LJ, Herman MM, Hanberg JW (1974) The relationship between differentiating medulloblastoma and dedifferentiating diffuse cerebellar astrocytoma. Light, electron microscopic, tissue, and organ culture observations. Cancer 33:675–690

Rudershausen V (1932) Über die Häufigkeit und Art der Hirngeschwülste an Hand des Sektionsmaterials des Pathologischen Institutes Heidelberg. Virchows Arch [A] 285:318–331

Ruggiero G, Grillo BA, Santoro G (1976) Two cases of glomus tumour treated by unusual embolization. Neuroradiology 11:265–269

Runnels JB, Hanbery JW (1974) Spontaneous subarachnoid hemorrhage associated with spinal cord tumor. Case report. J Neurosurg 39:252–254

Russell DS (1931) Vascular tumours of the brain and spinal cord. Proc R Soc Med 24:21–23

Russell DS (1932) The occurrence and distribution of intranuclear „inclusion bodies" in gliomas. J Pathol 35:625–634

Russell DS (1939) Histological technique for intracranial tumors. University Press, Oxford

Russell DS (1941) Angiectasias y angiomas de cerebro y medula espinal. Acta Espan Neurol Psyquiatr 2:133–152
Russell DS (1944) The pinealoma, its relationship to teratomas. J Pathol 56:145–150
Russell DS (1949) Observations on the pathology of hydrocephalus. Her Majesty's Stationery Office, London (Medical Research Council special report series no. 265)
Russell DS (1950) Meningeal tumours: a review. J Clin Pathol 3:191–211
Russell DS (1954a) Spontaneous intracranial haemorrhage. Proc R Soc Med 47:689–693
Russell DS (1954b) Ectopic pinealoma: its kinship to atypical teratoma of the pineal gland. Report of a case. J Pathol 68:125–129
Russell DS (1955) Polar spongioblastomas. Their place in the glioma series. Proceedings 2nd International Congress of Neuropathology, London vol 1. Excerpta Medica Foundation, Amsterdam, p 295
Russell DS (1960) A note on cerebral medullo-epithelioma. J Pathol Bacteriol 79:403–409
Russell DS, Bland JOW (1933) A study of gliomas by the method of tissue culture. J Pathol Bacteriol 36:273–283
Russell DS, Bland JOW (1934) Further notes on the tissue culture of gliomas with special reference to Bailey's spongioblastoma. J Pathol Bacteriol 39:375–380
Russell DS, Cairns H (1947a) Spinal metastases in a case of cerebral glioma of the type known as astrocytoma fibrillare. J Pathol 33:383–391
Russell DS, Cairns H (1947b) Polar spongioblastoma. Arch Histol (B. Aires) 3:423–441
Russell DS, Rubinstein LJ (1977) Pathology of tumours of the nervous system, IVth edn (1st edn 1959). Arnold, London
Russell DS, Rubinstein LJ (1962) Ganglioglioma: a case with long history and malignant evolution. J Neuropathol Exp Neurol 21:185–193
Russell DS, Marshall AHE, Smith FB (1948) Microgliomatosis: a form of reticulosis, affecting the brain. Brain 71:1–15
Russo LS Jr (1979) Multicentric glioma. A diagnostic problem. Arch Neurol 36:388
Ryzkow EV (1959) Zur Frage der diffusen Gliose des ZNS. (In Russian) Arkh Patol 21:54–59
Sachs E (1931) The diagnosis and treatment of brain tumors. Mosby, St. Louis
Sachs E (1954) The treatment of glioblastoma with radium. J Neurosurg 11:119–121
Sachs E, Horrax G (1949) A cervical and a lumbar pilonidal sinus communicating with intraspinal dermoids. Report of 2 cases and review of the literature. J Neurosurg 6:97–112
Sachs E Jr, Avman N, Fisher RG (1962) Meningiomas of pineal region and posterior part of 3rd ventricle. J Neurosurg 19:325–331
Sackett JF, Stenwig JT, Songsirikul P (1974) Meningeal and glial tumors in combination. Neuroradiology 7:153–160
Saeger W (1977) Morphologie der paraadenomatösen Adenohypophyse. Ein Beitrag zur Pathogenese der Hypophysenadenome. Virchows Arch [A] 372:299–314
Saeger W, Breuer H, Lüdecke D (1976) Zur Definition und Differentialdiagnose chromophober Hypophysenadenome. Licht- und elektronenmikroskopische Untersuchungen. Beitr Pathol 157:367–390
Sahs AL, Alexander L (1939) Vascular pattern of certain intracranial neoplasms. Studies with the benzidine stain. Arch Neurol Psychiatr 42:44–66
Sakai H, Nakamura N, Sekino H, Abe Y, Yasue M (1980) Midline oligodendroglioma: Definition, Pathogenesis and Symptomatology (In Japanese). No Shinkei Geka 8:827–836
Sakaki S, Mori Y, Motozaki T, Nakagawa K, Matsuoka K (1981a) A cerebral neuroblastoma with extracranial metastases. Surg Neurol 16:53–59
Sakaki S, Matsuo Y, Kuwabara H, Matsuoka K (1981b) Rupture of an aneurysm into a parasellar epidermoid cyst. Case report. J Neurosurg 55:629–632
Salazar OM, Rubin P (1976) The spread of glioblastoma multiforme as a determining factor in the radiation treated volume. Int J Radiat Oncol Biol Phys 1:627–637
Salcman M, Quest DO, Mount LA (1974) Histiocytosis-X of the spinal cord. J Neurosurg 41:383–386
Salerno TA, Munro DD, Little JR (1978) Surgical treatment of bronchogenic carcinoma with a brain metastasis. J Neurosurg 48:350–354
Saljman AJ (1949) Der unilokuläre und der multilokuläre Echinokokkus des Gehirns. (In Russian) Vopr Nevrochir 1:30–37

Salles M, Pecker J (1961) Gomme syphilitique cérébrale. Neurochirurgie 9:91–92
Salvati CA (1981) Metastatic meningioma. Clin Neurol Neurosurg 83:169–172
Samii M, Schürmann K, Schmitz P (1975) Report on one hundred pituitary adenomas. Adv Neurosurg 3:433–441
Samuelsson S-M, Werner I, Pontén J, Nathorst-Windahl G, Thorell J (1966) Reticuloendothelial (perivascular) sarcoma of the brain. Acta Neurol Scand 42:567–580
Sano K (1976) Diagnosis and treatment of tumours in the pineal region. Acta Neurochir (Wien) 34:153–157
Sano K (1983a) Pineal region tumors. Problems in pathology and treatment. Clin Neurosurg 30:59–91
Sano K (1983b) Integrative treatment of gliomas. Clin Neurosurg 30:93–124
Sano K (1985) Treatment of tumors in the pineal and posterior third ventricular region. Paper read on the International Symposium on Surgery in and Around the Brain Stem and the Third Ventricle, Hanover, 18–23 September 1985
Sansone ME, Liwnicz BH, Mandybur TI (1980) Giant pituitary cavernous hemangioma. Case report. J Neurosurg 53:124–126
Saravia-Gomez J (1978a) Aspergillosis of the central nervous system. In: Vinken PJ, Bruyn GW (eds) Infections of the nervous system. North-Holland, Amsterdam (Handbook of clinical neurology, vol 35, part III, pp 395–400)
Saravia-Gomez J (1978b) Paracoccidioidomycosis of the central nervous system. In: Vinken PJ, Bruyn GW (eds) Infections of the nervous system. North-Holland, Amsterdam (Handbook of clinical neurology, vol 35, part III, pp 531–539)
Sarhaddi S, Bravo E, Cyms AE (1973) Gliomatosis cerebri. South Med J 66:883–888
Sarwar M, McCormick WF (1978) Intracerebral venous angioma. Arch Neurol 35:323–325
Sassin JF (1974) Intracranial chordoma. In: Vinken PJ, Bruyn GW (eds) Tumors of the brain and skull. North-Holland, Amsterdam/American Elsevier, Oxford (Handbook of clinical neurology, vol 18, part III, pp 151–164
Sato K, Massing W, Zülch KJ (1971) Experimental concussion in the cat. Z Neurol 200:201–212
Sato M, Okamoto K, Handa J, Nakano Y (1980) Computed tomography in leptomeningeal and ventricular spread of primary brain tumors (In Japanese). No To Shinkei 32:847–854
Sato O, Sano K (1975) Brain tumors of children (In Japanese). No To Shinkei 27:185–193
Sato O, Takahashi H, Chien TC, Amano K (1973a) Spinal extradural meningiomas (In Japanese). No Shinkei Geka 1:513–518
Sato O, Tamura A, Sekino H, Sano K (1973b) Hirntumoren bei jungen Säuglingen (In Japanese). No To Shinkei 25:1447–1454
Sato O, Tamura A, Sano K (1975) Brain tumors of early infants. Childs Brain 1:121–125
Sato S, Sugimura T, Chien TC, Takakura K (1971) Adolase isozyme patterns of human brain tumors. Cancer 27:223–227
Sato S, Inaba K, Suematsu K (1977) Spinal cord tumor associated with papilledema (In Japanese). No Shinkei Geka 5:1375–1376
Sato T, Shimoda A, Takahashi T, Daita G, Goto S, Takamura H, Hirama M (1980) Congenital cerebellar neuroepithelial tumor with multiple divergent differentiations. Acta Neuropathol (Berl) 50:143–146
Sato T, Shimoda A, Takahashi T, Kurokawa H, Ando M, Goto S, Takamura H (1982) Congenital anaplastic ependymoma: a case report of familial glioma. Childs Brain 9:342–349
Savoiardo M, Lodrini S (1980) Hypodense area within a meningioma: metastasis from breast cancer. Neuroradiology 20:107–110
Saxer F (1902) Ependymepithel, Gliom and epitheliale Geschwülste des Zentralnervensystems. Beitr Pathol Anat 32:276–350
Sayk J (1960) Cytologie der Cerebrospinalflüssigkeit. Fischer, Jena
Sayk J (1974) The cerebrospinal fluid in brain tumors. In: Vinken PJ, Bruyn GW (eds) Tumors of the brain and skull. North-Holland, Amsterdam (Handbook of clinical neurology, vol 16, part I, pp 360–417)
Sayre GP (1964) The system of grading of gliomas. Acta Neurochir [Suppl] (Wien) X:98–106

Schachenmayr W, Friede RL (1979) Fine structure of arachnoid cysts. J Neuropathol Exp Neurol 38:434–446
Schaefer K (1965) Ein kasuistischer Beitrag zur Meningeomentstehung nach einem Trauma. Zentralbl Allg Pathol 107:476–480
Schär W, Christensen E (1939) Mißbildungstumoren des Großhirns. Zentralbl Neurochir 4:142–154
Schaffer K (1927) Bemerkungen zur Histopathologie des Hirnglioms. Monatsschr Psychiatr Neurol (Berl) 65:208–229
Schajowicz F, Ackerman LV, Sissons NA, Sobin LH, Torloni H (1972) Histological typing of bone tumours. International histological classification of tumours No. 6. World Health Organization, Geneva
Schaltenbrand G, Bailey P (1928) Die perivasculäre Pia-Gliamembran des Gehirns. J Psychol Neurol 35:199–278
Schaltenbrand G, Tönnis W (1936/1937) Traumatischer Hydrocephalus. Zentralbl Neurochir 1/2:42–51
Schaper A (1897) Die frühesten Differenzierungsvorgänge im ZNS. Arch Entwickl Mech Org 5:81–130
Scharrenberg K, Liss L (1969) Neuroectodermal tumors of the central and peripheral nervous system. Williams and Wilkins, Baltimore
Scharrer E, Brunngraber CV (1973) Gliome bei Vater und Sohn. J Neurol 205:287–295
Scharrer E, Brunngraber CV (1974) Über multiple Meningeome. Syndromgenetischer Beitrag zur Frage: Systemerkrankung oder Metastasierung? J Neurol 207:227–246
Scharrer VE, Heiming E (1974) Trabekulär-papilläres Ependymom über der Sakrokokzygealregion. Zentralbl Neurochir 35:131–161
Schattenfroh C (1962) Zur Klinik und Histologie der Caudaependymome. Acta Neurochir (Wien) 10:415–431
Schaumann J (1917) Etude sur le lupus pernio et ses rapports avec les sarcoides et la tuberculose. Ann Dermatol Syph 6:357
Schaumburg HH, Planck CR, Adams RI (1972) The reticulum cell sarcoma – microglioma group of brain tumours. A consideration of their clinical features and therapy. Brain 95:199–212
Schechter MM, Liebeskind AL, Asar-Kia B (1974) Intracranial chordomas. Neuroradiology 8:67–82
Scheid P (1938) Über Geschwulstbildung nach Schußverletzungen. Frankf Z Pathol 51:446–478
Scheidegger R (1954) Diffuse meningeale Sarkomatose. Oncologia 7:331–340
Scheidegger S (1939) Osteolipom des Gehirns. Virchows Arch [A] 303:423–435
Scheinberg LC, Taylor JM (1968) Immunological aspects of brain tumors. Prog Neurol Surg 2:267–291
Scheinker IM (1936) Beitrag zur Frage der diffusen Sclerose (diffuse Glioblastose des ZNS). Dtsch Z Nervenheilkd 139:253–264
Scheinker IM (1938a) Über die Umwandlung gutartiger Hirngliome (Astrocytome) in bösartige Glioblastome. Dtsch Z Nervenheilkd 145:54–69
Scheinker IM (1938b) Zur Frage der diffusen Glioblastose des Gehirns. Dtsch Z Nervenheilkd 145:70–82
Scheinker IM (1945) Subependymoma: A newly recognized tumor of subependymal derivation. J Neurosurg 2:232–240
Scheinker IM (1948) Neurosurgical pathology. Thomas, Springfield
Scheinker IM, Evans JP (1943) Diffuse cerebral gliomatosis. J Neuropathol Exp Neurol 2:178–189
Scheitauer BW (1978) Symptomatic subependymoma. Report of 21 cases with review of the literature. J Neurosurg 49:689–696
Schelin U (1962) Chromophobe and acidophil adenomas of the human pituitary gland. A light and electron microscopic study. Acta Pathol Microbiol Scand [Suppl] 158:1–80
Schenk VWD (1966) Congenital cavities of the posterior fossa. Acta Neuropathol (Berl) 6:117–126
Scherer E (1935a) Über Zystenbildung der weichen Häute der Sylviischen Furche mit hochgradiger Deformation des Gehirns. Z Gesamte Neurol Psychiatr 152:787–799

Scherer E (1935b) Über die pialen Lipome des Gehirns. Z Gesamte Neurol Psychiatr 154:45–61
Scherer E (1936) Die extramedullären pialen Lipome an der hinteren Wurzellinie des Rückenmarks. Z Gesamte Neurol Psychiatr 154:507–520
Scherer HJ (1933) Gliomstudien: I. Die Bedeutung des Mesenchyms in Gliomen. Virchows Arch [A] 291:321–340
Scherer HJ (1934) Untersuchungen über den geweblichen Aufbau der Geschwülste des peripheren Nervensystems. Virchows Arch [A] 292:479–553
Scherer HJ (1935) Gliomstudien II. Virchows Arch [A] 294:790–861
Scherer HJ (1938) La "glioblastomatose en plaques". Sur les limites anatomiques de la gliomatose et des processus sclérotiques progressifs (sclérose en plaques, sclérose diffuse de Schilder, sclérose concentrique). J Belge Neurol Psychiatr 38:1–17
Scherer HJ (1940a) The forms of growth in gliomas and their practical significance. Brain 63:1–35
Scherer HJ (1940b) A critical review: the pathology of cerebral gliomas. J Neurol Neurosurg Psychiatry 3:147–177
Scherer HJ (1941) Quelques résultats pratiques de l'étude anatomique complète de 135 cas de gliomes confrontés avec les expériences neurochirurgicales. Psychiatr Neurol Bl (Amst) 45:718–738
Scherer HJ (1944) Vergleichende Pathologie des Nervensystems der Säugetiere. Thieme, Leipzig
Schianchi P, Kraus-Ruppert R (1980) Familial brain tumors: Rhombencephalon – astrocytoma grade I in father and son. Acta Neuropathol 52:153–155
Schiefer B (1958) Über die experimentelle Erzeugung von Gehirntumoren mit Methylcholanthren. Zentralbl Neurochir 18:360–375
Schiefer B (1962) Zur Morphologie experimenteller Hirntumoren. Acta Neuropathol [Suppl] (Berl) 1:19–25
Schiefer B (1964) Morphology of experimental brain tumors. Acta Neurochir [Suppl] (Wien) 10:57–63
Schiefer B, Dahme E (1962) Primäre Geschwülste des ZNS bei Tieren. Acta Neuropathol (Berl) 2:202–212
Schiefer W (1969) Ein Beitrag zur extrakraniellen Metastasierung von Hirngeschwülsten. Bericht über ein in die Lunge metastasierendes Ependymom (unpublished paper)
Schiefer W, Udvarhelyi JB (1954) Das Glioblastoma multiforme im Serienangiogramm. Acta Neurochir (Wien) 4:76–105
Schiefer W, Rausch FJ, Udvarhelyi G (1955a) Zur Röntgendiagnostik intracerebraler Metastasen. Fortschr Roentgenstr 82:656–667
Schiefer W, Tönnis W, Udvarhelyi G (1955b) Die benignen Gliome im Serienbild. Zentralbl Neurochir 15:267–277
Schiffer D (1971) Calcification in nervous tissue. In: Minckler J (ed) Pathology of the nervous system, vol 2. McGraw-Hill, New York, pp 1342–1360
Schiffer D (1973) Histochemical observations on NDPase and TPPase in cerebral tumours. Acta Neuropathol (Berl) 23:112–117
Schiffer D, Fabiani A (1970) Patologia dei tumori cerebrali. Pensiero Scientifico, Rome
Schiffer D, Fabiani A (1975) I tumori cerebrali. Pensiero Scientifico, Rome
Schiffer D, Sibour F, Vesco C (1961) Calcifications in cerebral tumors, pathogenetic considerations. World Neurol (Minneap) 2:1069–1082
Schisano G, Tovi D (1962) Clivus chordomas. Neurochirurgia (Stuttg) 5:99–120
Schisano G, Tovi D, Nordenstam H (1963) Spongioblastoma polare of the cerebral hemisphere. J Neurosurg 20:241–251
Schleiden MJ (1838) Beiträge zur Phytogenesis. Arch Anat Physiol Wiss Med:137–176
Schlesinger H (1898) Beiträge zur Klinik der Rückenmarks- und Wirbeltumoren. Fischer, Jena
Schloffer H (1907) Erfolgreiche Operation eines Hypophysentumors auf nasalem Wege. Wien Klin Wochenschr :621–670; 1075
Schlote W (1964) Zur Ultrastructur der sog. Rosenthalschen Fasern im Zentralnervensystem. Naturwissenschaften 51:165–166
Schlote W (1966) Rosenthalsche Fasern und Spongioblasten im Zentralnervensystem. Beitr Pathol Anat 133:461–480

Schlote W (1967) Beitrag zum Vorkommen und zu Veränderungen an intracytoplasmatischen Filamenten in Gliomen. Acta Neuropathol (Berl) 8:108–112

Schlote W (1975) Piloide Astrocyten (Spongiocyten) und Rosenthalsche Fasern bei multipler Sclerose. Acta Neuropathol (Berl) 33:35–44

Schmaus H (1901) Vorlesungen über die pathologische Anatomie des Rückenmarks. Bergmann, Wiesbaden

Schmid AH (1973) A lipoma of the cerebellum. Acta Neuropathol (Berl) 26:75–80

Schmidek HH (1977) Pineal tumors. Masson, New York

Schmidt A (1904) Cyste der Dura mater spinalis, einen extramedullären Tumor vortäuschend, mit Erfolg operiert. Dtsch Z Nervenheilkd 26:318–323

Schmidt E, Hallervorden J, Spatz H (1958) Die Entstehung der Hamartome am Hypothalamus mit und ohne Pubertas praecox. Dtsch Z Nervenheilkd 177:235–262

Schmidt H, Jaquet G-H (1963) Meningeomentstehung und Fremdkörper. Zentralbl Neurochir 24:65–73

Schmidt MB (1900) Über seltene Spaltbildungen im Bereiche des mittleren Stirnfortsatzes. Virchows Arch [A] 162:340–370

Schmidt MB (1902) Über die Pacchionischen Granulationen und ihr Verhalten zu den Sarkomen und Psammomen der Dura mater. Virchows Arch [A] 170:429–464

Schmincke A (1909/1910) Beitrag zur Lehre der Ganglioneurome: Ein Ganglioneurom des Gehirns. Beitr Pathol Anat 47:354–371

Schmincke A (1914) Ein Ganglioneurom des Gehirns. Verh Dtsch Ges Pathol 17:537–543

Schmincke A (1921) Über lymphoepitheliale Geschwülste. Beitr Pathol Anat 68:161–170

Schmincke A (1924) Zur Kenntnis der diffusen meningealen Gliome des Kleinhirns. Z Gesamte Neurol Psychiatr 93:169–180

Schmincke A (1925) Beiträge zur Geschwulstpathologie. Beitr Pathol Anat 73:502–517

Schmincke A (1929) Zur Kenntnis der Zirbelgeschwülste. Ein Ganglioglioneurom der Zirbel. Beitr Pathol Anat 83:279–288

Schmincke A (1933) Statistik über Hirntumoren. MMW 1342

Schmitt R (1970) Pathologisch-anatomische Untersuchungen über neurologische Veränderungen bei akuten und chronischen Leukosen. Dissertation, Faculty of Medicine, University of Cologne

Schnabel R, Wuttke W-D (1966) Ein Meningeom der Zirbelregion. Med Bild (3):79–84

Schneck SA, Penn I (1970) Cerebral neoplasms associated with renal transplantation. Arch Neurol 22:226–233

Schneck SA, Penn I (1971) De-novo brain tumours in renal-transplant recipients. Lancet I:983–986

Schneider RC, Rand RW (1949) Actinomycotic brain abscess. Complete excision with recovery. J Neurosurg 6:255–259

Schneider P, Jänisch W, Schreiber D (1972) Zur Häufigkeit von Hypophysenmetastasen. Zentralbl Allg Pathol 114:159–167

Schnitzler ER, Richards MJS, Chun RWM (1978) Cerebellar medulloblastoma. An analysis of four cases of extraneural metastasis. Am J Dis Child 132:1004–1008

Schob F (1930) Pathologische Anatomie der Idiotie. In: Bumke O (ed) Die Anatomie der Psychosen. Springer, Berlin (Handbuch der Geisteskrankheiten, vol XI, part VII, pp 779–995)

Schochet SS Jr, Peters B, O'Neal J, McCormick WF (1975) Intracranial Esthesioneuroblastoma. Acta Neuropathol (Berl) 31:181–189

Schochet SS, Sarwar M, Kelly PJ, Masel BE (1980) Symptomatic cerebral histoplasmoma. Case report. J Neurosurg 52:273–275

Schöche J, Blinkov SM, Niebeling H-G, Konovalov AN, Puzillo MW (1980) Die Angioarchitektur der Gliome. Zentralbl Neurochir 41:287–302

Schoenberg BS, Christine BW (1970) Neoplasms of the brain and cranial meninges: a study of incidence, epidemiological trends and survival. Neurology (Minneap) 20:399

Schoenberg BS, Glista GG, Reagan TJ (1975) The familial occurrence of glioma. Surg Neurol 3:139–145

Schoenberg BS, Christine BW, Whisnant JP (1978) The resolution of discrepancies in the reported incidence of primary brain tumors. Neurology (Minneap) 28:817–823

Schöpe M (1938) Zur Frage Blastom-Encephalitis. Verhandlungen der Gesellschaft Deutscher Neurologen und Psychiater, Munich, 1937. Z Gesamte Neurol Psychiatr 161:177–183
Schöpe M (1939) Zur Frage „Blastom"-„Encephalitis". Arch Psychiatr Nervenkr 109:755–784
Schöpe M (1941) Ein Beitrag zur Klinik und Pathologie des Angioma racemosum des Rückenmarks und seiner Häute. Z Gesamte Neurol Psychiatr 171:799–810
Schöpe M (1942) Über ein Gangliogliom des Occipitallappens mit psychischen Veränderungen. Z Gesamte Neurol Psychiatr 174:522–533
Schöpe M (1951) Zur Pathogenese des Meningeoms und des zentralen Neurinoms bei der von Recklinghausen'schen Krankheit. Arch Psychiatr Nervenkr 186:603–622
Scholtz CL, Siu K (1976) Melanoma of the pituitary. Case report. J Neurosurg 45:101–103
Scholz V (1973) Difficulties of the differential diagnosis in a medulloblastoma. Eur Neurol 9:292–297
Scholz W (1934) Experimentelle Untersuchungen über die Einwirkung von Röntgenstrahlen auf das reife Gehirn. Z Gesamte Neurol Psychiatr 150:765–785
Scholz W, Hsü JK (1938) Late damage from roentgen irradiation of the human brain. Arch Neurol Psychiatry 40:928–936
Scholz W, Ducho EG, Breit A (1959) Experimentelle Röntgenspätschäden am Rückenmark des erwachsenen Kaninchens. Seishin Shinkeigaku Zasshi 61:417–442
Schrantz JL, Araoz CA (1972) Radiation-induced meningeal fibrosarcoma. Arch Pathol 93:26–31
Schreiber D, Jänisch W, Gerlach H (1982) CNS tumours in infancy, childhood and adolescence. In: Voth D, Gutjahr P, Langmaid C (eds) Tumours of the central nervous system in infancy and childhood. Springer, Berlin Heidelberg New York, pp 62–68
Schroeder AH, Médoc J (1951) Quiste hidático de cerebro. Proceedings of the Third Panamerican Congress of Pediatricians, Montevideo, vol 1, pp 687–708
Schröder JM, Brunngraber CV (1965) Über ein intramedulläres cavernöses Angiom. Acta Neurochir (Wien) 12:632–641
Schröder JM, Plogsties H-R (1966) Über das „umschriebene" Arachnoidalsarkom des Kleinhirns von Foerster und Gagel. Acta Neurochir (Wien) 14:264–277
Schröder JM, Wechsler W (1965) Ödem und Nekrose in der grauen und weißen Substanz beim experimentellen Hirntrauma (licht- und elektronenmikroskopische Untersuchungen). Acta Neuropathol (Berl) 5:82–111
Schröder R (1964) Die relative Häufigkeit atypischer Mitosen in Astrocytomen und Glioblastomen. Zentralbl Neurochir 24:289–299
Schröder R (1967) Unterschiedlicher Mitoseablauf bei neuroektodermalen und mesodermalen Tumoren. Naturwissenschaften 54:620
Schröder R, Kaess H (1972) Atypische Mitosen bei menschlichen Hirntumoren (Medulloblastome und Glioblastome). Acta Neuropathol (Berl) 20:171–173
Schröder R, Bonis G, Müller W, Vorreith M (1968a) Statistische Beiträge zum Grading der Gliome: I. Acta Neurochir (Wien) 18:43–56
Schröder R, Bonis G, Müller W, Vorreith M (1968b) Statistische Beiträge zum Grading der Gliome: II. Acta Neurochir (Wien) 18:186–200
Schröder R, Müller W, Bonis G, Vorreith M (1970) Statistische Beiträge zum Grading der Gliome: III. Acta Neurochir (Wien) 23:1–29
Schuback A (1927) Über die Angiomatosis des Zentralnervensystems (Lindau'sche Krankheit). Z Gesamte Neurol Psychiatr 110:359–371
Schubert JCF, Güllner HR, Fischer M, Kropp R (1971) Boecksches Sarkoid des Nervensystems. Dtsch Med Wochenschr 96:945–950
Schubiger O, Valavanis A, Menges H (1978) Computed tomography for small acoustic neuromas. Neuroradiology 15:287–290
Schürmeyer E, Bettmann M (1956) Melanoblastommetastase in der Hypophyse. Zentralbl Allg Pathol 95:180–182
Schuier F (1976) Is there an anaplastic type of oligodendroglioma? J Neurol 213:263–267
Schuier FJ, Vise WM, Hossmann K-A, Zülch KJ (1978) Cerebral microembolization. II. Morphological studies. Arch Neurol 35:264–270
Schultz OT (1926) Tumors of infancy and childhood. In: Abt's pediatrics, vol 8. Saunders, Philadelphia, pp 641–866

Schulze A, Bingas B (1968) Durch Fremdkörper induzierte Meningeombildung. Beitr Neurochir 15:297–301
Schulze E, Schnepper E (1967) Erfahrungen bei der Diagnose und Behandlung des eosinophilen Knochengranuloms mit besonderer Berücksichtigung der Telekobalt-Strahlentherapie. Strahlentherapie 132:173–183
Schulze HE (1954) Chondrom der mittleren und hinteren Schädelgrube. Ein Beitrag zur Diagnostik der seltenen Schädelbasisgeschwülste. Zentralbl Neurochir 14:113–128
Schumacher M, Gilsbach J, Friedrich H, Mennel HD (1978) Plexiform neurofibroma (Rankenneurofibrom) of the cauda equina. Neuroradiology 15:221–224
Schwann T (1839) Mikroskopische Untersuchungen über die Übereinstimmung in der Struktur und dem Wachstum der Tiere und Pflanzen. Berlin
Schwartz P (1932) Anatomische Typen der Hirngliome. Nervenarzt 5:449–456
Schwartz P (1936) Anatomische Typen der Hirngliome. Communications from the IInd International Congress on Cancer Research, pp 257–260
Schwartz P, Klauer HR (1927) Diffuse blastomatöse Wucherung des gliösen Apparates im Gehirn. Z Gesamte Neurol Psychiatr 109:438–452
Schwerdtfeger (1911) Beitrag zur Pathologie und Therapie der Chondrome der Nase und ihrer Nebenhöhlen. Z Laryngol Rhinol 3:581–595
Schwidde JT, Meyers R, Sweeney DB (1951) Intracerebral metastatic granular cell myoblastoma. J Neuropathol Exp Neurol 10:30–39
Scott M (1974) Infiltrating ependymomas of the cauda equina. Treatment by conservative surgery plus radiotherapy. J Neurosurg 41:446–448
Scott M, Ballantine HT Jr (1973) Cerebellar astrocytoma: malignant recurrence after prolonged postoperative survival. J Neurosurg 39:777–779
Scott M, Bentz R (1962) Intramedullary neurilemmoma (neurinoma) of the thoracic cord. A case report. J Neuropathol Exp Neurol 21:194–200
Scotti LN, Goldman RL, Rao GR, Heinz ER (1975) Cerebral venous angioma. Neuroradiology 9:125–128
Scoville WB, Manlapaz JS, Otis RD, Cabieses F (1963) Intraspinal enterogenous cyst. J Neurosurg 20:704–706
Sears RA, Burnett SW (1961) Angiographic appearance of a papilloma of the choroid plexus. J Neurosurg 18:822–825
Sehrbundt HJ, Schröder R (1968) Interferenzmikroskopische Untersuchungen an Medulloblastom- und Glioblastomzellen. Experientia 24:1232–1233
Seifarth G (1948) Das Neuroepitheliom des Rückenmarks im Lichte der organoiden Geschwulstbetrachtung. Virchows Arch [A] 316:149–186
Seiler RW, Greiner RH, Zimmerman A, Markwalder H (1978) Radiotherapy combined with procarbazine, bleomycin and CCNU in the treatment of high-grade supratentorial astrocytomas. J Neurosurg 48:861–865
Seitelberger F (1972) Die Phakomatosen. In: Opitz H, Schmidt F (eds) Lungen-Luftwege, Herz-Kreislauf, Nieren-Harnwege. Springer, Berlin Heidelberg New York (Handbuch der Kinderheilkunde, vol VII, pp 1ff.)
Seitz D, Kalm H (1957) Die diffuse Glioblastose. Dtsch Z Nervenheilkd 175:528–546
Seitz D, Kalm H (1958) Zur Diagnose der primären Hirnsarcome. Dtsch Z Nervenheilkd 177:597–617
Selby RC, Lopes NM (1973) Torulomas (cryptococcal granulomata) of the central nervous system. J Neurosurg 38:40–46
Seligman AM, Shear MJ (1939) Studies in carcinogenesis: VIII. Experimental production of brain tumors in mice with methylcholanthrene. Am J Cancer 37:364–399
Seur NH, Kooman A (1976) Arachnoid of the middle fossa with paradoxical changes of the bony structures. Neuroradiology 12:177–183
Sézary A (1938) La syphilis du système nerveux. Pathologie générale, traitement prophylactique. Masson, Paris
Shankar SK, Tandon PN, Roy S (1976) Third ventricular chromophobe adenoma with normal adenohypophysis. Acta Neuropathol (Berl) 35:353–356
Shanklin WM (1947) On the origin of tumorettes in human neurohypophysis. Anat Rec 99:297–327

Shanklin WM (1949) On the presence of cysts in the human pituitary. Anat Rec 104:379–407
Shapiro K, Shulman K (1976) Spinal cord seeding from cerebellar astrocytomas. Childs Brain 2:177–186
Shapiro K, Till K, Grant DN (1979) Craniopharyngiomas in childhood. J Neurosurg 50:617–623
Shapiro WR, Ausman JI (1969) The chemotherapy of brain tumors: A clinical and experimental review. In: Plum F (ed) Recent advances in neurology contemporary neurology series, vol 6. Davis, Philadelphia, pp 149–235
Shapiro WR, Ausman JI, Rall DP (1970) Studies on the chemotherapy of experimental brain tumors: Evaluation of 1,3-(2-chloroethyl-)1 nitrosourea, cyclophosphamide, mitramycin and methotrexate. Cancer Res 30:2401–2413
Sharpe JA, Deck JHN (1977) Neuroepithelial cyst of the fourth ventricle. J Neurosurg 46:820–824
Shaw C-M, Sumi M, Alvord EC, Gerdes AJ, Spence A, Parker RG (1978) Fast-neutron irradiation of glioblastoma multiforme. J Neurosurg 49:1–12
Sheldon WH, Galden A, Bondy PK (1954) Cushing's syndrome produced by a pituitary basophil carcinoma with hepatic metastases. Am J Med 17:134–142
Sheline GE, Boldrey E, Karlsberg P, Phillips T (1964) Therapeutic considerations in tumors affecting the central nervous system: Oligodendroglioma. Radiology 82:84–89
Shenkin HA (1965) The effect of roentgen-ray therapy on oligodendrogliomas of the brain. J Neurosurg 22:57–59
Shenkin HA, Alpers BJ (1944) Clinical and pathologic features of gliomas of the spinal cord. Arch Neurol Psychiatry 52:87–105
Sheps JG, Simon JL (1943) Solitary cerebral gumma. J Neuropathol Exp Neurol 2:353–364
Sherbet GV, Lakshmi MS (1974a) The surface properties of some human intracranial tumor cell lines in relation to their malignancy. Oncology 29:335–347
Sherbet GV, Lakshmi MS (1974b) Tumor grading by implantation in embryos: II Grading of some human astrocytomas. JNCI 52:687–692
Shima T, Ishikawa S, Okada Y et al. (1976) "Colloid cyst" of the lateral ventricle, report of a case (In Japanese). No Shinkei Geka 4:791–797
Shimidzu K (1935) Ein Operationsfall von Schistosomiasis cerebri. Arch Klin Chir 182:401–407
Shimura T, Ito Y, Ueda K, Nakazawa S, Yajima G (1980a) Widespread extracranial metastasis of primary intracerebral sarcoma. Neurol Surg 8:395–400
Shimura T, Ito Y, Nakazawa S, Yamada N, Aihara K (1980b) Extracranial metastasis of the glioblastoma multiforme. An ultrastructural study (In Japanese). No To Shinkei 32:601–609
Shin Woo-Yung, Laufer H, Lee Yin-Chen, Aftalion B, Hirano A, Zimmerman HM (1978) Fine structure of a cerebellar neuroblastoma. Acta Neuropathol (Berl) 42:11–13
Shinmura F, Sakakibara T, Takayasu K, Takagi S, Ariwa R (1980) A case of metastatic adenoid cystic carcinoma in left cerebellar hemisphere (In Japanese). No Shinkei Geka 8:571–577
Shuangshoti S (1973) Meningioma of the optic nerve. Br J Ophthalmol 57:265
Shuangshoti S, Netsky MG (1966a) Histogenesis of the choroid plexus in man. Am J Anat 118:283–316
Shuangshoti S, Netsky MG (1966b) Neuroepithelial colloid cysts of the nervous system: Further observations on pathogenesis, location, incidence and histochemistry. Neurology (Minneap) 16:887–903
Shuangshoti S, Netsky MG (1971) Neoplasms of mixed mesenchymal and neuroepithelial origin. J Neuropathol Exp Neurol 30:290–309
Shuangshoti S, Panyathanya R (1974) Neural neoplasms in Thailand: A study of 2897 cases. Neurology (Minneap) 24:1127–1134
Shuangshoti S, Piyaratn P, Viriyapanich PL (1968) Primary rhabdomyosarcoma of cerebellum. Necropsy report. Cancer 22:367–371
Shuangshoti S, Tangchai P, Netsky MG (1969) Neoplasms of the nervous system in Thailand. Cancer 23:493–496
Shuangshoti S, Hongsaprabhas C, Netsky MG (1970) Metastasizing meningioma. Cancer 26:832–841

Shuangshoti S, Tangchai P, Netsky MG (1971) Primary adenocarcinoma of choroid plexus. Arch Pathol Lab Med 91:101–106

Shuangshoti S, Phonprasert C, Suwanwela N, Netsky MG (1975) Combined neuroepithelial (colloid) cyst and xanthogranuloma (xanthoma) in the third ventricle. Neurology (Minneap) 25:547–552

Shuangshoti S, Rungruxsirivorn S, Netsky MG (1979) Combined occurrence of mucin-producing ependymoma and neuroepithelial (colloid) cysts. J Neuropathol Exp Neurol 38:72–79

Shuman RM, Alvord EC, Leech RW (1975) The biology of childhood ependymomas. Arch Neurol 32:701–739

Sibley WA, O'Brien JL (1956) Intracranial tuberculomas. A review of clinical features and treatment. Neurology (Minneap) 6:157–165

Sieben G, Sieben-Praet M, De Reuck J, De Coster W, Remouchamps A, Roels H, Van der Eecken H (1980) Dumb-bell sarcoma of the foramen jugulare with syringomyelia. A radio-induced tumour? J Neurol 222:219–225

Siegel GJ, Anderson PJ (1966) Extracalvarial meningioma. Case report. J Neurosurg 25:83–86

Siegler R, Pienta RJ (1962) Sarcoma of the brain. A study of two cases in children and experimental production of similar tumors in chick brain. J Neuropathol Exp Neurol 21:388–399

Siemssen S, Münster E, Lester I (1967) Ekstirpation at angiofibrom i rhinopharynx (Danish with English summary). Ugeskr Laeger 129:586–600

Silbert SW, Smitj KR, Horenstein S (1978) Primary leptomeningeal melanoma. Ultrastructural study. Cancer 41:519–528

Silvan (1914) Contributo allo studio delle metastasi neoplastiche nei centri nervosi, con una ventina di osservazioni. Policlinico (Sez Med) Roma 71

Silver ML, Hennigar G (1952) Cerebellar hemangioma (hemangioblastoma). J Neurosurg 9:484–494

Silverstein A, Feuer MM, Siltzbach LE (1965) Neurologic sarcoidosis. Arch Neurol 12:1–11

Sima AAF, Robertson DM (1979) Subependymal giant cell astrocytoma. J Neurosurg 50:240–245

Sima A, Kindblom L-G, Pellettieri L (1976) Liposarcoma of the meninges. Acta Pathol Microbiol Scand [A] 84:306–310

Simmonds M (1907) Über cysticercus racemosus der Hirnhäute. MMW 54:1346

Simmonds M (1919) Zwergwuchs bei Atrophie des Hypophysenvorderlappens. Dtsch Med Wochenschr 44:487

Simon E (1970) Gliosarcomas. Pol Med J 9:1466–1474

Simon T (1874) Das Spinnenzellen- und Pinselzellengliom. Virchows Arch [A] 61:90–100

Simpson D (1957) The recurrence of intracranial meningiomas after surgical treatment. J Neurol Neurosurg Psychiatry 20:22–39

Simson LR, Lampe I, Abell MR (1968) Suprasellar germinomas. Cancer 22:533–544

Singh R, Coerkamp G, Luyendijk W (1968) Spinal epidural meningiomas. Acta Neurochir (Wien) 18:237–245

Sinh G, Pandya SK, Dastur DK (1968) Pathogenesis of unusual intracranial tuberculomas and tuberculous space-occupying lesions. J Neurosurg 29:149–159

Sipe JC (1976) Gap junctions between human meningioma cells maintained in organ culture. Acta Neuropathol (Berl) 35:69–76

Sipe JC, Herman MM, Rubinstein LJ (1973) Electron microscopic observations on human glioblastomas and astrocytomas maintained in organ culture systems. Am J Pathol 73:589

Sivalingam S, Corkill G, Ellis WG, Claiche JR (1977) Focal eosinophilic granuloma of the temporal lobe. J Neurosurg 47:941–945

Siwe S (1956) Spinal cord tumors in children. Acta Paediatr Scand 45:437–439

Sjövall E (1910) Über eine Ependymzyste embryonalen Charakters (Paraphyse?) im 3. Ventrikel mit tödlichem Ausgang. Zugleich eine Beobachtung wahrer lipochromer Veränderungen mit Auftreten von Halbmondkörperchen. Beitr Pathol Anat 47:248–268

Skala O (1956) Über ein extraventriculäres Plexuspapillom. Zentralbl Allg Pathol 95:183–187

Skillicorn SA, Garrity RW (1955) Intracranial Boeck's sarcoid tumor resembling meningioma. J Neurosurg 12:407–413

Skolnick EM, Massari FS, Tenta LT (1966) Olfactory neuroepithelioma. Review of the world literature and presentation of 2 cases. Arch Otolaryngol 84:644–653

Šlais J (1968) Die Morphologie und histologische Diagnostik des Parasiten bei der Gehirncysticerkose. Acta Neuropathol (Berl) 10:295–307

Slansky BD, Mann-Kaplan RS, Reynolds AK Jr, Rosenblum ML, Walker MD (1974) 4-Demethylepipodophylotoxin-β-D-Thenylidene glucoside (PTG) in the treatment of malignant intracranial neoplasms. Cancer 33:460–467

Slooff JL, Kernohan JW, MacCarty CS (1964) Primary intramedullary tumors of the spinal cord and filum terminale. Saunders, Philadelphia

Slowik E, Pasztor E, Szöllösi B (1979) Subependymal gliomas. Neurosurg Rev 2:79–86

Slowik F, Balogh I (1980) Extracranial spreading of glioblastoma multiforme. Zentralbl Neurochir 41:57–68

Slowik T, Bittner-Manioka M, Grochowski W (1968) Chondroma of the cervical spine. Case reports and technical notes. J Neurosurg 29:276–279

Smink KWF, Hekster REM, Bots GTAM (1977) Clivus chordoma with distinct vascularity demonstrated by angiography. Neuroradiology 13:273–277

Smith CE, Long DM, Jones TK, Levitt SH (1973) Medulloblastoma: an analysis of time-dose relationships and recurrence patterns. Cancer 32:722–728

Smith FP, Slavik M, MacDonald JS (1978) Association of breast cancer with meningioma. Cancer 42:1992–1994

Smith KR Jr, Schwartz HG, Luse SA, Ogura JH (1963) Nasal gliomas. A report of five cases with electron microscopy of one. J Neurosurg 20:968–982

Smith RA III, Bucy PC (1953) Pituitary cyst lined with a single layer of columnar epithelium. J Neurosurg 10:540–543

Smith RA, Lampe I, Kahn E (1961) The prognosis of medulloblastoma in children. J Neurosurg 18:91–97

Smith TW, Tyler HR, Schoene WC (1975) Atypical astrocytes and Rosenthal fibers in a case of amyotrophic lateral sclerosis associated with a cerebral glioblastoma multiforme. Acta Neuropathol (Berl) 31:29–34

Smith VR, Stein PS, MacCarty CS (1975) Subarachnoid hemorrhage due to lateral ventricular meningiomas. Surg Neurol 4:241–243

Smith WT, Turner E (1968) Solitary intramedullary carcinomatous metastases in the spinal cord. J Neurosurg 29:648–651

Smitt WGS (1929) Über intracranielle chondrome. Dtsch Z Nervenheilkd 109:170–177

Snyder RA, Brady RO, Kornblith PL (1970) Ganglioside patterns of cultured human glioma cells. Neurology (Minneap) 20:412

Sobin LH (1981) The international histological classification of tumours. Bull WHO 59:813–819

Sobue H, Tanimura K, Terabayashi T, Minagawa M, Inoue K, Ueki K (1976) Immunological studies on patients with glioma. Changes of immunological responses in the course of treatments (In Japanese). No To Shinkei 28:87–93

Soejima T (1970) Fine structure of medulloblastoma. Gann 61:17–26

Soejima T, Fukui M, Kitamura K (1973) So-called arachnoidal sarcoma of the cerebellum, its histogenesis and clinical comparison with classical medulloblastoma (In Japanese). No To Shinkei 25:1275–1283

Soffer D, Brucher JM, Wechsler W (1970) Zur Feinstruktur menschlicher Chordome. Pathol Europ 5:420–441

Sogg RL, Donaldson SS, Yorke CH (1978) Malignant astrocytoma following radiotherapy of a craniopharyngioma. J Neurosurg 48:622–627

Soldatov PK, Kisilewskij VL, Grebenjuk VI (1954) Zur Frage des eosinophilen Granuloms der Schädelknochen. (In Russian). Vopr Nevrochir 18:20–26

Solitare GB (1962) Cerebellar and cerebral gliomas occurring in the same individual. J Neurosurg 29:1079–1084

Solomon A, Perret GE, McCormick WF (1969) Multicentric gliomas of the cerebral and cerebellar hemispheres. J Neurosurg 31:87–93

Sorgo W (1938) Weitere Mitteilung über die Klinik und Histologie des kongenitalen arteriovenösen Aneurysmas. Zentralbl Neurochir 3:64–87

Sorgo W (1940a) Kontrastmitteldiagnostik cerebraler Erkrankungen. Deuticke, Wien
Sorgo W (1940b) Über Hirntumoren des Kindesalters. Wien Med Wochenschr 1:259–261
Sorgo W (1942) Über den primären Wundverschluß bei der offenen Hirnverletzung. Zentralbl Neurochir 7:73–109
Sorgo W (1949) Klinik, Histologie und Operation eines Angioma arteriovenosum congenitale der Arteria cerebri posterior. Zentralbl Neurochir 9:108–114
Sorour O, Raafat M, El-Bolkainy N, Rifaat M (1975) Infiltrative potentiality of brain tumors in organ culture. J Neurosurg 43:742–749
Spaar FW, Wille H (1959) Zur vergleichenden Pathologie der Hypophysenadenome der Tiere. Zentralbl Veterinärmed 6:925–944
Sparling HJ Jr, Adams RD (1946) Primary Hodgkin's sarcoma of the brain. Case reports. Arch Pathol 42:338–344
Spataro J, Sacks O (1968) Oligodendrogliomas with remote metastases. Case report. J Neurosurg 28:373–379
Spatz H (1938) Über multizentrisch wachsende Gliome und zur Frage des Gliosarkoms. Z Gesamte Neurol Psychiatr 161:160–161
Spatz H, Hasenjäger T (1937) Über örtliche Veränderungen der Konfiguration des Gehirns bei Hirndruck. Arch Psychiatr 107:193
Spatz H, Laqueur G (1967) Transplacental induction of tumors in Sprague Dawley rats with crude cycad material. J Natl Cancer Inst 38:233–239
Spector GJ, Druck NS, Gado M (1976) Neurologic manifestations of glomus tumors in the head and neck. Arch Neurol 33:270–274
Spence AM, Rubinstein LJ (1975) Cerebellar capillary hemangioblastoma: its histogenesis studied by organ culture and electron microscopy. Cancer 35:326–341
Sperling SJ, Alpers BJ (1936) Lipoma and osteolipoma of the brain. J Nerv Ment Dis 83:13
Spielmeyer G (1969) Medicolegal problems of the head-injured: Causation in German law. In: Walker AE, Caveness WF, Critchley M (eds) The late effects of head injury. Thomas, Springfield, pp 447–452
Spielmeyer W (1922) Histopathologie des Nervensystems, vol I: Allgemeiner Teil. Springer, Berlin
Spielmeyer W (1927) Technik der mikroskopischen Untersuchung des Nervensystems. Springer, Berlin
Spigolon G, Gullotta F (1961) La patologia dei gliomi encefalici. Capelli, Bologna
Spina-França A, Mattosinho-França LC (1978) American trypanosomyasis (Chagas' disease). In: Vinken PJ, Bruyn GW (eds) Infections of the nervous system. North-Holland, Amsterdam (Handbook of clinical neurology, vol 35, part III, pp 85–114)
Spitz EB, Shenkin HA, Grant FC (1947) Cerebellar medulloblastoma in adults. Arch Neurol 57:417–422
Spota BB (1951) La aracnoiditis optoquiasmatica en su aspecto etiologico. Arch Neurocir (B. Aires) 8:17
Sprockhoff H (1940) Legal opinion. Neurochirurgische Universitätsklinik, Berlin
Staemmler M (1938) Hirngeschwulst und Unfall. Nervenarzt 19:427–431
Staemmler M (1939) Beiträge zur normalen und pathologischen Anatomie des Rückenmarks. Z Gesamte Neurol Psychiatr 164:179–194
Stage WS, Stein JJ (1974) Treatment of malignant astrocytomas. Am J Roentgenol 120:7–18
Stahlberger R, Friede RL (1977) Fine structure of myomedulloblastoma. Acta Neuropathol (Berl) 37:43–48
Staley NA, Polesky HF, Bensch KG (1967) Fine structural and biochemical studies on the malignant ganglioneuroma. J Neuropathol Exp Neurol 26:634–653
Starr A (1886) Brain tumors in childhood. Med Rec 29:174
Starr A (1889) Tumors of the brain in childhood. Med News 54:29–37
Starr A (1893) Brain surgery. Wood, New York
Starr A (1894) Hirnchirurgie. Deuticke, Vienna
Stavrou D, Haglid K, Weidenbach W (1971) The brain-specific proteins S-100 and 14.3.2. in experimental brain tumors of the rat. Z Gesamte Exp Med. 156:237–242
Stavrou D, Kredel M, Weidenbach W (1972) Vergleichende Aspekte bezüglich Aktivität und

Isobuzymmuster der Lactatdehydrogenase bei spontanen sowie experimentellen Hirngliomen. Neuropathol Pol 10:183–188
Stavrou D, Anzil AP, Weidenbach W, Rodt H (1977) Immunofluorescence study of lymphocytic infiltration in gliomas. J Neurol Sci 33:275–282
Stavrou D, Rieske E, Anzil AP, Haglid KG, Isenberg G (1980) Definition of a cell clone with astroglial characteristics derived from a chemically induced rabbit brain glioma. J Neurol Sci 45:287–301
Steegmann AT (1971) Chordomas. In: Minckler J (ed) Pathology of the nervous system, vol 2. McGraw-Hill, New York, pp 1917–1927
Steel GG (1978) Growth kinetics. In: Laerum OD, Bigner DD, Rajewsky MF (eds) Biology of brain tumors. UICC, Geneva (UICC technical report series, vol 30, no 5, pp 27–37)
Stefani FH, Mehralin P (1971) Beobachtung eines Gangliocytoms der medulla oblongata. Arch Psychiatr Nervenkr 214:107–115
Stefanko S, Grochmal S (1962) L'actinomycose cérébrale primitive. Rev Neurol (Paris) 106:730–731
Stefanko SZ, Mackay WM (1981) Papillary meningioma. Acta Neuropathol [Suppl] (Berl) 7:126–128
Stefanko SZ, Manschot WA (1979) Pinealoblastoma with retinoblastomatous differentiation. Brain 102:321–332
Stefanko SZ, Talerman A, Mackay WM, Vuzevski VD (1979) Infundibular germinoma. Acta Neurochir (Wien) 50:71–78
Steimlé R, Jaquet G, Bourghli A, et al. (1980) Suprasellar choristoma. Zentralbl Neurochir 41:49–56
Stein AA, Schilp AO, Whitefield RD (1960) The histogenesis of hemangioblastoma of the brain. A review of twenty-one cases. J Neurosurg 17:751–761
Stein BM, Leeds NE, Taveras JM, Pool JL (1963) Meningiomas of the foramen magnum. J Neurosurg 20:740–751
Steinberg JM, Gillespie JJ, MacKay B, Benjamin RS, Leavens ME (1978) Meningeal melanocytoma with invasion of the thoracic spinal cord. J Neurosurg 48:818–824
Steinbok P, Mahaley MS, Raymond U, Zinn DC, Lipper S, Mahaley JL, Bigner DD (1979) Synergism between BCNU and irradiation in the treatment of anaplastic gliomas. J Neurosurg 51:581–586
Steiner L (1982) Radiosurgery in intracranial tumours and arteriovenous malformations in children. In: Voth D, Gutjahr P, Langmaid C (eds) Tumors of the central nervous system in infancy and childhood. Springer, Berlin Heidelberg New York, pp 315–324
Steinheil SO (1895) Über einen Fall von Varix aneurismaticus im Bereich der Gehirngefäße. Dissertation, Faculty of Medicine, University of Würzburg
Steinke HJ, Eder M (1964) Rezidivierendes parasagittales Meningiom mit Lungenmetastase – ein Fallbericht. Zentralbl Neurochir 25:89–98
Stenberg B, Moberg A (1971) Radiotherapy of intracerebral astrocytomas. Acta Radiol [Ther] (Stockh) 10:27–32
Stender A (1937) Über fronto-orbitale Dermoidcysten. Zentralbl Neurochir 2:114–123
Stender A (1939) Zur Frage der operativen Behandlung der Arachnitis spinalis. Zentralbl Neurochir 4:214–233
Stender A, Zülch KJ (1943) Über die Ventrikeltumoren bei tuberöser Sklerose. Z Gesamte Neurol Psychiatr 176:556–578
Stepień L (1962) Cerebral cysticercosis in Poland. Clinical symptoms and operative results in 132 cases. J Neurosurg 19:505–513
Stepień L, Chorobski J (1949) Cysticercosis cerebri and its operative treatment. Arch Neurol Psychiatry 61:499–527
Stern RO (1937) Cerebral tumors in children. A pathologic report. Arch Dis Child 12:291–304
Sternberg C (1921) Ein Choristom der Neurohypophyse bei ausgebreiteten Ödemen. Zentralbl Allg Pathol 31:585–591
Sternberg C (1931) Zur Kenntnis der Aktinomykose des Gehirns. Z Hyg Infektionskr 113:151–159
Stevens H (1953) Actinomycosis of the nervous system. Neurology (Minneap) 3:761–772
Stevens JM, Ruiz JS, Kendall BE (1983) Observation on peritumoural oedema in meningioma:

1. Distribution, spread and resolution of vasogenic oedema seen on computed tomography. Neuroradiology 25:71–80
Stevenson L, Echlin F (1934) Nature and origin of some tumors of the cerebellum. Arch Neurol Psychiatry 31:93–109
Stewart FW, Copeland MM (1931) Neurogenic sarcoma. Cancer Res 15:1235–1320
Stewart G, Holmes G (1904) Symptomatology of cerebellar tumors. Brain 27:522–591
Stewart JM, Morin JE (1926) Chordoma. A review, with report of a new sacrococcygeal case. J Pathol 29:41–60
Stintz S (1974) Pathologisch-anatomische Untersuchungen über Tumormetastasen in der Hypophyse. Thesis, Faculty of Medicine, University of Halle
Stocker MGP (1975) Contributions of virology to oncology. Neoplasma 22:243
Störtebecker TP (1954) Metastatic tumors of the brain from a neurosurgical point of view. A follow-up study of 158 cases. J Neurosurg 11:84–111
Stoppani F (1937) Kraniopharyngeale und hypopharyngeale Tumoren. Fortschr Roentgenstr 55:375–406
Storch E (1899) Über die pathologischen Vorgänge am Stützgerüst des ZNS. Virchows Arch [A] 157:127–171
Storm-Mathisen A (1978) Syphilis. In: Vinken PJ, Bruyn GW (eds) Infections of the nervous system. North-Holland, Amsterdam (Handbook of clinical neurology, vol 33, part I, pp 337–394)
Storring FK, Duguid JB (1954) Vascular formations in glioblastoma. J Pathol Bacteriol 68:231–233
Stough DR, Hartzog JT, Fisher RG (1971) Unusual intradural spinal metastasis of a cranial chordoma. Case report. J Neurosurg 34:560–562
Stout AP (1949) Haemangiopericytoma: A study of twenty-five new cases. Cancer 2:1027–1054
Stout AP, Murray MR (1942) Haemangiopericytoma: a vascular tumor featuring Zimmerman's pericytes. Ann Surg 116:26–33
Stowell RE, Sachs E, Russell WD (1945) Primary intracranial chorioepithelioma with metastasis to the lungs. Am J Pathol 21:787–801
Strada F (1911) Beiträge zur Kenntnis der Geschwülste der Hypophyse und der Hypophysengegend. Virchows Arch [A] 203:1
Strang RR (1962) Metastatic tumor of the cervical cord. Med J Aust 49:205–206
Strang RR (1965) Metastasis of a breast carcinoma to an intracerebral oligodendroglioma. Zentralbl Neurochir 25:206–210
Strang RR, Nordenstam H (1962) Dumb-bell ganglioneuroma of the cervical spine. Acta Neurol Scand 38:60–66
Strang RR, Tovi D, Schisano G (1960) Teratomas of the posterior cranial fossa. Zentralbl Neurochir 20:359–372
Strauss I, Globus JH (1918) Spongioblastoma with unusually rapid growth following decompression. Neurol Bull NY 1:273–279
Stroebe H (1895) Über Entstehung und Bau der Hirngliome. Beitr Pathol Anat 18:405–485
Stroebe H (1904a) Krankhafte Veränderungen der knöchernen Kapsel und der Hüllen des Gehirns (ausschließlich Geschwülste, thierische Parasiten und Gefäßerkrankungen). In: Flatau E, Jacobsohn L, Minor L (eds) Handbuch der pathologischen Anatomie des Nervensystems, Chap VII. Karger, Berlin, pp 302–394
Stroebe H (1904b) Erkrankungen der Wirbelsäule und der Rückenmarkshüllen. In: Flatau E, Jacobsohn L, Minor L (eds) Handbuch der pathologischen Anatomie des Nervensystems, chap XVII. Karger, Berlin, pp 737–826
Strong AJ, Symon L, MacGregor BJL, O'Neill BP (1976) Coincidental meningioma and glioma. Report of two cases. J Neurosurg 45:455–458
Strong LC (1978) Primary tumors of the brain: B. Genetics and epidemiology (with special reference to retinoblastoma and neuroblastoma). In: Laerum OD, Bigner DD, Rajewsky MF (eds) Biology of brain tumors. UICC, Geneva (UICC technical report series, vol 30, pp 14–26)
Stroobandt G, Brucher JM (1968) Étude de tumeurs nerveuses obtenues par l'administration de méthylnitrosourée au rat. Neurochirugie 14:515–535

Studnička F (1900) Beiträge zur Kenntnis der Ganglienzellen. S-B Königl Böhm Ges Wiss, Prag
Stumpf R (1911) Histologische Beiträge zur Kenntnis des Glioms. Beitr Pathol Anat 51:1
Sturge WA (1879) A case of partial epilepsy, apparently due to a lesion of one of the vasomotor centers of the brain. Trans Clin Soc Lond 12:162–167
Sturm V, Georgi P, Netzeband G, et al (1982) Experiences with the treatment of cystic craniopharyngiomas by stereotactically injected radioisotopes. In: Voth D, Gutjahr P, Langmaid C (eds) Tumours of the central nervous system in infancy and childhood. Springer, Berlin Heidelberg New York, pp 310–314
Suchenwirth R (1963) Zur Klinik der Meningoenzephalitis Besnier-Boeck-Schaumann. Arch Psychiatr Nervenkr 204:370–388
Suchenwirth R (1968) Die Sarkoidose des Nervensystems. MMW 110:580–586
Suga H, Hirayama A, Uneoka K, Takaku A (1971) Meningioma in the 3rd ventricle. – A case report (In Japanese). No To Shinkei 23:1069–1074
Sugi T, Schuier FJ, Hossmann K-A, Zülch KJ (1980) The effect of mild microembolic injury on the energy metabolism of the cat brain. J Neurol 223:285–292
Sumra RS, Mongia SK, Roy DMS, Pathak SN (1973) Tuberculoma of the brain stem: control of relapses by steroid therapy. J Neurosurg 39:402–404
Sundaresan N, Galicich JH, Chu FCH, Huvos AG (1979) Spinal chordomas. J Neurosurg 50:312–319
Sunder-Plassmann M, Grunert V (1971) Infratentorielle Tumoren im Säuglingsalter. Monatsschr Kinderheilk 119:465–471
Sunder-Plassmann M, Jellinger K (1972) Großhirn-Glioblastom bei einem Säugling. Z Kinderchir 11:97–103
Sung DI, Harisiadis L, Chang CH (1978) Midline pineal tumors and suprasellar germinomas. Highly curable by irradiation. Radiology 128:745–751
Sung JH, Mastri AR, Segal EL (1973) Melanotic medulloblastoma of the cerebellum. Report of a case. J Neuropathol Exp Neurol 32:437–445
Suren E-G (1974) Metastasierende extracerebrale Ependymome. Nervenarzt 45:552–556
Suzuki H, Gilbert EF, Zimmermann B (1967) Primary extracranial meningioma. Arch Pathol 84:202–206
Svien HJ (1965) Surgical experiences with craniopharyngiomas. J Neurosurg 23:148–155
Svien HJ, Mabon RF, Kernohan JW, MckCraig W (1953) Ependymoma of the brain: Pathologic aspects. Neurology (Minneap) 3:1–15
Swaen GJV, Vossenaar T, Wyers HJG (1964) Abnormal mitosis in gliomas. J Pathol Bacteriol 87:75–78
Sweet WH, Javid M (1952) The possible use of neutron-capturing isotopes such as boron^{10} in the treatment of neoplasms: 1. Intracranial tumors. J Neurosurg 9:200–209
Swenberg JA (1976) Chemical induction of brain tumors. Adv Neurol 15:85–99
Swenberg JA, Hall TA, Harbach PR, Bigner DD (1975) Chemotherapy of experimental gliomas. California conference on brain tumor therapy. Monterey, California
Symon L, Ganz JC, Chir B, Burston J (1971) Granular cell myoblastoma of the neurohypophysis. J Neurosurg 35:82–89
Sypert GW, Leech RW, Harris AB (1973) Posttraumatic lumbar epidural true synovial cyst. Case report. J Neurosurg 39:246–248
Szegedy L, Huszár I (1966) Kliniko-pathologische Angaben zum Primärkarzinom des zentralen Nervensystems (mit dem Plexus choroideus als Ausgangspunkt). Psychiatr Neurol (Basel) 152:162–170
Szymas J, Hossmann K-A (1984a) Effect of dexamethasone on glial fibrillary acidic protein in peritumorous edema of cats: A morphometric study. Acta Neuropathol (Berl) 62:309–315
Szymas J, Hossmann K-A (1984b) Immunofluoroscopic investigation of extravasation of serum proteins in human brain tumors and adjacent structures. Acta Neurochir (Wien) 71:229–241
Szymas J, Gabryel P, Biczysko W (1980) Isomorphous and anaplastic (polymorphous) oligodendroglioma. An electron microscopic study. Neurosurg Rev 3:227–231
Tabaddor K, Shulman K, Dal Canto MC (1974) Neonatal craniopharyngioma. Am J Dis Child 128:381–383

Tabuchi K, Yamada O, Nishimoto A (1973) The ultrastructure of pinealomas. Acta Neuropathol (Berl) 24:117–127
Taggart JK, Walker AE (1942) Congenital atresia of the foramina of Luschka and Magendie. Arch Neurol Psychiatry 48:583–612
Takahashi S, Sonobe M, Nagamine Y (1980) Lipoma of corpus callosum with callosal agenesis (In Japanese). No Shinkei Geka 8:475–479
Takaku A, Mita R, Suzuki J (1973) Intracranial teratoma in early infancy. J Neurosurg 38:265–268
Takakura K, Sano K, Kobayashi F, Eda J (1973) Immunological diagnosis of brain tumors (In Japanese). No Shinkei Geka 1:219–224
Takakura K, Sano K, Hojo S, Hirano A (1982) Metastatic tumors of the central nervous system. Igaku-Shoin, Tokyo
Takaro T, Bond WM (1958) Pleuropulmonary, pericardial, and cerebral complications of amebiasis. A twenty-year survey. Int Abstr Surg 107:209–222
Takemi K, Ikeda M, Kimura K, Yonezawa T (1977) A case of intracranial rhabdomyosarcoma (In Japanese). No To Shinkey 29:971–976
Takeuchi J, Barnard RO (1976) Perivascular lymphocytic cuffing in astrocytomas. Acta Neuropathol (Berl) 35:265–271
Takeuchi J, Mori K, Moritake K, Tani F, Waga S, Handa H (1975) Teratomas in the suprasellar region: Report of 5 cases. Surg Neurol 3:247–255
Takeuchi J, Handa H, Nagata I (1978) Suprasellar germinoma. J Neurosurg 49:41–48
Takeuchi J, Handa H, Otsuka S, Takebe Y (1979) Neuroradiological aspects of suprasellar germinoma. Neuroradiology 17:153–159
Takeuchi K (1972) Treatment of brain tumors by intravenous injection of bleomycin. In: Hejzlar M, Semonsky M, Masak S (eds) Advances in antimicrobial and antineoplastic chemotherapy, vol II. Urban and Schwarzenberg, München, pp 657–662
Takeuchi K (1983) Natural history of glioma. Neurochirurgia (Stuttg) 26:42–46
Takeuchi K, Hoshino K (1975) Chemotherapy of glioblastoma (In Japanese). No To Shinkei 27:1160–1164
Takeuchi K, Hoshino K (1977) Statistical analysis of factors affecting survival after glioblastoma multiforme. Acta Neurochir (Wien) 37:57–73
Tamura M, Zülch KJ (1978) Experimental microembolism of the brain. Neurosurg Rev 1:111–117
Tamura M, Mennel HD, Zülch KJ (1979) Brain tumor chemotherapy using a rat glioma model. J Cancer Res Clin Oncol 94:39–46
Tan TJ (1972) Epidermoids and dermoids of the central nervous system. Acta Neurochir (Wien) 26:13–24
Tanaka Y, Takeuchi K, Maeda T (1975) Calcification in gliomas: First report with special reference to roentgenological calcification (In Japanese). No Shinkei Geka 3:219–225
Tandon PN, Roy S, Elvidge A (1972) Subarachnoid ependymal cyst. J Neurosurg 37:741–745
Tani E, Ametani T (1971) Membranous stacks in human glioblastoma multiforme. Acta Neuropathol (Berl) 18:248–256
Tani E, Higashi N (1972) Particle-lamella complex and lamellar crystalloid in human meningioma. J Ultrastruct Res 41:334–343
Tani E, Yamashita J, Takeuchi J, Handa H (1969) Polygonal crystalline structures and crystalline aggregates of cylindrical particles in human glioma. Acta Neuropathol (Berl) 13:324–337
Tani E, Takeuchi J, Ametani T (1970) Virus-like particles in cultured human glioma. Acta Neuropathol (Berl) 16:266–270
Tani E, Ametani T, Higashi N, Fujihara E (1972) Nuclear periphery of human glioma and meningioma cells. Acta Neuropathol (Berl) 20:32–42
Tani E, Nishiura M, Higashi N (1974) Freeze-fracture studies of gap junctions in human meningioma. Acta Neuropathol (Berl) 30:305–314
Tani E, Ikeda K, Kudo S, Yamagata S, Nishiura M, Higashi N (1974) Specialized intercellular junctions in human intracranial germinomas. Acta Neuropathol (Berl) 27:139–151
Tani E, Nakano M, Itagaki T, Fukumori T (1978) Cell membrane structure of human giant-celled glioblastoma. Acta Neuropathol (Berl) 41:61–67

Tannenberg J (1924) Über die Pathogenese der Syringomyelie, zugleich ein Beitrag zum Vorkommen von Capillarhämangiomen im Rückenmark. Z Gesamte Neurol Psychiatr 92:119–174
Taper HS, Brucher J-M, Fort L (1971) Activity of alkaline and acid nucleases in tumors of the central nervous system. Cancer 28:482–490
Taptas J-N, Andréadis A (1966) Papillome des plexus choroides développé dans l'angle ponto-cérébelleux et ayant subi une transformation maligne. Neurochirurgie 12:389–394
Tashiro K, Tachibana S, Tsuru M (1976) Spinal cord tumor with probable intracranial dissemination, presenting akinetic mutism (In Japanese). No To Shinkei 28:1311–1318
Taskiran N, Yenermen MH (1957) Le problème de malignité chez les neurilemomes (neurinomes). Acta Neurochir (Wien) 5:82–91
Taveras J, Wood E (1964) Diagnostic neuroradiology. Williams and Wilkins, Baltimore
Taylon C, Duff TA (1980) Giant cell granuloma involving the pituitary gland. Case report. J Neurosurg 52:584–587
Tedeschi F, Fragnito C, Brizzi R, Lecchi A, Trabattoni G, Pietrini V (1981a) On the pathology of meningiomas. A study of 412 cases. Acta Neuropathol [Suppl] (Berl) 7:119–121
Tedeschi F, Brizzi R, Lecchi A, Trabattoni G, Ferrari C, Tagliavini F (1981b) Meningiomas. A light and electron microscopy study. Acta Neuropathol [Suppl] (Berl) 7:122–125
Teilman K (1953) Hemangiomas of the pons. Arch Neurol Psychiatry 69:208–223
Teilum G (1959) Endodermal sinus tumors of the ovary and testis. Cancer 12:1092–1105
Teilum G (1965) Classification of endodermal sinus tumour (mesoblastoma vitellinum) and so-called "embryonal carcinoma" of the ovary. Acta Pathol Microbiol Scand 64:407–429
Teilum G (1971) Special tumors of the ovary and testis. Comparative pathology and histological identification. Munksgaard, Copenhagen/Lippincott, Philadelphia
Teltscharow L, Zülch KJ (1948) Das Astrocytom des Großhirns vom pathologisch-anatomischen Standpunkt aus. Arch Psychiatr Nervenkr 179:691–720
Terao H, Kobayashi S, Teraoka A, Okeda R (1978) Xanthogranulomas of the choroid plexus in a neuro-epileptic child. Case report. J Neurosurg 48:649–653
Terao H, Hori T, Matsutani M, Okeda R (1979) Detection of cryptic vascular malformations by computerized tomography. Report of two cases. J Neurosurg 51:546–551
Terry RD, Hyams VJ, Davidoff LM (1959) Combined non metastasizing fibrosarcoma and chromophobe tumor of the pituitary. Cancer 12:791–798
Theunissen J (1978) Über das Vorkommen von Tumoren des hämatopoetischen und lymphatischen Systems (Plasmocytome, Lymphogranulomatose, eosinophile Granulome) mit Einwirkung auf das ZNS. Dissertation, Faculty of Medicine, University of Cologne
Thibaut A (1963) Angiographie carotidienne élective dans les diagnostic et le traitement des angiofibromes nasopharyngiens. Acta Radiol [Diagn] (Stockh) 1:468–480
Thiem C (1912) Geschwülste und Unfall mit besonderer Berücksichtigung des Krebsgewächses. Unfallheilkunde 19:232
Thiem C (1916) Unfall und Invalidenwesen im Jahre 1915/16. Jahreskurse Ärztl Fortb 7
Thienemann H-H (1975) Atypische intracranielle Blutungen aus sogenannten Mikroangiomen. Dissertation, Faculty of Medicine, University of Cologne
Thierry A, Cortet P, Michiels R, Seigneuric C, Binnert D, Pelikan MC, Sautreaux JL (1978) Exérèse chirurgicale des localisations cérébrales de l'echinococcose multiloculaire. Neurochirurgie 24:123–128
Thies H, Kiefer H, Noetzel H (1961) Die neurologischen Komplikationen bei maligner Lymphogranulomatose. Dtsch Med Wochenschr 86:1908–1917; 1952–1956
Thijssen HOM, Marres EHM, Slooff JL (1976) Arachnoid cyst simulating intrameatal acoustic neuroma. Neuroradiology 11:205–207
Thomas HG, Dolman CL, Berry K (1981) Malignant meningioma: clinical and pathological features. J Neurosurg 55:929–934
Thomas JV, Schwartz PL, Gragoudas ES (1978) Von Hippel's disease in association with von Recklinghausen's neurofibromatosis. Br J Ophthalmol 62:604–608
Thompson RA, Green JR (1976) Neoplasia in the central nervous system. Raven, New York (Advances in neurology, vol 15)
Thompson RK (1946) Cystic cerebellar arachnoiditis. J Neurosurg 3:461–467
Thomson AF (1978) Other helminthous infections (echinococcus, ascariasis and hookworm).

In: Vinken PJ, Bruyn GW (eds) Infections of the nervous system. North-Holland, Amsterdam (Handbook of clinical Neurology, vol 35, part III, pp 343–370)
Thums K (1939) Die Brauchbarkeit der Zwillingsmethode für die Erblichkeitsforschung bei Gehirntumoren. IIIrd International Congress of Neurology. Copenhagen. Munksgaard, Copenhagen
Tibbs PA, Challa V, Mortara RH (1978) Isolated histiocytosis X of the hypothalamus. J Neurosurg 49:929–934
Tiberin P, Gruszkiewicz J (1961) Chronic arachnoidal cysts of the middle fossa and their relation to trauma. J Neurol Neurosurg Psychiatry 24:86–91
Tice GM, Irving NW (1950) Die Röntgentherapie als unterstützende Maßnahme für die Chirurgie in der Behandlung der Gliome. J Neurosurg 7:509–520
Tijssen CC, Halprin MR, Endtz LJ (1982) Ramilial brain tumors. A commented register. Nijhoff, The Hague Boston London
Tillman BP, Dahlin DC, Lipscomb PR, Stewart JR (1968) Aneurysmal bone cyst: An analysis of ninety-five cases. Mayo Clin Proc 43:478–495
Titrud LA (1973) Melanomatous meningiomas. Minn Med 56:23–25
Titrud LA, Peyton WT (1940) Nasopharyngeal tumours and their neural complications. J Nerv Ment Dis 92:727–747
Tobias F (1943) Metastatische Hirntumoren. Faculty of Medicine, Dissertation, University of Berlin
Tönnis W (1935) Die operative Behandlung der Geschwülste im hinteren Bereich der 3. Hirnkammer. Arch Klin Chir 183:426–429
Tönnis W (1936) Aseptische Arachnoiditis nach Hirnoperationen. Arch Klin Chir 186:375
Tönnis W (1937) Kongenitale Zysten der Zisternen. Zentralbl Neurochir 2:356
Tönnis W (1938) Über Hirngeschwülste. Z Gesamte Neurol Pschiatr 161:114–149
Tönnis W (1948) Die Chirurgie des Gehirns und seiner Häute. In: Kirschner N, Nordmann O (eds) Die Chirurgie des Kopfes, des Rückens und der Nerven, 2nd edn, vol III. Urban and Schwarzenberg, Vienna, pp 453–880
Tönnis W (1959) Pathophysiologie und Klinik der intrakraniellen Drucksteigerung. In: Olivecrona H, Tönnis W (eds) Grundlagen: I. Angewandte Anatomie, Physiologie, Pathophysiologie. Springer, Berlin Göttingen Heidelberg (Handbuch der Neurochirurgie, vol I/part 1, pp 304–445)
Tönnis W, Borck WF (1953) Großhirntumoren des Kindesalters. Zentralbl Neurochir 13:72–98
Tönnis W, Friedmann G (1964) Röntgenologische und klinische Befunde bei 23 Patienten mit Sturge-Weberscher Erkrankung. Zentralbl Neurochir 25:1–10
Tönnis W, Griponissiotis B (1939) Zur operativen Behandlung der posttraumatischen Spätepilepsie. Arch Klin Chir 196:515–533
Tönnis W, Nittner K (1957) Raumbeengende Prozesse im Spinalkanal (einschließlich Parasiten). In: Cobet R, Gutzeit K, Bock HE (eds) Klinik der Gegenwart. Urban and Schwarzenberg, Munich (Handbuch der praktischen Medizin, vol 4, pp 507–544)
Tönnis W, Nittner K (1968) Diagnostische Probleme bei Sanduhrgeschwülsten des Spinalkanals. Dtsch Z Nervenheilkd 194:219–231
Tönnis W, Schiefer W (1955) Zur Frage des Wachstums arteriovenöser Angiome. Zentralbl Neurochir 15:145–150
Tönnis W, Schürmann K (1951) Meningeome der Keilbeinflügel. Zentralbl Neurochir 11:1–13
Tönnis W, Walter W (1959) Das Glioblastoma multiforme. Acta Neurochir [Suppl] (Wien) VI:40–62
Tönnis W, Zülch KJ (1937) Das Ependymom der Großhirnhemisphären im Jugendalter. Zentralbl Neurochir 2:141–164
Tönnis W, Zülch KJ (1939) Intrakranielle Ganglienzellgeschwülste. Zentralbl Neurochir 4:273–307
Tönnis W, Müller W, Brilmayer H (1953) Zur Problematik der „mixed types" der Hypophysenadenome. Acta Endocrinol (Copenh) 13:227–230
Töppich G (1936) Über eine ausreifende Ganglienzellgeschwulst des Schläfenlappens. Z Gesamte Neurol Psychiatr 156:29–35
Törmä T (1957) Malignant tumors of the spine and the spinal extradural space: a study based on 250 histologically verified cases. Acta Chir Scand [Suppl] 225:1–176

Törmä T (1975) Benign osteogenic and chondrogenic tumours of the spine. In: Vinken PJ, Bruyn GW (eds) Tumors of the spine and spinal cord. North-Holland, Amsterdam/American Elsevier, Oxford (Handbook of clinical neurology, vol 19, part I, pp 293–312)
Törmä T, Heiskanen O (1961) Benign cerebral cysts. Acta Neurol Scand 37:145–156
Toga M (1976) Tumeurs du système nerveux ultrastructure. Laboratoire de Neuropathologie, Faculté de Medecine, Marseilles
Tokars PP, Sutton HG, Griem ML (1979) Cerebellar medulloblastoma. Results of a new method of radiation treatment. Cancer 43:129–136
Tolnai G, Campbell JC, Hill DP, Peterson EW, Hudson AJ, Luney FW (1966) Primary malignant melanomatosis of leptomeninges. Arch Neurol 15:404–409
Tolosa E (1954) Cysticercose cérébrale: Aspects cliniques et possibilités thérapeutiques. Rev Neurol (Paris) 90:187–208
Tomasello F, Albanese V, Iannotti F, Di Iorio G (1980) Supratentorial hemangioblastoma in a child. J Neurosurg 52:578–583
Tomatis L, Mohr U (1973) Transplacental carcinogenesis. WHO International Agency for Research on Cancer, Lyons (IARC scientific publications no. 4)
Tompkins VN, Haymaker W, Campbell EH (1950) Metastatic pineal tumors. A clinicopathological report of two cases. J Neurosurg 7:159–169
Tonning HO, Warren RF, Barrie HJ (1952) Familial haemangiomata of the cerebellum. J Neurosurg 9:124–132
Tooth HH (1912) Some observations on the growth and survival period of intracranial tumors. Brain 35:61–108
Touraine A (1949) Les mélanoses neurocutanées. Ann Dermatol Venereol 9:489–524
Trabant R, Mohr G (1979) Verkalktes Epidermoid im Interhemisphärenspalt. Nervenarzt 50:771–774
Treip CS (1957) A congenital medulloepithelioma of the midbrain. J Pathol Bacteriol 74:357–363
Trelles JO, Trelles L (1978) Cysticercosis of the nervous system. In: Vinken PJ, Bruyn GW (eds) Infections of the nervous system. North-Holland, Amsterdam (Handbook of clinical neurology, vol 35, part III, pp 291–320)
Trelles JO, Rocca ED, Franco J (1957) Cisticercosis racemosa del valle de silvio. Actas del VII. Congr. Latinoamericano de Neurocirugia, vol 2. Bedout, Medellin, pp 1–16
Tress B, Davis S (1979) Computed tomography of intracerebral toruloma. Neuroradiology 17:223–226
Trevisan C, Dettori P (1972) Diagnostic problems of cerebral metastases. Neuroradiology 3:216–223
Trimble GX (1973) Plasmocytoma primary in the brain. N Engl J Med 288:582
Tripier MF, Hassoun J, Toga M (1975) Étude ultrastructurale d'un chordome. J Neurol Sci 25:361–370
Trouillas P, Lapras U (1970) Immunothérapie active des tumeurs cérébrales. A propos de 20 cas. Neurochirurgie 16:143–170
Trowbridge WV, French JD (1952a) Benign arachnoid cysts of the posterior fossa. J Neurosurg 9:398–404
Trowbridge WV, French JD (1952b) Disseminated oligodendroglioma. J Neurosurg 9:643–648
Truelle JL, Ramée MP, Guy G, Adam Y, Jallet P, Allaert J (1976) Granulome hodgkinien cérébral hémisphérique. A propos d'une observation. Rev Neurol (Paris) 132:494–501
Trupp M, Sachs E (1948) Vascular tumors of the brain and spinal cord and their treatment. J Neurosurg 5:354–371
Ts'o MOM, Fine BS, Zimmermann LE, Vogel MH (1969) Photoreceptor elements in retinoblastoma: A preliminary report. Arch Ophthalmol 82:57–59
Ts'o MOM, Fine BS, Zimmermann LE (1970) The nature of retinoblastoma: II. Photoreceptor differentiation: An electron microscopic study. Am J Ophthalmol 69:350–359
Tsubokawa T, Richardson DH (1975) The sarcoma arising in glioblastoma: clinico-pathological report of two cases. Tohoku J Exp Med 115:85–93
Tsuchida T, Tanaka R, Kobayashi K, Ueki K, Koizumi R, Oyake Y (1976) A case of two cell pattern pinealoma developed 15 years after total removal of pineal teratoma (In Japanese). No To Shinkei 28:893–899

Tsukamoto Y, Muraoka I, Yoshimasu N, Yoshioka M (1976) A case of brain cysticercosis (In Japanese). No Shinkei Geka 4:811–815
Tucker HH, McKenzie KG, Linell EA (1955) Astrocytoma in the cerebral hemisphere of adults. Proceedings of the 2nd International Congress of Neuropathology, London. Excerpta Medica Foundation, Amsterdam, pp 163–164
Turnbull IM, Tom MI (1963) Pigmented meningioma. J Neurosurg 20:76–80
Turner OA (1954) Brain abscess caused by nocardia asteroides. J Neurosurg 11:312–318
Turner OA, Kernohan JW (1941) Vascular malformations and vascular tumors involving the spinal cord: A pathologic study of forty-six cases. Arch Neurol Psychiatry 46:444–463
Turner OA, Laird AT (1966) Meningioma with traumatic etiology. J Neurosurg 24:96–98
Turner OA, MckCraig W, Kernohan JW (1942) Malignant meningiomas. A clinical and pathologic study. Surgery 11:81–100
Tveten L (1965) Primary meningeal melanosis: a clinico-pathological report of two cases. Acta Pathol Microbiol Scand 63:1–10
Tveten L (1978) Candidiosis. In: Vinken PJ, Bruyn GW (eds) Infections of the nervous system. North-Holland, Amsterdam (Handbook of clinical neurology, vol 35, part III, pp 413–442)
Tym R (1961) Piloid gliomas of the anterior optic pathways. Br J Surg 49:322–331
Tyson G, Newman P, Strachan WE (1978) Tuberculous brain abscess. Arch Neurol 35:323–325
Tyson GW, Welsh JE, Butler AB, Jane JA, Winn HR (1979) Primary cerebellar nocardiosis. J Neurosurg 51:408–414
Tytus JS, Pennybacker J (1956) Pearly tumours in relation to the central nervous system. J Neurol Neurosurg Psychiatry 19:241–259
Tzonos T (1964) Über eine neue Methode zur Erzeugung von stereotypen Microembolien im Gehirn der Katze. Acta Neuropathol (Berl) 3:392–397
Tzonos T, Braun W (1965) Granulome mit sarkomatöser Entdifferenzierung im Chiasmabereich. Acta Neurochir (Wien) 13:427–440
Tzonos T, Brunngraber CV (1963a) Über ein Medulloblastom mit Riesenzellen. Zentralbl Neurochir 23:282–285
Tzonos T, Brunngraber CV (1963b) Über das melanoblastische Meningiom. Acta Neurochir (Wien) 11:416–421
Tzonos T, Müller W (1967) Beitrag zur Frage der gliösen Tumoren des Hypophysenhinterlappens. Acta Neurochir (Wien) 16:253–260
Tzonos T, Pfingst E (1964) Über einen seltenen Doppeltumor im Bereich der Hypophyse. Zentralbl Neurochir 25:108–111
Udvarhelyi BG, O'Connor JS, Walker AE, Laws ER Jr, Kranin S (1962) A histochemical study of tumors of the central nervous system. In: IV. International Congress of Neuropathology, vol I. Thieme, Stuttgart, pp 95–102
Udvarhelyi JB, Walter W, Schiefer W (1955) Die Gefäßstruktur des Glioblastoma multiforme in angiographischer und histologischer Darstellung. Acta Neurochir (Wien) 4:109–127
Ueda S, Hirose A, Miwa M, Sakai N (1975) Spinal cord tumor of children. – A cured case of infantile spinal cord tumor and review of domestic literature (In Japanese). No Shinkei Geka 3:501–507
Ueki K (1963) Diagnosis and treatment of the brain tumors. In: Proceedings of the 16th General Assembly of the Japan Medical Congress, vol 3. Igaku-Shoin, Tokyo, pp 183–187
Uemura S (1917) Zur normalen und pathologischen Anatomie der Glandula pinealis des Menschen und einiger Haustiere. Frankf Z Pathol 20:455–456
Ulbricht W (1966) Rückenmarkstumoren mit Stauungspapille. Acta Neurochir (Wien) 15:138–149
Ule G, Waidelich FW (1976) Neurosekretorisches Gangliencell-Choristom in der Adenohypophyse. Acta Neuropathol (Berl) 36:81–84
Ule G, Tschahargane C, Haag D, Berlet H, Volk B (1975) Maligner Granularzelltumor des Großhirnmarkes. Acta Neuropathol (Berl) 32:143–155
Ulrich J, Landolt A, Benini A (1974) Granularzelltumor im 3. Ventrikel des Großhirns. Acta Neuropathol (Berl) 27:215–223
Ulrich J, Lévy A, Pfister C (1978) Schwannoma of the olfactory groove. Case report and review of previous cases. Acta Neurochir (Wien) 40:315–321

Umbach G (1962) Klinik und Verlauf bei 192 spinalen Prozessen mit besonderer Berücksichtigung der Gefäßtumoren. Acta Neurochir (Wien) 10:167–187

Umbach W (1954) Neuere Erkenntnisse über Kleinhirnhämangiome (Lindau-Tumoren). Fortschr Neurol Psychiatr 22:357–368

Umbach W, Kunft HD (1976) Vascular tumours of the spinal cord. In: Vinken PJ, Bruyn GW (eds) Tumors of the spine and spinal cord. North-Holland, Amsterdam/American Elsevier, Oxford (Handbook of clinical neurology vol 20, part II, pp 435–480)

Unio Internationalis Contra Cancrum (1958) Histological nomenclature of human tumors. Acta Un Int Cancer 14.3:1–43

Unio Internationalis Contra Cancrum (1965) Illustrated tumor nomenclature. Springer, Berlin Heidelberg New York

Unio Internationalis Contra Cancrum (1966–1969) Cancer incidence in five continents, vol I. Springer, Berlin Heidelberg New York

Unsöld R (1982) Zur Computer-tomographischen Differentialdiagnose der Erkrankungen des Sehnerven. Graefe's Arch Clin Exp Ophthalmol 218:124–138

Unterharnscheidt FJ (1972) Routine tissue culture of CNS tumors and animal implantation. Prog Exp Tumor Res 17:111–150

Urban H (1936) Zur Klinik und Pathologie der Angioblastome im Zentralnervensystem. Z Gesamte Neurol Psychiatr 155:798–825

Utz JP (1967) Fungal infections of the central nervous system. Clin Neurosurg 14:86–100

Valavanis A, Schubiger O, Hayek J, Pouliadis G (1981) CT of meningiomas on the posterior surface of the petrous bone. Neuroradiology 22:111–121

Valdazo A, Theron J, Houtteville J-P, Lechevalier B (1978) Exerese d'une volumineuse tumeur du glomus jugulaire après embolisation préopératoire. Rev Otoneuroophthalmol 50:413–420

Valladares JB, Perry RH, Kalbag RM (1980) Malignant choroid plexus papilloma with extraneural metastasis. J Neurosurg 52:251–255

Van Bogaert L (1933) Sclérose tubéreuse et spongioblastome multiforme. J Belge Neurol Psychiatr 33:802–808

Van Bogaert L (1935) Les dysplasies neuro-ectodermiques congénitales. Rev Neurol (Paris) 63:373–398

Van Bogaert L (1949) Les dysplasies à tendance blastomateuse. In: Lemierre A, Lenormant C, Paniez P, Savy P, Fiessinger M, De Gennes L, Ravina A (eds) Traité de médicine, vol 16. Masson, Paris, pp 77–107

Van Bogaert L (1950) Pathologie des angiomatoses. Acta Neurol Psychiatr Belg 50:526–610

Van Bogaert L (1959) Aspect pseudotumoral d'affections neurologiques non-chirurgicales de connaissance récente. Acta Neurochir (Wien) 7:81–98

Van Bouwdijk-Bastiaanse FS (1914) Primäres, metastasierendes Gehirncarcinom. Z Gesamte Neurol Psychiatr 27:96–108

Van den Bergh R, Brucher JM (1970) L'abord transventriculaire dans les cranio-pharyngiomes du troisième ventricule. Aspects neurochirurgicaux et neuro-pathologiques. Neurochirurgie 16:51–65

Van den Herrewegen M (1954) Un cas curieux de kyste extracérébral à localisation parasagittale (kyste arachnoidien?). Acta Neurol Psychiatr Belg 51:291–303

Vandeputte M, Brucher JM (1962) Sarcomatose meningée experimentale provoquée chez le raton par le virus polyome. Acta Neuropathol (Berl) 1:397–405

Van der Drift JHA, Magnus O (1961) Space-occupying lesions in older patients. Psychiatr Neurol Neurochir 64:192–201

Van der Hoeve J (1933) Les phacomatoses de Bourneville, de Recklinghausen et de von Hippel-Lindau. Acta Neurol Psychiatr Belg 33:752–762

Van der Meulen JD, Houthoff HJ, Ebels EJ (1978) Glial fibrillary acidic protein in human gliomas. Neuropathol Appl Neurobiol 4:177–190

Van der Wiel HJ (1960) Inheritance of gliomas. The genetic aspects of cerebral glioma and its relation to status dysraphicus. Elsevier, Amsterdam

Van der Zwan A, Luyendijk W, Bots GTAM (1971) Metastasis of mammary carcinoma in a chromophobe adenoma of the hypophysis. Psychiatr Neurol Neurochir 74:369–377

Van Duinen MTA (1976) The ependymoma of the cauda equina. Trio, The Hague

Van Epps RR, Samuelson Dr, McCormick WF (1967) Cerebral medulloepithelioma. Case report. J Neurosurg 27:568–573

Van Gehuchten P, Brucher JM (1960) Sarcome cérébral à localisations multiples et à extension périvasculaire diffuse, pouvant donner l'aspect d'une encéphalite. Rev Neurol (Paris) 102:671–681

Van Gehuchten P, Brucher JM (1965) Evolution des gliomes des hémisphéres cérébraux d'après une statistique personelle de 245 cas. Bull Acad R Méd Belg 5:803–813

Van Gehuchten P, Brucher JM, Cornelis G (1967) Le diagnostic et le pronostic des gliomes des hémisphéres cérébraux d'après une étude de 245 observations. Acta Neurol Psychiatr Belg 67:797–813

Van Gilder JC, Schwartz HG (1967) Growth of dermoids from skin implants to the nervous system and surrounding spaces of the newborn rat. J Neurosurg 26:14–20

Van Hoytema GJ, Winkel WEF (1957) Zur Frage des primären Plexuskarzinoms. Zentralbl Neurochir 17:353–363

Van Veelen CWM, Verbiest H, Staal GEJ, Vlug AMC (1977) Alanine inhibition of pyruvate kinase in gliomas and meningiomas. Lancet II:384–385

Van Veelen CWM, Verbiest H, Veng AMC, Rijksen G, Staal GEJ (1978) Isozymes of pyruvate kinase from human brain, meningiomas and malignant gliomas. Cancer Res 38:4681–4687

Van Veelen CWM, Verbiest H, Zülch KJ et al. (1979) L-α-Alanine inhibition of pyruvate kinase from tumors of the human central nervous system. Cancer Res 39:4263–4269

Van Wagenen WP (1927) Tuberculomas of the brain: Its incidence among intracranial tumors and its surgical aspects. Arch Neurol 17:57–91

Van Wagenen WP (1930) Papillomas of the chorioid plexus. Arch Surg 20:199–231

Van Wagenen WP (1931) A surgical approach for the removal of certain pineal tumors. Surg Gynecol Obstet 53:216–220

Van Wagenen WP (1934) Verified brain tumors: end results of one hundred and forty-nine cases eight years after operation. JAMA 102:1454–1458

Vaquero J, Leunda G, Cabezudo JM, De Juan M, Herrero J, Bravo G (1979) Posterior fossa xanthogranuloma. J Neurosurg 51:718–722

Vaquero J, Carrillo R, Cabezudo J, Leunda G, Villoria F, Bravo G (1980) Cavernous angiomas of the pineal region. Report of two cases. J Neurosurg 53:833–835

Varadachari C, Palutke M, Climie ARW, Weise RW, Chason JL (1978) Immunoblastic sarcoma (histiocytic lymphoma) of the brain with B cell markers. J Neurosurg 49:887–892

Vara-Thorbeck R, Sanz-Esponera J (1970) Intrasacral ependymoma. Case report. J Neurosurg 32:589–592

Vasiliu DO, Oraseanu, Theodorescu (1937) Kystes congénitaux du 5ième ventricle. Rev Chir (Paris) 40:454–463

Vasquez JJ, Cervós-Navarro JC (1969) Intranucleäre stabförmige Gebilde bei einem Oligodendrogliom. Acta Neuropathol (Berl) 13:289–293

Vassilouthis J, Ambrose JAE (1978) Intraventricular meningioma in a child. Surg Neurol 10:105–107

Vaughan HG, Howard RG (1962) Intracranial hemorrhage due to metastatic chorionepithelioma. Neurology (Minneap) 12:771–777

Veiga-Pires JA, Dossetor RS, van Nieuwenhuizen O (1978) CT scanning for papilloma of choroid plexus. Neuroradiology 17:13–16

Velasco ME, Dahl D, Roessmann U, Gambetti P (1980) Immunohistochemical localization of glial fibrillary acidic protein in human glial neoplasms. Cancer 45:484–494

Venabble HP (1975) Pseudotumor cerebri, benign intracranial hypertension and otitic hydrocephalus, are they synonymous? Trans Am Ophthalmol Soc 1:166–173

Venes JL, McIntosh S, O'Brien RT, Schwartz AD (1979) Chemotherapy as an adjunct in the initial management of cerebellar medulloblastomas. J Neurosurg 50:721–724

Venzoni M (1942) Condromi endocranii. Encondroma gigante della dura madre encefalica. Dtsch Z Nervenheilkd 102:110–111

Verbiest H (1939) Die Epidermoide des Rückenmarks. Zentralbl Neurochir 4:129–141

Verbiest H (1951) Das intradurale arteriovenöse Aneurysma. Ned Tijdschr Geneeskd 95:1872–1880

Verbrugghen A, Learmonth JR (1932) Chondroma of the falx cerebri. J Nerv Ment Dis 76:463–466
Verhoeff FH (1922) Primary intraneural tumors of optic nerve. Arch Ophthalmol 51:120–140
Verhoeff FH (1932) Tumors of the optic nerve. In: Penfield W (ed) Cytology and cellular pathology of the nervous system, vol 3. Hoeber, New York, pp 1029–1039
Verity MA, Wolfson WL (1976) Cerebral lymphomatoid granulomatosis. Acta Neuropathol (Berl) 36:117–124
Verocay J (1908) Multiple Geschwülste als Systemerkrankungen am nervösen Apparat. Chiari Festschrift, Wien
Viale GL (1962) Histochemische Untersuchungen über die Cholinesterase in Hirngeschwülsten. Acta Neuropathol (Berl) 2:73–85
Viale GL, Ibba F (1964) Histochemische Untersuchungen über die Phosphorylasen in Hirngeschwülsten. Acta Neurochir (Wien) 3:475–485
Vick NA (1975) Discussion. In: Hekmatpanah J (ed) Gliomas. Current concepts in biology, diagnosis and therapy (recent results in cancer research). Springer, Berlin Heidelberg New York, pp 63–64
Vick NA, Khandekar JD, Bigner DD (1977) Chemotherapy of brain tumors. The blood-brain-barrier is not a factor. Arch Neurol 34:523–526
Victor J, Wolf A (1935) Metabolism of brain tumors. Ass Res Nerv Dis Proc 16:44–58
Vigouroux R, Choux M, Baurand C, Toga M, Mangiapan T (1963) Tumeurs intra-médullaires de l'enfant. A propos de 4 observations. Pediatrie 18:891–902
Vijayan N, Bhatt GP, Dreyfus PM (1971) Intraventricular cryptococcal granuloma. Neurology (Minneap) 21:728–734
Villar R del (1956) Astrocytomas of the nose. Arch Otolaryngol 63:466–473
Vincent C, Puech P, David M (1930) Haemangioblastome cérébrale. Rev Neurol (Paris) 37:769–779
Vincent C, Puech P, David M (1931) A propos de sept cas d'arachnoidite opto-chiasmatique. Rev Neurol (Paris) 38:760–767
Vincent FM, Bartone JR, Jones MZ (1980) Cerebellar astrocytoma presenting as a cerebellar hemorrhage in a child. Neurology 30:91–93
Vinken PJ, Slooff ACJ (1965) A case of carcinoma of the choroid plexus in a child. Zentralbl Neurochir 26:313–316
Virchow R (1847) Zur Entwicklungsgeschichte des Krebses. Virchows Arch [A] 1:94
Virchow R (1855) Über Perlgeschwülste. Virchows Arch [A] 8:371–418
Virchow R (1856) Über das granulierte Aussehen der Wandungen der Gehirnventrikel. Gesammelte Abhandlungen zur wissenschaftlichen Medizin. Medinger, Frankfurt
Virchow R (1857) Untersuchungen über die Entwicklung des Schädelgrundes im gesunden und krankhaften Zustand und über den Einfluß derselben auf Schädelform, Gesichtbildung und Gehirnbau. Reimer, Berlin
Virchow R (1859) Pigment und diffuse Melanose der Arachnoidea. Virchows Arch [A] 16:180–182
Virchow R (1860) Traubenhydatiden der weichen Hirnhaut. Virchows Arch [A] 18:528–536
Virchow R (1863–1865) Die krankhaften Geschwülste. Hirschwald, Berlin
Virchow R (1871) Die Cellularpathologie. Hirschwald, Berlin
Virchow R (1875) Über die Entstehung des Enchondroma und seine Beziehungen zur Enchondrosis und Exostosis cartilaginea. Monatsber Kgl Preuss Akad Wiss
Virchow R (1888) Zur Diagnose und Prognose des Carcinoms. Virchows Arch [A] 111:1–24
Virchow R (1900) Das Psammom. Virchows Arch (Pathol Anat) 160:32
Vise WM, Schuier F, Hossmann K-A, Takagi S, Zülch KJ (1977) Cerebral microembolization. I. Pathophysiological studies. Arch Neurol 34:660–665
Visudhiphan P, Bunyaratavej S, Khantanaphar S (1973) Cerebral aspergillosis. J Neurosurg 38:472–476
Vötisch B (1980) Das Retinoblastom. Übersicht über die humangenetischen Forschungsergebnisse der Jahre 1950–1977. Dissertation, Faculty of Medicine, University of Erlangen
Voigt K, Dietz V (1972) Granulome des Hypothalamus. Arch Psychiatr Nervenkr 216:343–357
Voigt K, Yasargil MG (1976) Cerebral cavernous haemangiomas or cavernomas. Neurochirurgia (Stuttg) 19:59–68

Voigt WH (1968) Elektronenmikroskopische Beobachtungen an menschlichen Medulloblastomen. Dtsch Z Nervenheilkd 192:290–309

Volland W (1938) Über multiple Chondrome der Dura mater spinalis. Zentralbl Allg Pathol 69:162–167

Volland W (1954) Aktuelle Melaninprobleme. Med Monatsschr 8:652–660

Vonderahe AR, Niemer WT (1944) Intracranial lipoma. J Neuropathol Exp Neurol 3:344–355

Vonwiller P (1911) Über das Epithel und die Geschwülste der Hirnkammern. Virchows Arch [A] 204:230

Vorderwinkler K (1951) Zur Histogenese von Krebsmetastasen im Gehirn. Zentralbl Neurochir 11:116–124

Vorreith M, Fuchsova M, Fryc O (1963) Tumors of the central nervous system in infants and children. Cesk Pediatr 18:193–199

Voth D, Gutjahr P, Langmaid C (1982) Tumours of the central nervous system in infancy and childhood. Springer, Berlin Heidelberg New York

Vraa-Jensen J (1974) Massive congenital intracranial teratoma. Acta Neuropathol (Berl) 30:271–276

Vuia O (1966) Das solitäre und multifokale polymorphe Granulom im Nervensystem. Arch Psychiatr Nervenkr 208:309–325

Vuia O (1973) Epidermoid und Dermoid des Zentralnervensystems vergesellschaftet mit dysraphischen Störungen, Spongioblastose und Rosenthalschen Fasern. J Neurol 203:279–298

Vuia O (1975) Primary cerebral reticulosis and plasma cell differentiation. Acta Neuropathol (Berl) 6:161–166

Vuia O, Mehraein P (1971) Primary reticulosis of the central nervous system. J Neurol Sci 14:469–482

Wada H, Kinoshita K, Yokota A, Matsukado Y (1975) Cerebral paragonimiasis. A report of three cases (In Japanese). No Shinkei Geka 3:1031–1038

Wätjen J (1930) Ein Ganglioneurom des ZNS. Virchows Arch [A] 277:441–465

Waga S (1965) A histological and electron microscopic study on medulloblastomas and cerebellar sarcomas (In Japanese). Nippon Geka Hokan 34:436–454

Waga S, Handa H (1976) Radiation-induced meningioma: with review of literature. Surg Neurol 5:215–219

Waga S, Nishikawa M, Ohtsubo K, Kamijyo Y, Handa H (1970) Extracalvarial meningiomas (2 cases). Neurology (Minneap) 20:368–372

Waga S, Matsushima M, Ando K, Morii S (1972) Intracranial chondrosarcoma with extracranial metastases. Case report. J Neurosurg 36:790–794

Waggener JD (1966) Ultrastructure of benign peripheral nerve sheath tumors. Cancer 19:699–709

Waggoner RW, Löwenberg K (1937) A clinico-pathologic study of astrocytomas. Arch Neurol 38:1208–1223

Wagner (1847) Chondrome. Virchows Arch [A] 1:10

Wagner G (1978) Zur Epidemiologie bösartiger Tumoren in der Bundesrepublik. Verh Dtsch Ges Inn Med 84:514–524

Wagner W (1889) Die temporäre Resektion des Schädeldaches an Stelle der Trepanation. Zentralbl Chir 16:833–838

Wagner W, Lange-Cosack H (1936) Zur Diagnose der Hirncysticerkose. Z Gesamte Neurol Psychiatr 156:660–676

Wahl RW, Dillard SH (1972) Multiple ganglioneuromas of the central nervous system. Arch Pathol 94:158–164

Wakai S, Matsutani M, Mizutani H, Sano K (1979) Tight junctions in choroid plexus papillomas. Acta Neuropathol (Berl) 45:159–160

Wakai S, Segawa H, Kitahara S, Asano T, Sano K, Ogihara R, Tomita S (1980) Teratoma in the pineal region in two brothers. J Neurosurg 53:239–243

Walker AE (1941) Astrocytosis arachnoideae cerebelli, a rare manifestation of v. Recklinghausen's neurofibromatosis. Arch Neurol 45:520–532

Walker AE (1945) Neurogenic polycythemia: Report of a case. Arch Neurol Psychiatr 53:251–253

Walker AE (1951) A history of neurological surgery. Williams and Wilkins, Baltimore

Walker AE (1969) Brain herniations. In: Vinken PJ, Bruyn GW (eds) Disturbances of nervous function. North-Holland, Amsterdam (Handbook of clinical neurology, vol 1, pp 550–573)

Walker AE, Adamkiewicz JJ (1964) Pseudotumor cerebri associated with prolonged corticosteroid therapy. JAMA 188:779–784

Walker AE, Johnson HC, Brown KM (1952) Hemangiomas of the fourth ventricle. J Neuropathol Exp Neurol 11:103–115

Walker JC, Horrax G (1947) Papilloma of the choroid plexus. J Neurosurg 4:387–391

Walker LG (1967) Intramedullary spinal cord metastasis from carcinoma of the colon. Am Surg 33:422–424

Walker MD, Weiss HD (1975) Chemotherapy in the treatment of malignant brain tumors. Adv Neurol 13:149–191

Walker MD, Alexander E, Hunt WE, et al (1978) Evaluation of BCNU and/or radiotherapy in the treatment of anaplastic gliomas. J Neurosurg 49:333–343

Wallach JB, Edberg S (1959) Metastases of cancer to primary intracranial tumor. Arch Neurol 1:191–194

Wallman H (1858) Eine Kolloidzyste im 3. Hirnventrikel und ein Lipom im Plexus chorioideus. Virchows Arch [A] 14:385–388

Walsh J, Gye R, Connelley TJ (1969) Meningioma, a late complication of head injury. Med J Aust 1:906–908

Walsh JW, Markesbery WR (1980) Histological features of congenital lipomas of the lower spinal canal. J Neurosurg 52:564–569

Walshe FMR (1961) Head injury as a factor in the aetiology of intracranial meningioma. Lancet II:993–996

Walter W (1955) Über die sogenannten Zylindrome an der Hirnbasis unter Hinweis auf eine besondere Gruppe am Ganglion gasseri. Zentralbl Allg Pathol 93:422

Walter W, Müller W (1959) Histologische Veränderungen an röntgenbestrahlten Gliomen. Zentralbl Neurochir 19:79–90

Walter W, Schettler G, Bischof W (1967) Klinik und Therapie der arteriovenösen Angiome im Bereich der hinteren Schädelgrube. Dtsch Z Nervenheilkd 191:39–73

Walther HE (1948) Krebs-Metastasen. Schwabe, Basel

Waltz TA, Brownell B (1966) Sarcoma: A possible late result of effective radiation therapy for pituitary adenoma. Report of two cases. J Neurosurg 24:901–907

Wara WM, Sheline GE, Newman H, Townsend JJ, Boldrey E (1976) Radiation therapy of meningiomas. AJR 123:453–458

Warecka K (1975) Immunological differential diagnosis of human brain tumours. J Neurol Sci 26:511–516

Warkany J (1977) Phakomatoses, hamartoses, and neurocristopathies: a personal view. In: Mulvihill JJ, Miller RW, Fraumeni JF (eds) Genetics of human cancer. Raven Press, New York (Progress in cancer research and therapy, vol 3, pp 199–204)

Warzok W, Arnold H (1972) Zur Problematik der intracraniellen Dysgerminome. Zentralbl Allg Pathol 115:67–73

Watt V (1968) Ependymoma of the cauda equina with distant metastasis. J Neurosurg 29:424–426

Waxweiler RJ, Stringer W, Wagoner JK, Jones I, Falk H, Carter C (1976) Neoplastic risk among workers exposed to vinyl chloride. Ann NY Acad Sci 271:40–48

Webb JH, Craig WM, Kernohan JW (1953) Intraspinal neoplasms in the cervical region. J Neurosurg 10:360–366

Weber E (1939) Die Teratome und Teratoide des Zentralnervensystems. Zentralbl Neurochir 4:47–57

Weber EL, Vogel FS, Odom GL (1970) Cysts of the sella turcica. J Neurosurg 33:48–53

Weber FP (1929) Note on association of extensive hemangiomatous naevus of skin with cerebral hemangioma. Proc R Soc Med 22:25–36

Weber O (1866) Zur Geschichte des Enchondroms namentlich in Bezug auf dessen hereditäres Vorkommen und secundäre Ausbreitung in inneren Organen durch Embolie. Virchows Arch [A] 35:501–522

Wechsler W (1964) Zur Feinstruktur normaler embryonaler, reaktiver und blastomatöser Zellen des Nervengewebes. Verh Dtsch Ges Pathol 48:129–134

Wechsler W (1972a) Teratogenic and oncogenic effects of ethylnitrosourea on the developing nervous system of rats. In: Cavanagh JB (ed) The brain in unclassified mental retardation. Churchill Livingstone, Edinburgh, pp 133–139

Wechsler W (1972b) Old and new concepts of oncogenesis in the nervous system of man and animals. Prog Exp Tumor Res 17:219–278

Wechsler W (1977) Differentiated functions of glial and Schwann cell clones. Arzneimittelforsch 28:447–458

Wechsler W, Hossmann K-A (1965a) Elektronenmikroskopische Untersuchungen chromophober Hypophysen-Adenome des Menschen. Zentralbl Neurochir 26:105–122

Wechsler W, Hossmann K-A (1965b) Zur Feinstruktur menschlicher Acusticusneurinome. Beitr Pathol Anat 132:319–343

Wechsler W, Zülch KJ (1974) Pathology of neurogenic tumors in childhood and adolescence. In: Bushe KA, Spoerri O, Shaw J (eds) Progress in paediatric neurosurgery. Hippokrates, Stuttgart, pp 13–18

Wechsler W, Riverson E, Schröder JM, Kleihues P, Palmeiro JF, Hossmann K-A (1967) Electron microscopic observations on different models of acute experimental brain edema. In: Klatzo I, Seitelberger F (eds) Brain edema. Springer, New York, pp 598–614

Wechsler W, Kleihues P, Matsumoto S, Zülch KJ, Ivankovic S, Preussmann R, Duckrey H (1969) Pathology of experimental neurogenic tumors chemically induced during prenatal and postnatal life. Ann NY Acad Sci 159:360–408

Wechsler W, Pfeiffer SE, Swenberg JA, Koestner A (1973) S-100 protein in methyl- and ethylnitrosourea induced tumors of the rat nervous system. Acta Neuropathol (Berl) 24:287–303

Weenink HR, Bruyn GW (1978) Cryptococcosis of the nervous system. In: Vinken PJ, Bruyn GW (eds) Infections of the nervous system. North-Holland, Amsterdam (Handbook of clinical neurology, vol 35, part III, pp 459–502)

Weibüll J-M (1961) On carotid body tumours. Acta Psychiatr Neurol Scand 36:497–511

Weickmann F (1969) Prognose intracranieller Tumoren des Kindesalters. Zentralbl Neurochir 30:227–240

Weigert C (1875) Zur Lehre von den Tumoren der Hirnanhänge. Virchows Arch [1] 65:212–219

Weil A, Rosenblum MP (1952) Astrocytoma of fifteen years duration. A case report. J Neuropathol Exp Neurol 11:409–420

Weinberger LM, Grant FC (1941) Precocious puberty and tumors of the hypothalamus. Report of a case and review of the literature with a pathophysiologic explanation of the precocious sexual syndrome. Arch Intern Med 67:762–792

Weiner LP, Anderson PN, Allen JC (1966) Cerebral plasmocytoma with myeloma protein in the cerebrospinal fluid. Neurology (Minneap) 16:615–618

Weinman DF (1965) Arachnoidal cysts in the Sylvian fissure of the brain. J Neurosurg 22:185–187

Weir B (1973) The relative significance of factors affecting postoperative survival in astrocytomas, grade 3 and 4. J Neurosurg 38:448–452

Weir B, Elvidge AR (1968) Oligodendrogliomas. An analysis of 63 cases. J Neurosurg 29:500–505

Weir B, Band P, Urtasun R, et al (1976) Radiotherapy and CCNU in the treatment of high-grade supratentorial astrocytomas. J Neurosurg 45:129–134

Weiss A (1932) Über einen Kombinationstumor des Gehirns. Dissertation, Faculty of Medicine, University of Hamburg

Weisse K, Krücke W (1953) Die Toxoplasma-Encephalitis. Z Kinderheilkd 72:597:624

Welcker E-R, Seidel K (1966) Kombination eines Angioma arteriovenosum aneurysmaticum mit einem Astrocytom. Dtsch Z Nervenheilkd 189:231–239

Wende S (1962) Sarkom der Schädelkalotte nach Röntgentherapie. Fortschr Röntgenstr 96:278–282

Wende S, Zieler E, Nakayama N (1974) Cerebral magnification angiography. Springer, Berlin Heidelberg New York

Wende S, Aulich A, Kretzschmar K, et al (1977) Die Computer-Tomography der Hirngeschwülste. Eine Sammelstudie über 1658 Tumoren. Radiologe 17:149–156

Wende S, Kazner E, Grumme T (1980) The diagnostic value of computed tomography in orbital diseases. Neurosurg Rev 3:43–49
Wendt F, Siedschlag W-D (1965) Zur Morphologie und Klinik der Glioblastome. Dtsch Gesundh Wes 20:1173–1177
Wendt F, Siedschlag W-D, Unger RR (1969) Zur Kenntnis der intracerebralen Tuberkulome. Zentralbl Neurochir 30:51–60
Werner T (1939) Ein Pinealom mit diffuser Metastasierung in die Meningen. Zentralbl Neurochir 4:155–160
Wernicke C, Hahn E (1882) Idiopathischer Abscess des Occipitallappens durch Trepanation entleert. Virchows Arch [A] 87:335–344
Wernicke R (1892) Über einen Protozoenbefund bei Mycosis fungoides. Zentralbl Bacteriol [I] Orig 12:859–861
West CGH (1979) Spinal subarachnoid metastatic spread from non-neuraxial primary neoplasms. J Neurosurg 51:251–253
Wettler H (1948) Das intrakranielle Epidermoid. Monatsschr Psychiatr Neurol 115:233–276
White JC, Bidwell RLeR, Kubik CS (1950) Meningioma of record size with unusual features. J Neurosurg 7:455–460
White TR, Colby MY Jr, Layton DD (1969) Radiation therapy of brain stem tumors. Radiology 93:413–416
Whitener DR (1978) Tuberculous brain abscess. Report of a case and review of the literature. Arch Neurol 35:148–155
Whiteside J, Philips F, Dargeon HW, Burchenal JH (1958) Intrathecal amethopterin in neurological manifestations of leukemia. Arch Intern Med 101:279–285
Whittaker LD, Pemberton J (1938) Tumors ventral to the sacrum. Ann Surg 107:69–106
Wieczorek V (1964) Erfahrungen mit der Tumorzelldiagnostik im Liquor cerebrospinalis bei primären und metastatischen Hirngeschwülsten. Dtsch Z Nervenheilkd 186:410–432
Wieczorek V (1965) Erfahrungen mit der Liquorzelldiagnostik. Eine Analyse von etwa 5000 liquorzytologischen Untersuchungen. Psychiatr Neurol (Basel) 150:42–55; 104–107
Wiederholt WC, Siekert RG (1965) Neurological manifestations of sarcoidosis. Neurology (Minneap) 15:1147–1154
Wiedersheim O, Herzog W (1952) Über Pseudogliom und Gliom (zur Frage der Entstehung des malignen Retinoblastoms). Albrecht Von Graefes Arch Ophthalmol 153:273–288
Wight PAL, Duff RH (1964) The histopathology of epizootic gliosis and astrocytomata of the domestic fowl. J Comp Pathol 74:373–380
Wilke G (1943) Zur Angioarchitektonik der gliomatösen Hirntumoren. Arch Psychiatr Nervenkr 116:658–720
Wilke G (1950) Über primäre Reticuloendotheliosen des Gehirns. J Neurol 164:332–380
Wilke G (1955) Granulomatous encephalitis, with reference to known and unknown aetiologies. Excerpta Med (Amst), Sect VIII, 824
Wilke G (1956) Die granulomatöse Encephalitis mit Bezug auf bekannte oder unbekannte Ätiologie. Nervenarzt 27:244–251
Wilkins RH, Brody IA (1971) Lindau's disease. Arch Neurol 25:472–477
Wilkins RH, Odom GL (1966) Cytological changes in cerebrospinal fluid associated with resections of intracranial neoplasms. J Neurosurg 25:24–34
Wilkins RH, Odom GL (1976) Spinal extradural cysts. In: Vinken PJ, Bruyn GW (eds) Tumors of the spine and spinal cord. North-Holland, Amsterdam (Handbook of clinical neurology, vol 20, part II, pp 137–175)
Wilkinson HA, Feris EJ, Muggia AL, Cantu RC (1971) Central nervous system tuberculosis: a persistent disease. J Neurosurg 34:15–22
Williams AO, Langundoye SB, Bankole MA (1970) Sacrococcygeal teratoma in Nigerian children. Arch Dis Child 45:110–113
Williams ED, Siebenmann RE, Sobin LH (1980) Histological typing of endocrine tumours. International histological classification of tumours No. 23. World Health Organization, Geneva
Willis RA (1960) Pathology of tumours, 3rd edn. Butterworths, London
Willis RA (1971) Nervous tissue in teratomas. In: Minckler J (ed) Pathology of the nervous system, vol II. McGraw-Hill, New York, pp 1937–1943

Wilmes F, Hossmann K-A (1979) A specific immunofluorescence technique for the demonstration of vasogenic brain edema in paraffin embedded material. Acta Neuropathol (Berl) 45:47–51
Wilson CB (1970) Medulloblastoma. Current views regarding the tumor and its treatment. Oncology 24:273–290
Wilson CB (1976) Chemotherapy of brain tumors. Adv Neurol 15:361–367
Wilson CB, Jenewein EP, Bryant LR (1967) Carcinoma of the lung metastatic to falx meningioma. Case report. J Neurosurg 27:161–165
Wilson CB, Kaufmann L, Barker M (1970) Chromosome analysis of glioblastoma multiforme. Neurology (Minneap) 20:821–828
Wilson G, Bartle H Jr, Dean JS (1940) Intradural spinal lipomas. Report of a case with remarks on their problematic origin and unusual pathological characteristics. J Nerv Ment Dis 91:745–753
Wilson WB, Grotta JC, Schold C, Fisher LE (1979) Cerebral mucormycosis. Arch Neurol 36:725–726
Winkelbauer A (1930) Duraendotheliom and Hyperostose. Wien Klin Wochenschr 43:748–752
Winkelman NW, Cassel C, Schlesinger B (1952) Intracranial tumors with extracranial metastases. J Neuropathol Exp Neurol 11:149–166
Winters WD, Rich JR (1975) Human meningioma antigens. Int J Cancer 15:815–822
Wintersteiner H (1897) Das Neuroepithelioma retinae. Deuticke, Leipzig
Wise BL, Malamud U, Boldrey EB (1953) Multiple intracranial tumors: Glioma associated with hypophyseal chromophobe adenoma. J Neuropathol Exp Neurol 12:224–231
Wishart J (1822) Cases of tumors in the skull, dura mater and brain. Edingburgh Med Surg J 18:393
Wisiol ES, Handler S, French LA (1962) Extracranial metastases of a glioblastoma multiforme. J Neurosurg 19:186–194
Wislocki GB, Putnam TJ (1924) Note on the anatomy of the area postrema. Anat Rec 27:151–156
Wisoff HS, Suzuki Y, Llena JF, Fine DIM (1978) Extramedullary hemangioblastoma of the spinal cord. Case report. J Neurosurg 48:461–464
Witte A (1979) Das monstrozelluläre Sarkom der Hingefäße. Dissertation, Faculty of Medicine, University of Cologne
Wittermann E (1936) Hypophysengangstumoren und vegetative Zentren des Zwischenhirns. Nervenarzt 9:441–516
Witthaut H (1959) Klinische Untersuchungen zur Frage einer biologisch prognostischen Einteilung der Astrocytome des Großhirns unter Zugrundelegung der histologischen Klassifikation nach dem Prinzip des „grading“. Internist (Berl) 14:725–730
Wohlwill F (1930) Zur pathologischen Anatomie der malignen medianen Kleinhirntumoren der Kinder (sogenannte „Medulloblastome“). Z Gesamte Neurol Psychiatr 128:587–614
Wohlwill FJ, Yakovlev PI (1957) Histopathology of meningofacial angiomatosis (Sturge-Weber's disease). Report of four cases. J Neuropathol Exp Neurol 16:341–364
Wojtek E (1949) Über Hirnmetastasen maligner Tumoren. Zentralbl Neurochir 9:294–307
Wolf A, Cowen D (1936) Angioblastic meningiomas. Bull Neurol Inst NY 5:485–503
Wolf A, Echlin F (1936) Osteochondrosarcoma of the falx invading the frontal lobes of the cerebrum. Bull Neurol Inst NY 5:515–525
Wolf A, Morton BF (1937) Ganglion cell tumors of the central nervous system. Bull Neurol Inst NY 6:453–488
Wolf A, Orton ST (1933) Intranuclear inclusions in brain tumors. Bull Neurol Inst NY 3:113–123
Wolf A, Cowen D, Graham S (1950) Xanthomas of the choroid plexus in man. J Neuropathol Exp Neurol 9:286–297
Wolf N (1951) Kriegsverletzung des Gehirns und Hirntumorentwicklung. Z Unfallmed Berufskr 44:279–284
Wolf PA, Rosman NP, New PFJ (1967) Multiple small cryptic venous angiomas of the brain mimicking cerebral metastases. Neurology (Minneap) 17:491–501
Wolff M, Santiago H, Duby MM (1972) Delayed distant metastasis from a subcutaneous

sacrococcygeal ependymoma. Case report, with tissue culture, ultrastructural observations, and review of the literature. Cancer 30:1046–1067
Wollemann M (1976) Biochemistry of tumours of the nervous system. In: Vinken PJ, Bruyn GW (eds) Metabolic and deficiency diseases of the nervous system. North-Holland, Amsterdam (Handbook of clinical neurology, vol 27, part I, pp 503–518)
Wolman L (1959) Infundibuloma. J Pathol Bacteriol 77:283–296
Wolman L, Balmforth GV (1963) Precocious puberty due to a hypothalamic hamartoma in a patient surviving to late middle age. J Neurol Neurosurg Pschiatry 26:275–280
Wolpert SM, Carter BL, Ferris EJ (1972) Lipoma of the corpus callosum. AJR 115:92–99
Woltman H (1922) Malignant tumors of the nasopharynx with involvement of the nervous system. Arch Neurol 8:412–429
Woltman HW, Kernohan JW, Adson AW, MckCraig W (1951) Intramedullary tumors of spinal cord and gliomas of intradural portion of filum terminale: Fate of patients who have these tumors. Arch Neurol Psychiatry 65:378–395
Wong T-W, Bennington JL (1962) Metastasis of a mammary carcinoma to an acoustic neuroma. Report of a case. J Neurosurg 19:1088–1093
Wood MW, White RJ, Kernohan JW (1957) One hundred intracranial meningiomas found incidentally at necropsy. J Neuropathol Exp Neurol 16:337–340
World Federation of Neurology (1966) Medulloblastomas and related tumors. Symposium of the Research Group on Neurooncology, Berne, 1965. Zentralbl Neurochir 27:50–53
World Health Organization (1973a) Immunity to cancer. Bull Wld Hlth Org 49:81–91
World Health Organization (1973b) Immunity to cancer. Bull Wld Hlth Org 49:205–213
World Health Organization (1976) International histological classification of tumours of domestic animals, parts I and II. WHO, Geneva
Woyke S, Domagala W, Olszewski W (1971) Same peculiar ultrastructural features of meningiomas. Pol Med J 10:975–1005
Wright JH (1910) Neurocytoma or neuroblastoma, a kind of tumor not generally recognized. J Exp Med 12:556–560
Wünscher W, Lehmann W (1960) Zur diffusen Glioblastose. Psychiatr Neurol Med Psychol (Leipz) 12:244–248
Wurtman RJ, Kammer H (1966) Melatonin synthesis by an ectopic pinealoma. N Engl J Med 274:1233–1237
Wurtman RJ, Axelrod J, Toch R (1964) Demonstration of hydroxyindole-*O*-methyl transferase, melatonin and serotonin in a metastatic parenchymatous pinealoma. Nature (Lond) 204:1323–1324
Wyburn-Mason R (1943) The vascular abnormalities and tumors of the spinal cord and its membranes. Kimpton, London
Yagishita S, Itoh Y, Chiba Y, Fujino H (1979) Primary rhabdomyosarcoma of the cerebrum. Acta Neuropathol (Berl) 45:111–115
Yamada H, Sakai N, Ando T, Nishimura Y, Kishimoto Y, Shimokawa K (1980) Trigeminal neurinoma with massive extracranial extension. Report of a case (In Japanese). No Shinkei Geka 8:469–474
Yamamoto M, Okino M, Beppu T, Kitamura K (1975) Melanoma of the spinal cord in pregnancy (In Japanese). No Shinkei Geka 3:415–422
Yamashita J, Gillingham FJ (1975) The effect of radiotherapy for glioblastoma. A review of 516 cases (In Japanese). No Shinkei Geka 3:329–336
Yamashita J, Maloney AFJ, Harris P (1973) Intradural spinal bronchiogenic cyst. J Neurosurg 39:240–245
Yamashita J, Handa H, Toyama M (1975) Medulloblastoma in two brothers. Surg Neurol 4:225–227
Yao Y-T, Lin W-S-J, Hung C-C, Liu K-N (1975) A case of glioblastoma multiforme with extracranial metastasis. Taiwan I Hsue Hui Tsa Chih 74:220–228
Yap H-Y, Yap B-S, Tashima CK, Di Stefano A, Blumenschein GR (1978) Meningeal carcinomatosis in breast cancer. Cancer 42:283–286
Yasargil MG (1976) Intradural spinal arteriovenous malformations. In: Vinken PJ, Bruyn GW (eds) Tumors of the spine and spinal cord. North-Holland, Amsterdam (Handbook of clinical neurology, vol 20, part II, pp 481–523)

Yenermen M (1955) Histological and topographical study of gliomas in Turkey. Excerpta Med (Amst), Sect VIII, 797
Yenermen MH, Bowerman CJ, Haymaker W (1958) Colloid cysts of the third ventricle. A clinical study of 54 cases in the light of previous publications. Acta Neuroveg (Wien) 17:211–277
Yohn DS (1972) Oncogenic viruses expectations and applications in neuropathology. Prog Exp Tumor Res 17:74
Yonemasu Y, Kitamura K, Okudera K (1975) Tumors in the pineal region. A clinico pathological study of 77 cases. Abstracts of the 5th Congress European Association of Neurosurgical Societies, Oxford, pp 124–126
Yoshida J, Kobayashi T, Kageyama N, Kanzaki M (1977) Symptomatic Rathke's cleft cyst. J Neurosurg 47:451–458
Yoshida N, Ohmaru YI, Sato T (1962) Electron microscopic studies on human brain tumor. In: Breese SS (ed) Electron microscopy, vol 2. Academic Press, New York, p 7
Young DG, Bahn RC, Randall RV (1965) Pituitary tumours associated with acromegaly. J Clin Endocrinol Metab 25:249–259
Young HF, Fu Y, Fratkin MJ (1976) Organ culture of craniopharyngioma and its cellular effects induced by colloidal chromic phosphate. J Neuropathol Exp Neurol 35:404–412
Young JL, Miller Ph, Miller RW (1975) Incidence of malignant tumors in US children. J Pediatr 86:254–258
Yuhl ET, Rand CW (1951) Tuberculous opticochiasmatic arachnoiditis. J Neurosurg 8:441–447
Zaaijer JH (1938) Über die Behandlung von metastatischen Tumoren. Zentralbl Neurochir 3:7–12
Zander E (1949) 6 Fälle von Papillomen des Plexus chorioideus. Monatsschr Psychiatr Neurol 118:321–363
Zander E, Khamlichi AE (1978) Étude d'une série opératoire homogène de 35 cas d'oligodendrogliomes. Neurochirurgie 24:37–46
Zang KD (1970) Cytological and cytogenetical studies on human meningiomas. Proceedings of the VIth International Congress of Neuropathology, Paris 1970. Masson, Paris, pp 982–983
Zankl H, Zang KD (1972) Cytological and cytogenetical studies on brain tumors. Hum Genet 14:167–169
Zapata JE (1963) Estudio histopatológico de los sarcomas de los hemisferios cerebrales. Trab Inst Cajal Invest Biol 55:193–227
Zapata JE, Iglesias RA (1964) Consideraciones acerca de los tumores benignos metastatisantes del tiroides. Acta Oncol (Madr) 3:3–11
Zehnder M (1938a) Echinokokken des Wirbelkanals. In: Sitzungsbericht über den Kongress der Neurologen und Psychiater, München 1937. Zentralbl Neurochir 3:51
Zehnder M (1938b) Subarachnoidalzysten des Gehirns. Zentralbl Neurochir 3:100–112
Zeitlin H (1935) Tumors in the region of the pineal body. Report of 3 cases. Arch Neurol 34:567–586
Zeitlin H (1942) Hemangioblastomas of the meninges and their relation to Lindau disease. J Neuropathol Exp Neurol 1:14–23
Zeman W (1952) Die Meningoenzephalitis Besnier-Boeck-Schaumann. Nervenarzt 23:43–52
Zeman W (1955) Veränderung durch ionisierende Strahlen. In: Scholz W (ed) Erkrankungen des zentralen Nervensystems. Springer, Berlin (Handbuch der speziellen Pathologischen Anatomie und Histologie, vol 13/3, pp 340–357)
Zeman W (1966) Pathogenesis of radiolesions in the mature central nervous system. Proceedings of the Vth International Congress of Neuropathology. Excerpta Medica Foundation, Amsterdam, pp 302–308
Zettner A, Netsky MG (1960) Lipoma of the corpus callosum. J Neuropathol Exp Neurol 19:305–319
Zimmerman HM (1943) Brain tumors produced with benzpyrene. Am J Pathol 19:939–955
Zimmerman HM (1955) The nature of gliomas as revealed by animal experimentation. Am J Pathol 31:1–29
Zimmerman HM (1961) The nature of experimental gliomas. Clin Neurosurg 7:247–260

Zimmerman HM (1962) Experimental brain tumors. In: Fields WS, Sharkey PC (eds) The biology and treatment of intracranial tumors. Thomas, Springfield, pp 49–74

Zimmerman HM (1967) The histopathology of experimental medulloblastoma. Acta Neuropathol (Berl) 8:69–75

Zimmerman HM (1969) Brain tumors: their incidence and classification in man and their experimental production. Ann NY Acad Sci 159:337–359

Zimmerman HM (1975) Malignant lymphomas of the nervous system. Acta Neuropathol (Berl) 6:69–74

Zimmerman HM, Arnold H (1940) Experimentally induced intracranial neoplasms. Trans Am Neurol Assoc 66:191–193

Zimmerman HM, Arnold H (1941) Experimental brain tumors: I. Tumors produced with methylcholanthrene. Cancer Res 1:919–938

Zimmerman HM, Arnold H (1943) Experimental brain tumors: II. Tumors produced with benzpyrene. Am J Pathol 19:939–955

Zimmerman HM, German WJ (1933) Colloid tumours of the third ventricle. Arch Neurol 30:309–325

Zimmerman HM, Netsky MD, Davidoff LM (1956) Atlas of tumors of the nervous system. Lea and Febiger, Philadelphia

Zlotnik EI, Sklyut IA, Smeyanovich AF, Stolkarts IZ (1979) Total removal of acoustic neurinomas. J Neurosurg 50:170–173

Zollinger HU (1941) Großzellig-granulomatöse Lymphangitis cerebri (morbus Boeck) unter dem Bild einer multiplen Sklerose verlaufend. Virchows Arch [A] 307:597–615

Zomzely-Neurath CE, Walker WA (1980) Nervous system specific protein 14.-3-2 protein, neuron specific enolase and S-100 protein. In: Bradshaw RA, Schneider DM (eds) Proteins of the nervous system. Raven, New York, pp 1–59

Zondek T (1952) A case of ependymoma of the aquaeduct of Sylvius. Monatsschr Psychiatr 123:323–328

Zschau H (1929) Beitrag zur Kenntnis der Cauda equina. Frankf Z Pathol 38:400–438

Zuccarello M, Pardatscher K, Andrioli GC, Fiore DL, Iavicoli R (1981) Brain tumours presenting as spontaneous intracerebral haemorrhage. Zentralbl Neurochir 42:1–6

Zucker DK, Katz R, Koto A, Horoupian DS (1978) Sarcomas metastatic to the brain. Case report of a metastatic fibrosarcoma, and review of literature. Surg Neurol 9:177–180

Zülch KJ (1937a) Zur histologischen Schnelldiagnose bei der Operation von Hirngeschwülsten. Arch Klin Chir 189:492–493

Zülch KJ (1937b) On the question of cerebellar astrocytomas. Zentralbl Neurochir 2:360

Zülch KJ (1937c) Zur Histopathologie der Großhirngliome in den ersten beiden Lebensjahrzehnten. Z Gesamte Neurol Psychiatr 158:369–374

Zülch KJ (1938a) Die Hirngeschwülste des Jugendalters. Z Gesamte Neurol Psychiatr 161:183–188

Zülch KJ (1938b) Multiple Papillome des Plexus chorioideus. Kongress der deutschen Neurologen und Psychiater, München 1937. Zentralbl Neurochir 3:51–52

Zülch KJ (1939a) Über die geschichtliche Entwicklung und den heutigen Stand der Klassifikation der Hirngeschwülste (unter besonderer Berücksichtigung der Gliome). Zentralbl Neurochir 4:251–272; 325–335

Zülch KJ (1939b) Die Gefäßversorgung der Gliome. Z Gesamte Neurol Psychiatr 167:585–592

Zülch KJ (1940a) Über das „sog." Kleinhirnastrocytom. Virchows Arch [A] 307:222–252

Zülch KJ (1940b) Hirngeschwülste im Jugendalter. Zentralbl Neurochir 5:238–274

Zülch KJ (1940c) Das Medulloblastom vom pathologisch-anatomischen Standpunkt aus. Arch Psychiatr Nervenkr 112:343–367

Zülch KJ (1940d) Über die morphologischen Folgen der Anwendung elektrischen Stromes zum Schneiden und Koagulieren des Hirn- und Geschwulstgewebes. Dtsch Z Nervenheilkd 151:141–145

Zülch KJ (1940e) Morphologische Befunde bei Hirnschwellung. Zentralbl Neurochir 5:166–175

Zülch KJ (1941a) Das Oligodendrogliom. Z Gesamte Neurol Psychiatr 172:407–482

Zülch KJ (1941b) Ein Medulloblastom mit glatten Muskelfasern. Arch Psychiatr Nervenkr 114:349–352

Zülch KJ (1941c) Die Entstehung des Hirndruckes, insbesondere des Prolapses bei der Hirnwunde und ihren Folgezuständen. Zentralbl Neurochir 6:212–232
Zülch KJ (1943) Hirnödem und Hirnschwellung. Virchows Arch [A] 310:1–58
Zülch KJ (1948) Primäre Hirnkarzinome. Zentralbl Allg Pathol 84:173–174
Zülch KJ (1949a) Plötzlicher Todesfall durch Einklemmung von Hirnteilen bei Massenverschiebungen. Hamburger Ärzteblatt, November: 242
Zülch KJ (1949b) Häufigkeit, Vorzugssitz und Erkrankungsalter bei Hirngeschwülsten. Zentralbl Neurochir 9:115–128
Zülch KJ (1950a) Über die „unklassifizierten" Hirngeschwülste. Acta Neurochir (Wien) 1:283–299
Zülch KJ (1950b) Zur Pathologie der äußeren Liquorräume: Beobachtungen über die Entstehung der Arachnoidalcysten und der liquormechanischen Vorgänge beim Hydrocephalus occlusus. Zentralbl Neurochir 10:25–38
Zülch KJ (1950c) Röntgendiagnostik beim cerebralen Anfall. Verh Dtsch Ges Inn Med 56:24–48
Zülch KJ (1951a) Diskussionsbemerkungen zu den Frontallappengeschwülsten. Zentralbl Neurochir 11:286–287
Zülch KJ (1951b) Die Hirngeschwülste in biologischer und morphologischer Darstellung, 1st edn. Barth, Leipzig (3rd edn 1958)
Zülch KJ (1951c) Hirnödem, Hirnschwellung, Hirndruck. Zentralbl Neurochir 11:350–355
Zülch KJ (1951d) Vorzugssitz, Erkrankungsalter und Geschlechtsbevorzugung bei Hirngeschwülsten als bisher ungeklärte Formen der Pathoklise. Dtsch Z Nervenheilkd 166:91–102
Zülch KJ (1952) Estado actual de la clasification de los tumores cerebrales. Folia Clin Int II, no. 5, 1–4
Zülch KJ (1953a) Über die primären Hirnsarkome. (Mit besonderer Berücksichtigung der monstrocellulären Formen). Arch Int Studi Neurol 2:1–35
Zülch KJ (1953b) Hirngeschwülste als Schädigungsfolge. Ärztl Forsch 7:535–543
Zülch KJ (1953c) Hirnschwellung und Hirnödem. Dtsch Z Nervenheilkd 170:179–208
Zülch KJ (1954) Betrachtungen über die Entstehung der frühkindlichen Hirnschäden auf Grund der klinischen und morphologischen Befunde. Arch Kinderheilkd 149:3–27
Zülch KJ (1955a) The problems in the diagnosis of oligodendrogliomas. Excerpta Med (Amst), Sect VIII:816–817
Zülch KJ (1955b) Genesis de los tumores cerebrales. Rev Esp Oncol 4:33–46
Zülch KJ (1955c) La malignidad de los tumores del encefalo y sus problemas. Rev Esp Oncol 4:47–59
Zülch KJ (1956) Biologie und Pathologie der Hirngeschwülste. Handbuch der Neurochirurgie, vol III. Springer, Berlin Göttingen Heidelberg
Zülch KJ (1957) Brain Tumors. Their biology and pathology, 1st edn. Springer, New York
Zülch KJ (1958a) Vascular polycystic astrocytoma (spongioblastoma?) of the temporal lobe. Cancer Seminar 2 (3):106–107
Zülch KJ (1958b) Geschwülste und Parasiten des Nervensystems. In: Kaufmann E, Staemmler M (eds) Lehrbuch der speziellen Anatomie. De Gruyter, Berlin, pp 427–574
Zülch KJ (1959a) Das Glioblastom, morphologisch und biologisch gesehen. Acta Neurochir [Suppl] (Wien) 6:1–30
Zülch KJ (1959b) Störungen des intrakraniellen Druckes. In: Olivecrona H, Tönnis W (eds) Angewandte Anatomie, Physiologie, Pathophysiologie. Springer, Berlin Göttingen Heidelberg (Handbuch der Neurochirurgie, vol I, part 1, pp 208–303)
Zülch KJ (1960a) The present state of the classification of intracranial tumours and its value for the neurosurgeon. Rev Brasil Chir 40:247–264
Zülch KJ (1960b) Über die Strahlensensibilität der Hirngeschwülste und die sogenannte Strahlen-Spätnekrose des Hirns. Dtsch Med Wochenschr 85:293–298; 309–310
Zülch KJ (1960c) Radiosensibilidad de los tumores cerebrales y la llamada radionecrosis tardia del cerebro. Med Alemana 1:11–23
Zülch KJ (1961) Die Pathologie und Biologie der Tumoren des dritten Ventrikels. Acta Neurochir (Wien) 9:277–296
Zülch KJ (1962a) The present state of the classification of intracranial tumors and its value

for the neurosurgeon. In: Fields WS, Sharkey P (eds) The biology and treatment of intracranial tumors. Thomas, Springfield, pp 157–177
Zülch KJ (1962 b) Neurinomas, meningiomas, and related tumors. In: Fields WS, Sharkey P (eds) The biology and treatment of intracranial tumors. Thomas Springfield, pp 218–247
Zülch KJ (1963a) La signification des fibres de Rosenthal. Coll. intern. sur les malformations congénitales de l'encéphale, Paris 1961. Masson, Paris, pp 61–63
Zülch KJ (1963b) Le spongioblastome et la maladie de Recklinghausen. Coll. intern. sur les malformations congénitales de l'encéphale, Paris 1961. Masson, Paris, pp 455–457
Zülch KJ (1963c) Morphologische Veränderungen an Geschwülsten nach Bestrahlung und Schädigungsmöglichkeit am normalen Hirn. In: Meyer H, Becker J (eds) Strahlenforschung und Strahlenbehandlung, vol IV. Urban and Schwarzenberg, Munich, pp 47–62
Zülch KJ (1964a) On the definition of the polymorphous oligodendroglioma. Acta Neurochir [Suppl] (Wien) 10:166–168
Zülch KJ (1964b) Neurologische Diagnostik bei endokraniellen Komplikationen von otorhinologischen Erkrankungen. Arch Ohr Nas Kehlk Heilkd 183:1–85
Zülch KJ (1965a) Brain tumors – their biology and pathology, 2nd edn. Springer, New York
Zülch KJ (1965b) Einige Besonderheiten der Hirngeschwülste in Alter und Sitz sowie im Geschlecht der Tumorträger. Zentralbl Chir 90:890–898
Zülch KJ (1966/1967) Morphologie, Biologie, Prognose der Hirntumoren. In: Landesausschuß Berlin für Krebsbekämpfung (ed) Probleme der Krebsbekämpfung III/IV. Hoffmann, Berlin, pp 108–123
Zülch KJ (1967a) Grading of intracranial tumors. Symposium International de Investigaciones Neurologicas, Lima/Peru 1967, Anales del XII Congreso Latinoamericano de Neurocirugia, pp 1103–1111
Zülch KJ (1967b) Neuropathological aspects and histological criteria of brain edema and brain swelling. In: Klatzo I, Seitelberger F (eds) Brain edema. Springer, New York, pp 95–116
Zülch KJ (1968) Soll man den Begriff des (unipolaren) Spongioblastoms beibehalten? Beitr Neurochir 15:373–382
Zülch KJ (1969a) Biology and morphology of glioblastoma multiforme. Acta Radiol Ther Phys Biol 8:65–77
Zülch KJ (1969b) Roentgen sensitivity of cerebral tumours and so-called late irradiation necrosis of the brain. Acta Radiol Ther Phys Biol 8:92–110
Zülch KJ (1969c) Medical causation. In: Walker AE, Caveness WF, Critchley M (eds) The late effects of head injury. Thomas, Springfield, pp 453–472
Zülch KJ (1969d) The newest development of experimental induced tumors of the central nervous system. J Genet Hum 17:511–529
Zülch KJ (1969e) Gibt es Beziehungen in den Befunden der experimentellen und spontanen neurogenen Tumoren? Arzneimittelforsch 19:1503–1508
Zülch KJ (1971a) Atlas of the histology of brain tumors. Springer, Berlin Heidelberg New York
Zülch KJ (1971b) Hemorrhage, thrombosis, embolism. In: Minckler J (ed) Pathology of the nervous system, vol 2. McGraw-Hill, New York, pp 1499–1536
Zülch KJ (1971c) Les angiomatoses médullaires et la maladie de Foix-Alajouanine. In: Michaux L, Chevreau J (eds) Les malformations congénitales du cervelet, de la moëlle épinière et du rachis. S.P.E.I., Paris, pp 115–124
Zülch KJ (1975a) Atlas of gross neurosurgical pathology. Springer, Berlin Heidelberg New York
Zülch KJ (1975b) Griff in die Medizingeschichte: Die erste Operation – Punktion – eines raumfordernden Prozesses, der von Wernicke rein neurologisch lokalisiert wurde. Zentralbl Neurochir 36:47–50
Zülch KJ (1978) Principles of the new WHO classification of brain tumors. J Neurosurg Sci 22:1–5
Zülch KJ (1979) Histological typing of tumours of the central nervous system. World Health Organization, Geneva (International histological classification of tumours, no. 21)
Zülch KJ (1980a) Principles of the new World Health Organization (WHO) classification of brain tumors. Neuroradiology 19:59–66

Zülch KJ (1980b) Pathologie und Biologie der raumfordernden Prozesse von Rückenmark und Wirbelsäule. Radiologe 20:459–465

Zülch KJ (1981a) Cerebrovascular pathology and pathogenesis as a basis of neuroradiological diagnosis. In: Diethelm L, Wende S (eds) Handbuch der medizinischen Radiologie, vol XIV, part 1A. Springer, Berlin Heidelberg New York, pp 1–192

Zülch KJ (1981b) Gleanings from medical history: Reflections on the surgery of the pineal gland (a glimpse into the past). Neurosurg Rev 4:159–162

Zülch KJ (1981c) Problems of the classification of tumors of the nervous system and the significance of electron microscopy. Folia Histochem Cytochem (Krakow) 19:171–178

Zülch KJ (1982a) Are there still unclassified cerebral tumours? Acta Neurochir (Wien) 61:139–144

Zülch KJ (1982b) Intracranial tumors of infancy and childhood. In: Voth D, Gutjahr P, Langmaid C (eds) Tumors of the central nervous system in infancy and childhood. Springer, Berlin Heidelberg New York, pp 1–16

Zülch KJ (1984) Trauma und Hirngeschwulst (traumatische Entstehung von Tumoren des zentralen Nervensystems). In: Rauschelbach HH, Jochheim KA (eds) Das neurologische Gutachten. Thieme, Stuttgart, pp 161–170

Zülch KJ (1985) Secondary changes in human and experimental brain infarction with particular consideration of microembolism. In: Baethman A, Go KG, Unterberg U (eds) Mechanisms of secondary brain damage. Plenum, New York

Zülch KJ, Bingas B (1963) Sôbre os sarcomas primitivos do cérebro. Rev Bras Cir 45:234–245

Zülch KJ, Borck WF (1952) Tafeln über die relative Häufigkeit der Hirngeschwülste in verschiedenen Altersklassen. Zentralbl Neurochir 12:93–97

Zülch KJ, Kleinsasser O (1957) Ortsgebundene Abweichungen in der Histologie und im biologischen Verhalten der Ependymome. Zentralbl Allg Pathol 97:59–66

Zülch KJ, Mennel HD (1970) Recent results on chemically induced tumors of the nervous system. In: VI. Congrés International de Neuropathologie, Paris 1970. Masson, Paris, pp 60–77

Zülch KJ, Mennel HD (1971a) Die Morphologie der durch alkylierende Substanzen erzeugten Tumoren des Nervensystems. Zentralbl Neurochir 32:225–243

Zülch KJ, Mennel HD (1971b) Gehirntumor und Trauma. Hefte Unfallheilkd 107:33–44

Zülch KJ, Mennel HD (1971c) Trauma und Hirntumor. Versorgungsbeamte 22:95–98

Zülch KJ, Mennel HD (1973) Recent results in new models of transplacental carcinogenesis in rats. In: Tomatis L, Mohr U (eds) Transplacental carcinogenesis. IARC, Lyons (Scientific publications, no. 4, pp 29–44)

Zülch KJ, Mennel HD (1974) The biology of brain tumours. In: Vinken PJ, Bruyn GW (eds) Tumours of the brain and skull. North-Holland, Amsterdam (Handbook of clinical neurology, vol 16, part I, pp 1–55)

Zülch KJ, Mennel HD (1975) Malignant meningiomas. Adv Neurosurg 2:3–11

Zülch KJ, Mennel HD (1977) New aspects of brain tumor research. J Neurol 214:241–250

Zülch KJ, Mennel HD (1978) History and problems of classification. In: Laerum OD, Bigner DD, Rajewsky MF (eds) Biology of brain tumors. UICC, Geneva (UICC technical report series, vol 30, no. 5, pp 1–13)

Zülch KJ, Milhaud M (1960) Etude de la fibre du neurinome, son origine schwannienne et sa nature neuroectodermique. Rev Neurol (Paris) 103:541:555

Zülch KJ, Nachtwey W (1958) Pathologie und Klinik des Aquäduktverschlusses. Zentralbl Neurochir 18:80–106

Zülch KJ, Nover A (1960) Die Spongioblastome des Sehnerven. Albrecht Von Graefes Arch Ophthalmol 161:405–419

Zülch KJ, Oeser H (1974) Delayed spinal radionecrosis – a juridical error? Neuroradiology 8:173–176

Zülch KJ, Schmid EE (1955) Über das Ependymom der Seitenkammern am Foramen Monro. Arch Psychiatr Nervenkr 193:214–228

Zülch KJ, Wechsler W (1968) Pathology and classification of gliomas. Prog Neurol Surg 2:1–84

Zülch KJ, Woolf AL (1964) Classification of brain tumors. The first Kölner Symposium. Acta Neurochir [Suppl] (Wien) 10

Zülch KJ, Tzonos T (1964) Transsudationsphänomene an den tiefen Hirnvenen nach Blockade von Arteriolen oder Kapillaren der Rinde durch Mikroembolien. Naturwissenschaften 51:539–540

Zülch KJ, Tzonos T (1965) Transudation phenomena at the deep veins after blockage of arterioles and capillaries by micro-emboli. Bibl Anat (Basel) 7:279–284

Zülch KJ, Pompeu F, Pinto F (1954) Über die Metastasierung der Meningeome. Zentralbl Neurochir 14:253–260

Zülch KJ, Behrend RC, Finkemeyer H (1973) The „early filling vein": Is „early venous filling" in an angiogram really a reliable sign of malignancy? Neuroradiology 5:111–113

Zülch KJ, Mennel HD, Zimmermann V (1974a) Intracranial hypertension. In: Vinken PJ, Bruyn GW (eds) Tumours of the brain and skull. North-Holland, Amsterdam (Handbook of clinical neurology, vol 16, part I, pp 89–149)

Zülch KJ, Dreesbach HA, Eschbach O (1974b) Occlusion of the middle cerebral artery with the formation of an abnormal arterial collateral system – moyamoya type – 23 months later. Neuroradiology 7:19–24

Zu Rhein GM, Varakis J (1975) Morphology of brain tumors induced in Syrian hamsters after inoculation with JC virus, a new human papovavirus. Proceedings of the VIth International Congress of Neuropathology, Budapest 1974. Excerpta Medica, Amsterdam

Subject Index